Bernard Regnauld

The Foot

Pathology, Aetiology, Semiology,
Clinical Investigation and Therapy

Edited and Translated by Reginald Elson

With 266 Figures in 2617 Separate Illustrations,
Some in Color

Springer-Verlag
Berlin Heidelberg New York Tokyo

Author
Bernard Regnauld, M.D.
2, Rue Camille-Berruyer
4000 Nantes, France

Editor and Translator
Reginald Elson, M.A., F.R.C.S.
Consultant Orthopaedic Surgeon
Northern General Hospital
Sheffield S5 7AU, Great Britain

Title of the original French edition: Le pied

ISBN 3-540-13223-6; 0-387-13223-6

ISBN 3-540-13222-8 Springer-Verlag Berlin Heidelberg New York Tokyo
ISBN 0-387-13222-8 Springer-Verlag New York Heidelberg Berlin Tokyo

Library of Congress Cataloging in Publication Data. Main entry under title:
Regnauld, Bernard. The foot: pathology, aetiology, semiology, clinical investigation and therapy. Includes bibliographies and index. 1. Podiatry. I. Title. [DNLM: 1. Foot. 2. Foot Diseases. WE 880 R339f] RD563.R42 1986 617'585 85-17312

Typesetting, Printing and Binding: G. Appl, Wemding
2124/3140-543210

Author's Preface

In orthopaedic surgery, the study of the foot has a special place. Familiarity with the congenital and acquired problems of inflammation and arthrosis must be blended with an understanding of the mechanics of support and propulsion before a sure choice of effective treatment can be made. There is involvement of bones, joints, tendons, ligaments, soft tissues and integument, none of which can be treated in isolation. Superficial appraisal can lead to the cardinal error of facile diagnosis, and ignorance of the physiology of the organ and of the differences of expert opinion with respect to pathogenesis and basic therapeutic concepts invites inevitably poor management.

In this book, I have attempted to interpret pathology, clinical presentation and treatment in the light of practical experience. I do not presume to be original, for many distinguished authors have written on the subject already. Lelièvre (1952), Viladot et al. (1956), de Doncker and Kowalski (1970) and many others, preceded by Hohmann (1951), Morton (1935), Hauser (1950) and Boehler (1944), have all contributed significantly to our basic knowledge and opened the way to understanding.

The philosopher Alain wrote succinctly: "When it is fully comprehended that there is no knowledge without experience and that one cannot conceive an idea unless there already exists a thought, no more need be said".

Thus my personal interpretation of the concepts of others may make some small increase to our understanding, to the benefit of our patients; that is my main aim here. In these pages, I recommend only what I have found to be genuinely useful.

November 1985 Bernard Regnauld

Editor's Preface

Podology is as much a specialty as hand surgery. As a general orthopaedic surgeon consulted by patients with foot disorders, the preparation of this English edition of Dr. Regnauld's book has provoked in me much doubt as to the accuracy of my previous management. In Great Britain at least, the concept used to prevail that the only good operations were those which were easy; an example is the routine Keller's arthoplasty for hallux valgus, which in fact yields a predictably mediocre result. It is debatable whether Dr. Regnauld's sophisticated procedure gives better results in the hands of the average orthopaedic surgeon, but the concept of easy techniques being better is no longer tenable in any branch of surgery; in the hands of the expert, beautiful results can be obtained from difficult operative procedures. Especially in the forefoot, I have already benefited from Dr. Regnauld's instruction.

The foot, in which the first signs of more widespread disease may manifest themselves, is treated not only by surgeons, but also by chiropodists, physiotherapists and general practitioners. It is for this reason that Dr. Regnauld has chosen to be comprehensive in his account, including some aspects which may at first appear to be unnecessary; for instance, mycotic infections may not seem very important to the surgeon, yet are seen every day in surgical patients.

It appears that in France, some doctors are able to specialise in podology alone, in contrast to the situation elsewhere. This narrower approach may be advantageous.

I have tried to convey the text accurately while preserving some of its French flavour. Problems of terminology and authorship must be expected, but the exchange of information with English-speaking practitioners can only be valuable. A short glossary is included.

I am grateful to Dr. Regnauld for allowing me to alter many aspects, and thank our publishers, Springer-Verlag, for their cooperation and understanding. My secretary, Mrs. Valerie Barclay, has made her usual valuable contribution, for which I am very indebted.

November 1985 — Reginald Elson

Foreword

To group in a single volume such topics as the anatomy and physiology of the foot, the disorders to which it is subject and the conservative and surgical treatment methods that can be brought to bear against them is a daring undertaking.
Dr. Regnauld has succeeded in this endeavour: hundreds of figures accompany the text, an abundance of authors are cited, yet the information is presented in a spirit of critical appraisal that sets the book utterly apart from a mere compilation of data.
In each chapter, the author indicates his preference, together with arguments justifying his choice, for specific treatment methods or techniques. In many instances, alongside conventional modes of treatment, he also presents techniques he himself has developed.
Congenital foot conditions and those resulting from trauma are described, and therapeutic measures are presented in detail. Unusual and intractable cases are also considered.
This volume represents a work of considerable import and will be of value not only to surgeons specialising in the foot, but also to orthopaedic surgeons in general.

January 1986 Jean Judet

Contents

Glossary

Antetarsus	The forefoot limited posteriorly by the Lisfranc joint linc
Arthrorisis	An operation to limit abnormal movement of a joint
Camptodactyly	Permanent flexion of a digit (e.g. claw toe)
Cavus	Increased hollowing of the plantar aspect: applied to the longitudinal arch (pes cavus) or transversely at the ball of the foot (forefoot cavus)
Chopart joint	The system comprising the talocalcaneo-navicular and calcaneocuboid joints
Clinodactyly	Permanent transverse deviation of a digit, e.g. hallux varus. In the text, these deformities are also referred to as transverse
Kinesitherapy	See under Physiotherapy
Lisfranc joint	The tarsometatarsal joint line
Onychauxis	Overgrowth in thickness of a nail
Onycholysis	Loosening of a nail
Onychomycosis	Mycotic infection of a nail
Orthopaedic	In French usage, "orthopaedic treatment" means conservative management
Physiotherapy	The French distinguish kinesitherapy (massage and manipulative therapy), re-education (physical exercises) and physiotherapy (application of agents such as heat, light and ultrasound)
Postural deformity	In French, the term "statique" applied to foot deformities implies an acquired idiopathic condition. Here the term "postural" is used

Subtalar complex	The joint system operating in motion between the calcaneum and the rest of the foot, comprising the subtalar, talocalcaneonavicular and calcaneocuboid joints

I Functional Structure, Diagnosis, and Cutaneous Infections

1 Functional Structure of the Foot

1.1 General Considerations

The static and dynamic forces operating in the foot relate to the weight of the body and the reactions from muscular contraction necessary for balance, movement and adaptation to the nature of the ground surface. Classically, forces are described as operating through two arch systems: the internal, which centres around the first metatarsal, and the outer, which operates through the fifth metatarsal. According to Pietrogrande (1965), the talus is the receiver, transmitter and distributor of these forces along two systems, posteriorly distributed towards the calcaneum, anteriorly through both internal and external pillars of the forefoot and above to the tibia. The magnitude of forces is increased when the foot is dorsiflexed or plantarflexed at the ankle joint. However, there is reason to believe that the distribution is not as simple as this description indicates. Tensile and compressive forces balance across different transmission systems of the foot, which may be likened to an aeroplane in flight rather than a car on the road; there is pitch, roll and yaw.

1.1.1 Tibiotalocalcaneal Complex

This complex transmits the forces generated during rising and falling (pitch), rolling (pronation and supination) and side-to-side motion (the internal and external cadences brought about by the pelvic muscles of the lower limb, peroneus brevis and tibialis posterior).

1.1.2 Subtalar Complex

Operating on the inner side, this complex comprises the subtalar joint and the talocalcaneonavicular joint, and on the outer side, the calcaneocuboid articulation. These joints stabilise forces of inclination (dorsiflexion and plantarflexion), augment or reduce the rolling forces of pronation and supination and distribute the side-to-side forces of abduction and adduction. At any given moment, the foot is stabilised according to the particular distribution of these forces.

1.1.3 Midtarsal Joints

This system comprises three parts: posteriorly the naviculocuneiform articulation, anteriorly the tarsometatarsal or Lisfranc joint and centrally the naviculocuboid joint. The system, being situated between the tarsus and the metatarsus, is analogous to the talus at its site between the tibia and the calcaneum. It assures perception, distribution and equilibrium of the different forces, proximally and distally as well as centrifugally and centripetally. The naviculocuneiform system adapts to side-to-side forces and to those of inclination (plantarflexion and dorsiflexion), and to a lesser degree to the movements of pronation and supination. The central part of the system adapts passively, while the tarsometatarsal joint line distributes and balances the forces of inclination and rolling.

1.1.4 Metatarsal System

With the toes, this system finally balances anterior-posterior and lateral movements, adapting to the forces acting during inclination, rolling and side-to-side movement which vary in distribution and intensity at the level of each of the metatarsal heads. The whole of this complex group is under the proprioceptive control of the proximal tibiotalocalcaneal and tarsomidtarsal system and under the more direct influence of the midtarsal and tarsometatarsal joints.

1.1.5 Ligaments

Certain ligaments are essential in maintaining the systems described above; their integrity should not be violated. The foremost are: the ligaments of the ankle, the talocalcaneal interosseous ligament, the bifurcate calcaneonavicular ligament, the interosseous cuneiform-metatarsal ligament (joining the medial cuneiform and the second metatarsal and described by Lisfranc), and the transverse metatarsal ligaments. To these must be added two "universal" ligaments spanning several joints, namely the long plantar ligament and the plantar aponeurosis.

1.1.6 Muscles

The restraining ligaments mentioned above are influenced by muscular control: plantarflexion and dorsiflexion by triceps surae and the long flexors and extensors; supination by flexor digitorum longus, tibialis posterior and tibialis anterior; pronation by peroneus brevis, peroneus longus, extensor digitorum longus, extensor digitorum brevis and peroneus tertius; and abduction-adduction, complementary to the action of leg muscles, by tibialis posterior and peroneus brevis.
These different systems relate to a series of joint lines of appropriate morphology: generally, each presents an internal plantar concavity, a transverse frontal convexity, and a general obliquity transversely, disposed forwards and inwards; the last-mentioned becomes more accentuated from behind and forwards, whose oblique axes converge towards the cuboid. Specifically, these features present at the Chopart joint (anterior base of the "triangle" of Ciardi-Dupré), at the naviculocuneiform joint, at the Lisfranc tarsometatarsal joint, at the line of application of load on the metatarsal heads, and at the toes, the line of distal propulsion.

1.2 The Foot Under Load

The considerations above lead to the following concepts: Under static loading, there are three points of pressure under the foot, namely the heel, a zone related to the cuboid and the base of the fifth metatarsal, and the forefoot. Under dynamic loading there are only two points of application, the heel and the forefoot.
To achieve stability while static it is necessary for three sites of pressure to prevail, and the morphology of the normal foot conforms to this principle. The outline of the footprint, the converging orientation of the joint lines towards the cuboid and the various transverse concavities of the articular systems of the foot, again relating and converging towards the cuboid, form a half-dome which has its summit at the navicular bone, where a complete medial longitudinal arch meets a transverse half arch orientated with its lowest part at the level of the joint between the cuboid and the fifth metatarsal. It is at this tarsometatarsal joint that the third point of application of pressure in the normal foot assures lateral equilibrium.
A different pattern presents in pes cavus, where there are only two points of pressure, the heel and the forefoot; this foot is unstable laterally, and while it may be supple, it fatigues easily because the muscles controlling eversion and inversion have to contract all the time. It is unusual for pressure symptoms not to develop at both anterior and posterior zones of pressure, and with increasing age, chronic discomfort is almost inevitable. Sometimes the cavus foot loses its dynamic control as a result of muscular fatigue, or imbalance may lead to a cavovalgus deformity. Maintenance of elevation of the cuboid leads to a lowering of the normally higher navicular, but cannot produce a useful third point of pressure. This valgus posture develops irreversibly into a flat foot in eversion.
A cavovarus foot may also result because of weakness of the evertors. The scaphoid summit elevates under unbalanced control of the internal muscles, resulting in a lowering of the cuboid summit as if in an effort to find a third point of pressure on the outer side of the foot; this leads to the appearance of a callosity under the cuboidometatarsal region.

1.3 Dynamic Considerations

Before any surgery is undertaken, it is essential to understand the dynamic physiology of the foot during gait and to recognise the interrelationship between the joints, which is altogether different from their apparent functions in isolation. The coordination of joint function entails a complex proprioceptive system, controlled particularly by the interosseous ligament of the sinus tarsi - the "eye of the foot" (Valenti 1980a, b).
De Doncker and Kowalski (1970) describe the foot as resting on two supports: the calcaneum and a median axial pallet composed of the central three metatarsals. The mechanism is flexible and loading is damped by the subcutaneous tissues of the sole, the medial ligament of the ankle, the anterior part of the heel and the torsion bar of Hendrix (1934). This torsion bar comprises the cuboid, the intermediate and lateral cuneiforms, the talonavicular "cushion" and two lever arms: posteriorly, the calcaneum, and anteriorly, the median pallet (I prefer to include the fourth metatarsal in the pallet, although Kowalski [de Doncker and Kowalski 1970]

mentioned only the second and third). The median pallet is balanced by the dynamic action of the more mobile first and fifth rays under muscular control of the peronei and tibialis muscles. Thus during propulsion the five metatarsal heads maintain equal pressure on the ground.

1.3.1 *Ankle Joint*

While the tibiotarsal joint apparently allows simple dorsiflexion and plantarflexion, it merits further consideration during dynamic loading:

a) Plantarflexion, as occurs on tiptoeing, results in:
   - Compression of the talus between the malleoli (Lecoeur 1938)
   - An equinus posture of the posterior tarsus under the action of triceps surae, flexor digitorum longus and flexor hallucis longus
   - Tension in the plantar fascial tie beam
   - Hollowing and lateral equilibrium of the dome of the intertarsal region by contraction of the tibialis and peroneal muscles
   - Dorsiflexion of the toes at the metatarsophalangeal joints while their prehensile action is maintained by the flexor muscles
   - A tendency towards supination of the calcaneum by contraction of tibialis posterior and flexor hallucis longus

   All of these muscle actions strengthen the general assembly of the foot and ensure its stability. Whenever one of the muscles is deficient or a bone deformed, some degree of disturbance will occur, this involving alterations in ligament tension, muscle imbalance, pain and joint disturbance.
b) Dorsiflexion at the ankle joint, as occurs in climbing stairs, includes:
   - A tendency to pronation of the calcaneum
   - A tendency for the midtarsal dome to flatten Initiation of flattening of the intertarsal dome
   - A tendency to internal and plantar displacement of the midtarsal joints

The foot in this posture tends to evert. Dorsiflexion must suffice to allow rolling of the forefoot on the ground, and loss of range of movement in this respect leads to lateral displacement and consequent signs of pressure at the metatarsal heads. Conversely, obstruction to dorsiflexion at the metatarsophalangeal joints results in compensatory lateral displacement of the midtarsal region, and can lead to compressive arthrosis of the ankle joint and contracture of peroneus brevis and extensor digitorum longus. Extreme tension develops in triceps surae in an effort to maintain pronation of the foot and hold the calcaneum in a horizontal position. Tibialis anterior contracts in an attempt to continue support of the medial longitudinal arch and prevent flattening and stiffness developing at the subtalar joint.

1.3.2 *Subtalar Joint*

At this articulation occur the following axes of motion.

a) *Inversion* (supination plus adduction). This movement results in supination of the midtarsus and a reflex pronation and adduction of the forefoot under the action of the long flexors and triceps surae. There is a hollowing of the midtarsus brought about by contraction of peroneus longus and tibialis anterior and posterior. These effects have been verified by Pisani (1977b) in his studies of the biomechanics of the foot.
b) *Eversion* (pronation plus abduction). Of smaller amplitude, this movement leads to pronation of the midtarsus and forefoot by contraction of peroneus brevis and extensor digitorum communis. This is counteracted by adduction of the midtarsus by tibialis posterior and elevation of the midtarsus by tibialis anterior, while plantarflexion of the first metatarsal is effected by peroneus longus.

In the normal foot these movements maintain balance of the arches, but when there is muscular deficiency, laxity of ligaments or osteoarticular displacement, the system fails, resulting in various functional disturbances such as tenosynovitis of the tibialis muscles and the peronei, abnormal loading of the second metatarsal head due to poor contraction of peroneus longus if it fails to depress the great metatarsal head, cavovarus deformity, and excessive loading under the fourth and fifth metatarsal heads and cuboid bones, especially when there is insufficiency of peroneus brevis and the long toe flexors so that they cannot restore balance.

1.3.4 *Antetarsal Joints*

Posteriorly, the tarsometatarsal joints play a role in longitudinal transmission of pressure, vertical damping and transverse balancing, influenced by their frontal convexity and their plantar concavity.

The median pallet and mobile first and fifth rays originate here.

Anteriorly, the five metatarsophalangeal joints are active in stance, propulsion and lateral balancing. This system is the final transmitter of forces; the enormous demands in terms of strength and mobility have been emphasised by Viladot (1969). It is sensitive, and is surgically a difficult area to treat. At all times, care must be taken to see that the five points of loading of the metatarsal condyles are aligned horizontally and conserve their suppleness relative to one another. The metatarsophalangeal joints display simple movement, dorsiflexion amounting to 90° and plantarflexion to 30°–40°. The zone of loading over which they operate, their amplitude and movement and general resilience allow the normal rolling action of the forefoot during propulsion.

1.3.5 Interphalangeal Joints

These joints, essentially prehensile in nature, distribute load and balance the forefoot. They protect the metatarsal heads, and failure to do so in the axes of the respective metatarsals always causes abnormal weight-bearing symptoms under them. They have no range of dorsiflexion.

A clearer understanding of the dynamic physiology of the foot demonstrates the importance and interdependence of the joints concerned and the dysfunction likely to be transmitted to adjacent articulations when one joint is disordered. Surgery aims to correct joint disorders by restoring mobility, re-establishing normal axes of motion, and restoring areas of disordered weight bearing. Arthrodesis is a procedure of last resort when articular surfaces are destroyed. Whenever possible, restoration of balance of antagonist muscles will guarantee the permanence of a corrective procedure.

2 Diagnosis of Disorders of the Foot

The predominant symptom causing the patient to consult a specialist is pain arising from disorders of loading of the foot during standing or walking. Congenital and acquired deformities are aggravated by fatigue, age, subsequent injury of the weight-bearing tissues, trauma, shoe pressure or even the complications of unsuccessful attempts at treatment. The symptom may relate directly to some obvious area of abnormality involving the integument, the skeleton, a joint or a vascular or neurological condition. Alternatively, the symptom can be diffuse without relation to any particular sign. A disciplined approach to diagnosis is essential.

2.1 History

Careful enquiry is important as to the mode and date of onset, the development up to the present time, the patient's general condition and any previous significant illnesses. In particular, details must be taken on inflammations of any type, rheumatism, mechanical disorders of the foot, infections, trauma and congenital conditions of a hereditary and familial nature.
An exact appraisal of all aspects of the pain is essential:

a) Time of onset, progressiveness, rapidity of progression, changes in severity during the day, relationship to any sort of trauma, relationship to shoes worn (especially height of heel), severity during work or onset after a long walk. Presence of pain, only or particularly in the morning, in the evening or at night may be significant.
b) Site of pain, presence or absence of radiation of pain and aggravating or ameliorating factors.
c) Character of pain. It is variously described as "shooting", "pricking", "sensation of tightness", "tingling", "like an electric shock" and so on, and the description may be useful in appraisal. Some idea of severity should be obtained.

2.2 Examination of Unloaded Foot

2.2.1 Integument

The integument includes the skin, subcutaneous tissue and underlying deep fascia. The skin should be assessed with particular regard to thickness, suppleness on the plantar aspect, dryness, general colour, pigmentation, and the axis of skin folds on the dorsal surface. Trophic conditions such as varicose ulcer, perforating ulcer, oedema, inflammation, local temperature, moistness and hyperhidrosis or anhidrosis should be noted. Skin rashes or corns, calluses or other local skin disease may be found.
Cutaneous tumours of many types can present on the foot, and irregularity of the surface, adherence to deep tissues or induration may arouse suspicion, indicating urgent biopsy.

2.2.2 Vascular Supply

The arterial pulses should be assessed, and in case of doubt, oscillography, arteriography and phlebography should be considered.

2.2.3 Nails

An exact description of the nail and subungual region is important in relation to congenital conditions such as onycholysis (loosening of the nail), onychauxis (thickening of the nail), onychogryphosis and other deformities. Mechanical disturbance of the nail due to trauma includes ingrowing toenail as well as onychogryphosis and onychauxis. Infections lead to abnormal staining, a friable, porous, thickened or striped condition of the nail, or even ingrowing. Examination of the subungual tissue may reveal a tumour, an exostosis or a subungual corn.

2.2.4 *Neurological Disorders*

Cutaneous sensibility to heat, pinprick, touch and pain should be tested in all areas, together with assessment of the tendon reflexes and cutaneous reflexes. A careful assessment of the power of all muscle groups should include bulk, tonicity, contracture or laxity, rupture or paralysis, weakness and pain provoked by compression of tendons.

2.2.5 *Joints*

Ankle Joint. The amplitude, quality and comfort of movement in each direction, should be recorded. The ankle normally displays 40° plantarflexion and 30° dorsiflexion.

Subtalar Complex. Pronation and supination of the calcaneum with the foot in a neutral position are each normally 10°, but the range should also be assessed in dorsiflexion and plantarflexion.

Chopart Joint Complex. The vertical mobility of the two components – the talonavicular joint and the calcaneocuboid joint – should be assessed in both dorsiflexion and plantarflexion with reference to the amplitude of pronation and supination and of inversion and eversion, together with assessment of the longitudinal axis of the midtarsus, the position of the head of the talus with respect to the navicular, any degree of cavus or planus, and the amount of convexity or concavity of the internal border of the foot which reflects valgus or varus arising at the tarsal region.

Naviculocuneiform Joint. Local pain on movement should be sought.

Lisfranc Joint Complex. Local palpation demonstrates mobility, the presence of any dorsal exostosis, lateral angulation or general equinus of the metatarsus or of a particular metatarsal and the site and degree of any pain on movement.

Metatarsophalangeal Joints. Normally, the range of movement amounts to 90° dorsiflexion and 30° plantarflexion. In each individual joint, mobility may be reduced by contracture or even ankylosis, and subluxation or complete dislocation of the phalangeal bases on the heads of the metatarsals may occur. Local pain associated with inflammation or effusion can sometimes be demonstrated. Each of the five metatarsal heads can display hypertrophy or displacement in the sagittal, frontal or horizontal plane.

In the horizontal plane, palpation can afford an initial assessment as to whether there is a sinking of one or several of the metatarsals. This affects, in ascending order of frequency, the second, third and fourth metatarsal heads. The degree of any such equinus deformity should be related to the form and size of the sesamoid bones, the presence of any hollowness, flatness or convexity of the forefoot and splayed posture of the forefoot. In the frontal plane, the disposition of the five metatarsal heads may be classified with respect to length as follows (Figs. 2.1, 2.2):

Greek type: $1<2\geqslant 3>4>5$
Egyptian type: $1>2>3>4>5$
Square type: $1=2=3\geqslant 4>5$

Protrusion of the second metatarsal head is very frequent, but protrusion of the second and third heads or the central three heads may also be present. Congenital aplasia most commonly affects the fourth head. It is immediately obvious on inspection from the under- or overriding of the toe with respect to its neighbours and from the longitudinal skin fold seen on the plantar aspect. There

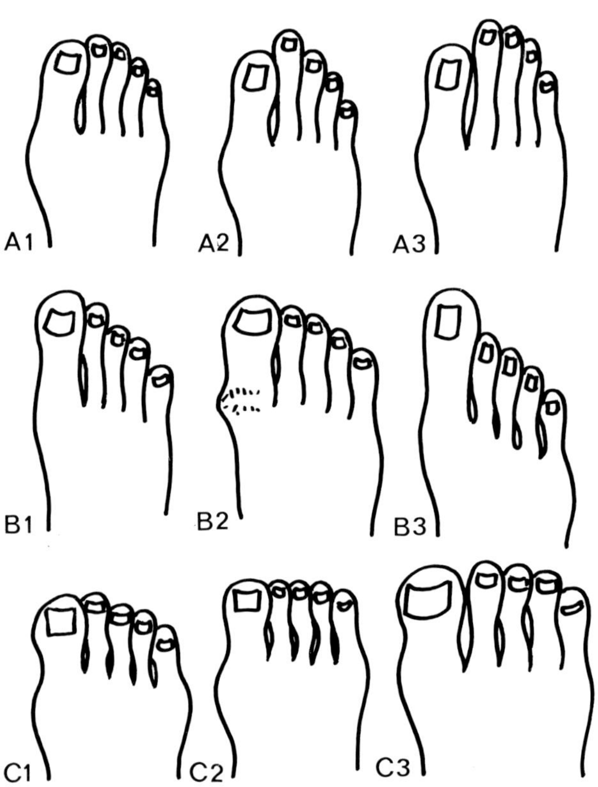

Fig. 2.1 A–C. Forefoot configurations. **A** Greek: *1, 2* Usual types; *3* unusually long toes. **B** Egyptian: *1, 2* Usual types; *3* hypertrophy of great toe. **C** Square: *1, 2* Usual types; *3* hypertrophy of lesser toes

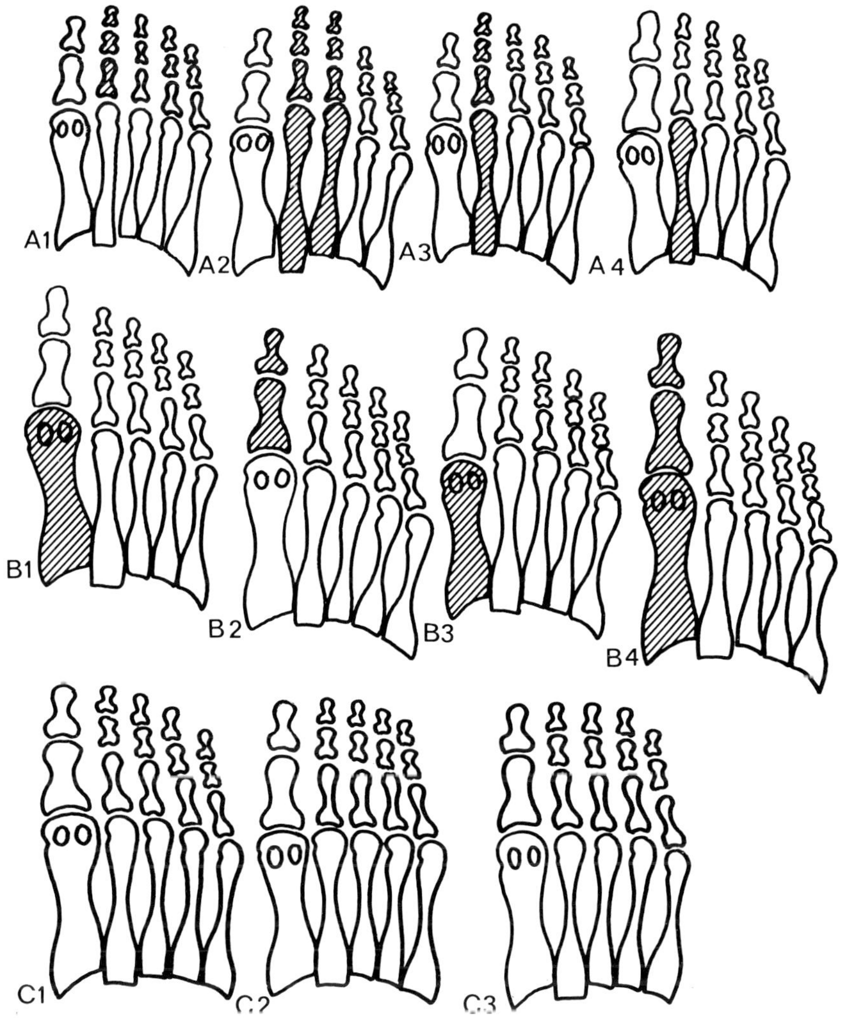

Fig. 2.2 A–C. Forefoot configuration: skeletal origin. **A** Greek: *1* Phalangeal; *2, 3* metatarsophalangeal; *4* metatarsal. **B** Egyptian: *1* Metatarsal; *2* phalangeal; *3* short first metatarsal; *4* metatarsophalangeal. **C** Square: *1* Phalangeal great and second toe; *2* metatarsophalangeal, all five metatarsals and first three phalanges; *3* metatarsophalangeal, all five metatarsals and four phalanges

may be general or irregular hypertrophy of one or several metatarsal heads.

Interphalangeal Joints. Mobility, amplitude and quality of movement, fixed flexion or tendency to flexion, and tension of the flexor and extensor tendons should be measured. Hyperextension of the distal interphalangeal joints may occur. Claw deformity involving the proximal or distal interphalangeal joints may be reducible, or may be fixed and associated with pressure signs on the plantar aspect of the tip of the toe or on the dorsum.

2.3 The Loaded Foot: Static

The podoscope yields valuable information with the patient seated or standing.

Seated. The posture of the foot under light loading can be assessed in this relatively relaxed position. Precise morphological classification of the foot can be made, and trophic signs, vertical subluxation of the tarsus, longitudinal subluxation in the midtarsal region, deformities of the sides of the metatarsus, exostoses and any digital deformities can be assessed. Podoscopy with the patient elevated and the examiner seated enables visualisation of the plantar weight-bearing pattern and accurate appraisal of the foot's posture in comfortable circumstances.

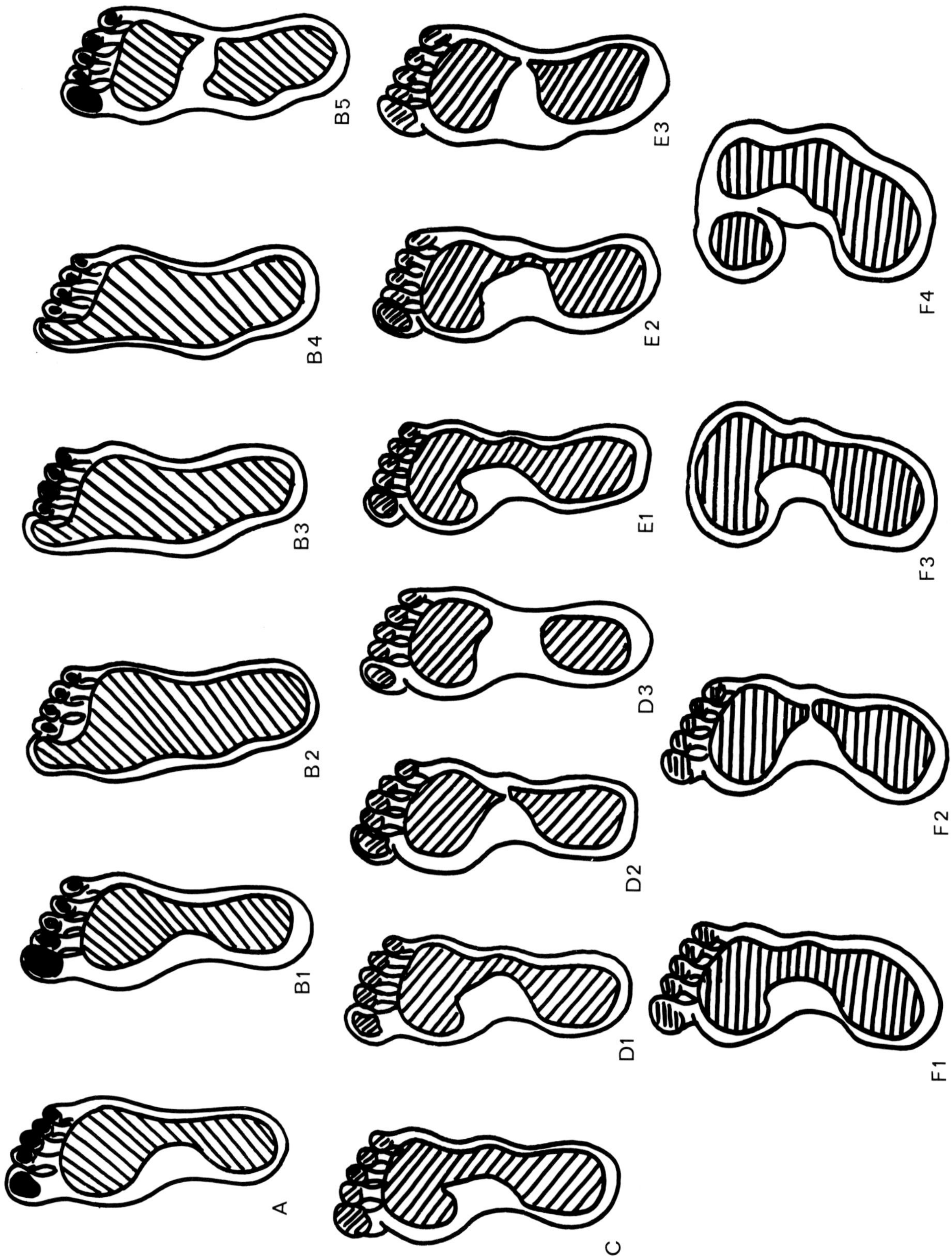

Fig. 2.3. **A** Normal foot. **B** Planovalgus foot: *1* First degree; *2* second degree; *3, 4* third degree; *5* contracted. **C** Precavus foot. **D** Balanced cavus foot: *1–3* First to third degree. **E** Cavovalgus foot: *1–3* First to third degree. **F** Cavovarus foot: *1–3* First to third degree; *4* third degree with forefoot cavus

Standing. With the patient standing on the podoscope, the foot should be viewed from its various aspects. When the patient stands on one foot, changes in the posture of the loaded side associated with efforts to balance may become very obvious (Fig. 2.3).

The general stance of the body, the configuration of the vertebral column, the relative level of the shoulders, the upper border of the iliac wings, the buttock folds and the popliteal fossa are scrutinised from behind. In the foot itself, any varus or valgus of the heel, indicating pronation or supination of the calcaneum, can be clearly seen. Also apparent are the configuration of the midtarsal region with respect to its height (in the normal foot the height of the arch, measured conveniently with a wedge inserted firmly from the medial aspect, approximates to 13-14 mm), any internal displacement with prominence of the talonavicular or Lisfranc joints, and any sinking of the arch of the foot. Conversely, a cavus foot may present. The general degree of eversion or inversion of the foot should be noted. The height of the plantar arch in millimetres should be measured, together with the degree of angulation of the medial aspect of the tarsus internally.

The print of the foot is important. Attention is paid to the general longitudinal axis, general form, and the size and shape (or occasional absence) of an isthmus of contact along the midtarsal region on the outer side of the foot.

The podoscopic examination of the footprint should be conducted in both bipedal and monopedal stance. Normally, the print is characterised by harmony, with a regularity of outline of the points of pressure both in the anterior and posterior parts. Thus, the plantar surfaces of the toes show regular outlines, the anterior band under the metatarsal heads spreads transversely and the heel presents a regular oval. These areas are joined by an external band which narrows in its middle section, is lightly concave interiorly and outwardly and usually measures 1-1½ cm in breadth. Its internal limit blends with the transverse band under the metatarsal heads and reaches in front to between the second and third metatarsal heads: at this site a hollow is seen behind the mid-part of the metatarsal heads. The overall axis of the forefoot and heel normally follows a line from the centre of the heel to the second interspace.

When the patient is viewed from in front on the podoscope, the general form of the body, the quality of the abdominal musculature, the axes of the femur and tibia and any degree of rotation of the lower limb can be assessed. A note should be made of abnormal genu valgum or genu varum. In the foot, longitudinal alignment at the tarsometatarsal joints, subluxations at the metatarsophalangeal joints, the spread of the forefoot and the positions of the toes relative to each other are apparent. The toes may be parallel, individually valgus or varus, or there may be overriding (superductus), underriding (infraductus) or flexion deformities, of which the suppleness or rigidity will already have been assessed. Overloading or underloading of metatarsal heads may be accompanied by callus formation or even plantar keratoses. The zone of metatarsal loading can be seen and the general aspect of the forefoot confirmed.

If the footprints are abnormal, photographic recording is useful.

2.4 The Loaded Foot: Dynamic

During gait, the foot is inspected with regard to the attitude of the heel on striking the ground, the reactions in the midtarsal and tarsometatarsal region during progress of the step, and the normal or abnormal supination or pronation of the forefoot towards the end of the step. During the stance phase, the moment of development of a limp should be noted. The fashion in which the patient plants his foot on the ground may be relevant to the difficulty or pain he experiences. Subluxations of the tarsus or tarsometatarsal joints may persist or disappear during loading. It may be that a particular movement is limited by a mechanical obstacle or by pain. By the close of the clinical examination efforts should have been made to localise precisely the source, site and cause of the commonest symptom, pain.

2.5 Special Investigations

Certain further investigations refine the clinical findings and in many instances prove indispensable.

2.5.1 *Podometry*

Rocher (1942) made the important observation, contrary to accepted ideas at that time, that the anterior transverse arch does not exist under load and that the heads of the five metatarsals should share load equally.

Thus the transverse anterior arch only exists when the foot is unloaded. During bipedal stance, a trapezoidal area is outlined by the heels, the cuboids and the forefeet. During monopedal loading, during elevation of the heel up to 5 cm, the foot rests on the calcaneum, the cuboidometatarsal joint and the five metatarsal heads. Of the latter, the three middle heads give rigid support, while the first and fifth metatarsals, because of their great range of movement, contribute to collateral balance (de Doncker and Kowalski 1970; Courriades 1971; Rocher 1974), while during propulsion, the main thrust comes from the three central, more rigid metatarsal heads then on to the toes, not on to the first metatarsal head as has commonly been thought.

Clinical examination can establish only the regularity of the zone of pressure of the metatarsus or of gross anomalies of high loading due to frontal protrusions or equinus, not the details of vertical loading, which can be of great importance. However, podometric investigation is of great value, as it allows precise measurement of pressure exercised under each of the five metatarsal heads and enables more exact assessment and planning of orthotic and surgical measures.

Of the various pieces of apparatus available, the reader's attention is directed to the baropodometric machine developed by Martorell Martorell (1963), which was the prototype, the later podometric apparatus of Stroescu (1971) and the electronic device of Steinfort (1975). The information gained is especially valuable in metatarsalgia, and includes accurate localisation of the frontal alignment of the forefoot under load together with a precise understanding of the pressure changes due to adaptation of the foot to ground irregularities. An objective map of the distribution of pressure under the heads of the metatarsals (Martorell, Steinfort) can be made, affording an objective evaluation of disharmony between the metatarsal heads which can easily escape attention in a clinical examination. The exact relative heights of the metatarsal heads can be assessed. The length of resection required to correct an equinus posture of one or several metatarsals can be calculated with precision.

Resections may be by basal osteotomy, or more distally when there is isolated protrusion of a metatarsal head. A corrective insole must be prepared for each individual case. Most importantly, choice of the wrong surgical procedure is minimised.

2.5.2 *Radiography*

The choice of radiographic view depends on the clinical condition.

Standard dorsoplantar[1], anteroposterior and lateral views should be taken of the whole foot when weight-bearing and when relaxed, with the centre beam directed to the midtarsal region. From these views a study of the internal and external longitudinal arches can be made, together with the angulations occurring at the tarsometatarsal region, orientation of all bony axes, and the height and level of the various skeletal elements with respect to each other.

Standard dorsoplantar and oblique views of the forefoot centred on the metatarsophalangeal joints show the transverse line of the five metatarsal heads and their respective lengths, epiphyseal structure, shape, distortion if present and size, together with any lysis or necrosis. Articular alignment and subluxation if present may be dorsal, lateral or display varus of a "windswept" appearance. Müller (1927), Güntz (1939), Blondin-Walter (1949), Rocher (1962), Delagoutte and Hoeffel (1976), Chevrot (1981) and Chaigneau (1981) described tangential anteroposterior radiographic views of the loaded metatarsal heads which show the relative heights of each of these and the position of sesamoid bones at the condyles of the metatarsals. These views are taken on a thick felt pad measuring 3 by 4 cm. The calcaneum rests on a heelpiece 3 cm higher; the blocks of material are permeable to the X-rays.

Views of the foot and ankle under static load comprise an anteroposterior projection of the ankle joint (Meary) which outlines the mortice and determines the frontal axis of the hindfoot under any angle of valgus. The axial view of the subtalar joint described by Milton-Lewis may be valuable.

Special views for particular points of bony interest may be necessary.

2.5.3 *Other Special Investigations*

Angiography, phlebography, lymphangiography and electromyography can be ordered if indicated, and scintigraphy may also be valuable. Finally, special investigations related to the patient's general condition will include cardiovascular assessment and routine laboratory examinations.

---

1 The dorsoplantar view is frequently and erroneously called "anteroposterior of the foot"; it is taken with the loaded foot on the cassette, the tube directed vertically downwards at right angles to the plate, and the leg dorsiflexed 10°

3 Painful Syndromes of the Foot and Other Parts

It will be seen that a number of systemic diseases may present local pathology in the foot. In addition, there is an undoubted relationship between postural abnormalities in the lower limbs and in the vertebral column. The uncertainty as to which is the primary abnormality may remain, but it is useful to give some indication of the possible relationships of lumbago, sacralgia and pain in the knee with transverse and longitudinal postural abnormalities in the foot.

3.1 Muscle Pains

Diffuse aching due to abnormal strain or tension arising in muscle masses may arise in the following ways:

1. Diffuse myalgia of a dull fatiguing character experienced in the postero-internal aspect of the calf, which can be associated with pes planovalgus, is due to chronic strain of tibialis anterior and posterior and triceps surae.
2. Pes cavus, especially with a varus component, leads to strain of the peroneal and long extensor muscles.
3. In any valgus posture of the foot, especially with pes planus but also sometimes with pes cavus, a cramp-like fatigued sensation in triceps surae can be experienced.
4. In longitudinal pes cavus, the intrinsic muscles of the foot can suffer cramps which spread into the leg.

The proof of a mechanical etiology for these muscle pains is given by the effectiveness of suitable insoles. When these re-establish lateral equilibrium of the foot, support a pes planus or extend a pes cavus, the muscle pains tend to disappear.

3.2 Tendinitis

The classic Achilles tendinitis, affecting the child or adult with pes planovalgus or pes cavus, is well established. In the cavovarus foot there is frequently tendinitis of the peronei, while in pes planovalgus it is not rare for tendinitis to establish itself at the insertions of the tibialis posterior and anterior tendons. In some instances, the cause-and-effect relationship of the painful tendon with the displacement of the foot may be uncertain. The painful tendon insertion can produce a reactive hypertonia and consequent displacement of the foot. Again, the relationship is proved by effective use of an appropriate insole.

3.3 Pain in Knee, Hip and Vertebral Column

Displacement of the foot into valgus or varus entails modification of the lines of transmission of forces throughout the lower limb and may manifest with symptoms at higher levels. Invariably, the symptoms are aggravated by standing, stamping and walking and are relieved by rest. At the outset they are described as diffuse syndromes of fatigue, muscle tension and cramps affecting almost any vertebral level with diffuse arthralgias at the hip or the knee. They are of an "inflammatory" character, like arthrosis, or of varying intensity, like neuralgia. Usually they occur towards the end of the day but the time of onset becomes progressively earlier, until finally the pains are permanent. The pains are not relieved by anti-inflammatory or anti-arthrosic treatment, bur can be controlled by the use of an insole, again indicating the foot as being the primary source of the disorder.

3.4 Neuralgias

Two particular syndromes, sciatica and pain in the base of the neck, appear to be frequently related to bilateral pes planovalgus in which the lowering of the medial longitudinal arch is more marked on one side. This lowering of the midtarsal mass asymmetrically is accompanied by a more valgus calcaneal posture on the side concerned, a swelling of the retromalleolar gutter and a tilting of the pelvis towards the side most affected. A scoliotic dorsolumbar posture is adopted. Podoscopic examination is therefore particularly valuable in the differential diagnosis of sciatica, which may be due to a postural abnormality of the foot when it presents characteristics other than those of pain due to nerve root irritation at a lumbar disc. It should be noted that a trial of corrective insole is valuable for the low cervicalgia, but that it should not consist of a simple compensating heel raise, as this leads to anteversion of the pelvis rather than true correction of the lateral tilting caused by the asymmetrical low plantar arch on one side. A supporting insole correcting a planovalgus deformity may bring surprising relief of the neck pain.

3.5 Classification of Relevant Foot Displacements

The term "longitudinal displacements" refers to pes planus and pes cavus, while "lateral displacements" indicates valgus or varus components. The two are frequently associated.

3.5.1 Balanced Pes Cavus

Balanced pes cavus (i.e. without valgus or varus) leads to augmentation of calcaneal inclination and hypertonia of the posterior calf muscles and anterior muscles of the thigh with a forward tilting of the pelvis. There is compensatory increased lumbar lordosis, and the syndrome of calf muscle pains and cramps, pains at the back of the knee, lumbago and sacralgia are possible results.
Treatment includes measures to strengthen the abdominal muscles, a shoe with a raised heel of 3–4 cm if calf muscle pain is predominant, the use of a retrocapital bar insole to relax the cavus and anti-inflammatory agents.

3.5.2 Bilateral Pes Planus

In this condition there is diminution of the angle of inclination of the calcaneum and a lowering of the medial plantar arch. Tibialis posterior is strained, leading to calf pain, while internal rotation of the ankle mortice and therefore of the knee must follow. Achilles and tibialis tendinitis, posterior myalgia in the calf muscle, and pain, most frequently on the inner side of the knee, may be accompanied by discomfort in the hip, the low back and the base of the neck. A genu valgum may be apparent. These various pains will be relieved by an appropriate insole supporting the plantar arch.

3.5.3 Pes Cavovarus

This more frequent association is accompanied by inversion of the midtarsal mass. On account of the supination of the calcaneum there is external rotation of the ankle mortice, which reflects on the knee and leads to peroneal tendinitis, and a genu varum accompanied by pain of an arthrosic type on the outer side of the knee radiating to the hip and the dorsolumbar region.
Correction of the varus of the tarsus and general inversion of the foot and relaxation of the cavus deformity by an appropriate insole attenuates the skeletal pains detailed above and will be sufficient provided there is no fixed structural abnormality in the foot.

As in generalised systemic disease of a medical nature, these brief remarks indicate the importance of the podologist having a more widespread understanding of generalised disorders and not confining examination purely to the presenting organ, the foot.

4 Mycoses

Fungal infections of the foot affect the cornified epidermal layer and the nails. The organisms responsible are yeasts or dermatophytes. The conditions are chronic with exacerbations during the summer, the acute phases being favoured by sweating or a humid environment. While other parts of the body can be affected without alteration of a general healthy state, Grigoriu (1975 a) has estimated that 15% of cutaneous diseases of the foot are due to mycoses. Sabouraud (1910), Emmons (1910) and Kaufmann and Woef (1914) all isolated dermatophytic organisms, while Haren and Brown (1950) extracted nystatin and actidione from the mycelia of *Streptomyces noursei.* Achten (1964) contributed specifically to the onychomycoses, with specific reference to the histopathology of the nail.

Sabouraud and Emmons (1910) classified the responsible organisms into three main groups:

Microsporum audouini, M. gypseum, M. ferrugineum and M. carus

Epidermatophyton floccosum

Trichophyton rubrum (most frequently), *T. mentographytes* interdigitale asteroide, and more rarely, *T. megnini* and *T. persicolor.* Among yeasts, *Candida albicans* filament was the most frequent.

Previously, 70% of mycoses were of a *Candida* origin, but nowadays the majority are due to trichophytes or epidermophytes, especially *Trichophyton rubrum* (Beurey, Weber, Percebois, Franquey). Numerous names have been given to the digital epidermatophytoses, e.g. tinea pedis, athlete's foot and Hong Kong foot. The superficial nature of the mycotic infections involving the cornified epidermic layer, the hair and the nails is in contrast with the subcutaneous mycoses developing in the deeper layers of the dermis which can provoke cutaneous manifestations due to myectomata (madura foot), chromoblastomycomata, sporotrichoses and histoplasmoses.

Infection gains access through microscopic breaches in the epidermis, propagates slowly and eventually manifests as interdigital intertrigo, mycoses of the plantar aspect of the foot, or onychomycosis and onyxis of the nail. Adolescents and adults, usually males, are afflicted, and Kligmann and Rosenthal have drawn attention to the relevance of the extreme variability between individual subjects in contracting the infection, with particular reference to the epidermophytes. The seasonal recrudescences occur during the first warmth of spring and again at the beginning of autumn when subjects go back to wearing closed shoes. Direct transmission is rare (Grigoriu 1975), and most infections result from walking in bare feet in swimming pools (40% of swimmers according to Van ken Seghem and 62% according to Alteras et al.), sauna baths, gymnasia, hotel bathrooms, and barracks where socks and shoes are changed. Lack of hygiene, and paradoxically an excess of bathing not followed by careful drying of the feet and interdigital spaces in an optimum temperature of 10°-15°, predispose to infection, as do warmth and humidity, wind, fog, rain, and other climatic factors. Sweating, the use of alkaline soaps, poor drying of the feet and failure to use talc all favour the development of mycoses in poorly ventilated regions. Grigoriu (1975) stated that some subjects are more prone to infection, e.g. those who sweat excessively, diabetics, those with circulatory disorders, those with pes planus, and those who have just been treated with antibiotics and corticoids.

4.1 Clinical Features

4.1.1 Interdigital Intertrigo

This condition presents in one of the interdigital commissures (usually the fourth) as a whitish macerated desquamating area. The sides of the surfaces of the toes can become involved and the surrounding skin appears pinker and moister than normal. The lesions are pruritic and may become painful when the subject wears a closed shoe or performs vigorous exercise. The interdigital itching becomes smarting in nature. In the absence of subsequent hygienic measures - drying and ventilation of the shoes - the affectation becomes chronic and lasts for years, extending progressively into the forefoot, either on the dorsum or, more frequently, the proximal plantar aspect. It then assumes one of two clinical forms.

Erythematous-Squamous Intertrigo. This is usually due to *Trichophyton*. On the plantar aspect, an erythematous plaque forms which is clearly delineated and characterised by the skin becoming shiny, losing its folds and developing a pink violaceous or deep red coloration. The area is covered by little dry scales which are greyish in colour and very irritating. The condition is worsened by the subject scratching the pruritic area.

Vesicular Bullous Intertrigo. The lesion in the commissure is from the outset fissured, macerated and of a damp, bright red, fatty appearance spreading on to the collateral aspects of the adjacent toes. It extends further onto the dorsal and lateral aspect of the foot. The erythematous fatty appearance is due to a lemon-yellowish exudate from tiny vesicles which are noted more frequently towards the periphery of the lesions. Again, superinfection from scratching is common. Digital oedema of the foot can become severe and the toes generally develop a podgy, pink violaceous appearance with thin stretched skin on the dorsal aspects, which seem to be separated from the forefoot by transverse furrows. There is a pain described as a cooking or burning sensation, together with the pruritis. Lymphangitis and lymphadenopathy with fever may develop.
The foot becomes voluminous, and considerable disability and immobilisation may ensue. Treatment is usually effective but must be pursued rigorously.

4.1.2 Plantar Mycoses

These mycoses usually begin insidiously on the plantar aspect of the foot under the arch, although they can follow from digital intertrigo. Combination of the two sites is not unusual. *Trichophyton rubrum* and *T. mentagrophytes* are the organisms most commonly responsible. Two presentations can be distinguished:

a) The vesiculobullous or pustulous form of Djeladdin-Mouktar is usually caused by *T. mentagrophytes* (Bazex et al. 1966) and begins on the medial aspect of the plantar arch as a plaque of varying extent and erythematous appearance associated with severe pruritis, pain and functional disability as a result of the presence of multiple small vesicles which rapidly become confluent in a bulla of varying size filled with yellowish fluid and bulging the epidermis. Gradually the plaque spreads to involve the whole of the plantar aspect of the foot. Generalised oedema becomes significant spreading on to the dorsum and into the malleolar area. Superinfection can lead to athlete's foot or evolve towards the desquamative form.
b) The dry or scaly (erythematous-squamous or hyperkeratotic) form has been well studied by Bazex et al. (1966). This type of mycosis, predominantly caused by *T. rubrum* (Bazex et al. 1966), is usually unilateral but can affect both feet. From the outset there is a hyperkeratotic lesion with thick scales which confer a pseudokeratotic form to the isolated plaques, surrounded by painful crevices. It is difficult to differentiate from the plantar lesions of keratodermia and psoriasis and may be succeeded by vesiculobullous mycosis or the lesions of plantar dyshydrosis. The plaques are reddish with rounded contours, very clearly delineated and covered with thick dry greyish or dirty-white scales progressively spreading to the plantar aspect of the forefoot, the toes, the borders of the foot and the dorsal aspect. Untreated, it spreads inexorably, becoming complicated by superinfection (lymphangitis, folliculitis or erysipelas according to Grigoriu), invasion and progressive destruction of the nails and the development of allergic manifestations. Natural seasonal remissions may give a false impression of the efficacy of treatment. Eczematous reactions and lichenification can occur (Grigoriu 1975; Bazex et al. 1963). The clinical diagnosis is confirmed by the clear delineation of the circular plaques, perhaps with a protruding, red-infiltrated or pink violaceous collarette, the eccentric extension of the lesions, the coexistence of intertriginous lesions and desquamative lesions of the plantar aspect of the foot, the intensity of the pruritis, which ceases only after several days of treatment, the chronic development over years and the equally slow regression, and the association of mycotic infections at other sites (trunk, beard and hands).

Laboratory examination is essential for final diagnosis.

4.1.3 Ungual Mycosis or Onyxis of Toes

Mycotic involvement of the nail is characterised by changes in coloration and opacification; the nail loses its translucent appearance, becoming yellowish or dirty grey. This is accompanied by progressive thickening of the nail plate and by invasion, onycholysis, or total destruction with cornified subungual maceration and swelling. One or more toes may be involved. The condition may follow from an intertriginous digital lesion or from a plantar mycosis developing into an epidermal disease. Whatever the presentation, the onset is extremely slow and initially passes unperceived by the patient (See Fig. 17.3; I).

Epidermatophytes [most commonly *Trichophyton rubrum* (Achten 1964) and *T. mentagrophytes*] are often responsible, but moulds *(Scopulariopsis, Cephalosporium, Aspergillus* and *Fusarium)* and yeasts *(Candida albicans, C. parapsilosis* and *C. tropicale)* can also cause perhaps up to 50% of cases (Baran 1981). Only laboratory study will determine which organism is responsible.

Baran (1978), in his remarkable study of onyxis, distinguished four forms, and valuable information can be gained from Pierre's book *The Nail* (1978).

Subungual Distal Onychomycosis. There is retrograde invasion of the extremity of the nail plate spreading towards its root, comprising a loss of transparency, with red, green or greyish coloration, and a friable consistency like old rotten wood. The onyxis sometimes ends in onycholysis or with keratosis in the subungual region, which elevates the free border of the nail. According to Pierre (1978) and Baran (1978), 50% of cases are due to moulds *(Scopulariopsis)* and yeasts *(Candida albicans* or *C. tropicale),* 25% to dermatophytes *(Trichophyton rubrum, T. mentagrophytes interdigitale)* and 25% to bacteria.

Leuconychomycosis Superficialae. This condition (Pierre 1978; Baran 1978) is characterised by the appearance of little opaque specks, whitish in colour and clearly delineated, which spread to involve the whole of the nail surface with progressive modification in consistency and colour of the nail, which becomes rugose, softer and then friable, and takes on a yellowish colour.

It is always produced by *T. rubrum* and *T. mentagrophytes,* except in rare instances in which the causative agents are moulds.

Subungual Proximal Onychomycosis. This affects the deeper layers of the nail and is manifested by the appearance under the lunule and then under the nail fold of little white zones which extend progressively towards the distal extremity of the nail.

Primary Onychomycodystrophy. This condition is also known as candida granuloma, and according to Pierre (1978) and Baran (1978) is exceptional in that it involves the whole of the nail. The nail plate becomes brownish with opaque thickening and whitish longitudinal streaks, but is not friable. The infection is associated with inflammatory reactions in the neighbourhood: perionyxis, thickening of the nail bed and the hyponychium. It is due to the yeast *C. albicans.*

4.2 Laboratory Examination

Identification of the etiological organism is essential for efficacious treatment and for determining when the mycosis, especially of the nail, has been finally controlled. Specimens must be taken under rigorous aseptic conditions, ideally in the laboratory performing the examination, and are obtained using a vaccination lance or a Brocq curette which takes an effective biopsy sample from the periphery of a lesion in the region of the desquamative collarettes. The examination must be performed before the institution of general or local treatment; if any form of treatment has been commenced, it should be interrupted for at least a week before specimens are taken.

Direct microscopic examination of the specimen in a lactophenolic solution gives information with regard to the squames and the nail shavings (Achten 1964), allowing distinction between mycelia and ramifying filaments or the fragmented filaments in arthrospores; dermatophytes, pseudofilaments, and yeast cells can also be distinguished. Sometimes there may be association of a dermatophyte with a yeast.

Culture is performed on Sabouraud medium complemented by chloramphenicol or actidione, to control bacterial growth. This examination can be amplified by subculture using special media in a suspended drop technique. Identification of dermatophytes is made from the speed of growth (5 days to 4 weeks), the appearance of the colonies, the production of pigment and the vitamin requirements for growth, while the identification of yeasts such as *Candida albicans* (taking 24–48 h) is made by the appearance of the colonies, which develop by budding of blastophores.

Tests on *Candida albicans* grown in protein agar and Tween 80 may reveal the presence of chlamydospore. Achten (1964) described histological examination of nail fragments in which specimens embedded in paraffin (not fixed or dehydrated) demonstrate bright red filaments and spores after staining with PAS, allowing differentiation between dermatophytes and yeasts.

4.3 Treatment

Management should be directed towards prophylaxis and cure of the established condition.

4.3.1 Prophylaxis

Good hygiene is the basis of avoiding mycotic infections. After bathing or showering, the following should be carried out: careful drying of the feet, friction with 90% alcohol and powdering with talc on the plantar aspect of the foot and between the toes. Socks should be light and should be changed each day, and shoes should have a leather insole or an aerated leather upper. Open or woven shoes should be worn during the summer, and impermeable shoes should be avoided altogether.

4.3.2 Treatment of the Established Condition

In general, both local and systemic treatment is indicated and is directed simultaneously against trichophytes and yeasts because of the frequency of overlap of the infections.

4.3.2.1 General Treatment

Antitrichophytic treatment includes the use of griseofulvin, which exercises a fungostatic action on the epidermis and deeper layers, with specific action against the mycelia of the cutaneous and nail dermatophytes, and is particularly active against the trichophytes and therefore against mycotic intertrigo. Daily oral administration continues for several months.
Antilevuric agents include nystatin and amphotericin β, which inhibit the growth of *Candida albicans*. They are fungostatic and fungicidal. Nystatin is administered at a dose of 3-4 mega-units/day by local application in a cream. Amphotericin β dosage is 1.5 g/day by intravenous administration in an infusion. Both are effective against *Candida* and *Aspergillus fumigatus*.

4.3.2.2 Local Treatment

Many valuable local agents have been described, among them the following:

60% silver nitrate
Potassium iodide solution
Acid soaps for dermatoses of the skin folds
Undecylenic fatty acids of the types active against *Candida* infections
Quaternary ammonium compounds with antifungal action against *Candida* and the trichophytes (e.g. Fongeryl[1])
Benzthiazide, which has a fungistatic action against dermatophytes and a kerolytic action against *Trichophyton rubrum*.

4.3.2.3 Some Specific Treatments

Trichophyte Mycoses. General treatment comprises administration of griseofulvin 500 mg to 1 g/day for 4 weeks. Locally, the appropriate treatment is cleaning with dilute acid soap, irrigation with iodinated alcohol, Betadine, or Fongeryl coupled with antimycotic cream dressings both in the morning and at night. Hewit cream and other preparations such as Fongeryl, buclosamide and Mycodecyl are valuable.

Candida *Mycoses.* General treatment comprises nystatin; in very severely septicaemic forms, amphotericin β by intravenous infusion may be necessary. Local treatment involves cleaning with dilute acid soap (e.g. Dermacide, a soap combined with benzoic acid, salicylic acid and tartaric acid) and application of a solution of Fongeryl, Mycostatin cream containing nystatin, triamcinolone, and neomycin, which exercises a triple action against *Candida*, inflammation and other bacteria.

Mycotic Onyxis. In the first instance a firm laboratory examination result is necessary, and then griseofulvin or another anti-yeast agent such as nystatin is administered systemically for some 4-5 months. Locally, treatment must continue for months or even years until the smallest nail lesion disappears completely; it comprises chiropodial management of the nail once a week with filing and drilling, and dressing of the nails with a cream base adapted to the infecting organism.

---

1 Fongeryl (Laboratoire Clin Midy, 20, rue des Fossés Saint Jacques - 75240 Paris)

Athlete's Foot. General treatment must include periods of rest with the leg elevated. Secondary infection with bacteria is common and necessitates systemic antibiotic therapy with oleandomycin, tetramycin or erythromycin. Local treatment comprises permanganate of potash baths (1:4000) and damp dressings after irrigation with antimycotic solution. After 8 days, this may be succeeded by 3 weeks treatment with agents specifically directed against the causative organism, perhaps antidermatophytic (griseofulvin), or against a yeast infection (Mycostatin, or perhaps Fungizone intravenously).

II Functional and Structural Disorders of the Forefoot

5 Painful Syndromes of the Forefoot*

5.1 Causes

The following mechanisms, which may occur singly or in combination, appear to contribute to pain in the forefoot:

Muscular weakness or incoordination
Modifications to the plantar, longitudinal and transverse arches
Modifications in the degree of frontal curvature of the Lisfranc joint line

5.1.1 Muscular Weakness and Incoordination

The three central metatarsals are relatively immobile compared with the outer and inner components (Hendrix 1934; de Doncker and Kowalski 1970). Irrespective of the metatarsal formula (Egyptian, Greek or square) a painful syndrome may result if there is incoordination or weakness of the muscles inserted into the first and fifth rays. In one subject, overlong central metatarsals with respect to the outer and inner rays may cause no problems of loading, whereas in another, specific painful syndromes may result, relating entirely to the loss of uniformity of loading of the metatarsal heads in rolling of the forefoot during the stance phase. As this phase progresses, increased loading on the central metatarsal heads, which act relatively as a unit, is accompanied by adaptation of the more mobile first and fifth metatarsal heads to the ground and by a transverse rolling movement which becomes more and more marked towards the medial side of the foot towards the end of the stance. The adaptability of the more mobile extreme metatarsal heads ensures uniformity of loading throughout.

The harmonious action is under the influence of reflex muscle control, and it is clear that as the heel rises, given a normal frontal convexity of the metatarsal heads of the formula $1<2\geqslant 3\geqslant 4>5$, the first and fifth metatarsals must accentuate their plantar flexion relative to the central rays. Further, their movement is directed towards the mid-axis of the foot so as to tend to produce an excavated plantar outline which could be likened to a horseshoe. The extrinsic muscles of the foot (the long toe flexors, tibialis posterior and anterior, and the peronei) and the intrinsic muscles of the foot are all involved in this dynamic control. The concept of uniformity of loading of the metatarsal heads throughout the stance phase or during standing is crucial to an understanding of the painful forefoot.

When there is a disadvantageous configuration of the metatarsal heads, the likelihood of muscular control being able to compensate for the changing pattern of loading must be decreased. If the power of plantar flexion of the first and fifth metatarsals is deficient, overloading will result centrally. Conversely, if there is overaction of the plantar flexors of the first and fifth metatarsals, underloading of the central metatarsal heads can occur, producing a *cavus forefoot*. The ability of the first and fifth metatarsal heads to compensate for loading, especially in the presence of a disadvantageous metatarsal head formula (see below), must be regarded as the main influence in protecting the weight-bearing tissues of the ball of the foot; failure of the mechanism is the most important cause of the painful syndromes of the forefoot which will be described later.

5.1.2 Modifications of Longitudinal and Transverse Arches of Foot

These modifications relate to the relative plantar inclinations of the metatarsals and the frontal configuration of the Lisfranc joint line.

Hendrix (1934) regarded the talonavicular complex as the key to both the plantar longitudinal arch and the transverse arch; he called it the talonavicular cushion. Its key position between the calcaneum posteriorly, the cuboid laterally and the

* This material was published in *Chirurgia del Piede* vol. 2 no.3 pp. 121–136 (1978) and is reproduced by courtesy of Editions Minerva Medica

Lisfranc joint anteriorly is influenced by the load of the body weight acting through the talus. The balance of its mechanism is conditioned by the concavity of the longitudinal and plantar arches, through which it controls the action of the forefoot. It relates immediately to the overall degree of frontal convexity of the Lisfranc joint line, which controls the relative positions of the five metatarsal heads. Without entering into the etiology of the various deformations which can occur, they may be broadly classified as follows:
(a) the flat triangular forefoot (Locke); (b) the simple convex forefoot; (c) the convex triangular forefoot; (d) the cavus forefoot.

a) *The flat triangular forefoot* has initially a metatarsal head formula of the Greek type, in which the frontal protrusion of the second, third and fourth metatarsal heads is not accompanied by any selective equinus thereof. The five metatarsal heads are situated in the same horizontal plane.
b) *The simple convex forefoot* is associated with a longitudinal balanced cavus foot related to one or both of the following causes:
   - Frontal protrusion of the middle metatarsal heads of the Greek type
   - Equinus of the middle metatarsals with a normal horizontal position of the first and fifth metatarsal heads
c) *The convex triangular forefoot* is produced by a longitudinal cavovalgus configuration associated with internal midtarsal displacement. The valgus imposed on the cavus foot results in a loss of height of the plantar longitudinal and transverse arches and an augmentation of the frontal convexity of the Lisfranc joint configuration. The latter leads to frontal protrusion of the central metatarsal heads together with equinus and divergence of the first and fifth metatarsals.
d) *The cavus forefoot* occurs in a balanced longitudinal cavus foot or one with a varus posture. Only the first and fifth metatarsals are lowered, the three central metatarsal heads being in a more elevated position than normal. The first and fifth metatarsals become relatively shorter.

5.1.3 Modifications of Frontal Configuration of Lisfranc Joint

There is an interrelationship between the frontal convex curve of the Lisfranc joint, the longitudinal arch and the transverse arch of the foot. The configuration of the foot as a whole can be likened to an English Gothic arch which widens fanwise from behind forwards. A series of joint lines, convex forwards, develop progressively from the talonavicular level: the naviculocuneiform, the tarsometatarsal, the metatarsophalangeal and the interphalangeal joints (Fig. 5.1). Going forwards, there is augmentation of curvature, and any change in the degree of frontal convexity will develop progressively towards the front of the foot. It is in this light that the configuration of the forefoot should be understood, with respect to both the frontal anterior convexities of the joint lines and the plantar transverse concavity. The morphology of the forefoot is modified accordingly, as follows:

- Increased concavity of the plantar longitudinal arch is accompanied by increased concavity of the transverse arch, as in pes cavus (Fig. 5.2).
- Increased concavity of the transverse arch is accompanied by reduction of the forward frontal convexity of the Lisfranc joint line (pes cavus) (Fig. 5.3).
- Diminished convexity of the Lisfranc joint line is accompanied by reduced divergence of the metatarsals (Fig. 5.4).

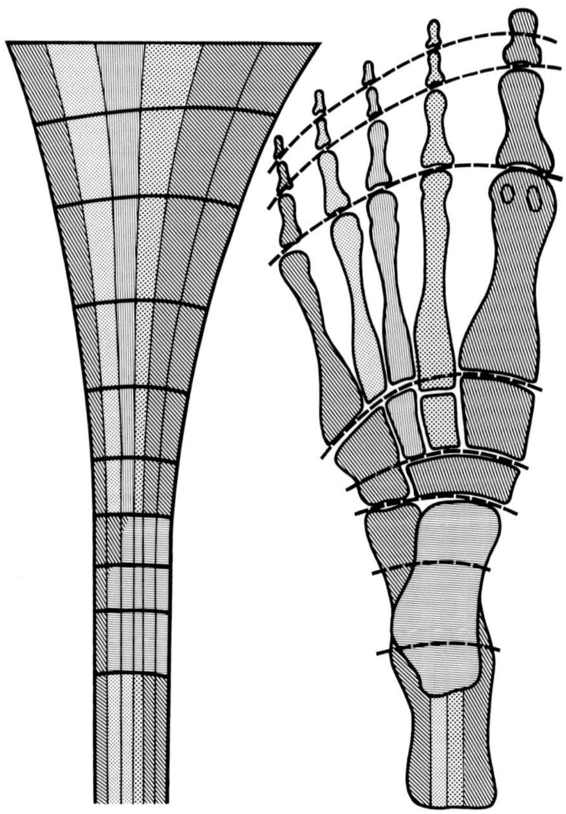

Fig. 5.1. The Anglo-Gothic arch (Regnauld)

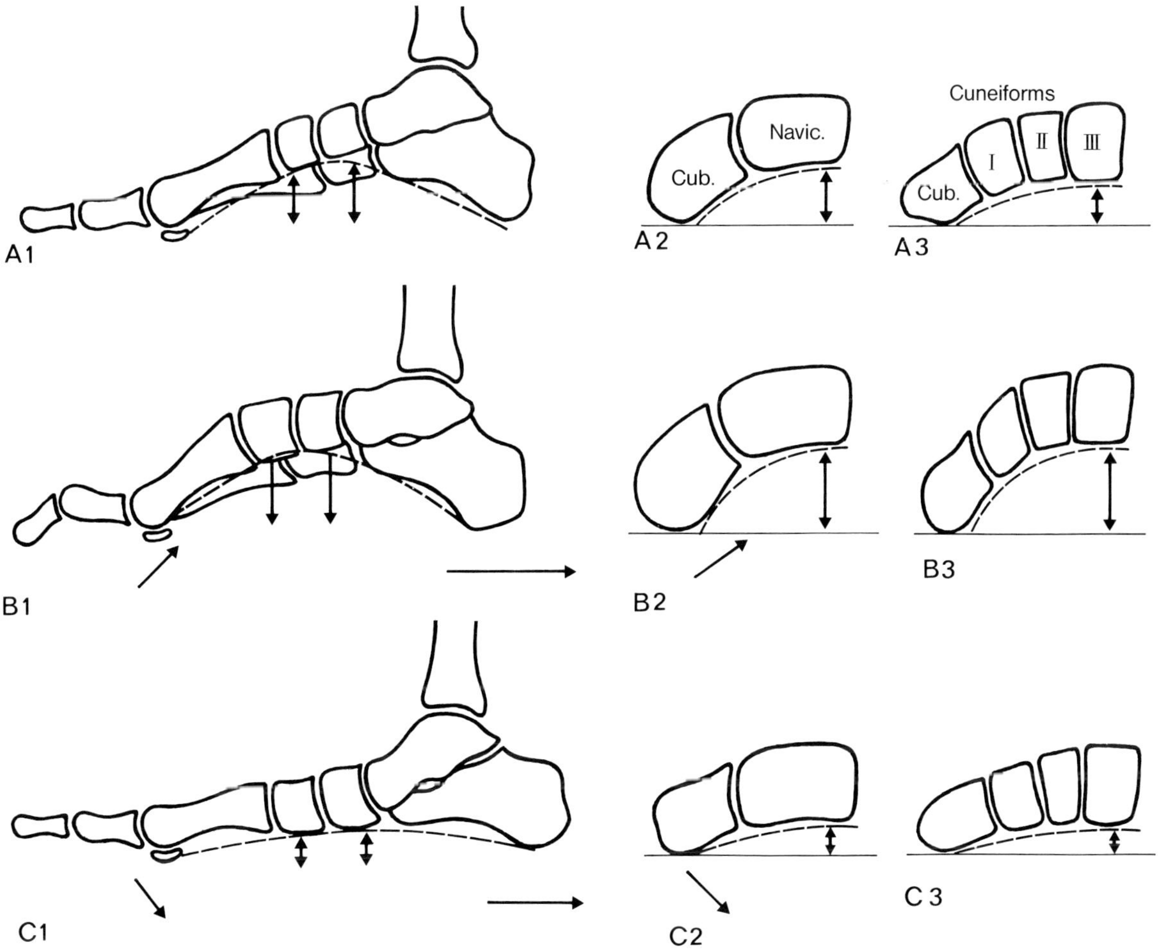

Fig. 5.2 A–C. Longitudinal arch *(1)* and transverse arch at midtarsus *(2)* and Lisfranc joint *(3)* in **A** a normal foot, **B** a cavus foot, and **C** a planus foot

The converse also applies:

- Diminished longitudinal concavity of the foot is accompanied by diminution of the transverse plantar concavity (pes planus) (Fig. 5.2).
- Diminished plantar transverse concavity of the foot corresponds with the augmentation of the frontal anterior convexity of the Lisfranc joint line (pes planus) (Fig. 5.3).
- Augmented frontal convexity of the tarsometatarsal joint line is accompanied by augmentation of divergence of the five metatarsals (the flat forefoot) (Fig. 5.4).

In the normal foot, the longitudinal and plantar concavities develop progressively (a) in the midtarsal region at the talonavicular cushion, and (b) at the torsion bar of the Lisfranc joints where the intermediate and lateral cuneiforms, between the medial cuneiform and the cuboid, articulate with the second and third metatarsals and the navicular respectively (Fig. 5.5).

When the talonavicular cushion is elevated, as in the cavus foot, it provokes movement of the intermediate and lateral cuneiform upwards and backwards, resulting in a diminution of the frontal transverse convexity of the Lisfranc joint line. It follows that the metatarsals augment their equinus and diminish their divergence, leading to either the convex or the cavus forefoot.

Conversely, when the talonavicular cushion is lowered, as in the flat foot, there is downward and forward displacement of the intermediate and lateral cuneiforms, resulting in augmentation of the frontal anterior convexity of the Lisfranc joint; the metatarsals diminish their equinus, augment their frontal protrusion and augment their divergence leading to a triangular forefoot which may be simple, flat or convex.

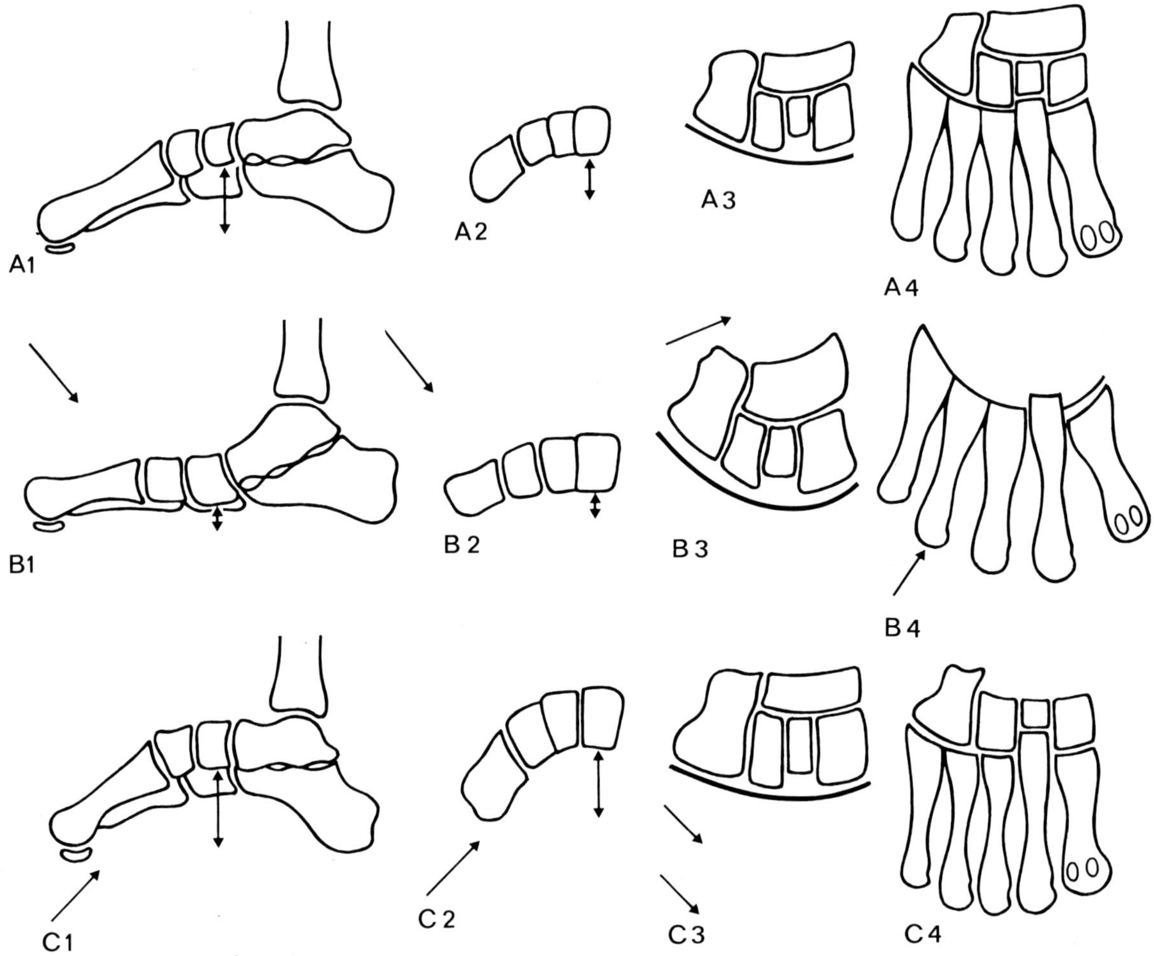
A1
A2
A3
A4
B1
B2
B3
B4
C1
C2
C3
C4

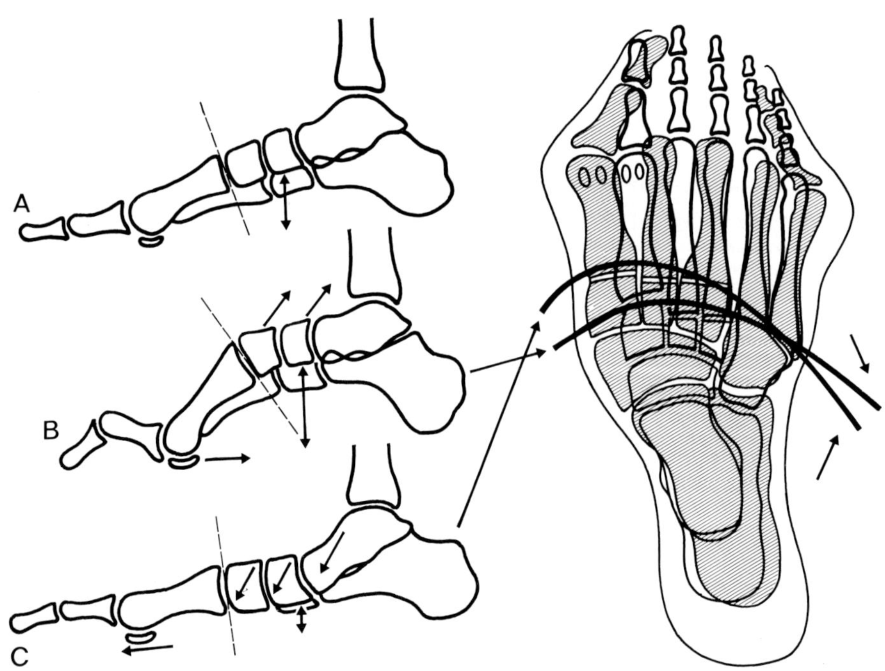
A
B
C

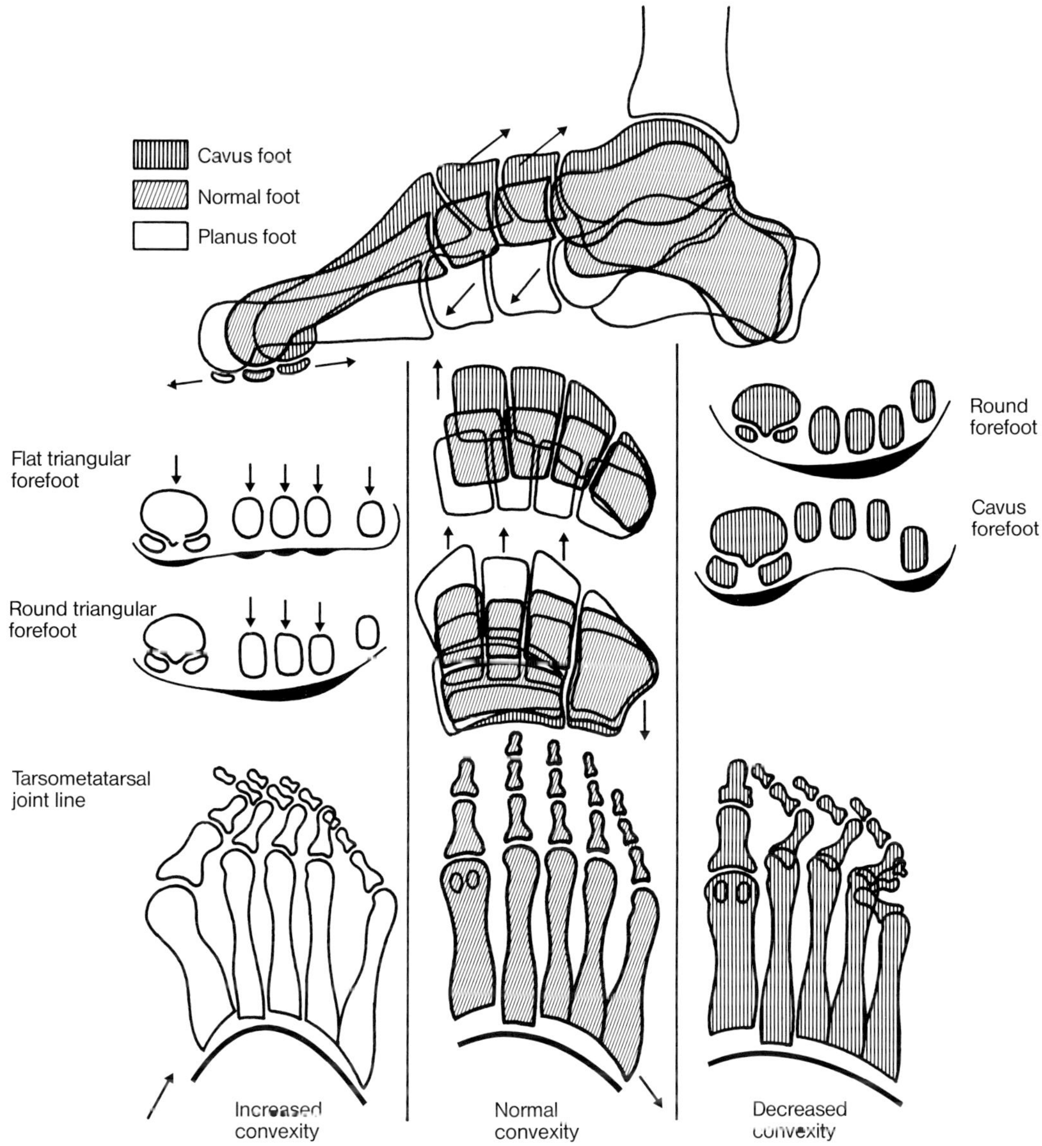

Fig. 5.5. Displacements of skeletal elements occurring in syndromes of the forefoot

◁ **Fig. 5.3 A–C** *(Above)*. Alteration of longitudinal arch and transverse convexity. **A** Normal foot. **B** Planus foot: *1* Lowering of longitudinal arch; *2* lowering of transverse arch; *3* increase in frontal transverse convexity; *4* increase in metatarsal divergence. **C** Cavus foot: *1* Raising of longitudinal arch; *2* raising of transverse arch; *3* decrease in frontal transverse convexity; *4* decrease in metatarsal divergence

Fig. 5.4 A–C *(Below)*. Alteration of transverse plane of tarsometatarsal joints. **A** Normal foot. **B** Cavus foot: increased inclination, increased metatarsal equinus, reduced frontal convexity. **C** Planus foot: decreased inclination, decreased metatarsal equinus, increased frontal convexity in pes planovalgus

The result of lowering of the transverse arch of the foot, formed by the Lisfranc joint line, is a change in position downwards and forwards of the intermediate and lateral cuneiforms, associated with depression and inward direction of the medial metatarsals and outward direction of the fourth and fifth metatarsals.
The first and fifth metatarsals cannot diminish or augment their equinus without a change in their divergence. This is relevant to the fitting of the foot to a shoe. If the fit is perfect, the foot not being compressed in the relaxed state, as soon as it is loaded, during stance and propulsion there is a diminution of the longitudinal and transverse concavities which must be accompanied by augmentation of the frontal anterior convexity of the joint lines and consequent divergence of the metatarsals, which produces compression of the forefoot by the margins of the shoe upper; the foot is now said to fill the shoe. This sensation of compression under load is a result of the divergence of the metatarsus. In a foot model, Ombredanne and Mathieu (1937) showed this progressive reverberation of effect from segment to segment, i.e. from the tarsometatarsal region to the metatarsal heads. Modification of the longitudinal orientation of the metatarsals leads to changes at the metatarsophalangeal joints and in the position of the toes. The toes especially are affected by the constraints of containment in the shoe and by the wearing of a high heel. Progressive deformities are associated with the various unequal pressures, but these are influenced fundamentally by the vertical and lateral orientations of the metatarsals themselves. Muscular overaction is succeeded by stretching of the joint ligaments and contractures of the tendons which become progressively irreversible. Irreducibility of the soft tissues is accompanied by osteoarticular displacements which are also permanent.

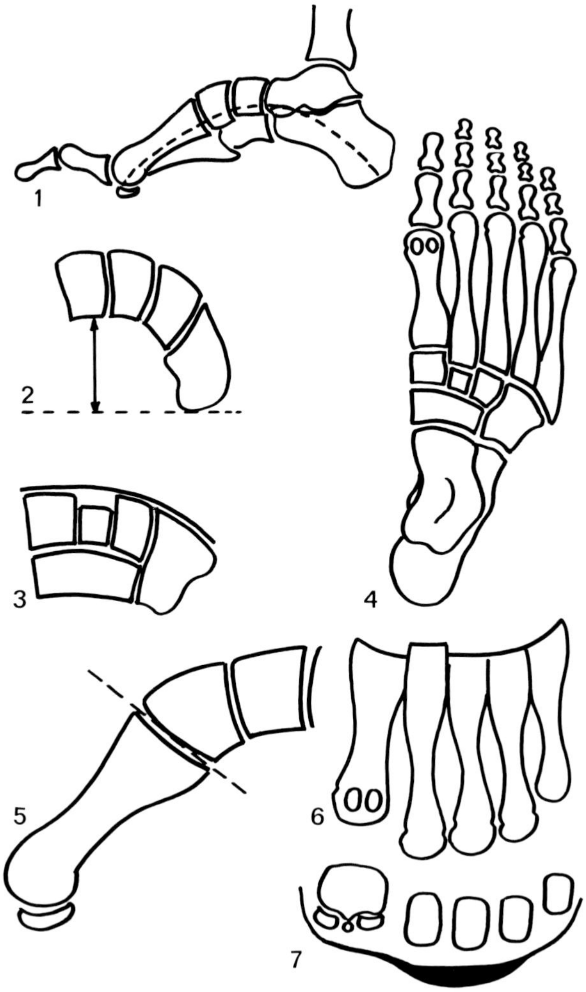

Fig. 5.6. Simple convex forefoot. The longitudinal arch *(1)* and transverse arch *(2)* are augmented. The transverse convexity of the metatarsophalangeal joint line is reduced *(3)* and there is no metatarsal divergence *(4)*. The increased height and backward displacement respectively of the longitudinal and transverse arches lead to equinus and protrusion of the central three metatarsals *(6, 7)*. There is equinus of the first metatarsal *(5)*

The importance of the foot as a whole to the loading of the metatarsus and forefoot should be understood clearly.
In the normal or balanced foot the metatarsal fan stays a little open, and both the transverse concavities at different levels and the metatarsal obliquity are normal. There is no pathological divergence of the metatarsus.
In the balanced cavus foot the metatarsal fan is less divergent and the transverse concavities are more marked. There is no divergence of the metatarsus, but if the longitudinal cavus is associated with the anatomical disposition of the Greek type of forefoot, the resulting backward and upward displacement of the cuneiforms leads to selective equinus of the middle metatarsals and overloading at their heads. This overloading will be strongly related to any congenital shortness of the first and fifth metatarsals. A convex forefoot results (Fig. 5.6).
In a cavovarus foot the metatarsal fan is closed, while the transverse concavity at different levels is much more marked. There is a diminution of the forward frontal convexity of the Lisfranc joint due to backward displacement of the cuneiforms while the first and fifth metatarsals develop relative equinus (Fig. 5.7). The latter are in effect involuted like a Provence tile nail deformity and the metatarsal formula is usually of the Egyptian or square type.

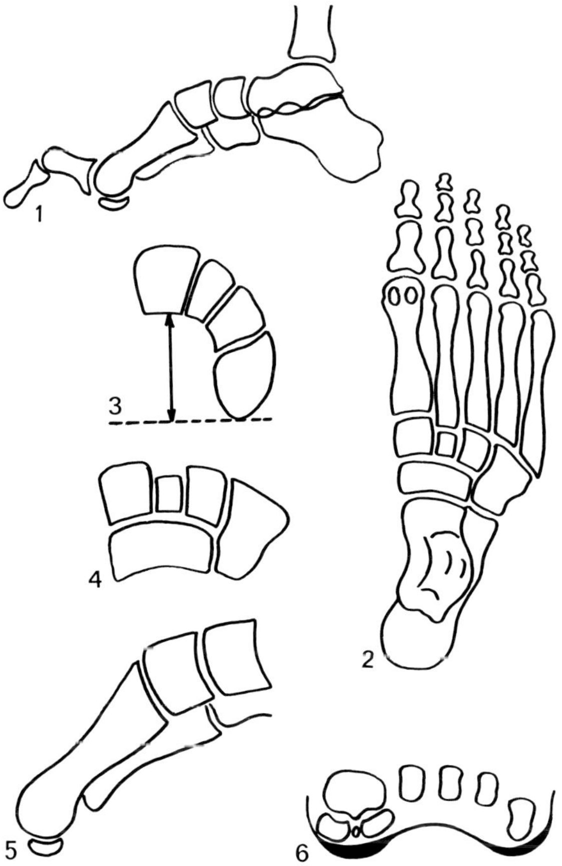

Fig. 5.7. Cavus forefoot. There is metatarsal equinus *(1)* and the metatarsals are parallel *(2)*. The longitudinal arch is augmented and there is a varus posture of the midtarsus. These two factors produce backward displacement and elevation of the tarsometatarsal joint line *(3, 4)*. There is loss of vertical mobility of the first and fifth metatarsals *(5)*. Transverse cavus leads to callus formation under the first and fifth metatarsal heads *(6)*

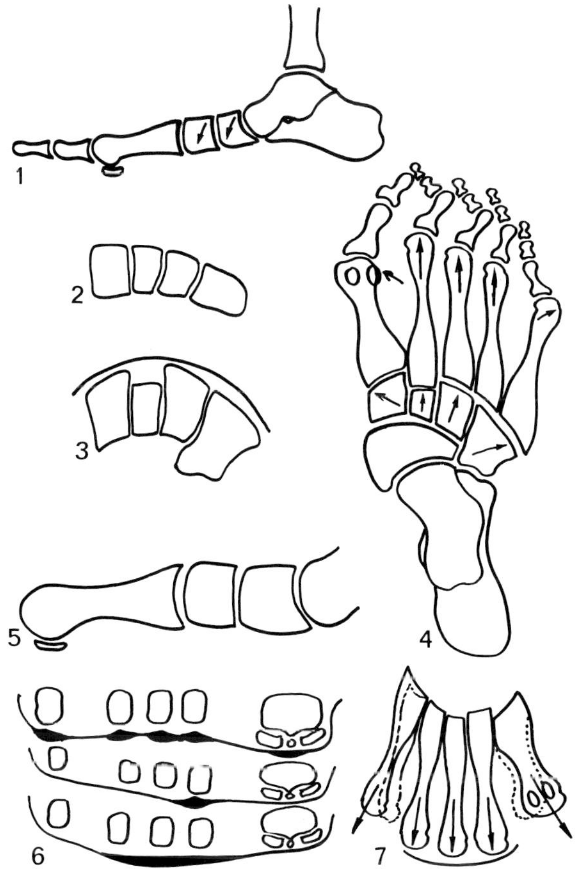

Fig. 5.8. Flat triangular forefoot and convex triangular forefoot. The longitudinal arch and the transverse arch are reduced *(1, 2)*, and the lateral cuneiforms are displaced forwards *(3)*. Collapse of the transverse arch leads to increased divergence of the medial cuneiform and the cuboid *(4)*. Increased convexity of the transverse plane of the tarsometatarsal joints line causes loss of metatarsal equinus *(5)*, increased divergence of the first and fifth metatarsals and protrusion of the central three metatarsal heads *(6, 7)*

This is the mechanism of development of the cavus forefoot.

In the cavovalgus foot the metatarsal fan is less open. The longitudinal concavity is less marked, while the transverse concavities at different levels are more developed than normal. The development of a valgus component on the cavus foot, however, leads to lowering of the longitudinal arch and diminution of the transverse plantar concavity at different levels (Fig. 5.8). The metatarsal fan then opens progressively in relation to the plantar longitudinal arch, while the plantar transverse concavity diminishes. This results in an increase of the frontal convexity of the tarsometatarsal joint and an augmentation of metatarsal divergence, most marked at the first and fifth rays. The middle metatarsals also diverge, but less markedly. The metatarsal formula of the Greek type with shortening of the first and fifth metatarsals results, and the middle metatarsal heads protrude and are also in equinus, thereby leading to a convex triangular forefoot.

In a planovalgus foot the longitudinal arch is lowered at all levels (Chopart, midtarsal and Lisfranc); the plantar transverse concavity is also diminished, but its degree of frontal curvature is augmented. This increased frontal convexity at the Lisfranc joint line leads to a spreading of the metatarsal fan, most marked in the first and fifth rays, but is accompanied, significantly, by reduced equinus of the metatarsus as a whole, so that the longitudinal axis becomes more horizontally inclined and a

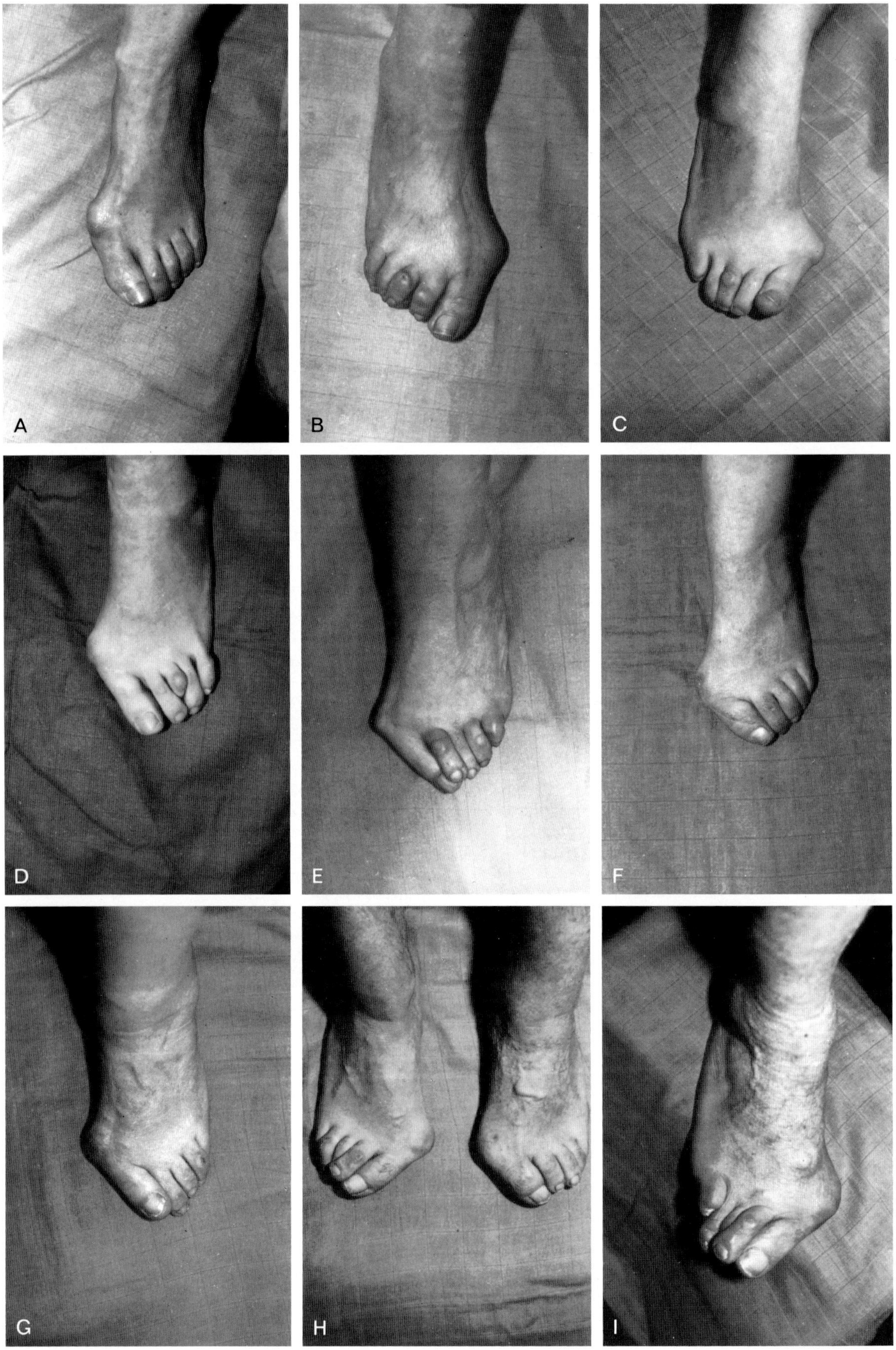
A
B
C
D
E
F
G
H
I

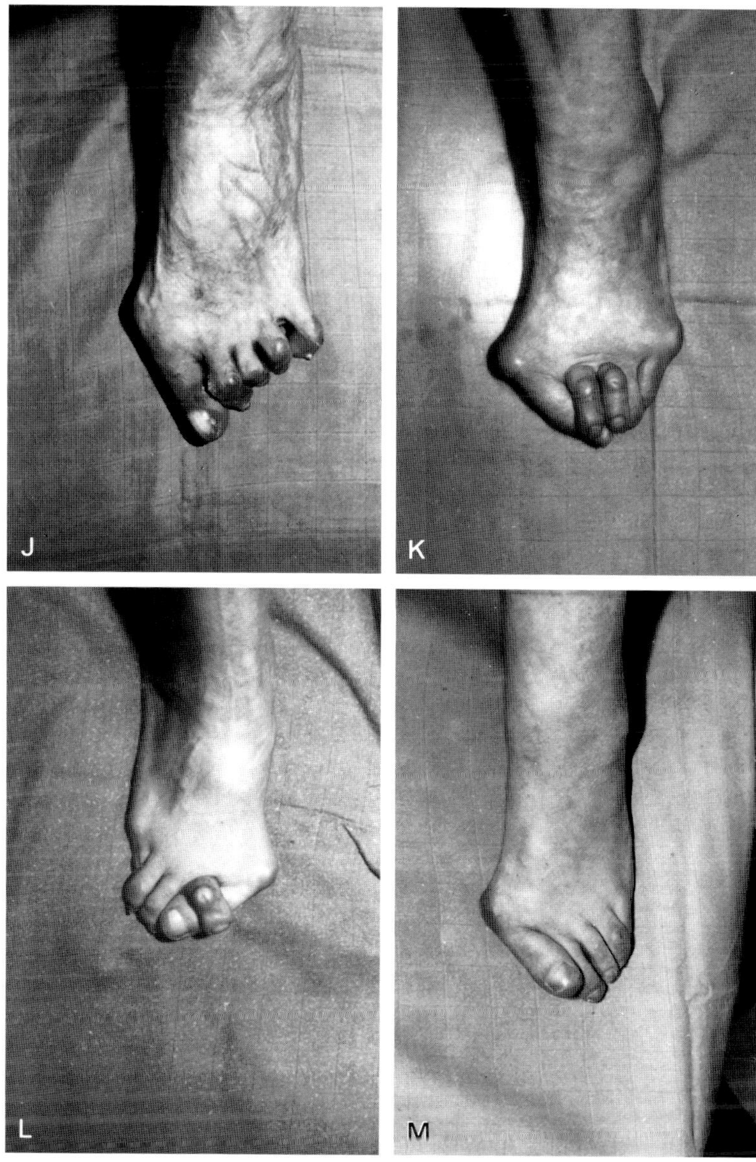

◁ **Fig. 5.9 A–M.** Windswept and irregular displacement of the toes. **A–H** Lateral windswept deformities becoming progressively accentuated in a convex triangular forefoot. **I–L** Irregular deformities in a convex triangular forefoot. **I** Valgus displacement with infraductus of third toe and clawing of fifth toe. **J** Rigid clawing in slight valgus. **K** Third-degree hallux valgus with clawing of second and third toes and supraductus with varus deformity of fifth toe (simple triangular forefoot: Locke syndrome). **L, M** Third-degree hallux valgus, clawing with varus supraductus of second toe, clawing and valgus posture of third and fourth toes and varus infraductus of fifth toe

simple triangular or convex triangular forefoot results.

The above mechanisms, complicated to understand, relate the modifications of the plantar longitudinal and transverse arches to the frontal anterior convexities, of the Lisfranc joint in particular. An appreciation of the various types of forefoot deformities and consequent painful syndromes is essential for appropriate therapy.

5.2 Relationship Between Morphological and Clinical Features

In this section brief summaries of the morphological and functional abnormalities found in the painful syndromes of the forefoot are related to the clinical presentations. The deformities may be congenital in origin or acquired - of rheumatic origin, from inflammation or arthrosis, due to static phenomena, post-traumatic or iatrogenic (the result of failure of previous surgery). The following brief descriptions of each type of syndrome relate to the particular appearance of the plantar zone of the forefoot, specific displacements of the metatarsophalangeal and interphalangeal joints, the soft tissue contractures involving tendon, capsule and skin, and the types of metatarsalgia produced. In subsequent chapters these features will be amplified, but in the interests of an overall understanding of this important group of syndromes, it is desirable that the reader should at this stage grasp the logical contrasts in presentation and development which relate them.

5.2.1 Flat Triangular Forefoot Syndrome

This condition usually involves a flat valgus forefoot. There is general divergence of the antetarsus including the first and fifth rays, general convergence of the first and fifth toes with various deformations of the central three, horizontal alignment of the metatarsal heads and significant atrophy of the weight-bearing soft tissues with individual calluses under each metatarsal head. The absence of convexity of the plantar aspect of the forefoot should be noted (Fig. 5.9 C, E, J, K; see pp. 30–31).

5.2.2 Convex Triangular Forefoot

This condition occurs in the cavovalgus foot. There is frontal protrusion and equinus of the central three metatarsals associated with shortening and divergence of the first and fifth metatarsals. The first and fifth toes converge, while there is clawing of the central three toes. Inspection of the forefoot reveals both anteroposterior and transverse convexity with the development of either a central localised callus formation underlying the second and third metatarsal heads or, alternatively, two discrete callus formations, one under each of these heads. As in the simple triangular forefoot, subluxation or dislocation of the metatarsophalangeal joints occurs together with infraductus or supraductus of the fifth toe. Clawing, swan-neck deformity and transverse deformities can also occur (Fig. 5.9 B, F, G, I, L).

5.2.3 Simple Convex Forefoot

This condition is associated with a cavus balanced foot (see Figs. 7.1, 8.1). There is accentuated equinus of the central metatarsals, sometimes with frontal protrusion and relative shortening of the first and fifth metatarsals. The first and fifth metatarsals do not diverge. Clawing affects all toes, and there is both longitudinal and transverse convexity of the ball of the foot. A large central callosity develops with a general globular appearance of the forefoot. The skin under the first and fifth metatarsal heads tends to be thinner and red. Perforating lesions can develop in the overloaded central area.

5.2.4 Cavus Forefoot

Although this condition occurs in a balanced cavus foot, there is frequently an additional tendency to varus (see Fig. 9.1). There is general equinus of the antetarsus, together with absence of divergence of the metatarsals, which lie parallel or even tend to converge. The equinus is most marked in the first and fifth metatarsals, in which there is an abnormal reduction in mobility. Various claw deformities of the toes develop, and the transverse concavity under the ball of the foot can be very marked. Localised callus formation is likely under the first and fifth metatarsal heads.

5.3 Symptoms

The predominant symptom is pain – pain arising from distortion of the joints, especially in the metatarsophalangeal region, metatarsalgia of overloading of metatarsal heads associated with corns and callosities, painful toe deformities with pressure areas at various sites, depending on configuration, or Morton's neuralgia related to compression of the nerves in their intermetatarsal sites or sometimes to the development of a neuroma.

5.4 Principles of Treatment

Of paramount importance is the need to recognise and classify the painful forefoot syndrome. This enables a rational choice of operative procedure or conservative management. Operative treatment, if indicated, will be directed primarily at realignment of the metatarsals to their correct positions, preserving the metatarsophalangeal joints if they are not too damaged but incorporating arthroplastic procedures if they are irreversibly distorted or altered. Much will depend on the etiology, especially if it is rheumatic or post-traumatic or if the range of movement of the metatarsals at the Lisfranc joint line is disturbed. The basic five corrective proce-

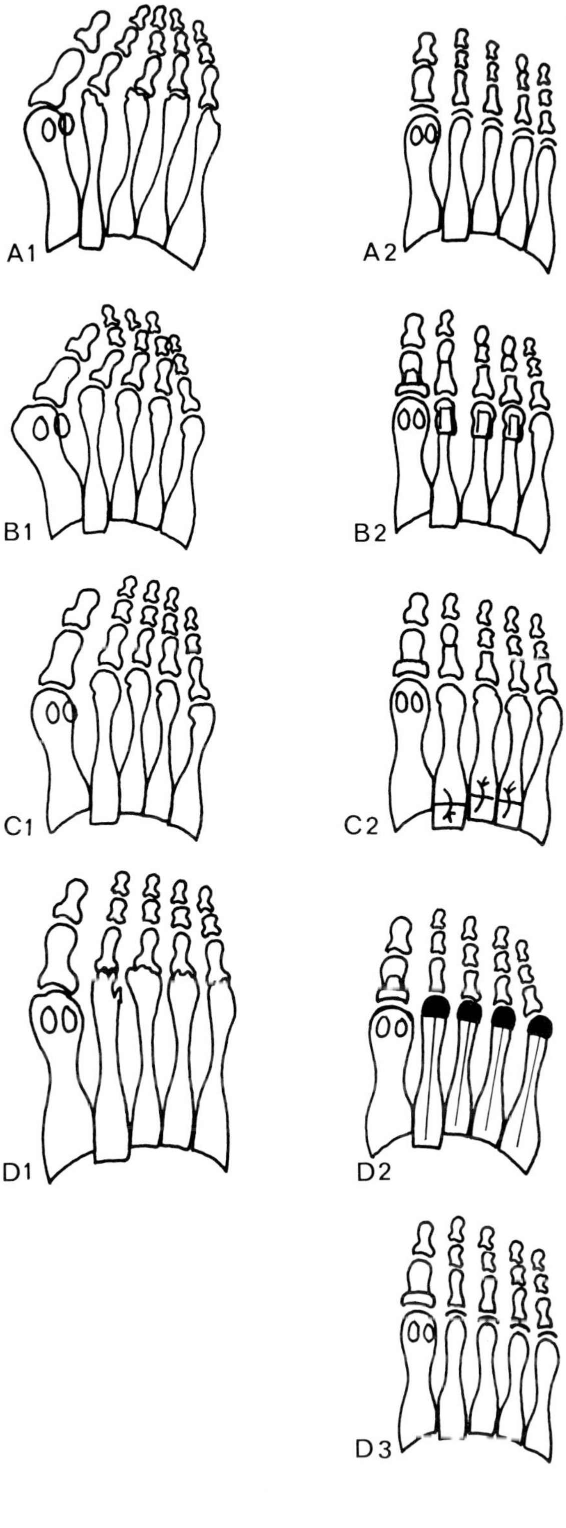

◁ **Fig. 5.10 A–D.** Scheme illustrating various operative procedures for realignment of metatarsals and management of damaged metatarsophalangeal joints. **A** *1* Before treatment; *2* after realignment (Lelièvre) and cup arthroplasties (Regnauld). **B** *1* Before treatment; *2* after shaft-head metatarsal enclavement (Regnauld). **C** *1* Before treatment; *2* after basal metatarsal osteotomies (Thys and Martorell). **D** *1* Before treatment; *2* after realignment of metatarsals with prosthetic replacement of heads for 1 year; *3* after removal of prostheses, realignment of metatarsals (Clayton) and cup arthroplasties (Regnauld)

dures are summarised in Fig. 5.10. It may be necessary to supplement these by corrections for hallux valgus or metatarsus primus varus, comparable deformities of the fifth ray, clawing of the toes or contractures of the soft tissue. The long tendons may have to be corrected if they are too short. Occasionally plantar keratomata must be excised.

The operative procedures found most satisfactory by the author are described in detail in Chap. 42, but it can be stated briefly here that the universal aims are correction of disordered loading of the metatarsal heads, alignment of the toes, and preservation of comfortable joint mobility. The operations described are applicable in various combinations under different conditions, and particular recommendations will be made in the subsequent chapters describing the painful syndromes of the forefoot in detail.

6 The Flat Triangular Forefoot

It was Locke who identified the flat triangular forefoot as a separate entity, describing a triangular appearance of the forefoot with transverse splaying of the metatarsals in the same horizontal plane associated with atrophy of the loading area. It becomes accompanied by irreducible complex joint displacements maintained by contractures of the soft tissues and consequent development of metatarsalgia. The convergence of the toes is striking (see Figs. 5.9C, E, I, K, L; 18.2D; 18.7B, G, H, J, L).

The condition develops in a generally lax foot, especially in the presence of a planovalgus posture, shortness or insufficiency of the first ray or selective laxity of the midtarsal region (Fgi. 6.1). There may be a contributing etiology such as rheumatoid arthritis, ankylosing spondylitis, a prolonged period of recumbency following some other disease, or hormonal disbalance. Alternatively, overloading from prolonged standing, trauma or muscle weakness may be responsible. Each has the consequence of lowering the plantar and longitudinal arches of the foot, which determines the formation of the flat triangular configuration. It appears that in the majority of cases, the triangular shape of the upper of the shoe is responsible for the progressive deterioration seen once the development has begun.

There is general divergence of the antetarsus, the first and fifth rays deviating from the central axis maintained by the middle metatarsals. The latter may protrude frontally. The first and fourth intercapital spaces are abnormally widened.

In contrast, the toes converge. In the normal infant, the toes are parallel and it is the use of shoes which tends to bring about convergence of the first and fifth toes. This convergence becomes much more significant if divergence of the metatarsals exists or develops. Camptodactyly or clinodactyly in various combinations affect predominantly the three middle toes.

Atrophy of the sole at the ball of the foot appears late, and it may be that there is some vasomotor effect, produced in a reflex manner by displacement of the whole tarsus or the midtarsus, which encourages malnutrition of the integument and aggravates the process. A progressive thinning of the subcutaneous tissue occurs, robbing the skin of its normal protective padding from above and thereby exposing it to the trauma from the metatarsal heads during loading which produces the plantar calluses that develop individually under each metatarsal head.

The horizontal alignment of the metatarsal heads stems from the Lisfranc joint line, and the diminution of transverse plantar concavity, together with the generalised laxity of this type of foot, produces the flattening of the anterior zone of loading. Sinking of the transverse concavity of the Lisfranc joint line is accompanied by augmentation of the frontal anterior convexity of the same joint line and leads to flattening and divergence of the five metatarsals.

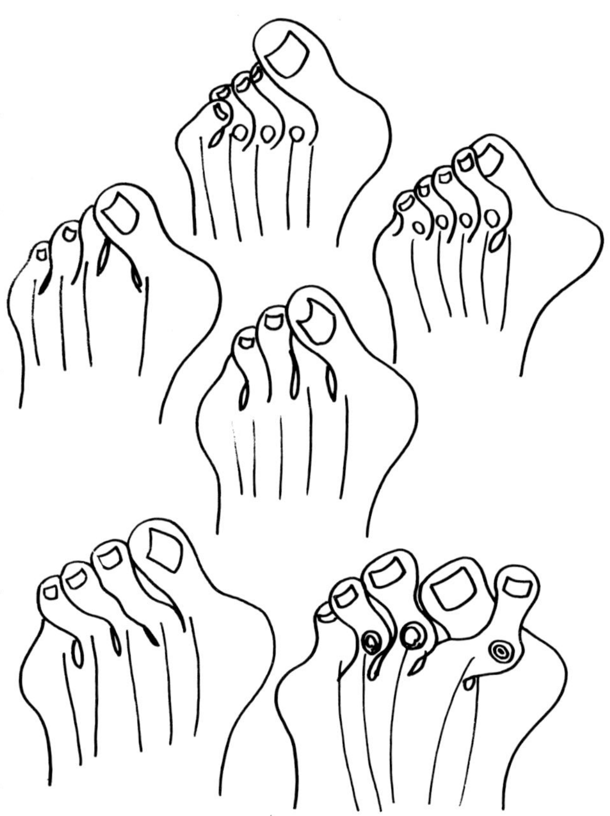

Fig. 6.1. Types of flat triangular forefoot

Axial disturbances at the metatarsophalangeal joints are the result of imbalance between the intrinsic and the extrinsic muscles together with the convergence of the toes provoked by the triangular form of the shoe upper. Hallux valgus and quintus varus are inevitable, while the development of clawing and the form it takes depend on the exact forces acting on the central three toes.
The essential feature in the development of this painful syndrome with its fixed osteoarticular displacements is the longitudinal lowering of the midtarsal region which induces the characteristic triangular shape of the forefoot.

6.1 Clinical Features

The flat triangular forefoot is seen most commonly in women from about 50 years of age, but when induced by a condition such as rheumatoid arthritis it can be seen towards the 30th year. It evolves progressively and becomes irreducible as destructive arthropathy advances; infection and ulceration of corns and calluses occur and vascular and trophic complications supervene, all contributing to metatarsalgia and digitalgia. Pain may render the patient almost unable to walk. While contractures of the integument, osteoarticular displacements and metatarsalgia are not peculiar to the triangular forefoot syndrome, they do present a particular individuality: an irregular lozenge-shaped forefoot, discrete callus formations and grossly irregular deformities of all the toes. Contractures involve skin, tendons and joint capsules.
On the dorsal aspect, the skin becomes thin, stretched and marked by the underlying extensor tendons, having lost its suppleness and subcutaneous tissue. In most instances it becomes grey or violaceous and dorsal corns develop on the toes. On the plantar aspect, the skin is again stretched and thin, coming in to direct contact with the metatarsal heads, which can easily be palpated. The individual plantar calluses are prominent, becoming delineated by folds in the skin under the intercapital areas (Fig. 6.2). The plantar calluses may be simple, or conical formations may develop, resulting in painful contact with the metatarsal condyles above them. Ulceration and infection can occur.
Individual callus formation is characteristic of this syndrome, although the calluses under the second and third metatarsal heads can become confluent, this being commoner in the convex forefoot. Occasionally, local formations occur under the second or third metatarsal heads together with one under the first and fifth.

The long extensor tendons become contracted and encourage irreducible osteoarticular displacements, bridging under the dorsal skin. The long and short flexor tendons of the second, third and fourth toes are contracted, producing clawing. It is only during operation that one establishes contracture of the dorsal interossei and the lumbricales, which develop a paradoxical action due to subluxation in the central toes.
Capsular contracture and related distension result in fixed dorsiflexion at the metatarsophalangeal joints of the central three toes, while in the great and fifth toes there is central transverse deviation. The deformities at the metatarsophalangeal joints are accompanied by infraductus or supraductus, especially of the second toe with respect to the great toe, and irreducible clawing, swan-neck deformity, transverse deformities, or inverse clawing of the lesser toes. Quintus varus with infraductus or supraductus is likely. The multiplicity and variability of the deformities characterise this syndrome (Fig. 5.9 C, E, K, L).

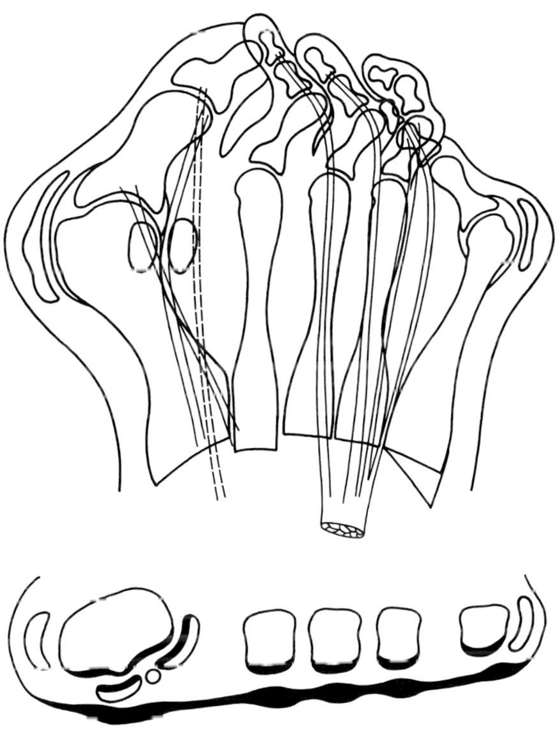

Fig. 6.2. Flat triangular forefoot (Locke syndrome). The features include clinodactyly of all rays, frontal protrusion of the three central metatarsal heads, irregular displacement of all toes, contracture of tendons, capsules and skin, atrophy of plantar subcutaneous tissue and localised callus formation under each metatarsal head

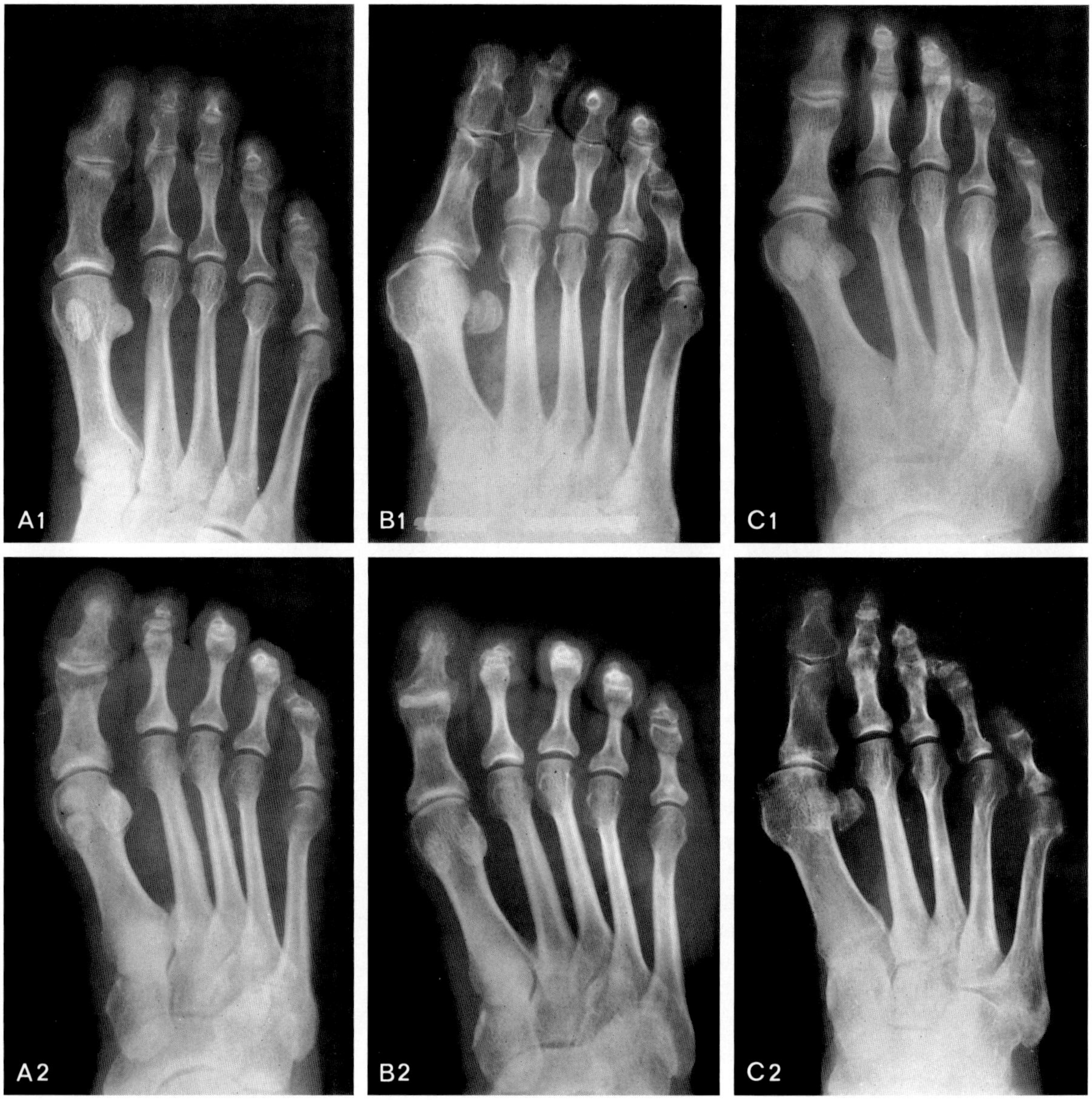

Fig. 6.3 A–F. Convex forefoot, convex triangular forefoot, and simple triangular forefoot. **A** Convex forefoot. *1* Onset: no hallux valgus, frontal protusion of second, third and fourth metatarsals, no digital clawing; *2* more advanced: onset of hallux valgus, frontal protrusion of second, third and fourth metatarsals, supple clawing of toes. **B** Convex triangular forefoot. *1* Hallux valgus, quintus varus, frontal protrusion of second, third and fourth metatarsals, clawing of toes; *2* absence of hallux valgus, frontal protrusion of second, third and fourth metatarsals, clawing of toes, onset of dorsolateral displacement. **C** Convex triangular forefoot. *1, 2* Hallux valgus, quintus varus, frontal protrusion of second, third and fourth metatarsal heads, various digital clawing. ▷ **D** Convex triangular forefoot. Hallux valgus, frontal protrusion of second, third and fourth metatarsal heads, lateral displacement of clawed toes, which remain supple. **E** Congenital simple triangular forefoot. Dystrophy of first metatarsal head, third-degree hallux valgus, frontal protrusion of second, third and fourth metatarsal heads, distal digital clawing. **F** Flat triangular forefoot (Locke syndrome) in adult. Hallux valgus, quintus varus, divergence of first and fifth metatarsals, no frontal protrusion of central metatarsal heads, lateral displacement of toes. **D–F** see p. 37

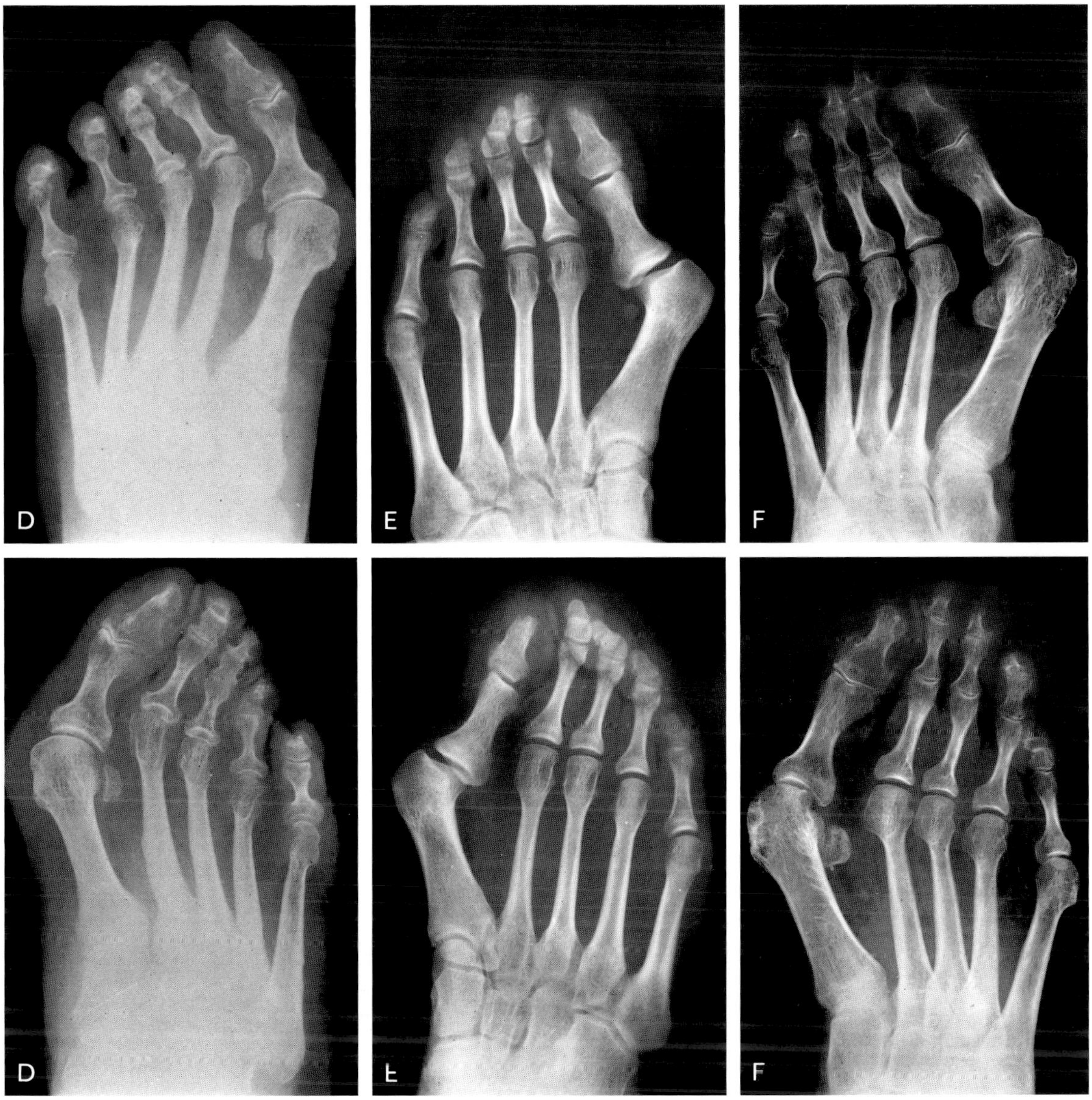

Fig. 6.3 D–F. Legend see p. 36

Displacements of the first ray comprise varus of second or third degree of the metatarsal and the development of an extra-articular exostosis, associated with hallux valgus of second or third degree. The angulation becomes fixed irreducibly and provokes obliquity of the plane of the base of the proximal phalanx. Bridging of the long extensor and short extensor tendons under the skin becomes obvious (Fig. 6.3). The painful bursitis over the medial aspect of the first metatarsal head is exacerbated by episodes of inflammation or frank infection and ulceration; sometimes here there is a keratotic punctiform or elongated lesion at the junction of the plantar and internal aspects due to overloading and friction at this point. The sesamoids are displaced posteriorly and dislocate into the first interspace. The great toe may develop an axial rotation of varying degree, causing its medial surface to face downwards. This can be observed well on axial inspection of the nail.

Exactly comparable deformities of the fifth ray occur, with development of a tailor's bunion, a dorsal digital corn, traumatic onyxis (which must never be treated in isolation) and abnormal loading on the lateral surface due to the axial rotation. Subluxation of the long tendons into the fourth intercapital space and fixity of the deformity develop progressively.

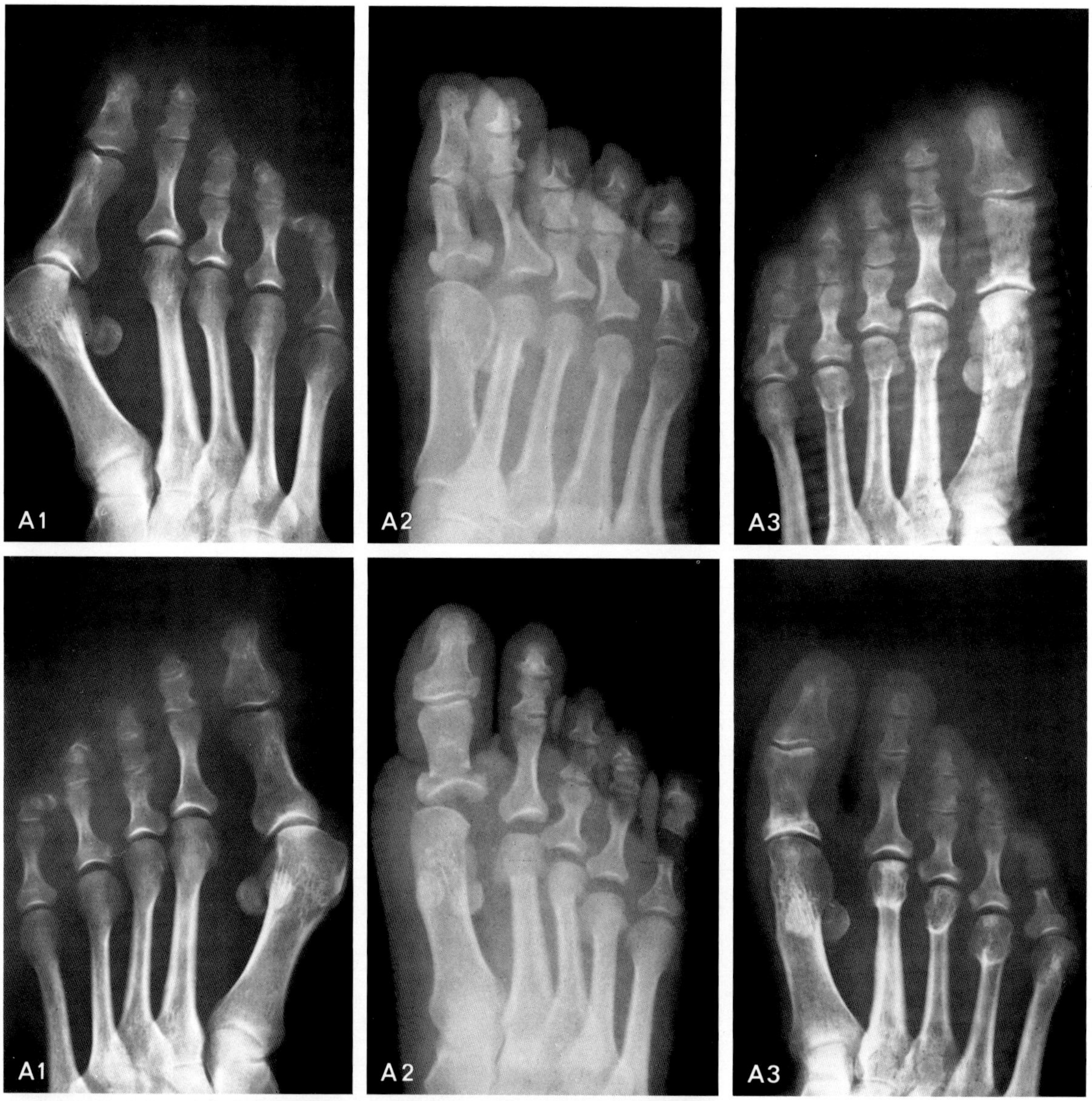

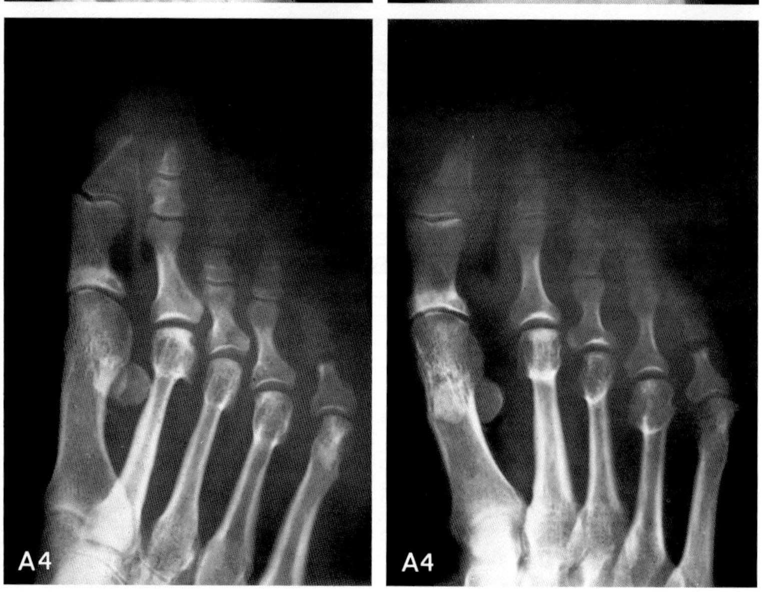

Fig. 6.5 A. Legend see p. 39

The deformity seen at the metatarsophalangeal joints of the central three toes varies. They may be in dorsiflexion accompanied by either internal or external deviation. The toes become abnormally compressed, abutting against the shoe upper, and various configurations occur. For example, there may be an association of swan-neck deformity of the second toe or clawed supra ductus with hallux valgus of the great toe while the third, fourth and fifth toes are in varus and infraductus (the crossed transverse deformity). Occasionally a typical windswept external angulation of the central toes accompanies hallux valgus and quintus varus. A simple, dorsal, somewhat externally directed clawing may occur, but it should be noted that pure dorsal clawing of the central three toes is exceptional in the flat or convex triangular type of forefoot.

Fig. 6.4 A, B see p. 42

The metatarsophalangeal joints of the middle toes become subluxed or dislocated dorsolateraly under the influence of tendinous contractures and capsular stretching, so that there is reduced vertical suppleness of the metatarsals with consequent loss of resilience on loading accompanied by pain.

Podoscopy and podometry confirm and define the abnormal loading and disturbed equilibrium of the foot.

Radiography plainly shows the severity of joint displacements and reveals the metatarsal formula (most frequently Greek). The lines of loading of the metatarsal heads can be identified, especially with respect to protrusion of the central rays. The condition of the involved joints and the underlying displacements must be defined clearly before treatment is commenced.

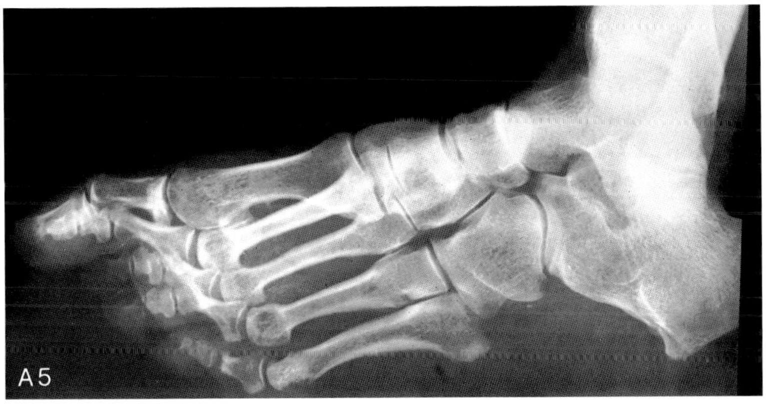

◁ **Fig. 6.5 A–C.** Simple triangular and convex triangular forefoot: treatment by head-shaft enclavement of metatarsals (Regnauld). **A** Bilateral simple triangular forefoot. *1* Third-degree hallux valgus, marked metatarsus primus varus; *2* operation in 1974: head-shaft enclavement of metatarsals, correction of hallux valgus using hat-shaped graft, arthroplasty with shortening of the fifth toe; *3* appearance 2 years postoperatively: normal alignment of metatarsophalangeal joint lines; *4* three years postoperatively; *5* three years postoperatively: perfect reconstruction and good alignment of metatarsal heads. **B** Simple triangular forefoot. *1* Spreading of forefoot, divergence of first and fifth metatarsals, hallux valgus; *2* operation in 1974 and 1975: head-shaft enclavement of second, third and fourth metatarsals, correction of hallux valgus with hat-shaped graft, arthroplasty of fifth toe; *3* both feet 3 years postoperatively; *4* left foot 3 years postoperatively: oblique view showing perfect reconstruction and consolidation; *5* right foot 3 years postoperatively: graft of great toe, good realignment of enclaved second, third and fourth metatarsal heads. **C** Convex triangular forefoot. *1* Hallux valgus, quintus varus, divergence of first and fifth metatarsals, frontal protusion and equinus of second, third and fourth metatarsal heads; *2* operation in 1978: head-shaft enclavement of metatarsals, correction of hallux valgus with cork-shaped graft, orthroplasty with shortening of fifth toe; *3* one year postoperatively; *4* two years postoperatively: good reconstruction of enclaved metatarsal heads and of graft in first metatarsophangeal joint. **B, C** see pp. 40, 41

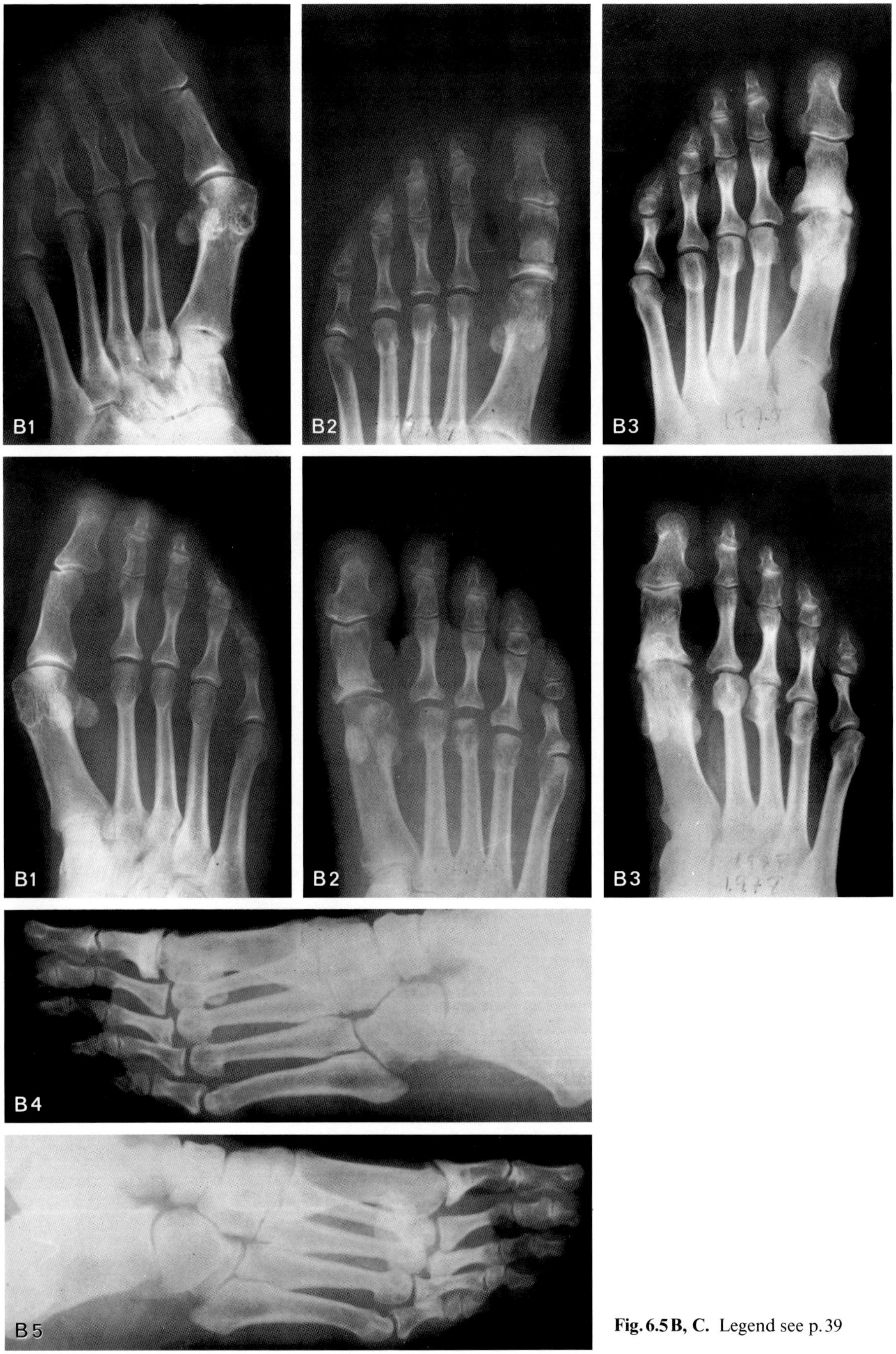

Fig. 6.5 B, C. Legend see p. 39

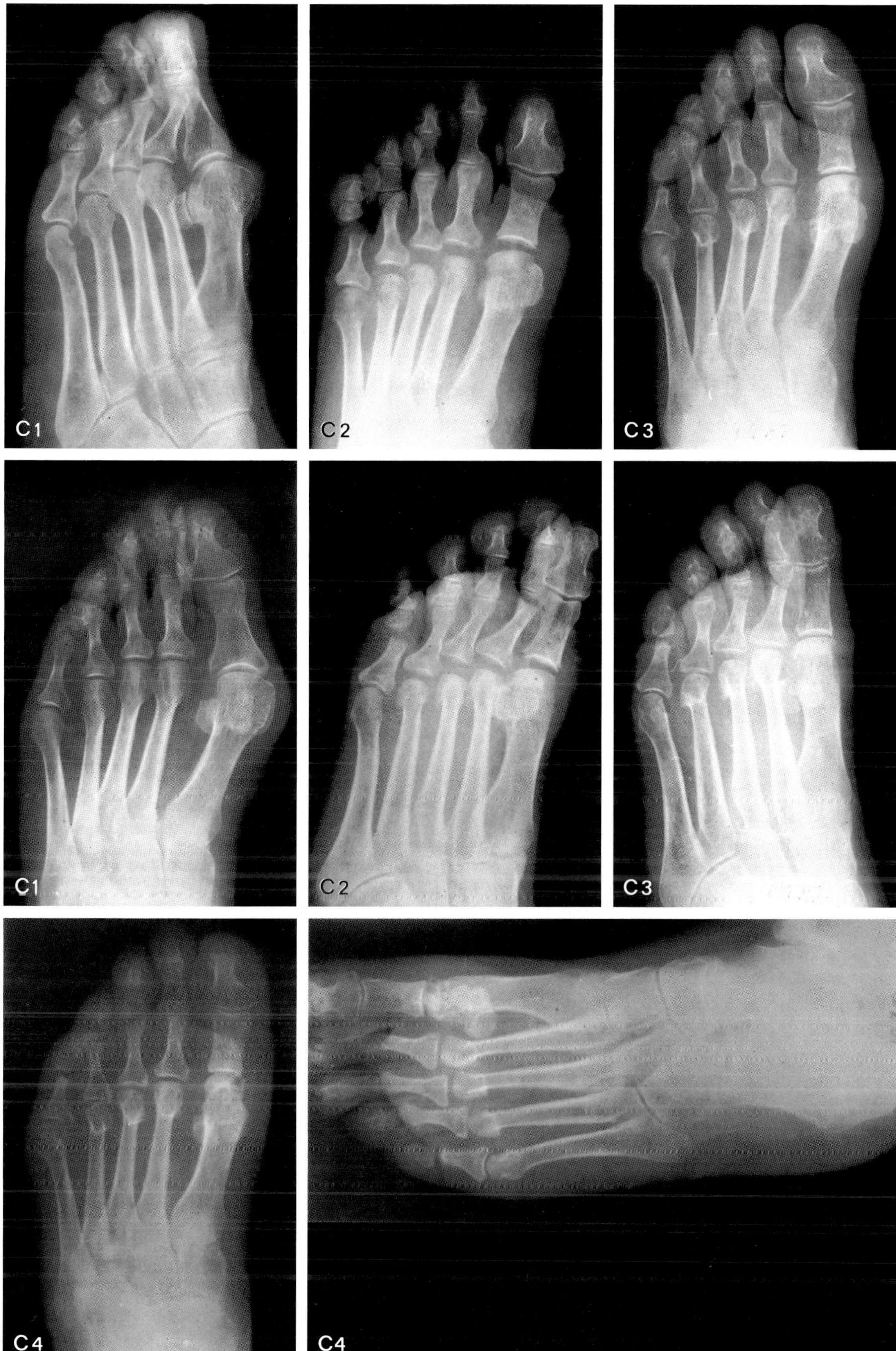
C1
C2
C3
C1
C2
C3
C4
C4

6.2 Treatment

6.2.1 Conservative

Conservative treatment is purely palliative for the relief of pain. A supportive insole made from compliant material should be excavated appropriately to accomodate the protruding metatarsal heads; it may incorporate subcapital and retrocapital bars or comprise a physiological monoblock type with a retrocapital bar (see Chap. 40).

6.2.2 Operative

Assuming the age and general condition of the patient are suitable, treatment is operative (Fig. 6.4). It includes the following components although the emphasis will be different in each individual case:

Correction of hallux valgus and varus of the first metatarsal (see Chap. 18)
Correction of quintus varus and valgus of the fifth metatarsal (see Chap. 19)
Elongation of the long extensor and flexor tendons (Figs. 6.3, 8.5 A1–A3)
Capsulotomies on the dorsal and, as appropriate, internal or external aspects of the metatarsophalangeal joints (Fig. 6.5 A, B).
Correction of excessive frontal protrusion of the central metatarsal heads by head shaft enclavement if the joint surfaces are intact or by interposition cup prostheses if they are too damaged (see Chap. 42)
Correction of claw toes by arthroplasty or appropriate arthrodesis (see Chap. 17)
Release of skin contractures by V-, W-, or Y-plasties, as appropriate

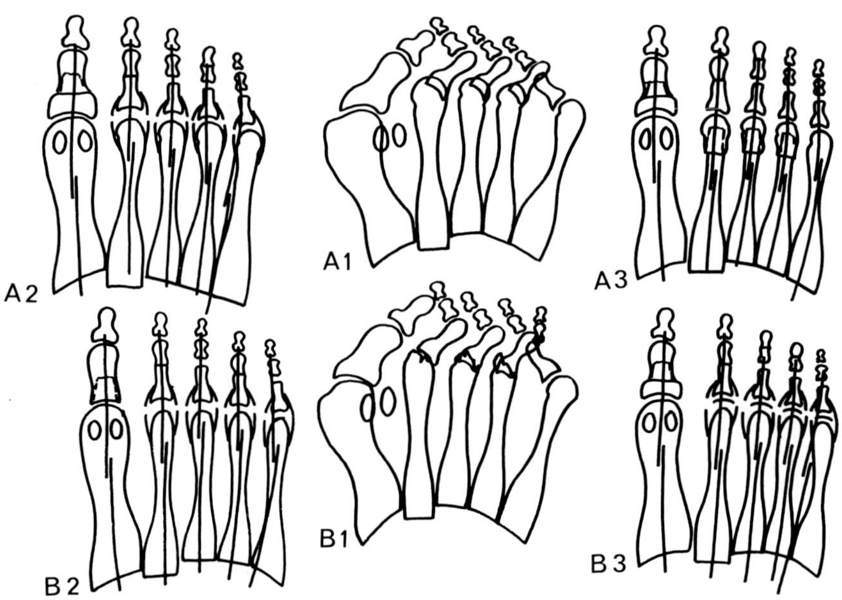

Fig. 6.4 A, B. Treatment of flat triangular forefoot. **A** Metatarsal and phalangeal cartilages intact: *1* Before treatment; *2* after reduction of metatarsophalangeal joints by arthrotomy; *3* after metatarsal shaft-head enclavements. **B** Arthrosic or arthritic damage of metatarsal cartilages: *1* Before treatment; *2* after Lelièvre metatarsal realignments; *3* after Lelièvre metatarsal realignments with cup arthroplasties (Regnauld). All procedures accompanied by correction of hallux valgus and quintus varus, metatarsophalangeal capsulotomies, elongation of tendons and any necessary interphalangeal arthrodeses

7 The Simple Convex Forefoot

The second commonest of the painful forefoot syndromes, the flat convex forefoot, supervenes on a metatarsal formula of the Greek type ($1 < 2 \geqslant 3 \geqslant 4 > 5$). Protrusion, equinus or both may affect the middle metatarsal heads (see Fig. 11.8).

The condition occurs most commonly in a balanced precavus or balanced cavus foot with neutral longitudinal tarsometatarsal axis; the relative shortness and normal posture of the first and fifth metatarsals accentuates the effect of the overlong, depressed middle metatarsals.

The cavus foot embodies augmentation of the plantar longitudinal and transverse arches, the summits of which are located at the intermediate and lateral cuneiforms. Augmentation of curvature of the plantar concavities is accompanied, as always, by reduced frontal convexity of the Lisfranc joint configuration. Thus the increased equinus of the middle metatarsals results from the elevated position of the intermediate and lateral cuneiforms, accentuated by a downward inclination of the metatarsal articular surfaces of these bones. The diminished frontal anterior convexity of the Lisfranc joint line leads to absence of divergence of the metatarsals, which are kept pressed together (Fig. 7.2).

The increased length, equinus and absence of divergence of the middle metatarsals contribute to the overloading of the affected metatarsal heads and the convex appearance of the ball of the foot. The progressive overloading disturbs the balance of muscle forces, and overaction of the extensor muscles ensues; they shorten progressively, become irreducibly contracted and lead to dorsal displacements at the metatarsophalangeal joints with secondary capsular contracture. The toes become irreducibly clawed and secondary contracture of the flexor tendons occurs. There is a marked contrast between the thin dorsal skin, tented by the contracted underlying tendons, and the thickened and yet stretched plantar skin under the protruding metatarsal heads.

7.1 Clinical Features

The condition predominantly affects women between the ages of 30 and 40 years, exceptionally before the age of 20 years. There is frequently a history of injudicious use of high heels during adolescence, especially in younger individuals.

7.1.1 Symptoms

The patient seeks advice because of pain and a large persistent plantar callosity which can no longer be controlled by conservative means. Occasionally a serous bursa develops in the ball of the foot at an early stage, but more usually, thick callus formation on the plantar aspect of the foot associated with metatarsalgia is the presenting sign (Fig. 7.1).

Pain is aggravated by walking and standing, especially in shoes, and is relieved by rest. There are three types.

a) Continuous pain of a burning, pricking character when the foot is loaded, essentially plantar metatarsalgia, of varying intensity and often severe, located under the three central metatarsal heads, all of which are sensitive to pressure. Pain also results from compression of dorsal corns on the toes and terminal corns related to deformation and hypertrophy of the nails.
b) Intermittent pain, occurring only on certain days, relates to arthralgia of the distorted metatarsophalangeal joints, but is less common in this particular type of forefoot. When present, the pain is of a tension type, exacerbated by passive mobilisation and plantarflexion of the metatarsophalangeal joints, this explaining the fact that patients state they are unable to walk in shoes without heels. Sometimes other joint complexes in the foot are painful, although they are not primarily involved with the disease process; they are strained by the longitudinal disbalance of the foot as a whole.

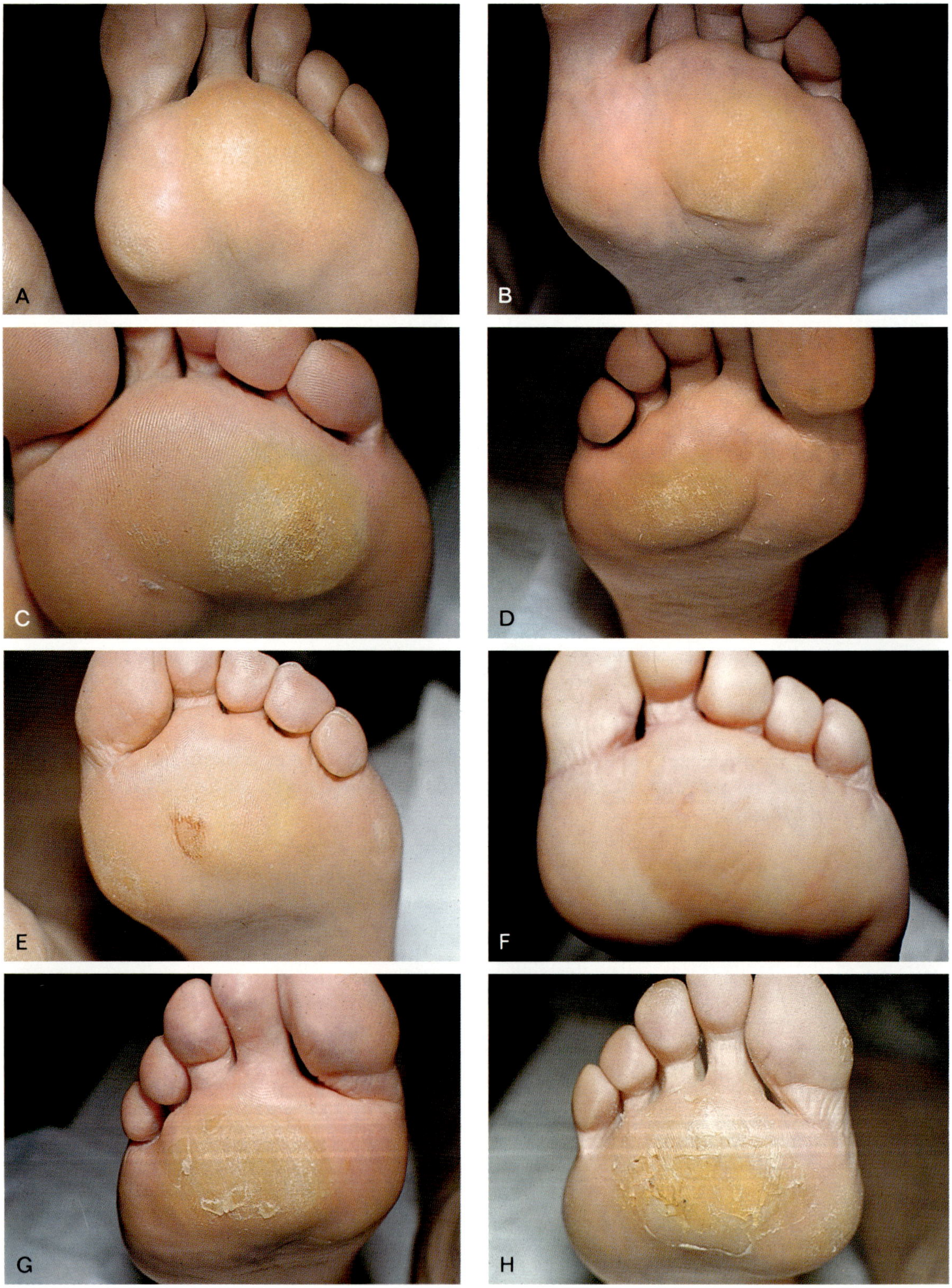

Fig. 7.1 A–H. Simple convex forefoot. **A** With lowering and protrusion of second metatarsal head. **B** With lowering and protrusion of third metatarsal head. **C** With equinus of fourth metatarsal. **D** With equinus of third and fourth metatarsals. **E–F** With frontal protrusion and equinus of second, third and fourth metatarsals

c) More frequent is pain from neuralgias of compression of the nerves in the intermetatarsal spaces, due probably to the parallel alignment of the metatarsal shafts. The pain is fleeting and of sudden appearance, similar to that from Morton's neuroma but of different etiology.

7.1.2 Physical Signs

Early in the development of the convex forefoot syndrome, there is a fixed plantar swelling in the mid-part of the ball of the foot, accentuated sometimes by a serous bursa which may be inflamed and distended intermittently (Fig. 7.2). The bursa may be palpable and is tender; it is accompanied by complaints of pain of a lancing or pricking type, but rarely burning, during early development. The pain appears first at the end of the day after standing or prolonged walking, and then progressively earlier as the bursa develops. At this early stage the joints remain supple, but the protrusion or equinus of the central metatarsal heads is palpable, and early clawing, which is correctable, may be apparent (see Fig. 6.3 A). When the foot is loaded, the early clawing reduces completely except for slight bowstringing of the extensor tendons visible under the skin on the dorsum of the foot.

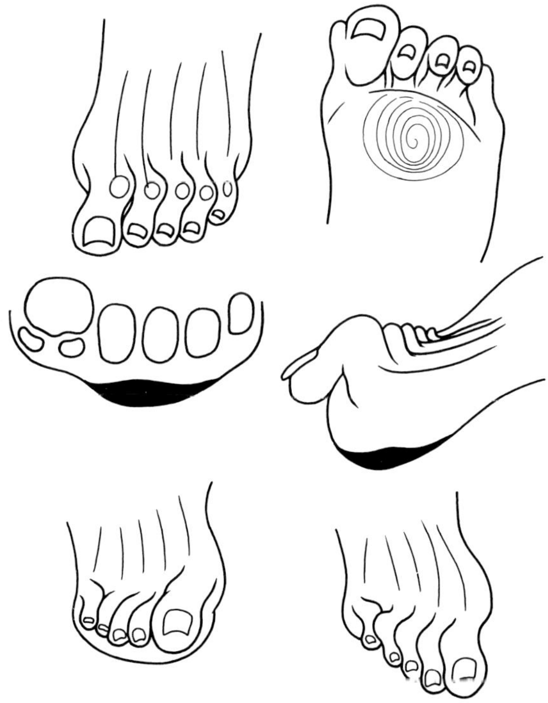

Fig. 7.2. Simple convex forefoot with longitudinal cavus. There is a central plantar callosity, irreducible clawing of toes, dorsal subluxation of metatarsophalangeal joints and contracture of long extensor and flexor tendons

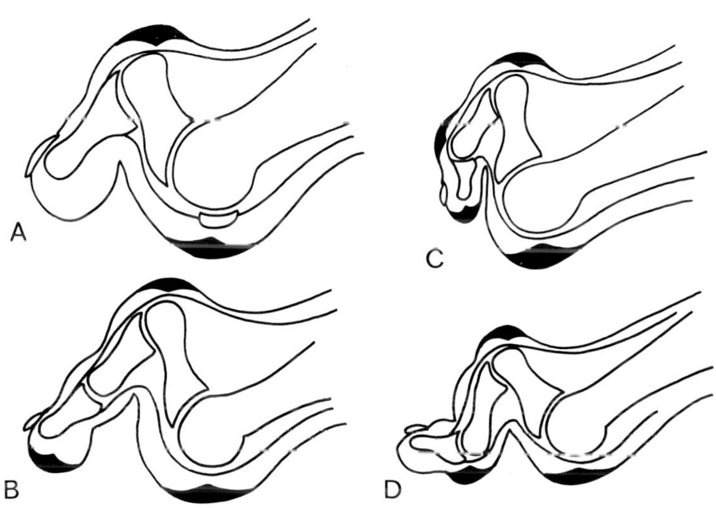

Fig. 7.3 A–D. Clawing of toes. **A** Great toe. **B** Involving the proximal interphalangeal joint. **C** Involving both interphalangeal joints. **D** Inverted clawing with dorsiflexion of proximal interphalangeal joint and plantarflexion of distal interphalangeal joint

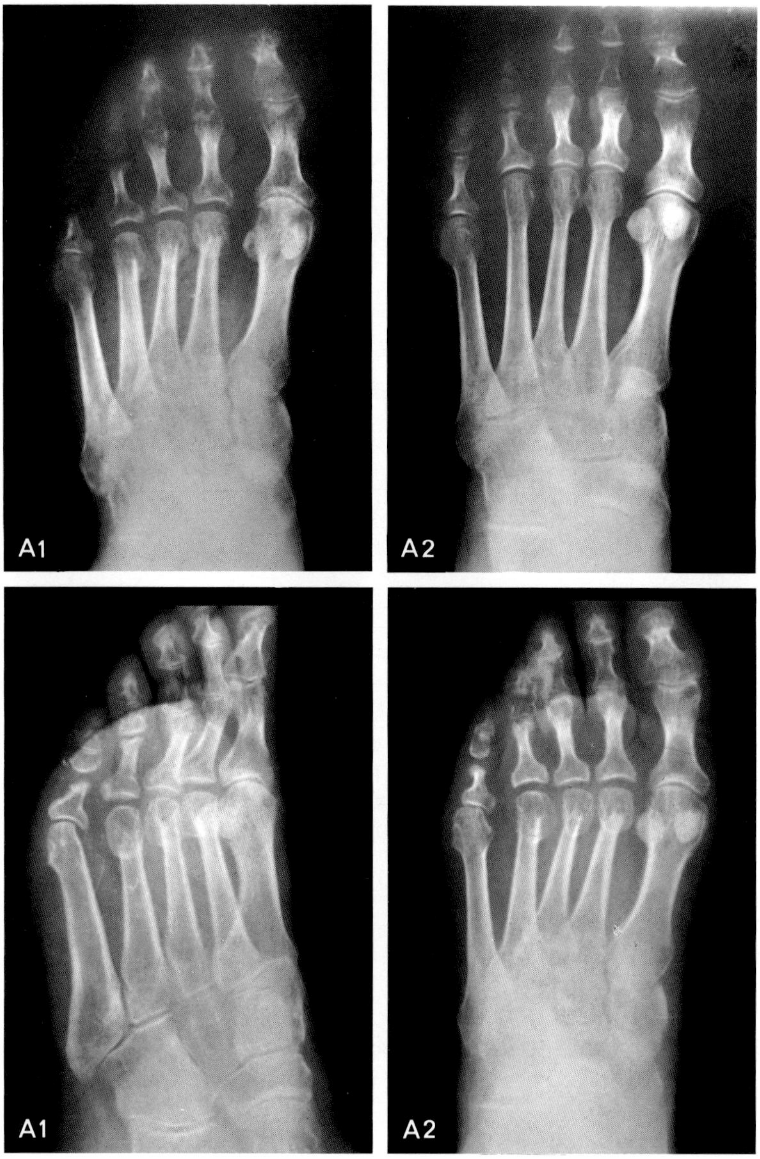

Fig. 7.4 A–C. Painful convex forefoot: treatment by head-shaft enclavement of second, third and fourth metatarsals (Regnauld). **A** *1* Left foot, dorsoplantar *(above)* and oblique *(below)* views: convex forefoot, protrusion and equinus of second, third, and fourth metatarsals, absence of divergence of first and fifth metatarsals, no hallux valgus or quintus varus; *2* one week *(above)* and 3 months *(below)* after enclavement of second, third, and fourth metatarsals. **B** *1* Left foot, dorsoplantar view: convex forefoot, protrusion and equinus of second, third and fourth metatarsals, absence of divergence of metatarsals, absence of hallux valgus and quintus varus; *2* oblique view before treatment; *3, 4* oblique and dorsoplantar views 6 months postoperatively: incomplete correction of realigned metatarsophalangeal joints. **C** *1* Right foot: convex forefoot, protrusion and equinus of second, third and fourth metatarsals, absence of divergence of first and fifth metatarsals, absence of hallux valgus and quintus varus, rigid clawing of fourth and fifth toes, supple clawing of second and third toes; *2* three months after enclavement of second, third and fourth metatarsal heads and arthroplasty of proximal interphalangeal joints of fourth and fifth toes; *3* six months postoperatively. **B, C** see p. 47 ▷

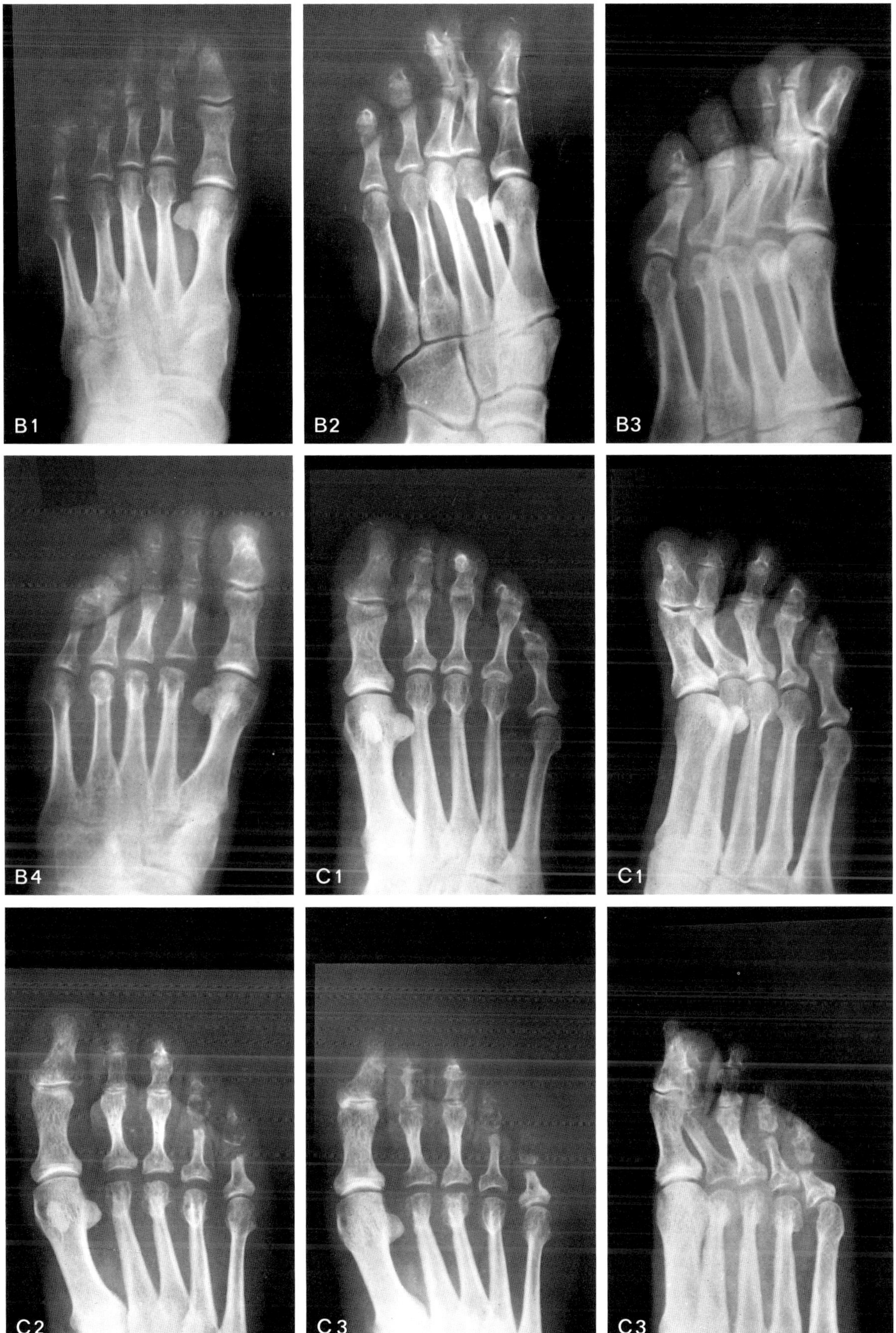
B1
B2
B3
B4
C1
C1
C2
C3
C3

Progressively, and at a variable rate depending to some extent on the daily activity of the subject and the type of shoes worn, there develops the irreducible syndrome in which the callus under the convex ball forms a rigid glass-like plaque. This, together with the contracted toes, gives the appearance of a boxing glove and the forefoot rests on the ground only at the level of the middle metatarsal heads (Fig. 7.3). The tips of the contracted toes do not reach the ground and may actually indent the anterior part of the prominent ball of the foot.

The dorsal aspect of the foot, when viewed from the side, presents an S-shaped outline due to the convexity of the Lisfranc joint region, the concavity overlying the metatarsophalangeal joints and the clawed toes. The dorsal skin is contracted and tented by the subcutaneous cords of the extensor tendons. Due to retraction of the dorsal skin, the commissures between the toes often become situated at the level of the proximal interphalangeal joints, the proximal phalanges in a dorsiflexion posture being submerged under the dorsal soft tissues. This sign indicates that the round foot syndrome has existed for a significant period of time.

From above, the forefoot is of normal breadth and there is no clinical evidence of divergence of the first or fifth metatarsals.

Palpation reveals that the characteristic outlines of the foot are produced by the equinus posture of the metatarsals and the fixed dorsiflexion of the proximal phalanges. Later dorsal subluxation of the metatarsophalangeal joints may amount to frank dislocation, and the contracted metatarsophalangeal and interphalangeal joints are rigid and uncorrectable. All five rays are affected. In one paradoxical exception, inverse clawing of toes can occur due to an isolated contracture of the short plantar flexor; the toe assumes an inverted Z-form in which the proximal phalanx is dorsiflexed, the middle phalanx is plantarflexed and the distal phalanx is in acute dorsiflexion. In the more normal type of clawing, traumatic onychogryphosis can occur and be responsible for pain and inflammation.

Selective evaluation of the soft tissues confirms the contracture of tendons and skin. Progressively, the extensor hallucis longus, then the extensor communis and short extensor tendons and finally the flexors are involved. The dorsal tendons bowstring under the dorsal skin, which they elevate in longitudinal crests, contrasting with the grooves over the joint interspaces; they appear to insert directly into the proximal interphalangeal joint and drag the toes into the fixed irreducible clawing which is so characteristic. Some of the tension in the extensor tendons disappears when the ankle is dorsiflexed, but is accentuated in plantarflexion. In contrast, the flexor tendons do not relax under the influence of ankle posture.

Contracture of the flexor tendons is secondary to that of the extensors, and it is as a result of the acute dorsiflexion at the metatarsophalangeal joints that the length of the tendon is taken up at the expense of plantarflexion at the interphalangeal joints. This becomes progressively irreducible, depending on the stage of the condition.

Capsular involvement, with stretching on the convex surfaces and contracture on the concave surfaces follows inevitably. Atrophy of the extensors is very marked at exploration.

Podoscopy and podometry make the characteristic zones of overloading very clear. Podoscopy indicates the imprint of a cavus foot, while podometry confirms predominant overloading of the middle metatarsal heads.

Radiography should include anteroposterior, oblique and Müller-Güntz (Müller 1927; Güntz 1938) or Chevrot (1981) and Chaigneau (1981) views, which identify the metatarsal formula, the exact degree of frontal protrusion of the middle metatarsal heads and the degree of equinus of the middle metatarsals, especially as regards the lowering of the middle metatarsal condyles with respect to the first and fifth condyles (Fig. 7.4 A1, B1, C1). Any damage to the joint surfaces may be apparent, although this is rare in the convex forefoot. Absence of divergence of the metatarsals is confirmed. In relation to treatment, radiography is essential for evaluation of the degree of shortening or elevation of the metatarsals necessary for correction of the condition.

7.2 Treatment

7.2.1 Conservative

In the early case, chiropody and orthotic measures will control the condition to some extent. Chiropody comprises care of plantar corns and treatment of inflammation.

Orthotic treatment involves the use of one of three different types of orthopaedic insole; care must be taken to choose the correct type. In die *precavus foot* an insole with a retrocapital bar exercises a relaxing effect on the longitudinal cavus and corrects digital clawing (Fig. 7.5); it raises the forefoot and balances pressure behind the five metatarsal heads.

It must be complemented by a supinating wedge under the heel if there is a tendency towards a valgus posture of the heel, and also by a pronating band on the external side if there is a tendency to wards general varus of the foot. In *longitudinal pes cavus* the convex forefoot is relieved by a monoblock insole including a retrocapital bar. The object of this insole is to distribute the body weight over the whole plantar surface of the forefoot. In addition, it stabilises the foot by restricting forward and backward movement during walking, thereby lessening plantar metatarsalgia of loading. Sometimes the convex forefoot leads to a *reactionary varus* posture due to reflex spasm, and if this is the case the insoles must be complemented by a pronating bar or an external pronating wedge so as to restore neutral balance and relieve the strain on the joints which accompanies this varus posture, at whatever level of the foot it originates.

7.2.2 *Operative*

In the established condition, chiropody and other conservative measures are ineffective. Operative treatment is indicated and is designed to establish a new line of metatarsal loading and restore normal phalangeal propulsion. It is usual for the joint surfaces to remain well preserved.

When there is no contracture of the soft tissue or displacement of the joints, simple metatarsal V-osteotomies of Mau (1940) or Thys (1974b) may be effective (Figs. 7.6, 7.7).

The author finds head-shaft enclavement of the metatarsals (Fig. 7.7 D, E) an easier procedure to perform in that the basal osteotomy is difficult to align exactly, whereas at the time of enclavement it is relatively easy to ensure that the horizontal plane has been restored under the metatarsal heads. However, in particular cases where there is a selective equinus of one of the middle metatarsals, it is sometimes necessary to complement an enclavement procedure with a basal osteotomy.

In the first ray, if there is no hallux valgus, only a clawing of the great toe, correction may be achieved by metatarsophalangeal arthroplasty with a graft (Fig. 7.8). If the clawing of the great toe is supple without hallux valgus, metatarsophalangeal and interphalangeal arthrotomies associated with elongation of the extensor tendons may suffice. If, however, there is irreducible clawing of the great toe at the interphalangeal joint, metatarsal arthrotomy associated with elongation of the extensor tendons and arthrodesis of the interphalangeal joint become necessary (Fig. 7.4).

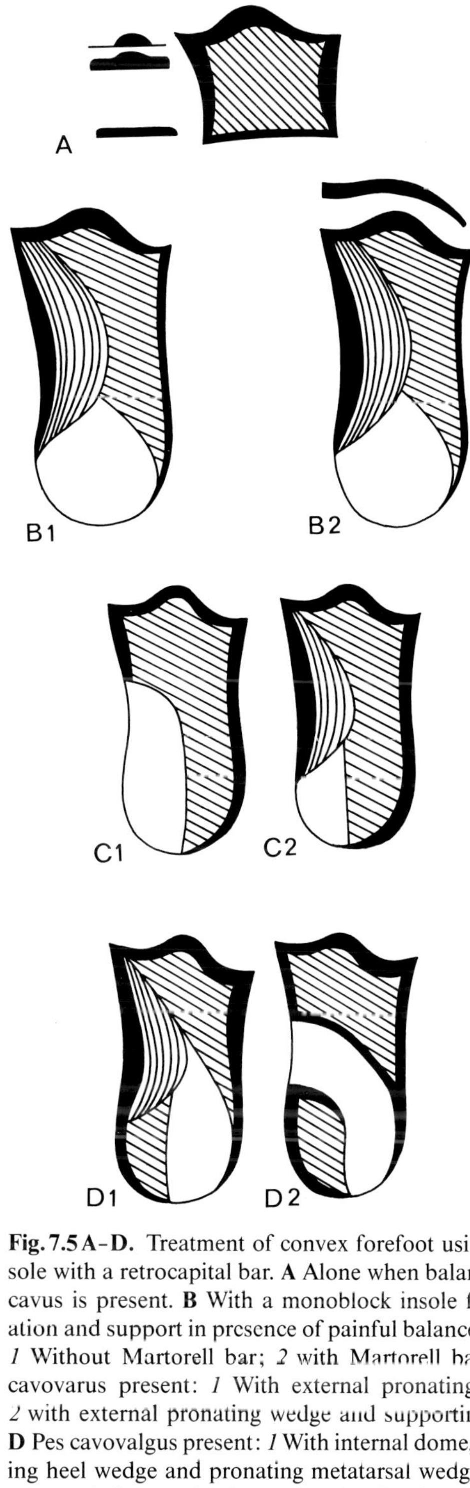

Fig. 7.5 A–D. Treatment of convex forefoot using an insole with a retrocapital bar. **A** Alone when balanced precavus is present. **B** With a monoblock insole for relaxation and support in presence of painful balanced cavus: *1* Without Martorell bar; *2* with Martorell bar. **C** Pes cavovarus present: *1* With external pronating wedge; *2* with external pronating wedge and supporting dome. **D** Pes cavovalgus present: *1* With internal dome, supinating heel wedge and pronating metatarsal wedge; *2* with retrocapital pronating bar and supinating heel wedge

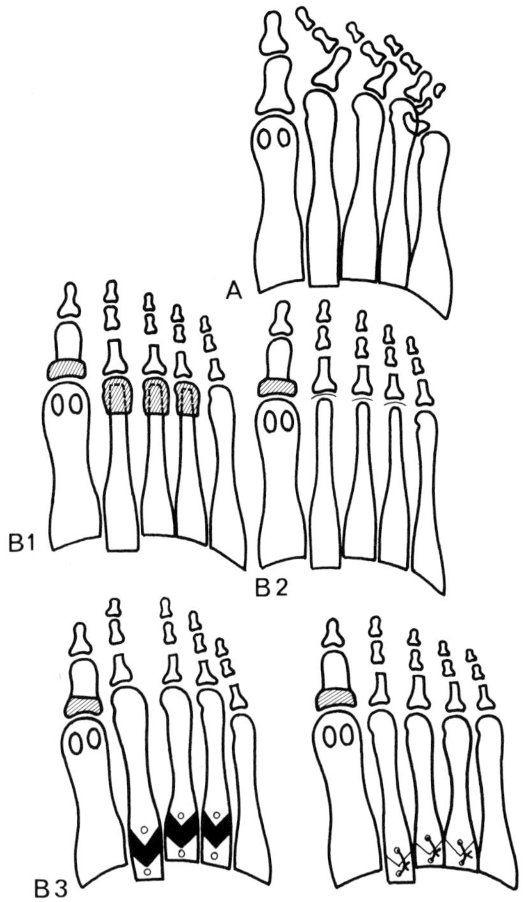

Fig. 7.6 A, B. Treatment of convex forefoot. **A** Before treatment: metatarsal configuration is I < II ⩾ III ⩾ IV > V. **B** Correction of hallux valgus, interphalangeal arthroplasties and elongation of tendons are accompanied by one of the following: enclavement of second to fourth metatarsal heads *(1)*, Lelièvre realignment with cup arthroplastic *(2)*, or basal metatarsal V-osteotomies *(3)*

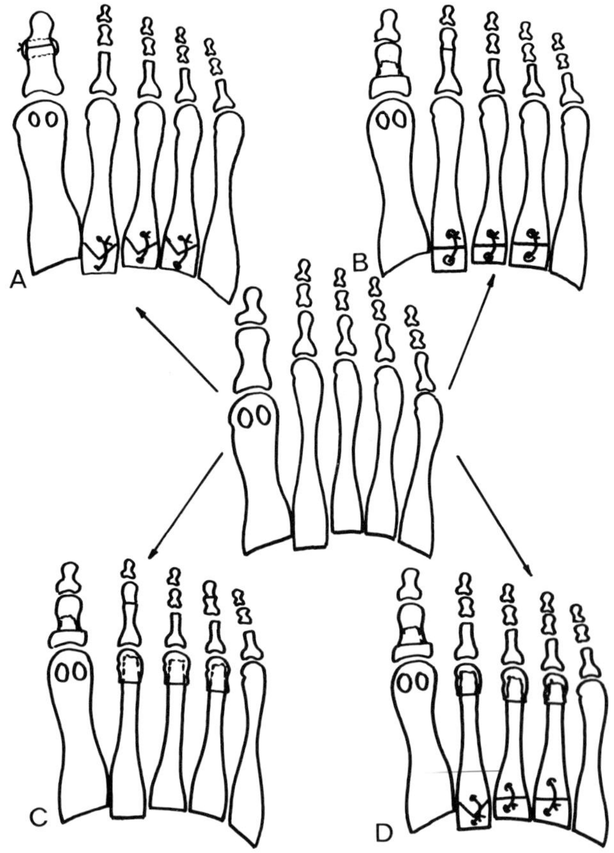

Fig. 7.7 A–D. Treatment of convex forefoot displaying central overloading. **A** Basal ostectomy of central three metatarsals and interphalangeal arthrodesis of great toe. **B** Thys-Martorell basal ostectomy of central three metatarsals and metatarsophalangeal arthroplasty of great toe. **C** Metatarsal shaft-head enclavements with interphalangeal arthrodeses as indicated and metatarsophalangeal arthroplasty of great toe. **D** Metatarsal shaft-head enclavements with basal ostectomies of great toe as indicated and metatarsophalangeal arthroplasty

Finally, it should be emphasised that it is never necessary to perform realignment of the metatarsals as described by Lelièvre (1952); this intervention should be reserved for metatarsophalangeal arthropathies with destruction of joint cartilage, as may occur in rheumatoid arthropathy or trauma with lysis of the metatarsal heads. The presence of longitudinal cavus contra-indicates this procedure most definitely. The procedure described by T. Judet (1972), comprising plastic elongation and transposition of the extensors onto the metatarsal heads, should be avoided, as it accentuates the clawing of the toes and does not correct the round forefoot configuration.

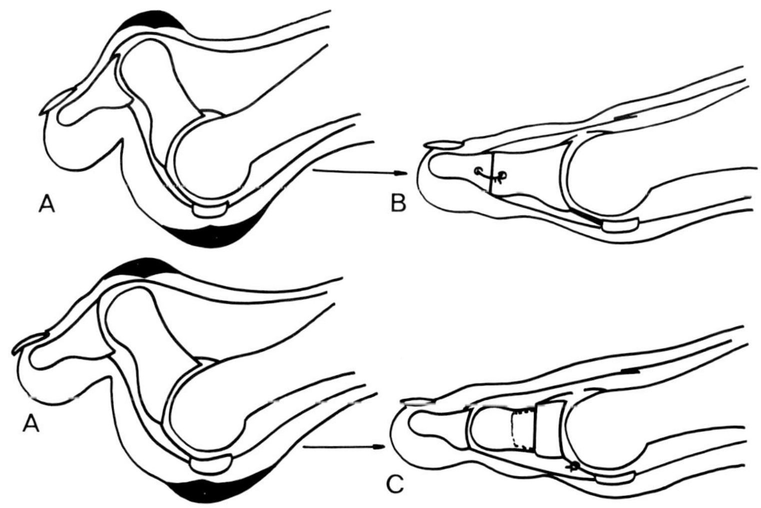

Fig. 7.8 A–C. Treatment of claw deformity of great toe. **A** Before treatment. **B** After interphalangeal arthrodesis. **C** After metatarsophalangeal arthroplasty. Both procedures are accompanied by elongation of extensor hallucis langus and dorsal capsulotomy of metatarsophalangeal joint

8 The Convex Triangular Forefoot

The convex triangular forefoot arises in a cavovalgus foot and is characterised by a triangular convex appearance of the ball of the foot due to an equinus posture of the central three metatarsals associated with frontal protrusion of the same metatarsal heads. The first and fifth metatarsals are short and diverge. The toes are compressed together; the first and fifth converge, while the central three develop claw deformities. Joint displacements and contractures involving tendons, capsules and skin render the condition irreversible.

The metatarsal formula is of the Greek type ($1 < 2 > 3 > 4 > 5$), and the foot initially exhibits a precavus or established cavus shape. At first supple, it later becomes unbalanced laterally at the midtarsus on account of a valgus posture of the heel. This results in internal and plantar displacement of the midtarsus which affects the balance of the Lisfranc joint line, modifying its frontal anterior convexity. Both plantar concavities, longitudinal and transverse, are accentuated, and the second and third metatarsals, grasped by the cuneiform metatarsal joints, are fixed in excessive equinus from this level. The normal relative immobility of the central metatarsals is accentuated by their posture and length. Because they are relatively shorter, the first and fifth metatarsals are unable to compensate for the central protrusion, and the cavus foot is in unstable equilibrium, balancing on the heel and the central part of the metatarsal paddle like a bicycle on its two wheels. Because of the longitudinal cavus, the base of the fifth metatarsal has no contact with the ground (see Fig. 11.8 N). As a result of this unbalanced situation, there is a valgus posture of the midtarsus, which sinks medially and downwards. There follows a diminution of the plantar longitudinal and transverse cavities of the midtarsus which is more significant at the second and third cuneiform-metatarsal joints, this adding to the excessive protrusion of the second and third metatarsals. The diminution of the plantar concavities at the midtarsus favours an increase in the frontal convexity of the Lisfranc joint line and has two consequences: increased frontal protrusion of the central metatarsal heads and divergence of the first and fifth metatarsals. The convergence of the toes is secondary to this configuration of the metatarsal heads.

8.1 Clinical Features

The syndrome develops at about the age of 40, predominantly in women. It is rarely seen in men except when associated with constant wearing of poor shoes, prolonged standing or overweight.

8.1.1 Symptoms

The onset of metatarsalgia precedes the development of obvious displacements or the formation of calluses. The pain may arise from the early displacements of hallux valgus or quintus varus, or may be localised to the second metatarsal head, when it is nearly always associated with a valgus heel; slight thickening may be noted in the skin under the second or third metatarsal head. There may be evidence of compression of the second intermetatarsal space as described by Serre et al. (1972), which may have symptoms similar to those of Morton's metatarsalgia (1876) but of different etiology. The pain seems to have an inflammatory character, but its mechanical etiology is evidenced by the fact that it is aggravated by standing and walking but relieved at resting. Initially it may be well controlled by the use of an insole or anti-inflammatory drugs, but this is likely to be only temporary.

The patient may first attend because of first-degree hallux valgus with early pain from pressure, or because of metatarsus quintus valgus. These displacements make shoe-fitting difficult and walking often painful. The pain described is of the tension type, with fatigue and with tightness in the weight-bearing zone of the foot. It is aggravated by a fleeting, burning pain after prolonged standing, walking or sport.

Later, the convex triangular appearance is much more obvious and is accompanied by metatarsophalangeal and interphalangeal joint displacements (Fig. 8.1). At this stage the patient complains of troublesome callus or corn formation, increasingly resistant to ordinary chiropodical management. The onset of overloading pain in the prominent ball of the foot, at first most significant towards the end of the day, gradually becomes earlier. The pain is episodic, aggravated by walking and especially a high-heeled shoe. It gradually becomes continuous during the day and even at night; patients complain that their feet are too hot in bed.

8.1.2 Physical Signs

At the early stage, while there may be some local tenderness under the second or third metatarsal heads, it is the triangular appearance, associated with the valgus heel and the progressive onset of transverse convexity of the ball of the foot, which is more likely to be evident. Once fully established, the metatarsophalangeal joint and interphalangeal joint displacements become more noticeable, with contractures of the soft tissues. Characteristically, a large plantar corn, sometimes oval in shape, underlies the affected metatarsal heads, its white, yellowish or violaceous appearance contrasting with the normal reddish colour of the plantar skin under the first and fifth metatarsal heads. There is atrophy of the weight-bearing subcutaneous tissue.

Palpation reveals from the outset the relative shortness of the first and fifth metatarsals together with the prominence of the central three. The abnormal breadth of the first and fourth intercapital spaces may be striking. The broad forefoot can be compressed manually, giving the palpating hand the impression of a median bony block due to intercapital apposition at the first and fourth interspaces.

The hallux valgus, accentuated in appearance by varus of the first metatarsal, may reach second or third degree. The great toe may develop slight dorsiflexion associated with the claw contractures of the central toes. The sesamoids sublux laterally, and there is contracture of the long and short extensor tendons, which form a cord in the angle of the metatarsophalangeal joint, tenting the overlying dorsal skin.

The quintus varus is frequently associated with an external bursa and a tailor's bunion provoked by friction against the shoe. Usually the fifth toe develops a supraductus or infraductus relative to the fourth toe. The long extensor tendon subluxes laterally, tenting the dorsal skin markedly.

The central three toes, initally longer, develop flexion contractures, partly because they abut against the toecap of the shoe. The condition leads eventually to dorsal dislocation of the associated metatarsophalangeal joints. This aggravates the depressed posture of the metatarsal heads and is fixed by capsular and cutaneous contractures and shortening of the long tendons. The action of the intrinsic muscles is reversed. Trauma from the shoes leads to various clinodactylies or camptodactylies.

Initially, the skin on the dorsum of the foot remains normal and pink but the subcutaneous tissue is increased in thickness. With the development of the obvious convex triangular syndrome, however, abnormal tension contributing to the fixation of the toes leads eventually to an apparent disappearance of the proximal segments of the three central toes. As mentioned earlier, the contrast in the appearance of the skin under the first and fifth metatarsal heads with that of the central zone is striking.

Podoscopy shows, even in the early stages, the print of a precavus or cavus foot with a light valgus spreading of the heel. *Podometry* provides useful information on the abnormal loading of the second, third and fourth metatarsal heads.

Radiography: Standard radiographs confirm the severity of the cavus of the foot and the general equinus of the antetarsus. Displacements of the joints are revealed, and the degree of frontal protrusion of the central metatarsal heads can be measured (see Fig. 6.3 D).

8.2 Treatment

8.2.1 Conservative

Conservative measures are the same as for the simple convex forefoot syndrome; failure to ease discomfort indicates the need for operative treatment.

8.2.2 Operative

Any longitudinal and fixed cavus deformity of the foot must be corrected, either by osteotomies near the tarsometatarsal joints or, better, by extra-articular cuneiform-cuboidal osteotomies of the midtarsus (Figs. 8.2, 8.3). This component must be corrected before any intervention in the forefoot itself. Osteotomies of the proximal metatarsals as described by Thys (1974) can be successful when performed exactly as described.

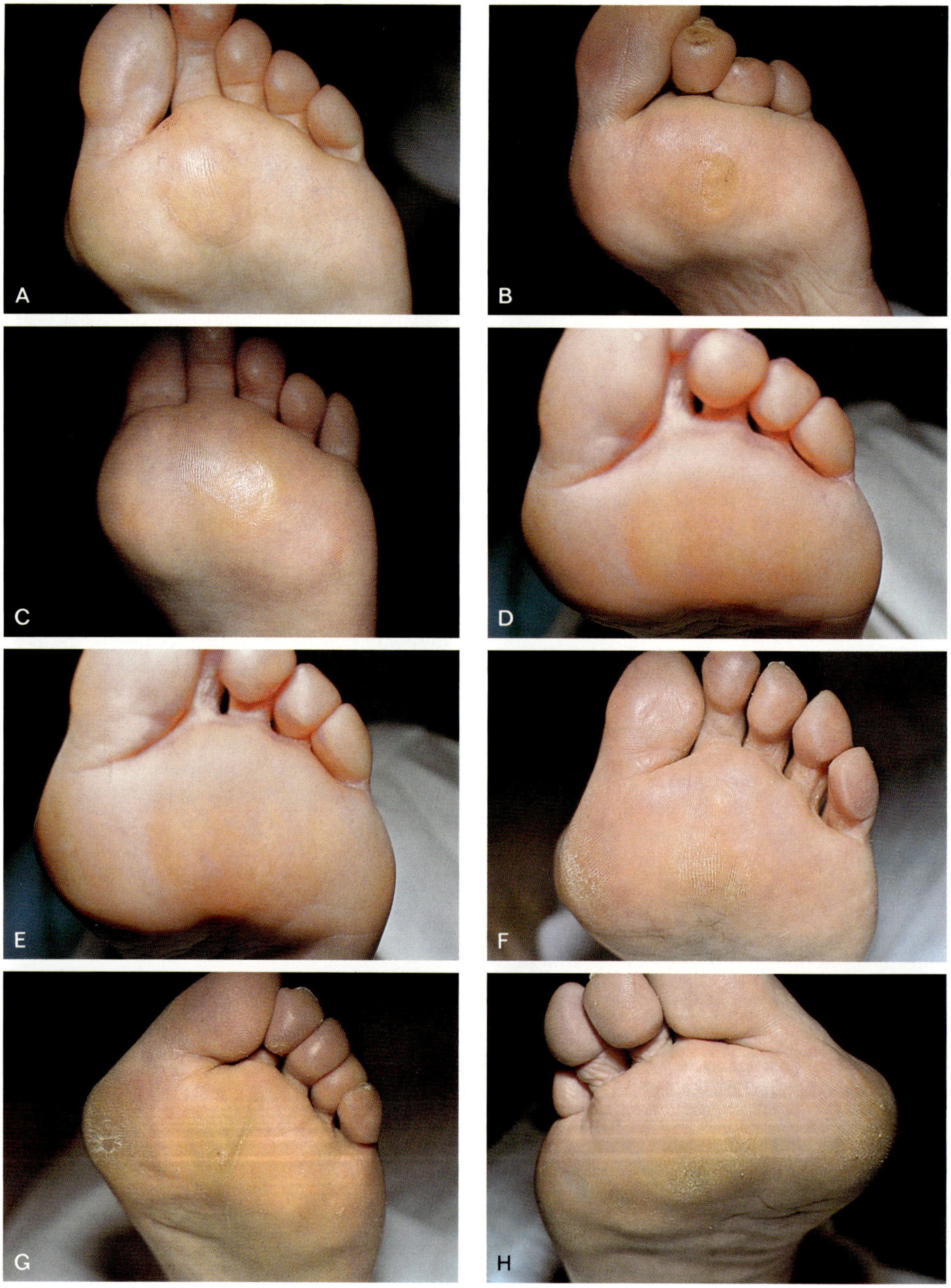

Fig. 8.1 A–I. Convex triangular forefoot. **A** First degree centred on second metatarsal. **B** First degree centred on third metatarsal. **C** First degree centred on second and third metatarsals. **D, E** Second degree centred on second, third and fourth metatarsals. **F–I** Third degree. **I** see p. 55 ▷

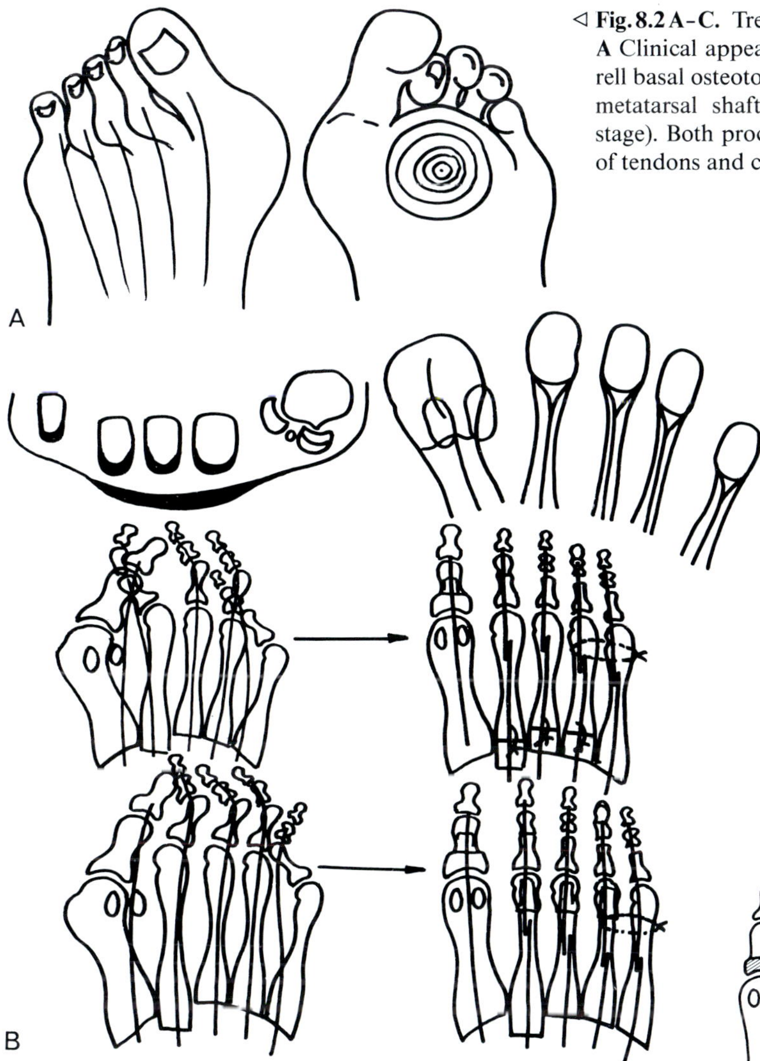

◁ **Fig. 8.2 A–C.** Treatment of convex triangular forefoot. **A** Clinical appearance. **B** Before and after Thys-Martorell basal osteotomies (in early stage). **C** Before and after metatarsal shaft-head enclavements (in early or late stage). Both procedures are accompanied by elongation of tendons and correction of toes

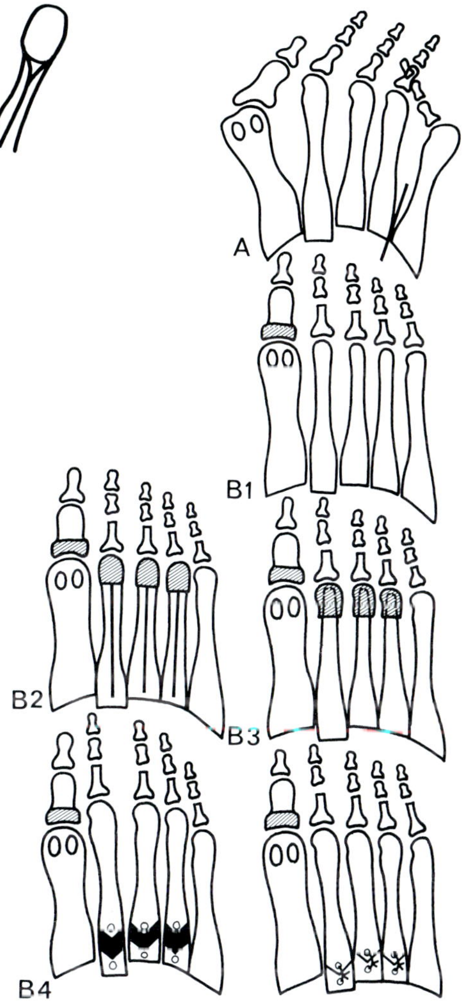

Fig. 8.3 A, B. Treatment of flat triangular forefoot and convex triangular forefoot. **A** Before treatment: metatarsal configuration is I $<$ II $>$ III $>$ IV $>$ V. **B** Correction of hallux valgus and metatarsus quintus valgus, elongation of tendons, interphalangeal arthroplasties and osteotomy between fourth and fifth metatarsals *(1)* are accompanied by one of the following: Lelièvre realignment, realignment with implantation of prostheses *(2)*, enclavement of second to fourth metatarsal heads *(3)* or Thys-Martorell basal osteotomies of metatarsals *(4)*

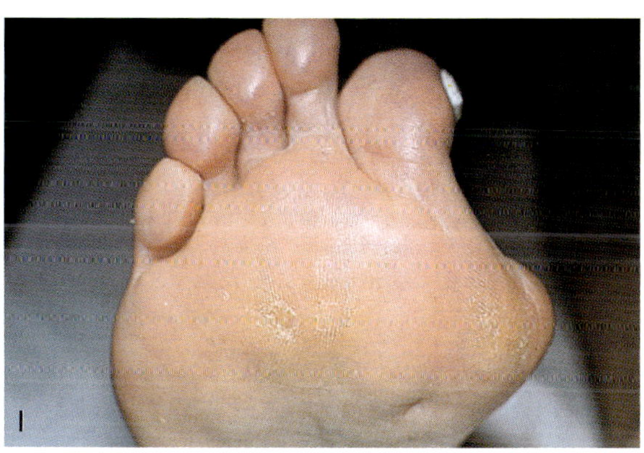

Fig. 8.1 I. Legend see p. 54

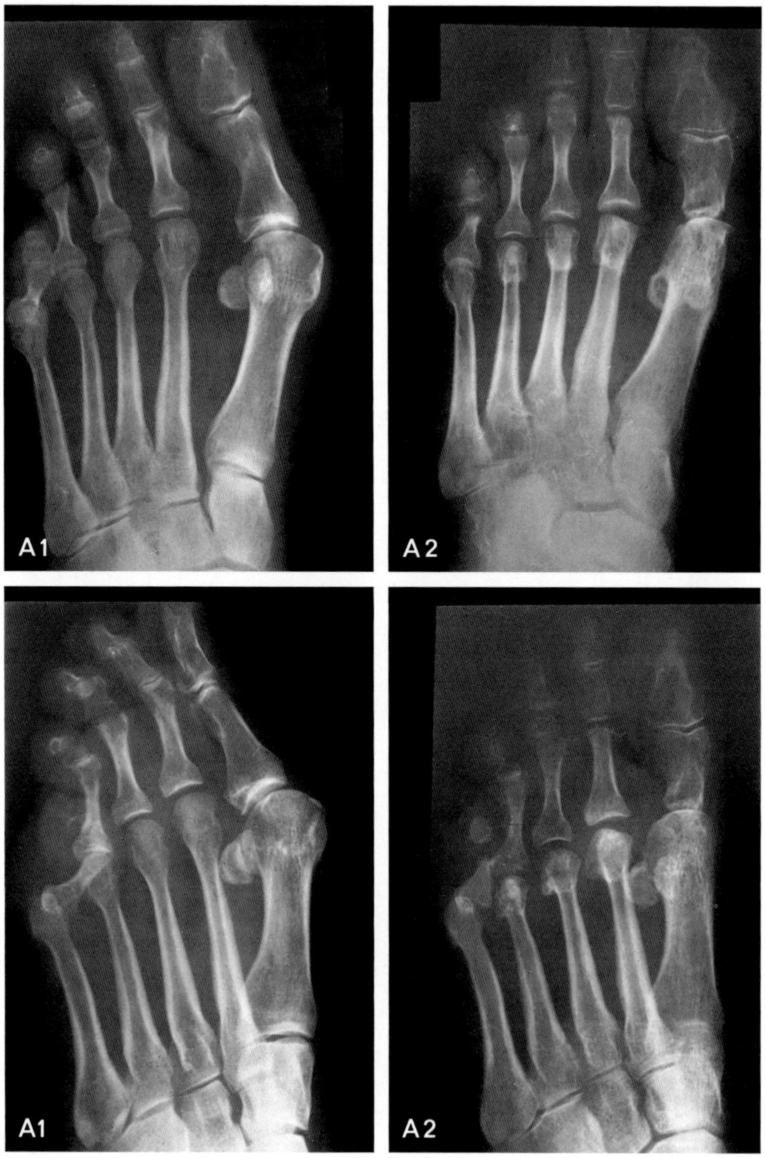

Fig. 8.4 A–C. Convex triangular forefoot and flat triangular forefoot: treatment by realignment head-shaft enclavement of metatarsals. **A** Convex triangular forefoot. *1* Hallux valgus, quintus varus, frontal protusion of second, third and fourth metatarsal heads; *2* realignment head-shaft enclavement of central three metatarsals, correction of hallux valgus with cork-shaped graft, arthroplasty of second and fifth toes. **B** Convex triangular forefoot. *1* Protrusion of central three metatarsal heads, hallux valgus, quintus varus, divergence of first and fifth metatarsals; *2* appearance after realignment by head-shaft enclavement of central three metatarsals, correction of hallux valgus by arthroplasty with graft; *3* oblique view showing postoperative appearance of all metatarsophalangeal joints. **C** Flat triangular forefoot. *1* Second-degree hallux valgus, quintus varus, divergence of first and fifth metatarsals, frontal protrusion of central three metatarsal heads, absence of equinus of central three metatarsals; *2* oblique and dorsoplantar views showing appearance after correction of hallux valgus with cork-shaped graft and arthroplasty, realignment head-shaft enclavement of central metatarsal heads, arthroplasty with shortening of fifth toe. **B, C** see p. 57

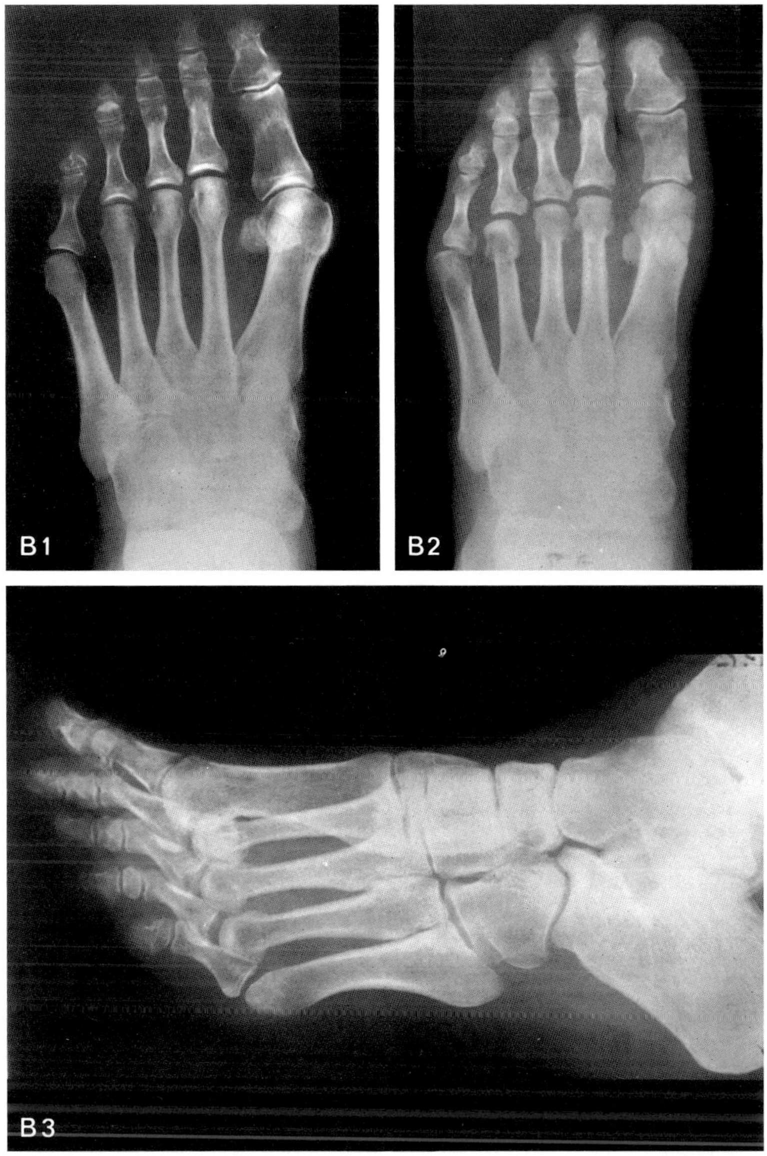

Fig. 8.4 B, C. Legend see p. 56

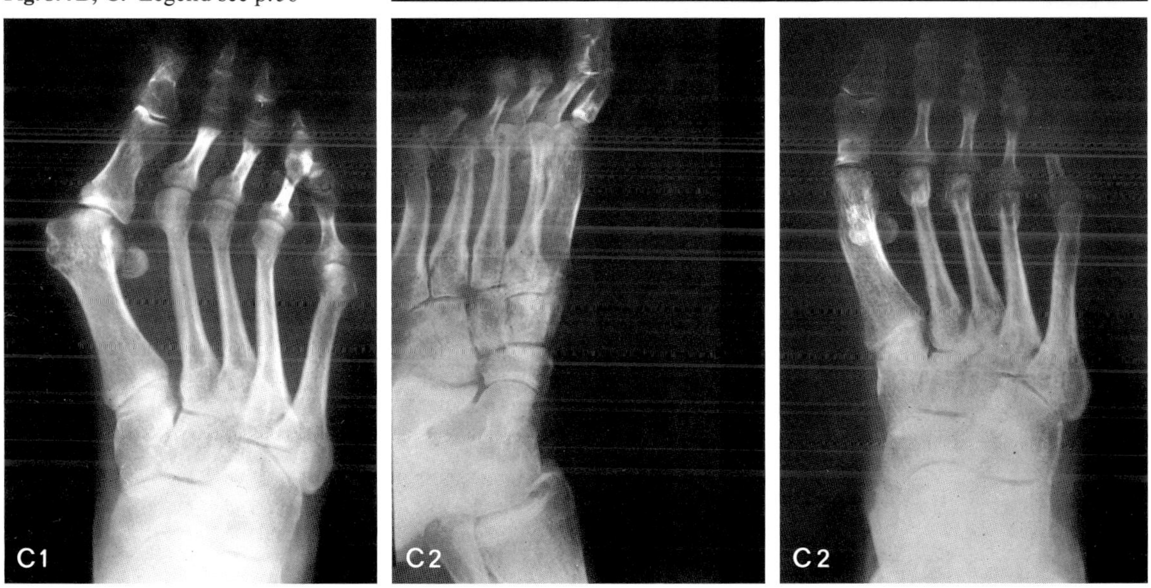

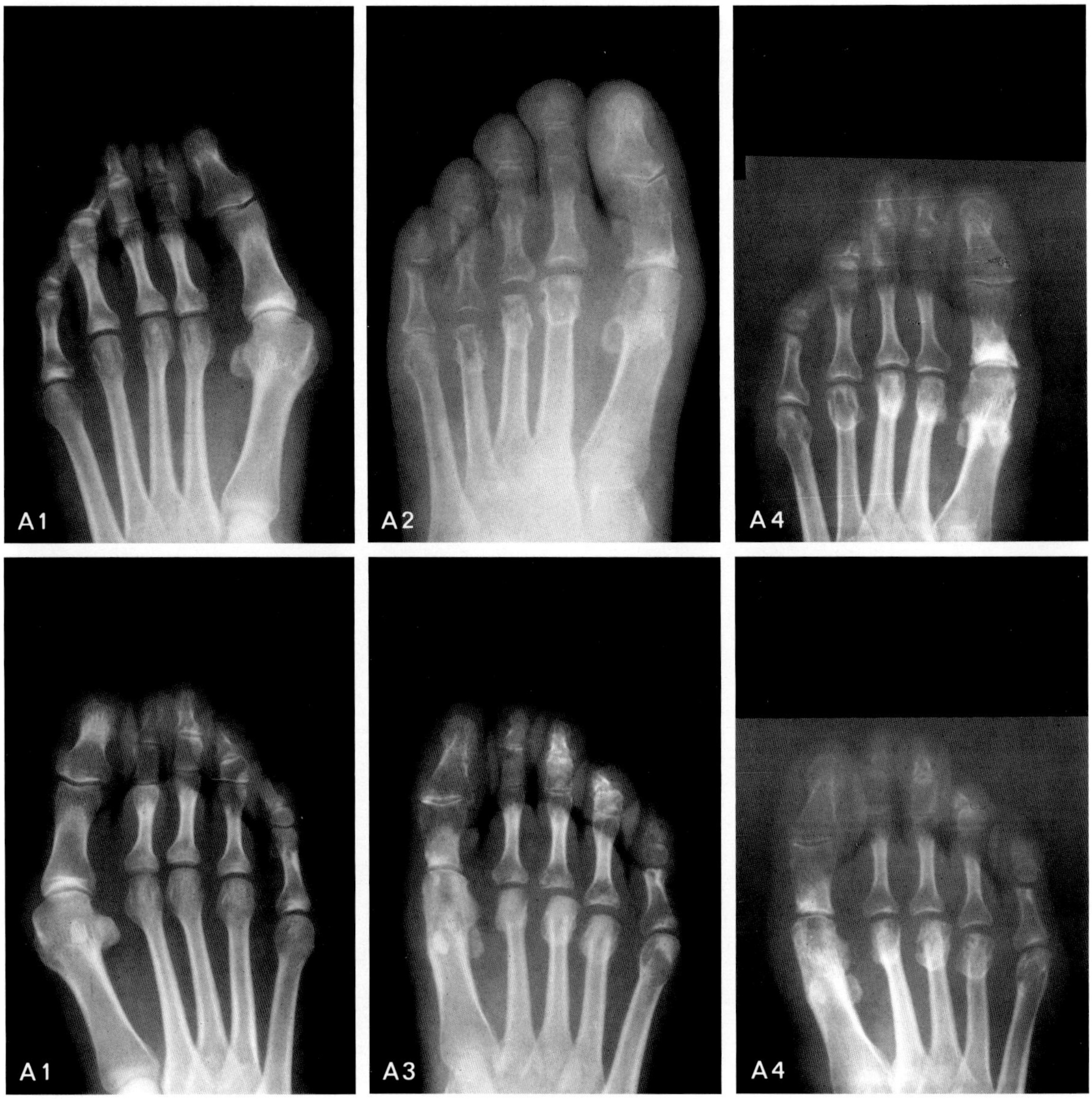

Fig. 8.5 A–D. Painful convex triangular forefoot and simple triangular forefoot: treatment by correction of hallux valgus, enclavement, arthroplasties of toes and tendinous elongations. **A** Simple triangular forefoot. *1* Metatarsal divergence, hallux valgus, varus of terminal phalanges of fifth toe, protrusion of central three metatarsal heads; *2* six months after head-shaft enclavement, correction of hallux valgus with hat-shaped graft, arthroplasty of fifth toe; *3* six months after head-shaft enclavement, correction of hallux valgus with cork-shaped graft, shortening; *4* appearance 1 year postoperatively. **B** Convex triangular forefoot. *1* Divergence of metatarsals, protrusion with equinus of central metatarsal heads, supple claw toes; *2* left foot: appearance 1 year after head-shaft enclavement of central metatarsal heads, correction of hallux valgus with hat-shaped graft, arthroplasty of fifth toe. Right foot: convex triangular forefoot; *3* left foot 4 months later: note that the capsular contracture is not completely corrected. Right foot: appearance 1 year after head-shaft enclavement of central metatarsal head, correction of hallux valgus, with hat-shaped graft, arthroplasty of fifth toe. **B–D** see pp. 59–61 ▷

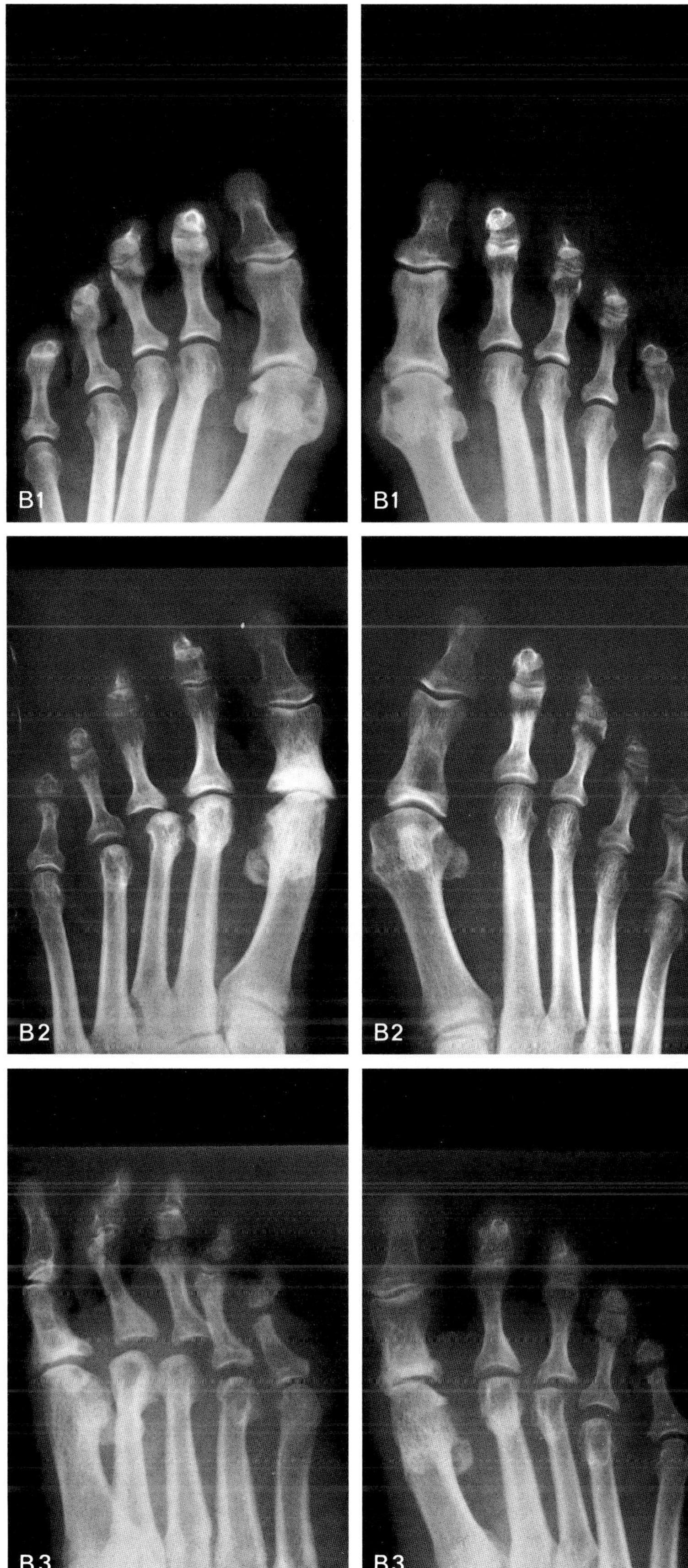

Fig. 8.5 B. Legend see p. 58

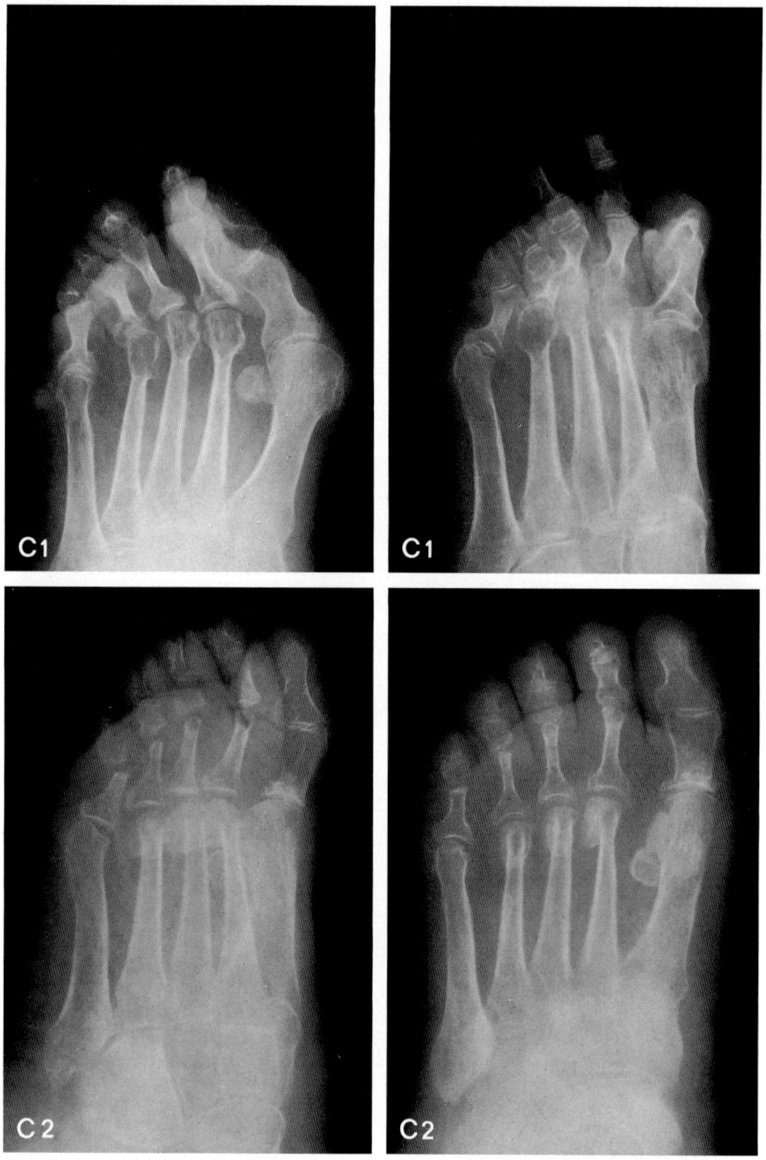

Fig. 8.5 *(continued)*. **C** Convex forefoot. *1* Absence of divergence of metatarsals, significant protrusion of central three metatarsal heads, hallux valgus, disordered claw formations; *2* head-shaft enclavement of central three metatarsal heads, correction of hallux valgus with hat-shaped graft, intraphalangeal arthroplasties and tendinous elongations. **D** Convex forefoot. *1* Absence of divergence of first and fifth metatarsals, first-degree hallux valgus, protrusion and equinus of central three metatarsals; *2* three months after enclavement, correction of hallux valgus with hat-shaped graft; *3* eight months postoperatively: very good incorporation of condylar graft, but capsular contracture of metatarsophalangeal joint not completely corrected. **D** see p. 61 ▷

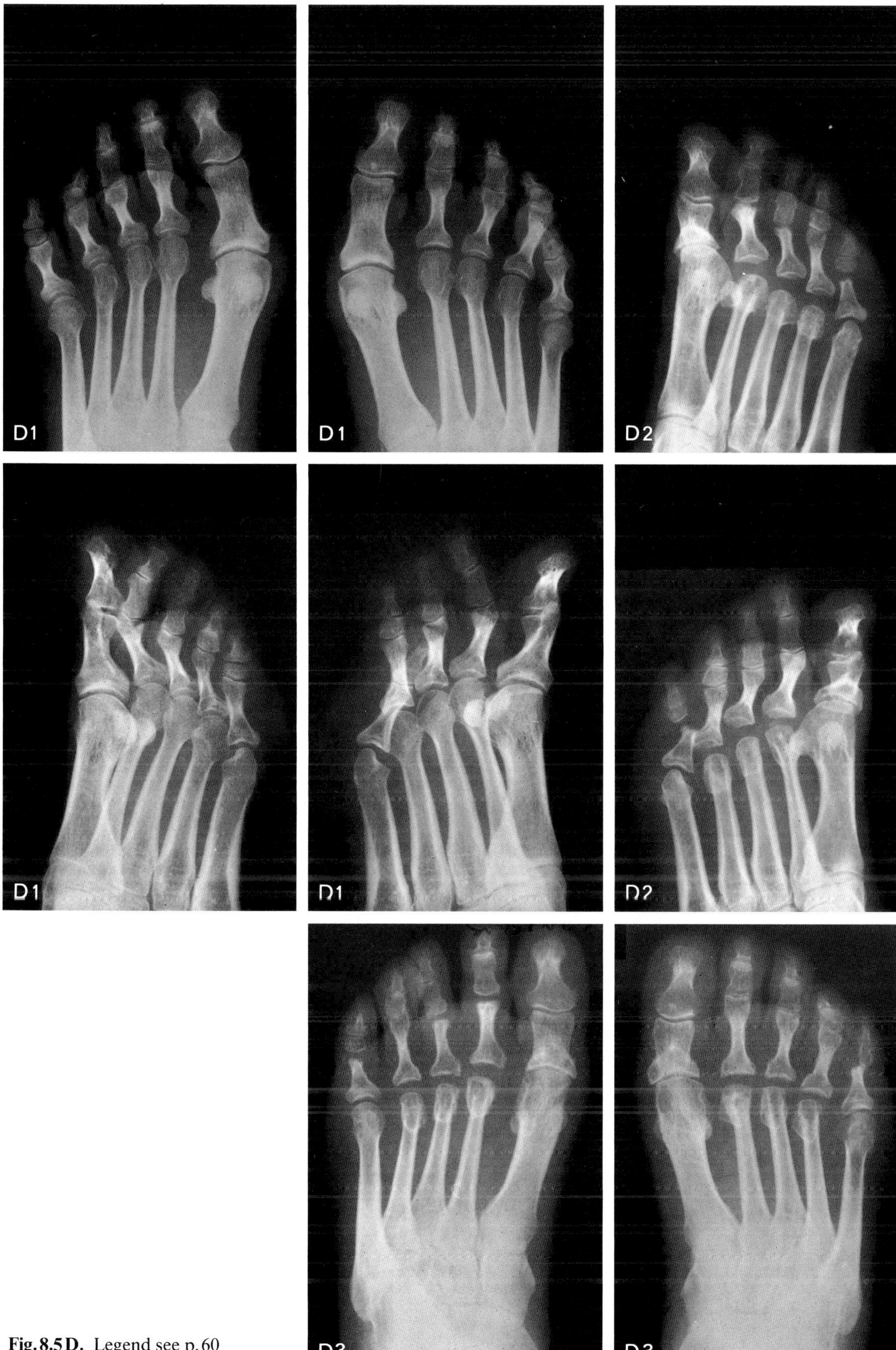

Fig. 8.5 D. Legend see p. 60

They must be accompanied by elongations of the tendons to allow correction of the claw toes. However, the author has abandoned this technique because of the difficulty of exact measurement of the degree of elevation or shortening of the metatarsals and the danger of converting the convex forefoot into a cavus forefoot. It is only in the very early stages that basal trapezoidal osteotomy should be considered.

The author recommends that in the established condition with contractures present, operative treatment should comprise correction of the hallux valgus and quintus varus associated with realignment head-shaft enclavement of the central metatarsal heads, tendon elongations, capsulotomies of the lateral and dorsal aspects of the metatarsophalangeal joints to correct the subluxations or dislocations, and finally, arthroplasties or arthrodeses of the interphalangeal joints as appropriate. Head-shaft enclavement allows precise frontal and horizontal realignment. An isolated equinus persisting in one metatarsal can be corrected by an osteotomy at the base of this bone as a final procedure if necessary (Figs. 6.5C, 8.4, 8.5).

9 The Cavus Forefoot

The metatarsal formula is usually of square, occasionally of Greek or Egyptian configuration. There is longitudinal balanced or varus pes cavus and the condition is characterised by the appearance of a transverse concavity under the ball of the foot associated with typical callus formation under the first and fifth metatarsal heads, displacements at the tarsometatarsal joint line and displacements of the metatarsophalangeal joints with contractures of the integument and capsulotendinous structures. Initially the foot may be supple with a precavus shape, but the longitudinal cavus progressively increases and deviates into valgus or varus. Rarely, the condition may be associated with a flat contracted foot. As well as the transverse concavity at the metatarsal heads, there may be increased cavus at the level of the talonavicular joint line or at the midtarsus corresponding to the cuneiforms and the cuboid. Increased cavus at the midtarsal level results in a reduction in frontal convexity at the Lisfranc joint line; there follows an associated increase in equinus of the antetarsus generally and an absence of divergence of the metatarsals, so that the antetarsus is maintained compressed as well as in equinus. The metatarsals are parallel, and in the majority of cases, they are of equal length; the central three exhibit a relatively reduced equinus. In these circumstances the cavus of the foot is balanced. In some instances, there is congenital shortening of the first metatarsal, increasing the degree of equinus necessary for the head to reach the ground and achieve collateral stability, in which case the cavus becomes accompanied by a varus posture.

The development of the cavus forefoot syndrome merits close attention. It stems from the alignment of the cuneiform and cuboid bones; the summit of curvature is at the level of the intermediate and lateral cuneiforms, the bases of the five metatarsals correspond, and accordingly, the second, third and fourth are in a more elevated position. Because of the equal length of the first to fourth metatarsals and perhaps a general inversion of the foot into varus, the condyles of the central three metatarsals do not make contact with the ground when the first and fifth heads are loaded. This will apply in the cavus balanced foot. In the cavovarus foot, the fact that the base of the fifth metatarsal is lower than that of the first metatarsal induces a progressive increase of equinus of the first metatarsal, accentuating the cavus forefoot.

It is a combination of the elevation of the second and third metatarsals, the lengths of the second, third and fourth metatarsals with respect to the first and the diminution of the frontal transverse convexity of the Lisfranc joint line which determine the equinus of the first and fifth metatarsals and the consequent overloading of their heads. In the balanced cavus foot the overloading is symmetrical; in the cavovarus foot, it is initially more marked under the fifth metatarsal head, but subsequently, due to progressive increase of equinus of the first metatarsal, appears under its head as well. Serous bursae form and calluses develop, and a reactionary sesamoid hypertrophy may occur.

In order to relieve pain under the first metatarsal head, the patient tends to walk with the foot in varus and supination. This is established by action of tibialis anterior and tibialis posterior, so the varus is seen in both tarsal and midtarsal regions. Permanent contraction of peroneus longus accentuates the equinus, while contraction of extensor hallucis longus produces clawing of the great toe; both increase the supination of the forefoot. The varus tarsus and supination of the forefoot have two further consequences: Firstly, there is an increase of the already present overloading of the fifth metatarsal head, aggravated further by the action of peroneus brevis and the long flexors in response to the general excessive loading of the outer side of the foot. These factors progressively augment the equinus, so establishing a vicious circle of increasing overloading. Secondly, the first metatarsal increases its degree of equinus in order to continue to bear weight on its head despite the supination of the forefoot. Contraction of peroneus longus achieves this at the expense of raising the medial cuneiform while depressing the first metatarsal. This supinating effect on the foot increases the equinus of the first metatarsal further and is accompanied by permanent contraction of the long and short extensors. The latter causes clawing of the toes and progressive subluxation and dislocation of the metatarsophalangeal joints.

This vicious circle of pain leads to a supinating reaction, then a pronating reaction and finally dorsiflexion of the toes; it accentuates the cavus posture of the forefoot and leads to the irreversible changes described.

9.1 Clinical Features

The cavus forefoot can appear between the ages of 20 and 50 years and is more common in men, especially when accentuated by prolonged standing at work (Fig. 9.1).

9.1.1 Symptoms

Pain, the presenting symptom, is directly due to the overloading of the first and fifth metatarsal heads and the distortion in the midtarsal region and subtalar joint when a varus component accompanies the cavus of the forefoot.

Initially the metatarsalgia is localised in the overloaded areas and is of a burning or pricking character; it is accentuated by standing and walking, relieved by rest. It becomes increasingly continuous, and may become intolerable on the development of bursitis or infection of the calluses. Rarely, there may be pain of a neuralgic type, like Morton metatarsalgia, of a more sudden, tense quality, aggravated by mechanical pressure and supination of the forefoot; this affects the first and fourth intercapital spaces.

The subtalar joint may be the site of arthralgic pain, usually along its external aspect; the midtarsal and tarsometatarsal joint lines may also hurt. Pain in the toes is due to local pressure from clawing and terminal corns.

9.1.2 Physical Signs

The calluses under the first and fifth metatarsal heads are fusiform, yellowish and often prominent from keratoma formation. The central skin remains pink and supple, being grooved by folds between the central metatarsal heads. The elevated position of the central metatarsals can be palpated. The clawing of the toes is typical, with an S-shaped profile when viewed from the side due to subluxation or dislocation dorsally of the metatarsophalangeal joints and to the flexion contractures, which sometimes involve only the proximal, but more commonly also the distal, interphalangeal joints; this is more marked in the central three toes. In early cases, the clawing is supple and can be corrected, but it soon becomes fixed by soft tissue contractures and has the effect of augmenting the longitudinal cavus of the foot.

The joint displacements and the longitudinal cavus result in a loss of balance of the antagonist muscles with contracture of both extensors and flexors. While slight at first, the long extensor contractures become fixed and then bridge the skin over the metatarsophalangeal joints. The fixed clawing is due to the flexor muscles but is augmented by a paradoxical action of the interossei and lumbricales which occurs on dislocation of the metatarsophalangeal joints. The accompanying capsular contractures complete the fixation of the joints in their deformed position. The cutaneous layer is equally affected.

In untreated cases, infection of the calluses and a general chronic inflammatory process with oedema may be accompanied by joint involvement or even osteitis. The bunched-up toes may display inflamed dorsal corns over the interphalangeal joints, and the nails may be adversely affected by pressure, as evidenced by a greyish or dirty-yellow appearance, or the development of onychogryphosis or onychomycosis.

Podoscopy shows a very characteristic bifocal appearance of the forefoot. *Podometry* provides final proof of overloading of the first and fifth metatarsal heads, even in early cases.

Radiography: Routine views confirm the cavus foot, the metatarsal formula, the joint displacements, and the transverse concavity affecting the five metatarsal heads. A longitudinal crest may be visible on the sesamoid bones due to hypertrophy from overloading.

9.2 Treatment

9.2.1 Conservative

In the early stages the longitudinal cavus of the foot is still supple, and similarly the posture of the toes can be corrected easily (Fig. 9.2). In such cases, an insole with a retrocapital bar, augmented in the case of the varus foot by a pronating wedge, controls the progressive development of the condition and, with appropriate chiropody for the corns and calluses, may keep the patient comfortable. It is, however, unlikely to cure the condition. Progres-

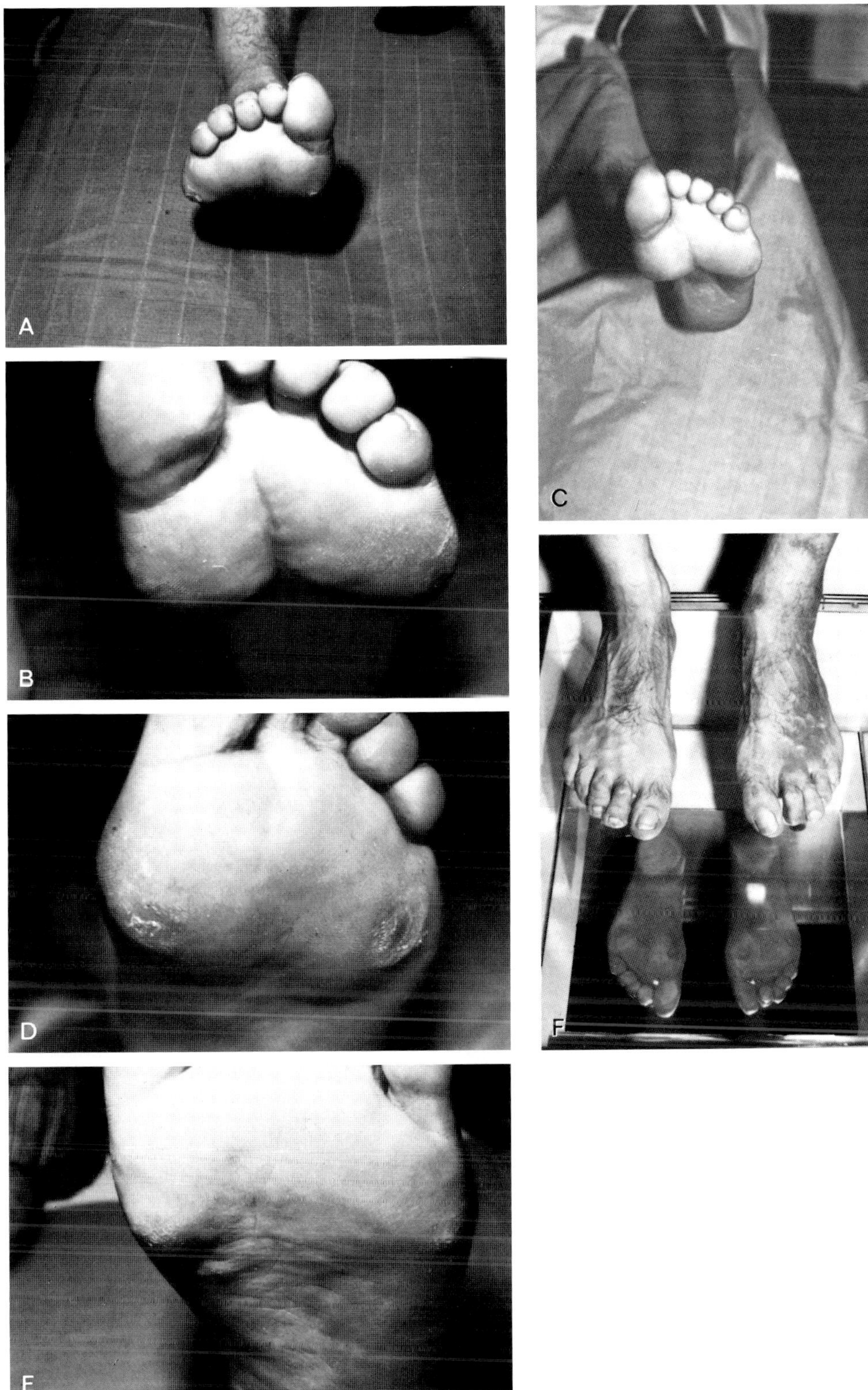

Fig. 9.1 A–F. Forefoot cavus. **A** Transverse concavity of ball of foot. **B, C** Central longitudinal furrow. **D, E** Callus or keratoma under first and fifth metatarsal heads. **F** Footprint of pes cavus and forefoot cavus

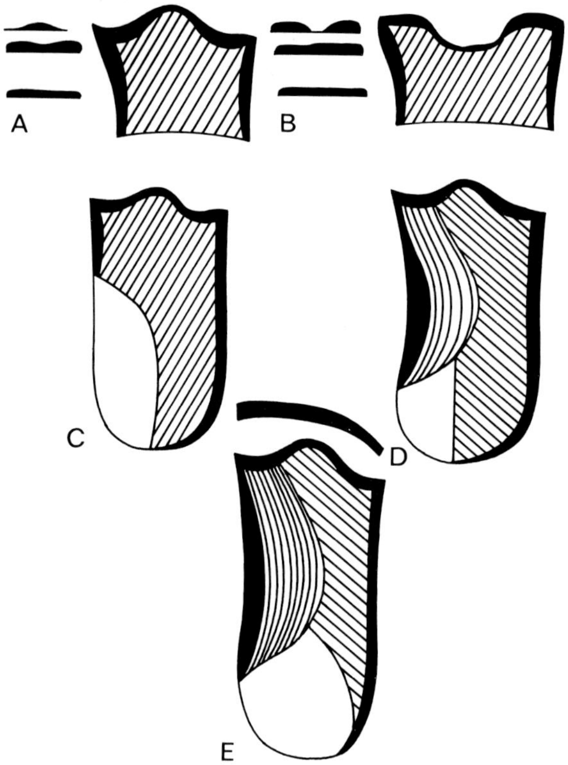

Fig. 9.2 A–E. Corrective insoles for cavus forefoot. **A** Retrocapital bar. **B** Subcapital bar with central excavation. **C** Retrocapital bar with external pronating wedge. **D** Retrocapital bar with external pronating wedge and internal dome. **E** Retrocapital bar with monoblock insole and Martorell antecapital bar

sion or fixity of the various deformities described can respond only to surgical management.

9.2.2 Operative

Operative procedures must be chosen according to whether the syndrome has developed in a cavus foot in which the deformity is the result of selective equinus of the first and fifth metatarsals, or in association with an irreducible fixed longitudinal cavus stemming from the midtarsal region.

9.2.2.1 Cavus Due to Equinus of First and Fifth Metatarsals

Procedures are limited to the forefoot and are designed to restore horizontal alignment of the five metatarsal heads while maintaining strength for loading of the first and fifth components:

- Basal semicircular osteotomy of the first metatarsal, correcting equinus (Regnauld; Fig. 9.3).
- Flattening of a hypertrophied sesamoid bone by removing the crest or diminishing the thickness of both sesamoids.
- Correction of the fifth metatarsal with respect to its fixed equinus, which is associated with loss of movement at the bases of the fourth and fifth metatarsals (Fig. 9.4). Proximally, a longitudinal capsulotomy between the fourth and fifth metatarsal bases releases the fifth metatarsal, allowing some vertical movement as well as lateral mobility. If movement is not restored, it is necessary to perform a transverse V-shaped osteotomy at the base of the fifth metatarsal. Distally, the hypertrophied condyle should be flattened.
- At a second stage, the metatarsophalangeal joints require capsulotomy together with elongation of the associated tendons, thereby allowing reduction of the dorsal dislocation. The contracted interphalangeal joints may be treated by arthroplasty or arthrodesis, supplemented by tenotomy of the long and short flexor tendons as necessary.

9.2.2.2 Forefoot Cavus Associated with Longitudinal Cavus Foot

Surgical treatment is more complex and demands attention to both the midtarsal and the antetarsal regions which, as explained earlier, are particularly intimately related in this syndrome. The longitudinal cavus with its varus or valgus components must be corrected first with appropriate osteotomies, and then attention can be devoted to the forefoot. In the midtarsal or tarsal region the fixed deformities and their site dictate in which cases osteotomy is appropriate. This is performed at the summit of the longitudinal arch, adapted according to whether there is a varus or valgus component. Thus it may be that arthrodesis of the Chopart joint line with removal of a wedge of bone based dorsally, together with arthrodesis of the subtalar joint, will be the procedure of choice. The configuration of the excised bone must be calculated exactly. Alternatively, a midtarsal naviculocuneiform resection extended to an intracuboid osteotomy, with the wedge of bone based dorsally and externally, may be more suited to the individual case. Finally, osteotomy at the Lisfranc joint region may be indicated, in which case the wedge of bone removed must accentuate the correction predominantly of the first and fifth metatarsals. The angle of resection must be wider at the first cuneiform-metatarsal

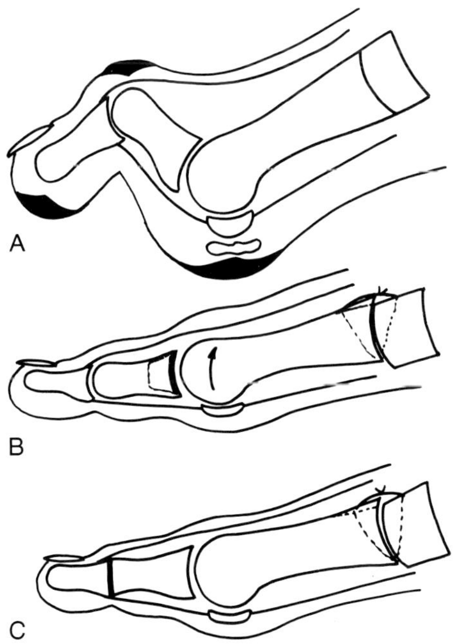

Fig. 9.3 A–C. First ray in cavus forefoot. **A** Before treatment. There is equinus of metatarsal, clawing of toe and callus formation under metatarsal head, on dorsal aspect of interphalangeal joint and on terminal aspect of toe. **B** After basal dome osteotomy of metatarsal and metatarsophalangeal arthroplasty with graft (Regnauld). **C** After basal dome osteotomy of metatarsal and interphalangeal arthrodesis (Regnauld)

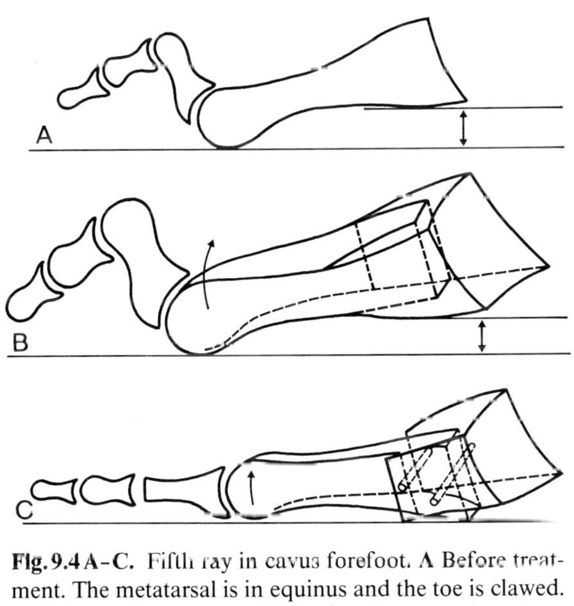

Fig. 9.4 A–C. Fifth ray in cavus forefoot. **A** Before treatment. The metatarsal is in equinus and the toe is clawed. **B, C** Stages in treatment. The procedures employed are elevating basal osteotomy (Regnauld), metatarsophalangeal arthrolysis, elongation of tendons and proximal interphalangeal arthroplasty (Regnauld)

joint so as to establish an exactly horizontal alignment of the five metatarsal heads. The supination of the forefoot must be corrected, and if necessary correction can be completed by a transcalcaneal osteotomy as described by Dwyer (1959), with the wedge of bone based externally, correcting varus of the calcaneum.

These osteotomy-arthrodeses must not be performed in patients over the age of 40 years or in whom the longitudinal cavus of the foot and the varus displacement are so accentuated that they make the foot rigid without any chance of recovery after correction of cavus.

In the young adult, extra-articular osteotomies of the first and fifth metatarsals may be applicable when the longitudinal cavus is mild and still supple (Fig. 9.5). Osteotomy of the first metatarsal is easy if it is performed using a semicircular technique which allows exact correction under direct vision. Flattening of the hypertrophied plantar surface of the two sesamoids may be a useful supplement. Basal osteotomy of the fifth metatarsal, which may be by removal of a wedge of bone or by the semicircular technique, sometimes creates a problem of coaptation of the cut surfaces of the bone on account of the considerable tension exerted by peroneus brevis on its base. The author recommends a diaphyseo-epiphyseal osteotomy, which avoids this problem.

Following operation, a plaster of Paris insole should be used for 6 weeks and progressive weight bearing allowed from about the 4th week.

In the forefoot cavus syndrome the choice of surgical technique is highly individual. Often, for example, the three central metatarsal heads are not in the same horizontal plane, and it is then necessary to adjust these selectively by basal osteotomies (Fig. 9.6).

Following correction of the hind- and midfoot, the cavus forefoot correction may be completed by attention to the deformed joints. Arthrotomy of the metatarsophalangeal joints, elongation of the extensor tendons and detachment of the long and short flexor tendons at their digital insertions will allow correction there, while arthrodeses or arthroplasties of the interphalangeal joints are necessary to re-establish straightness of the toes. Finally, correction is completed by adjustment of the length of the tibialis posterior tendon and the long flexor tendons of the toes, while if there is persistent varus of the foot, hemitransplantation of tibialis anterior to the lateral cuneiform bone can re-establish excellent balance.

Attention to the skin is general in all cases. Plantar keratomata, especially if they have suppurated,

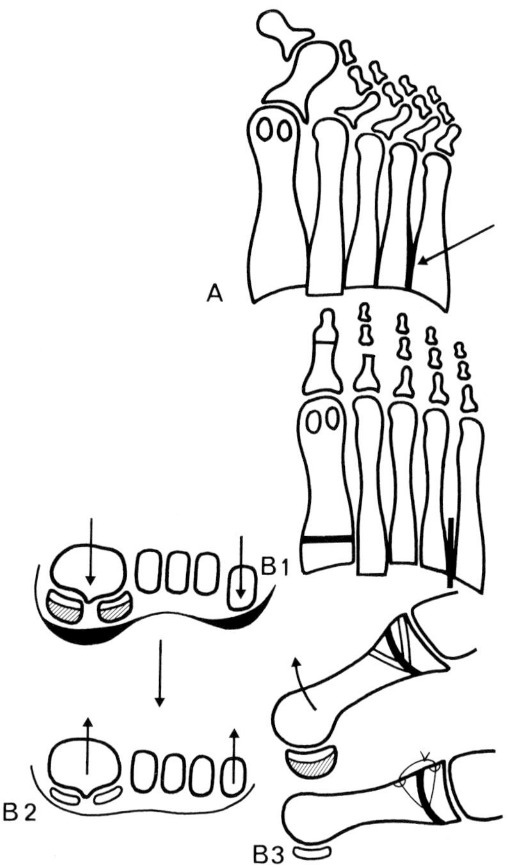

Fig. 9.5 A, B. Treatment of cavus forefoot. **A** Before treatment: metatarsal configuration is I > II > III > IV > V. **B** Correction of hallux valgus or of clawing of great toe, interphalangeal arthroplasties and elongation of tendons *(1)* are accompanied in a *flexible* foot by dome osteotomy, reduction of sesamoids and plastic resection of plantar keratoma in the great toe *(2)* and by osteotomy between fourth and fifth metatarsals including reduction of condylar prominence of fifth metatarsal *(1)*, in a *rigid* foot by osteotomy adjacent to or through tarsometatarsal joint line *(3)* and correction of forefoot cavus

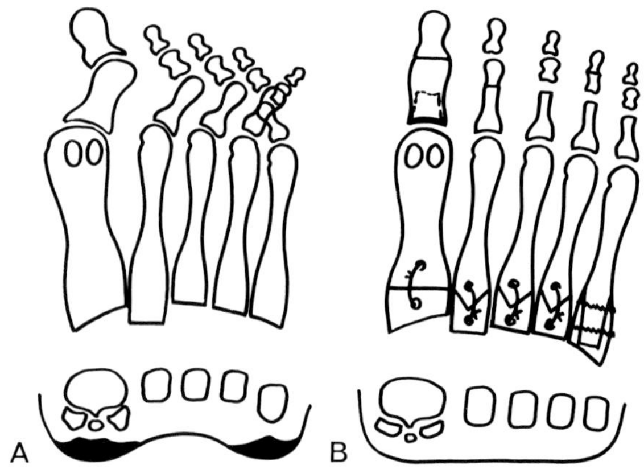

Fig. 9.6 A, B. Cavus forefoot with callus formation under first and fifth metatarsal heads. **A** Before treatment. **B** After elevating basal osteotomies of first and fifth metatarsals and lowering basal osteotomies of second to fourth metatarsals

persist despite excellent correction of the contours of the foot. Plastic surgical procedures involving local transposition flaps may be indicated.

9.3 Iatrogenic Cavus Forefoot

The particular problem posed by the iatrogenic cavus forefoot usually relates to previous excision of the central three metatarsal heads. While the normal vertical mobility of the first and fifth metatarsals is retained, this cannot compensate for the inevitable overloading to which they are subjected. The empty area where the resected heads used to be is accompanied by calluses under the first and fifth heads. The central three toes are retracted and bound to the dorsal aspects of the metatarsal stumps, and the great and fifth toes develop clinodactylies with infraductus. The dorsally displaced central toes press painfully against the toecap of the shoe and develop dorsal callosities.
Operative treatment should be considered, and after elongation of the shortened tendons and clawed toes, three possibilities exist:

1. Shortening of the first and fifth metatarsals, although this leads to overall shortening of the foot
2. Implantation of metatarsal head prostheses, restoring foot length, with occasional additional shortening of the first and fifth metatarsals
3. Implantation of metatarsal head homografts.

10 Convex Forefoot with Insufficiency of the First Ray

There is a group of forefoot syndromes characterised by convexity of the plantar weight-bearing surface associated with insufficiency of action of the first ray. They may be subdivided as follows:

1. Short first metatarsal
   a) Relative: due to congenital overlengthening of the second metatarsal in a planovalgus foot (Duddley Morton 1924a)
   b) Absolute: congenital shortening of first metatarsal
   c) Acquired: iatrogenic
2. Short great toe: acquired, usually iatrogenic
3. Hypermobility of first metatarsal, described by Courriades (1971)

10.1 Congenital Familial Forefoot of Duddley Morton

This entity (Duddley Morton 1924a) has been termed the "atavistic foot" or "Neanderthal foot" (Fig. 10.1).

10.1.1 Etiology

There is hypertrophy in length and volume of the second metatarsal with abnormal divergence of the neighbouring metatarsals away from the second metatarsal's longitudinal axis. The divergence is most significant in the first and fifth metatarsals, relating to the congenital planovalgus deformity which is part of the syndrome. In the infant it is striking how the five toes are splayed in line with their metatarsals. In contrast, by adulthood the wearing of shoes has constricted the toes towards the midline, so that they converge progressively and also exercise some restraint on the splaying of the metatarsals, which tend to group together at their heads encouraging the development of convexity of the ball of the foot. These structural disorders become associated with tendinous contractures, joint involvements, cutaneous manifestations and metatarsalgia. Clinical symptoms may be precipitated as a result of a Deutschländer fatigue fracture of the second metatarsal (Deutschländer 1921).

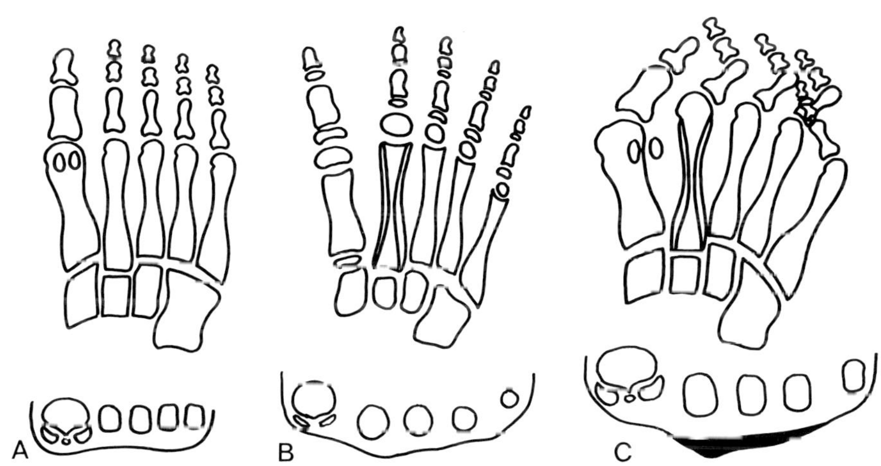

Fig. 10.1 A–C. Congenital convex forefoot of Duddley Morton. **A** Normal foot for comparison. **B** In the infant. **C** In the adult

10.1.2 Clinical Presentation

In the *first ray,* the metatarsophalangeal angulation amounts to first- or second-degree hallux valgus, with shortening of the first metatarsal, which is in significant varus. There is usually an increase in amplitude of vertical and lateral movement of the first metatarsal, stemming from hypermobility at the first cuneiform-metatarsal joint, a feature stressed by Lelièvre and Courriades. The insufficiency of the first ray originates in the majority of cases primarily in the shortening, in contrast with ordinary hallux valgus of the adult.

In conjunction with radiographic changes, there is evident abnormal widening of the first intercapital space and posterior displacement of the sesamoid bones, which on palpation reveal abnormal anteroposterior mobility. The plane of the first cuneiform-metatarsal joint is directed more obliquely forwards, downwards, and inwards with respect to the cuneiform, while the articular surface of the base of the first metatarsal is almost perpendicular to the long axis of this bone (normally the basal plane of the metatarsal presents an obliquity with respect to the long axis, and it is the distortion here which perhaps explains the accentuated varus of the first metatarsal).

In the *fifth ray,* the metatarsal is again hypermobile, like a piano key, and is very much influenced by the constraint exercised by the shoe. On its external face there may be a serous bursa which becomes inflamed or infected, together with a painful callus. Supraductus or infraductus of the fifth toe develops in its varus posture. The fourth intercapital space is widened, amounting to a triangular dehiscence of which the base is formed by the fourth ray and the two sides by the angulation of the metatarsophalangeal joint. The extensor longus tendon to the fifth toe bowstrings laterally and may be contracted.

With respect to the *second ray,* it is unusual for initial inspection in the adult to detect its abnormal length. This is because of the constraint of the shoe, which very soon provokes a semiflexed position leading eventually to fixed clawing. Palpation however reveals the true length of the second metatarsal and its lowered position, together with the consequent keratotic cornified skin under the head. The flexion or clawing of the second toe may become marked, and the displacement at the metatarsophalangeal joint fixed by a contracture of the extensor tendon, leading eventually to dorsal subluxation.

In the *third and fourth rays,* angulations at the metatarsophalangeal and interphalangeal joints are the consequence of local compression from the shoe, leading to camptodactyly or clinodactyly variable both in direction and suppleness.

Tendinous involvement is less significant in the young adult. With increasing age, contracture occurs, with bowstringing of the extensors under the dorsal skin of the forefoot. At a more advanced stage, there is also inverse action of the plantar interossei secondary to the displacements at the metatarsophalangeal and interphalangeal joints. The joints become irreducibly fixed.

The skin is affected predominantly on the plantar aspect, where a sometimes very extensive median rounded or oval callosity develops selectively under the second metatarsal head. A serous bursa sometimes forms, and can ulcerate or become infected. Digital corns appear dorsally and distally as a result of the clawing.

Metatarsalgia arises from overloading and is aggressive. At first it occurs only towards the end of the day, but the onset becomes increasingly early, and finally the pain is permanent. It is provoked by standing, walking and sport and is usually of a burning character with a sensation of tension, localised to the second metatarsal head region. Together with this pain from overloading, arthralgia occurs at the second cuneiform-metatarsal joint region, provoked by the hypermobility of the joint, which can be seen to enlarge. This pain is itself sometimes a presenting symptom.

Neuralgia results from compression of plantar nerves between the shoe upper and a hypertrophic cuneiform bone. The pain associated with a Deutschländer fatigue fracture of the second metatarsal has already been mentioned (Sect. 10.1.1).

Podoscopy reveals a loss of lateral balance of the foot. The peculiar form of the footprint shows overloading under the second metatarsal head. *Podometry* confirms the disturbance of pressure distribution.

Radiography: The metatarsal formula $1<2>3>4>5$ confirms the morphology of the loading zone of the metatarsal heads. Characteristic signs are the protrusion of the middle metatarsal heads, especially the second, and the latter's increase in volume and density with thickening of the diaphyseal cortex and diminution or obliteration of the medullary canal. The displacements at the metatarsophalangeal joints determine the degree of hallux valgus, metatarsus varus and quintus varus, together with any subluxations and clawing. There is abnormal widening of the first and fourth intercapital spaces, and examination of the position of the sesamoid bones of the first ray confirms their retropulsion. The degree of abnormality of the plane of the first cuneiform-metatarsal joint, described above, can be measured.

10.1.3 Treatment

Conservative. In the presence of a planovalgus foot and supple involvement of the metatarsophalangeal joints, an insole somprising an internal supporting dome and a supinating wedge under the heel, with a retrocapital pronating bar, may suffice to control the situation. If the planovalgus component is fairly well balanced, so that it is only the distal and basal metatarsalgias which trouble the patient, a monoblock insole is preferred.
If inflammatory features related to the central callosity become more frequent or if the symptoms are related more to the hallux valgus component and the angulation of the fifth ray, surgery is indicated.

Operative. The aim must be to correct all components of the disorder (Fig. 10.2). This may be achieved by:

- Correction of the hallux valgus
- Metatarsal head-shaft enclavement of the middle three rays, or basal osteotomies of the three central metatarsals, very carefully calculated, as described by Thys (1974b)
- When protrusion of the second metatarsal head is the predominant feature, a V-ostectomy
- Z-elongation of the long and short extensor tendons, completed by arthroplasties or arthrodeses of the interphalangeal joints

Operative treatment means that the patient must cease work for at least 2 months, but the results can be most gratifying and worthwhile.

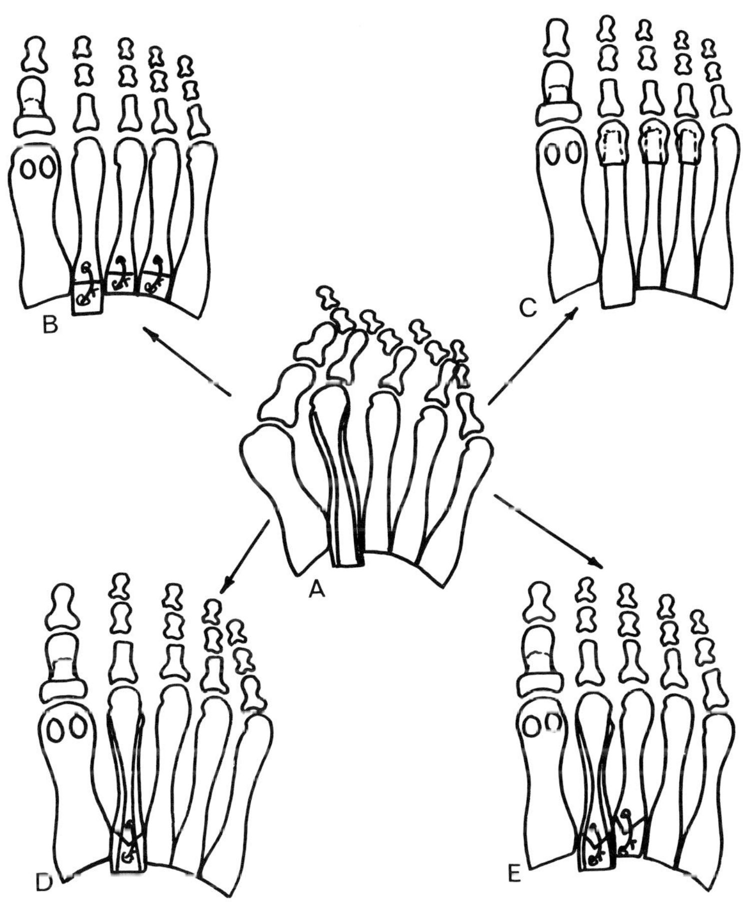

Fig. 10.2 A–E. Congenital convex forefoot of Duddley Morton in the adult. **A** Before treatment. **B** Mau or Thys-Martorell basal osteotomies in central three metatarsals, correction of first and fifth rays, realignment of metatarsal heads in frontal and horizontal planes by coaptation of osteotomies (Thys-Martorell). **C** Realignment by enclavement of central metatarsal heads, redistribution of loading, correction of digital displacements. **D, E** Overloading of second (or second and third) metatarsal head present: correction of digital displacements, basal V-osteotomy of second (or second and third) metatarsal

10.2 Congenital Short First Metatarsal

10.2.1 Etiology

Incompetence of the great ray is due to its shortness, which cannot be compensated by the normal plantar flexion during walking. The condition is progressive, resulting in selective overloading of the second metatarsal head, but in contrast with the familial forefoot of Duddley Morton, planovalgus is not a feature. The mechanism of pain, however, is analogous.

10.2.2 Clinical Presentation

On the plantar aspect, a zone of redness or whiteness is seen under the second metatarsal head at the onset of failure. Progressively, fixed deformities develop with tenderness and capsular contracture and the great toe deviates into valgus or develops clawing (Fig. 27.1 A–D).
Metatarsalgia is confined to overloading symptoms under the second metatarsal head, sometimes accompanied by neuralgic symptoms from the second space as described by Serre et al. (1972). Later, pain from displacement of the metatarsophalangeal joints generally increases and pressure signs from clawing of the toes complete the symptomatology.
Podoscopy and *podometry* confirm the overloading of the second metatarsal head. *Radiography* reveals the difference in length of the metatarsals and the diverse clinodactylies of the five rays (see Fig. 11.8 U).

10.2.3 Treatment

Conservative. A monoblock insole with a retrocapital bar controls the early phases of development. Callus formation and progressive displacement at the metatarsophalangeal joints which cannot be reduced are indications for surgery.

Operative. If the second metatarsal is predominantly overlong, simple correction is achieved by basal osteotomy to elevate the metatarsal, or by basal osteotomy-ostectomy according to Thys (1974b) or Mau (1940) to both elevate and shorten the bone (Fig. 10.3). Extensor tendon elongation, metatarsophalangeal arthrotomy, and arthroplasty or arthro-

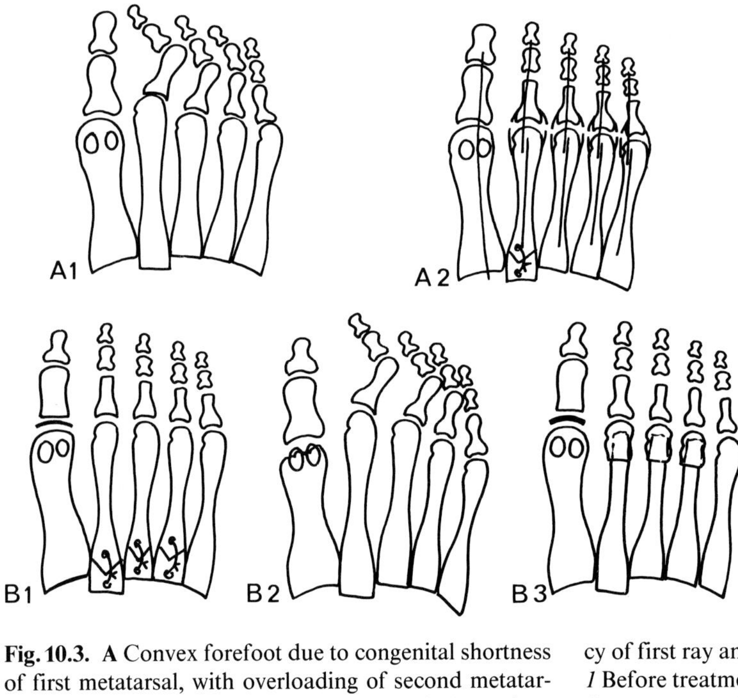

Fig. 10.3. A Convex forefoot due to congenital shortness of first metatarsal, with overloading of second metatarsal: *1* Before treatment; *2* after metatarsophalangeal arthrotomies, elongation of extensor tendons, V basal osteotomy of second metatarsal if indicated and metatarsophalangeal capsulotomies. **B** Convex forefoot due to iatrogenic shortening of first metatarsal, with insufficiency of first ray and overloading of outer metatarsal heads: *1* Before treatment; *2* after V basal osteotomies of central three metatarsals and metatarsophalangeal cup arthroplasty of first ray; *3* after realignment enclavement of central three metatarsal heads and metatarsophangeal cup arthroplasty of first ray (Regnauld)

desis of the interphalangeal joint may also be necessary. If the frontal protrusion affects all three central metatarsals, isolated treatment of the second ray risks provocation of overloading of the adjacent third and fourth metatarsal heads. In this circumstance, metatarsal head-shaft enclavement or the more critical trapezoidal ostectomy at the bases of the metatarsals (Thys 1974b) is the appropriate procedure. These operations aim to compensate for the shortness of the first metatarsal; an alternative approach is a lengthening operation for the primary shortness (Burutaran 1976).

10.3 Acquired Short First Metatarsal

This condition which is usually the result of a previous operative resection of the first metatarsal head, leads to incompetence of loading of the first ray and severe overloading of the second metatarsal head, with consequent toe deformities (cf. Fig. 25.1 A–H). In addition to the metatarsalgia of overloading, the remnant of the first metatarsophalangeal joint is frequently painful. The patient walks with the foot in slight supination and is unable to roll the forefoot normally.

Conservative treatment with an insole is usually ineffective if arthrosis of the first metatarsophalangeal joint remnant is significant.

Operative treatment aims at compensation by means of metatarsal head-shaft enclavement in the middle three rays or by basal osteotomies as described above.

An effort should be made to restore function at the great metatarsophalangeal joint. This may be achieved by excision of osteophytes and insertion of a cup prosthesis (Regnauld and Grassin 1975), or if the articular cartilage is preserved, an osteoarticular graft can be inserted.

10.4 Short Great Toe

In this condition, which is commonly associated with previous surgery to the great metatarsophalangeal joint, the toe becomes shortened and is fixed in dorsiflexion or even in an erect posture by capsular contracture and shortening of both extensor tendons. The toe loses its prehensile and rolling function during gait with consequent overloading of the middle metatarsal heads. A convex forefoot develops, with contracture and clawing of the lesser toes and painful callus formation.

Treatment comprises reconstitution of the great metatarsophalangeal joint by arthroplasty, using a cup prosthesis, a replacement prosthesis for the base of the phalanx, or a cutaneous interposition arthroplasty in the young adult (de Wulf 1978). Realignment metatarsal head-shaft enclavement may be necessary, or occasionally basal ostectomy. The contractures of the soft tissues must be relieved by appropriate tendinous elongations and the claw toes must be flattened by arthroplasties or arthrodeses.

10.5 Hypermobility of First Metatarsal

In contrast with the length and posture deficiencies affecting the first metatarsal, this syndrome relates to incompetence due to hypermobility at the Lisfranc joint line (Courriades 1971).

It is characterised by a metatarsal head formula of $1 \geqslant 2 \geqslant 3 > 4 > 5$, hypermobility of the first metatarsal with diminution of the angle of inclination with the ground during loading (normally 18°), separation between the first and second cuneiform-metatarsal joint lines, insufficiency of peroneus longus and lowering of the plantar longitudinal arch along its inner border amounting to a flat foot with an accompanying plantar displacement of the neck of the talus (Larichellière 1962). There is a consequent overloading syndrome of the second or middle metatarsal head.

10.5.1 Clinical Presentation

In the *forefoot*, the amplitude of vertical movement of the first metatarsal is considerably augmented during loading and on palpation. Crepitus may be palpable at the first and second cuneiform-metatarsophalangeal joints, and the elevated position of the condyle of the first metatarsal with respect to the second may be marked. Callus under the second metatarsal head or a more diffuse convexity affecting the central three metatarsals may be apparent. Occasionally, fatigue fracture of the second metatarsal occurs.

In the *midtarsal region*, palpation and manipulation of the first and second cuneiform-metatarsal joints may be painful due to primary involvement there, and the joints may be clinically arthrosic with swelling and osteophyte formation. Local pain at the site of insertion of peroneus longus may be detected.

Metatarsalgia arises from overloading of the second metatarsal head or of all three central metatarsal heads; the patient may also complain of arthralgic pain at the tarsometatarsal joint line, pain from peroneus longus tendinitis or general aching of a myalgic source due to lowering of the plantar arch.

Radiography. In the dorsoplantar view the gap between the first and second metatarsals and the absence of shortness of the first metatarsal are characteristic. Arthrosis in the first and second cuneiform-metatarsal joints may predominate. Occasionally, the callus from an old fatigue fracture of the second metatarsal may be apparent. In the lateral view under load, there is a noticeably reduced angle of declination of the first metatarsal (less than 15°) with plantar displacement of the midtarsus generally. An exostosis or osteophytes may be obvious on the dorsal aspect of the tarsometatarsal joint line.

10.5.3 Treatment

Conservative. The insole appropriate for this condition is of the monoblock type with a supporting internal dome and a retrocapital bar. If the pes planus component is marked, an insole with an internal supporting dome, a supinating wedge under the heel and a pronating wedge joined to the retrocapital bar may be more appropriate. The use of insoles is not usually acceptable to the young patient and may fail for this reason, and it will certainly be ineffective in the more advanced case with arthrosis of the tarsometatarsal joint line.

Operative. Courriades (1971) proposed arthrodesis of the cuneiform-metatarsal joints, but this, while at first sight logical, does not take into account the arthrosis which will have developed adjacently. For this reason, the author is strongly of the opinion that hypermobility of the first metatarsal should be treated selectively by basal semicircular osteotomy, thereby lowering its inclination, and that any planovalgus component, depending upon its severity and the age of the subject, should also be corrected. With progressing age and severity, arthrorisis of the subtalar joint, midtarsal extra-articular osteotomy or plastic shortening of the talocalcaneonavicular ligament may be indicated, possibly supplemented by transplantation of tibialis posterior more anteriorly or a tenodesis (Albanese 1948, cited by Niederecker 1959, pp. 186, 190) between tibialis anterior and tibialis posterior.
The author maintains that partial arthrodesis of a joint line like the Lisfranc will lead to distortion and subsequent progressive arthrosis in that part which has been left free. This is a general principle in foot surgery. If any doubt exists as to the advisability of surgery, it is wiser to limit treatment to use of an insole.

11 Selective Overloading of Metatarsal Heads

Selective overloading may be due to any one or a combination of a multitude of factors affecting each metatarsal head and it is important that the etiology should be understood in each individual case so that treatment can be planned accordingly. Arbitrary management without reference to the cause is likely to prove unsuccessful. Some overlap with conditions described in other chapters is inevitable but it is useful to consider this group of conditions together in the interests of complete understanding.

11.1 First Metatarsal

11.1.1 Congenital Hypertrophy

11.1.1.1 Etiology

The metatarsal formula is of the Egyptian type, and the increased length of the first ray is accompanied by pressure signs under the head and a progressive clinodactyly of the great toe, which goes into valgus, encouraging external angulation of the adjacent toes (Fig. 11.1). Frequently there is coexisting hallux rigidus, in which there is naturally a restricted range of movement. In this instance, a varus component in the alignment of the first metatarsal does not occur.

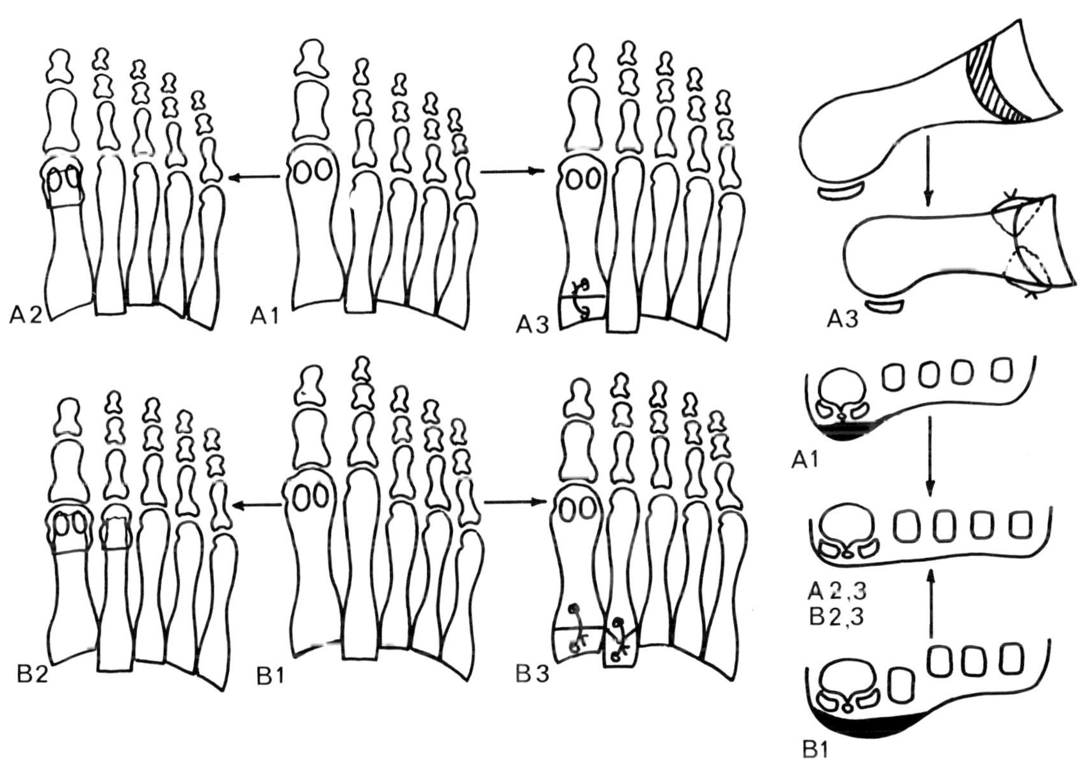

Fig. 11.1. A Congenital overloading of first metatarsal head: *1* Before treatment; *2* after metatarsal head-shaft enclavement (Regnauld); *3* after basal dome osteotomy and shortening of metatarsal (Regnauld). **B** Congenital overloading of first and second metatarsal heads: *1* Before treatment; *2* after metatarsal head-shaft enclavements; *3* after basal dome osteotomy of first metatarsal and Thys-Martorell osteotomy of second metatarsal

11.1.1.2 Clinical Presentation

There is metatarsalgia of selective overloading and pain in the metatarsophalangeal joint, especially in the presence of hallux rigidus and pressure symptoms from the shoe.
Radiography reveals the increased length of the first ray with respect to its neighbours and, in lateral view, the depression of the first head. The hallux valgus or hallux rigidus may be marked, according to the stage of the condition.

11.1.1.3 Treatment

Conservative management may be effective before the development of fixed deformity of irreversible damage of the weight-bearing or compressed soft tissues. A physiological monoblock insole with an internal dome and a retrocapital bar must be complemented in the presence of a varus component by a pronating external wedge, thereby re-establishing lateral balance of the foot.
Operative treatment may comprise most effectively a realignment first metatarsal head-shaft enclavement, or alternatively osteotomy of the first metatarsal base by the semicircular technique of Regnauld (1974). Correction of the digital clawing and hallux valgus may be necessary.

11.1.2 Acquired Equinus Deformity

11.1.2.1 Etiology

Selective equinus of the first metatarsal relates to shortness of the first ray. This may at first seem paradoxical but it appears in the majority of cases in a precavus foot with the metatarsal formula of the Greek type. The Greek forefoot provokes initially a lateral imbalance of the forefoot. Lateral balance is in part restored onto the median metatarsal heads by a supinating reflex action of the forefoot and by exaggeration of the longitudinal covus of the internal border. Later, a permanent plantarflexed posture of the great metatarsal is effected by hypertonia of peroneus longus and subsequent contracture of the plantar aponeurosis in an effort to bring the first metatarsal head into contact with the ground and maintain lateral balance. In a young subject, especially a girl wearing high heels, the condition may develop rapidly.

11.1.2.2 Clinical Presentation

The patient is often a girl of 12–18 years of age or a young rather heavy woman with a high heel who presents with painful swelling under the plantar region confined to the great metatarsal head and a longitudinal cavus foot of varying degree but remaining supple in the early phases (Fig. 11.2). The adolescent complains in most cases because of a serous bursa which inflames intermittently. The plantar skin overlying such a bursa is thickened, sometimes with a thin pastille-shaped cornified bed. The pain is characteristically of a burning, lancing or tense type, and is exaggerated by walking, standing and wearing of a high heel. At first it occurs only towards the end of the day, but the onset becomes progressively earlier.
The longitudinal cavus is most marked on the inner border of the foot, accentuated by the prominence of the metatarsal head, to which the patient may draw attention. Inspection reveals that the configuration under the outer four metatarsal heads is flat, but the plantar surface seems to inflate towards its medial margin. The degree of suppleness remaining in the precavus condition should be assessed carefully. The serous bursa, so characteristic, may be very tender. The sesamoid bones, which may be hypertrophic, augment the prominence of the medial ball of the foot. Varying degrees of inflammation or exceptionally suppuration may be present. The lateral equilibrium of the hindfoot may be disturbed, with a varus calcaneum which deteriorates progressively. A varus posture frequently remains supple in the young woman but becomes irreducible when the supinated attitude of the foot has become fixed over a long period, fixation perhaps occurring by the age of 40 years in those who have neglected their symptoms.
Radiography: The lateral view confirms the accentuated equinus of the first metatarsal and any accompanying hypertrophy of the sesamoids, the plantar face of which can be markedly pointed. The Müller view confirms the depressed position of the first metatarsal head.

11.1.2.2 Treatment

Choice of management relates very much to the age of the patient and the suppleness of the foot.

Conservative. In the adolescent, conservative management with an insole is essential and no surgery should be envisaged. Obviously, there must be judicious choice of footwear.

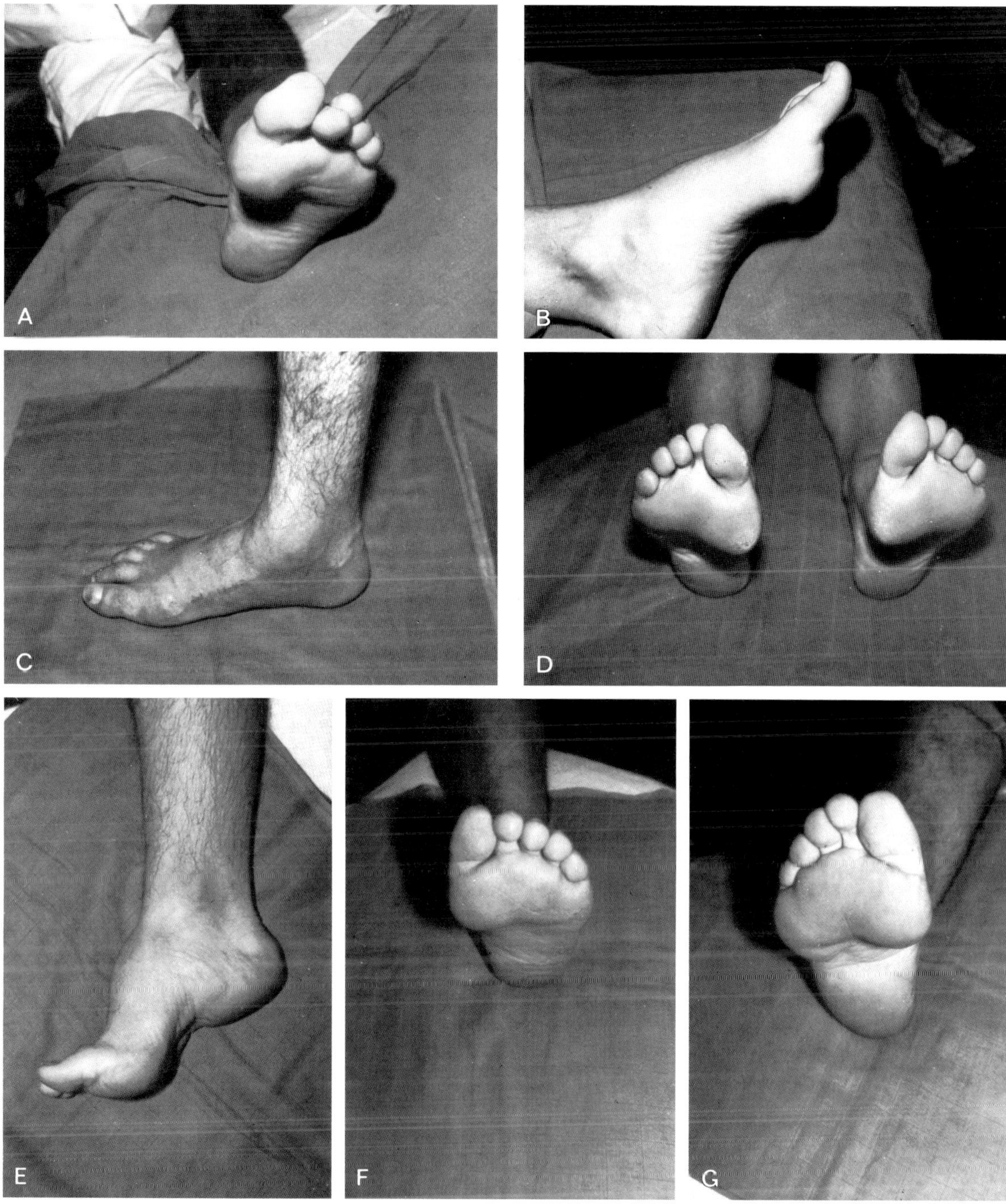

Fig. 11.2 A–G. Isolated equinus of first metatarsal. **A, B** Displacement of first metatarsal head. **C** Same foot as **A, B** after basal osteotomy of first metatarsal. **D, E** Equinus displacement of first metatarsal head. **F, G** Same foot as **D, E** after basal osteotomy of first metatarsal

Operative. In the young adult woman, operative treatment should be considered. Before corrective osteotomy is performed, it is necessary to verify the balance of the hindfoot. A supple varus posture of the calcaneum can be reduced by the use of a pronating wedge in an insole under the heel. Accompanied by basal semicircular osteotomy (Regnauld 1974) of the first metatarsal, this will afford stable and permanent correction (Fig. 11.3). However, when the equinus of the first metatarsal is accompanied by a fixed, supinated calcaneum, basal osteotomy of the first metatarsal must be supplemented by transcalcaneal osteotomy (Dwyer 1959) with elongation of tibialis anterior and tibialis posterior, thereby restoring the general equilibrium of the foot. The osteotomy of the base of the first metatarsal must correct the equinus without including any shortening of the metatarsal. For this reason, a wedge resection should be avoided and the semicircular technique used. Precise realignment can be achieved.

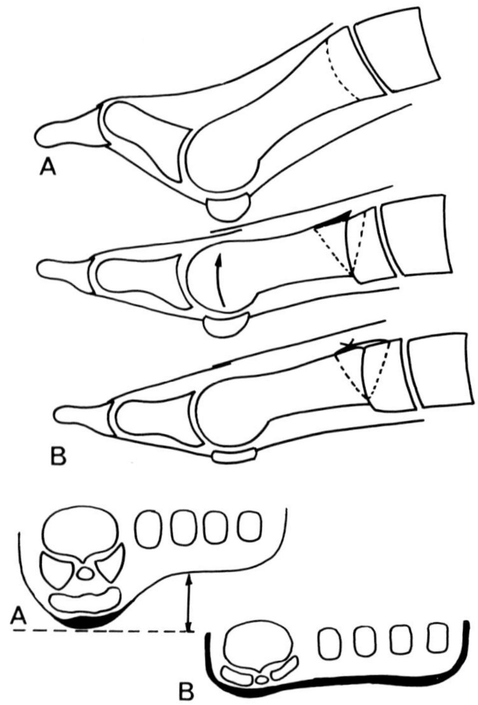

Fig. 11.3 A, B. Overloading of first metatarsal head due to equinus and hypertrophy of sesamoids. **A** Before treatment. **B** After basal dome osteotomy and trimming of sesamoids (Regnauld)

11.1.3 Hypertrophy of Sesamoids

11.1.3.1 Etiology

Increased size of the sesamoid bones from any cause will produce overloading of the medial side of the ball of the foot. It may augment abnormalities of the metatarsals or be the primary cause; thus there may be an equinus posture of the metatarsal or a normal posture. Sometimes there is a past history of trauma or a sesamoiditis during adolescence. The sesamoid may become pointed (Fig. 11.4) losing its normal rounded surface and bearing a longitudinally disposed crest.

11.1.3.2 Clinical Presentation

Whatever the cause, there is evidence of overloading with callus formation and tenderness impeding normal rolling action during walking. Bursitis may be obvious.

Podoscopic examination reveals an antalgic supinated posture, the varus component being fully correctable.

Radiography: The horizontal views of Chevrot (1981), Chaigneau (1981) and Blondin-Walter (1949) clearly demonstrate the accumination and the longitudinal groove.

11.1.3.3 Treatment

Conservative. An insole is usually effective provided a correct pattern is fitted. For the balanced foot, a physiological monoblock type should incorporate a retrocapital bar and an internal dome of the same height as the medial longitudinal arch. A Martorell antecapital supporting bar may help further. In the presence of pes cavus, the insole for the young person should incorporate a retrocapital support, and an extended pronating wedge; for the older person with loss of suppleness, an internal dome, slightly less than the height of the internal longitudinal arch, together with retrocapital and antecapital supports, are necessary.

Operative. Failure of the insole is an indication for surgical treatment, but excision should be avoided except for partial ablation in the case of old fracture or bipartitism (Figs. 11.5, 11.6). Flattening of the prominent surface suffices, perhaps accompanied by elevation of an equinus metatarsal by curvilinear basal osteotomy (Regnauld 1974) (see Chap. 13).

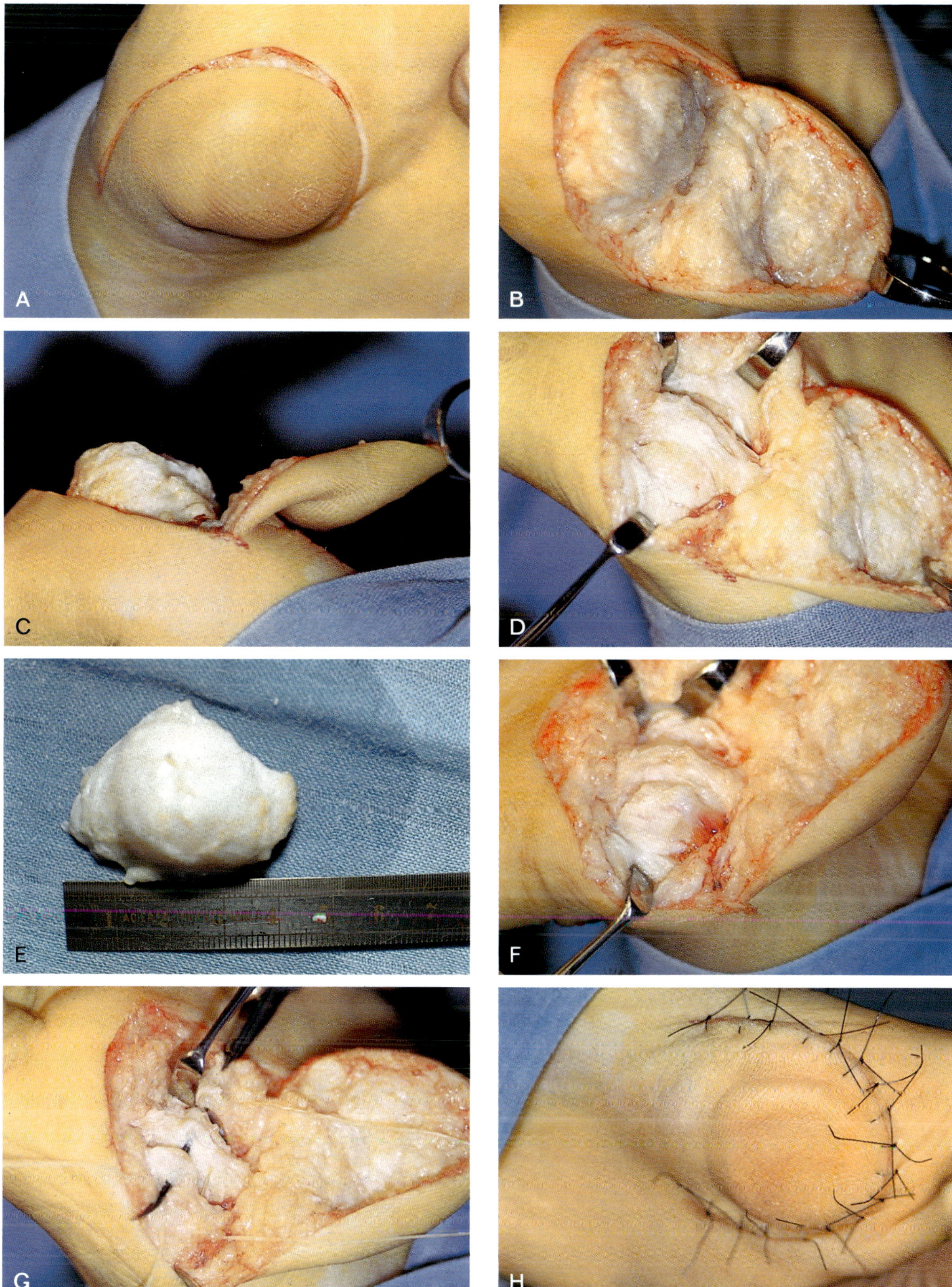

Fig. 11.4 A–K. Treatment of sesamoid hypertrophy. **A** Sesamoid hypertrophy with plantar serous bursa formation. Horseshoe-shaped incision skirting load-bearing area. **B** Reflection of cutaneous layer. **C** Serous bursa. **D** Excision of serous bursa and detachment of periosteum from plantar aspect of the two sesamoids. **E** Serous bursa. **F** Flattening of sesamoids. **G** Essential repair of capsuloperiosteum. **H** Skin suture. **I–K** see p. 80

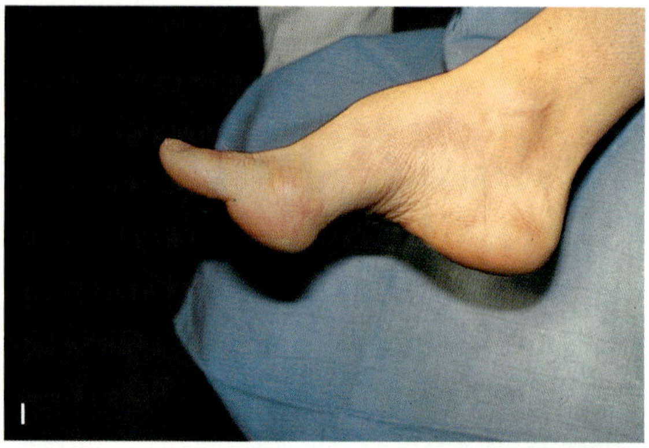

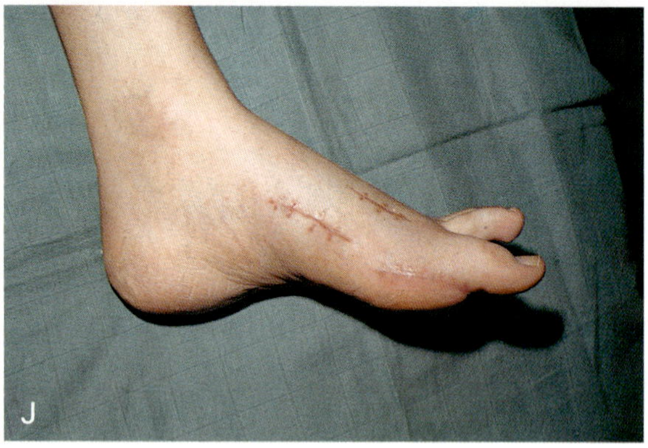

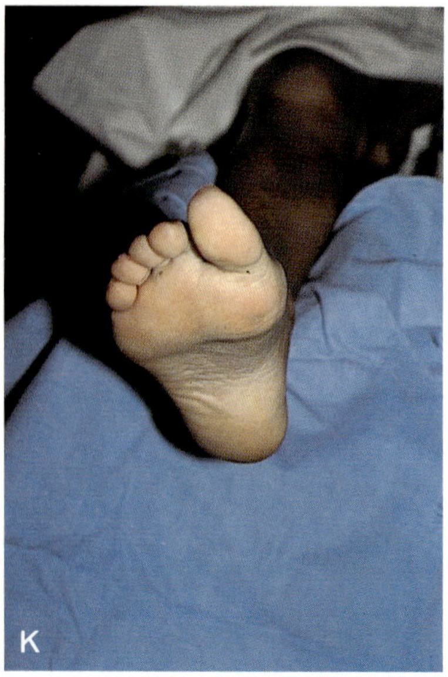

Fig. 11.4 *(continued)*. **I** Serous bursa in plantar region under sesamoids with isolated equinus of first metatarsal. **J** Postoperative result after semicircular basal osteotomy of first metatarsal, excision of serous bursa and elongation of extensor hallucis longus. **K** Correction of load bearing achieved in forefoot

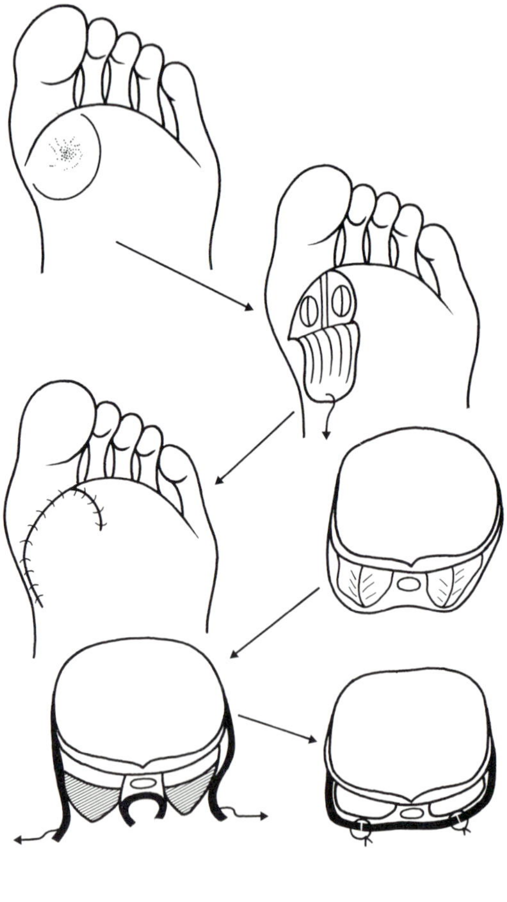

◁ **Fig. 11.5.** Overloading of first metatarsal head due to sesamoid hypertrophy: stages in trimming of sesamoids (Regnauld)

11.1.4 Iatrogenic Conditions

Resection of the three middle metatarsal heads leads to overloading of the remaining heads or perhaps a cavus forefoot syndrome (Fig. 11.7) (see Chap. 9.3).

Almost inevitably, clawing of the related toe develops due to absence of proper support, and secondary clinodactylies of the first and fifth rays will occur. These transverse deviations may become gross, amounting to 80° for the great toe and 50° for the fifth toe. Painful scarring of the central metatarsophalangeal joints or the residual pseudarthroses are common, and deformities are quickly fixed by contractures of the soft tissue, tendons, capsules and skin.

Treatment. Conservative management may be indicated in the older patient, but in the younger subject it is worthwhile considering efforts to restore the situation surgically. Hallux valgus and angulation of the fifth toe must be dealt with, and digital clawing and tendinous contractures must be corrected by appropriate releases and perhaps arthrodeses, but the crux of correction is restoration of load bearing to the amputated metatarsal heads. This may be achieved by an appropriate head-shaft enclavement or by introduction of a homograft; occasionally, three metatarsal head prostheses have been inserted. Some compensatory improvement can be achieved by shortening and realignment enclavement of the first and fifth metatarsals. It is possible to insert cup prostheses onto the stumps of the middle metatarsals and secure some mechanical stability. No two cases are the same.

11.2 Congenital Hypertrophy of First and Second Metatarsals

This condition results in a special metatarsal formula: 1=2>3>4>5. Congenital overlength of the first and second metatarsals produces change comparable to that of the isolated first metatarsal condition described above (Sect. 11.1.1) except that the callus or serous bursa of overloading is shifted somewhat and, as is so often the case, the somewhat greater length of the second toe leads to compression from the upper of the shoe and early claw formation. Either metatarsal head can be the primary source of metatarsalgia due to pressure, recurrent inflammation, or arthrosis.

Treatment is similar to that of the isolated first metatarsal hypertrophy except that the second ray must also be treated, most probably with basal osteotomy as described by Mau or Thys. Digital clawing may be more marked.

11.3 Second, Third, and Fourth Metatarsals

11.3.1 Etiology

Overloading of the central metatarsals alone may be due to congenital overlength, or may be acquired, either as an isolated phenomenon or consecutive to longitudinal displacement in a cavovalgus or planovalgus foot. In the latter instances, it most often affects the second metatarsal, less often the third or fourth. Conversely, in a varus foot it is the fourth head or more rarely the third which is involved. In a cavus foot the second, third and fourth heads are affected with equal frequency.

Overloading can also arise from fracture of a diaphyseal shaft which has been badly reduced in plantarflexion or from fracture near the base of the condyle itself. Depending on the cause, this condition may appear at any time between the ages of 30 and 50 years, with equal frequency in men and women.

The association of localised metatarsalgia affecting the third or fourth rays with very slight lateral displacement into valgus or varus of the tarsus is significant, for the use of an insole which re-establishes equilibrium of the tarsus can frequently suppress the metatarsalgia (Pisani 1975 a, b). Thus, in the planovalgus foot, the cavovalgus foot, or simple valgus of the calcaneum, overloading under the second or third metatarsal heads is explained by the lowering of the plantar concavity longitudinally and transversely which results from calcaneal pronation. The lowering of the longitudinal arch leads to augmentation of the frontal convexity of the Lisfranc joint line and, by way of consequence, advancement of the second and third cuneiforms and relative elongation (due to metatarsal lowering) of the second and third metatarsals. In the cavus balanced foot, this may advance further to the development of a convex forefoot syndrome, whereas in the cavus foot with a varus tendency, the midtarsal distortion seems to reflect mostly onto the fourth metatarsal, which becomes selectively depressed. This may extend with time to affect the fifth metatarsal head. In the precavus and cavus foot, the excessive loading of the forefoot is more externally orientated, but again predominantly the fourth metatarsal head is affected. The coexistence of varus, however slight, accentuates the phenomenon. Certainly, osteotomies for elective equinus of metatarsals have been most frequently conducted on the fourth ray.

The possibility of overloading due to malunion of fractures is obvious.

11.3.2 Clinical Presentation

The patient presents with pain confined to a precise area in the forefoot, occasionally with features of neuralgia. The projection of the metatarsal head may be obvious, and there may be associated claw ing of the corresponding toe.

The typical burning, tension type of metatarsalgia from overloading comes on progressively earlier in the day and is aggravated by standing or walking, whereas Morton neuralgia in one of the intercapital spaces has more of a lancing, electric shock character due to compression of the digital nerve. As always, it is important to distinguish between the types of pain and not, for example, treat a neuralgia by isolated attention to the digital nerve. It is the depression of the metatarsal head which is important.

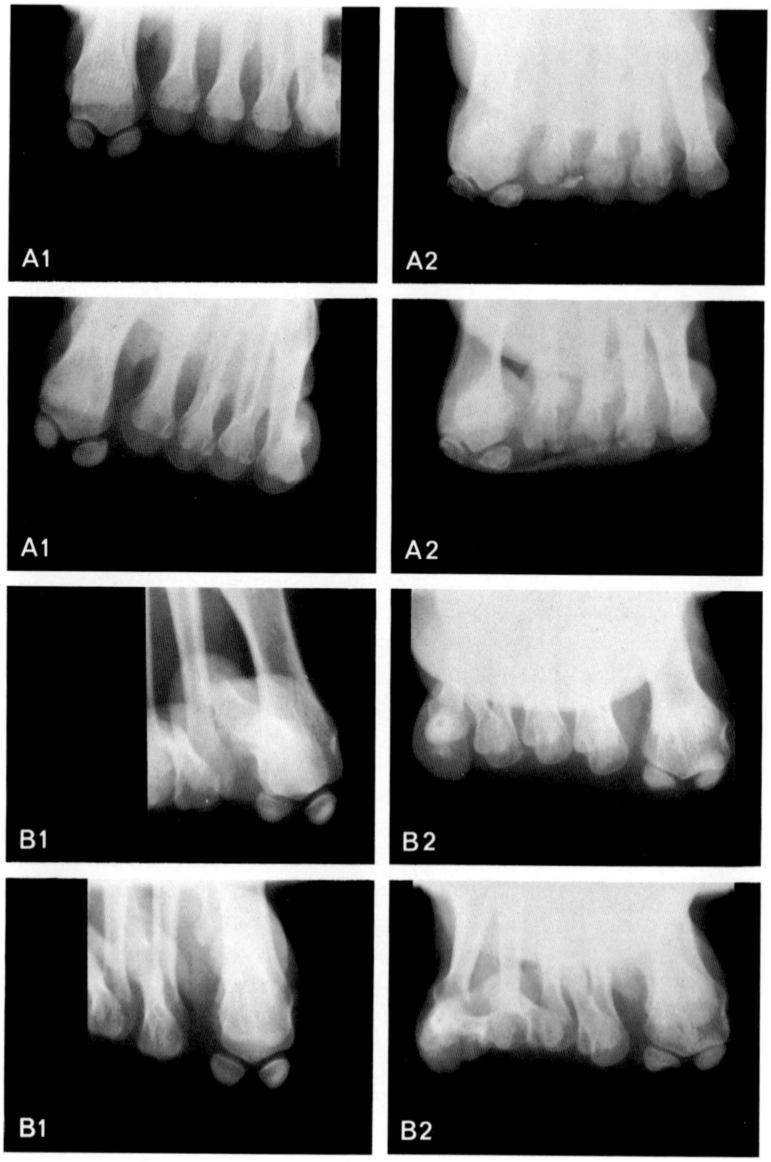

Fig. 11.6 A–D. Isolated equinus of first metatarsal: correction by curvilinear basal osteotomy and flattening of sesamoids. **A** *1* Preoperative appearance: prominent head of first metatarsal; *2* postoperative appearance after flattening of sesamoids. **B** *1* Preoperative appearance: equinus of first metatarsal, prominent metatarsosesamoid joint, sesamoid crest; *2* postoperative appearance after flattening of sesamoids; *3* left foot: isolated equinus of first metatarsal, plantar prominence of sesamoids; ▷ *4* right foot: isolated equinus of first metatarsal, prominent sesamoids; *5* left foot: basal curvilinear osteotomy of first metatarsal, flattening of sesamoids. *6* Right foot: basal curvilinear osteotomy of first metatarsal, flattenting of sesamoids. *7, 8* Both feet: dorsoplantar views after osteotomy at base of first metatarsal. *8* Right foot: Same. **B** *3–8*–**D** see pp. 83–86

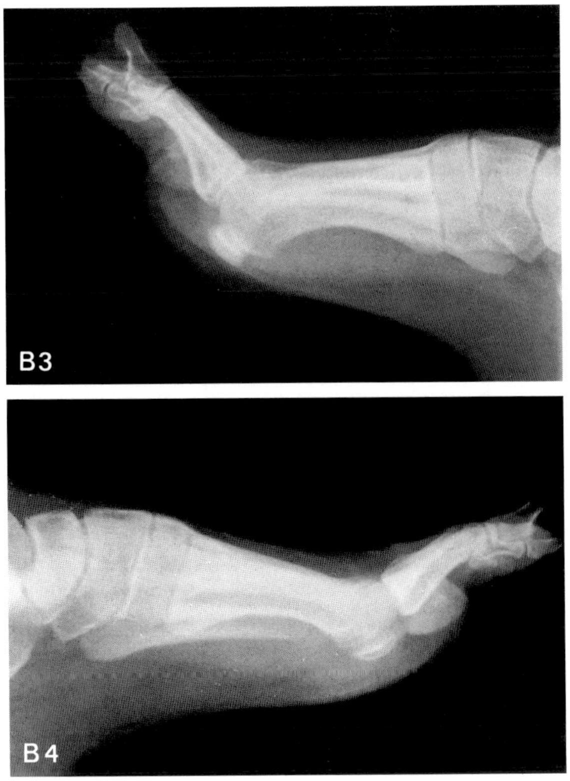

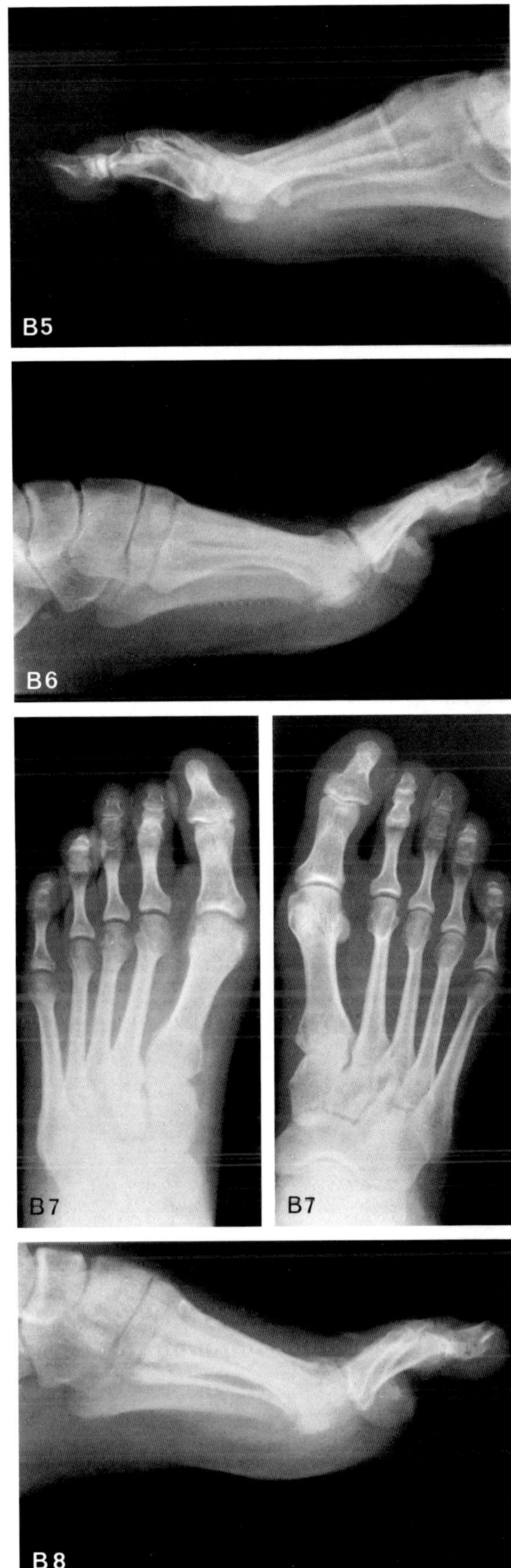

Fig. 11.6 B *3–8.* Legend see p. 82

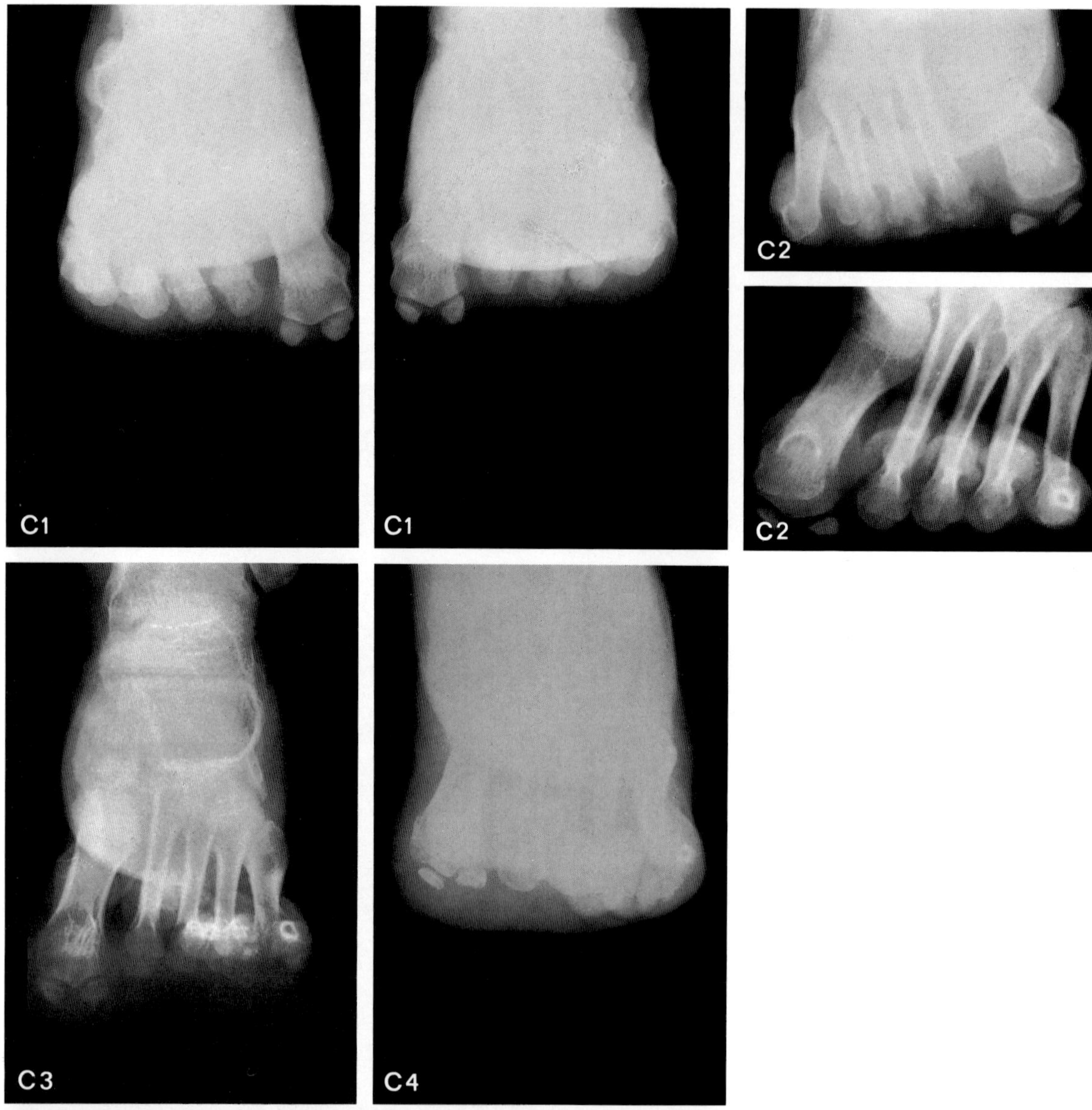

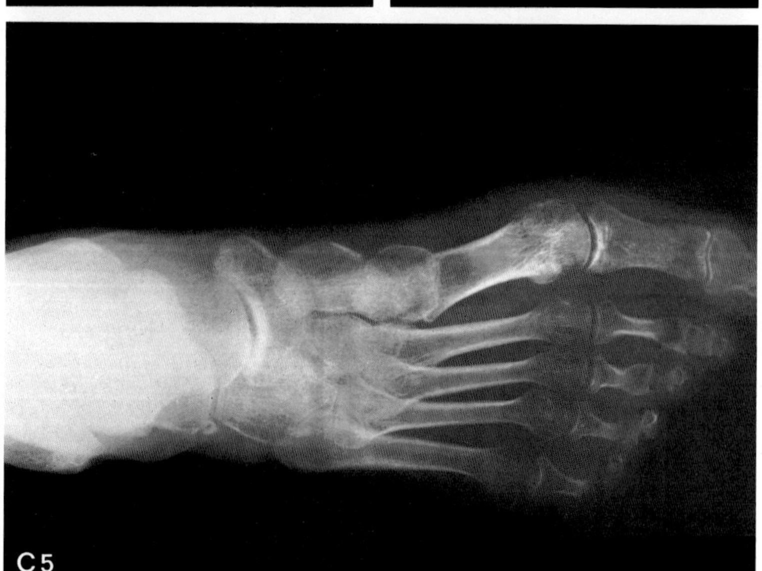

Fig. 11.6 C *1–5*. Legend see p. 85

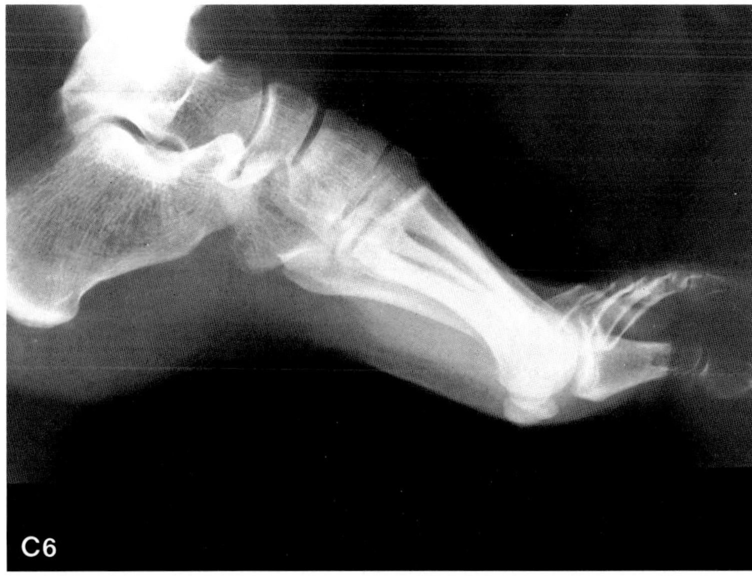

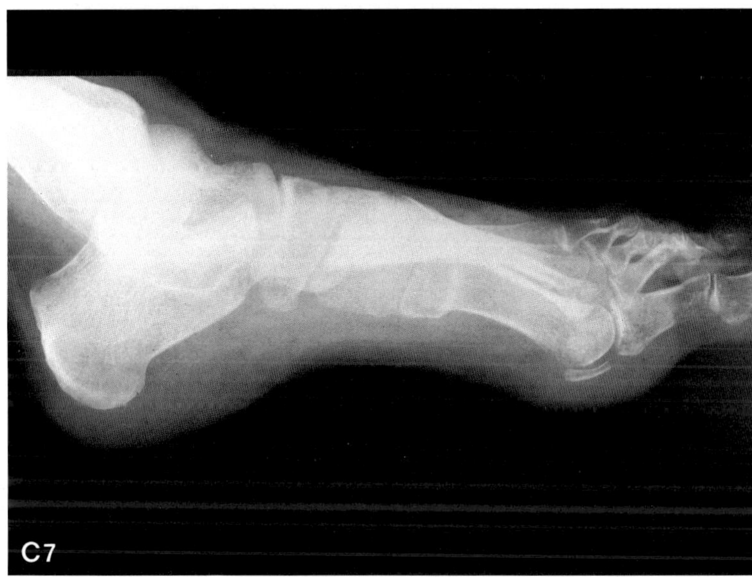

◁ **Fig. 11.6** *(continued).* **C** *1* Right and left foot, preoperative appearance: isolated equinus of first metatarsal, prominent sesamoids. *2* Right and left foot: basal curvilinear osteotomy of first metatarsal, flattening of sesamoids. *3* Correction of equinus of first metatarsal, flattening of sesamoids. *4* Isolated equinus of first metatarsal. *5* Dorsoplantar view after osteotomy at base of first metatarsal.

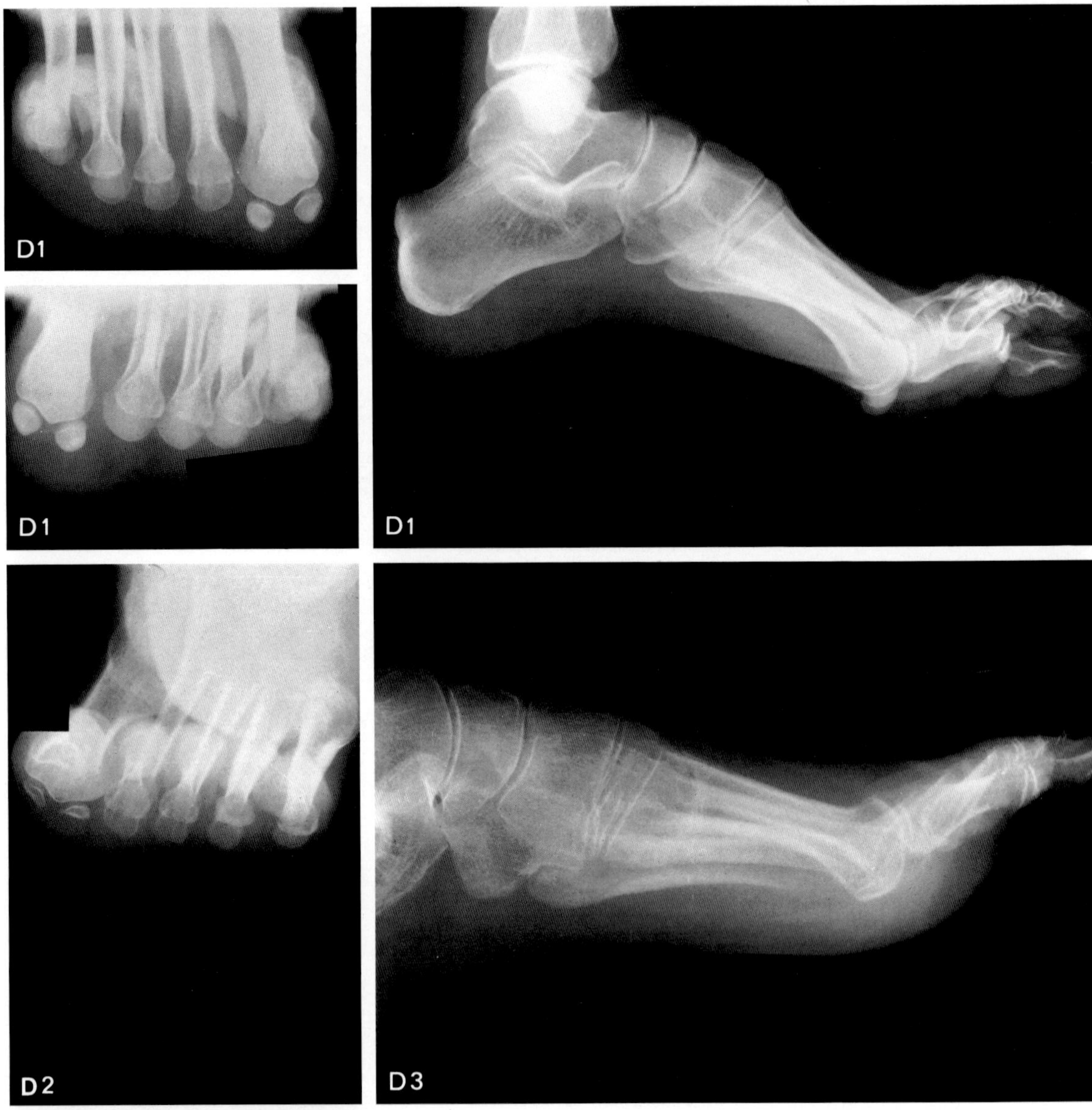

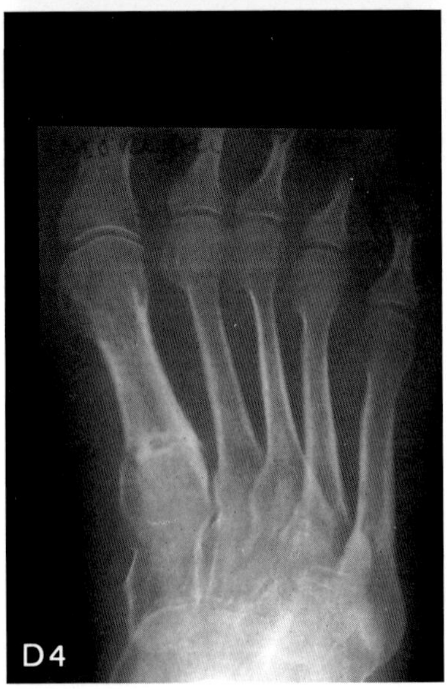

Fig. 11.6 *(continued).* **D** *1* Isolated equinus of first metatarsal, plantar prominence of sesamoids; *2* postoperative appearance after flattening of sesamoids; *3* lateral view after curvilinear basal osteotomy of first metatarsal, flattening of sesamoids; *4* dorsoplantar view following basal osteotomy of first metatarsal

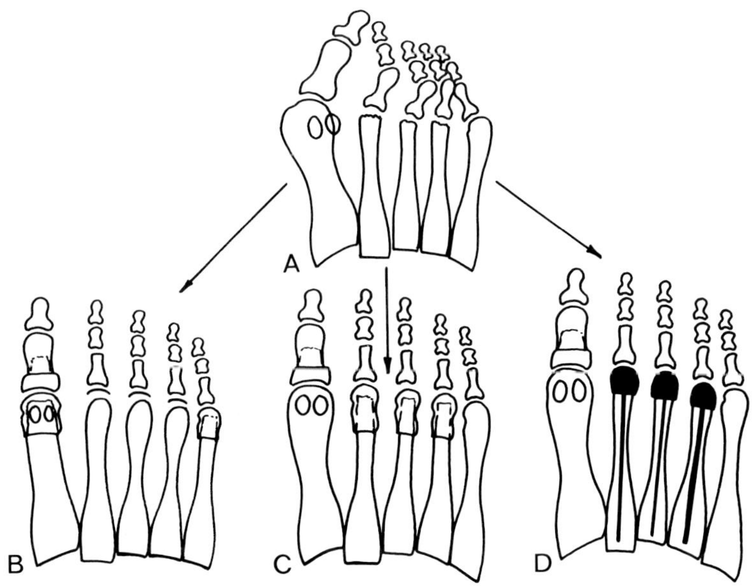

Fig. 11.7 A–D. Overloading of first and fifth metatarsal heads resulting from operative failure (resection of metatarsal heads). **A** Before reoperation. **B** After correction of hallux valgus and claw toes, enclavement of first and fifth metatarsal heads and metatarsophalangeal cup arthroplasties in central three rays. **C** After correction of hallux valgus and claw toes and enclavement of metatarsal heads using homografts. **D** After correction of hallux valgus and claw toes and implantation of head prostheses in central three metatarsals

Inspection of the foot confirms the isolated depression of the metatarsal, under which there may be a comma-shaped keratoma related to callus. A degree of frontal protrusion may be obvious. The associated clawing of the toe is accompanied by tendinous contracture. *Podology* and *podometry* confirm the clinical findings and overloading.
Radiography: The dorsoplantar, oblique and Walter views do not always show the isolated equinus of the metatarsal clearly unless it relates to a traumatic lesion (Fig. 11.8). The Cherrot or Chaigneau tangential view affords a better display of the equinus. The anteroposterior view plainly shows the frontal protrusion of the metatarsal head.

11.3.3 Treatment

Conservative. Management using an insole may be permanently successful. A monoblock physiological insole under the retrocapital area is appropriate for the balanced precavus forefoot, with a subcapital elevating pad appropriate to the neighbouring metatarsal heads. If there is a cavovarus of the foot, an insole with a retrocapital bar associated with a pronating external wedge at the forefoot is appropriate, whereas in cavovalgus a supinating wedge under the heel is indicated. For a planovalgus foot, a pronating wedge anterolaterally and a supinating wedge under the heel should be complemented if necessary by an internal supporting dome in the patient aged 50 years or over who will not tolerate a more dynamic type of orthosis.

Operative. Surgery is indicated for the young subject who rejects the use of insoles or the younger adult who wishes to indulge in sport or wear safety shoes at work. The choice of operation depends upon the exact etiology.
In congenital localised hypertrophy of length, head-shaft enclavement of the metatarsal restores regularity of loading (Fig. 11.9). There is never any indication for amputation of a metatarsal head. The basal osteotomy of Thys (1974) can correct the equinus, but if there is overcorrection, a syndrome of insufficiency will be produced (Fig. 11.10). In some instances this basal osteotomy can be combined very effectively with head-shaft enclavement, especially in the case of an irreducible fixed clinodactyly due to capsular contracture at the metatarsophalangeal and interphalangeal joints (Fig. 11.10). Appropriate lengthening of the long tendons and capsulotomy are essential. An isolated overloading syndrome due to a malunited fracture may be treated directly by osteotomy and fixation with an axial screw in the case of the neck of the metatarsal (see Chap. 22), or by compensatory basal V-osteotomy in the case of a diaphyseal fracture.

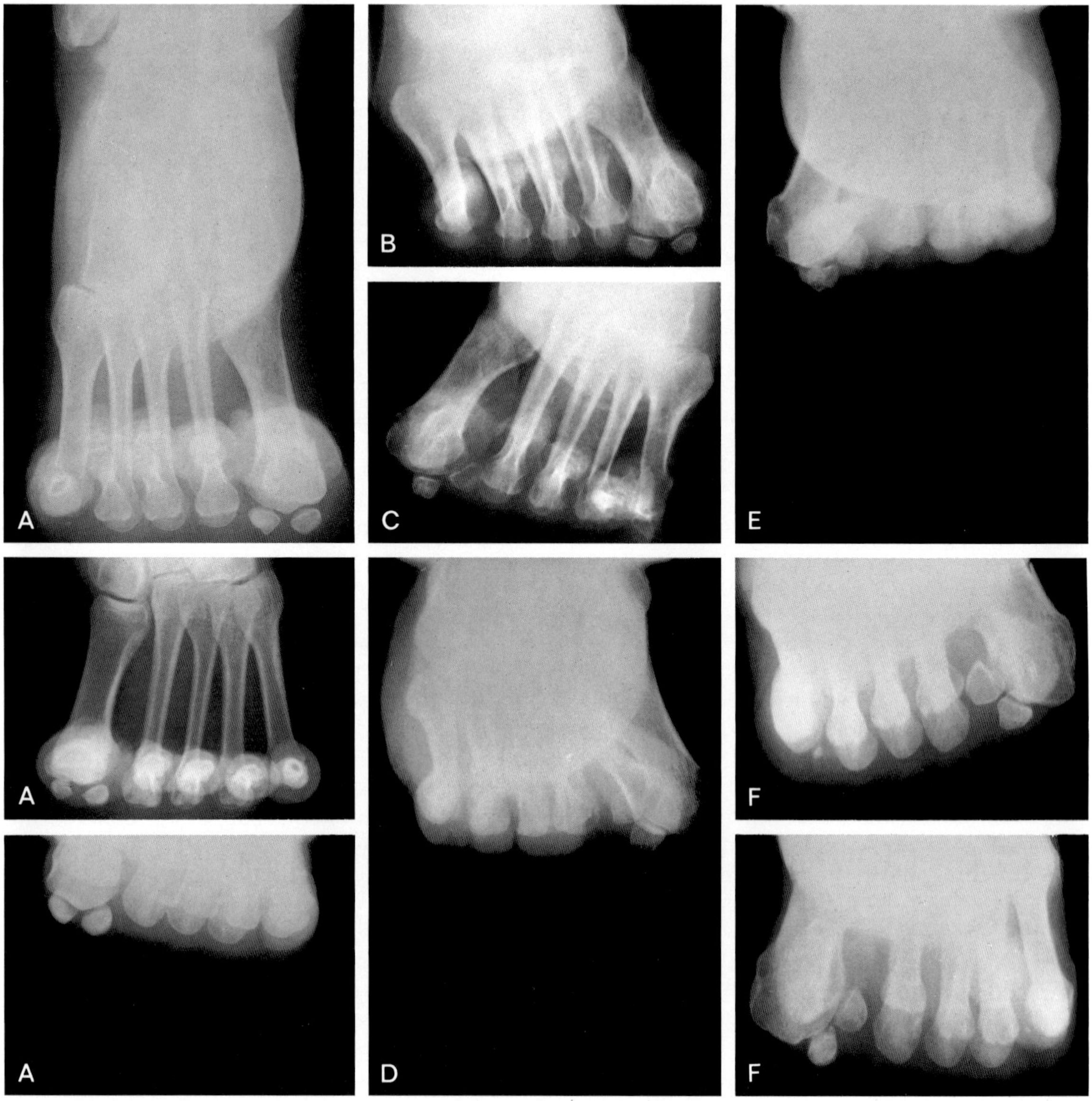

Fig. 11.8. **A** Normal forefoot. **B** Onset of sesamoid subluxation. **C** Lateral subluxation of sesamoids. **D** Third-degree hallux valgus lateral subluxation of sesamoids into first intercapital space. **E** Second-degree hallux valgus, dislocation of outer sesamoid into first intercapital space, subluxation of medial sesamoid. **F** Lateral dislocation of both sesamoids. **G** Underloading of second metatarsal head, overloading of third and fourth metatarsal heads. **H** Overloading of fourth metatarsal head due to isolated equinus of fourth metatarsal. **I** Brachydactyly of first metatarsal, congenital convex forefoot, frontal protrusion and equinus of three central metatarsals. **J** Overloading of medial sesamoid. **K** Congenital macropodia due to involvement of second and third metatarsals. **L** Acumination of plantar aspect of sesamoids. **M** Lateral sesamoid dystrophy. **N** Convex triangular forefoot. **O** Isolated equinus of first metatarsal leading to overloading of first metatarsal head. **P** Simple convex forefoot. **Q** Overloading of second and third metatarsal heads. **G–U** see pp. 89, 90

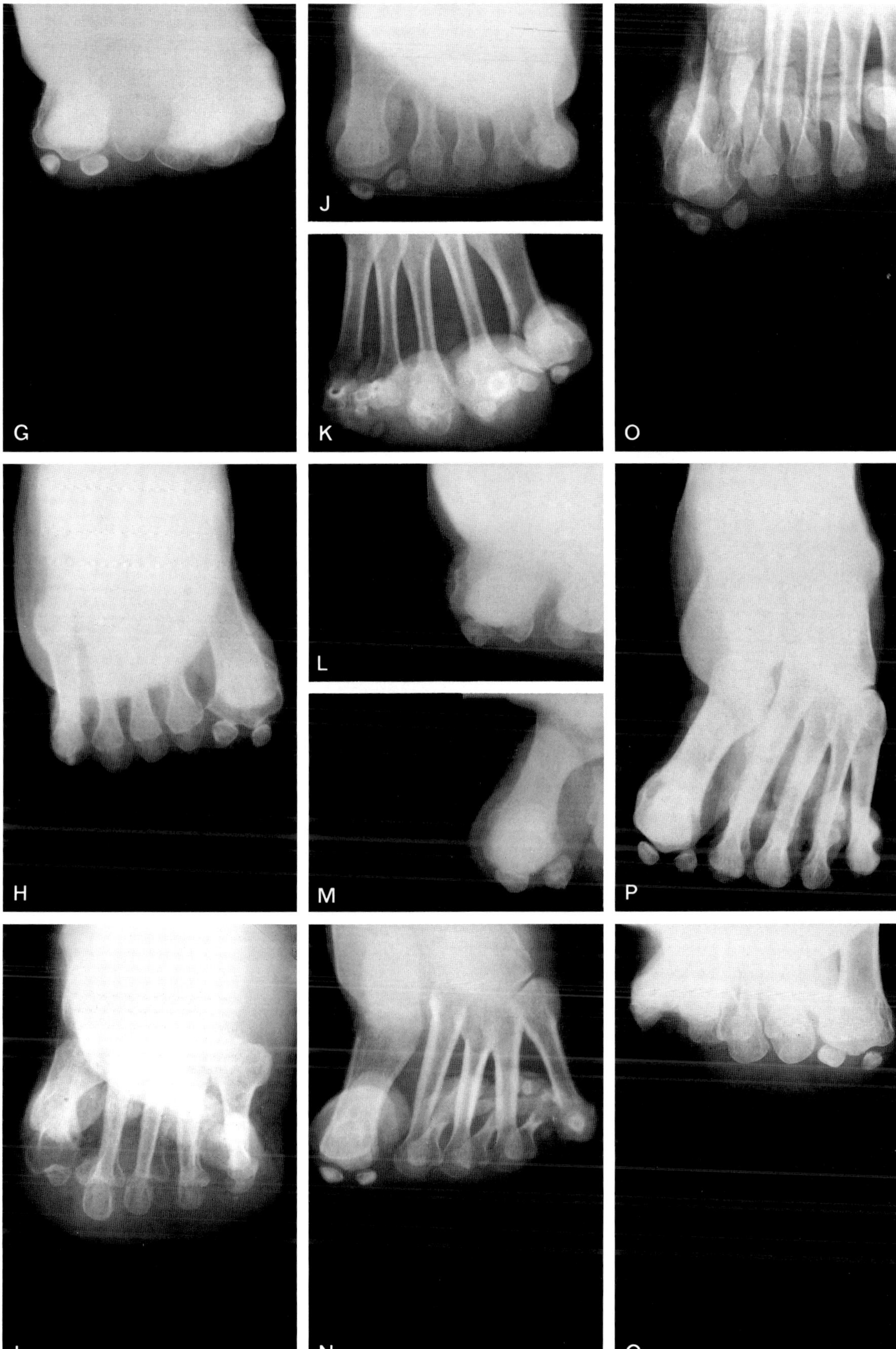
G
J
K
O
H
L
M
P
I
N
Q

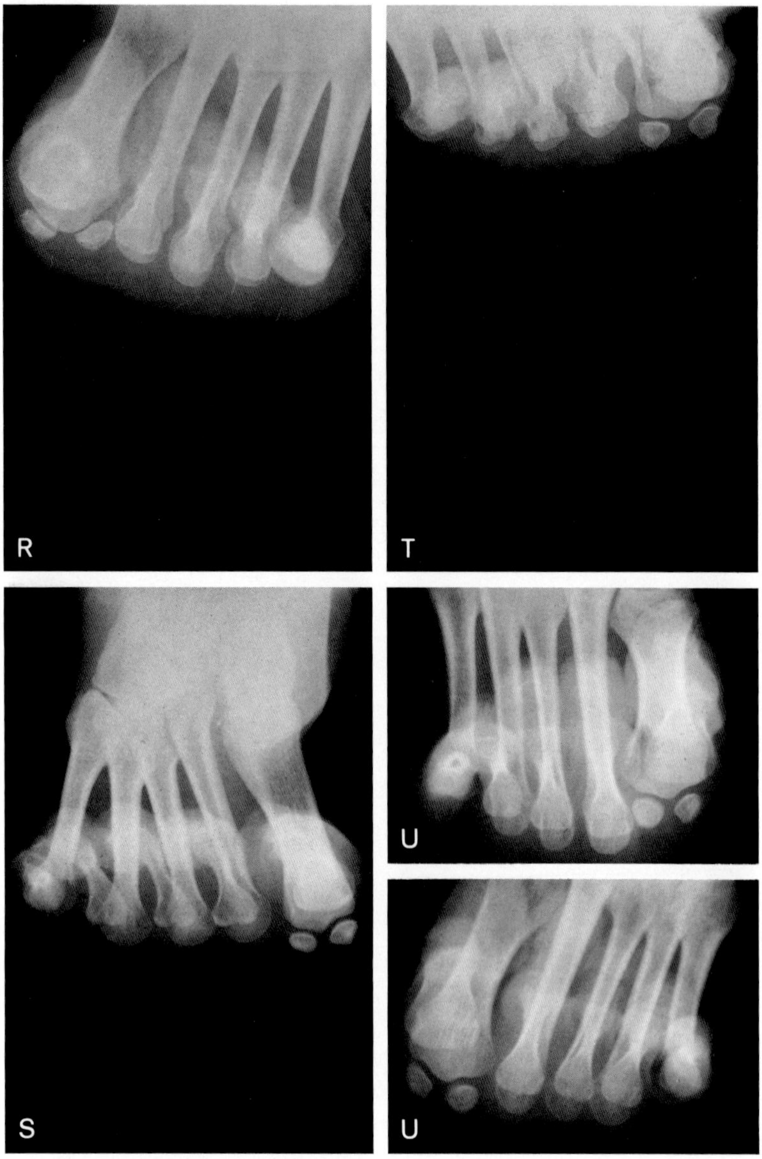

Fig. 11.8 *(continued)*. **R** Overloading of third metatarsal. **S** Overloading of fourth metatarsal head due to isolated equinus. **T** Overloading of third and fourth metatarsal heads. **U** Congenital shortness of first metatarsals. Overloading of central metatarsal heads

Fig. 11.9 A–I see pp. 92–94

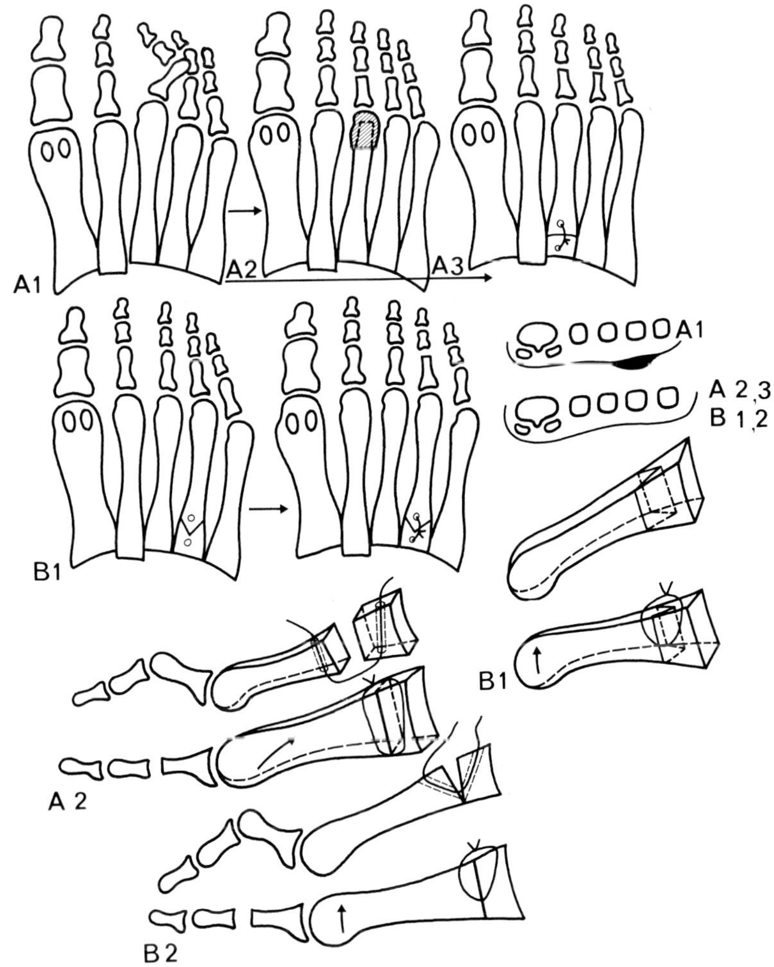

Fig. 11.10. A Overloading of a metatarsal head due to protrusion or excessive length of metatarsal: *1* Before treatment; *2* after realignment head-shaft enclavement; *3* after Thys-Martorell basal osteotomy. **B** Overloading of a metatarsal due to isolated equinus is treated by V-osteotomy *(1)* or Thys-Martorell *(2)* basal osteotomy

A diaphyseal fracture correction treated locally can be fixed with a Müller plate. In all instances digital clawing must be corrected by interphalangeal arthrodesis, and punctiform keratoma formation may indicate local excision here. Usually a callus without keratoma resolves after the cause of overloading has been removed. It should be obvious that overloading relates to protrusion, equinus or both and that the corrective procedure must be selected accordingly.

11.4 Fifth Metatarsal

Isolated overloading of the fifth metatarsal head is infrequent because of the relatively protected position it occupies behind the fourth metatarsal head. A primary syndrome of overloading does exist, but it must be clearly distinguished from much commoner iatrogenic causes (see Chap. 9). Broadly, it occurs when reduced vertical mobility of the fifth metatarsal is accompanied by some lateral imbalance, as seen in the cavovarus foot. Alternatively, in a rigid contracted foot of any origin associated with pes planus, longitudinal cavus, various arthritic conditions, or in polyneuritis, subcutaneous tissue atrophy is seen. Abnormal hypertrophy of the plantar aspect of the condyle can occur if it is subjected to compression and rubbing by the shoe due to lateral hypermobility or valgus of the metatarsal shaft.

The condition is divided below into four basic etiological types, but these have certain clinical features in common. There is overloading metatarsalgia under the fifth metatarsal head, accompanied only rarely by serous bursitis but often by a sensitive, whitish, localised thick callus or keratoma.

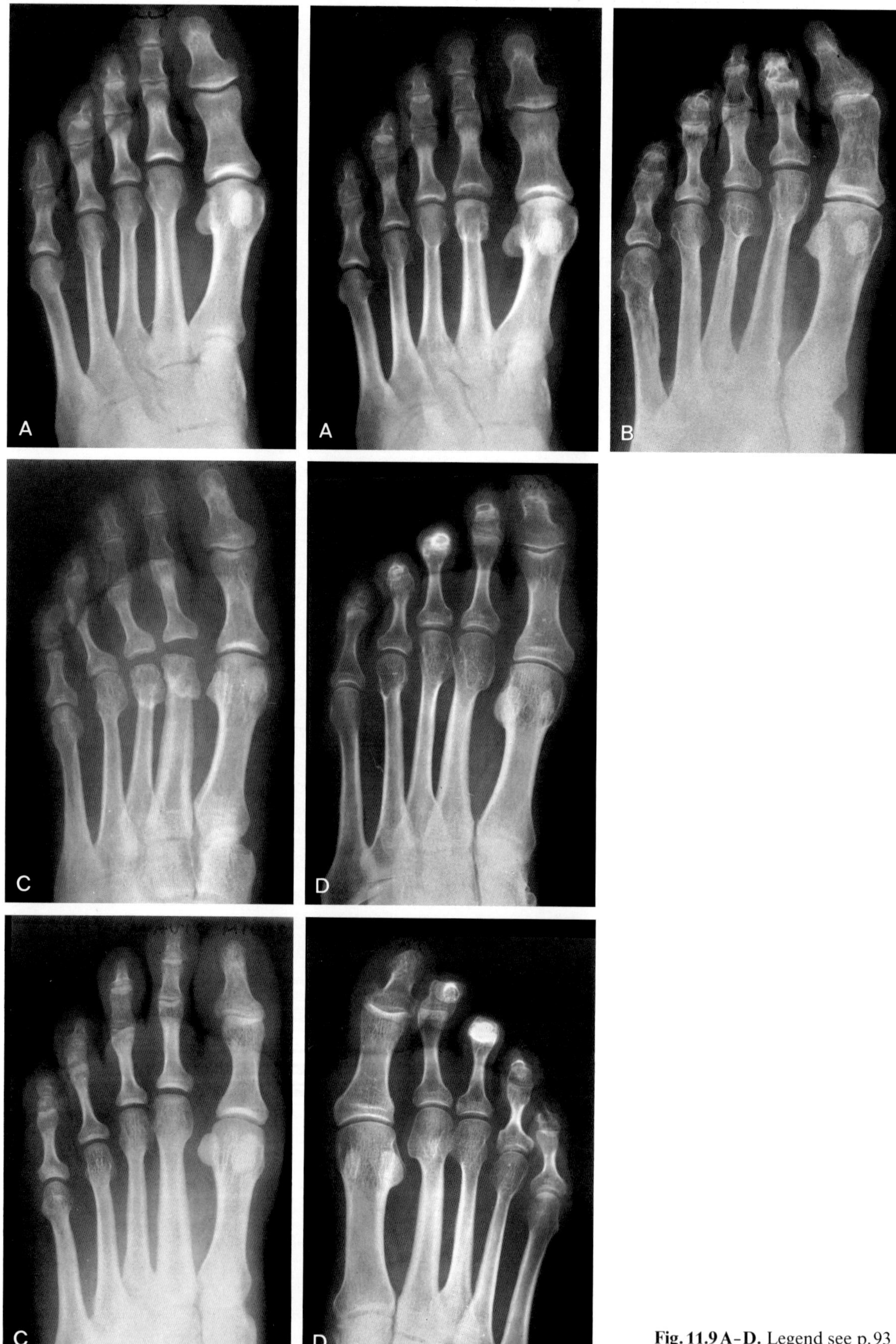

Fig. 11.9 A–D. Legend see p. 93

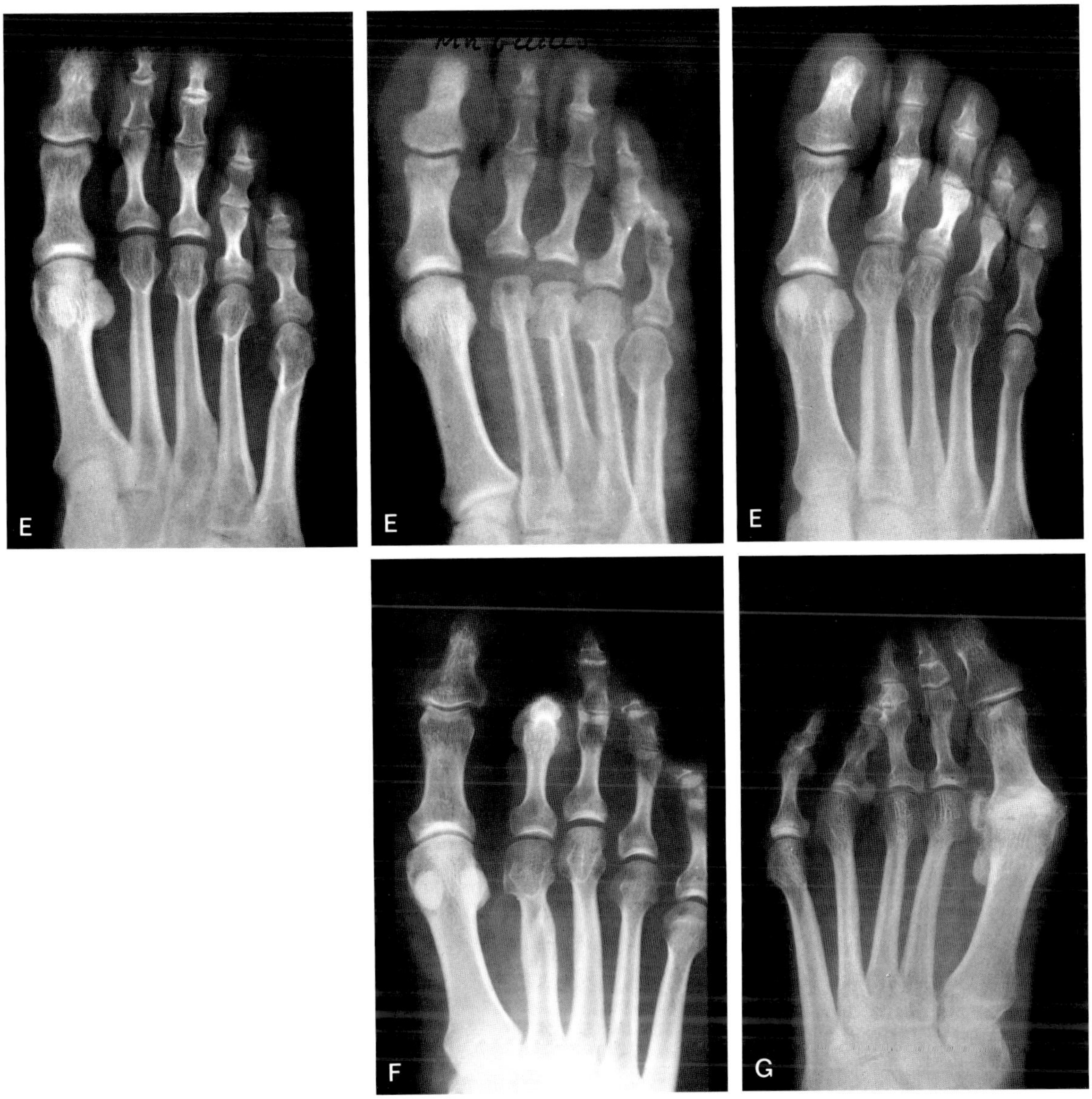

◁ **Fig. 11.9 A–I.** Overloading of one or more metatarsal heads due to frontal protrusion. **A** Overloading of second metatarsal head, hypertrophy in length of second metatarsal, thickening of diaphyseal cortex. Treatment: Realignment of second metatarsal head by head-shaft enclavement. **B** Hypertrophy in length and overloading of second metatarsal, protrusion of second, third and fourth metatarsal heads. Treatment: Head-shaft enclavement. **C** Overloading of second and third metatarsal heads. Treatment: Realignment by head-shaft enclavement of second and third metatarsals. **D** Overloading of third metatarsal due to frontal protrusion of three central metatarsals. Treatment: Realignment head-shaft enclavement of second, third and fourth metatarsals. **E** Overloading of second and third metatarsal heads due to hypertrophy in length. Treatment: Realignment by head-shaft enclavement of second and third metatarsals. **F** Overloading of third metatarsal head. Treatment: Realignment by head-shaft enclavement of third metatarsal. **G** Overloading of fourth metatarsal head. Treatment: Realignment by head-shaft enclavement of fourth metatarsal. **H, I** see p. 94

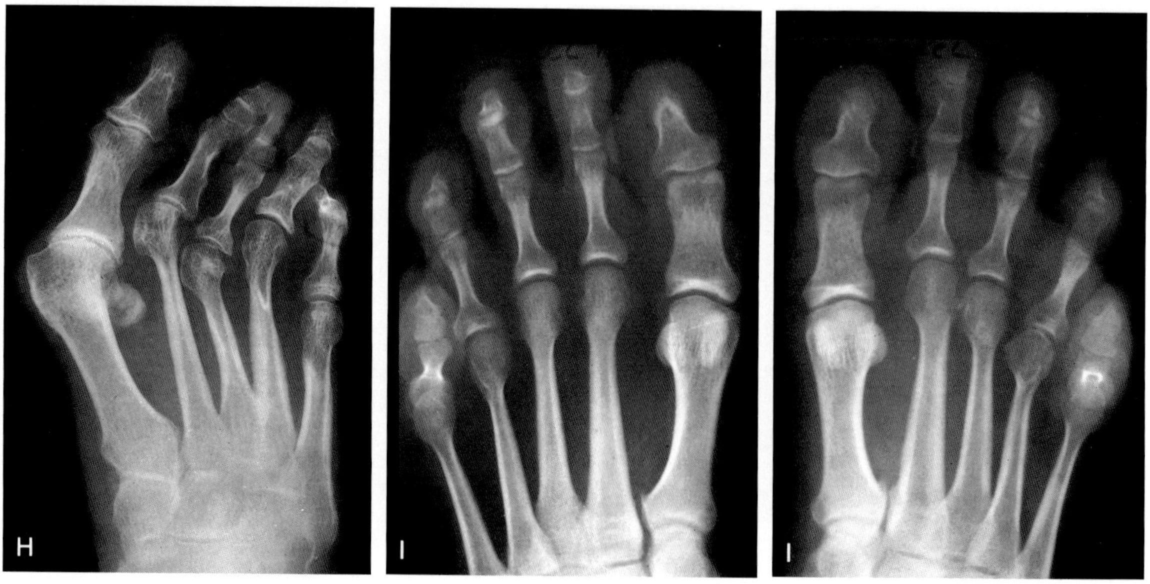

Fig. 11.9 *(continued)*. **H** Overloading of second and fourth metatarsal heads. Treatment: Realignment of second and fourth metatarsal heads by head-shaft enclavement. **I** Convex forefoot from protrusion of three central metatarsal heads due to hypertrophy in length, callus formation under second and third metatarsal heads. Treatment: Realignment by head-shaft enclavement of second and third metatarsals

The tendency to inflammation is greater in the fifth metatorsal head than in the others because of its small size and exposed situation in the shoe. Longstanding examples are common, presenting with ulceration or even underlying infective osteonecrosis (Fig. 31.1 G).

11.4.1 With Clawing of Toe

The fifth ray has a clinodactyly like a sharp hook (Fig. 11.11). The fifth metatarsal is in light equinus and the proximal phalanx is directed upwards and inwards with its base entirely dislocated onto the dorsal or dorsomedial aspect of the metatarsal head, while the middle and distal phalanges are hyperflexed plantarwards. This total clawing is rigid and irreducible, fixed by capsular contracture and the bridging of the extensor tendons under the dorsal skin. A callus or plantar keratoma forms on the plantar aspect of the metatarsal head and a large keratoma lies over the head of the proximal phalanx. The flexor tendon is tightly contracted. The fifth toe usually adopts a supraductus, forming a partridge-eye lesion on its internal aspect.
The clawing of the toe induces overloading of the underlying metatarsal head because of the bulk of tissue which presses against the upper of the shoe, but the patient complains of as much pain from the plantar callus as from the digital corns.

11.4.1.1 Treatment

Conservative. Chiropodial treatment or the use of an insole does little to improve the condition and operation is always indicated, except in the very elderly.

Operative. Surgical treatment comprises elongation of the contracted extensor tendon, arthroplasty of the proximal interphalangeal joint by generous resection of the condyles of the proximal phalanx, and detachment of the flexor tendon from the bases of the middle and distal phalanges. At the metatarsophalangeal joint, dorsal and lateral capsulotomy allow correction. Shortening of the proximal phalanx may be needed in order to restore the proper position of the metatarsophalangeal joint. A VY-plasty of the dorsal skin is frequently necessary.
It should be recognised that clawing of the fifth toe may accompany other abnormalities and that its correction may therefore be complementary to more basic problems.

11.4.2 With Reduced Vertical Mobility

Overloading is in this case due to rigidity arising from fibrosis at the contiguous surfaces of the faces of the fourth and fifth metatarsals. Courriades

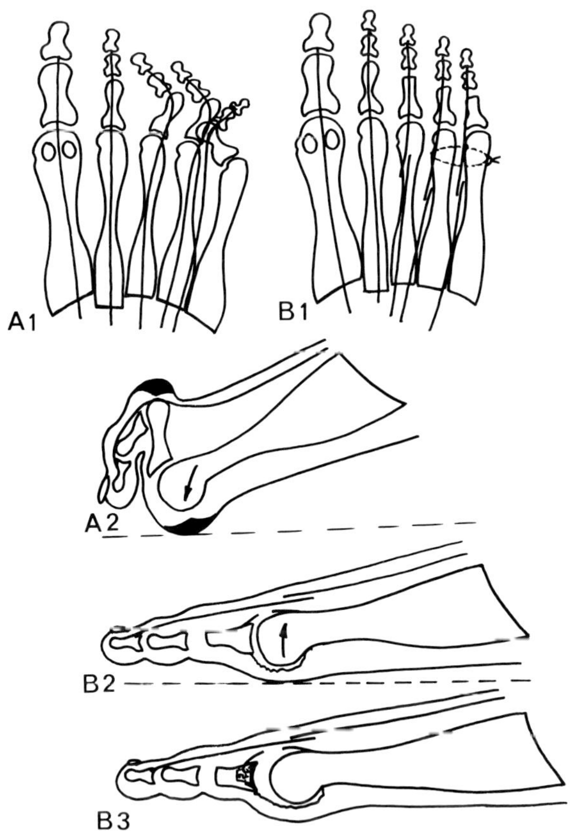

Fig. 11.11 A, B. Overloading of fifth metatarsal head due to clawing of fifth toe. **A** Before treatment. **B** *1* Intercapsulorraphy of fourth and fifth metatarsophalangeal joints, elongation of extensor tendons and metatarsophalangeal arthrotomy; *2* proximal interphalangeal arthroplasty; *3* proximal interphalangeal arthroplasty and metatarsophalangeal graft arthroplasty

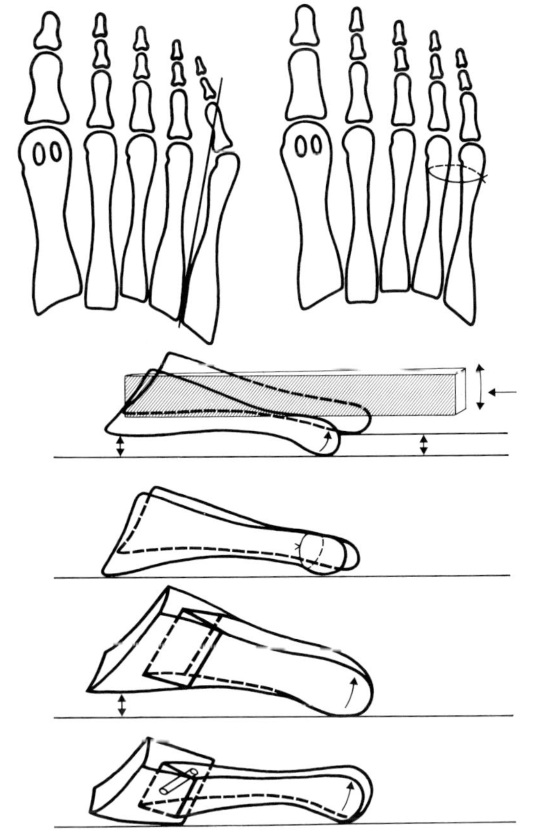

Fig. 11.12. Overloading of fifth metatarsal head associated with loss of vertical range of motion of metatarsal. Treatment includes intermetatarsal osteotomy between bases of fourth and fifth metatarsals, intercapsulorraphy of fourth and fifth metatarsophalangeal joints, correction of inclination of fifth metatarsal and elevating basal osteotomy (Thys-Martorell) of fifth metarsal

(1971) described how the external portion of the cuboidometatarsal component of the Lisfranc joint line could be relatively fixed with an articular plane orientated obliquely forwards and outwards perpendicular to the axis of loading of the foot along the calcaneum-cuboid-fifth metatarsal axis. In this syndrome of overloading, the orientation of this part of the joint line is more accentuated, so that the basal apophysis of the fifth metatarsal finds itself below that of the fourth metatarsal. There follows a significant diminution of mobility or even total rigidity of the interline between the fourth and fifth metatarsals.

The inability of the fifth ray to elevate when loaded during the rolling phase of the step leads to overloading at its distal extremity and the formation of a local plantar callus. When this metatarsal malposition and fibrous rigidity supervene in a precavus foot, the malposition is accentuated, partly by the augmentation of the plantar transverse concavity at the Lisfranc joint line and partly by the accompanying diminution of the frontal transverse convexity.

11.4.2.1 Treatment

Treatment is *operative* and includes mobilisation of the base of the fifth metatarsal and excision of the exostosis at the head of the bone which always develops (Fig. 11.12). Tendinous elongations are necessary and it is usually possible to relocate the fifth metatarsal head onto the same horizontal level as its neighbouring fourth. Correction is usually stable, but if this is not so, distal capsulorrhaphy of the fourth and fifth metatarsals is necessary. Additionally, the long extensor tendon can be transplanted through a tunnel onto the neck of the metatarsal so as to maintain the elevated position.

Operative Technique (Regnauld 1974). With tourniquet applied, a curvilinear incision commences on the outer aspect of the fifth toe, crosses onto the dorsal aspect of the metatarsophalangeal joint, then returns to the outer aspect and passes proximally overlying the anterior half of the metatarsal shaft. The long extensor tendon is elongated and the capsule of the exposed joint divided completely. The head of the metatarsal is trimmed of osteophytes and introduced along the inner aspect of the metatarsal shaft. The ligaments between the bases of the fourth and fifth metatarsals are divided, restoring freedom of vertical movement of the fifth metatarsal. This in turn restores horizontal alignment of the head, which is maintained by distal capsulorrhaphy to the fourth metatarsal. The capsule and the elongated long extensor tendon are sutured and the skin closed. Weight bearing recommences about 3 weeks postoperatively and increases progressively.

11.4.3 With Equinus of Metatarsal Associated with Longitudinal or Forefoot Cavus or of Iatrogenic Origin

In a *cavus foot,* the metatarsalgia and overloading are provoked by augmentation of the angle of declination of the fifth metatarsal. The base of the bone does not rest on the ground, there being a gap of several millimetres. The appearance is confirmed on podoscopy, which gives a typically bifocal imprint with loss of the external band.

When the longitudinal cavus is supple in the midtarsal region, an insole may control the pain of overloading at the level of the callus. If not, surgical treatment is designed to correct the equinus. A V-osteotomy is carried out at the base of the metatarsal with internal fixation, using a screw or a staple, so as to resist displacement of the proximal segment under the traction of peroneus brevis.

If the cavus is fixed, wedge osteotomy should be performed at the summit of the curve, sometimes at the Lisfranc joint line but more frequently in the midtarsal region. The wedge is based dorsally and is somewhat more generous in its external part when there is general varus of the foot. If the varus is present in the calcaneum, a transcalcaneal osteotomy (Dwyer 1959) should be performed, with removal of a wedge based externally. These procedures must re-establish lateral balance as well as achieve longitudinal correction of the foot while preserving the subtalar joint. The triple arthrodesis involving the midtarsal and subtalar joints described by Bertrand and Launay should be avoided, as it robs the foot of one of its most important joint systems; Valenti (1980a, b) in his description of "the eye of the foot", stresses the importance of the subtalar joint in adaptation to rough ground. Subtalar arthrodesis is appropriate *only* in a very severe and irreducible cavovarus foot.

In the presence of *forefoot cavus,* operative measures vary according to the significance of the accompanying longitudinal cavus (Fig. 11.13). Thus, when the longitudinal cavus remains supple, basal intra-osseous osteotomy at the fourth and fifth metatarsals is appropriate. This can take the form of semicircular osteotomy at the base of the fifth metatarsal and V-osteotomies in the third and fourth metatarsals.

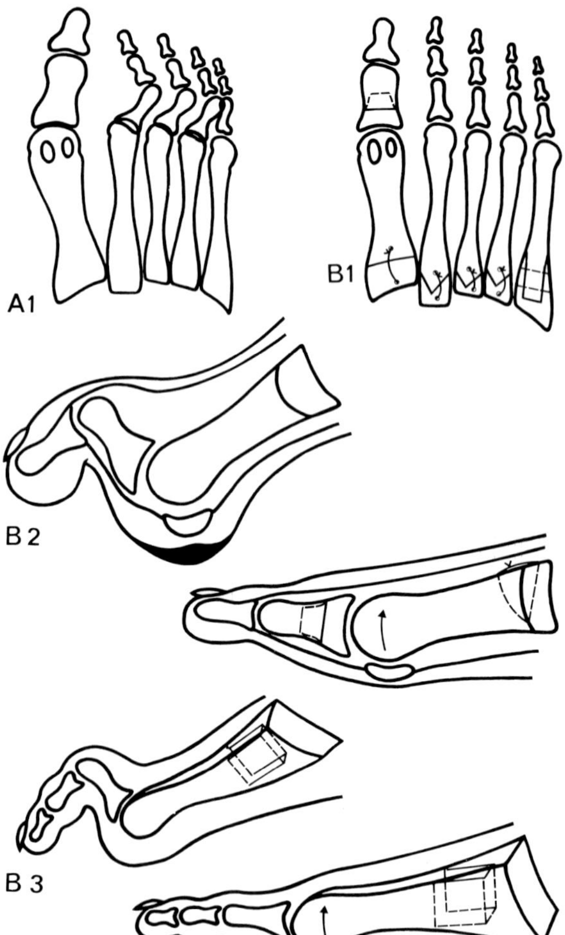

Fig. 11.13 A, B. Overloading of first and fifth metatarsal heads in pes cavus. **A** Before treatment. **B** Treatment comprises correction of hallux valgus, if present *(1, 2),* lowering basal osteotomy of central three metatarsals *(1)* and elevating basal osteomy of first *(2)* and fifth *(3)* metatarsals

If the longitudinal cavus is irreducible, transverse wedge osteotomies at the Lisfranc joint line with the bases dorsally can reduce the deformity in one stage and correct the overloading of the first and fifth metatarsals, provided the section is a little more generous at the outer and inner extremes of the joint line.

If the forefoot is in supination with a planovalgus posture, treatment should be limited to the use of an insole, incorparating an internal supporting dome, a supinating wedge under the heel and an anterior pronating wedge leading to a well-shaped retrocapital bar. Surgical procedures in the fifth ray for the planovalgus foot should be avoided in the adult; if operation for planovalgus is necessary, it must be performed in the midtarsal region.

11.4.4 *With Plantar Cutaneous Atrophy*

Loss of resilience of the subcutaneous tissue under the fifth metatarsal head is common in senility, vascular disease, neurovascular disorders of polyneuritis or toxaemia (especially alcoholic polyneuritis), paralytic conditions and inflammatory rheumatoid arthritis.

Treatment is essentially conservative, with the use of a monoblock insole including a retrocapital bar, well padded and protecting the points of painful loading (Fig. 11.14). Surgery is contra-indicated except in the case of rheumatoid arthritis.

One of the difficult aspects of this condition is its association with displacements at the midtarsus or tarsus, and it may not be possible to ascertain which is the primary cause of the overall condition. In the absence of treatment, the metatarsalgia provokes permanent contracture of the foot, digital clawing, cavus forefoot, cavovarus or cavovalgus foot deformity or even a club-shaped deformity. It is impossible to foresee whether these deformities will become controlled, and even after the most minute study it may be difficult to identify the occasional indication for surgery. Whenever in doubt, conservative management is wiser.

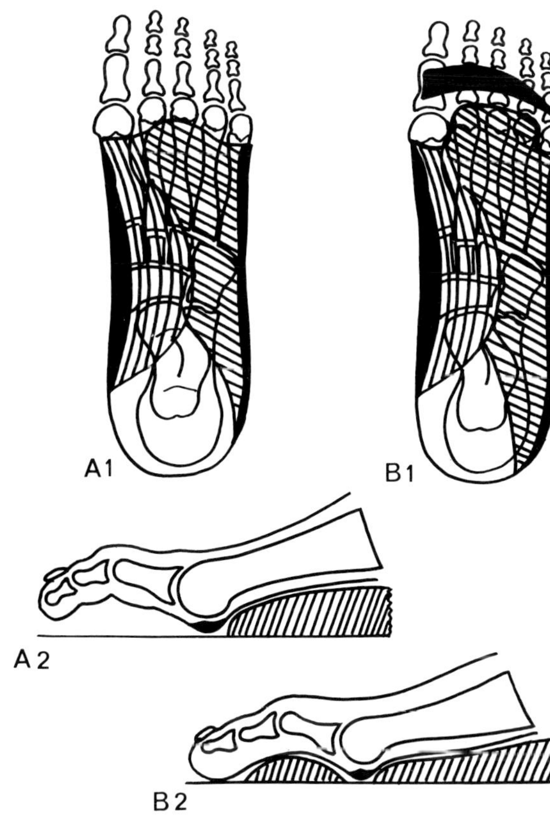

Fig. 11.14 A, B. Overloading of fifth metatarsal head with atrophy of plantar soft tissues: treatment with monoblock insoles. **A** With retrocapital bar. **B** With elevation under central three metatarsal heads, elevation behind first and fifth heads, excavation under fifth head and Martorell antecapital bar

12 Insufficiency of the Central Metatarsals

Insufficiency of loading of one or more rays results in overloading of the adjacent heads. The condition can be congenital (aplasia of a metatarsal) or acquired (trauma, infection, or following operation, such as amputation of a metatarsal head).

12.1 Etiology

Whatever the cause of the incompetence of loading it is under the neighbouring metatarsal heads that relative overloading occurs, with the development of all the characteristics of mechanical metatarsalgia. In the acquired forms, there may also be symptoms from the disordered joint primarily concerned, which may assume various deformities with corresponding toe involvement, most frequently resulting in clawing; the toe tends to be backwardly displaced with respect to its neighbours and develops pressure areas on exposed projecting surfaces, with the development in most cases of a varus supraductus. In time, clinodactylies of neighbouring toes develop as they try to fill the gap created by the metatarsal aplasia and displacement of the associated toe.
In acquired insufficiency due to trauma or infection, the appearance of retropulsion of the affected toe stems from the articular lesions at the metatarsophalangeal joint which limit the amplitude of movement and result in a fixed clawed deformity from fibrous ankylosis of the metatarsophalangeal joint with accompanying tendinous contracture.
The loss of a metatarsal head by surgical excision can result in gross examples of this underloading syndrome.

12.2 Clinical Presentation

The patient presents with pain of overloading under the neighbouring metatarsal heads, a characteristic burning provoked by standing and exaggerated by walking or the use of a high heel. The pain improves with rest and begins progressively earlier in the day. Examination of the primary aplastic case reveals loss of prehensile function and dorsal displacement of the toe, which lies in supraductus. On the plantar surface there is a longitudinal fold which separates the areas of plantar callus from adjacent overloading. Palpation reveals lack of resistance at the site of metatarsal insufficiency.
In the acquired cases, when a remnant of joint remains, the toe is stiffer, being fixed in an attitude of acute dorsiflexion, and the tendons which help to anchor it in its deformed position are easily palpable (see Fig. 27.5 G–I). Calluses over the acutely flexed interphalangeal joint are evident from shoe pressure.
Podology, podometry and *radiography* confirm the clinical findings and demonstrate the degree of destruction of the joint.

12.3 Treatment

12.3.1 Conservative

In some instances the definitive method of treatment can be a suitably adapted insole, comprising a simple retrocapital bar or a physiological monoblock with a retrocapital bar. If there is no gross contracture of the toe or formation of a dorsal digital corn, this may suffice.

12.3.2 Operative

In more advanced cases of deformity, surgery is indicated, with the aim of re-establishing normal loading of the incompetent metatarsal head. The toe must be reduced into its proper position and restored to its normal length relative to its neighbours.

12.3.2.1 Congenital Insufficiency

In this instance the shortened metatarsal is intact, presenting a metatarsal condyle which although well formed is more slender than usual. The metatarsophalangeal joint is somewhat displaced vertically. The situation can be corrected by elongation of the metatarsal and its extensor and flexor tendons.

Operative Technique. With tourniquet applied, a longitudinal incision is made over the dorsal aspect of the metatarsal concerned, capsular arthrolysis of the metatarsophalangeal joint performed and the long and short extensor tendons prepared, Z-fashion, for lengthening (Fig. 12.1). Using an oscillating saw, the metatarsal is sectioned transversely about 6 mm from its base and freed from its soft tissue attachments collaterally. By traction, a gap is created corresponding in dimension to the degree of shortening measured from previous radiographs. A

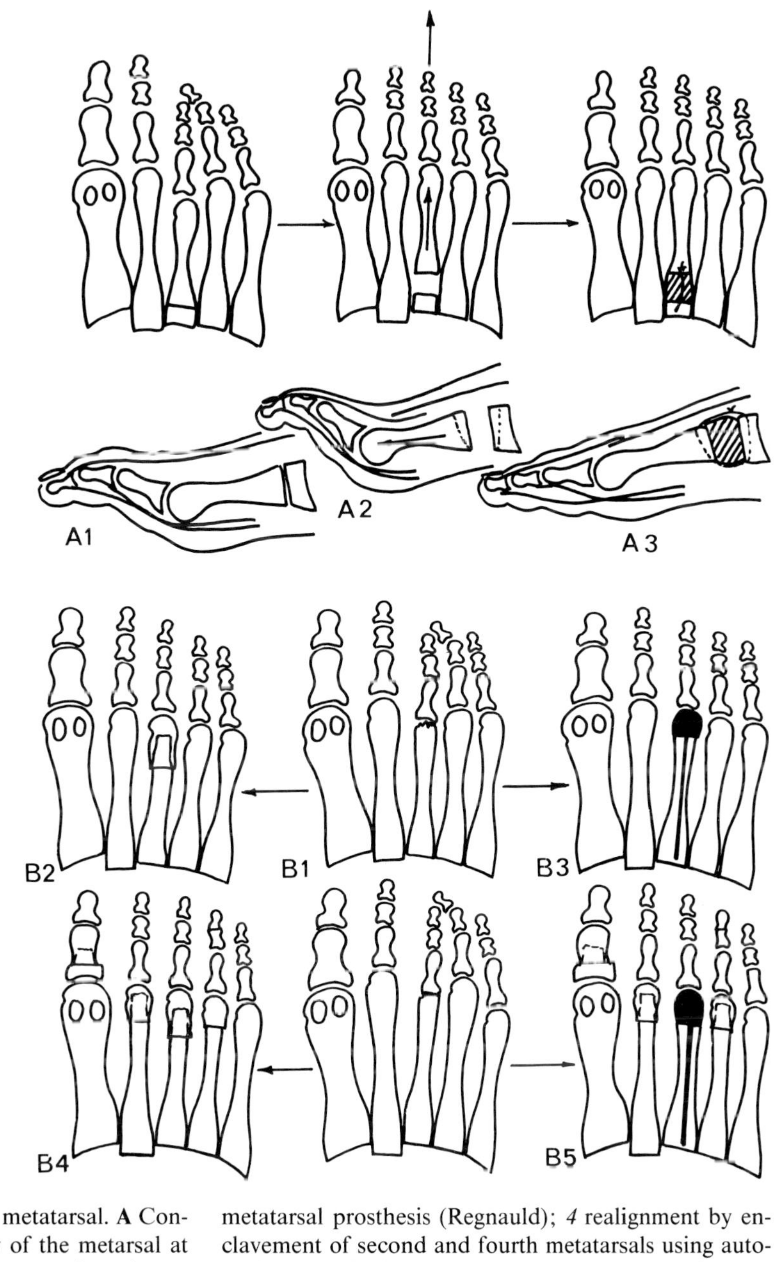

Fig. 12.1 A, B. Underloading of third metatarsal. **A** Congenital shortness: *1* Basal osteotomy of the metarsal at the diaphyseo-epiphyseal junction; *2* separation of osteotomy surfaces; *3* insertion of bone graft to bring metatarsal to desired length. **B** Iatrogenic insufficiency: *1* Before reoperation; *2* realignment by enclavement using a homograft (Regnauld); *3* realignment by implantation of metatarsal prosthesis (Regnauld); *4* realignment by enclavement of second and fourth metatarsals using autografts and of third metatarsal using a homograft; *5* realignment by enclavement of second and fourth metatarsals using autografts and implantation of a metatarsal prosthesis in third metatarsal

cube-shaped bone graft taken from the iliac crest or the tibia is inserted between the two fragments and anchored by suture of the periosteum. A below-knee plaster cast is applied for approximately 2 months, depending upon radiological assessment of union.

12.3.2.2 Trauma

In cases of traumatic involvement associated with fracture of a metatarsal head, choice of operation will depend upon the condition of the injured part. If the state of the condylar head is adequate, after exposure it can be trimmed of deforming osteophytes and reimplanted using a secret-screw technique (Regnauld 1968), thereby re-establishing a normal position for the metatarsal head (Fig. 12.2).

Operative Technique. With tourniquet applied, the site of fracture is exposed and the surface freshened with minimum excision of bone. A pin or screw of suitable size is introduced provisionally into the medullary canal, and the head of the screw (if used) is cut off with shears. A hole is fashioned in the distal fragment using a drill slightly smaller in diameter than the screw or pin, which is coaxed distally so as to fix the fracture site. The toe is repositioned and the capsule and tendons are repaired. Healing is assessed radiologically and loading avoided until union is assured.

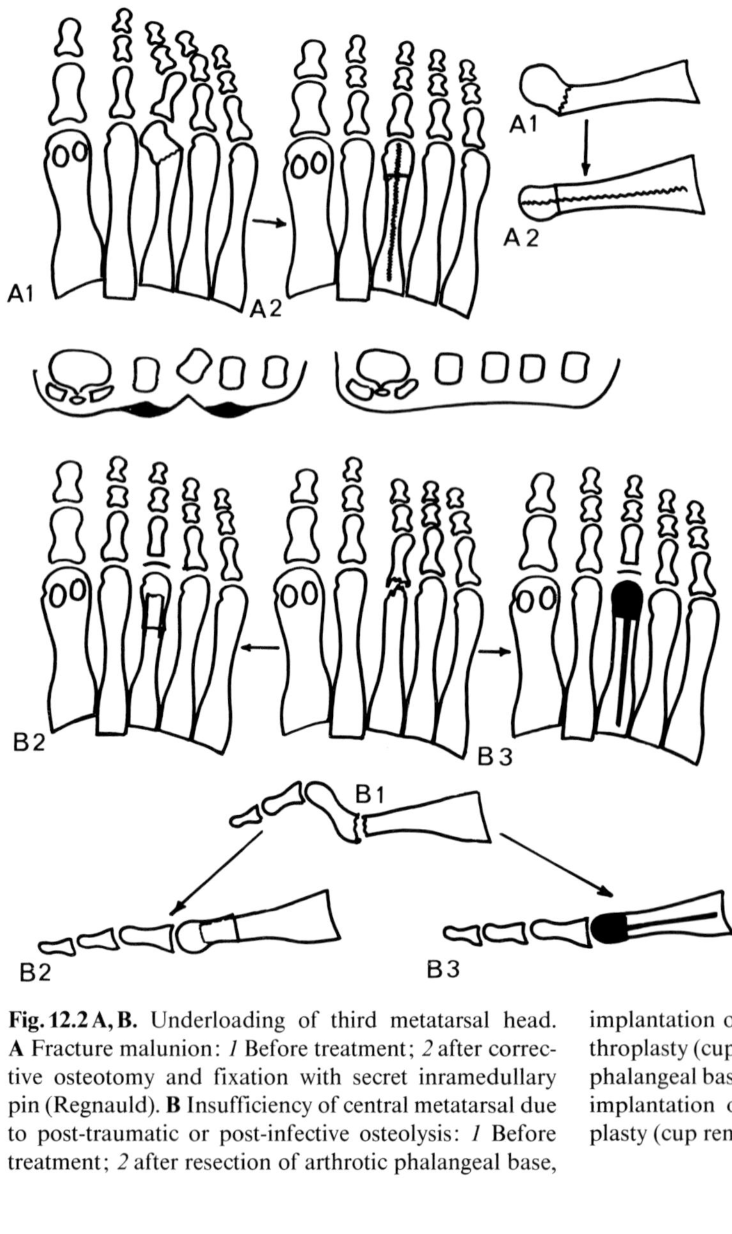

Fig. 12.2 A, B. Underloading of third metatarsal head. **A** Fracture malunion: *1* Before treatment; *2* after corrective osteotomy and fixation with secret inramedullary pin (Regnauld). **B** Insufficiency of central metatarsal due to post-traumatic or post-infective osteolysis: *1* Before treatment; *2* after resection of arthrotic phalangeal base, implantation of metatarsal head homograft and cup arthroplasty (cup removed after a year); *3* after resection of phalangeal base, resection of distal portion of metatarsal, implantation of metatarsal prosthesis and cup arthroplasty (cup removed after a year)

If this technique is impossible, due to the state of the metatarsal head, metatarsal head-shaft enclavement of the adjacent metatarsals may be preferable. Alternatively, implantation of a metatarsal head prosthesis is necessary in necrosis of the head or when osteoporosis is so advanced that reimplantation is impossible. The implant must be exactly aligned. A metatarsal head homograft associated with enclavement as demanded by the metatarsal formula of the forefoot is a further possibility.

12.3.2.3 Localised Insufficiency of Infectious Origin

This condition is exceptional but has been met in osteolysis of the head in rheumatoid arthritis and in tuberculosis of the metatarsophalangeal joint. Operative treatment comprises excision of the affected metatarsophalangeal joint after section through the neck of the metatarsal and the base of the proximal phalanx. The joint is replaced with a homograft or cup prosthesis, followed by reduction of any digital clawing by appropriate capsulotomies, arthoplasties or arthrodeses of the interphalangeal joints.

12.3.2.4 Iatrogenic Metatarsal Head Insufficiency

This condition may be corrected by metatarsal head homograft (Regnauld 1971 b).

Operative Technique. With tourniquet applied, a longitudinal incision is made over the metatarsophalangeal joint concerned and longitudinal arthrotomy is performed alongside the tendons which may require division, Z-fashion, for lengthening. The capsule is detached from the dorsal plantar and lateral surfaces of the metatarsal epiphyseal region. The elongation of the tendons and the capsules allow, by distal traction, the reposition of the toe in its proper place with respect to its neighbours. Arthroplasties or arthrodeses, as appropriate, may be necessary in the interphalangeal joints of the neighbouring toes if there is camptodactyly. With traction on the affected toe, access to the end of the affected metatarsal is possible, and a quadrangular tendon is fashioned with rongeurs. A metatarsal homograft head is prepared with a mortice of comparable dimensions, giving firm fixation and good alignment when applied to the prepared end of the metatarsal. The fibroperiosteum is sutured and the capsule closed. After careful haemostasis the skin is sutured. Progressively active movements are commenced on the 2nd day, but osseous fusion is slow and full weight bearing is not possible until about 6 months after operation.

If a convex forefoot has become associated with insufficiency of a metatarsal, adjacent head-shaft metatarsal enclavement may be necessary.

13 Disorders of the Sesamoids

These little bones shaped like sesame seeds were described by Sommering in his treatise on posteology. Gillette (1874), Retterer (1884), Pfitzner (1890), Tedeschi (1891) (all cited by Testut 1904) and Inge and Ferguson (1933) all contributed to an understanding of their significance. Inge and Ferguson regarded the sesamoids as skeletal structures rather than true bones. They appear early, at about the 12th week of intra-uterine life, and appear to arise by ossification in cartilage. Later, they become surrounded by flexor hallucis brevis. Ossification is completed between the ages of 8 and 11 years.

The sesamoids should be regarded as supernumerary bones on the plantar aspect of the forefoot underlying the condyles of the first, second, third and fifth metatarsals and the head of the proximal phalanx of the great toe (Fig. 13.1 A, K–M). They are most constantly present under the first metatarsal. Those of the outer rays are relatively immune to pathological change, becoming involved only occasionally in the pathology of overloading. In contrast, those of the first metatarsal or proximal phalanx of the great toe, as a result of their volume and position, are frequently involved. Overloading syndrome related to the sesamoids manifests itself by the presence of a plantar callosity with sharp lancing pain similar to that associated with a foreign body in the tissues, experienced during loading and relieved by rest. Callus becomes keratinised in a punctiform manner and is very painful, being prone to serous inflammatory bursitis and making choice of footwear most difficult. If the corn so formed is pared, palpation reveals a sharp hard swelling associated with the sesamoid.

The causes of pain, which can be congenital or acquired, associated with the sesamoid bones relate to joint involvement or overloading.

13.1 Congenital Bipartite or Tripartite Sesamoid

The sesamoid bones can be congenitally separated into two, three, or even four parts along a transverse axis or in Y-form (Fig. 13.1 B). Inge and Ferguson state that this is a normal finding in 10% of individuals. This partitism is normally symptom free but may be diagnosed following trauma, either directly or indirectly.

Pain is of inflammatory or mechanical origin, aggravated by pressure and loading and relieved by rest or anti-inflammatory agents. It is usually of a sharp, cutting type, like the sensation of a nail in the shoe, or of a tearing nature, and is localised to the part concerned and aggravated by dorsiflexion of the great toe. There may be local warmth on palpation.

Treatment may be conservative, comprising rest, anti-inflammatory agents and an elastic support, and occassionally an appropriate insole helps. Cases that do not resolve require surgical management, comprising meticulous local excision of one or two portions of the sesamoids with an attempt to leave the major part in situ. Excision must be limited to the osseous tissue; the capsule of the joint must be preserved.

13.2 Dystrophy or Aseptic Necrosis (Renander's Disease)

Usually it is a young subject indulging in sport who develops sesamoid metatarsalgia, often intense at the beginning, without apparent precipitating cause. The pain appears almost like gout, with nocturnal fluctuation, and is associated with slight local swelling. It is exacerbated by loading, walking or local pressure [Renander 1924, cited by Hohmann (1951), Natiello (1971) and Denis (1975 a)]. Radiography reveals apparent fragmentation of the sesamoids with apparent loss of continuity in stellate form (Fig. 13.1 C). Irregular zones of rarefaction with eburnated condensations are seen.

The pain associated with the condition evolves over several weeks and is often relieved by medical treatment comprising local rest, a supporting dressing of Unna's paste (G. Bureau 1982), a physiological monoblock insole and anti-inflammatory agents (Denis 1975 a). Rarely is surgery necessary. The cause of this condition is not certain.

Denis (1975 a) regards it as a primary fracture with patchy necrosis and residual islands of cartilage. Wisbrun regards sesamoiditis as a traumatic osteochondritis. The transverse fissuring can be likened to an old fracture leading to osteoarthritic lesion. Inge and Ferguson (1933) state that the condition may be an osteomalacia of the sesamoids, but this seems unlikely because of the presence of sesamoid-metatarsal arthritis, subsesamoid bursitis, and dislocations of these bones outwards or behind the metatarsal head. G. Bureau (1982) attributes the aseptic necrosis to ischaemia which has led to localised necrosis, lysis and fracture of the sesamoid (Fig. 13.1 G–I).

13.3 Fracture

Fracture of the sesamoids can result from direct or indirect trauma: a fall, a crush injury or perhaps lo-

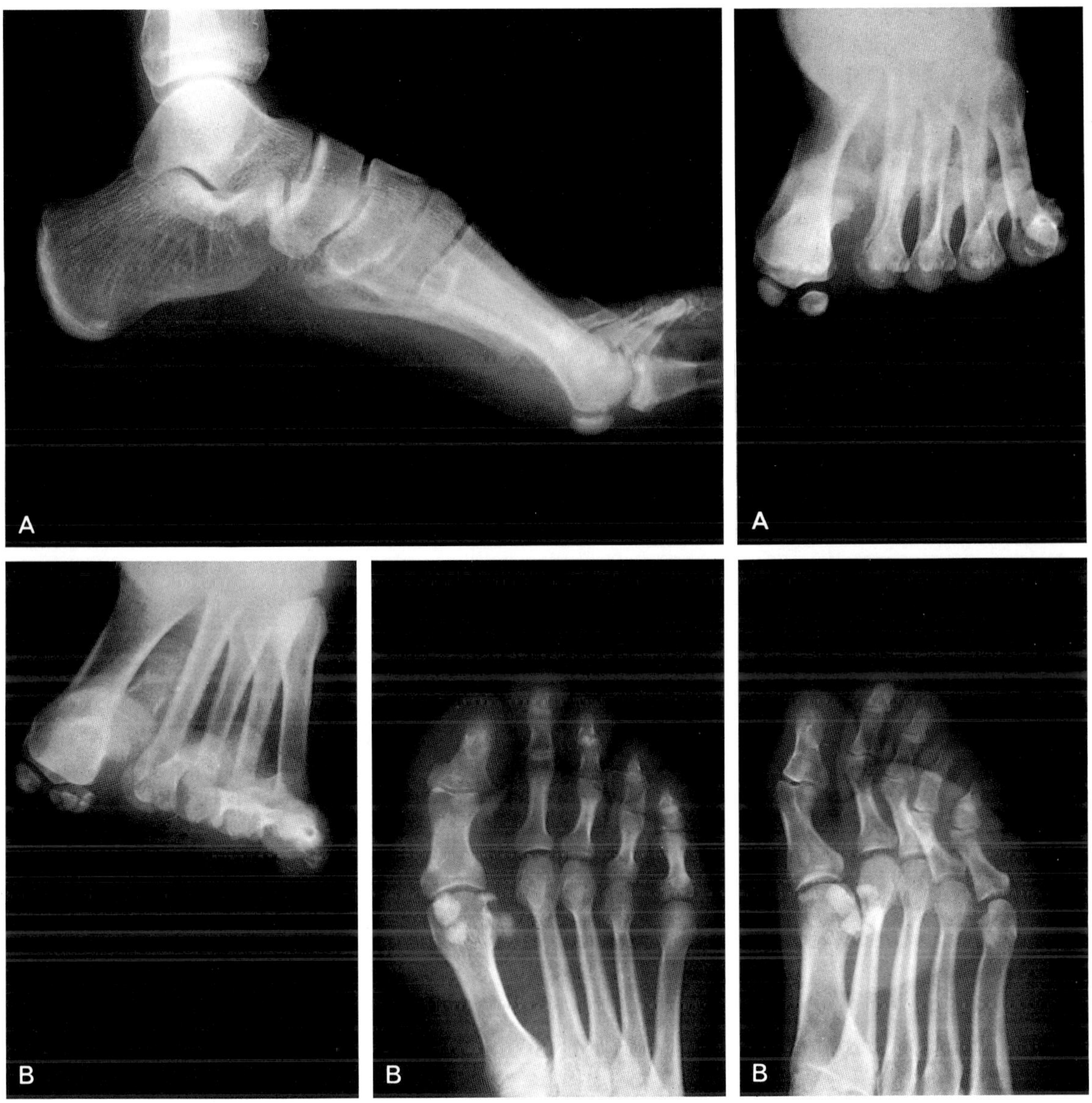

Fig. 13.1 A–M. The sesamoids. **A** Normal first metatarsal sesamoids. **B** Bipartite sesamoids. **C** Renander's sesamoiditis. **D** Post-traumatic osteolysis of sesamoids. **E** Lateral sesamoiditis due to fracture. **F** Fracture of medial sesamoid. **G** Osteonecrosis of medial sesamoid. **H, I** Sesamoiditis. **J** Acumination of plantar aspect of sesamoids. **K** Sesamoids associated with all five metatarsal heads. **L** Sesamoids associated with first, second, third and fifth metatarsal heads. **M** Plantar sesamoids associated with interphalangeal joint of great toe. **C–M** see pp. 104–106

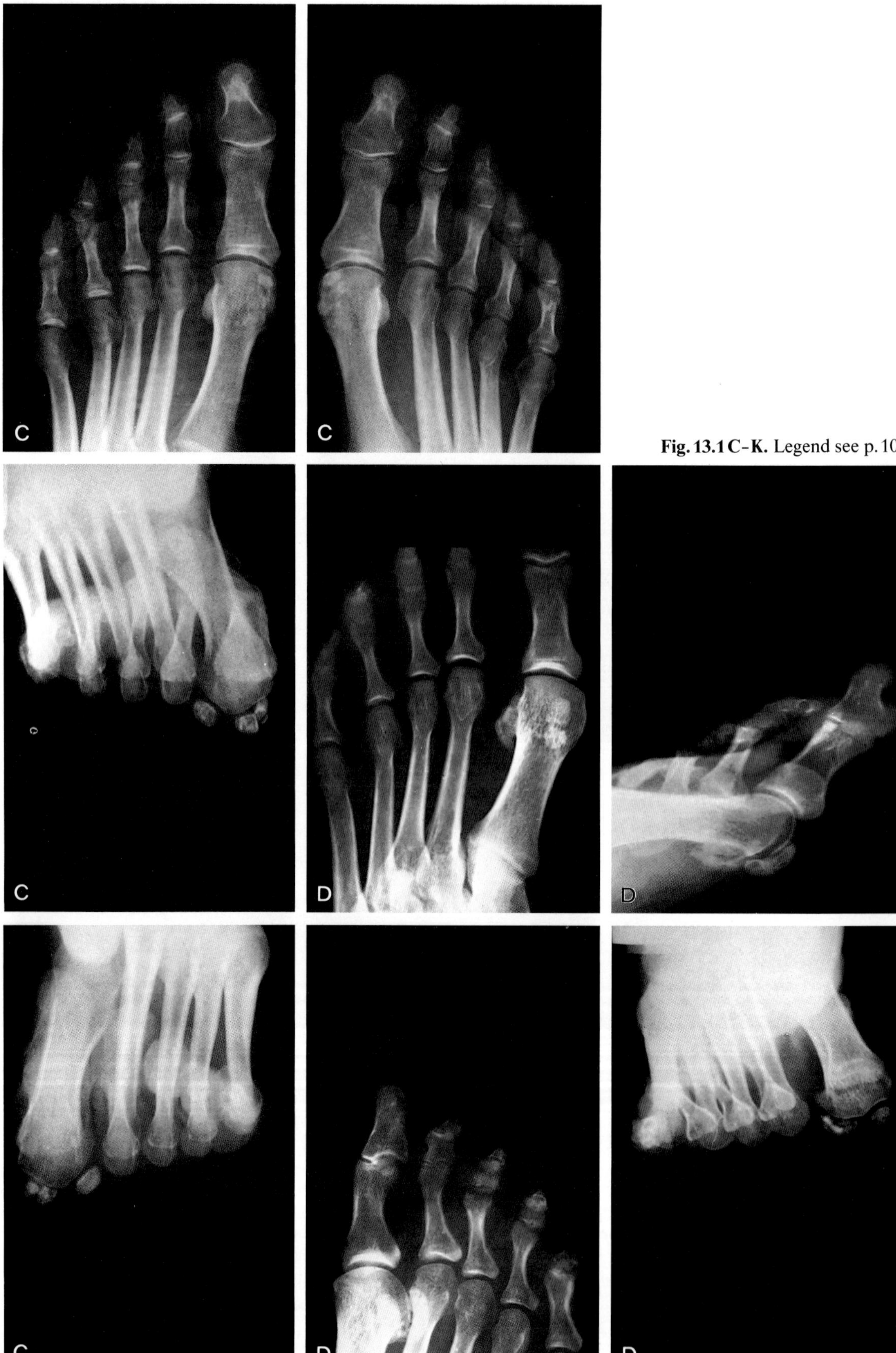

Fig. 13.1 C–K. Legend see p. 103

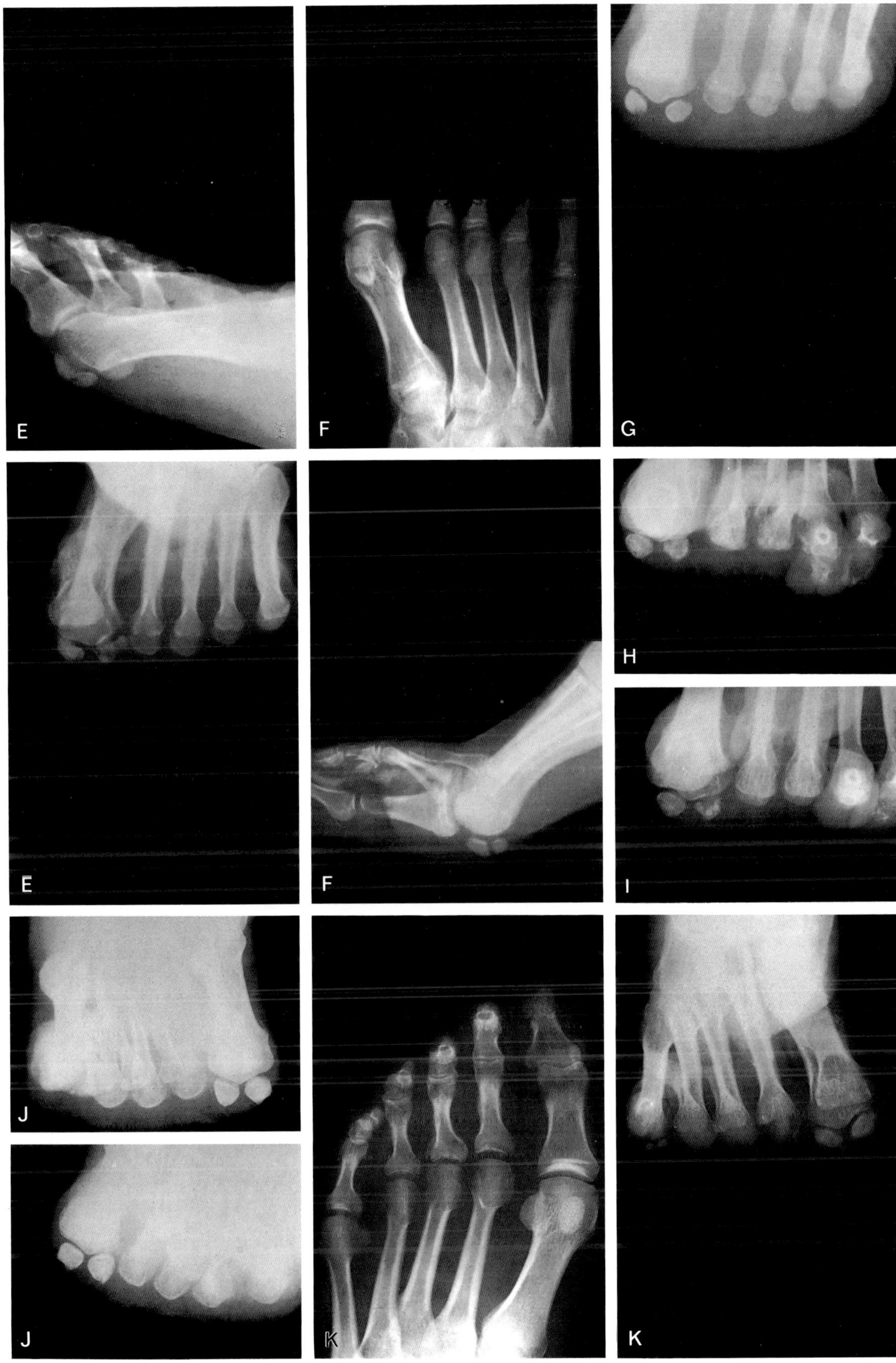
E
F
G
E
F
H
I
J
J
K
K

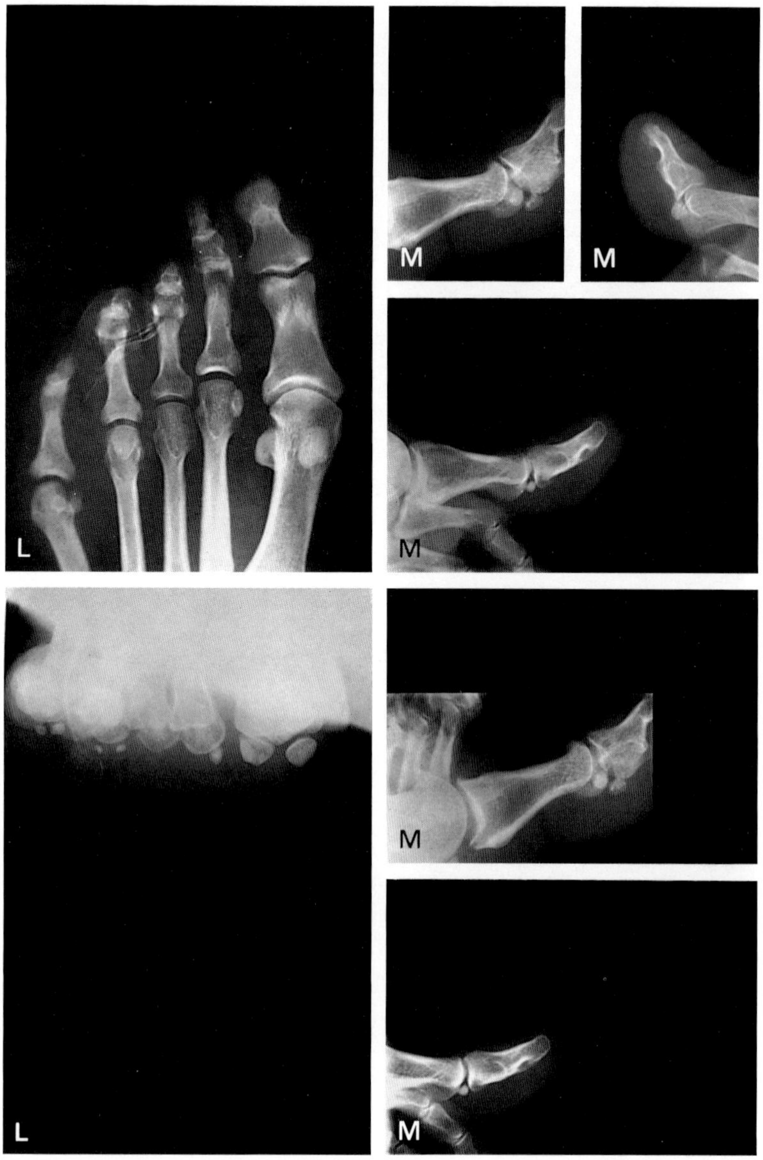

Fig. 13.1 L–M. Legend see p. 103

cal indirect traction from violent straining of the foot. Very frequently, minimal trauma or a stumble can produce changes suggestive of fracture or fragmentation (G. Bureau 1982). The internal sesamoid is most often affected.

Radiography confirms a single or multiple fracture line and sometimes a simple displacement of the outer portion of the inner sesamoid (Fig. 13.1 D–F). Pain can be exquisite. It is exacerbated by any local pressure, and relived by rest.

In the absence of treatment, metatarsalgia persists and leads eventually to sesamoid-metatarsal arthrosis with accompanying surrounding osteophytosis and localised patchy osteoporosis. More rarely, complete lysis of the bone can occur (Fig. 13.1 D).

Treatment may be conservative, involving rest, anti-inflammatory agents, analgesics and splinting. A physiological monoblock insole with excavation under the metatarsal head concerned is useful.

Failure to respond indicates a need for surgical excision of a fragment or several fragments leaving intact the capsuloperiosteal layer which must be reconstituted most carefully.

13.4 Exostosis

Exostoses of the sesamoid are rare, but G. Bureau (1982) described several cases. The condition leads to pain on loading and sometimes development of a plantar keratoma. Occasionally it is discovered incidentally on radiographs taken for some other reason. Usually there is a past history of trauma. In the event of sufficiently severe symptoms, local excision of the exostosis must be undertaken.

13.5 Sesamoiditis from Overloading

This condition results from hypertrophy of the sesamoid and may be associated with the arthrosis of hallux rigidus in which case treatment will consist of management of the primary condition together with partial excision of the plantar part of the two sesamoids and trimming of any surrounding osteophytes. Another cause is elective equinus of the great metatarsal, exceptionally associated with hypertrophy of length.

There is typical metatarsalgia of overloading, with sharp, lancing pains and painful tension under the great metatarsal head. Often there is a plantar inflammatory bursa. Usually the patient is a young woman complaining of these symptoms, which are aggravated by loading, walking, sport, and high heels and relieved by rest. The condition is progressive, becoming more acute and complicated by episodes of inflammation and possibly infection and ulceration. Localised equinus of the great metatarsal and hypertrophy of the sesamoid coexist, and the configuration of the hypertrophy is usually pointed. The undersurface loses its regular rounded convexity and presents with two obliquely disposed faces separated by a longitudinal crest which corresponds exactly to the subjacent plantar keratoma.

Conservative treatment with an insole may be successful provided the great metatarsal remains reducible and supple. The insole must incorporate a retrocapital bar, a platform under the central metatarsal heads and, in the region of the irritable first metatarsal head, an anterocapital bar of Martorell (1968).

Failure indicates the need for surgery, comprising curvilinear basal osteotomy of the great metatarsal to reduce the equinus of the bone, trimming of the plantar crest of the sesamoid and removal of a serous bursa or excision of a keratoma, which may require a plantar flap if the skin is too damaged (see Fig. 11.4).

Sesamoid overloading associated with cavus forefoot syndrome is described in Chap. 9.

The condition may occur in association with pes planus, in which abduction of the forefoot is associated with local overloading and leads to a reactionary hyperostosis on the plantar aspect. Use of a corrective insole and stabilisation of the pes planus may bring improvement, but if this fails, local excision followed by further conservative measures is necessary.

Overloading from iatrogenic causes, notably amputation of the second, third and fourth metatarsal heads in the Hohmann-Wallet operation (Hohmann 1951) can provoke a severe degree of pain and keratotic changes in the local skin. Treatment is initially by an insole with a retrocapital and anterocapital bar as described by Martorell (1968). Failure indicates surgery, which comprises realignment head-shaft enclavement of the first and fifth metatarsals with some adjustment of the central three amputated metatarsals. Realignment by implantation of metatarsal prostheses or homografts may also be employed.

External subluxation of the sesamoids occurs in association with hallux valgus and is discussed in Chap. 18.

14 Metatarsalgia

14.1 General Considerations and Classification

Pain in the forefoot accounts for about half the patients presenting with disorders of the foot. Of these cases, three-quarters present in women and are due to an alteration of the biomechanics of the forefoot, sometimes with primary pathology, sometimes secondary to disorders of the hindfoot. There is variation in the site of the pain, its degree of localisation, its severity and its mode of appearance. Common features are aggravation on standing and walking, progressiveness and irreversibility. The foot becomes increasingly disturbed during static weight bearing and loses its normal rolling action during gait. Secondary effects are produced more proximally. Without effective treatment, the irreversibility of changes will ruin this organ of static loading and propulsion. Etiology, diagnosis and consequent therapy are intricately related.
Metatarsalgia may be classified as follows:

- Diffuse: affecting the general assembly of the forefoot, which is displaced as a whole
- Localised: there is a precise source of pain within the metatarsus
- Non-mechanical: originating in the soft tissues, independent of loading

Treatment of metatarsalgia is fraught with uncertainty if the surgeon does not take into consideration the following points:

- The pain in the metatarsus must not be considered in isolation.
- The forefoot is not an isolated element of the foot, but must always be considered in relation to the hindfoot and leg.
- A clear understanding of the mechanism of the foot as outlined in earlier chapters is essential.
- Conservative treatment with insoles and other simple measures should usually be tried first.
- The necessity and the time for surgery should be decided when it is clear that conservative measures are not efficacious.
- An apparently simple lesion may be secondary to some more widespread disorder necessitating perhaps a more major operation. The patient may have difficulty in appreciating this.
- Reduction of loading of the foot is an essential part of postoperative care. Physiotherapy and use of an adapted shoe are important adjuncts.

14.2 Diffuse Metatarsalgia

14.2.1 Clinical Presentation

General Features. There is pain related to the anterior zone of weight bearing generally or to a portion thereof. It is intermittent when the subject is standing and may disappear completely at rest, but may be aggravated by wearing of shoes, walking and sport. Initially pain is commoner in the evenings, but tends to start progressively earlier in the day as the irreversible situation is approached. Local heat, oedema and redness of overlying skin indicates the inflammatory character seen most frequently. These general pains respond progressively, or even rapidly, to appropriate treatment.

Specific Symptoms Related to Etiology. Pain of a pricking, tingling type most frequently suggests a medical - vascular, neurological or cellular - origin. Anaesthesia, hypo-aesthesia and hyperaesthesia all suggest a neurological cause, and may be enhanced by electric-shock-like sensations when a nerve is directly irritated, perhaps under the forefoot locally or more proximally in the tarsal tunnel syndrome or sciatica. A sensation of constriction, tension or grinding indicates an articular source of the pain, which may be rheumatic, iatrogenic, traumatic or functional in origin. Lancing, pricking, heavy, tense or burning pain may indicate a congenital or acquired condition resulting in disordered mechanical function. Obviously a great overlap exists between the individual characteristics of these symptoms.

Diffuse metatarsalgia will now be considered according to the following classification:

- Longitudinal displacements of elements of the foot

- Displacements of the metatarsal heads
- Functional disorders
- Medical causes

14.2.2 Longitudinal Displacement

Normal action of the foot entails passage of pressure from propulsion at the midtarsus to the medial four metatarsal heads (Paparella-Treccia 1977; Pisani 1975b). Deformity of the medial longitudinal arch of the foot may result in pes planus, cavovalgus, or cavovarus.

In *pes planus* or *cavovalgus* deformity, the calcaneum is pronated while the medial longitudinal arch is lowered or raised. Load transfer is displaced to the internal border of the midtarsal region, and there is accompanying abduction of the forefoot. This results in excessive pressure under the heads of the second and third metatarsals and foot strain aggravated by rotation of the forefoot during propulsion. The great metatarsal is more mobile (Courriades 1971, 1973b) and in the valgus posture supports relatively little of the force of propulsion, in contrast to its function in the normally balanced foot. However, the great toe is the final load-bearing element, and because of the valgus posture it tends to be driven into abduction, explaining the frequent appearance of hallux valgus in valgoid feet.

In the *varus* or *cavovarus* foot, the calcaneum is supinated, leading to metatarsalgia arising from the fourth and fifth rays. This pain is of a constrictive, pricking, pins-and-needles or grinding character and is brought about by compression of the neurovascular bundles between the heads of the metatarsals, most frequently between the condyles of the third and fourth metatarsals; this imbalance stems predominantly from the tarsal region. Metatarsalgia in the region of the third and especially the fourth metatarsal head should lead to careful assessment of the heel for this reason. In general, the evolution of metatarsalgia due to displacement of the medial longitudinal arch reflects any static disturbance of the tarsus or midtarsus, which must always result in secondary disturbance of the normal uniformity of metatarsal head loadbearing.

In the supple foot, the use of an insole is usually effective. The correct pattern will restore balance and relieve the source of pain. In contrast, in a fixed deformity an insole is likely to be ineffective, but is nevertheless worth trying as on occasion surprising relief of symptoms can be achieved. When this is not the case, operative treatment is indicated and must be based on a clear understanding of the mechanisms involved.

14.2.2.1 Treatment of Diffuse Metatarsalgia in the Cavus Foot

Supple Cavus Foot. An insole should be chosen according to the type of foot concerned. In the balanced cavus foot, a bar behind the metatarsal heads relaxes the plantar arch by protecting the metatarsal load-bearing zone and allowing some correction of supple claw toes, thereby restoring normal function at the metatarsophalangeal joints. In the suppple cavovarus foot, the bar behind the metatarsal heads should be extended laterally to exert a pronating effect on the foot. The rebalancing of the varus heel restores uniformity of pressure during propulsion to the five metatarsal heads. In the adult with midtarsal pain, further support is necessary by means of a longitudinal physiological arch support, otherwise the bar behind the metatarsal heads and its lateral extension will tend to produce a hypercorrection in the midtarsal region.

Irreducible Cavus Foot. An insole is likely to be ineffective, callus formation under the overloaded metatarsal heads causing intolerable pain, usually of a tense, burning type aggravated during standing and walking by a shoe with a heel. Cessation of weight bearing and chiropodical removal of the hard skin give temporary relief, but if the metatarsophalangeal articular surfaces become involved, pain will be present during day and night. Clawing of the toes becomes irreducible, with subluxation or dorsal dislocation at the metatarsophalangeal joints, fixed by tendinous and capsular contracture. In the convex forefoot, the callosities under the metatarsal heads tend to be in the central part, whereas they are more diffuse in the convex triangular or flat triangular forefoot. In a cavus forefoot there may be skin thickenings specifically under the first or fifth metatarsal heads.

In this type of fixed cavus foot, operation is indicated and must aim to correct, in one intervention, the longitudinal cavus, the tarsal displacement (pronated, supinated or calcanear), and the deformities of the forefoot itself. In the balanced cavus foot, cuneiform osteotomy at the summit of the dorsal convexity in the midtarsal region should be performed at the tarsometatarsal joint line or at the midtarsal naviculocuneiform and calcaneocuboid joints. Alternatively an extra-articular transcunei-

form-transcuboidal corrective osteotomy may be possible.
When the cavus foot is in varus, midtarsal osteotomy-arthrodesis by the dorsal approach should be orientated with the base dorsolaterally. Curvilinear osteotomies are preferred because they allow a more accurate realignment of the foot with better adaptation of the bony surfaces; the cavus, midtarsal varus, adduction and supination of the forefoot can be corrected. Extra-articular curvilinear osteotomies of the midtarsal region are however much preferred to osteotomy-arthrodesis, because some degree of freedom of movement is preserved. They may be transnaviculocuboidal or transcuneiform-cuboidal and should be accompanied by plantar fasciotomy, elongation of the long flexor tendons and the tendons of tibialis anterior and posterior and sometimes those of extensor communis and extensor brevis, and correction of any displacement at the metatarsophalangeal joints. If the cavus foot is in valgus, osteotomy-arthrodesis of the midtarsal region is indicated in the exceptional cases where there is irreversible arthrosis.
When the general abduction of the metatarsus stems from an angulation in the midtarsal region, arthrodesis of the tarsometatarsal joint is indicated; a wedge of bone based dorsally and medially is removed so as to correct both the cavus and the abduction of the metatarsal region. Preferable again is the curvilinear osteotomy performed outside the joints through a medial approach. The zone of resection involves the intercuneiform-cuboidal or naviculocuboidal bone stock. It is necessary to transfer the insertion of tibialis anterior distally onto the medial cuneiform bone so as to maintain reduction of the midtarsal correction.
Once the tarsomidtarsal region has been corrected, it is necessary in a second operation to deal with deformity of the forefoot. The nature of the operation chosen depends on the suppleness of the part: if apart from the clawing of the toes the forefoot is normal with respect to metatarsal alignment, correction of the toes can be achieved by elongation of the shortened flexor and extensor tendons. The flexors should never be elongated without accompanying correction of the long extensor and extensor brevis tendons, because such isolated action will create an unbalanced situation leading to further digital displacement. Also the extensor tendon should never be transposed onto the heads of the metatarsal: this is a disastrous operation with respect to balance of the forefoot and totally unphysiological. Capsulotomy of the metatarsophalangeal joints allows complete correction of the axes of the parts, and good balance of the forefoot can be restored.
In a convex or simple triangular forefoot, enclavement of the shafts into the heads of the metatarsals together with correction of hallux valgus and of the claw toes is very effective. Both metatarsal displacements and clawing can be corrected accurately and this procedure is preferred to the bony procedures of the metatarsal bases described by Mau (1940) and Thys (1974b), which in a fixed cavus foot do not allow good correction of the claw toes or of the dislocations of the metatarsophalangeal joints.
In a square or Egyptian metatarsus with cavus, osteotomies of the first and fifth metatarsals are performed at the same time as correction of the claw toes.

14.2.2.2 Treatment of Diffuse Metatarsalgia in the Planovalgus Foot

As in the foregoing cavus foot, the two elements, correction of the general planovalgus posture and correction of the forefoot itself, must be integrated. The valgus posture of the heel results in metatarsalgia specifically from the region of the second metatarsal head. Frequently, discomfort in this region is the first clinical sign in the adult before the development of discomfort in the medial aspect of the tarsometatarsal level; in the child, however, pain in the region of the talus may be the first symptom. The development of the symptoms can be explained logically by the pronation of the calcaneum provoking relative weakness of peroneus longus and as a consequence an elevation of the first metatarsal, allowed by its greater mobility, resulting in deficient load bearing under the first metatarsal head; this leads to relative elongation of the second metatarsal. Excessive loading of the second metatarsal head in its more prominent position (cf. Chap. 5) is due to a prehensile insufficiency of the first metatarsal as emphasised by Courriades (1973b). The localised metatarsalgia in the region of the second metatarsal head comes from the joint and from distortion with protrusion of the condyle, as evidenced by the formation of callosity which is often heard and keratinised.
Treatment must begin with a trial of orthopaedic insole. If the planovalgus foot is of first or second degree, the insole must incorporate a wedge underneath the heel exerting a supinating effect and a support on the outer aspect of the metatarsus which will re-establish balance, especially in the adolescent or the young adult. In the adult and in the elderly, it is necessary to supplement these two elements by a plantar dome supporting the midtarsal region.

In second-degree planovalgus in a young adult, surgery is indicated if improvement is not achieved. Operations limiting movement of the subtalar joint are valuable in such cases because the midtarsal joint remains supple and correction of the valgus calcaneum re-establishes good midtarsal balance. The Grice operation (1952), in which an extra-articular arthrodesis blocking movement of the subtalar joint is performed, should be reserved for the paralytic foot.
Arthrorisis procedures through the sinus tarsi are valuable and a number of techniques have been described. The operation of Voutey (1970a, 1972), in which a bone block taken from the phalangeal base is used, is the preferred procedure. Alternatively, the technique of Valenti (1976a) may be employed. In the former, the valgus is corrected by external distraction, but the latter employs a prosthesis inserted between the head of the talus and the calcaneum. A screw or metallic prosthesis can risk collapse of the roof of the sinus tarsi later. Additionally, operation may be supplemented by an internal plantar wedge resection internal of the plantar talonavicular ligament accompanied by a transposition of tibialis posterior, comparable to the ligamentoplasty of the plantar calcaneonavicular ligament of Rodgvelle (1976, cited by Pisani (1979a) (see Cap. 16).
In the planovalgus foot, the choice of operative procedure depends on the location of the summit of the midtarsal angulation (see Chap. 16). Isolated correction of calcaneal pronation by fixation of the subtalar joint does not suffice to correct the sunken medial arch or the medial midtarsal angulation, which becomes fixed by osteoarticular hypertrophy in this region. Operation must correct the midtarsus and re-establish the midtarsal arch, thereby restoring general alignment of the forefoot.

14.2.3 *Displacement of Metatarsal Heads*

14.2.3.1 Congenital

Duddley Morton Metatarsalgia. As a consequence of divergence of the metatarsals, the second metatarsal supports the greatest load as evidenced by its thickened diaphyseal cortex. This can be accentuated by selective abnormal depression stemming from the second cuneiform-metatarsal joint.
Conservative treatment with an insole may be adequate. The insole may be of any of several types, designed according to the specific case: thus simple elevation of the middle metatarsal heads and a bar behind the metatarsal heads if the cavus foot is supple, perhaps accompanied by a pronating outer extension if there is a cavovarus component. A bar behind the metatarsal heads pronating the metatarsus with a supinating raise under the calcaneum is more appropriate for the cavovalgus foot, a stabilising insole for the planovalgus foot.
Specifically, in a valgus flat foot which is supple, the insole bears a supinating subcalcaneal wedge and a pronating external elevation for the metatarsus exerting pressure on a zone behind the middle metatarsal head; in the fixed valgus flat foot, the insole is made with a supinating wedge under the heel, a pronating wedge anteriorly under the outer metatarsals, a medial arch support and a central support behind the metatarsal heads. If the foot is balanced, all that is necessary is a retrocapital bar support behind the metatarsal heads.
In the irreducibly fixed case, Morton metatarsalgia becomes intolerable with intense burning pain. Central callosities or even a serous plantar bursa may develop, with periodic episodes of inflammation. Surgical treatment is now essential. The aim is to reduce the varus of the first metatarsal, correct any valgus of the fifth metatarsal and realign the axes of the second, third and fourth metatarsals according to the line of weight bearing described by Lelièvre (1952), thereby regularising the pressures under the five metatarsal heads. The realignment of the metatarsal heads must be correct in both horizontal and frontal planes. The procedure of choice may be the osteotomy described by Mau (1940) or that of Thys (1974b) (cf. Chap. 42) provided there is no displacement at the metatarsophalangeal joints due to capsulotendinous or cutaneous contracture. Alternatively, enclavement of the second, third and fourth metatarsal heads (cf. Chap. 42) is preferable when there are claw toe deformities which are fixed by tissue contractures. Both procedures will abolish the metatarsalgia.

Convex Forefoot. See Cap. 7.

Local Gigantism. One or several bones of the forefoot may be enlarged (Fig. 27.5 F, M). This will result in a forefoot augmented in volume, generally centred about hypertrophy in the metatarsophalangeal region; metatarsalgia due to disorders of weight bearing and local pressure, hypertrophy of metatarsophalangeal or phalangeal joints; hyperplasia of the soft tissues, especially on the plantar aspect of the foot, where callosity develops under the hypertrophied metatarsal head; and difficulty with footwear which restricts patients to unattractive models. The nature of local gigantism may be

macrometatarsia, macrodactyly or macromelia, in which the hypertrophy relates to a whole ray.
Conservative treatment has little to offer, while operative management has to be adapted to the particular case, always aiming to re-establish uniformity of loading of the forefoot by realignment of the metatarsal heads as necessary. In principle, surgical treatment consists of shortening of the phalanges and realignment and enclavement of one or more metatarsal hypertrophied heads with reduction of their volume, perhaps completed by metatarsal basal osteotomy or basal ostectomy as described by Thys (1974b). Soft tissue procedures may also be necessary - longitudinal division of the toe and resection of the soft parts and of the hypertrophied nail.

Longitudinal Reduction Deformities. These include a whole range of possibilities (see Chap. 27). Lobster-claw deformity comprises aplasia of the middle rays of the metatarsus with complete absence of the associated toes; only the outer and inner rays are developed. Various degrees may present: a phalanx may be absent, or the reduction may include a metatarsal and be accompanied by syndactyly or a synostosis of two metatarsals. There may be disparity in length or general hypertrophy of the middle metatarsals, in which case symptoms from local overloading will affect the first, fifth or perhaps both fourth and fifth metatarsal head regions. Painful callosities may develop as a result.
Operative treatment can correct digital displacements and selective equinus of the metatarsals. Special footwear adapted to the various displacements can be used in an effort to equalise pressure under the midtarsus and support the metatarsal heads, possibly incorporating a plantar dome or a bar behind the metatarsal heads. In the situation where five metatarsals are present and the reduction deformity affects the middle toes, there may be relative lengthening of the middle metatarsals, possibly hypertrophic. Realignment of these by enclavement or by shortening at the metatarsal base will create a new line of loading of the metatarsal heads, thereby equalising pressure.

14.2.3.2 Acquired Mechanical Disorders

There are five basic types of acquired mechanical disorders.

Displacement of Anterior Transverse Arch. This is seen in the simple convex and triangular forefeet, the cavus forefoot, and the relative shortening of the first ray in hallux valgus (see Chaps. 6-9, 18).

Inflammatory Conditions. In general these are rheumatoid in type, manifested by development of pain in one or more joints progressively. Women are affected more often than men. The actual source of pain is frequently complex, relating to abnormal loading, displacements at the metatarsophalangeal joints, atrophy of the soft tissues of the ball of the foot and thickening of the skin. Joint pains may be due to dislocation, destruction of the articular surface and fibrosis of the metatarsophalangeal joints secondary to the evolving inflammatory process. Progressive deformation of the joint surfaces together with fibrous contracture produces complicated displacements. Characteristically, the inflammatory pain results in local heat, stiffness, pain first thing in the morning and swelling of the joints with effusions and oedema. Rheumatoid arthritis, psoriatic arthritis and gout present with similar features. Florid deformities, including hallux valgus, claw toes, windswept configuration of the lesser toes in valgus and more irregular disturbances, may be seen. Final destruction is due to progressive invasion of the epiphyses by hypertrophied synovial reaction, deformity of the forefoot from the ligamentous and tendinous contractures, and fibrous ankylosis.
The diagnosis having been confirmed, appropriate medical treatment underlies any surgical measures employed. Operation as necessary should be delayed until control of the systemic condition as evidenced by improvement of the erythrocyte sedimentation rate. During this period, conservative measures are valuable. From the outset, an insole prepared carefully according to the individual case will give great relief to the sensitive foot. The most useful type is a monoblock supporting the midtarsal region completed by a bar behind the metatarsal heads, with excavations accurately situated underneath the sensitive skin thickenings perhaps aided by pads in front of the metatarsal heads. Correction by the insole of valgus or varus in the tarsal region should be prudent, because undue stress on the sensitive joints will only aggravate symptoms. The insole should be made of supple material like cork or India rubber lined with compliant felt, rubber or Bullatex, the whole supported on a supple copper plate (see Chap. 40).
Surgical treatment may involve from the outset synovectomy of as many joints as necessary. Later, the type of surgery selected will depend largely on the stage of osteocartilaginous destruction. It is unusual for patients to be referred before this stage is

reached but there are examples of misaligned metatarsophalangeal joints which are appropriate for realignment by an enclavement procedure. Irreversible destruction of a metatarsal head, or, in the burned-out case, fixed deformities and severe symptoms constitute indications for surgical measures designed specifically to restore regular pressure under the five metatarsal heads. The procedures may be complex, involving a realignment as described by Lelièvre (1952) or the use of interposition cup prostheses, made necessary by lysis of the distal end of the metatarsals which renders impossible any enclavement procedure. Plastic procedures including the skin, tendons and joint capsules require accurate execution if the four outer metatarsophalangeal joints are to be balanced correctly; there is no place for isolated procedures on joints unless this measure can be achieved (see Chap. 36).

Infections. Tuberculous arthritis of a metatarsophalangeal joint may not be recognised for some time, and initial treatment may be for non-specific arthritis. Periodic inflammation with abscess and sinus formation pursues a chronic course, and it is unusual for the diagnosis to be made before suppuration occurs. Radiology exhibits erosion and loss of joint space with marked local patchy osteoporosis. Tuberculosis is not specifically responsible for these appearances. Treatment comprises general antituberculous therapy, which once instituted allows resection of the infected joint. Other specific infections include *Staphylococcus aureus,* gonorrhoea and pneumococcal arthritis.

Iatrogenic Conditions. Surgical intervention may have been poorly chosen with respect to the causal deformity or may have been complicated by infection. Pain may be due to arthrosis or to contractures at the metatarsophalangeal joints associated with recurring displacements. Insufficiency of the first ray may be due to overgenerous resection in amputation of the head of the metatarsal (Mayo 1908). It should be recognised that *any* surgical procedure can lead to disordered alignment of the metatarsal heads (see also Chap. 25).

Trauma. Fracture of the metatarsal shafts or of the epiphyseal region and fatigue fracture of Deutschländer (1921) are typical causes of pain in the forefoot. Treatment is by relief of weight bearing, later supplemented with support from an elastic bandage together with physiotherapy. The overuse of the foot which leads to fatigue fracture may be evidenced later by the appearance of pseudarthrosis on X-rays. The choice of surgery is specific to the nature of the injury (Chap. 22).

14.2.4 Functional Disorders

14.2.4.1 Ligamentous Laxity

Longitudinal ligamentous laxity results in a pes cavus or cavovalgus deformity. A comparable laxity may exist transversely across the tarsometatarsal joint line.

Metatarsalgias from *longitudinal laxity.* are associated with displacements in the frontal and horizontal planes of the zone of metatarsal loading largely on account of hypermobility of the first ray (Courriades 1971). This hypermobility can entail an elevation of the great metatarsal and favours the appearance of a valgus flat foot or a cavovalgus foot with general suppleness (cf. Chap. 5.1.3). Metatarsalgias due to overloading of the central part of the ball of the foot have been discussed already. These relate predominantly to the condyles of the second and third metatarsal heads and cause discomfort of a lancing, tense quality and then a burning sensation at the site of development of serous bursitis with or without callosities. Frequently, there is frontal protrusion of the second and third metatarsal heads, alone in a valgus flat foot or with additional plantar direction in the cavovalgus foot. Initially, the situation will be corrected by the use of an orthopaedic insole comprising a bar behind the metatarsal heads with a pronating wedge on the outer part of the metatarsus associated with a supinating wedge under the calcaneum when the latter is associated with a cavovalgus deformity. The insole for a planovalgus foot constitutes a raise under the inner aspect of the heel and another under the outer aspect of the metatarsal region together with a central bar behind the middle three metatarsal heads. Additionally, an arch support under the midtarsal region may be advantageous. Surgery is indicated when the insole is ineffective, and has two aims. (a) The valgus posture of the calcaneum must be corrected by means of release of the subtalar joint or by cuneiform resection of the talonavicular ligament accompanied by anterior transposition of the tibialis anterior insertion onto the first cuneiform bone. If during operation correction of the valgus calcaneum appears insufficient, extra-articular curvilinear osteotomy in the midtarsus may be completed by release of the subtalar joint and anterior transposition of tibialis anterior. (b) The heads of the middle metatarsals must be realigned, perhaps by basal osteotomies

(Thys 1974b) or by enclavement of the second, third and fourth metatarsals.

Laxity of Tarsometatarsal Joint. This may result in metatarsalgia due to transverse instability in the talus foot. Pain is located over the head of the first metatarsal and over the heads of the fourth and fifth metatarsals. Unstable skin thickening occurs, almost always centred on a plantar keratoma underneath the sesamoids of the first metatarsophalangeal joint and the fourth and fifth metatarsophalangeal joints or, in the presence of a triangular forefoot, under each of the metatarsal heads. Pains are of a pricking type, like having a stone in the shoe. They appear as soon as the foot is loaded in the plantigrade posture and are exacerbated and rendered intolerable during walking, which may become impossible. Transverse instability of the cavus foot may be associated with a valgus or varus posture of the heel. The planovalgus configuration may be associated with a triangular forefoot, while a cavovalgus foot is found with a convex triangular forefoot. The basic deformity occurs at the tarsometatarsal joints (cf. Chap. 5.1.3). In the planovalgus situation, metatarsalgias are the consequences of the triangular flat foot or the Locke syndrome. The metatarsals diverge, especially the first, which is in varus, and the fifth, in valgus. These two extreme pillars, already hypermobile, increase their prehensile action and induce callus formation over their medial and lateral aspects in addition to the specific skin thickenings under the three central metatarsals.
Initial treatment is with an insole of the planovalgus pattern (an internal dome, a supinating wedge, an anterior pronating wedge and a retrocapital bar), but if this conservative measure does not improve symptoms, operative treatment to correct the planovalgus and the triangular forefoot becomes necessary.
In the cavovalgus foot, medial angulation at the midtarsal region augments the frontal anterior convexity of the Lisfranc joint line and leads to the formation of a round triangular forefoot. Again, an insole with a retrocapital bar, an external metatarsal pronating corner and a supinating corner under the calcaneum should be tried first, otherwise operative treatment as for the round triangular forefoot syndrome is necessary.
A mobile cavus foot, balanced initially, may develop a valgus or varus deformity resisted by the prehensile action of the first and fifth metatarsals. As the rigidity of the load-bearing area of the central metatarsal heads increases progressively, in addition to the longitudinal cavus, hypermobility and prehensile plantarflexion of the first and fifth metatarsal pillars of the foot diminish. At the same time, the transverse plantar concavity of the Lisfranc joint line increases while the frontal anterior convexity diminishes. The consequence of these deformities is a tendency for the first and fifth metatarsals to converge in a plantar direction, producing a cavus forefoot. In the absence of successful management with an insole, this can develop into a cavovarus foot. The appearance is typical, with skin thickenings and keratoma formation under the fifth metatarsal head together with a progressive painful cavovarus deformity. At first, the condition may be relieved by an insole incorporating a retrocapital bar completed in the presence of a general varus of the foot by a pronating band externally. This distributes loading of the foot more effectively, and lowers the plantar arch while blocking the posture of the heel. Some of the shearing in an anteroposterior direction is impeded at the level of the metatarsal heads. Martorell Martorell (1963) incorporates a subdigital bar which allows even greater efficacy in this respect. Surgery is indicated in the event of failure of conservative measures and must include correction of the longitudinal imbalance and of the forefoot condition itself.

14.2.4.2 Disordered Muscular Control

Two patterns may be recognised:

- Insufficiency of action of peroneus longus, tibialis anterior and tibialis posterior leads to a planovalgus posture allowed by the increased mobility of the first ray, the metatarsal becoming elevated.
- Hypertonus of triceps surae and flexor digitorum longus associated with weakness of the short muscles of the foot leads to a cavovarus deformity.

The treatment is initially conservative and comprises muscle strengthening and re-educational exercises, an orthopaedic insole and perhaps elongation of contracted tendons.
The metatarsalgias produced in these cases are due to overloading under the second and third metatarsal heads in the case of the planovalgus foot, under the outer metatarsal heads in the case of the cavovarus variety.

14.2.4.3 *Abnormalities of Ankle Joint*

Abnormalities of the ankle may lead to metatarsalgia in the following circumstances:

- Limitation of dorsiflexion of the foot due to hypertonia or contraction of the muscles of the posterior compartment of the leg.
- Equinus posture of the talus due to arthrosis or a fixed arthrodesis in a poor position.
- Pseudarthrosis after fracture of the malleoli.
- Hypertrophy of the antero-external portion of the articular surface of the talus, as may occur in congenital talipes equinovarus or following trauma. This hypertrophy prevents the talus entering the mortice fully, so impeding dorsiflexion.

The metatarsalgias secondary to disorders in the region of the ankle result in overloading of the metatarsal heads secondary to an equinus posture and are accompanied by callus formation in various places, usually towards the outer side of the foot. The resilience afforded by the midtarsal joints is not sufficient to compensate for the loss of dorsiflexion during walking.

Except in cases involving hypertrophy of the antero-external part of the articular surface of the talus, which always requires surgery, metatarsalgias secondary to abnormal posture imposed by the ankle may respond to an insole. A simple retrocapital bar is usually insufficient, except for very mild degrees of plantarflexion of the foot. A physiological insole of the monoblock type incorporating a retrocapital bar and perhaps a digital bar, as described by Martorell Martorell (1963), is likely to be more effective. This supportive measure, associated with appropriate shoes, is especially appropriate for metatarsalgia related to a stiff ankle following either progressive arthrosis or arthrodesis. However, it will be useless for a foot fixed in equinus, where revision of the ankle posture is necessary. If there is a malunion in the region of the ankle joint producing a valgus or varus component, the same type of insole associated with a pronating band on the outer side or a supinating wedge under the heel can allay the painful metatarsalgia to some extent. More commonly, however, it is desirable to proceed to operative treatment, osteotomy of the malunion being performed so as to re-establish the normal transverse axis of the ankle and facilitate the correct rolling action of the forefoot during gait.

Arthrosis of the ankle joint may respond to conservative measures, otherwise operative treatment is necessary: arthrodesis, soft tissue release in cases where the articular surfaces are intact, osteotomy as described by H. Judet (1976) or ankle arthroplasty may be employed.

With regard to ankle arthroplasty, Viladot (1976c), Buchholz et al. (1973), Lord and Marotte (1979) and Regnauld and Saudreau (1978) have described prostheses. Personal experience indicates that results are imperfect in terms of duration, function and control of pain. Failure appears to relate to the thickness of the prosthesis, which prevents freedom of motion by causing loss of play of the talus in the mortice, associated with the complex effects of tightening and separation of the malleoli and abduction and adduction of the body of the talus. Originally, I utilised a metal prosthesis in two parts mated by a central groove, which allowed good mobility but caused pain. I abandoned this in 1975 in favour of a thin (1-mm) interpositional prosthesis between the surfaces of the talus and tibia, inserted after the joint surfaces have been cleared of cartilage debris and exostoses trimmed. It is still too early to judge the long-term efficacy of this prosthesis, but the minimum amount of bony resection entailed enables a salvage arthrodesis to be performed without undue shortening. The operation is easy, but postoperative re-education must be intensive and lasts at least 6 months.

According to Lecoeur (1938), prosthetic replacement of the ankle allows recovery of walking after 4 weeks and a functional mobility compatible with a normal rolling step. Nevertheless, discomfort is common and the inferior tibiofibular joint line may become tight. Lelièvre (1968a) performed several arthroplasties of the ankle joint involving resection of a significant amount of the tibia without any interpositional prosthesis and had a good result in one case; however, while the idea may seem satisfactory, the result was painful for a long time and necessitated a very long period of re-education.

In view of the uncertainties of ankle arthroplasty, whenever articular cartilage remains I prefer to perform a release of the ankle joint and of the inferior tibiofibular joint together with rebalancing of tendons and ligaments.

The metatarsalgias produced by contraction or hypertonia of the posterior calf muscles can be relieved by elongation of these structures, but afterwards an insole should be used permanently so as to avoid recurrence of these tendinous contractures.

14.2.4.4 *Overloading of Metatarsal Heads*

Constitutional factors like obesity or overactivity can result in discomfort in the foot, chiefly in the

tarsometatarsal region and under the metatarsal heads. Workers who stand continuously are prone to this overloading.
Treatment consists partly of the use of an orthopaedic insole of the monoblock type supporting the midtarsal region, with a retro- or subcapital metatarsal support with a pronating wedge or a supinating wedge at the heel depending on whether there is a varus or valgus posture. Obvious etiologies may indicate the need for dietary weight loss or re-education in work habits.

14.2.4.5 Metatarsalgia from High-Heeled Shoes

While much has been said on this subject, it must be recognised that in 75% of normal feet in women with balanced precavus posture, lifelong wearing of heels 4–5 cm high may be tolerated without the appearance of further deformity or displacement leading to metatarsalgia. When normal, the feet adapt precisely to shoes in which the arch has a physiological curvature appropriate to the height of the heel. In shoes of good quality, most of the loading can be taken by the tarsus, and it is important that the arch of the shoe should be reinforced corresponding to that of the foot. This is a matter of education in the choice of shoes with heels. The majority of female patients wear poor shoes, with a high heel of which the arch forms a disastrous incline, and it is not surprising that metatarsalgia can result from overloading of the forefoot. In these instances the high heel must be avoided and an adapted shoe with a heel not exceeding 4 cm will ameliorate the discomforts, provided the foot has remained supple and there is no metatarsal or midtarsal deformity. In addition to the height of the heel, the shoe should be modified by a central support in the retrocapital area, thereby rebalancing the first and fifth metatarsals, and by a metatarsal support behind the heads in the precavus type of foot if it is supple and well balanced. When there is a tendency to varus posture, a pronating external raise should be placed under the metatarsal heads (Berthet and Charry 1945), perhaps under the outer part of the shoe in the region of the base of the fifth metatarsal, so as to suppress a tendency to varus and rebalance the forefoot.
Midtarsal and metatarsal irreducible deformities can be treated initially by the monoblock insole with an internal dome in the midtarsal region, a retrocapital bar or a retro- and subcapital bar matching those metatarsal condyles which are associated with painful keratoses. In addition, a pronating raise or a supinating stabilisation of the tarsus can be added if there exists a varus or valgus deformity. Surgical treatment becomes occasionally necessary. This is the case from painful irreducible deformity of the midtarsal regions and in the metatarsus of the young adult. Each case is individual and usually comprises a midtarsal correction and a reconstitution of the forefoot.

14.2.5 Medical Causes

Metatarsalgias from medical causes usually present as one symptom of the general illness. They may be called plantalgias, and are not accompanied by structural displacements except in the case of a neurological disorder. They include:

- Vascular disease (arteritis, Raynaud's phenomenon, acrocyanosis, erythromelalgia, frostbite, erythema pernio and gangrene)
- Neurological conditions (spina bifida, polyneuritis, hemiplegia, syringomyelia, spastic paralysis, parkinsonism, Friedreich's ataxia and dystrophia myotonica)
- Cutaneous conditions (scleroderma, hyperhidrosis, senile atrophy of the weight-bearing tissues and heat rash)

Treatment is for the causal condition, supplemented perhaps by an insole, and chiropody. Occasionally surgical treatment is indicated, as in the case of hemiplegia, spastic paralysis or fixed cavus deformity from neurological involvement.

14.3 Localised Metatarsalgia

In contradistinction to diffuse metatarsalgia, localised metatarsalgia relates to a specific condyle, intercapital space, metatarsal shaft or metatarsophalangeal joint.

14.3.1 Clinical Presentation

The character of the pain depends on the cause and may relate to pressure under the metatarsal heads or nerve compression, or be associated with arthrosis, restricted movement and dislocations of joints from various causes. The metatarsals are individual with respect to their function in the foot. There are certain features in common with the diffuse metatarsalgias described earlier. For example, discomfort is exaggerated by standing, walking, sport and certain types of work, and may be relieved to various extents by rest and prosthetic treatment. The metatarsalgia becomes progressively irreversible, due to bony displacements or damage to the associated joints. Treatment depends upon which metatarsal is involved. For each metatarsal, individual etiologies can be distinguished.

14.3.2 Congenital

Hypertrophy in Length (Macropodia and Macromelia). Any metatarsal head can become selectively overloaded in the event of disproportional length (see Chap. 27).

Metatarsal Aplasia (Simple Aplasia and Reduction Deformities). This condition involves the middle part of the metatarsal. It may occassionally be acquired as a result of ill-chosen excision of the head of a middle metatarsal to deal with a painful callosity, leading inevitably to metatarsalgias from overloading of the adjacent metatarsal heads (see Chap. 27).

Syndactyly. This produces metatarsalgia only in the presence of a supernumerary metatarsal.

14.3.3 Acquired

14.3.3.1 Joint Disorders

Localised metatarsalgia can result from hallux valgus, hallux rigidus, Köhler's epiphysitis, tuberculous arthritis, rheumatoid arthritis, metabolic conditions associated with perforating ulcer or iatrogenic arthrosis following amputation of a metatarsal head (Mayo 1908), and can occur after metatarsophalangeal arthroplasty (Keller 1904; Hohmann 1951).

14.3.3.2 Osseous Disorders

Selective Equinus of a Metatarsal. This condition particularly involves the second, third or fourth metatarsal.

Conditions Involving First Metatarsal. Equinus posture, sesamoid hypertrophy, prominence of the sesamoids, sesamoiditis, exostosis and Renander's disease [Renander 1924, citet by Hohmann (1951), Natiello (1971) and Denis (1975a)] can all lead to localised metatarsalgia.

Second Metatarsal Syndrome. This specific metatarsalgia localised to the second metatarsal head is often the first sign of the onset of pes planus. The cause is primarily a pronation of the calcaneum which provokes hypotonia of peroneus longus, leading to supination of the forefoot and resulting in insufficiency of power of depression of the first metatarsal head. The loss of effective load bearing of the first metatarsal leads to distortion of the forefoot and overloading at the second metatarsal head. The matter is discussed more fully in Chap. 16.

Metatarsalgia involving the second metatarsal head often appears at the same time as hallux valgus. Broadening of the forefoot associated with increased varus of the first metatarsal provokes rupture of the zone of loading under the metatarsal heads, particularly affecting the second ray. Correction of the hallux valgus and basal osteotomy of the second metatarsal controls this localised overloading.

Selective overloading of the third and fourth metatarsal heads relates to specific equinus or protrusion of these metatarsals and is often related to imbalance of the tarsus supervening on a precavus or cavus foot. Basal osteotomy of the metatarsals concerned re-establishes normal distribution of loading.

14.3.3.3 Traumatic Metatarsalgia

This includes metatarsalgias from sprains, dislocations, and fractures.

14.4 Subcutaneous Soft Tissue Metatarsaliga

1.4.1 Hygroma

A hygroma (a serous bursa) can develop under the plantar aspect of a metatarsal head. In the middle three metatarsals the condition is related to equinus posture, whereas on the first metatarsal head it can be associated with hallux valgus or be located on the dorsal aspect relative to a hallux flexus or hallux rigidus. On the fifth metatarsal head it may be on the lateral aspect and associated with valgus angulation (tailor's bunion). Contracture of an associated tendon can lead to irritation from pressure at the free border of the toecap of a shoe.

These conditions are provoked by compression of the subcutaneous tissue, either extrinsic, commonly from the hard sole or the upper of a shoe, or intrinsic, associated with a metatarsal condyle, a tendon, hypertrophied sesamoids or a fixed claw toe. The hygroma comprises a rounded swelling bulging under the skin, sometimes multilocular, and varying in tension. The pain produced is burning, tight, tense or lancing in character. Intermittent at first, it becomes continuous when the more florid signs of inflammation are seen. It is aggravated by standing, walking or other activity.

Treatment comprises relief of the compression, e.g. by correction of a prominent condyle, cure of hallux valgus or fifth metatarsal valgus, correction of a specific equinus deformity of a metatarsal, removal or correction of an abnormal position of a sesamoid, resection of the dorsal exostosis found in hallux rigidus, or elongation of a tendon which as a result of bowstringing is producing painful pressure against the shoe upper.

14.4.2 Articular Synovial Cyst

Cysts of this type commonly produce compression of a neurovascular bundle due to generalised increase in volume of the forefoot. The commonest site is between the first and second metatarsals, whence the irradiation of pain, with perhaps vascular features, will be typical. The cyst is usually multilocular roughly elongated, and occupies most of the interspace, pushing aside the neurovascular bundle. It may be prominent on both dorsal and plantar aspects, the main bulk lying proximal to the metatarsal heads.

Involvement of the second intermetatarsal space is analogous to that in Morton's syndrome (1876).

14.4.3 Intermetatarsal Syndrome of Claustre

This syndrome (Claustre et al. 1983) is a local metatarsalgia without irradiation into the toes which is due to local inflammation. It is associated with shortness of the first ray. Symptoms may be relieved by local infiltration with a corticosteroid.

14.4.4 Morton's Neuroma

For information on this condition (Morton 1876) see Chap. 35.

14.4.5 Neoplasm

Development is usually slow, without inflammation, and in the case of malignancy a bosselated, indurated swelling is characteristic. Diagnosis is by operative exploration and histological examination.

14.5 Cutaneous Metatarsalgia

14.5.1 Callus

Callus formation is regularly provoked by overloading of the skin from abnormal prominence of some osseous structure. The cornified mass of tissue may develop in a variety of ways: for example, those under the second to fourth metatarsal heads are frequently localised and convex, rounded or oval, whereas overlying an exostosis on the medial aspect of the first metatarsal head or on the outer aspect of the fifth metatarsal head, they may reach 1–2 cm in diameter.

A *keratoma* is a small lesion varying from 1 to 10 mm in circumference. It is constituted by an avascular mass of white or dirty-yellow tissue limited by a clearer halo circumferentially, being conical in general form. It penetrates into the dermis and causes a particular type of pain due to involvement of the sensitive nerve filaments located there. It is painful on direct pressure or on compression during walking and standing. Located under a metatarsal condyle or sesamoid, it may be secondary to some disturbance of equilibrium of the foot. Treatment is either by complete excision followed by suture, or by swinging of a small skin flap after removal of the prominent base of the metatarsal concerned.

Another type of lesion is the *miliary corn*, an avascular mass about 1 mm in diameter arising from a blocked sweat gland. It may be isolated, or occur in groups elongated longitudinally under an intercapital space. Treatment is usually by chiropody, although exceptionally surgical curettage or excision by suture is necessary.

14.5.2 Verruca

A verruca is a papilloma which arises in the epidermis and never invades the dermis (Fig. 17.5 A–H). It is a contagious viral infection, and there is a risk of frequent recrudescence if treatment is incomplete and/or not followed by adequate precautions. The lesion involves nerve filaments, which explains its particular tenderness, most frequently noticeable first thing in the morning and aggravated by walking or lateral compression. It tends to be covered superficially by surrounding cornified epidermis. When this has been removed, the verruca presents as a regular, rounded or oval mass well defined by a clearer surrounding halo which is softer in consistency. The surface may be villous in appearance, greyish or yellowish-white in colour, translucent and marked by tiny brown flecks which correspond to hypertrophied papillae and become more apparent after application of silver nitrate alcohol-soaked cotton wool.

Initial therapy is medical and is successful in 95% of cases after 3–5 weeks. The following treatment is recommended: Friction of the verruca, morning and evening, with cotton wool soaked in 90% alcohol, compresses three times a day with magnesium chloride, and oral administration of two drops of tincture of thuya in a little water. The verruca usually becomes dark brown, dries and falls off without leaving any scar. Thereafter, in order to avoid recurrence, the patient should replace the insole of a contaminated shoe with sheepskin.

If medical treatment fails, more vigorous chiropody, comprising abrasion, cauterisation with silver nitrate or hydrochloric acid and subsequent dressing with Oxyplastine, may be effective.

As a final resort, electrocoagulation should be employed. Excision and suture should be avoided because of the risk of a keratotic scar on the plantar aspect of the foot, which may be painful. The electrocoagulation should be performed under local anaesthesia when only one or a few papillomas are present, general anaesthesia if they are numerous. In order to avoid scarring of the skin, which may be painful, the subjacent dermis should be spared, the electrocoagulation being confined to the clear circumferential halo around the papilloma. If the dermis is injured, the likely result is a painful scar which may require excision followed by a plastic skin procedure in order to cover the raw area. Alternatively, the thick margins of cornified shin can be trimmed with a scalpel under local anaesthesia; after careful curettage (avoiding the dermis), a dressing of tulle gras and cotton wool should be applied. The dressing should be changed after 1 day and thereafter twice a week until healing is complete. During this period, weight bearing on the affected area should not be allowed.

14.5.3 Perforating Plantar Ulcer

Perforating plantar ulcer is described in Chap. 31.

14.5.4 Plantar Fistula

A plantar fistula can result either from a foreign body embedded in the plantar tissues or from abnormality of subjacent bone.

14.5.5 Radiodermatitis

Radiodermatitis was relatively frequent 30 years ago due to the widespread use of radiotherapy for inflammatory conditions. Lelièvre (1959) detailed 200 cases. Verruca, corns and keratoma taken for papilloma were treated in this way, particularly on the plantar aspect of the foot, and decreased vascularity or frank ischaemia subsequently developed at sites of loading. Lelièvre divided radiodermatitis into *acute* (presenting as a simple erythema, occurring during anti-inflammatory radiotherapy under the heel or developing as a little star-shaped ulcer involving the dermis) and *chronic* (presenting as sclerosis, necrosis or exceptionally with malignant change). Nowadays, the rarity of the lesion is due to prudence in the use of radiotherapy on the plantar aspect of the foot, an improved understanding of the limits of use of this treatment for the above lesions, and a better diagnosis of them. In general, radiotherapy in the foot is avoided. Acute radiodermatitis is very rare, but some chronic lesions may still be met (Fig. 14.1).

Radiosclerosis is a painful keratotic condition involving the dermis and epidermis. The lesion may be round, pale yellow or pink, from a few millimetres to a centimetre across, of varying thickness and induration, sometimes linear and irregular, sometimes star-shaped, with typical scarred points surrounded by a yellowish-pink or haemorrhagic-appearing area. Radiosclerosis develops in scar tissue in an area of loading a number of years after treatment by irradiation.

Thus a metatarsal condyle, a sesamoid, the base of the fifth metatarsal or the plantar aspect or sides of the heel may be involved (Fig. 14.1).

Radionecrosis results in frank ulceration of a specific type which differs in character from the classic perforation ulcer described by Nélaton (1851). The ulcer is of variable size, most frequently small (5–10 mm in diameter), and exceptionally extended. It is surrounded by flat margins which are not raised but delineate a small central crater with a pale-grey, moist, purulent floor (Fig. 14.1).

Three signs characterise radiosclerosis and radionecrosis: (a) permanent, localised, intense, burning or gnawing pain, impeding all contact with the ground; (b) refractory healing; and (c) gradual ex-

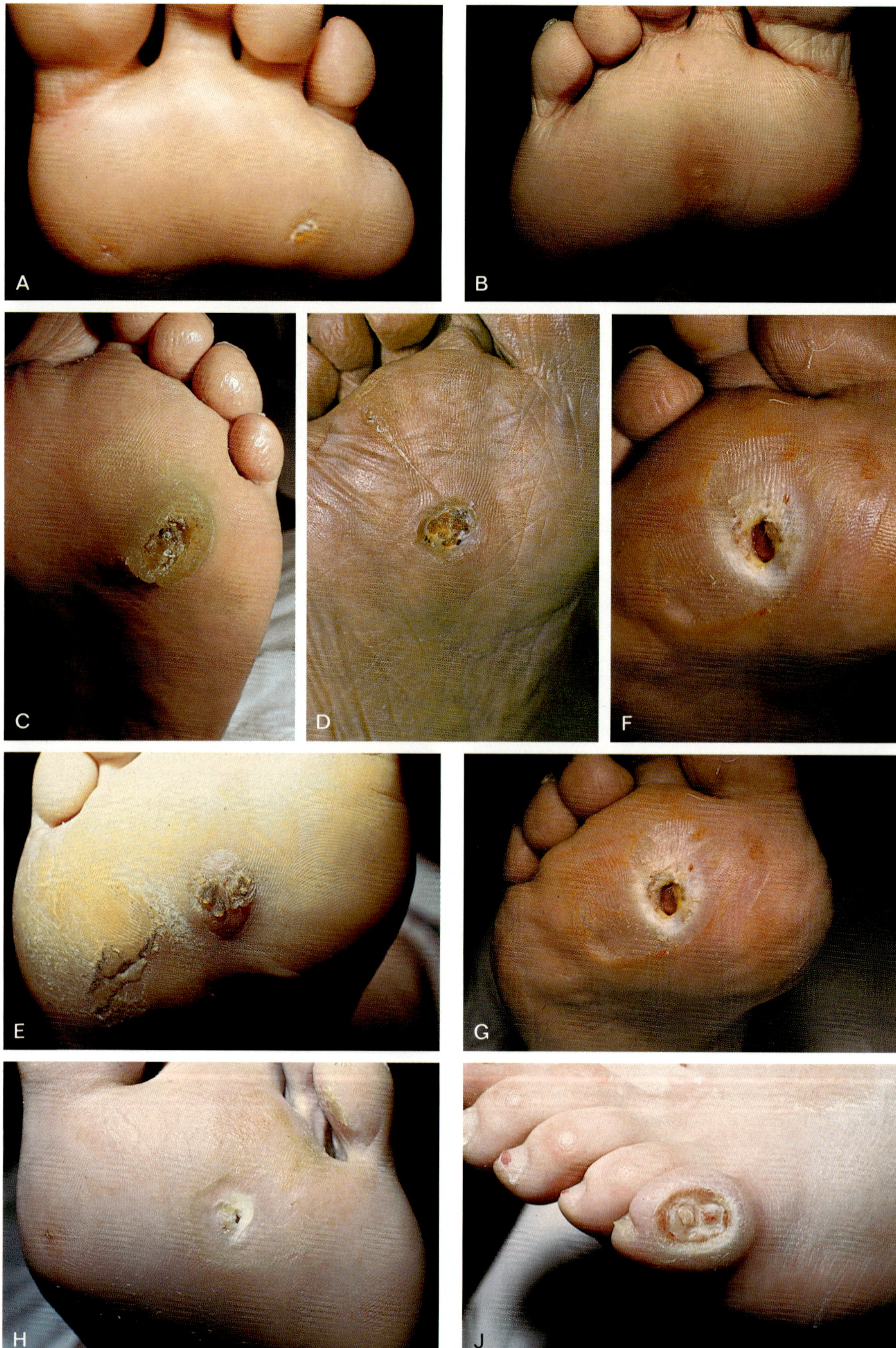
A
B
C
D
F
E
G
H
J

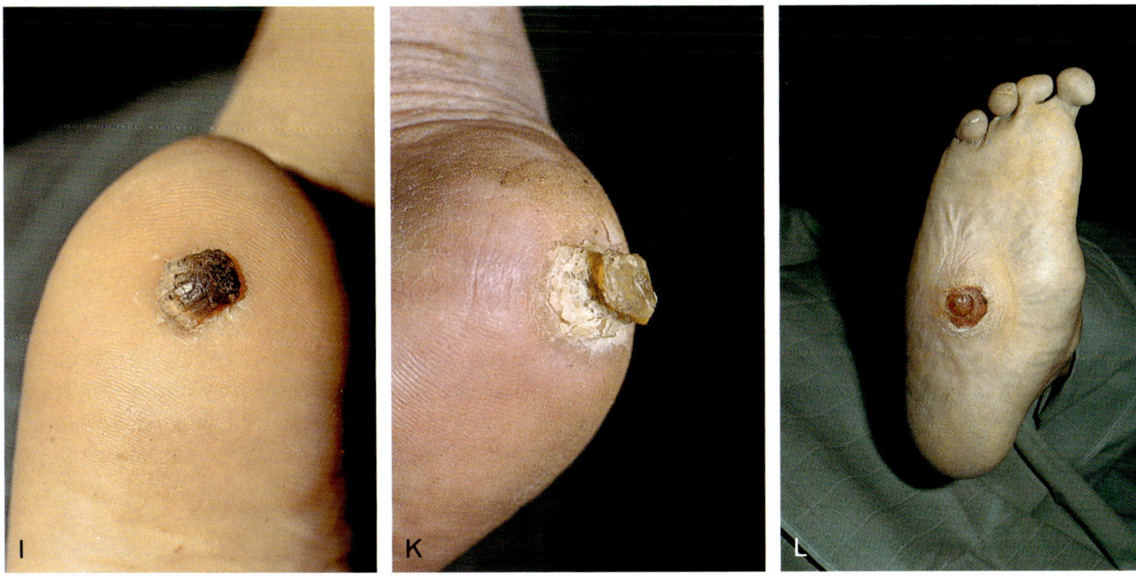

◁ **Fig. 14.1 A–L.** Radiosclerosis, radionecrosis and plantar radiodermatitis. **A–D** Radiosclerosis. **E–H** Radionecrosis. **I–L** Radiodermatits

tension both in depth and size. The lesions of the dermis extending into the subcutaneous tissue are deceptively large compared with the appearance of ulcer. For this reason, local excision, even with plastic procedures, may not succeed in eradicating the necrotic tissue completely.

Treatment. Wide excision of the lesion is necessary, followed by appropriate plastic procedures to achieve cover. There should then be correction of any abnormality of local overloading, such as equinus of a metatarsal, prominence of a sesamoid or correction of a forefoot syndrome. A valgus or varus foot should be rebalanced by the use of appropriate insoles and, in the case of the heel, the area concerned should be spared by means of a compensating insole. Prolonged relief of weight bearing is necessary, together with ancillary vasodilators, local massage and the permanent use of a compliant well-fitted insole.

15 Pes Cavus

The term cavus refers to an increased concavity or hollowness of the plantar longitudinal arch and the transverse arch located in the tarsometatarsal region, as well as under the metatarsal heads. In this chapter, *transverse* cavus relates to the tarsometatarsal region, *longitudinal* cavus can refer to the whole arch or its medial or lateral margins, while the term *forefoot* cavus describes a particular configuration of the metatarsal heads (cf. Chap. 9). Cavus may be accompanied by a coronal (transverse) imbalance of the foot into *valgus* or *varus*. Many structural combinations occur, and the etiology is diverse. The following broad classification is convenient for descriptive purposes both from the point of view of origin and treatment:

- Physiological pes cavus
- Idiopathic acquired pes cavus in infancy or adulthood
- Neurological pes cavus due to hypertonia or spasticity
- Pes equinocavus in specific neurological conditions

It should be stated from the outset that the infantile and adolescent forms are only exceptionally treated by surgery before the age of 18 years, whereas, in contrast, the established adult forms constitute a strong indication for operation. The use of an orthosis, or insole, has a place in the mobile foot and is a complement to surgery.

15.1 General Considerations

Whatever the type or stage of the cavus foot, certain general characteristics are present (Fig. 15.1).

15.1.1 Longitudinal Cavus

Longitudinal cavus varies in general form, orientation, suppleness and reducibility. In the physiological cavus foot, the longitudinal arch is relatively flaccid and balanced. In the fixed idiopathic cavus foot, the contraction relates mostly to the midtarsus, increasing the angles of declination of all the metatarsals but having less effect on the posture of the calcaneum; this pattern is unstable, tending to go into either valgus or varus disbalance (Fig. 15.2). In the neurological cavus foot, muscle imbalance determines the degree of equinus of the metatarsus with or without change of the calcaneal posture; thus in posterior paralysis, the cavus arises from change in position of the calcaneum and by overunbalanced action of the intrinsic muscles. The spastic cavus variety tends to affect both the

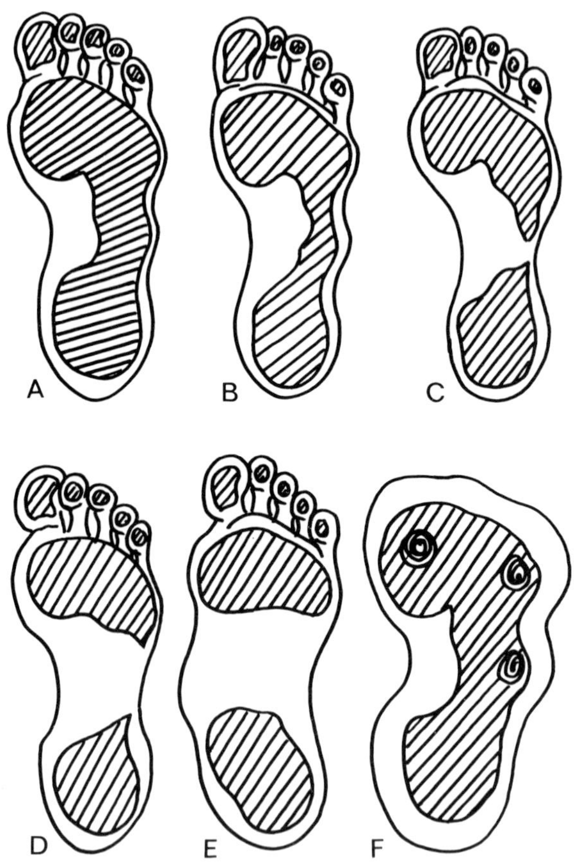

Fig. 15.1 A–F. Loading in various degrees of pes cavus. **A** Normal foot for comparison. **B** First-degree cavus. **C** Second-degree cavus. **D** Balanced third-degree cavus. **E** Pes cavovalgus. **F** Pes cavovarus

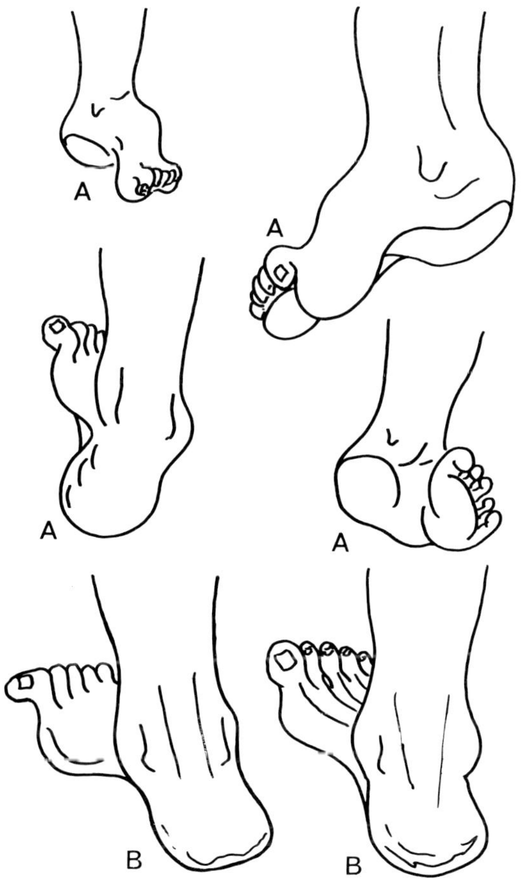

Fig. 15.2. **A** A cavovarus foot and **B** a cavovalgus foot viewed from various angles

downward angle of the metatarsus as well as the calcaneal inclination both of which can become very augmented. The equinocavus foot, as its name indicates, is one in which a general equinus of the whole foot prevails and the cavus is really secondary.

15.1.2 Dorsal Longitudinal Arch

The summit of the arch as seen from its dorsal aspect varies in position, although hard and fast rules cannot be made. In the idiopathic fixed cavus foot it may be at the navicular, cuneiform, or tarsometatarsal joint line. In a hypertonic neurological cavus foot, it is likely to be at the tarsometatarsal joint line, but in the spastic neurological type it lies more posteriorly, at the navicular. The talonavicular joint is more likely to be the summit in the direct equinocavus foot or in posterior paralysis.

15.1.3 Disordered Loading of Forefoot and Hindfoot

Lelièvre (1952) ascertained the degree of loss of congruent loading normally present between the heel and the ball of the foot by measurement of the angle of a tangent to the plantar surfaces of these parts. While this gives an appreciation of the extent of disturbance, it must be recognised that it is the degree of suppleness and correctability of the cavus, rather than its shape, which will determine the onset of symptoms. The supple cavus foot is compliant and absorbs the shock of loading. It is around appreciation of these facts that choice of conservative or operative treatment revolves.

15.1.4 Transverse Displacement

In addition to the sagittal or longitudinal displacement described, the foot may go into varus or valgus. This component may relate to the calcaneum, with augmentation or diminution of the angle of declination of the neck of the talus. In the midtarsus, varus results in lowering and supination of the cuboid-fifth metatarsal ensemble and elevation and inversion of the nvaiculocuneiform mass, and valgus with angulation at the talonavicular-cuneiform mass leads to relative lowering of this part and elevation of the cuboidometatarsal region. Finally, the forefoot may be distorted into either varus with inversion, the supination and adduction of the antetarsus arising at the Lisfranc joint line, or valgus with eversion, i. e. pronation and abduction of the forefoot. There are two corollaries, namely relative lowering of the internal part of the Lisfranc joint line and external angulation at the cuneiform-metatarsal junction, which is characteristic.
The final character of the displacements of the forefoot depends on the type of cavus component – balanced, varus or valgus – and the metatarsal head formula.
The symptoms which may arise in any of the types of cavus forefoot to be described relate to disorders of the ligaments, metatarsalgias of loading, and arthralgias of subluxation or dislocation at the metatarsophalangeal joints. Clawing of the toes may be the presenting symptom of this painful state.
Successful treatment depends totally on an overall understanding of the mechanism, which may have to be viewed from several aspects.

15.2 Pathological Changes in Tissues

Changes in the soft tissues, the bones and the joints all contribute to the disorder.

15.2.1 Soft Tissues

The subcutaneous connective tissue under the ball of the foot becomes atrophied and serous bursae develop under the condyles. The short plantar muscles are contracted, painful, and sometimes ridge the plantar skin of the foot. The plantar aponeurosis is contracted, and its internal cord forms an indurated bridge which is sometimes tender and uncompliant. The plantar ligaments are generally hypertrophied and contracted, as are the anterior capsule of the ankle joint and the dorsal aspect of the capsules of the metatarsophalangeal joints. The apposing ligamentous structures are, in contrast, atrophied and stretched.

The state of the tendons varies according to the clinical form. Extensor digitorum longus and extensor hallucis longus remain supple in the early stages, but contract progressively to a state of irreversible bowstringing under the dorsal skin over the metatarsophalangeal region, resulting in the provocation of claw toes. At the end of the development of the permanent cavus foot the long and short flexor tendons also become retracted, fixing the clawing. Tibialis posterior and flexor digitorum longus, and to a lesser degree the tendons of tibialis anterior, are contracted in the cavovarus foot. If at the outset the cause is equinus of the foot due to paralysis of the anterior muscles, the triceps surae becomes contracted, whereas if triceps surae is the primarily weakened component, a posterior cavus foot is created by the predominance of the dorsiflexors and plantar flexors.

15.2.2 Bones

During growth in a foot where the soft tissue influence has established cavus, the plantar aspects of the growth plates are subjected to compression, thereby reducing growth in length inferiorly according to the law of Delpech. Hypertrophy of the dorsal aspect occurs and the articular surfaces are distorted.

Thus the neck of the talus does not grow normally in length, but hypertrophies in thickness and contributes to the augmentation of the dorsal curvature. Its dorsal aspect forms a "hog's back", the maximum protrusion of which is marked by a transverse ridge from the anterior border of the articular surface of the tibia. Abutment of the area against the margin of the tibia causes the latter to hypertrophy and maintain the equinus of the foot, impeding dorsiflexion.

The anterosuperior apophysis of the calcaneum is hypertrophied in length, and together with the hypoplasia of the inferior cuboidal surface of the bone, this causes an augmented plantar orientation of the calcaneocuboid joint.

The navicular becomes wedge-shaped, its two articular surfaces, anterior and posterior, no longer parallel.

The cuboid and the cuneiforms behave similarly, with hypertrophy in length of their dorsal surfaces. The changes in the shapes of the bones contribute to the respective angles of declination and inclination of the antetarsus and tarsus.

15.2.3 Joints

The ankle joint is modified in its shape and function by hypertrophy of the tibial anterior margin abutting the hog's back feature on the talus. The subtalar joint augments its concavity.

The calcaneocuboid joint line accentuates its normal italic S form in the frontal plane and becomes orientated markedly lower and forwards.

The naviculocuneiform joint is distorted so that dorsally its margins protrude, producing local pressure symptoms.

The planes of the metatarsophalangeal joints are more plantarwards disposed than normal. The phalangeal bases tend to sublux or dislocate onto the dorsal faces of the metatarsal heads.

The interphalangeal joints cause clawing, the heads of the proximal phalanges become dislocated and the clawing itself serves to accentuate the depression of the metatarsal heads.

15.3 Physiological Pes Cavus

Fortunately, the physiological variety of pes cavus is the most frequent. The foot is normally formed, functions well, and is balanced with respect to muscle control (Fig. 15.3). Its suppleness is maintained and there is no disturbance of function. Indeed, this form of pes cavus is seen in dancers, sportsmen and women who wear high-heeled shoes, and has been recorded in many famous people throughout history. The importance of this foot lies only in our ability to recognise it!

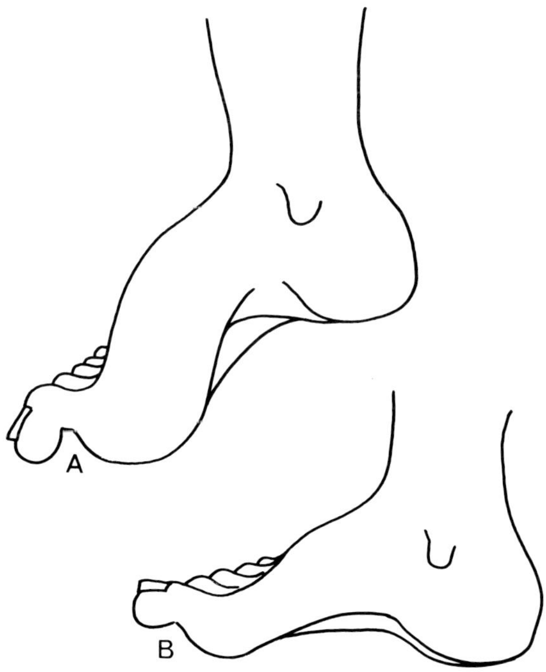

Fig. 15.3 A, B. Physiological cavus foot. **A** Unloaded. **B** Loaded

15.4 Idiopathic Acquired Pes Cavus

15.4.1 Etiology

Idiopathic acquired pes cavus first appears during childhood, between the 5th and 7th years, but is met in patients of all ages. If it is left untreated, there is progressive loss of suppleness and trophic symptoms appear from overloading and distortion in the tarsus, midtarsus and metatarsophalangeal regions. It ends with transverse displacement, either cavovalgus or cavovarus, developing from the initially balanced cavus foot configuration.

As in the planovalgus foot, but inversely, the condition seems to relate mostly to the talocalcaneal region, in which the general axis of inclination and a degree of convergence are more marked than normal. There is hypertrophy of the sustentaculum tali which coincides with decreased length of the talus and calcaneum (as opposed to the elongated appearance of these zones in the flat foot).

The shortness of the posterior tarsal elements leads physiologically and mechanically to augmentation of its angle of inclination tending to elevate the midtarsal mass and thus the height of the plantar arch. By way of consequence, the antetarsus is "dragged up" and is functionally short. These changes seem to relate to loss of balance between the extrinsic muscles and hypertonicity of the intrinsic muscles, as well as contracture of the plantar ligaments and aponeuroses.

Graceau and Brahms (1956) believed that it was the hypertonicity of the intrinsic muscles of the foot which led to this variety of cavus deformity. I believe, however, that this hypertonia is a consequence of the alteration of position of the talocalcaneal complex and is relative to the imbalance of the extrinsic muscles.

Whatever the cause, the hypertonia of the intrinsic short muscles renders the foot transversely unbalanced. It rests, like a bicycle, on only two points - one posterior and narrow (the posterior apophysis of the calcaneum), the other anterior, wider and inherently unstable because of inability of the outer and inner lever arms comprised by the first and fifth metatarsals to assure equilibrium. The normal third point of external loading under the base of the fifth metatarsal is lost. Three consequences are possible:

- Maintenance of transverse equilibrium by augmentation of tonicity of all muscles, notably tibialis anterior, tibialis posterior and the peronei. The cavus remains balanced and to some extent physiological.
- Alternatively, progressive loss of synergic control by the extrinsic muscles as a result of growth, the use of inappropriate shoes, and temporary overweight in the prepubertal period. When the posteromedial muscle groups (the tibialis muscles, triceps surae and the long flexors) are worst afflicted, the antero-external muscles (the extensors and peronei) are dominant, producing a cavovalgus foot in eversion. If the antero-external muscles are more severely affected, the posteromedial muscles predominate and a cavovarus foot in inversion results.

This idiopathic cavus foot remains supple until about the age of 18 years and then becomes progressively fixed, with resulting symptoms.

15.4.2 Balanced Cavus Foot

15.4.2.1 Infant

In the infant the condition presents as a longitudinal cavus with elevation of up to 30 mm with respect to weight bearing on the outer band (elevation in excess of this amount gives ground for suspicion of a neurological origin). The condition is correctable, and the accompanying digital clawing is supple. No callus formation is visible, but there may already be indications of a cavus forefoot component or a convex forefoot component.

Podoscopy shows a variable degree of disappearance of the external band of loading.
Radiography at this stage does not reveal any morphological change of the skeletal structures, but shows a vertical alignment of the talus with respect to the calcaneum and sometimes, on lateral view, incipient convergence.

15.4.2.2 Adult

In the adult the elevation of the lateral border does not exceed 35 mm. The condition becomes increasingly rigid and irreducible. There is anterior loading disturbance with the beginnings of a median callus formation in a convex forefoot (with a Greek metatarsal formula) or sometimes thick callus or keratoma formation under the first and fourth or fifth metatarsal heads in the cavus forefoot (with a square metatarsal formula). In untreated cases and in subjects who stand continually or neglect foot hygiene, classical ulceration and inflammation are engendered by the fixity of the longitudinal cavus.

15.4.2.3 Treatment

Conservative. Management of a conservative nature is appropriate for the *infant* and the *adolescent.* An insole with a retrocapital bar exercises a stretching effect on the plantar structures and seems in this way to exercise a secondary form of relaxation. If this type of insole is not tolerated, a physiological monoblock pattern with a retrocapital bar and a plantar dome of support may be acceptable. The height of the dome must be less than that of the plantar arch of the foot concerned, in order to avoid coronal imbalance, which may occur during growth and result in cavovalgus or cavovarus posture. In the *adult,* orthotic treatment may also be successful in some cases and must always be complemented by proper chiropody.

Operative. In the otherwise supple cavus foot, disorders of loading can still develop if there is a convex or cavus forefoot component. These conditions demand realignment by appropriate enclavement operations or basal osteotomies, as described in earlier chapters. It would be disastous to perform a resection arthroplasty of the tarsometatarsal joints or arthrodese a midtarsal component in the supple cavus balanced foot.
In the rigid cavus foot, the loading disorder at the metatarsus and toes and the arthralgias from distorted joints demand overall appraisal. It is unlikely that chiropody or orthotic treatment, even with a monoblock orthopaedic insole with a retrocapital bar and excavations under the calluses, will be appropriate except in the elderly patient. Operation may again be confined to correction of forefoot loading by enclavement or basal osteotomies, but occasionally the severity of the cavus may demand metatarsectomy as described by Lelièvre (1952), cuneiform-metatarsal osteotomy at the Lisfranc joint line or cuneiform-cuboidal wedge osteotomy as described by Meary et al. (1976). The choice of procedure will depend on the individual case.

15.4.3 Cavovalgus Foot

In addition to the longitudinal cavus, the external cuboidal fifth metatarsal mass is elevated, together with a valgoid posture of the heel, protrusion of the calcaneum laterally and abduction of the metatarsus (Figs. 15.4, 15.5). This is a "false flat foot"; on podoscopy, the imprint is that of a cavus foot in that the lateral border is elevated with the formation of an external longitudinal arch and a valgus tarsometatarsal angulation with convexity of the medial border of the forefoot. The external border is seen to be concave. This foot is unstable and prone to injury both at the ankle joint and in the subtalar and midtarsal elements. In the adult, it is accompanied by the formation of a convex triangular or flat triangular metatarsus.

15.4.3.1 Infant and Adolescent

In the infant and adolescent, symptoms relate to the hindfoot, due to the calcaneal pronation. Pain is localised to the posterior apophysis and is exaggerated by standing, walking or sport. There may be local tenderness and sometimes local heat lateral to the apophysis. The inflammatory elements should not be confused with the posterior apophysitis which occurs during growth. Sometimes pain is felt at the navicular or at the insertion of the tibialis posterior tendon due to tenosynovitis or tendinitis.

15.4.3.2 Adult

In the adult the predominant symptoms arise from distortion at the midtarsal joints due to ligament irritability. The pain is of a sharp, boiling or constricting character with a sensation of pinching of the tissues or spasm, sometimes located over the

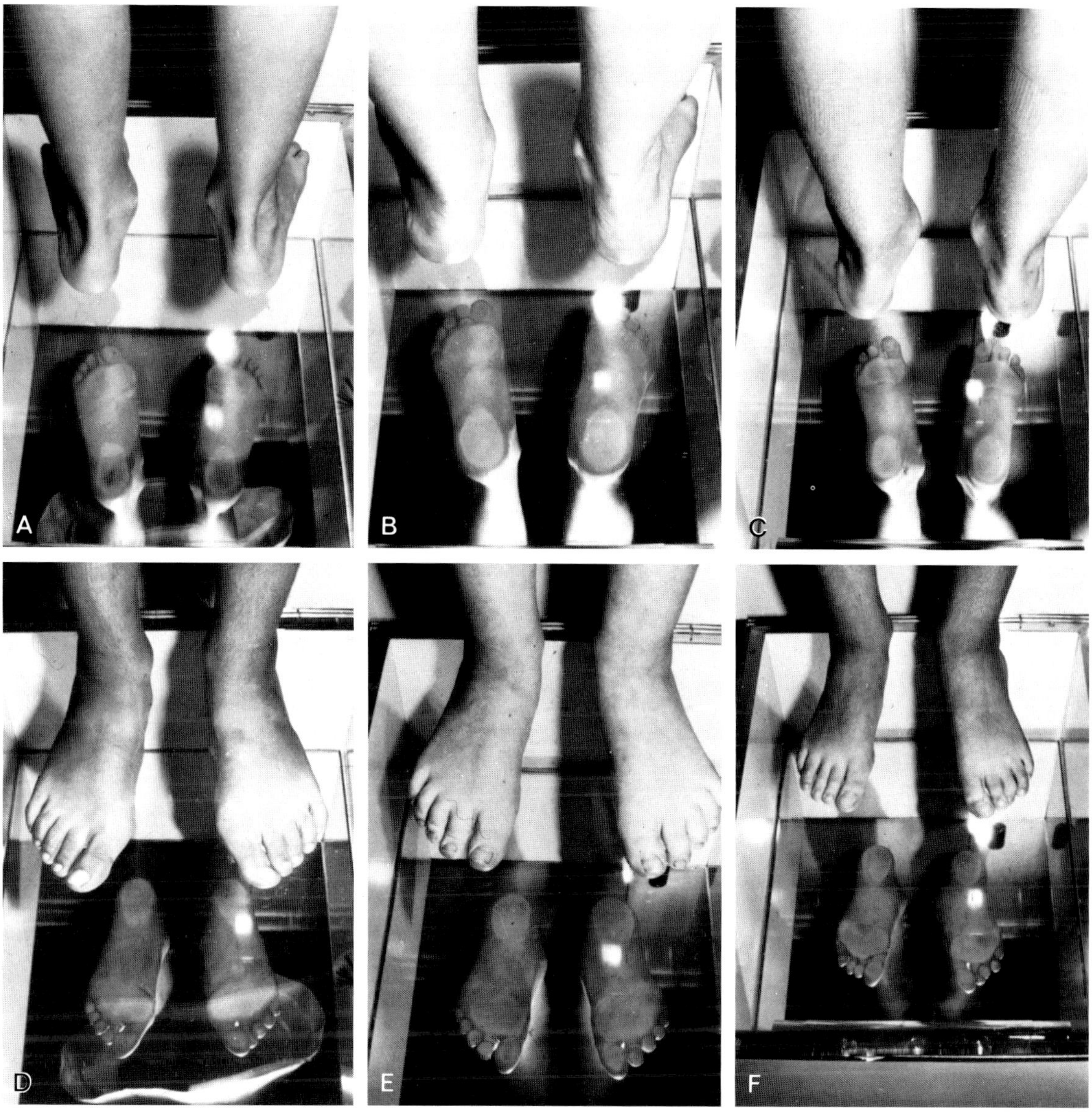

Fig. 15.4 A–F. Pes cavovalgus in infancy. **A–C** Valgus posture of tarsus, medial displacement of midtarsus, angulation of outer border of foot, abduction of forefoot, displacement increasing from first to third rays. **D–F** Adducted heel component of footprint, medial displacement of midtarsus, abduction and pronation of forefoot

external orifice of the sinus tarsi or at the calcaneocuboidal joint. Metatarsalgia from overloading and callus formation under the first and second rays are common. The foot may become increasingly contracted, and pain may be exaggerated by attempts to mobilise it, even gently, with an insole. The foot takes on a dystrophic appearance.

Podoscopic examination shows two points of loading, on the heel and the metatarsus, with narrowness or absence of the external longitudinal band as a result of elevation of the cuboid. The adduction of the longitudinal axis of the heel print is accompanied by abduction of the forefoot print (Fig. 15.1).

Radiography: The anteroposterior view reveals the external angulation of the tarsometatarsal region, the variable abduction of the metatarsus and the internal subluxation of the navicular. The lateral view reveals moderate raising of the plantar arch contrasting with the degree of clinical cavus.

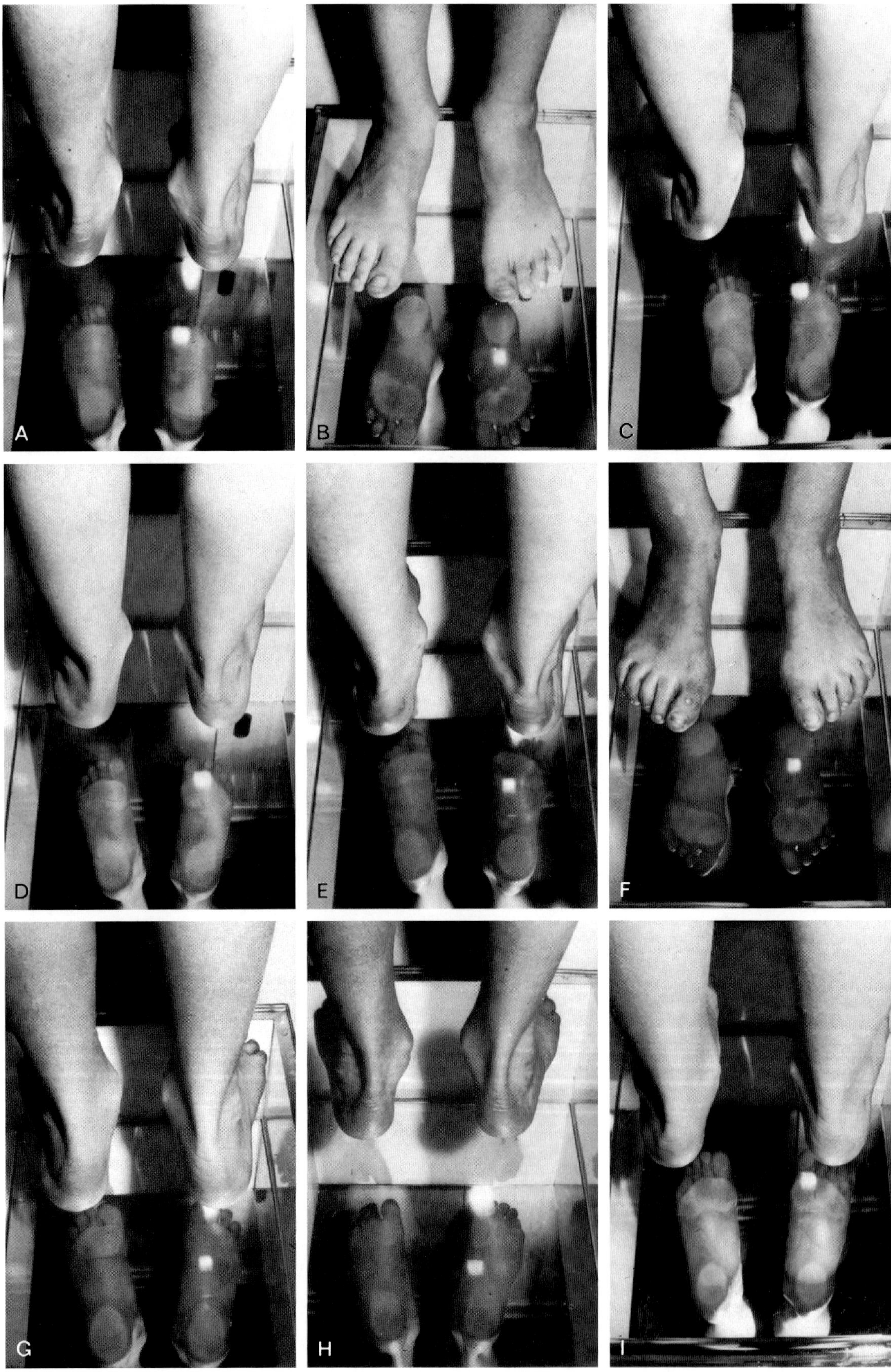
A
B
C
D
E
F
G
H
I

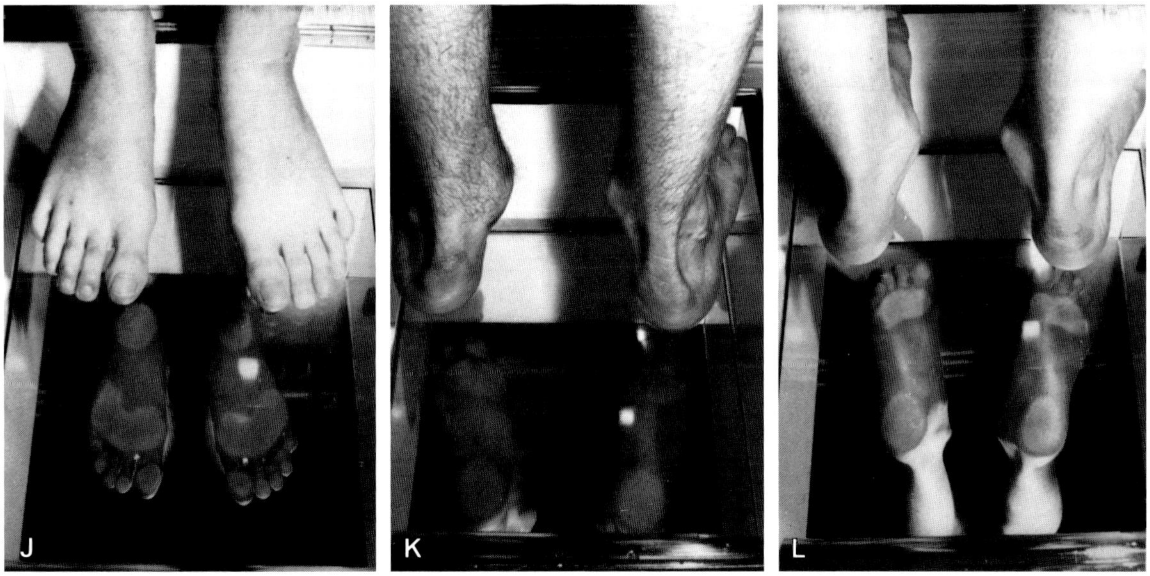

◁ **Fig. 15.5 A–L.** Pes cavovalgus in adolescence and adulthood. **A–H** Adolescence: **A–D** First degree: occasional persistence of load bearing under cuboid, tarsal valgus, light midtarsal displacement; **E–H** second degree: disappearance of load bearing under cuboid, slight accentuation of tarsal valgus, medial midtarsal displacement leading in absence of treatment to plantar collapse, incipient abduction of forefoot. **I–L** Adulthood: **I, J** First degree: insignificant valgus, light midtarsal displacement; **K, L** second degree: valgus more accentuated, medial displacement of midtarsus, concave angulation of outer border of foot, abduction of forefoot

15.4.3.3 Treatment

Conservative. In the *infant* and *adolescent* the use of an insole is usually sufficient to relax, correct and stabilise the foot. The insole should comprise a supinating wedge at the heel and a retrocapital pronating bar. In the adolescent or young adult, a plantar arch support should be added. In the *adult*, however, the insole is unlikely to be successful.

Operative. Arthrodesis of the Lisfranc joint, the naviculocuneiform and cuboidal joints or the talonavicular joint line may be necessary in the presence of arthrosis (Figs. 15.6, 15.7 A). When no arthrosic changes have occurred, extra-articular curvilinear transverse ostectomies, excising more bone dorsally and internally, may correct the cavus and the valgus (Regnauld 1974). They should be chosen according to the summit of the displacement, which can be naviculocuboidal or cuneiform-cuboidal.
The ostectomy should comprise resection of a bony block shaped like a crescent moon, concave from behind with the base facing medially and the apex reaching the outer aspect of the cuboid (Fig. 15.7 B). It may cross the transcuneiform-cuboidal region, or in some instances the trans-naviculocuboidal zone must be selected.

Operative Technique. A medial longitudinal incision is made centred over the navicular or cuneiforms as selected. For transcuneiform resection, the soft tissues are separated by sharp dissection from the dorsal surface of the other cuneiforms and the cuboid, carefully protecting the dorsalis pedis artery and the extensor tendons, and bone levers are inserted. For the navicular resection, it is necessary to detach the insertion of tibialis posterior in order to expose the required bone surface. Under direct vision, the orientation of the bone cuts necessary is estimated and the curvilinear ostectomies are performed, initially with Volkmann nibblers and then with curved Smith-Petersen rongeurs. The bone block is excised and the wedge coapted, being held by a nylon stitch passed through anterior and posterior tunnels through the contiguous bone surfaces. Tibialis posterior should be transposed to a more anterior position on the medial cuneiform bone.

15.4.4 Cavovarus Foot

Overaction of the postero-internal leg muscles and triceps surae predominates and drags the tarsus into supination and inversion, which reflect on the midtarsus and the metatarsus.

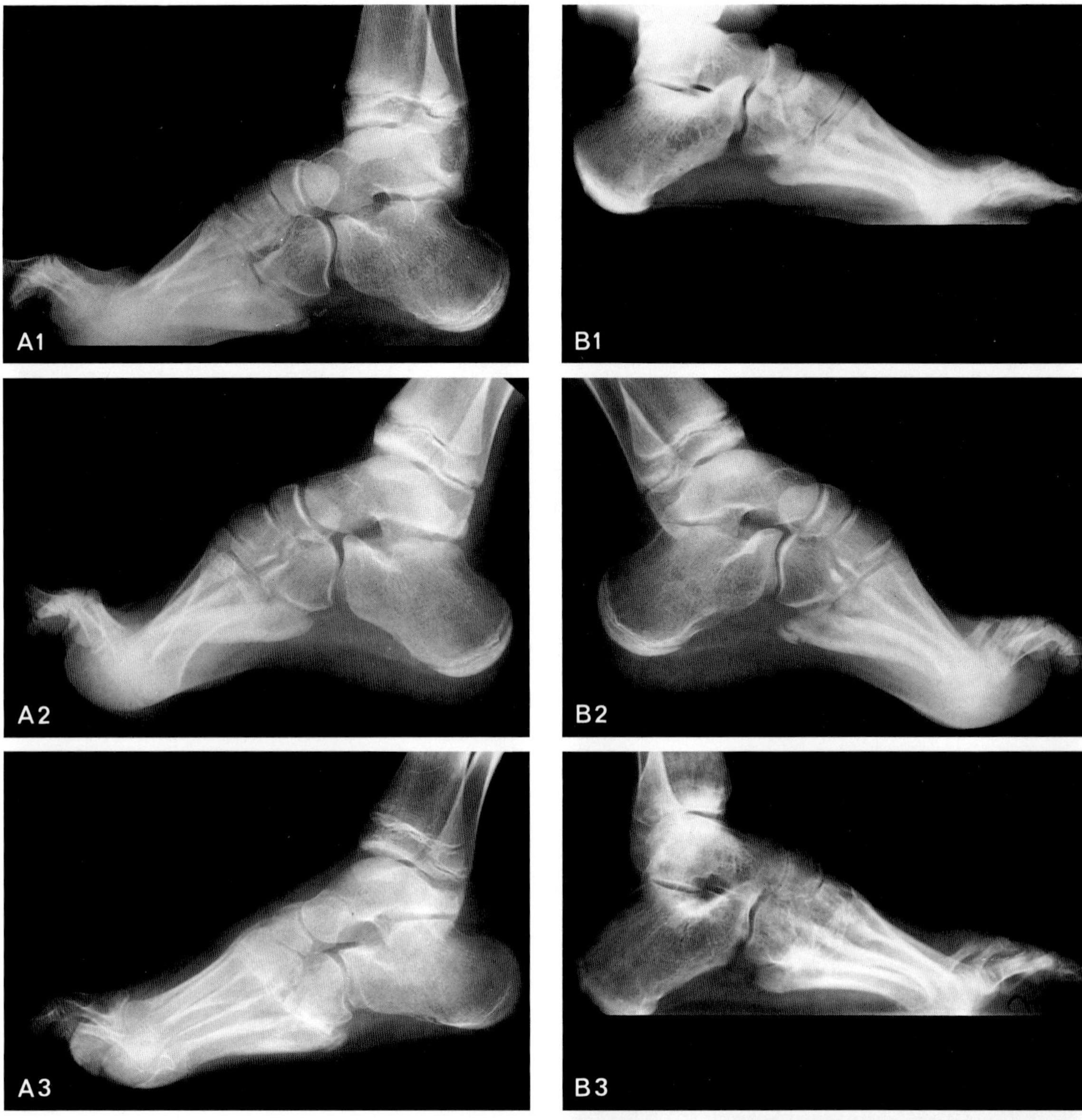

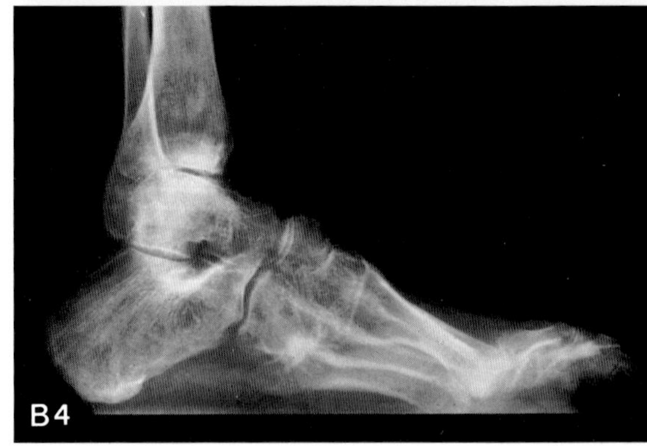

Fig. 15.6 A–D. Pes cavus: preoperative state and postoperative appearance after arthrodesis of tarsometatarsal joint line (Lisfranc). **A** Idiopathic pes cavus, left foot, lateral views. *1* Weight bearing, preoperative; *2* non-weight bearing, preoperative; *3* non-weight bearing after osteotomy-arthrodesis of tarsometatarsal joint line. **B** Right foot, lateral views. *1* Weight bearing, preoperative; *2* non-weight bearing, preoperative; *3* weight bearing after osteotomy-arthrodesis of tarsometatarsal joint line; *4* non-weight bearing after arthrodesis of tarsometatarsal joint line. **C, D** see p. 131

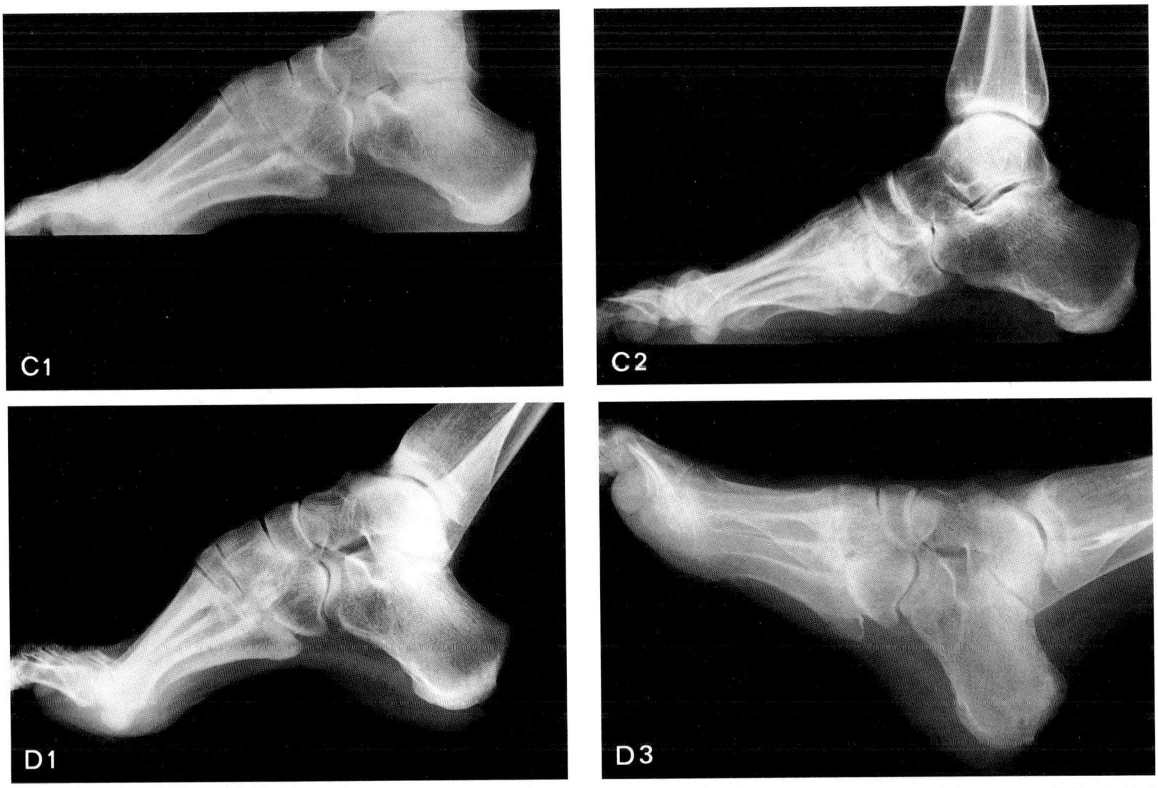

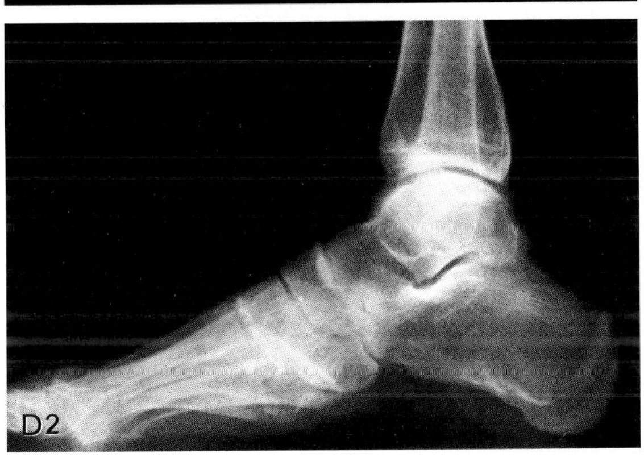

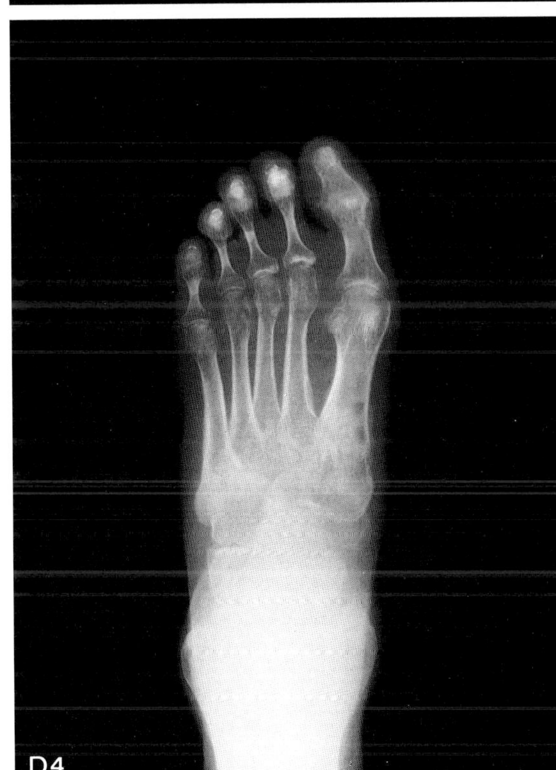

Fig. 15.6 *(continued)*. **C** Left foot, lateral views. *1* Weight bearing, preoperative; *2* weight bearing after osteotomy-arthrodesis of tarsometatarsal joint line. **D** Pes cavus in Friedreich's ataxia, left foot. *1* Non-weight-bearing preoperative lateral view; *2* weight-bearing lateral view after osteotomy-arthrodesis of tarsometatarsal joint line; *3* non-weight-bearing postoperative lateral view. *4* Postoperative dorsoplantar view

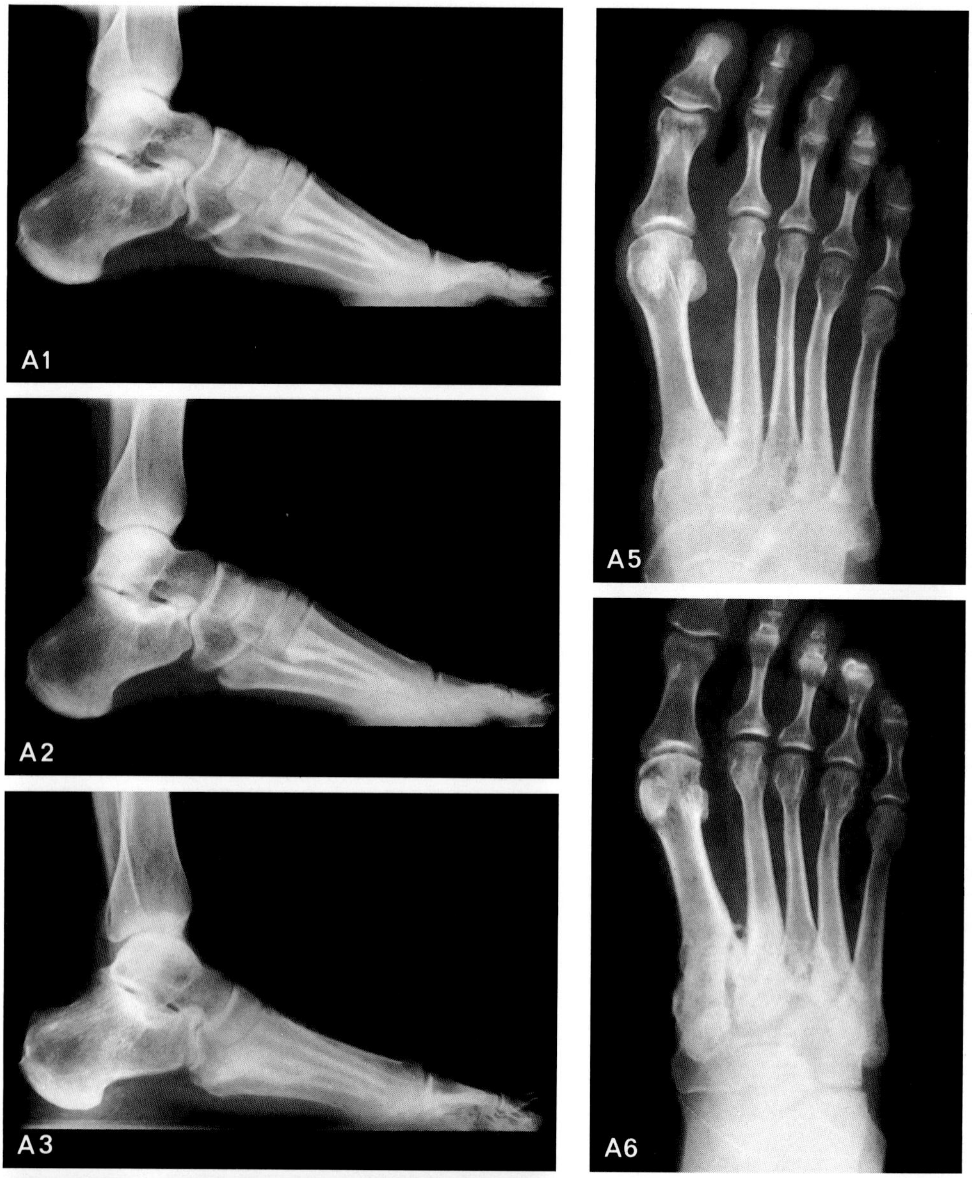

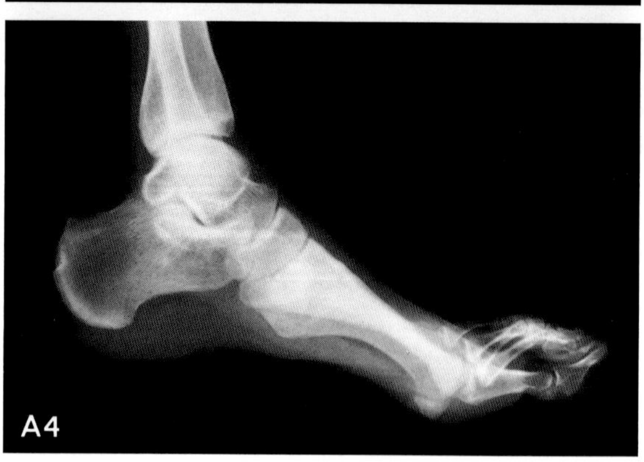

Fig. 15.7 A, B. Idiopathic anterior pes cavus before and ▷ after treatment. **A** Right foot. *1* Non-weight-bearing preoperative lateral view: absence of superimposition of navicular and cuboid, which appear clearly separated, indicating longitudinal cavus; *2* weight-bearing, preoperative lateral view; *3* weight-bearing lateral view after osteotomy-arthrodesis of cuneiform-metatarsal joints and correction of longitudinal vavus; *4* lateral view after osteotomy-arthrodesis of cuneiform metatarsal joints; *5* weight-bearing dorsoplantar view after osteotomy-arthrodesis of tarsometatarsal joint line; *6* non-weight-bearing dorsoplantar view after osteotomy-arthrodesis of tarsometatarsal joint line. **B** see p. 133

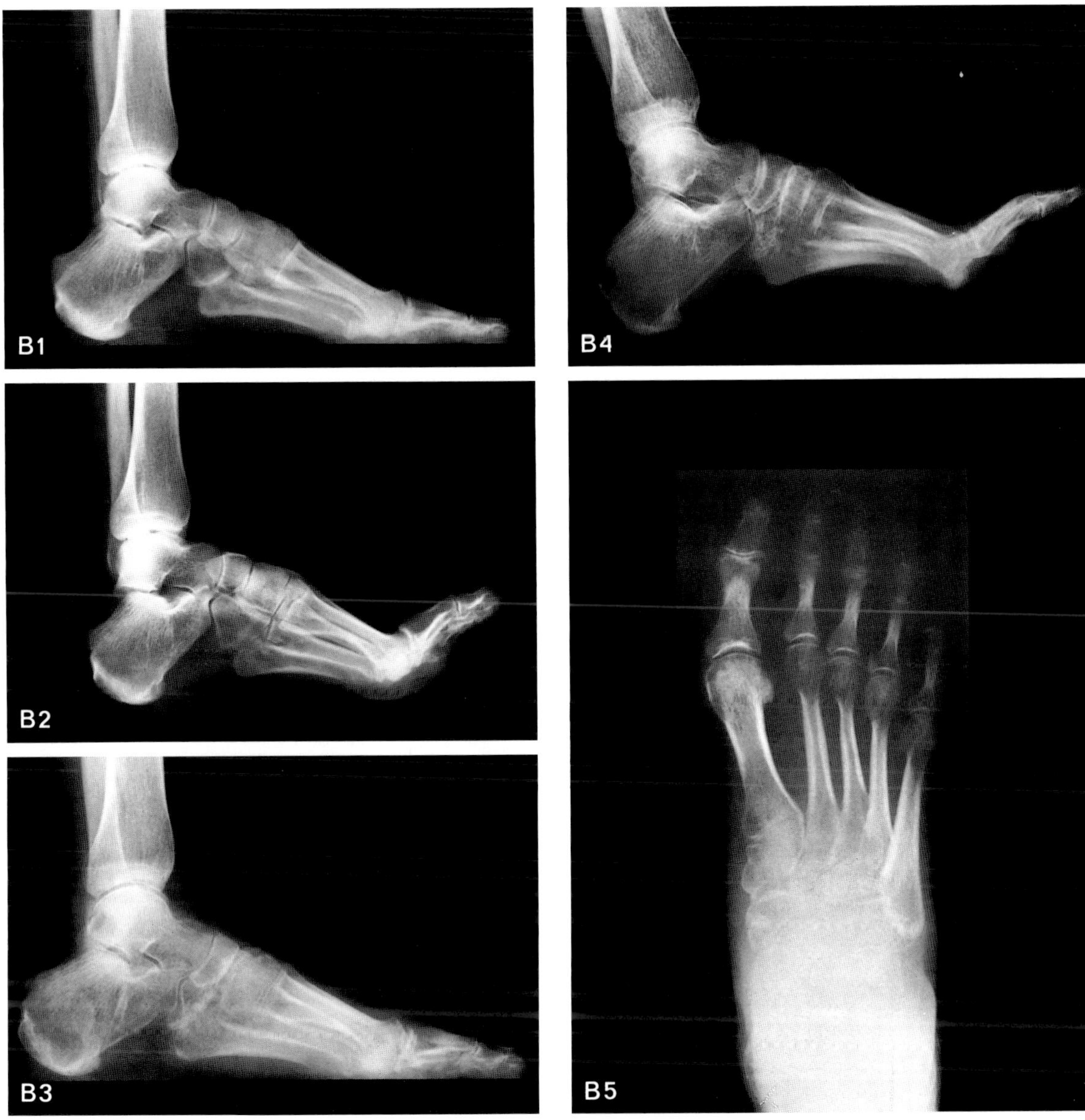

Fig. 15.7 *(continued)*. **B** *1* Right foot. Weight-bearing preoperative lateral view: compound pes cavus with augmentation of angle of inclination of calcaneum and metatarsus, longitudinal cavus with summit at cuneiform region; *2* non-weight-bearing preoperative view: lateral dorsal summit at cuneiform region with loss of regularity; *3* weight-bearing lateral view after midtarsal osteotomy at naviculocuneiform and intracuboidal regions; *4* non-weight-bearing lateral view after midtarsal osteotomy at naviculocuneiform and intracuboidal regions; *5* postoperative dorsoplantar view

This leads to a swivelling of the foot externally and plantarwards, that is to say, inversion of the midtarsal mass by elevation of the navicular and lowering of the cuboid. The eventual appearance is similar to that of a varus club foot, but the condition differs in its acquired character and also in the absence of significant modifications of the bony structure.

Especially medially, with the varus of the tarsus and the supination of the metatarsus, the longitudinal cavus becomes rapidly irreducible and fixed by contracture of the aponeurosis, which bowstrings under the plantar aspect of the foot. Some compensatory varus and inversion of the foot occurs, maintained by contracture of tibialis posterior and triceps surae.

Pain is related to the outer side of the tarsus, especially at the lateral ligament of the ankle, and the outer side of the subtalar joint, and consists of a sensation of tension accentuated by standing and walking. The forefoot develops a thick wide tender callus under the fifth metatarsal head and later under the base of the fifth metatarsal. Contracture of the extensor tendons leads to clawing of the toes. The deformed foot bulges the external upper of the shoe and causes wear of the outer part of the sole. *Podoscopic examination* reveals a characteristic print in which the heel and metatarsal loading areas are connected by a thick band of overloading in the subcuboidal region (Fig. 15.8). A hollowing occurs in the mid-part of the metatarsal print, indicating the tendency for cavus forefoot to develop due to the equinus posture of the first metatarsal. *Radiography:* In the dorsoplantar view, the lateral convergence of the talus and calcaneum, the inversion of the midtarsus and the external involution and adduction of the metatarsus are all visible. The lateral view reveals the elevation of the internal plantar arch, notably involving the navicular, as well as augmentation of the calcaneal angle of inclination. The equinus of the inner metatarsals is marked. The outer metatarsals become progressively horizontal.

15.4.4.1 Treatment

Conservative. Management with an insole, comprising a pronating external bar and a retrocapital pronating bar, is appropriate for the *adolescent* and

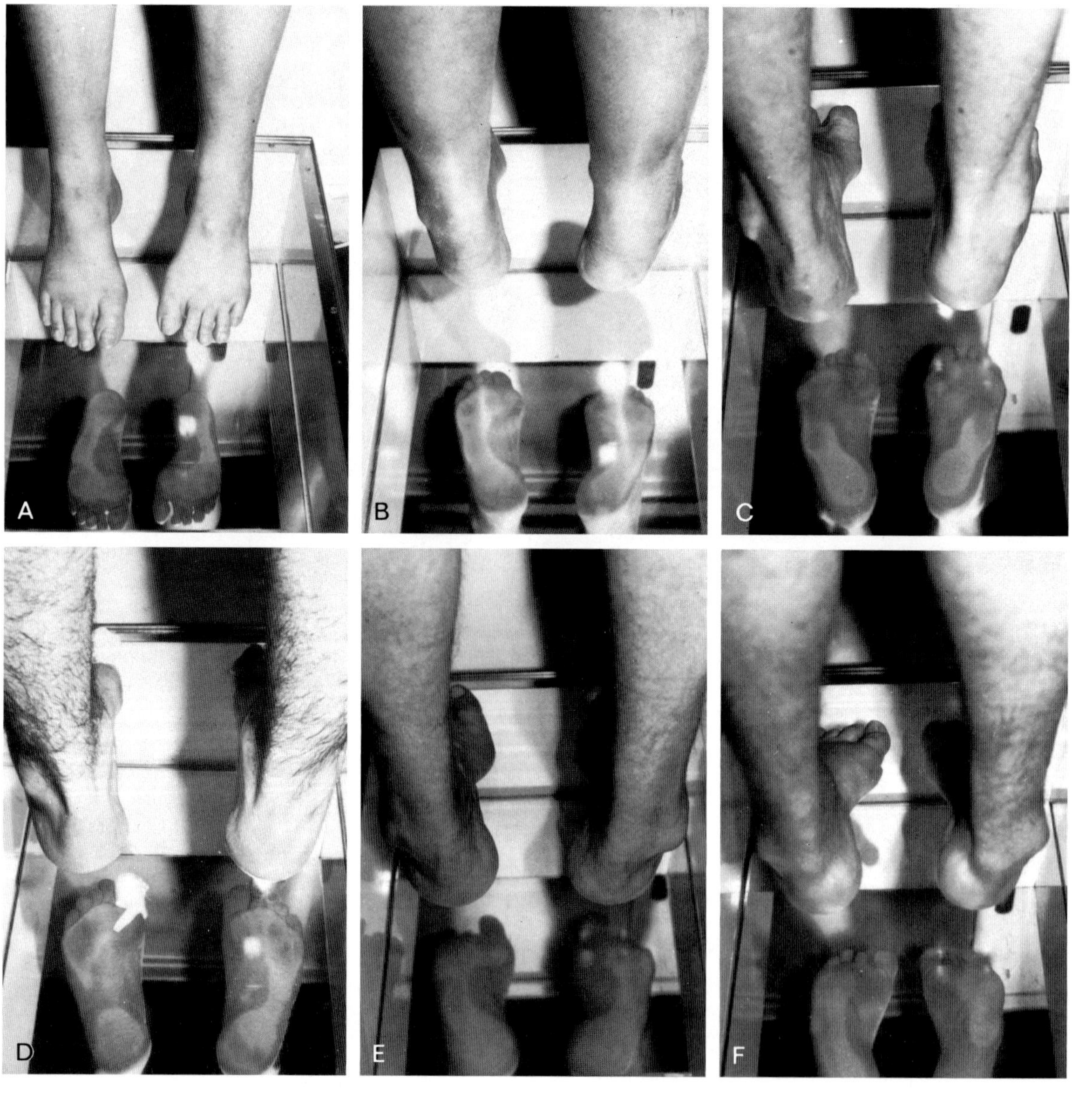

the *young adult*. In the *adult*, this insole may be tolerated but it is sometimes necessary to supplement support by an internal plantar dome a few millimetres less in height than the elevated position of the internal plantar arch. Generally, in the adult, the rigidity will not correct and surgery is necessary.

Operative. Surgery comprises midtarsal osteotomy with removal of a wedge based dorsally and externally situated across the naviculo-cuneiform joint and transecting the cuboid; it corrects in one act the cavus and the adduction of the metatarsus. The orientation and size of wedge removed must be carefully calculated. If there is coexisting irreducible calcaneal supination, calcaneal osteotomy (Dwyer 1959) will correct the tarsal varus. The presence of arthrosic lesions in the older adult (50 years or more) indicates the need for arthrodesis of the midtarsal and subtalar regions with appropriate wedge resections. Triple arthrodesis should only exceptionally be necessary. In the presence of undamaged joints, an extra-articular curvilinear midtarsal osteotomy is possible (see above).

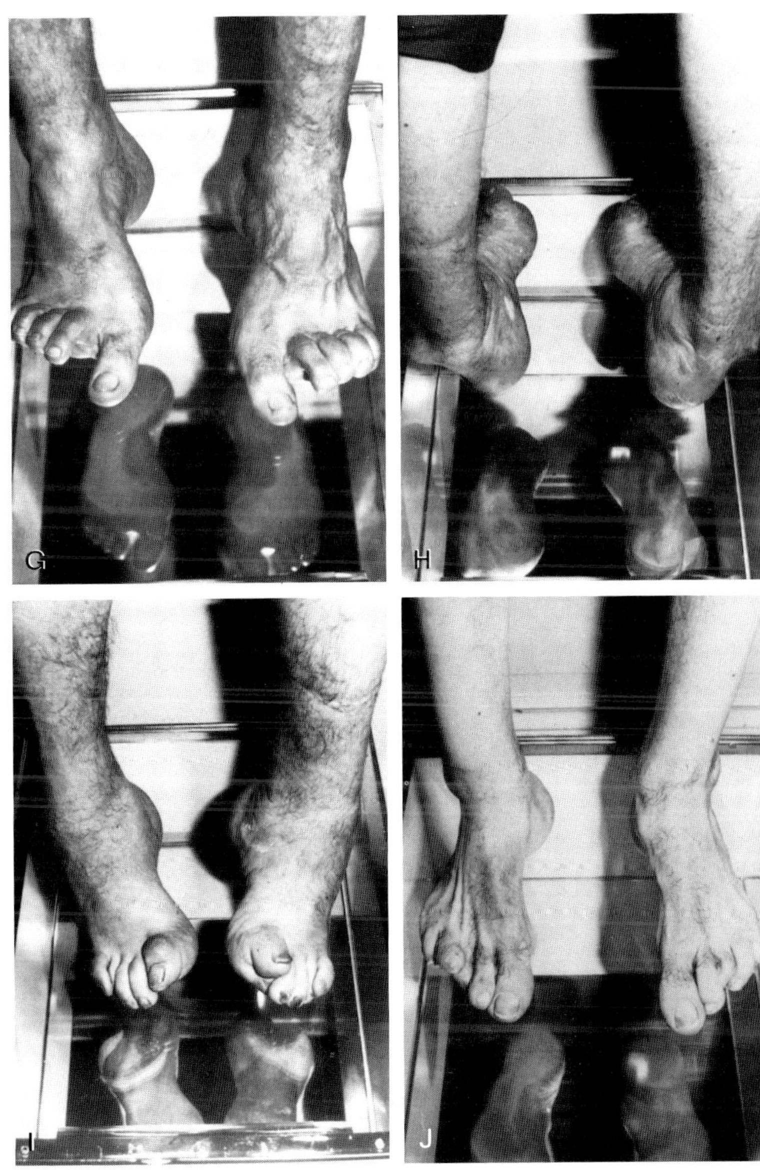

◁ **Fig. 15.8 A–J.** Pes cavovarus of different degrees. **A** Child. **B, C** Adolescent. **D–J** Adult

15.5 Neurological Pes Cavus

Neurological cavus deformity, whatever the cause, typically presents as a progressive condition due to muscle imbalance of some sort. The deformity may be gross, and rapidly becomes irreducible and fixed. There is frequently a familial history, but some acquired neurological conditions are occasionally manifested first in the foot. According to Courriades (1979) there are two main etiological forms:

Hypertonic. By hypertonia, Courriades means excessive action of some muscle group, possibly by direct excitation of the gamma motor neuron system. An example is the familial cavus foot of Friedreich (1863), but the definition also includes the cavus foot associated with shortening of the lower limb due to congenital unilateral dislocation of the hip in which the equinocavus posture is in part compensatory or may derive from direct excitation of muscle function by painfully sensitive nervous pathways. Old trauma of the lower limb with fracture of the long bones, especially after prolonged plaster cast immobilisation or after an overtight cast, can result in the same deformity, analogous to the Volkmann syndrome of the forearm. Other sources of irritation inducing muscle imbalance include persistent use of overhigh heels and excessive use of the feet in heavy manual workers who stand all the time.

Fig. 15.9 A–D see pp. 137–139

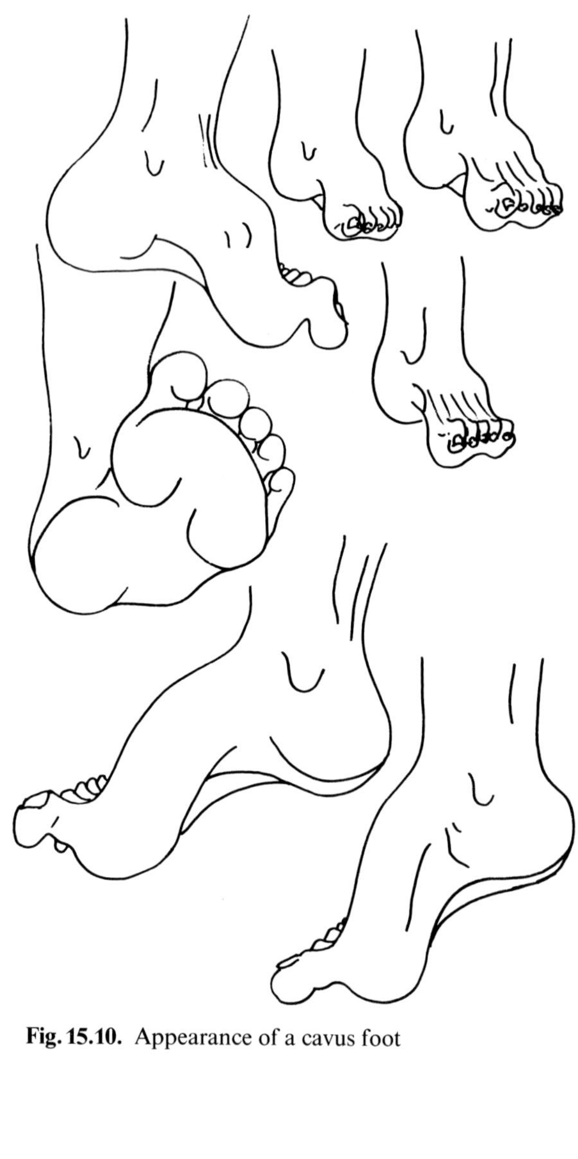

Fig. 15.10. Appearance of a cavus foot

Spastic. This again is a rapidly irreducible progressive condition associated with neurological deficit from encephalitis, spinocerebellar disease or disorder of the pyramidal pathway.

These two neurological origins, hypertonic and spastic, are reflected in different configurations of the cavus. Anterior cavus indicates predominant equinus of the antetarsus; posterior cavus is the term used for hindfoot calcaneus position. Whatever the form, the majority of authors agree that the cause is imbalance between the intrinsic and extrinsic muscles of the foot which leads to the progressive cavus and subsequent fixation by soft tissues. In the growing foot, the inevitable changes in bone growth contribute to the problem.

It should be emphasized that hypertonia of the intrinsic muscles is a common denominator; differences between cases are an expression of the variability of the imbalance of the extrinsic muscles above.

Four types may be distinguished: anterior, posterior, equinus and various combinations of these (Fig. 15.9).

15.5.1 Anterior Cavus

This is the most common variety and was described fully by Lelièvre. There are five subtypes (Figs. 15.10, 15.11):

a) Antero-internal cavus
b) Supinated cavovarus
c) Anterior longitudinal cavus with forefoot cavus
d) Anterior longitudinal balanced cavus with convex forefoot
e) Anterior cavovalgus

Anterior longitudinal cavus with forefoot cavus is a combination of the two preceding forms and results from a failure to treat them.

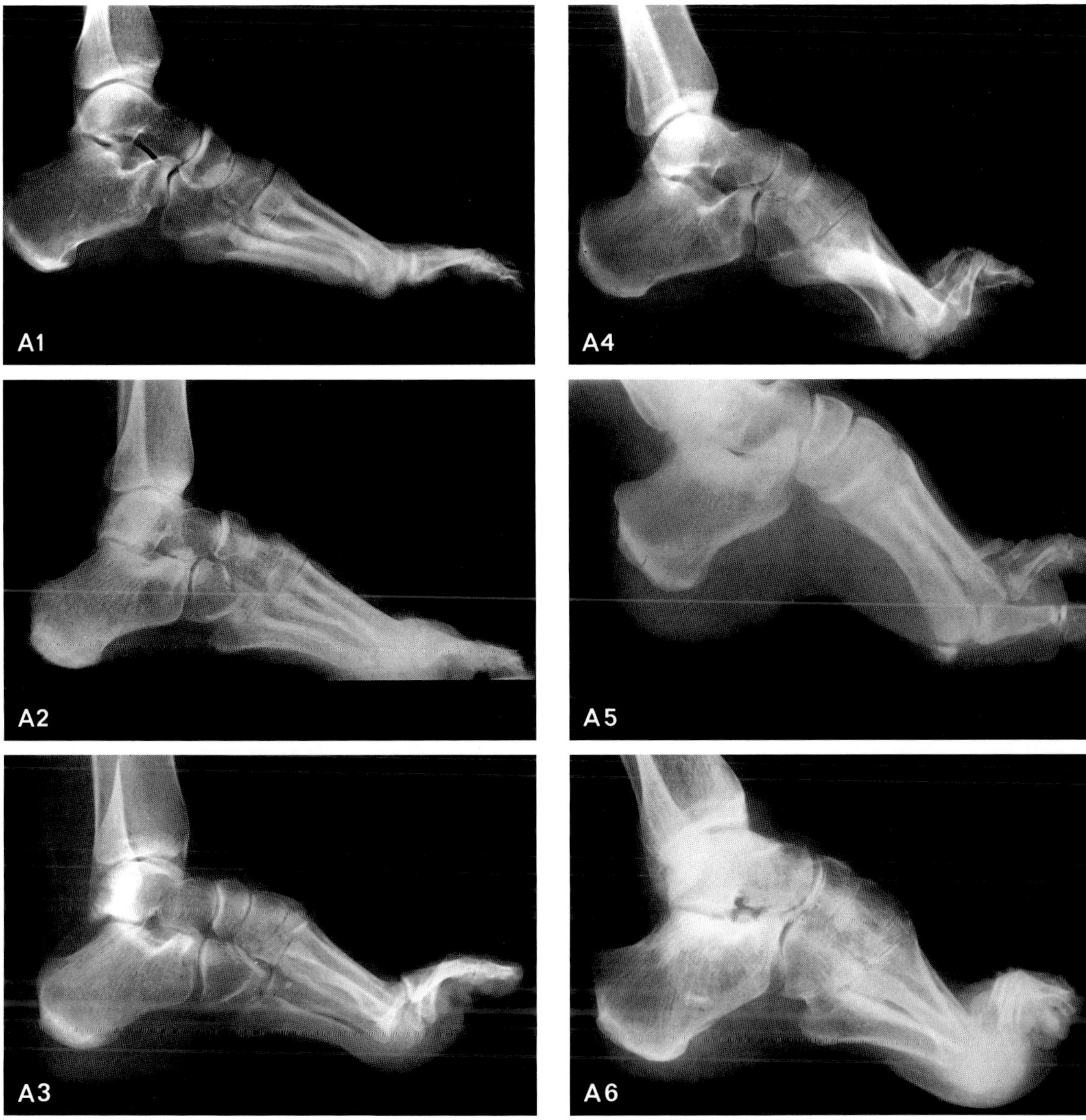

Fig. 15.9 A–D. Pes cavus: anterior, posterior, mixed and varus. **A** Anterior pes cavus. *1* Onset; *2* augmentation of angulation at cuneiform-metatarsal region; *3* dorsal angulation of cuneiform-metatarsal region; *4* dorsal angulation of midtarsal mass and equinus of antetarsus; *5* marked dorsal angulation with accentuated equinus at the naviculo-cuneiform-metatarsal region; *6* anterior pes cavus. **B–D** see pp. 138, 139

The variety in the types of anterior cavus foot is the result of variable imbalance between the extrinsic muscles imposed on the same intrinsic patterns. Tonicity of triceps surae maintains a normal sagittal attitude of the talocalcaneal complex under the ankle joint, but dominance of the tibialis muscles, flexor hallucis longus and flexor digitorum longus draws the antetarsus into equinus while hypertonia of the extensor muscles drags the toes into clawing. These muscle tensions markedly lower the metatarsals, the angulation tending to occur at the tarsometatarsal joint, where the hypertonic tibialis anterior maintains and elevates the cuneiforms. For this reason, the summit of the arch of anterior cavus is only rarely situated as far back as the navicular.
The talus is held in a neutral position in the ankle mortice, while the calcaneum can yield either into varus or valgus. *Varus* will be induced by predominance of hypertonia in the triceps and tibialis muscles, and depending upon the metatarsal formula, a convex forefoot or a supinated forefoot will result. The latter develops finally into a cavus forefoot

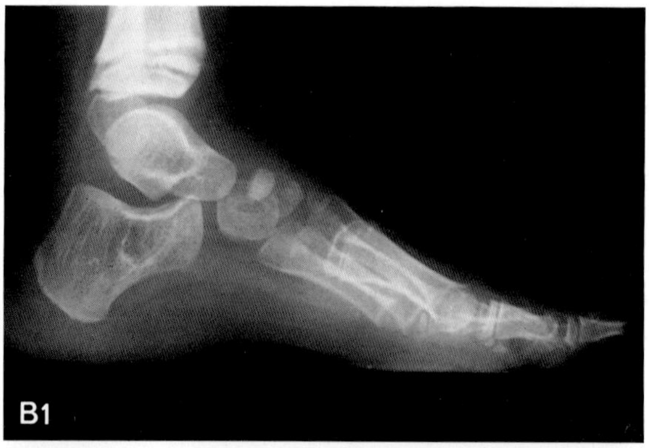

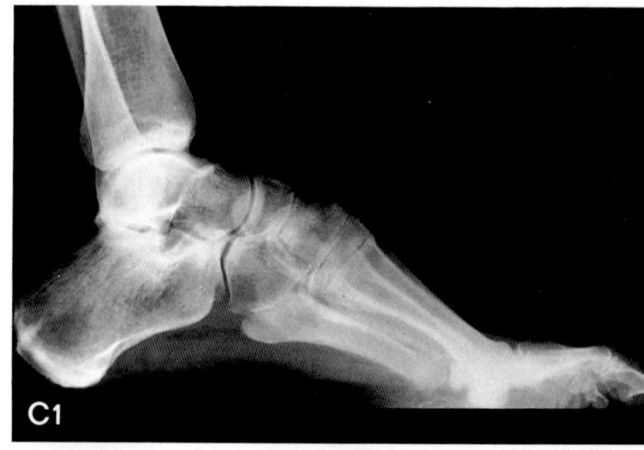

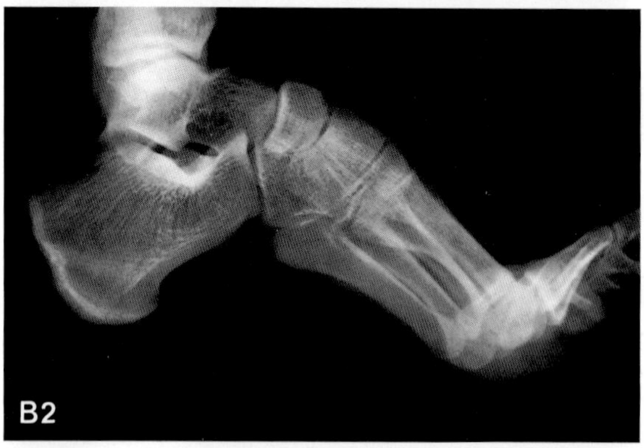

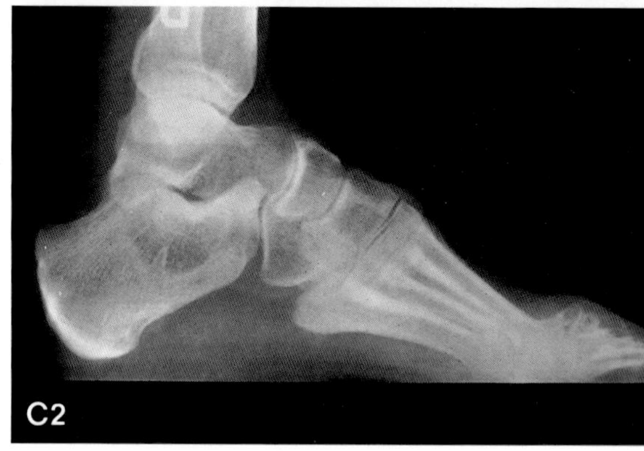

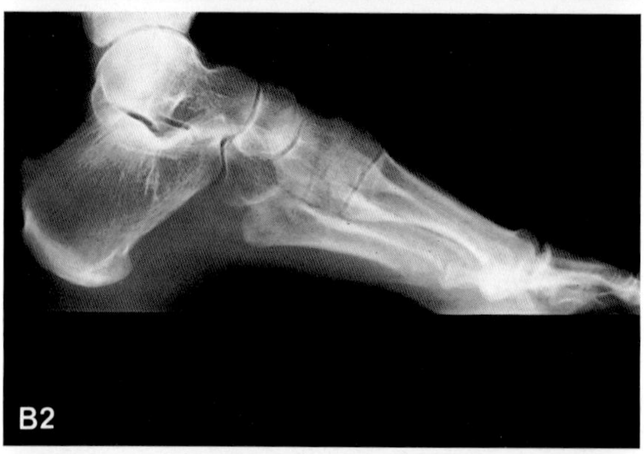

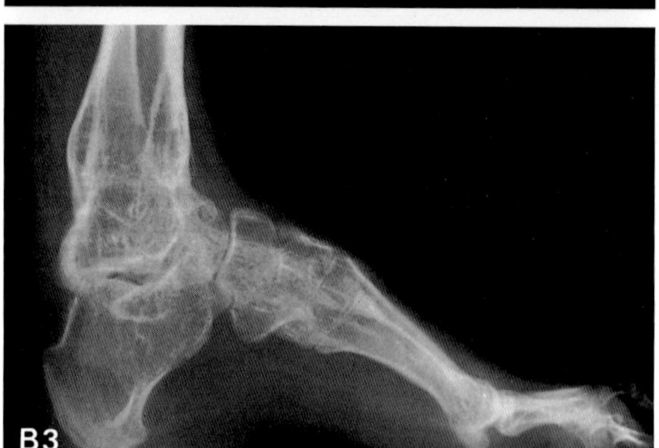

Fig. 15.9 *(continued)*. **B** Posterior pes cavus. *1* Posterior equinocavus in poliomyelitis in childhood; *2* posterior pes cavus with marked tarsal equinus; *3* posterior paralytic pes cavus; **C** *1, 2* combined pes cavus

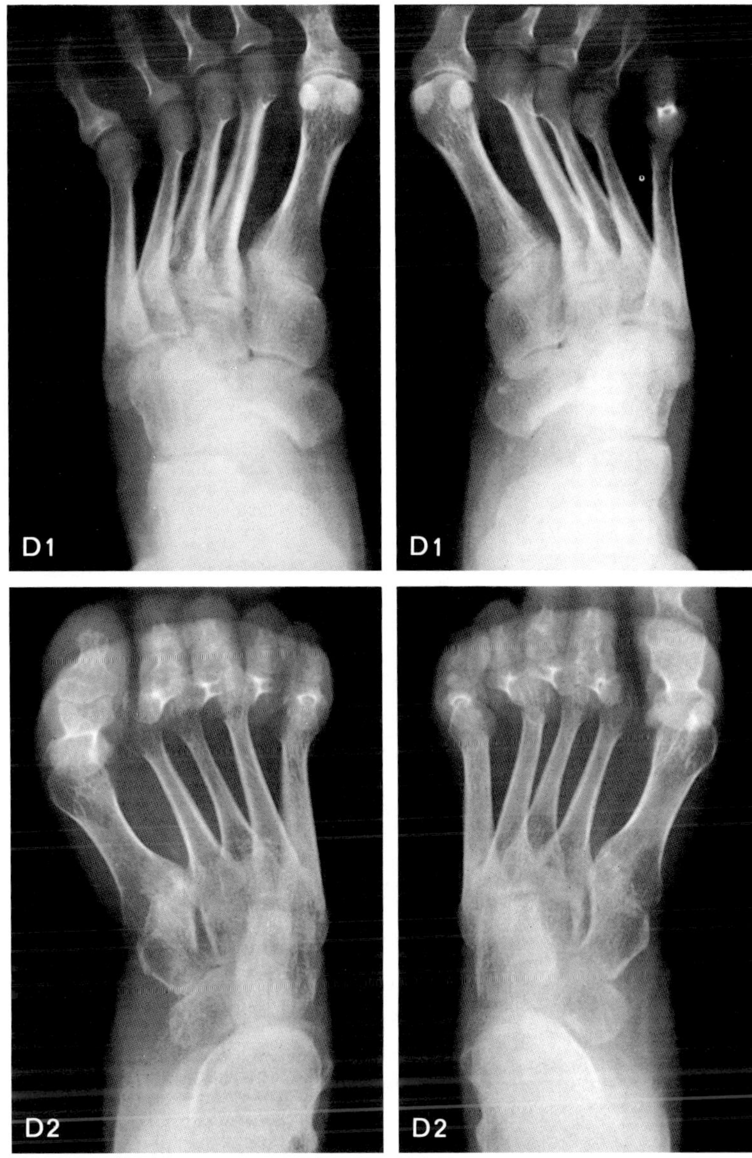

Fig. 15.9 *(continued)*. **D** Pes cavovarus. *1* Midtarsal inversion; *2* adduction of antetarsus

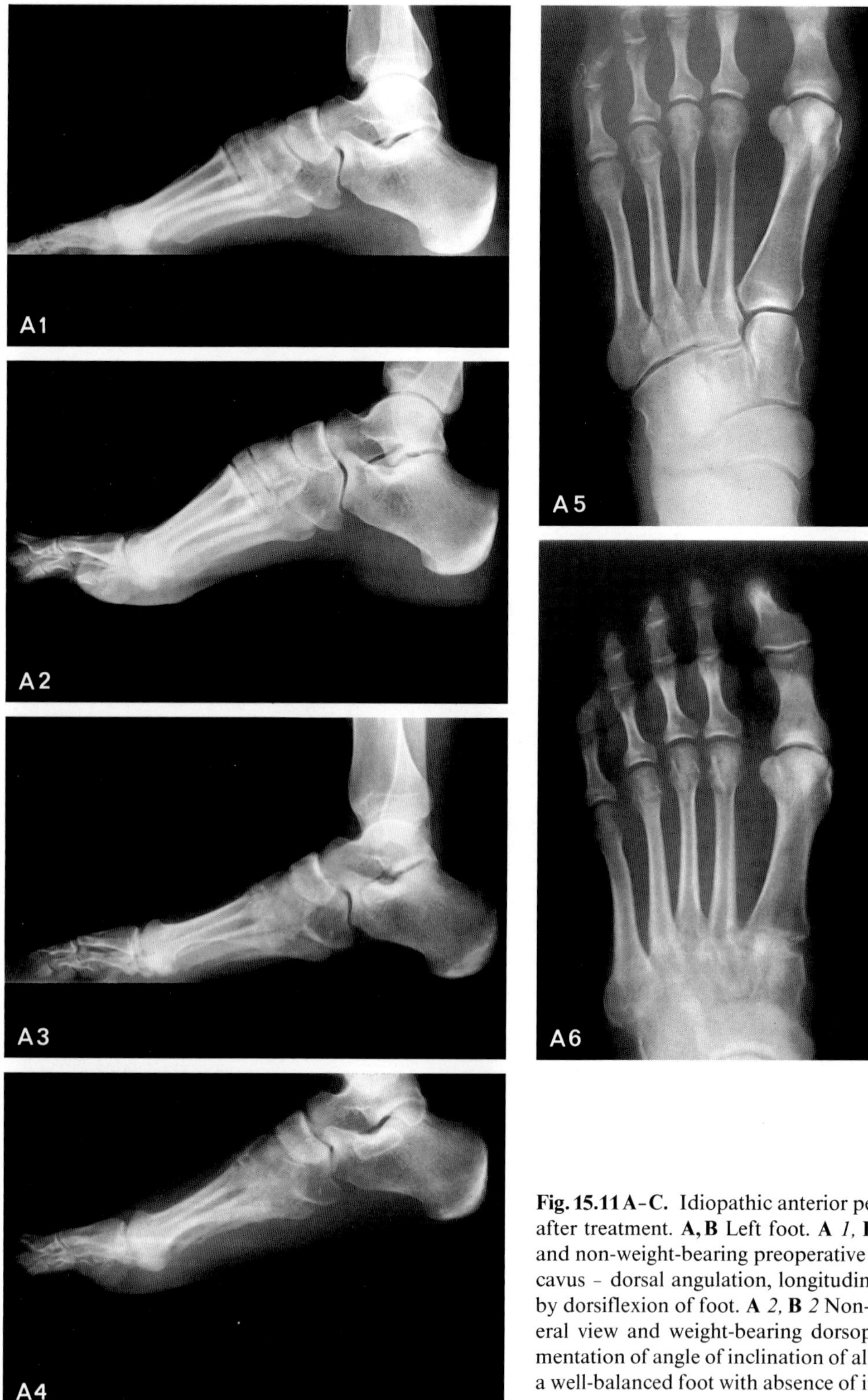

Fig. 15.11 A–C. Idiopathic anterior pes cavus before and ▷ after treatment. **A, B** Left foot. **A** *1*, **B** *1* Weight-bearing and non-weight-bearing preoperative views: anterior pes cavus – dorsal angulation, longitudinal cavus, reducible by dorsiflexion of foot. **A** *2*, **B** *2* Non-weight-bearing lateral view and weight-bearing dorsoplantar views: augmentation of angle of inclination of all five metatarsals in a well-balanced foot with absence of inversion of midtarsus

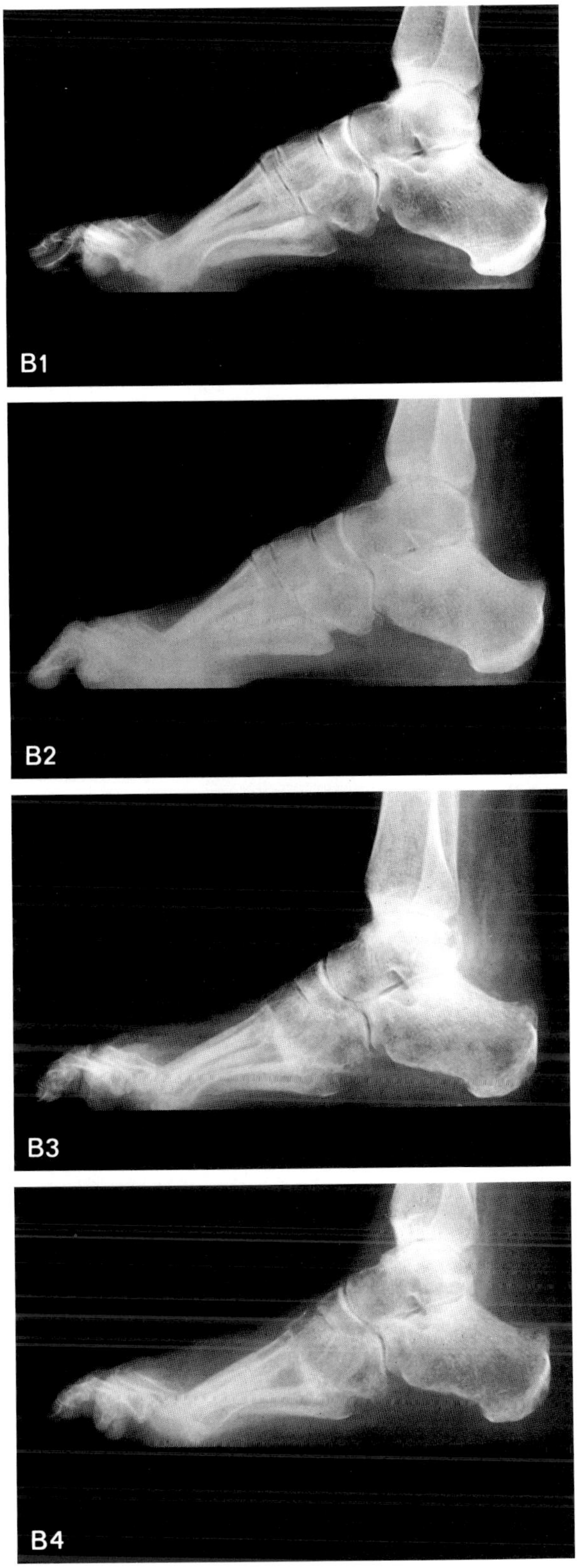

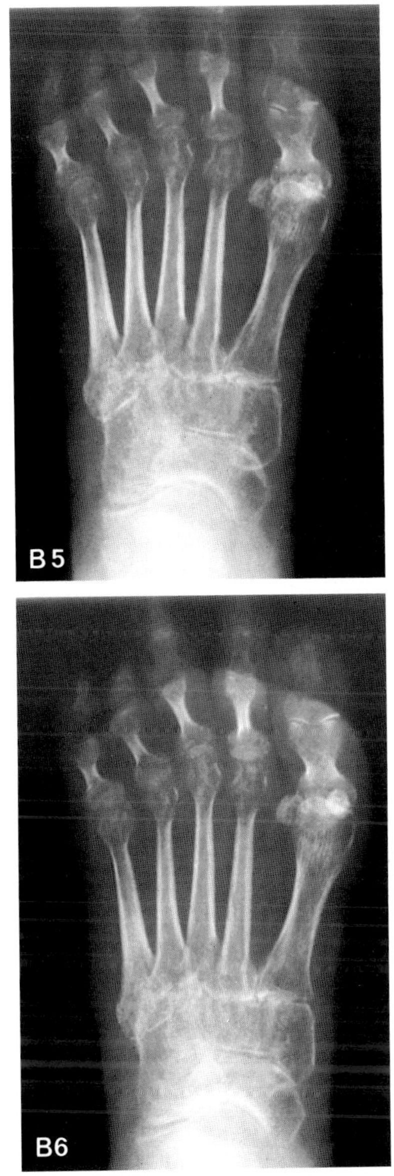

Fig. 15.11 *(continued)*. **A** *3*, **B** *3* Weight-bearing lateral views after osteotomy at tarsometatarsal joint line *(Lisfranc)*. **A** *4*, **B** *4* Non-weight-bearing lateral views after osteotomy of tarsometatarsal joint line. **A** *5, 6* Dorsoplantar views before and after osteotomy of cuneiform and cuboidometatarsal joints. **B** *5, 6* Weight-bearing and non-weight-bearing dorsoplantar views after osteotomy at tarsometatarsal joint line. **C** see p. 142

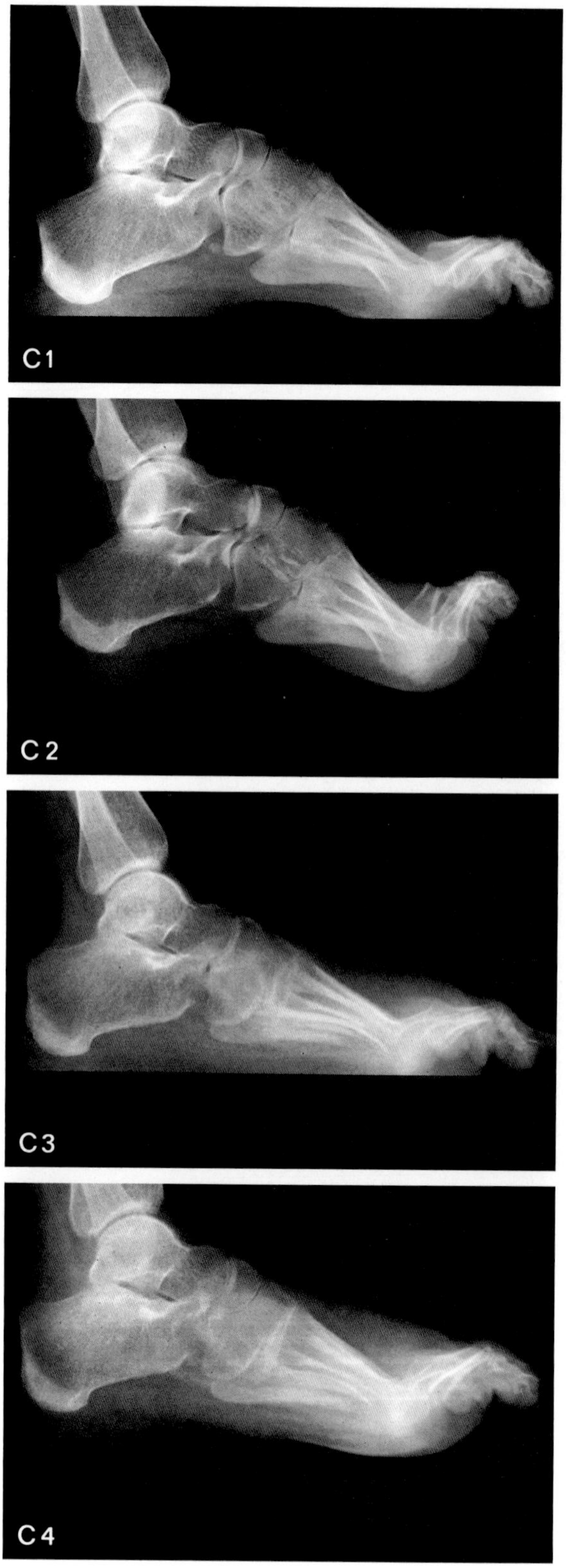

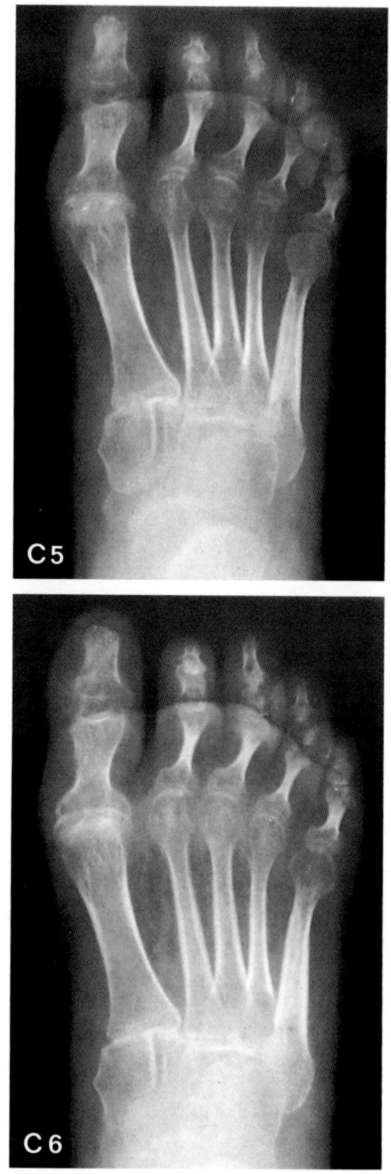

Fig. 15.11 *(continued)*. **C** Right foot. *1* Weight-bearing, preoperative lateral view: anterior pes cavus with irreducible deformity, cavus and marked augmentation of arch, augmentation of angle of inclination of metatarsus. Onset of inversion of midtarsus is detected; *2* non-weight-bearing, preoperative lateral view; *3, 4* weight-bearing and non-weight-bearing lateral views after osteotomy at cuneiform-cuboidometatarsal joint line; *5, 6* weight-bearing and non-weight-bearing dorsoplantar views after osteotomy at cuneiform-cuboidometatarsal joint line

due to excessive pronation of the first ray, which follows because the first metatarsal head has lost its contact with the ground. *Valgus* displacement appears when hypertonia of the peronei predominates so that the inner border yields at the level of the medial cuneiform or at the Lisfranc joint line and becomes convex with abduction of the metatarsus. This determines the appearance of a convex triangular forefoot.

When transverse equilibrium of the talocalcaneal complex is maintained by equal hypertonia of the internal and external extrinsic muscle groups, the generalised quinus of the metatarsals results in a convex forefoot or a cavus forefoot, depending upon the initial metatarsal formula.

The angle between the tibia and the calcaneum remains a little more than 90°. The varieties of anterior longitudinal cavus show the following features:

a) *Longitudinal cavus,* constituted by depression of the anterior segment with the posterior limb in the proper position with respect to the axis of the tibia. The posterior tibiotarsal angle is normal or slightly increased. The summit of the cavus is more anterior in location, being at the level of the cuneiforms or the tarsometatarsal joint lines, and may be accompanied from the beginning by selective equinus accentuated in the first metatarsal (a reaction to valgus or varus disbalance of the tarsus in the adolescent or young adult, especially when provoked by the wearing of high heels). This results in the antero-internal cavus foot, which in the absence of correction progresses to the anterior supinated cavus foot or the anterior cavovarus foot. Alternatively, when the tarsus remains balanced there may be equinus and protrusion of the second and third metatarsals. This amounts to the formation of either the balanced cavus foot with convex forefoot or an anterior cavovalgus foot from imbalance in the tarsometatarsal region.
b) *The dorsal arch configuration* is characterised by a sudden angular change at the level of the cuneiforms, these bones tending to protrude beyond the metatarsal bases.
c) *Elevation of the lateral band,* which may exceed 50 mm.
d) *Symptoms* of tarsalgia externally in the anterior cavovarus foot and internally in the anterior cavovalgus foot. General pains from the tarsometatarsal joint lines are accompanied by typical metatarsalgia and painful clawed toes.

The *clinical presentations* of the five types of anterior cavus may be summarised as follows.

15.5.1.1 Antero-internal Cavus

This, the first stage of anterior cavus, is associated with accentuated deformity along the inner border of the foot. The summit of the dorsal arch is situated at the level of the first cuneiform-metatarsal joint and it is only the medial side of the foot which is noticeably elevated, the outer border resting on the ground normally. The heel is balanced and pronation and supination of the calcaneum are normal. Digital clawing is fixed only in the great toe, remaining supple in the other toes. Keratoma, callus or a serous bursa develops under the first metatarsal head and may be associated with sesamoid hypertrophy. The sesamoids may develop a longitudinal crest, their retracted position accentuating the claw posture of the toe. The great metatarsal head is markedly lowered with respect to its neighbours, which remain normally aligned.

Radiography confirms the clinical findings, the equinus of the great metatarsal and the normal orientation of the outer four metatarsals.

Conservative treatment with an insole is indicated when the condition remains supple. The insole may comprise a retrocapital bar supplemented in the presence of valgus or varus of the tarsus by a supinating or a pronating subcalcaneal wedge. Alternatively a monoblock insole with a retrocapital bar may be appropriate for the adult who cannot tolerate the corrective insole.

Operative treatment is usually indicated beyond the age of 18 years. It is directed towards correction of the antero-internal cavus, this being achieved by a semicircular basal osteotomy perhaps associated with the excision of a serous bursa or flattening of a hypertrophied sesamoid. Occasionally a plantar cutaneous rotation flap is necessary after excision of an isolated keratoma, but the thickening of a callus disappears spontaneously after correction of the equinus of the first metatarsal. Extensor hallucis longus and brevis may require elongation if the clawing of the great toe is marked, together with arthrodesis of the interphalangeal joint if it is irreducible.

15.5.1.2 Anterior Supinated Cavovarus

This condition represents an evolution of the antero-internal cavus foot in which permanent metatarsalgia under the great metatarsal head induces supination of the foot so as to reduce this painful loading. The transfer of more and more load externally leads to metatarsalgias under the fourth and fifth metatarsal heads, where callus and keratomata form. The metatarsal equinus and overall longitudinal cavus tend to extend to the outer side of the foot, and the convexity of the dorsal arch is maximal at the level of the intermediate and lateral cuneiforms.

This condition can arise spontaneously, when it is characterised by rigidity of the fourth metatarsal and consequent overloading of its head. It becomes associated with varus posture of the calcaneum, as well as the supination of the forefoot which leads inevitably to overloading of the fifth metatarsal heads. Digital clawing produces the usual symptoms, and pain develops over the outer part of the midtarsal region, with a tension component localised to the calcaneocuboid joint space and to the lateral ligaments of the subtalar joint.

Radiography reveals the longitudinal cavus and the varus inversion of the metatarsus.

Conservative treatment may be tried in the supple foot, using an insole with a retrocapital bar and a pronating external band. Surgery is indicated for the rigid foot.

Operative treatment comprises basal osteotomy of the fourth and fifth metatarsals together with possible transcuneiform-cuboidal wedge osteotomy with the base dorso-externally, completed if necessary by plantar fasciotomy. The re-establishment of calcaneal balance can be maintained by external transposition of tibialis anterior onto the lateral cuneiform, or even the cuboid, together with elongation of tibialis posterior.

15.5.1.3 Anterior Longitudinal Cavus with Forefoot Cavus

This is a combination of the two preceding forms. Occasionally it can appear at the outset, particularly when induced by trauma from a shoe with an excessively rigid sole. The forefoot cavus arises from an attempt to rebalance a supinated forefoot by depression of the great metatarsal so as to re-establish contact with the ground. This is brought about by hypertonia of the peronei, which tend to correct the varus of the foot and at the same time influence the position of the first metatarsal. Overloading occurs under the first and perhaps fourth and fifth metatarsal heads.

In contrast with the two preceding forms, this foot becomes rigid early. The longitudinal cavus and bulging of the dorsal arch occur at the intermediate and lateral cuneiforms, while the contracture of the plantar aponeurosis is marked by a rigid cord which is palpable under the skin, especially when the great toe is dorsiflexed. Early contracture of the long extensor and flexor tendons of the toes provokes irreducible digital clawing with subluxation or dislocation of the metatarsophalangeal joints, associated capsular contractions, and atrophy of the dorsal skin.

Conservative treatment has little to offer.

Operative treatment comprises calcaneal osteotomy (Dwyer 1959) to correct the varus of the foot and transverse osteotomy at the Lisfranc joint line in which more bone is removed at the bases of the first and fifth rays, accompanied when necessary by external transposition of tibialis anterior in order to consolidate the rebalanced foot (Fig. 15.12). Clawing of the toes is treated subsequently.

15.5.1.4 Anterior Longitudinal Balanced Cavus with Convex Forefoot

In this condition, hypertonia of the medial and lateral extrinsic muscle groups is balanced but occurs in a foot with a metatarsal formula of the Greek type, there being protrusion of the central metatarsal heads. Overloading occurs, with formation of a large callosity in the centre of the ball of the forefoot, and in severe cases the deformity can be gross, amounting to 40 or 50 mm of depression. The maximum angulation of the longitudinal arch occurs at the intermediate and lateral cuneiforms, while clawing of the toes is very severe and fixed.

Radiography strikingly shows the parallel alignment of the five metatarsals with anterior protrusion of the central three rays. In the Müller view, the depression of the metatarsal heads is evident.

Conservative management with an insole can be attempted, using a retrocapital bar or more frequently a monoblock insole with a retrocapital bar; however, it is not likely to succeed in such a fixed foot.

Operative treatment by means of Lelièvre basal metatarsectomy procedure has been advocated, but I prefer correction at the Lisfranc joint line with greater resection at the middle three rays. The convex forefoot has to be realigned distally by enclavement of the second, third and fourth metatarsal heads, this being frequently necessary because of dislocation at the metatarsophalangeal joints. The clawing of the toes is corrected simultaneously by appropriate tendinous elongations or arthrodeses of the interphalangeal joints. In cases where the forefoot happens to remain supple, V-osteotomies of the metatarsal bases can be considered.

While ostectomies of Mau (1940) or Thys (1974b) correct the round forefoot element very well, there is the usual problem of the need for extreme precision in their fashioning; overresection will result in a cavus forefoot.

15.5.1.5 Anterior Cavovalgus

During the supple phase of the developing longitudinal cavus, loss of loading under the base of the fifth metatarsal renders the foot unstable, so that the forefoot tends to supinate, bringing the lateral border nearer to the ground; this becomes accompanied by a valgus deformity in the hindfoot. Calcaneal pronation is a result of predominance of the peronei over tibialis posterior.

The anterior cavovalgus foot is therefore characterised by progressive loss of contact with the ground along the lateral border of the foot. The height of the plantar arch decreases internally at the same rate as it increases externally, with a relative difference of some 2-4 mm between the extremes. Eventually there is a contracted cavovalgus foot with a residual dorsal arch at the Lisfranc joint line and cuneiforms which protrude beyond the bases of the metatarsals. The calcaneum becomes valgoid. The abduction of the metatarsus may become a very significant component and is accompanied by marked angulation at the Lisfranc joint line arising at the medial cuneiform bone. The external border of the foot, in contrast, presents a sharp concavity at the angulation, again at the Lisfranc joint line. In the forefoot, a convex triangular or cavus deformity develops.

Conservative treatment should be employed when the condition is seen early in the infant or adolescent. Management should be with an insole bearing a pronating band in the retrocapital area and a supinating wedge under the heel. In the older patient this will prove intolerable unless supplemented by a plantar dome.

Operative treatment is usually indicated in the adult and comprises extra-articular semicircular transverse cuneiform-cuboidal osteotomy or osteotomy-arthrodesis at the Lisfranc joint line (Figs. 15.13, 15.14). With appropriate trapezoid wedges, the bases lying dorsally and medially, it is possible to correct the longitudinal cavus and the abduction of the metatarsus (Regnauld 1974) at one and the same time.

15.5.2 Posterior Longitudinal Pes Cavus

15.5.2.1 Etiology

This condition nearly always arises from neuromuscular paralysis, most frequently from poliomyelitis or as a sequel of trauma, much less commonly from a spastic condition. The posterior cavus is a consequence of relative weakness of triceps surae, as a result of which the calcaneum is not maintained in a balanced position sagittally and augments its angle of inclination significantly. The talus becomes fully dorsiflexed in the ankle mortice and a secondary equinus of the antetarsus develops. The summit of the angulation constituting the longitudinal cavus is at the Chopart or talonavicular joint line.

The inclination of the calcaneum is markedly augmented, sometimes exceeding 130°, and this, together with the elevated midtarsus and equinus metatarsus, leads to the pronounced cavus deformity. The heel is square and in varus (or rarely in valgus when overaction of the peronei is accompanied by paralysis of triceps surae and the tibialis muscles) (Fig. 15.14).

The functional disability associated with the elevated midtarsal mass and equinus of the antetarsus may be severe, the subject finding it impossible to walk on tiptoe or climb stairs. In addition to the deformity, these actions are impeded by the weakness of triceps surae.

When the *longitudinal cavus* is viewed laterally, it can be seen that the inclination of the calcaneum forms an angle of some 60° with the ground, more than 130° with the tibia. From the talonavicular joint, the antetarsus presents a straight line. The cavus is irreducible, fixed initially by a contracture of the intrinsic muscles and then by osteoarticular deformity, especially at the talocalcaneal junction. Depending on further details of muscle imbalance, the longitudinal cavus may take one of three forms:

Balanced: This will occur when the lateral muscles are equally competent and the general axis of the foot is preserved. However, depending on muscle balance, the loading of the heel and forefoot will vary. Thus, if with the paralysis of triceps surae there is relative weakness of the long flexors, the forefoot may not reach the ground, with the result that most loading occurs at the heel, which then hypertrophies. Conversely, if there is dominance of the flexors of the forefoot and weakness of the extensors and triceps surae, overloading of the forefoot may occur, with callus formation and clawing of the toes.

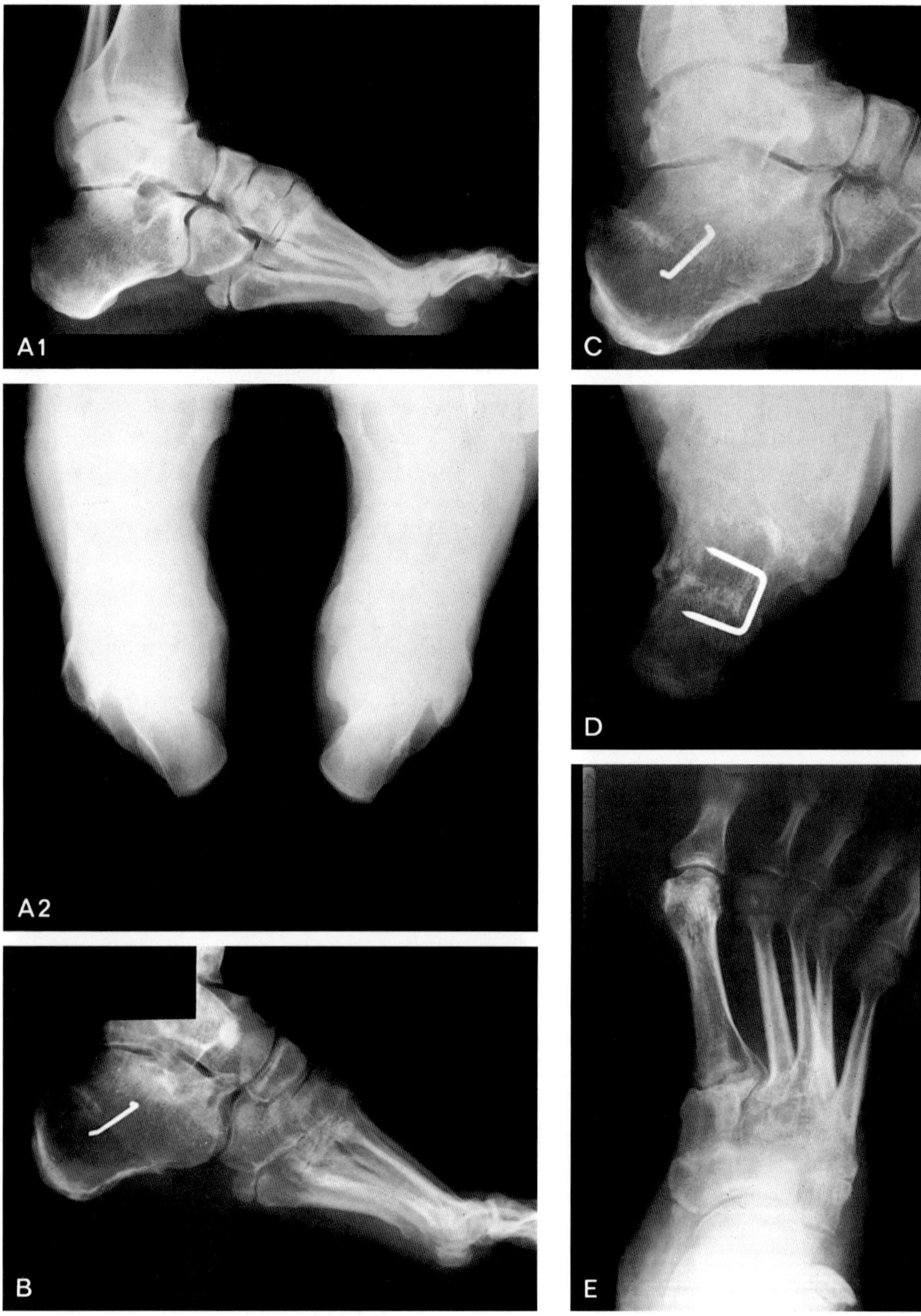

Fig. 15.12 A–H. Pes cavovarus. **A** Right foot. *1* Preoperative lateral view showing pes cavovarus. The longitudinal cavus has its summit at angulation seen at level of tarsometatarsal joint line. There is deformation of ankle; *2* marked varus or supination of calcaneum. **B** Lateral view after postoperative osteotomy of tarsometatarsal joint line with calcaneal osteotomy (Dwyer) correcting ▷ varus posture of calcaneum. **C, D** Lateral and posterior views of calcaneal osteotomy. **E** Dorsoplantar view after osteotomy at cuneiform-metatarsal joint correcting both cavus and varus. **F–H** see p. 147

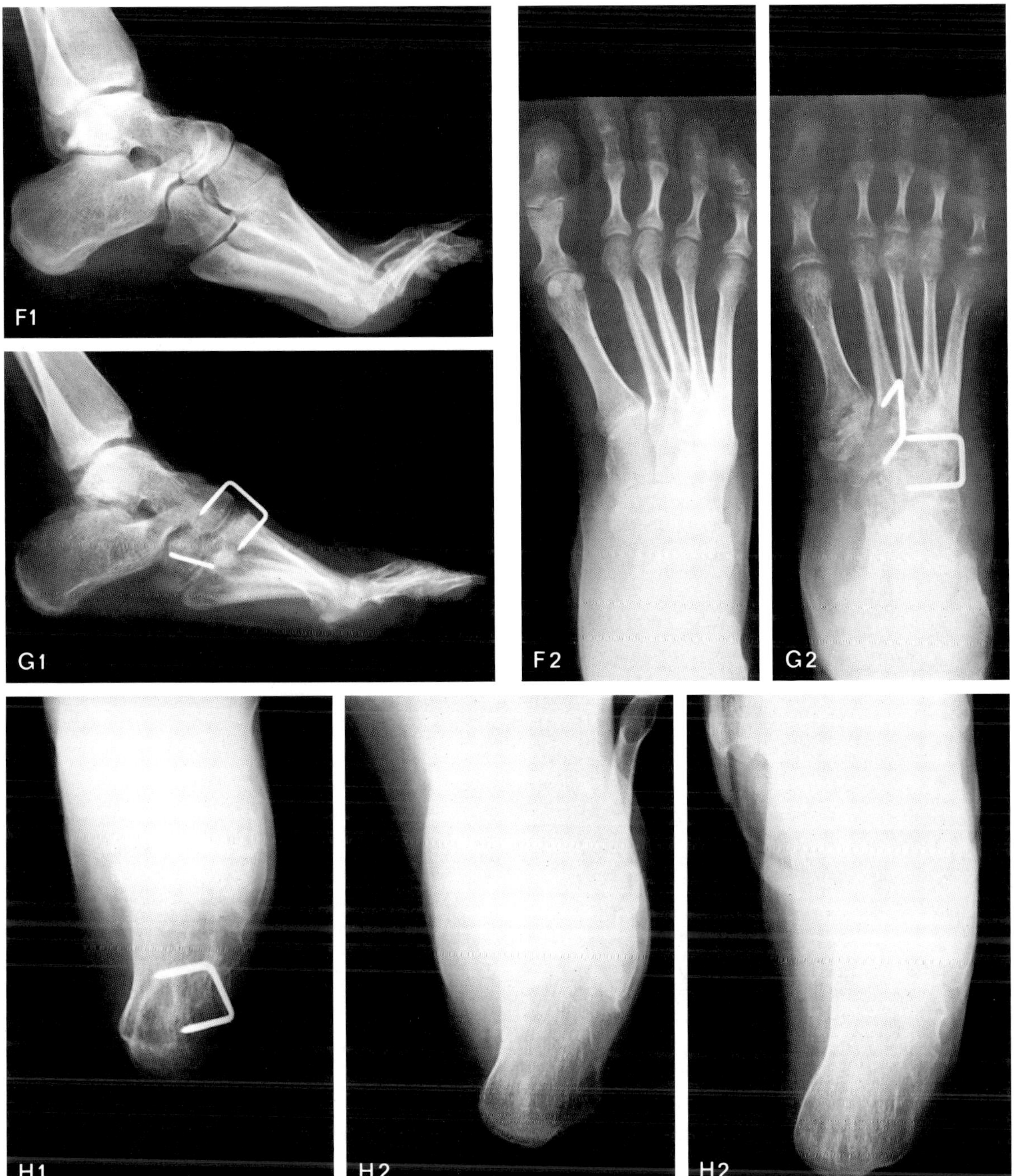

Fig. 15.12 *(continued)* **F** Right foot. *1* Lateral view: cavovarus deformity with longitudinal component at level of navicular; *2* dorsoplantar view: pes cavus with inversion and adduction of the antetarsus. **G** Right foot. *1* Lateral view after osteotomy at naviculocuneiform region correcting cavus and anterior varus as well as adduction component; *2* dorsoplantar view after osteotomy across navicular cuneiform joint line and into cuboid correcting longitudinal cavus, varus of midtarsus and adduction of antetarsus. **H** *1* Dwyer osteotomy of calcaneum correcting varus posture; *2* supination of tarsus: both varus and calcaneal supination

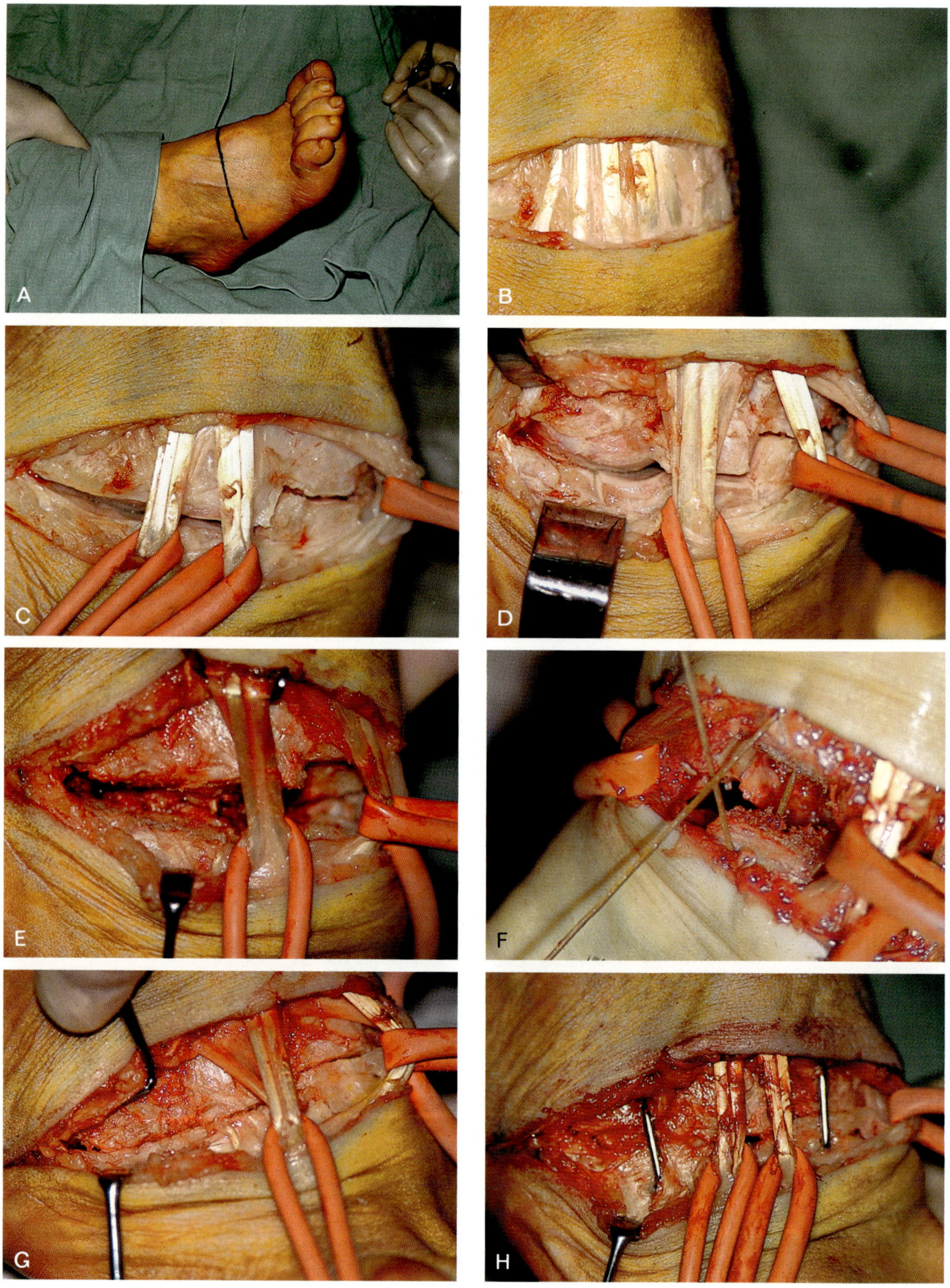

Fig. 15.13 A–F. Correction of anterior pes cavus by osteotomy-arthrodesis at the Lisfranc joint line. **A–C** Incisions. **D–F** Wedge resection with base dorsally at the cuneiform-metatarsal joint line. **G–L** Resection and coaptation of bone surfaces. **M, N** Fixation by staple ▷ or intra-osseous suture. **O, P** Closure of the two layers.

I–P see p. 149

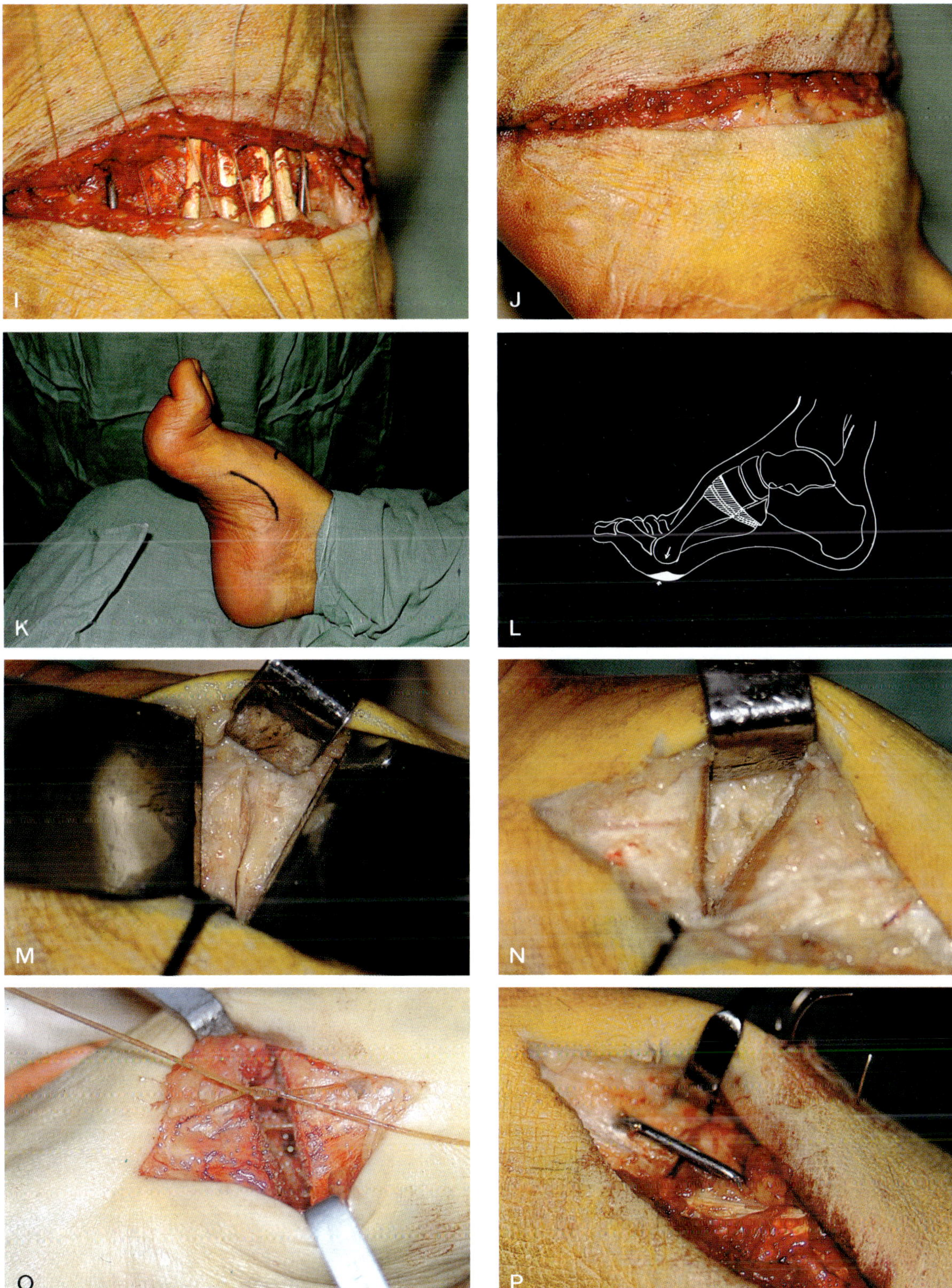

Fig. 15.13 I–P. Legend see p. 148

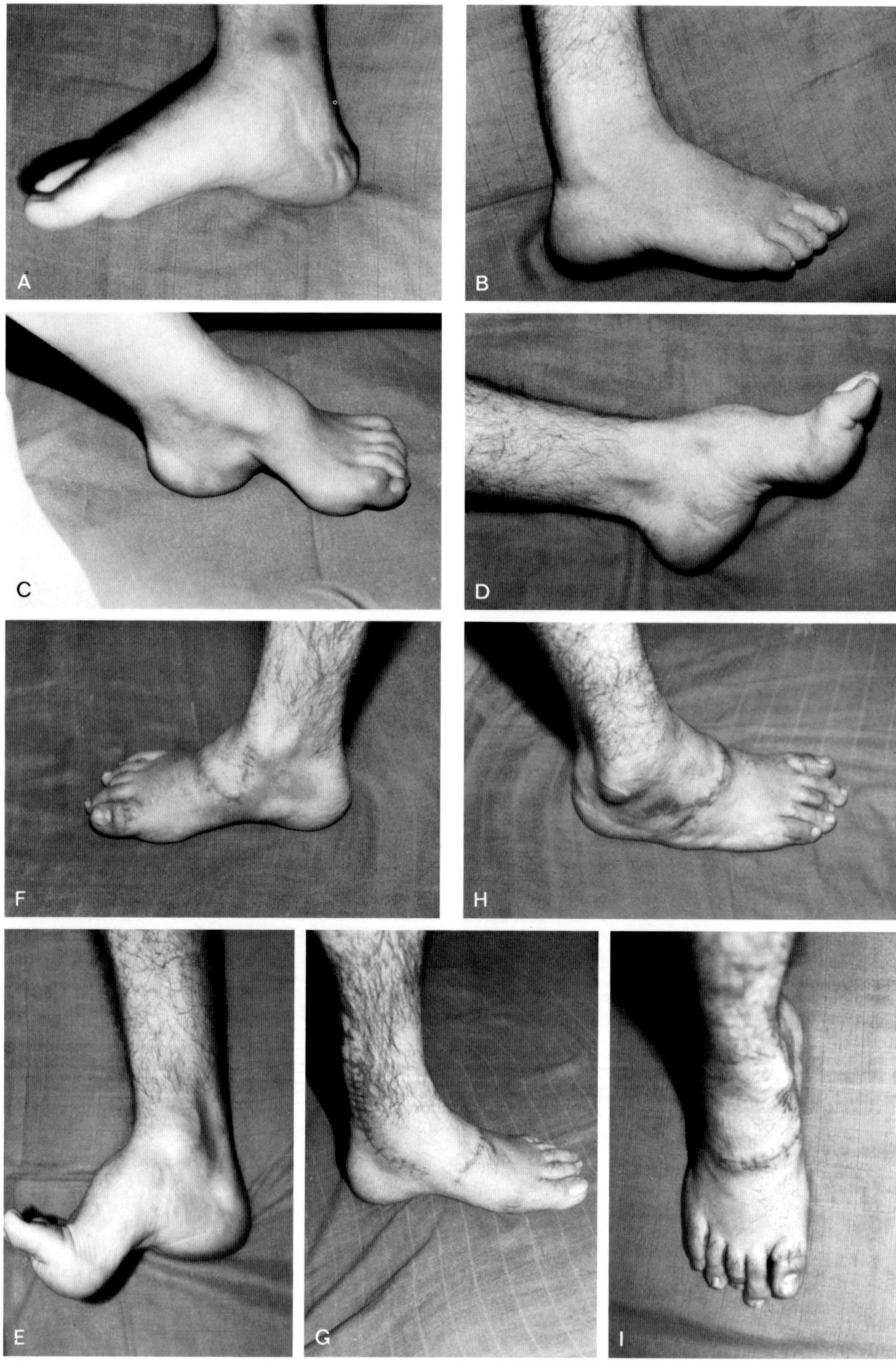
A
B
C
D
F
H
E
G
I

Varus: The foot may develop internal deviation when there is imbalance between the medial and lateral muscles. A plantar internal concavity develops, associated with a fold in the skin at the medial aspect of the navicular. This is the most frequent configuration. Tibialis anterior, tibialis posterior and flexor hallucis longus are dominant. As a result of the cavovarus deformity, there is overloading with painful callus formation under the fifth metatarsal head and further symptoms from tension in the lateral aspect of the ankle joint.
Valgus: This rare form is the result of weakness of triceps surae and the tibialis muscles. Significant valgus of the tarsus with abduction of the metatarsus and development of an external angulation at the level of the cuboid coexists with dorsiflexion posture of the ankle joint. This is maintained by overaction of the peroneal muscles and of the extensors, the tendons of which bowstring noticeably under the skin. Despite the longitudinal accentuated cavus, the foot rests on the ground almost only at the heel.
In all three forms, the elevation of the midtarsal region may be gross, up to 50 mm from the ground. *Forefoot displacements* are variable according to the type of displacement into valgus or varus of the longitudinal arch. Clawing of the toes with metatarsophalangeal dorsal disorganisation will be exaggerated if the long extensor action preponderates, and will become fixed by shortening of the interossei and lumbricales. Cavus forefoot or convex forefoot will be associated with the usual callus formations.

15.5.2.2 Clinical Features

These are logical in terms of the mechanism and development of the deformity described above. Pain is experienced at the anterior aspect of the ankle joint, and the patient may say that he finds more comfort in a higher heel. Walking without shoes aggravates the pain progressively. There may be discomfort over the outer aspect of the ankle and subtalar joints, perhaps located at the sinus tarsi. This is particularly so in the cavovarus variety, whereas in posterior cavovalgus, pain is located along the inner aspect of the ankle and subtalar joint. Arthrosic pains in the midtarsal region are unusual. Together with the hindfoot pains, the symptoms from metatarsalgia of disordered loading complete the presentation.
Radiography: In the lateral view, the calcaneus posture of the talus and the vertical alignment of the calcaneum are obvious. The fully dorsiflexed position of the ankle joint may be striking, and on the dorsal aspect of the neck of the talus, a hog's back may develop. The site of maximum longitudinal cavus at the talonavicular or naviculocuneiform levels can be identified and the degree of loss of contact with the ground measured in weight-bearing views. Dorsal dislocations of the metatarsophalangeal joints are identified (Fig. 15.15). A frontal view shows the levels of the five metatarsal heads, and the metatarsal formula can be identified in the dorsoplantar view.

◁ **Fig. 15.14 A–I.** Posterior and combined pes cavus. **A, B** Posterior pes cavus with paralysis of triceps surae. **C** Posterior pes cavus. **D, E** Combined pes cavus, preoperative. **F–I** Combined pes cavus after operative correction

15.5.2.3 Treatment

Operation is the treatment of choice. The procedure will vary according to the exact sites of deformity; perhaps a pantalar arthrodesis of the ankle, subtalar and midtarsal joints or a triple arthrodesis of the subtalar and midtarsal joints. Tendo Achillis may be shortened or tenodesed. Flexor hallucis longus and peroneus brevis may be transplanted onto tendo Achillis, while the tibialis anterior tendon may be elongated. Anterior capsulotomy of the ankle joint and lateral arthrolysis can restore movement here.
In the presence of a varus calcaneum, the elongation of tibialis anterior tendon should be accompanied by lateral transplantation onto the intermediate or lateral cuneiforms. Bony correction may be achieved by extra-articular osteotomy (intracuneiform-cuboidal) wedge resection with the base situated dorso-externally or by arthrodesis of the naviculocuneiform joint and osteotomy of the cuboid. A Dwyer (1959) calcaneal osteotomy can be associated to advantage with plantar release. Subsequent to surgical management, a corrective insole with a varus wedge under the heel should be used.

15.6 Pes Equinocavus

Pes equinocavus is a distinct entity which may be of neurological origin following encephalitis of infancy, paralysis of tibialis anterior in poliomyelitis, complete sciatic palsy associated with flail foot, lateral popliteal nerve palsy when it produces an equinovarus foot, or selective weakness of the peronei leading to a varus posture (Figs. 15.16, 15.17).

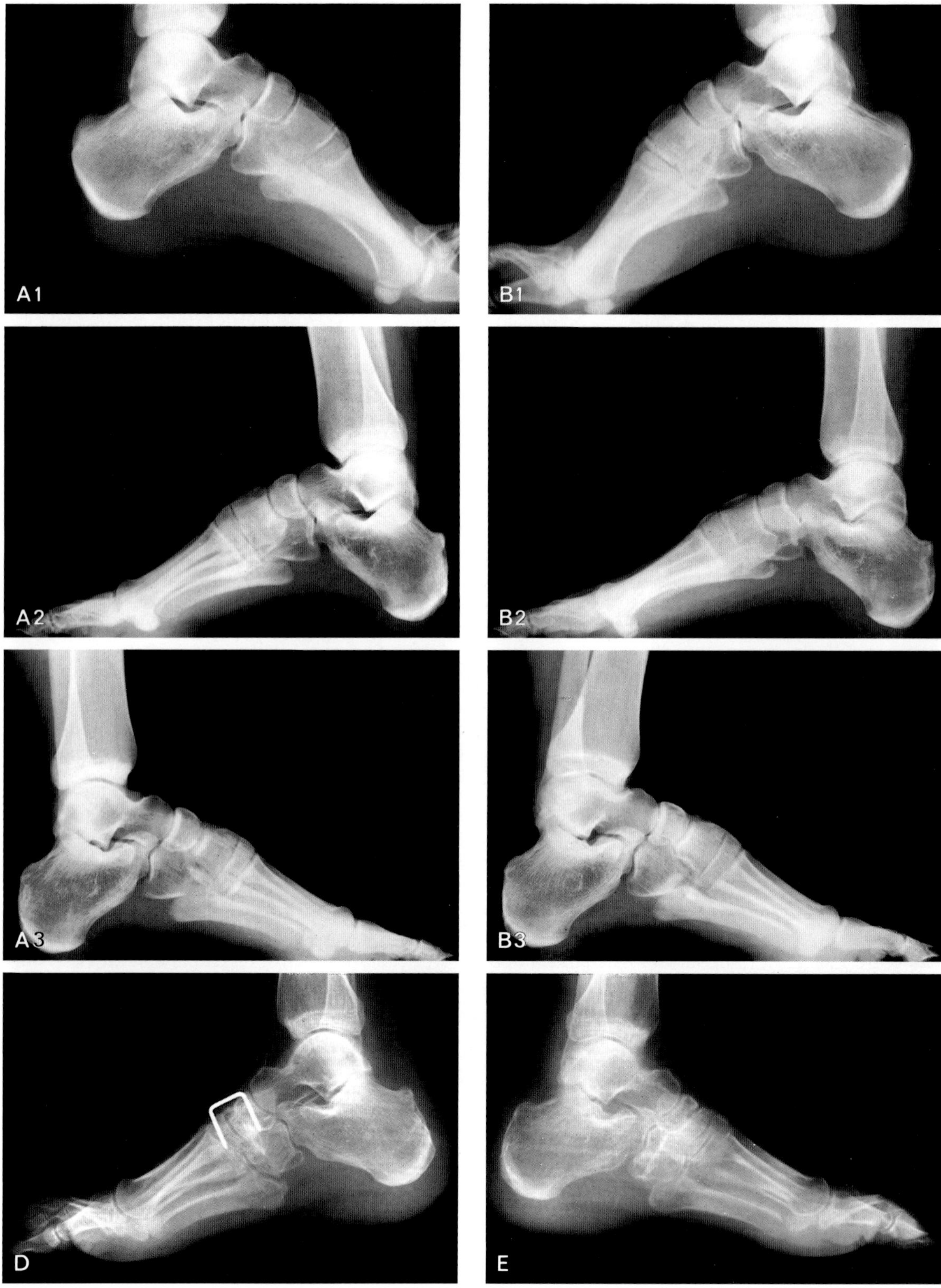

Fig. 15.15 A–E. Legend see p. 153

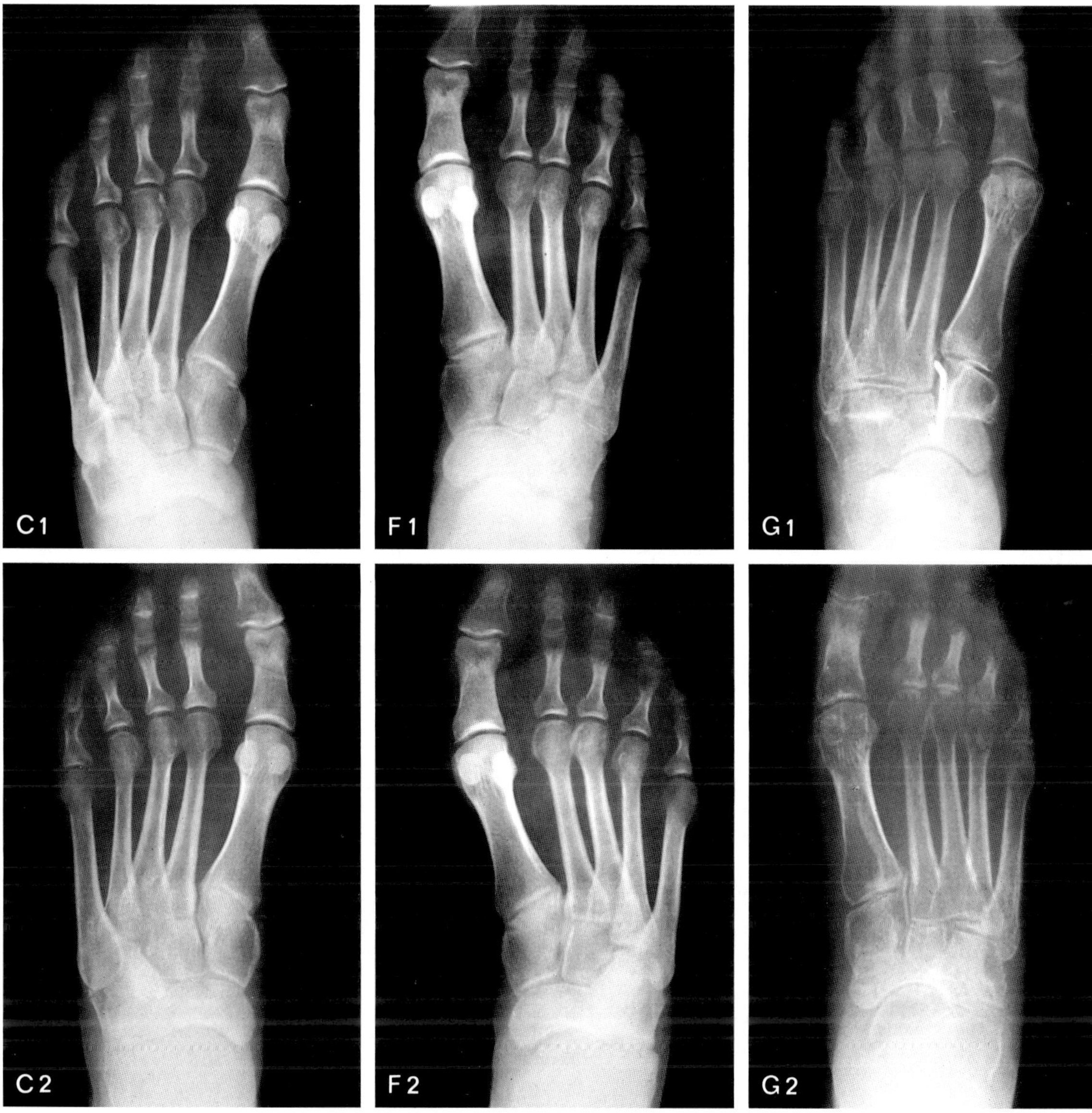

◁ **Fig. 15.15 A–G.** A case of posterior pes cavus. **A** *1, 2* Non-weight-bearing lateral views of right foot and left foot respectively; *3* weight-bearing lateral view of right foot: three images show disturbed loading, longitudinal cavus, dorsal angulation and calcaneal equinus with augmentation of angle of inclination of calcaneum. **B** *1* Non-weight-bearing lateral view of left foot: dorsal angulation, plantar cavus, disturbance of loading; *2, 3* weight-bearing lateral views of left and right foot: significant augmentation of angle of inclination of calcaneum. **C** *1, 2* Weight-bearing and non-weight-bearing preoperative dorsoplantar views of left foot. **D, E** Non-weight-bearing lateral views of left and right foot after osteotomy at naviculocuneiform region extended to cuboidal region. **F** *1, 2* Weight-bearing and non-weight-bearing preoperative dorsoplantar views of right foot. **G** *1, 2* Dorsoplantar views of left and right foot after transmidtarsal osteotomy at naviculocuneiform and intracuboidal regions

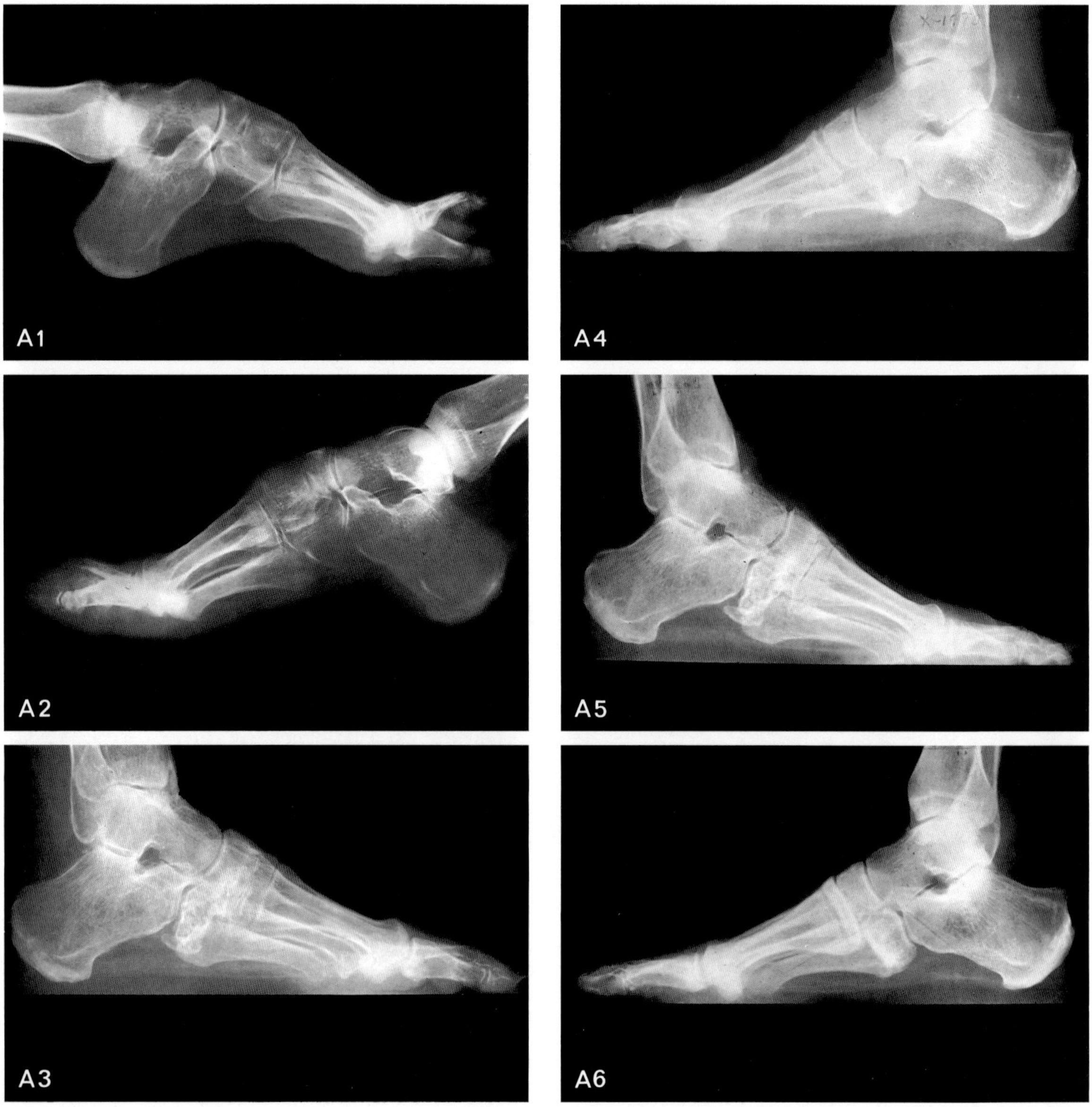

Fig. 15.16 A–C. Pes equinocavus and combined pes cavus. **A** Pes equinocavus with summit at level of navicular. *1, 2* Preoperative lateral views of left foot and right foot respectively; *3, 4* three months after naviculocuneiform ▷ and transcuboidal osteotomy; *5, 6* eight months postoperatively. **B, C** see pp. 155, 156

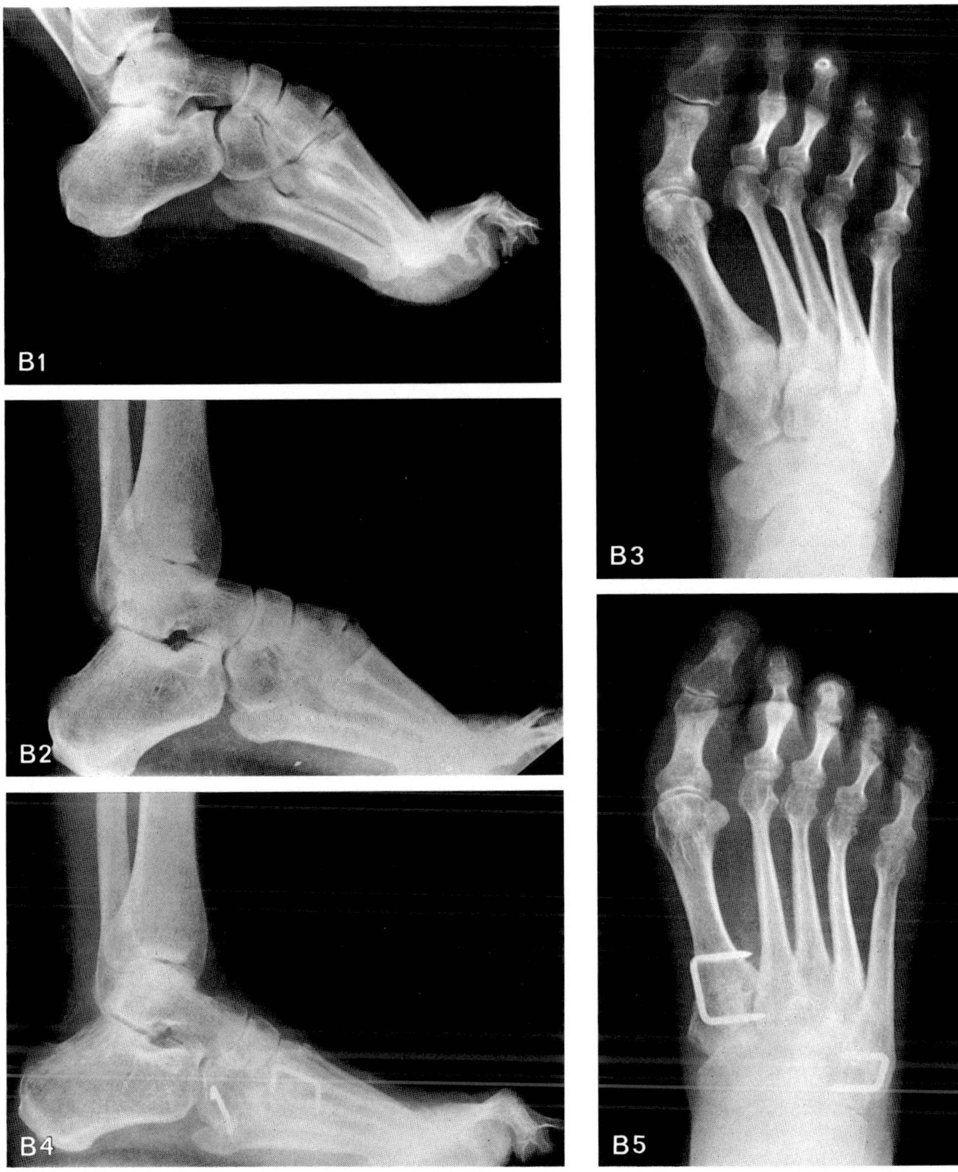

Fig. 15.16 *(continued).* **B** Combined varus and cavus foot with summit at tarsometatarsal joint line. *1, 2* Non-weight-bearing and weight-bearing views; *3* dorsoplantar view: adduction of antetarsus and inversion of midtarsus; *4* lateral view after osteotomy-arthrodesis of tarsometatarsal joint line correcting varus, inversion and adduction of metatarsus; *5* dorsoplantar view after osteotomy-arthrodesis of tarsometatarsal joint line achieving good longitudinal realignment of foot

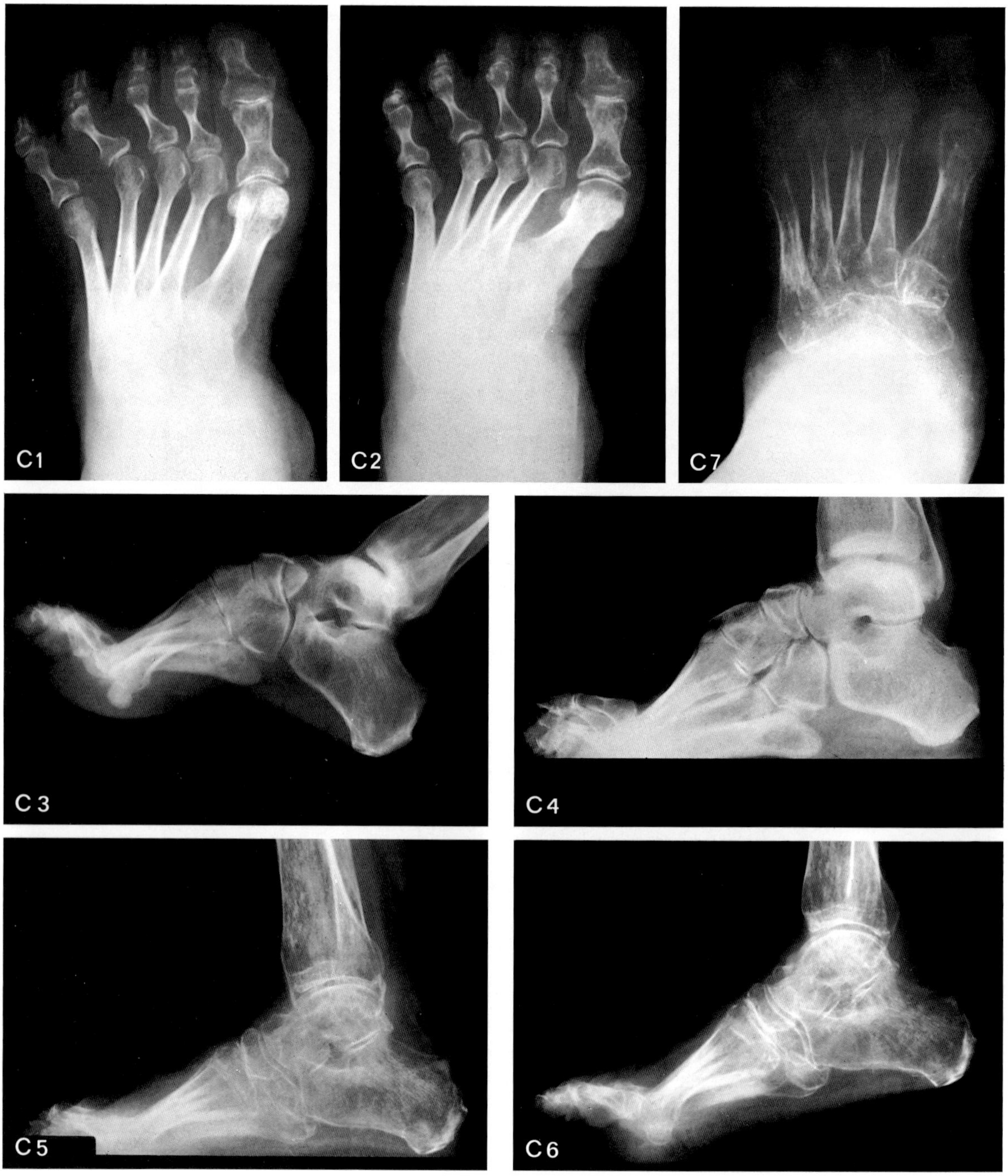

Fig. 15.16 *(continued)*. **C** Combined pes cavus with summit at naviculocuneiform joint. *1, 2* Weight-bearing and non-weight-bearing dorsoplantar views: adduction of antetarsus; *3, 4* non-weight-bearing and weight-bearing lateral views; *5, 6, 7* after osteotomy-arthrodesis at naviculocuneiform and transcuboidal regions correcting cavus, inversion and adduction of forefoot

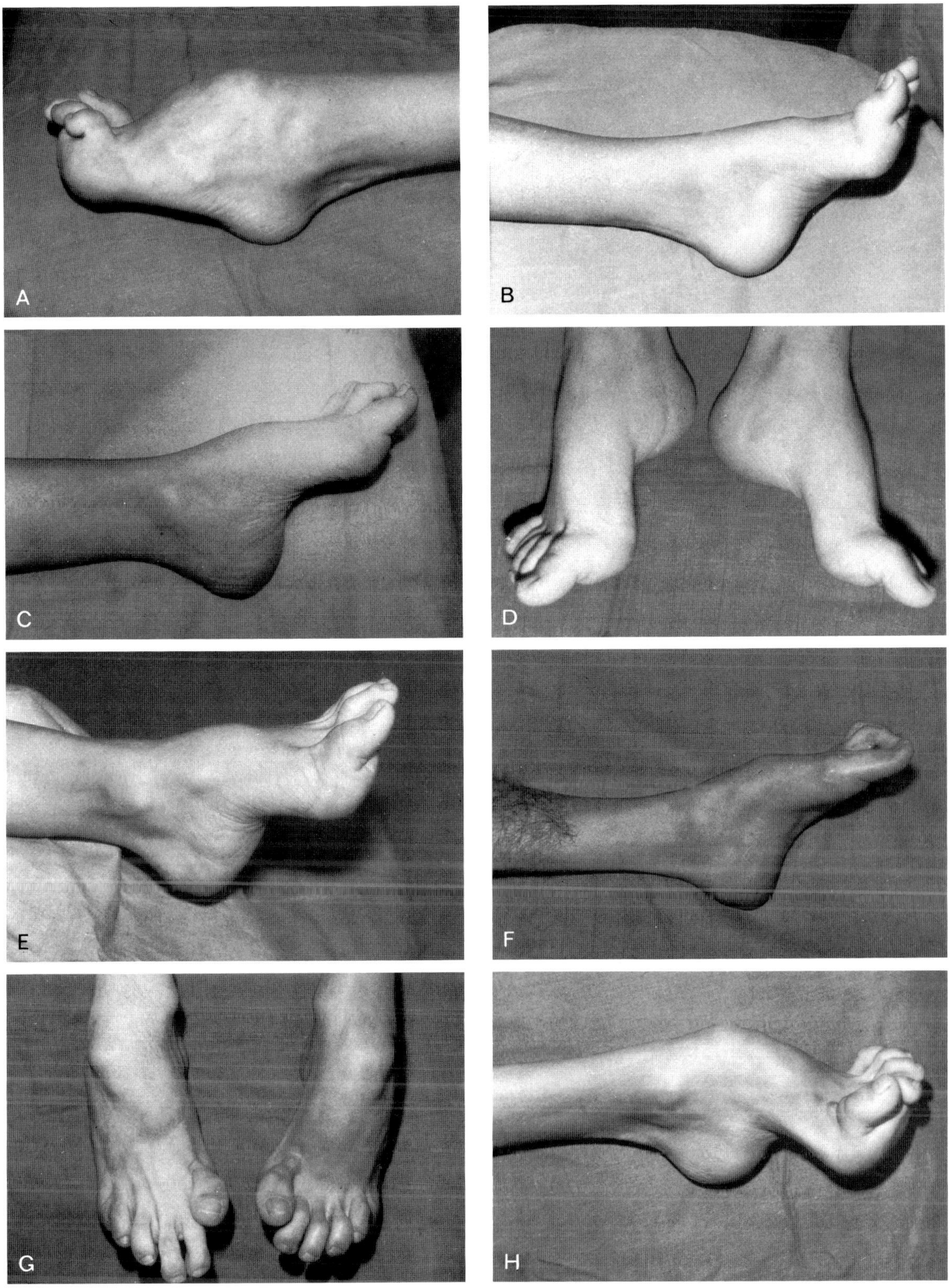

Fig. 15.17 A–I. Pes equinocavus. **A–F** Neutral alignment. **G–H** Varus alignment

It can also arise from efforts to compensate for shortening of the lower limb on account of, for example, congenital dislocation of the hip or poliomyelitis of infancy. Even fracture of the femoral shaft or of the tibia and fibula with loss of length can lead to this condition.

The foot is characterised by longitudinal cavus affecting both the forefoot and hindfoot analogous to the longitudinal cavus which can be produced from dancing on the points of the toes. Contracture of triceps surae fixes the foot in overall equinus, and the ankle is permanently plantarflexed. The posterior tibiocalcaneal angle may be normal or reduced. The maximum convexity of the dorsal arch is in the midtarsal region, and overloading of the forefoot results either in a median callosity or in scattered callosities under various metatarsal heads. Irreverisble digital clawing occurs.

Clinical examination must include an appreciation of any lower limb shortening, and it is wise to assess muscle power electromyographically in planning appropriate tendon transfers.

Radiography confirms the structural description given (Fig. 15.18).

Treatment is operative, most frequently comprising osteotomy of the midtarsal region, preserving the talonavicular joint line whenever possible (Fig. 15.19). It may have to be associated with midtarsal arthrodesis and subtalar arthrodesis. Tendinous elongations may be necessary for tendo Achillis, flexor hallucis longus and flexor digitorum longus, while arthrolysis of the ankle joint and selective treatment for dislocated metatarsophalangeal joints are essential. If there is a convex forefoot this should be corrected by enclavement procedures after management of the hindfoot. Finally, compensation for shortening of the ipsilateral lower limb should be ensured.

15.7 Other Forms of Pes Cavus

The foregoing part of this chapter has classified pes cavus on a structural basis, but there are numerous etiologies which are difficult to individualise and can best be simply catalogued. They are often important in that their presence leads to diagnosis of a more fundamental disorder elsewhere.

15.7.1 Encephalitic Pes Cavus

15.7.1.1 Pyramidal

Flaccid hemiplegia in general leads to pes planus, whereas the spastic variety tends to cavus. Various syndromes exist.

Spastic hemiplegia in the infant or the adult leads to equinovarus with predominance of supination. Its early treatment before the age of 10 years comprises Steindler (1929) plantar release and elongation of tendo Achillis by the Green technique. After the age of 10 years, the soft tissue procedures are supplemented as appropriate by corrective osteotomies for cavus deformity, by wedge tarsectomy or by midtarsal and subtalar arthrodesis. Also necessary are (a) either elongation of the posterior tendons behind the medial malleolus or distal tenotomy of the long flexor tendons, and (b) hemitransplantation laterally of tibialis anterior to peroneus brevis.

Acute encephalitis may lead to a balanced cavus or equinovarus cavus foot (Fig. 15.18 C).

Spastic paraplegia (Little 1861): This pyramidal syndrome leads to muscular contracture secondary to exaggeration of tonus. When the spastic hypertonia is posterior in distribution, it involves primarily triceps surae and leads to a balanced or straight equinocavus foot. If there is postero-internal predominance, tibialis anterior drags the foot into inversion and adduction and leads to a varus equinocavus foot; this is the most frequent form. Should the predominance be antero-external, there appears at first a cavus foot with anterior pronation of the forefoot and a valgus metatarsal, and then, secondarily as a result of loading of the foot, a paralytic valgus flat foot, i.e. an everted cavovalgus foot. The foot disorder is associated with internal rotation of the hip and genu recurvatum, both of which may require correction in addition to the treatment of the foot, which is similar to that of the encephalitic form.

15.7.1.2 Extrapyramidal

The three main extrapyramidal conditions are:

1. *Parkinson's disease,* which in its encephalatic form may result at an early stage in a neutral cavus foot and later in development of a varus component (Fig. 15.18). The muscular rigidity and hypertonia causes fixity of the deformity while other features are permanent extension of the great toe and clawing of the lesser toes.
2. *Progressive lenticular degeneration* (Wilson 1912), which sometimes leads to a neutral equinocavus foot.
3. The *athetoid foot* described by Hammond (1879), which results in a hypertonic cavus foot.

These conditions have in common a neurological deficit associated with overaction of the extrapyramidal system.

15.7.2 Medullary Syndromes

Cavus deformities of the feet may result from acquired conditions such as poliomyelitis or from familial neurological disorders.

15.7.2.1 Poliomyelitis

Described by Heine (1840) and Medin (1890) poliomyelitis was responsible over many years for cavus deformities of the feet (Fig. 15.20). Immunisation has led to diminution of incidence, but occasionally examples are met of anterior internal cavus foot with equinus of the great metatarsal due to previous subclinical infections. The scattered segmental involvement of the anterior horn cells is a characteristic feature, but consistent patterns of muscle imbalance are common. These have been described in Sect. 15.5.3.

15.7.2.2 Friedreich's Ataxia

In this condition, spinocerebellar tract degeneration leads to locomotor ataxia and is accompanied most frequently by an anterior cavus foot (Fig. 15.18 B, 15.19 B, 15.21, 15.22). Initially this is neutral, but with progressive postero-internal predominance becomes cavus and then equinocavovarus. The main site of deformity is in the midtarsal region. The foot condition may be the presenting sign of the disease and is most frequently bilateral. Despite the early appearance and the familial origin, this should not be called a congenital foot disorder because the foot is normal at birth. It should be remembered that some generations may be spared.
The first signs of the disease may be mild effects of muscular hypertonia; gait abnormality [a tendency to walk on the points of the toes and a high stepping action (Estève 1971)], difficulty in getting the heels to the ground due to excessive tension in the triceps, abnormal wear of the anterior shoe, instability, frequent falls, and incoordination. Then develops progressive pes cavus, which is correctable at first, but later, associated with rigid clawing of the toes and contracture of the soft tissues, becomes fixed, usually with a varus component (Fig. 15.22). Sometimes there is predominating anterior cavus, the dorsal summit of which is located at the Lisfranc joint line or the cuneiforms or more rarely at the talonavicular joint (Fig. 15.23). The bridging of the medial cord of the plantar aponeurosis under the skin may be marked. When cavus is present, usually in the adolescent, compensation for the equinus occurs at the ankle joint, which becomes hyperdorsiflexed, tending to accentuate the inversion of the antetarsus beginning at the midtarsal level. Deformities of the forefoot accompany the cavus, with calluses under the first and fifth metatarsal heads when there is cavus forefoot, and a median callosity when there is a round forefoot configuration. Occasionally calluses of overloading form under the cuboid region, but this is exceptional. At this stage the plantar print is that of a cavovarus foot.
Neurological abnormalities manifesting before the fixed deformities of the foot are evident comprise those due to cerebellar involvement (loss of balance, dysmetria, asynergy, involuntary movements, dysarthria and nystagmus), posterior cord involvement (ataxia and tendinous areflexia) and pyramidal syndromes (weakness and an extensor plantar response).
Conservative treatment must be employed under the age of 18 years. During infancy and adolescence, an insole may delay progress, the aim being to rebalance the foot coronally and relax the cavus by damping the overloading of the forefoot and relaxing the claw toes. However, an insole will not completely arrest the deterioration.
Operative treatment is valuable, but it must be recognised that in a progressive condition, permanence of effect cannot be guaranteed. During infancy and adolescence, soft tissue release of the plantar fascia and internal side of the foot [the plantar calcaneonavicular ligament and tendinous elongations of the adductor and tibialis muscles, of which the plantar extensions must be sectioned (Estève 1971)] may be indicated, together with release for digital clawing. After the age of 18 years, simultaneous bony procedures may be contemplated, comprising osteotomy-arthrodesis of the tarsometatarsal joint line (Lelièvre 1962b) and midtarsal osteotomy by cuneiform resection with the wedge based dorsally or dorso-externally, which can correct cavus and varus. Varus of the calcaneum will require a Dwyer (1959) osteotomy based laterally. The subsequent use of corrective insoles is essential.

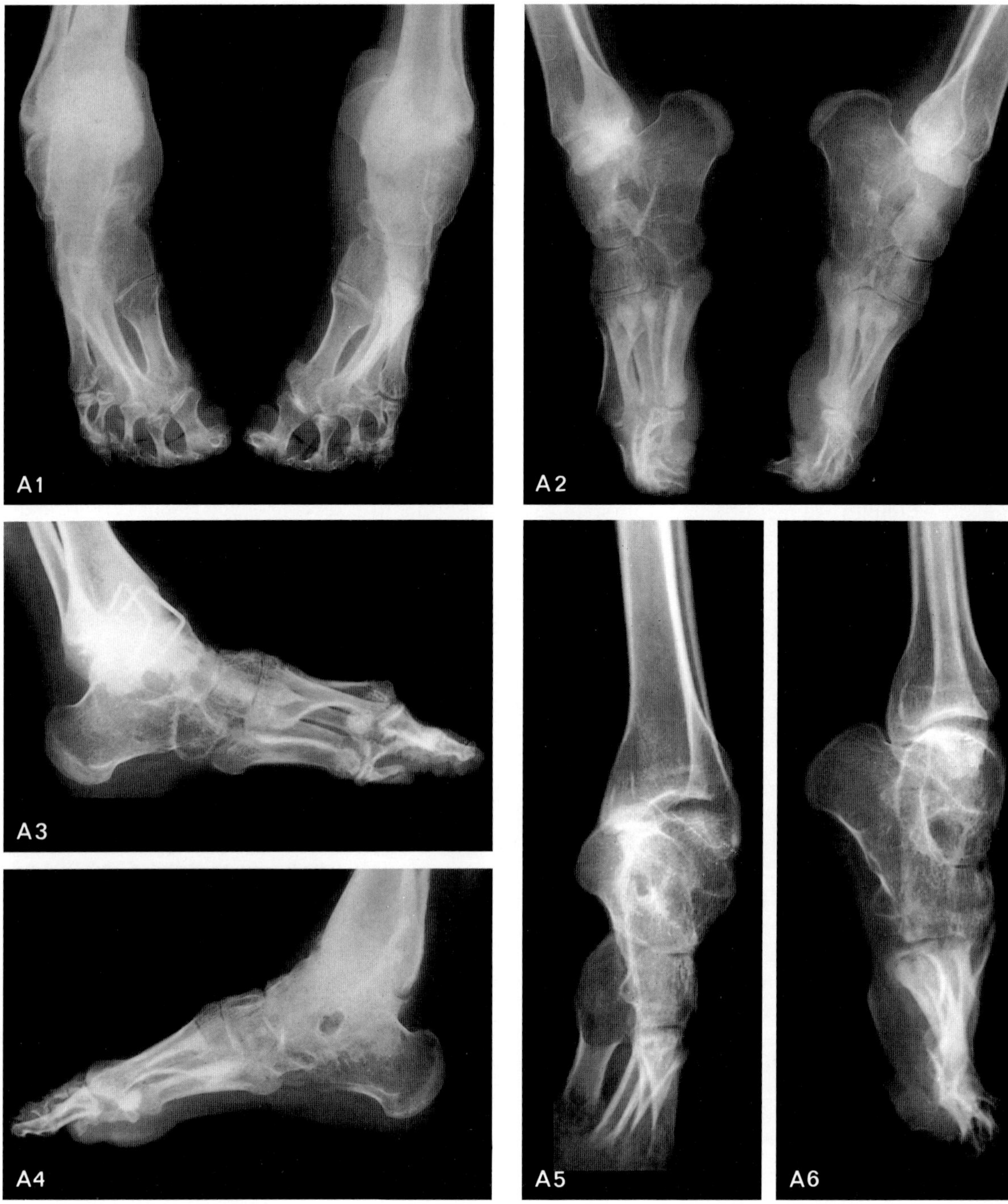

Fig. 15.18. A Rigid equinus posture in arthrogryphosis associated with amyotrophic lateral sclerosis. *1, 2* Preoperative; *3–6* after arthrodesis of ankle joint. **B** Pes cavus in Friedreich's ataxia. **C** Pes cavus in encephalitis. **D** Pes cavus in Parkinson's disease. **E** Paralytic pes cavus ▷ (poliomyelitis). **F, G** Pes equinocavus in poliomyelitis. **B–G** see p. 161

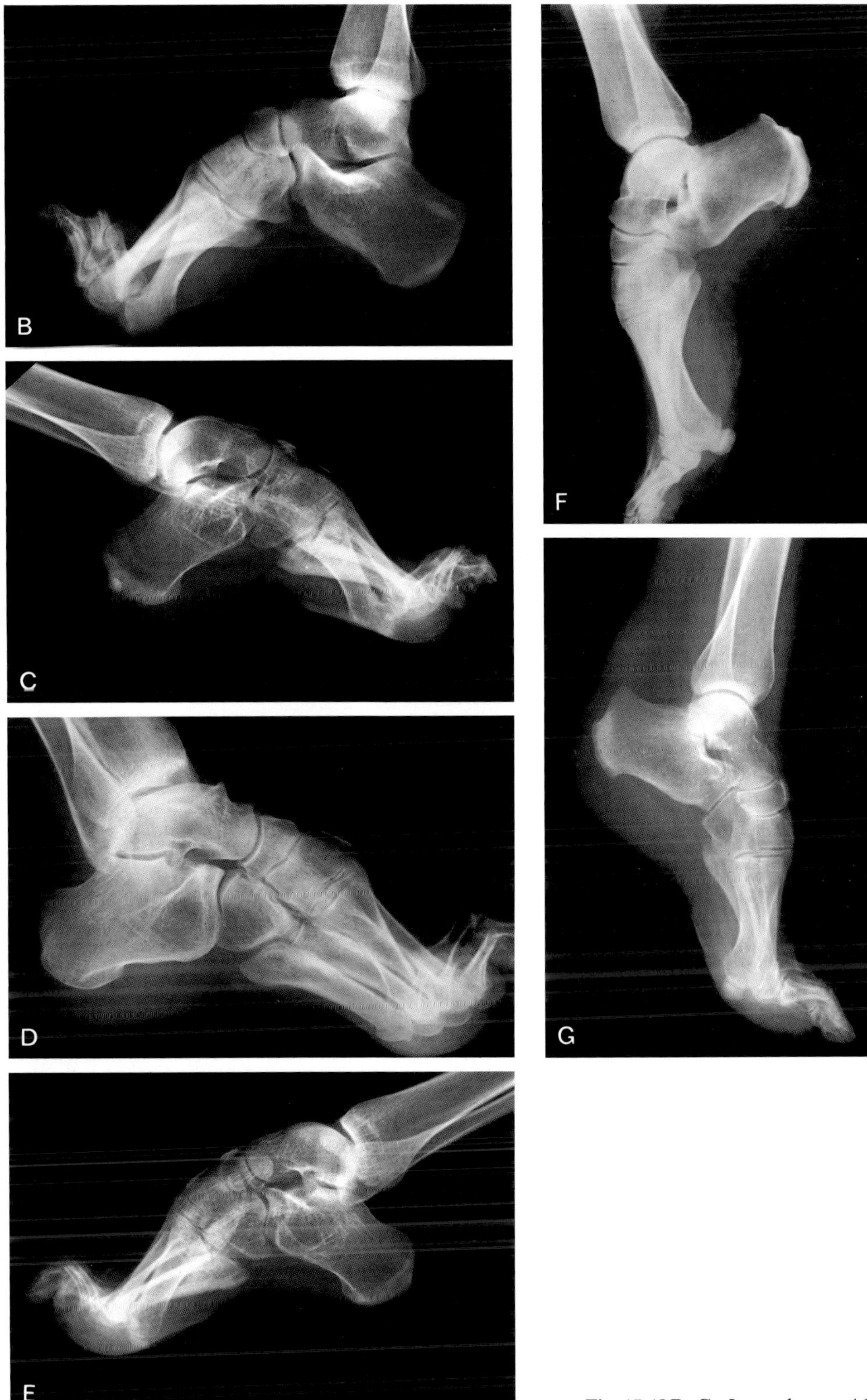

Fig. 15.18 B–G. Legend see p. 160

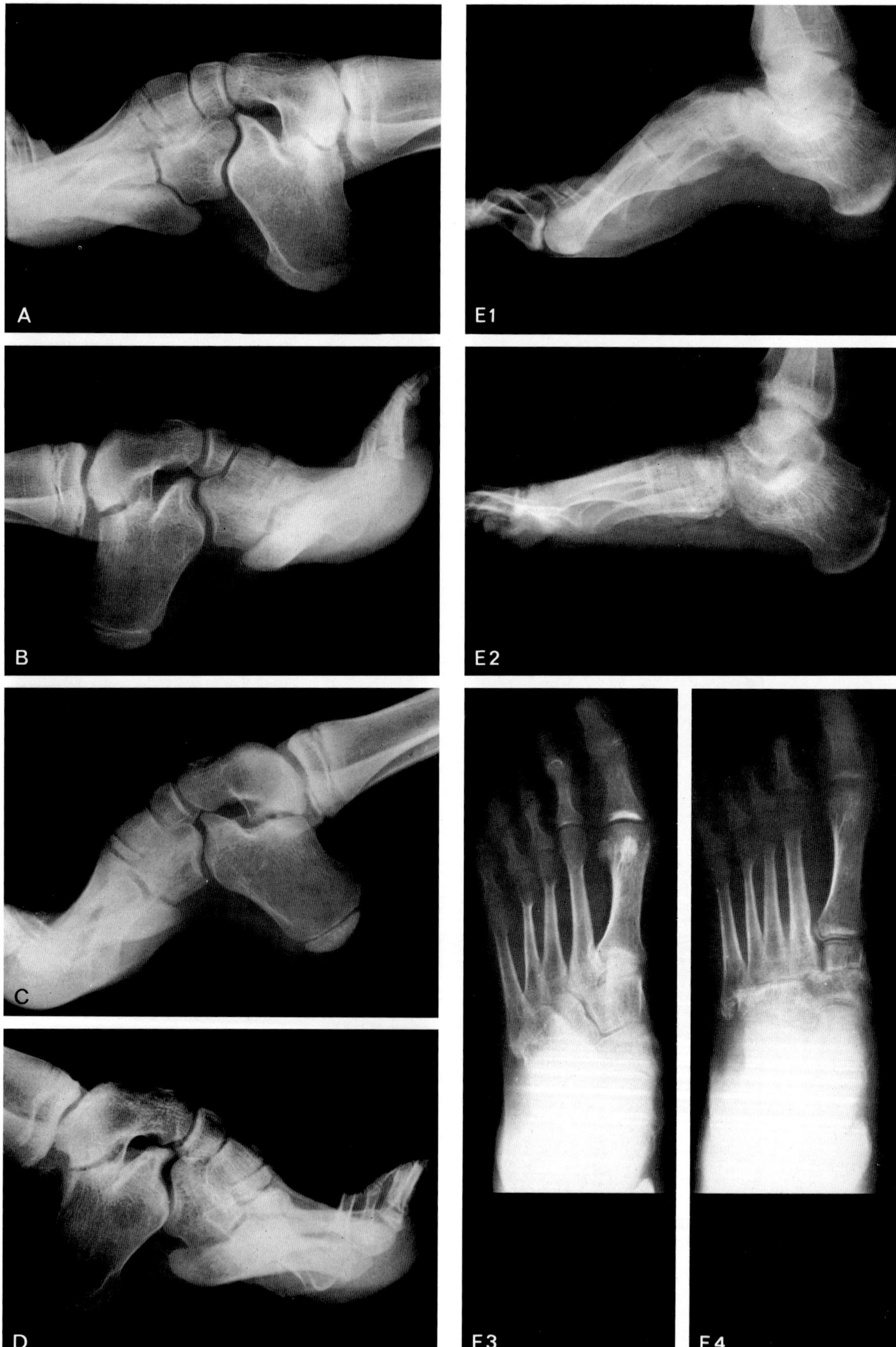
A
E1
B
E2
C
D
E3
E4

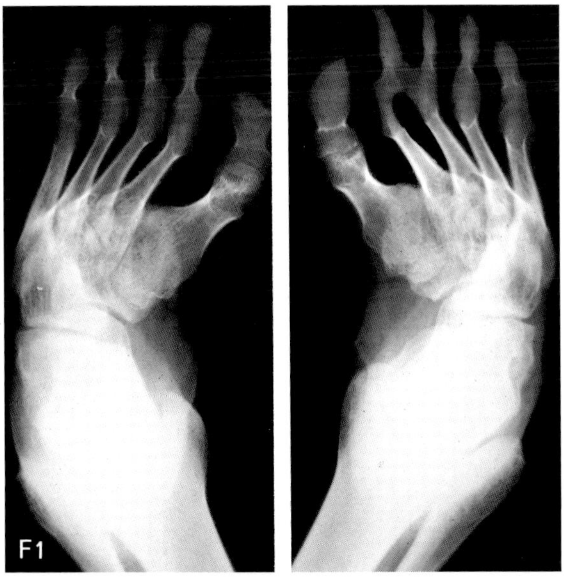

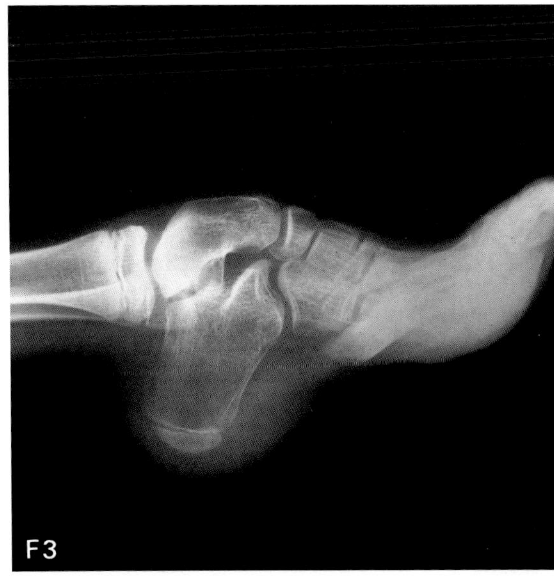

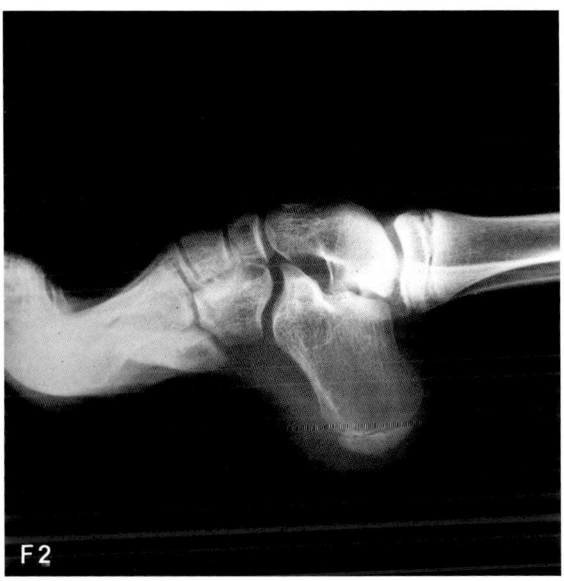

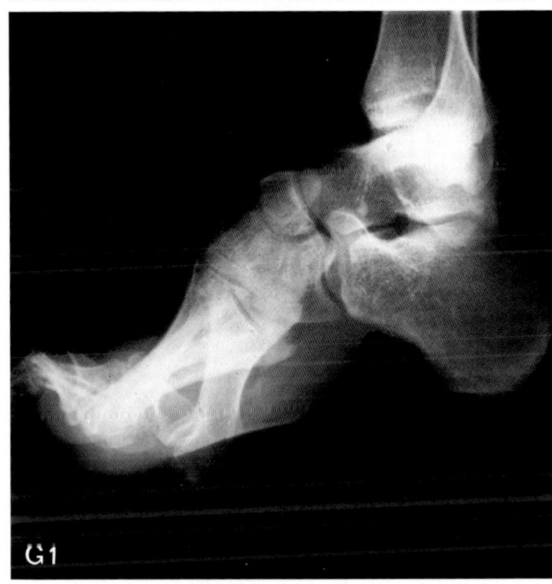

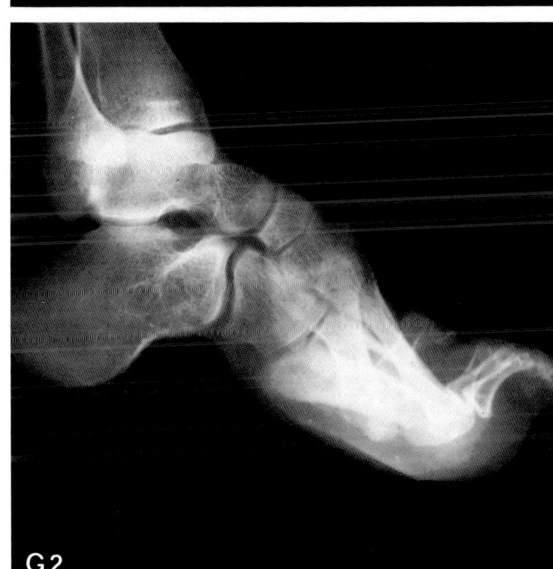

◁ **Fig. 15.19. A–D** Pes equinocavus. **E** Pes cavovalgus. *1, 2* Weight-bearing pre- and postoperative lateral views; *3, 4* dorsoplantar views before and after osteotomy of midtarsus at naviculocuneiform, cuneiform and cuneiform-cuboidomidtarsal joints. **F** *1–3* Pes equinocavovarus in Friedreich's ataxia. **G** *1, 2* Pes cavovarus resulting from equinovarus club foot. **A–E** see p. 162

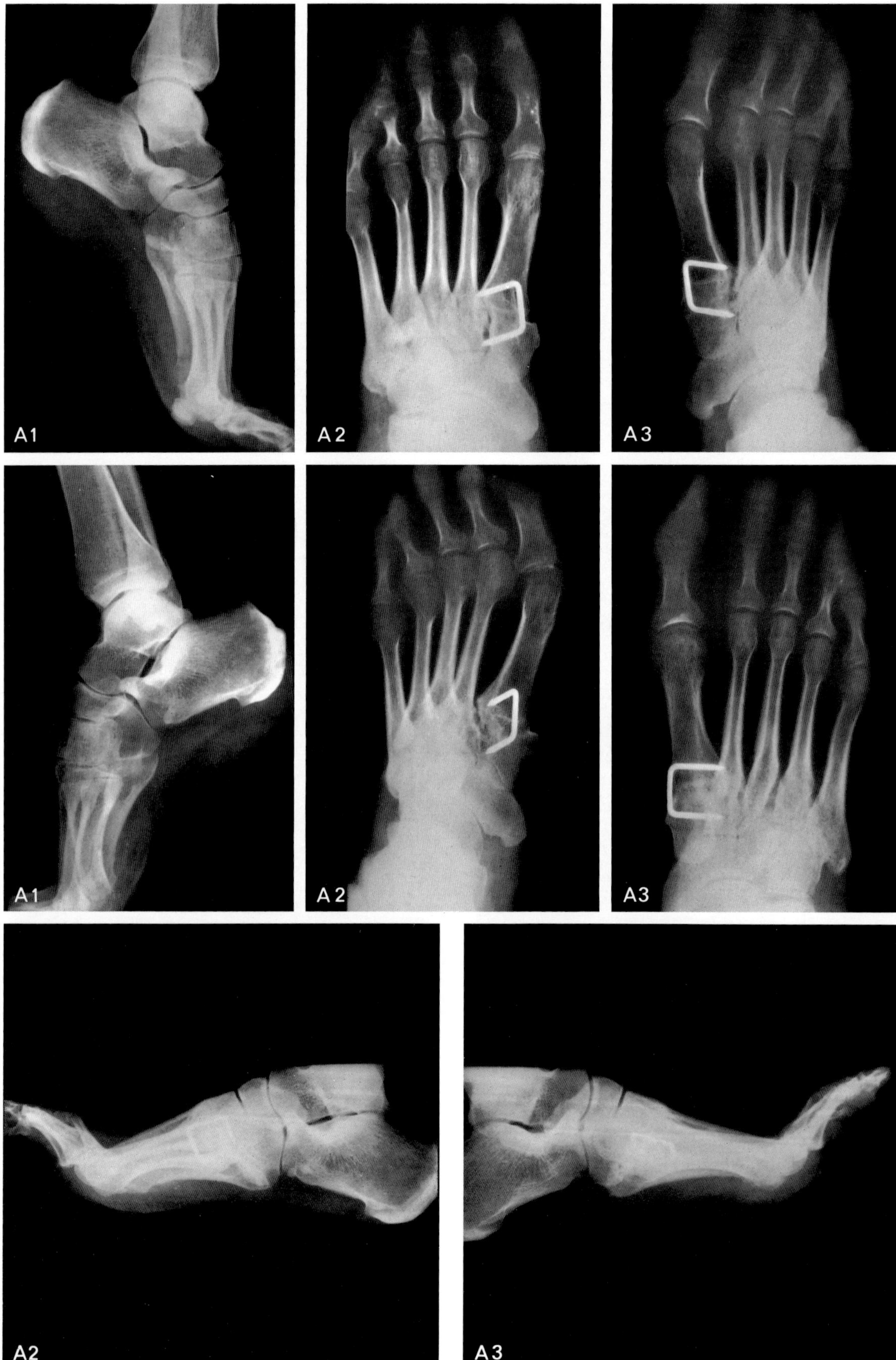
A1
A2
A3
A1
A2
A3
A2
A3

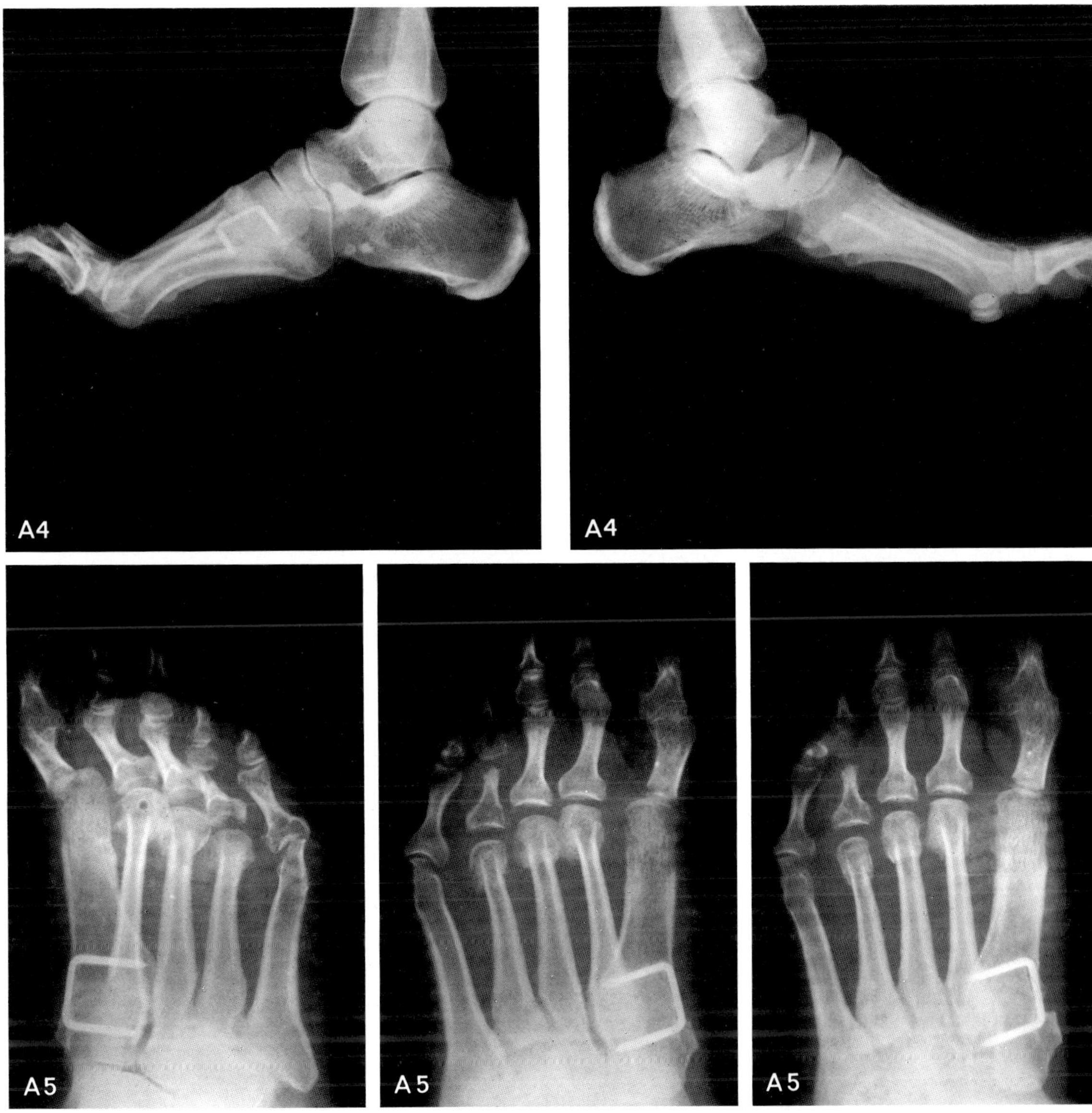

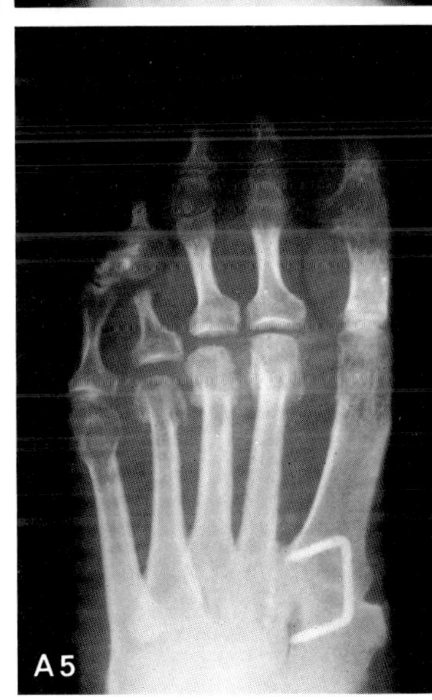

◁ **Fig. 15.20 A–C.** Pes equinocavus in poliomyelitis before and after treatment. **A** *1* Non-weight-bearing preoperative lateral views of both feet: pes equinocavus with convex forefoot; *2* left foot after osteotomy at cuneiform-metatarsal joints to correct cavus; *3* right foot after same operation; *4* both feet after operation; *5* left foot after correction of convex forefoot by head-shaft enclavement of metatarsals. **B, C** see p. 166

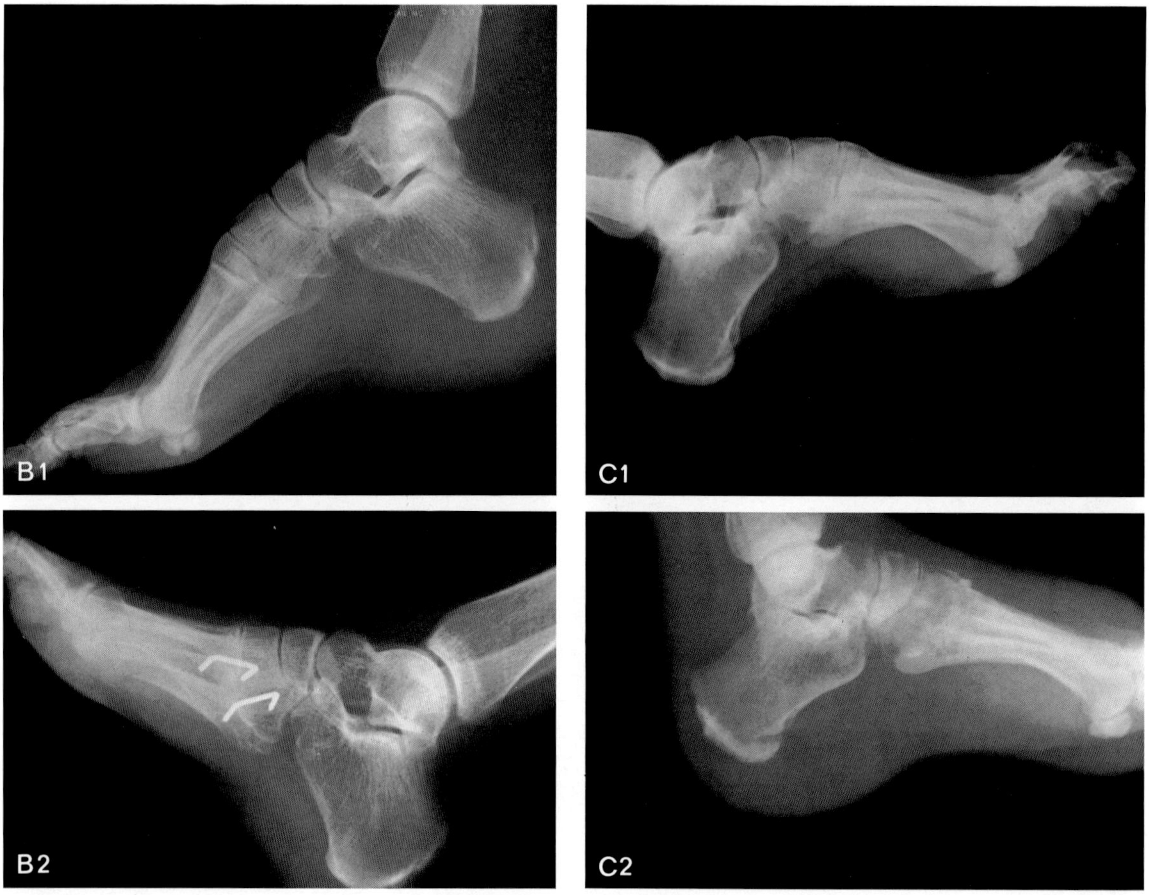

Fig. 15.20 *(continued)*. **B** Left foot, non-weight-bearing lateral views. *1* Preoperative: equinus, disturbance of loading, dorsal angulation at level of tarsometatarsal joint line; *2* after osteotomy-arthrodesis of tarsometatarsal joint line (Lisfranc). **C** Right foot, non-weight-bearing lateral view. *1* Preoperative: pes equinocavus; *2* after osteotomy-arthrodesis of tarsometatarsal joint line

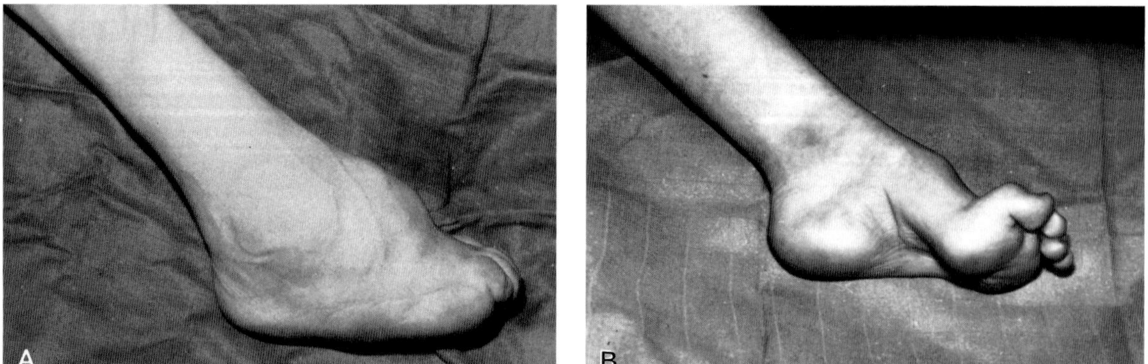

Fig. 15.21 A–J. Neurogenic pes cavus. **A** Charcot. **B–C** Friedreich. **D** Marfan. **E, G** Poliomyelitis. **F** Roussy-Ley. ▷ **H–J** Parkinson. **C–J** see p. 167

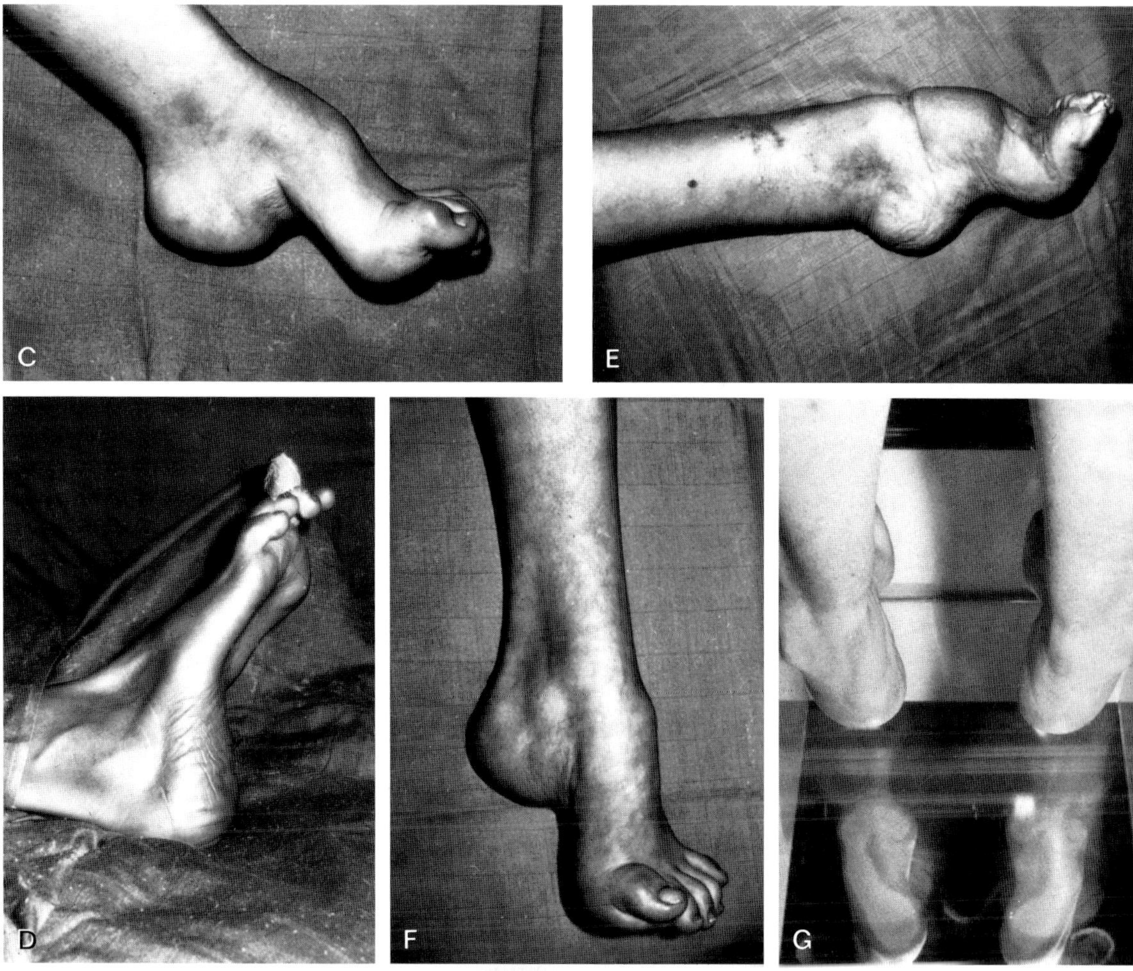

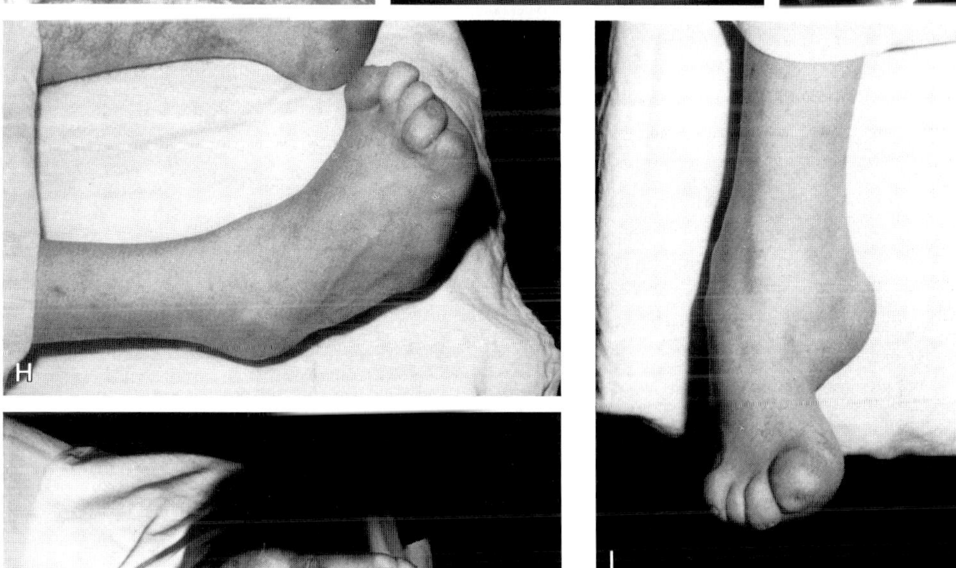

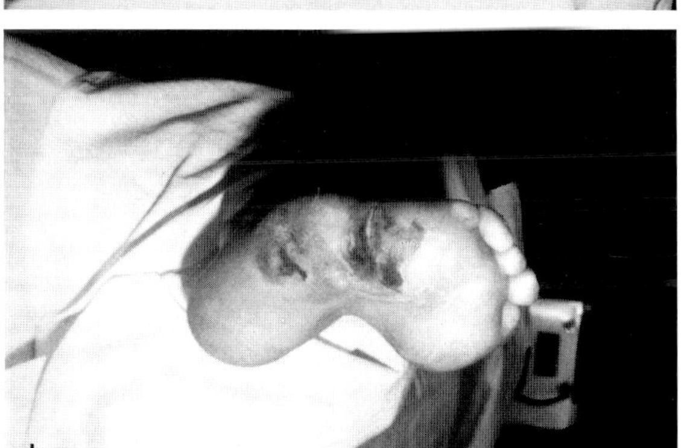

Fig. 15.21 C–J. Legend see p. 166

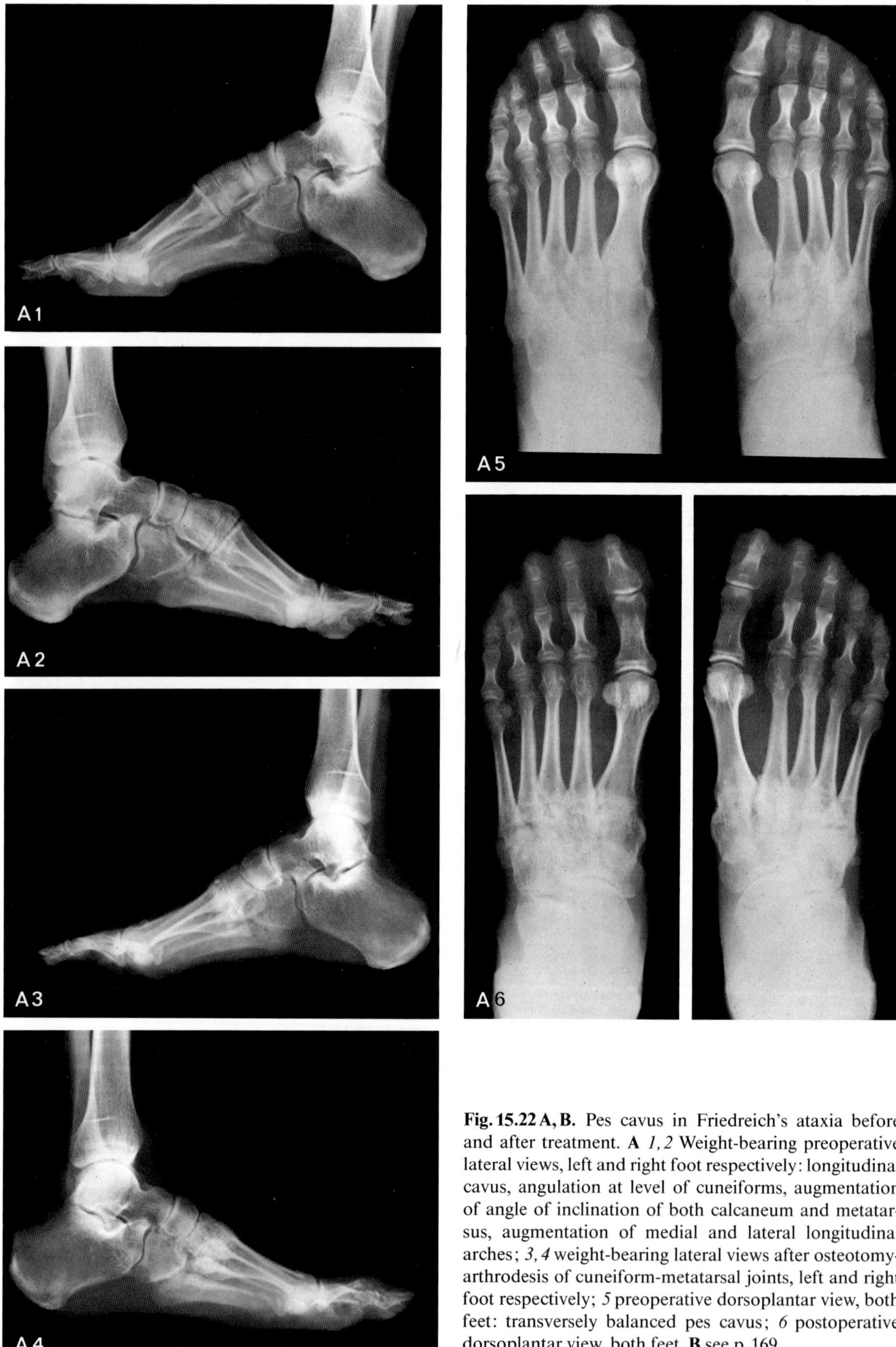

Fig. 15.22 A, B. Pes cavus in Friedreich's ataxia before and after treatment. **A** *1, 2* Weight-bearing preoperative lateral views, left and right foot respectively: longitudinal cavus, angulation at level of cuneiforms, augmentation of angle of inclination of both calcaneum and metatarsus, augmentation of medial and lateral longitudinal arches; *3, 4* weight-bearing lateral views after osteotomy-arthrodesis of cuneiform-metatarsal joints, left and right foot respectively; *5* preoperative dorsoplantar view, both feet: transversely balanced pes cavus; *6* postoperative dorsoplantar view, both feet. **B** see p. 169

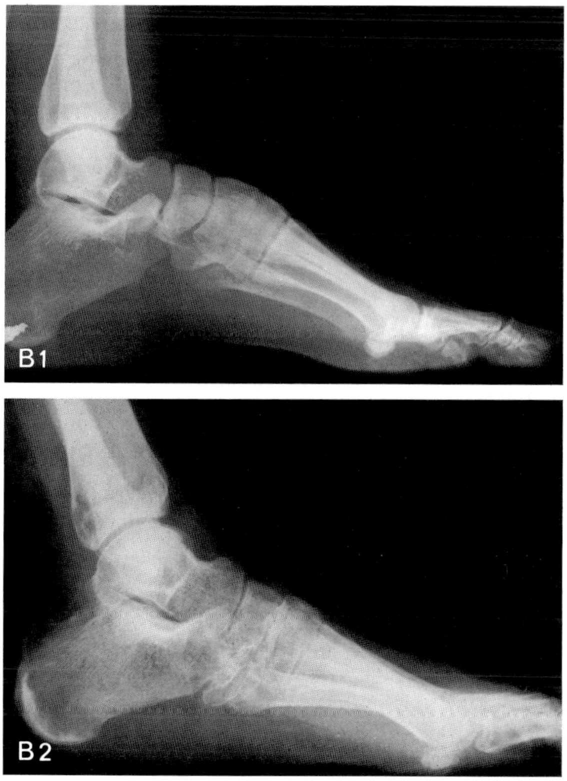

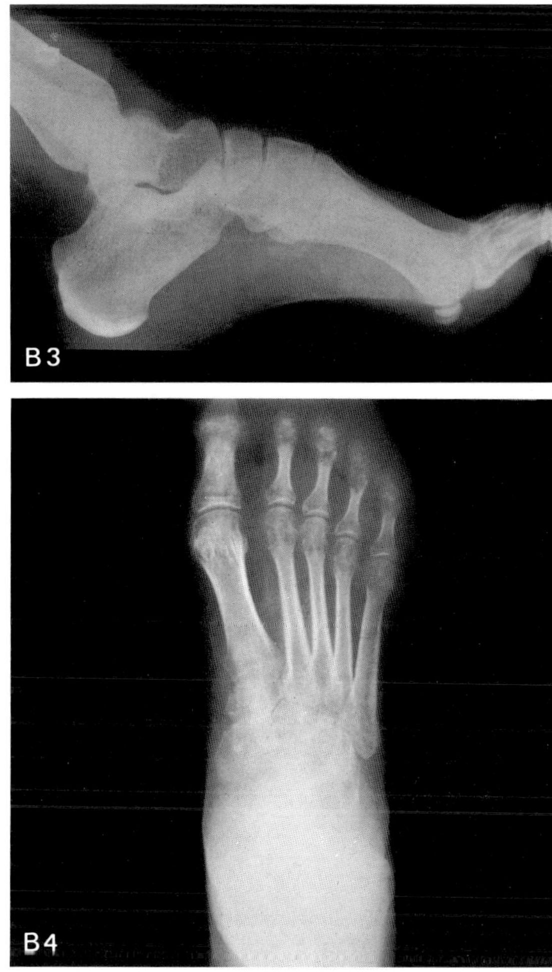

Fig. 15.22 *(continued)*. **B** Right foot. *1* Weight-bearing lateral view: dorsal angulation at cuneiform region, longitudinal cavus; *2* non-weight-bearing lateral view: disturbance of loading; *3, 4* lateral and dorsoplantar views after midtarsal osteotomy across cuneiforms and cuboid

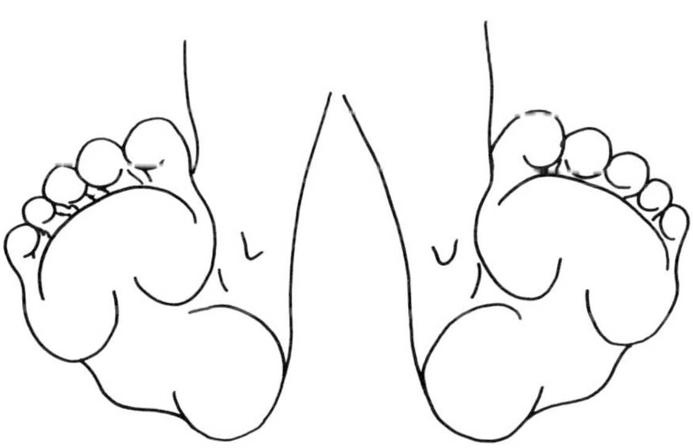

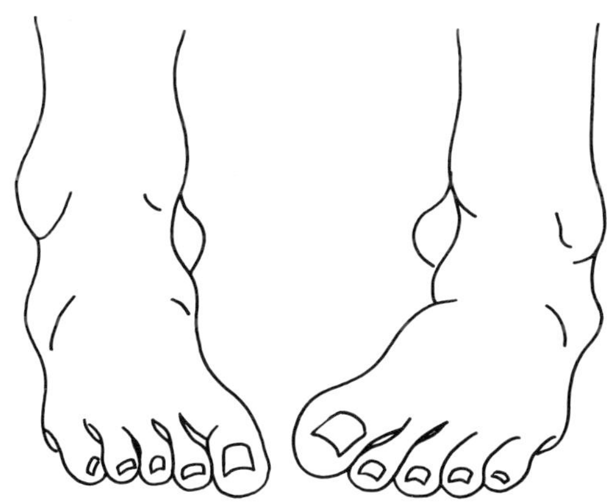

Fig. 15.23. Pes cavus in Friedreich's ataxia

15.7.2.3 Roussy-Levy Syndrome

This condition (Roussy-Levy 1926) comprises progressive neuropathic (peroneal) muscular atrophy with scoliosis and cerebellar ataxia. The foot disorder appears much earlier than that in Friedreich's ataxia, at about the age of 4–5 years. It takes the form of a cavus club foot (cavo-equinovarus) and, again in contrast with Friedreich's ataxia, is unilateral in the majority of cases. The cavus component is mainly anterior and its progression arrests at about the age of 30 years. By this time the displacements are fixed, but they do sometimes show a tendency to regress.

Treatment should be conservative. An insole to balance and relax the foot, correcting lateral displacement, should be supplemented by vitamin C, E and B_1 therapy. It is only in the fixed cavovarus equinus foot with painful callus formation that corrective surgery is indicated.

15.7.2.4 Spina Bifida

Estève (1971) has distinguished types of foot deformity according to the level of the myelomeningocele. Thus in the high variety (T 12 to L 3) there is a paralytic foot with sinking of the forefoot into light equinus and the absence of valgus or varus. In contrast, when the neurological deficit is at L 5 and the spine above is normal, there is paralysis of the extensors but preservation of unbalanced action of tibialis anterior and posterior. At S 3, equinovarus deformity of the foot develops due to paralysis of the short plantar flexors. The cavus foot of spina bifida is characterised by slow progressive development during growth, the progressively fixed cavus deformity and a tendency to relapse after any form of correction. Corrective surgery must be associated with efforts at re-education, manipulation and the use of insoles.

15.7.3 Myopathic Pes Cavus

The myopathies are usually hereditary, sometimes being transmitted by an asymptomatic mother, and develop more frequently in males. The symmetrical cavus feet are at first balanced but then develop varus and equinus components, becoming fixed with the forefoot in adduction and supination. There are essentially two broad etiological types, hypertrophic and atrophic.

15.7.3.1 Hypertrophic Myopathy

This condition (Thomsen 1876) is characterised by the contrast between the hypertrophy of the muscle and the diminution of muscle power, delay in relaxation, and hypo-excitability. It leads to planovalgus or often cavovarus foot. A cavus component is usually anterior and the condition bilateral and symmetrical. The family history is usually well established. The deformity usually begins at about the age of 10 years but can appear after the 20th year. Initially a pure cavus, it lapses into varus at the tarsal region and then equinus during later development, subsequently involving the forefoot in adduction and supination. The forefoot deformity may become significant, but tends to stay mild for a long period of time.

15.7.3.2 Atrophic Myopathy

This condition (Steinert 1909) presents the same hereditary characteristics and bilateral occurrence as hypertrophic myopathy. It is distinguished, however, by the more rapid and early development of varus and inversion in the foot and deformities elsewhere. It involves three main clinical syndromes:

1. An atrophic muscular syndrome, most severe in the antero-external musculature of the leg and foot, with a positive myotonic reaction and delay in relaxation of the muscle (Erb 1868)
2. An endocrine sympathetic syndrome including premature balding, nail disorders, peripheral vasomotor disorders, hyperlaxity of joints, bone fragility (with consequent fractures) and ocular disorders, predominantly cataracts
3. A neurological aspect comprising loss of tendon reflexes, disorders of superficial sensation and coordination and, in particular, psychiatric disturbance

These three aspects confer the predominantly symmetrical deformities of the feet, difficulty in coordination, hyperlaxity and general fragility.

With regard to the feet, as stated earlier the progress towards tarsal varus, adduction and supination of the forefoot and then equinovarus is more rapid than in hypertrophic myopathy. The result is an equinovarus lax club foot comprising accentuated cavus with the maximum curvature in the midtarsal region; displacement of the talus, which, while in its normal position in the ankle mortice, deforms so that its head points more forwards and outwards than usual; and adduction of the meta-

tarsus, which confers a plantar internal angulation on the developing longitudinal cavus.
There is general equinus of the foot which limits the possibility of dorsiflexion and encourages compensatory supination of the forefoot. The general muscular laxity in the thigh and leg and the stretching of ligaments produce an incoordinated gait characterised by lateral movements of the trunk, a high stepping action and a tendency for initial loading of the foot along its external border, which leads to unusual callus formation under the cuboid region.

The *treatment* of myopathic feet is generally conservative, involving use of appropriate shoes and insoles. Surgery can exceptionally be indicated for hypertrophic myopathy, but never for the atrophic type, on account of the bone fragility and hyperlaxity.

15.7.4 Polyneuritis

Polyneuritis is met most frequently in alcoholic women and sufferers from diabetes mellitus. The usual configuration is one of fixed anterior cavus with rigid clawing of the toes as a result of hypertonic contracture of the long flexor tendons due to the flaccid paralysis of the extensors, which may be painful. It is symmetrical, of progressive nature and predominantly involves the extensors and peronei. Pain arises from the atrophy of the plantar tissues, which become progressively inflamed, and later the development of ulceration (described in Chap. 31). The diabetic cavus foot is described in Chap. 32.

15.7.5 Post-Traumatic Pes Cavus

Post-traumatic pes cavus arises in one of two ways.

15.7.5.1 Compression Syndrome Leading to Volkmann's Contracture

Many conditions can cause muscle necrosis associated with trauma of different types - local damage to tissues, heamatoma, swelling and oedema in the fascial compartments of the leg, arterial damage, complications of operations involving use of a tourniquet. Subsequent immobilisation in a plaster cast or in prolonged traction may lead to further deterioration. The atrophic foot presents muscle contractures and general rigidity of the joint at all levels. Osteoporosis, which may be severe, is indicated by a violaceous appearance of the thin contracted skin with bridging over tendinous cords moulded to the bony outlines and with frequent disorders of the nails, which are grey, cyanotic, thickened or friable, often with fungal disease or onychogryphosis. The foot is painful on loading and on mobilisation due to the articular rigidity, while corns and calluses in the plantar region are frequent.
The general configuration is cavus with some equinus. Clawing of the toes is usually fixed, with dislocation of the metatarsophalangeal joints dorsally. The metatarsal heads are usually very prominent in the atrophied soft tissues of the ball of the foot. The cavus is usually balanced, but sometimes it is in varus; it is never seen in valgus because the neuromuscular involvement is predominantly in the posterior and postero-internal muscles.
The *podoscopic* appearance is typically cavus (less commonly the cavovarus, the result of an effort to compensate in a cavus foot left untreated for a long period of time).
Treatment is essentially *conservative*. Medical care comprises calcium therapy, vasodilators, analgesics and anti-inflammatory agents, local injections of topical steroid at the area of induration (Voutey 1970), physiotherapy (massage and gentle stretching) and an insole comprising a monoblock ante-antalgic support with protected areas for the painful joints rebalancing the foot coronally if necessary. The insoles should be made of felt or supple supporting material.
Operative treatment should be delayed until improvement in vasomotor function and in osteoporosis is achieved. Only then should irreducible claw toes or the cavovarus deformity be corrected. Operative correction of the cavus may be by arthrodesis at the midtarsal region or tarsometatarsal region associated with tendon elongations as necessary and correction of the dislocated metatarsophalangeal joints and claw toes. Persistent contracture due to tension in flexor hallucis longus sometimes produces a hallux flexus, and this may be improved by Z-elongation of the tendon. Postoperative immobilisation should not be in a complete plaster cast but in a back splint supporting the foot in a neutral position. Further conservative measures should be taken thereafter.

15.7.5.2 Lateral Popliteal Nerve Palsy

This condition can produce an equinovarus paralytic foot characterised by weakness of dorsiflexion and abduction, a high stepping gait, progressive fixed plantarflexion of the foot at the ankle and interphalangeal joints and unbalanced action of the postero-internal muscles (supplied by the medial popliteal nerve) drawing the foot into equinus and varus.

Treatment is operative and is carried out in the absence of signs of regeneration of the nerve at least 3 months after local treatment. Lambrinudi arthrodesis (1927) associated with transposition of the tibialis posterior tendon through the interosseous membrane in front of the annular ligament and onto the intermediate cuneiform can improve dorsiflexion and gait. Tendo Achillis, flexor hallucis longus and flexor digitorum may require elongation, accompanied by posterior capsulotomy of the ankle and subtalar joint. Interphalangeal arthrodesis to correct the claw toes may be necessary. Three months of plaster immobilisation is necessary postoperatively.

16 Pes Planovalgus

Abnormal lowering of the plantar longitudinal arch may be associated with obvious neuromuscular deficiency or congenital abnormalities, but must otherwise be labelled idiopathic. The subject is complex and it is difficult to reconcile varying opinions on the chain of events which lead to the abnormality. This applies especially in the idiopathic variety.

It may aid the reader to mention here a number of important normal parameters to which reference will be made:

a) In the sagittal plane, the tarsometatarsal joints are aligned in a straight line.
b) The internal longitudinal arch varies in height from 13 to 16 mm.
c) The balance of loading on the metatarsal heads is controlled by the mobility of the first and fifth metatarsals.
d) Coronal (transverse) equilibrium of the hindfoot depends on vertical alignment of the talus and calcaneum, although slight valgus of the calcaneum (less than 10°) may exist normally. As the limit of 10° is approached, the internal longitudinal arch sinks to 13 mm in the adult or even to as low as 9 mm in the infant, but this is still within a normal range.
e) The axis of the neck of the talus forms an angle of 115° - 120° with that of the body of the calcaneum - the angle of declination - and an angle of 150° - 160° with the anteroposterior axis of the talus-ankle articular mass - the angle of medial deviation.
f) The calcaneal axis inclines upwards, forming an angle of 5° with the horizontal in the newborn, increasing to 14° in the adult man and 16° in the adult woman.
g) The first metatarsal declines, forming an angle of 18° with the horizontal.
h) The obtuse angle formed at the summit of the plantar arch varies with age (Volkow 1902):
   Infant before walking: 130° - 150°
   Child 1-6 years old: 120° - 135° (from increasing inclination of the calcaneum)
   Child 6-13 years old: 120°
   Adolescent and adult: 130° - 140°
i) The bimalleolar axis of the ankle joint forms an angle of 20° with the neutral frontal plane and corresponds to the normal external rotation of the tibiofibular alignment.
j) The neck-shaft alignment of the normal femur may be taken as 120° of valgus and 20° of anteversion.

Normal alignment and balance of the foot are maintained during static and dynamic loading. This is associated with normal posture of the vertebral column and other lower limb segments.

16.1 Idiopathic Pes Planovalgus

There is disturbance of all the parameters listed above.

In the *vertebral column* there is augmentation or diminution of the normal sagittal curves.

The *neck-shaft angle* of the femur is disturbed, usually tending to retroversion and coxa vara.

Examination of the *ankle joint* reveals (a) ligamentous laxity with impaired stability of the talus in its mortice; (b) reduced external rotation of the transverse bimalleolar axis, which leads to increased adduction of the neck of the talus; and (c) increase in the angle of declination of the talus.

In the hindfoot are found (a) increased inclination of the talus relative to the vertical axis of the tibia, i.e. an equinus posture; (b) reduced inclination of the axis of the calcaneum; (c) increase in the inferior plantar angle of the vault of the inner arch, amounting to 170°; (d) reduced height of the plantar longitudinal arch, which may disappear; (e) in the lateral radiograph, superimposition of the scaphoid on the cuboid under load (a basic diagnostic feature); and (f) external deviation into abduction occurring at the naviculocuneiform and talonavicular joint levels.

The metatarsus displays (a) reduced angle of declination of the metatarsals and (b) disturbance of the axis of the metatarsus into abduction, arising at the Lisfranc or Chopart joint line. This is augmented by an abducted posture of the toes.

Loading of the foot (Chiappara and Berardi 1963) is so distributed that the calcaneum and the forefoot each bear one half. The load normally borne by the hindfoot is shared equally between (a) the anterior process of the calcaneum, the cuboid and the fourth and fifth metatarsals (the lateral column) and (b) the head of the talus, the navicular and the medial three metatarsals (the medial column). In idiopathic pes planus, the horizontal and valgus alignment of the calcaneum, which is associated with some degree of pronation, and the adducted plantar flexed attitude of the talus are accompanied by an abnormal sharing of the load between these columns - an estimated 40% on the inside and only 10% on the outside. The degree of valgus and pronation of the calcaneum is reflected by the severity of subluxation of the midtarsal joints.

These fundamental features of the pes planovalgus deformity relate to intrinsic factors in the foot itself and extrinsic factors from above. The intrinsic factors are plantar ligamentous laxity, hypotonia or muscle disbalance and various osteoarticular abnormalities, while the extrinsic factors are linked with postural abnormalities of the vertebral column, the attitude of the pelvis and hip, genu valgum and genu varum and a variety of suggested muscle imbalances. The overlap among the many descriptions of extrinsic and intrinsic causes needs to be appraised if any understanding is to be achieved, and it is a useful exercise to summarise certain important contributions:

Duchenne de Boulogne (1867) regarded "impotence" of the peroneus longus as the prime originator of pes planovalgus.

Lorenz and Modernes described a sequence of events comprising (a) valgus posture of the calcaneum leading to pronation of the fifth metatarsal and lowering of the external arch of the foot together with (b) rotation of the head of the talus and sinking of the medial longitudinal arch together with divergence of the metatarsals.

Lelièvre (1952) stated that pronation of the calcaneum is the originator, accompanied by downward and inward displacement of the talar head and laxity of the plantar calcaneal ligament.

Judet (1966) described the talus as maintaining its normal position in the ankle mortice while the calcaneum became pronated and directed forwards and outwards. This posture of the calcaneum was primary, leading to valgus of the hindfoot and abduction of the forefoot.

Viladot et al. (1956) regarded the stability of the talocalcaneal joints as dependent on balance between tendo Achillis and the plantar muscles. Predominance of the tendo Achillis action leads to loss of tonus of the short flexor muscles, increased ligamentous laxity, progressive shortening of tendo Achillis and horizontal posture of the calcaneum. The last-named also causes pronation of the calcaneum and tends to make the talus slide forwards and its head sink, this being allowed by the lax calcaneonavicular ligaments and loss of tone of tibialis posterior and the long flexors.

Roig Puerta (1965) described laxity of the tibiotalar-calcaneal complex, involving hypotonia of tibialis posterior and flexor hallucis longus and the tibiotalar and tibiocalcaneal ligaments.

Barry and Courriades (1963) noted that planovalgus foot supervened in children of a particular type, characterised by general hypotonia (floppiness), sometimes with scoliosis, genu valgum or incurved legs, accompanied in 75% of cases with chronic respiratory disease, prognathism of the upper jaw and retrognathism of the lower jaw and deformities of the hard palate.

Besse (1979) noted an association of pes planovalgus with failure of the neck-shaft angle of the femur to develop normally. Persistent coxa valga with anteversion was accompanied by genu valgum and an inward foot posture, while coxa vara with retroversion was accompanied by pes planovalgus.

Poinot (1962) [cited by Besse (1969)] and Lecoeur (1938) stressed that abnormalities of the head-shaft angle of the femur reflected not only on the knee joint, producing genu varum and genu valgum, but also on the axis of the ankle mortice. This could result in reduced external torsion (normally some 20°) and separation of the malleoli, the latter leading to loss of stability.

Reduced external rotation of the malleolar axis affects the posture of the talus (Besse 1979), which becomes significantly and abnormally adducted. The mechanism has been explained by Megret (1966): in the normal subject, the neck of the talus has an angle of declination of 150°-160° and is in minimal adduction, but in pes planus, as well as displaying more adduction, it is hypertrophied in length, perhaps according to the law of Delpech.

I am of the opinion that the increased length of the neck of the talus, undoubtedly seen in some forms of pes planus, is of great importance, being associated with an increased angle of declination of the neck and a less vertical posture of the talus. Conversely, a small angle of declination of the neck corresponds to a normal or short talar neck with a more vertical posture. The posture of the talar neck determines the horizontality of the calcaneum, i.e. reduced declination and extreme equinus of the talar neck lead to loss of inclination of the calcaneum so that it is horizontally orientated.

Lecoeur's very important contribution (1938, 1976) to the understanding of the ankle mortice and its influence on the formation of the pes planus merits close attention:

In the *normal subject,* the talus in full dorsiflexion occupies the entire width of the ankle mortice because of the shape of its articular surface, broader anteriorly. Thus it would seem that in plantarflexion, the talus is likely to be unstable in the mortice. However, this potential instability is controlled by changes in position of the lateral malleolus under the influence of the crural muscles in the following manner. The extensors of the foot and ankle originate largely on the tibia and their contraction has no influence on the fibula. Thus, during dorsiflexion of the ankle under the influence of the extensors, the fibula remains mobile and can separate from the tibia, thereby accommodating the anterior portion of the talar mass into the mortice. In contrast, the posterior muscles controlling plantarflexion originate mostly from the fibula and the tibia and the fibula together during their contraction. Further, they backwardly displace the fibular malleolus and control the position of the talus so that its angle of declination is reduced during plantarflexion. Lecoeur stresses that it is tibialis posterior which causes most compression and backward displacement of the fibula, at the same time influencing adduction of the navicular distally and favouring a rise of the arch and general stabilisation of the foot. This free play of separation and pressing together of the mortice elements is only possible if the ankle joint is orientated properly, that is to say with its bimalleolar axis forming an angle of about 20° with the frontal plane. In these circumstances, the talus is well stabilised both longitudinally and transversely during all positions of dorsiflexion and plantarflexion. Further, the mechanism explains how the midtarsus and the calcaneum also remain balanced.

In *pes planus,* if the normal external orientation of the bimalleolar axis is diminished or absent, the mechanism fails and the ankle mortice is permanently widened. Relative stability occurs only during full dorsiflexion, and there is a tendency to eversion sprains affecting the medial ligament of the ankle, seen so commonly in pes planovalgus. The fibular malleolus lies more anteriorly, and because of the loss of normal external torsion of the ankle mortice, the longitudinal axis of the talus is orientated noticeably inwardly and downwardly, i. e. in plantarflexion relative to the foot and adducted with respect to the longitudinal axis of the tarsometatarsal axis. The special action of the long flexors is lost, while extensor hallucis longus, extensor digitorum longus and tibialis anterior exercise their normal effect of dorsiflexion and abduction of the midtarsus. Because of the increased angle of declination of the talar neck, they exaggerate their abducting effect on the metatarsus and cause internal displacement of the midtarsus with lowering.

In *pes planovalgus,* when the foot is fully plantarflexed, the talus is adducted and in full plantarflexion and the forefoot is dorsiflexed relative to the midtarsus, and solely the posterior portion of the talus articular surface is found to be engaged under the tibial shaft in the mortice. Because of the incompetent mechanism engendered by the loss of external orientation of the bimalleolar axis, the posterior tibial muscles cannot stabilise the talus and consequently cannot reduce the tendency of the talar neck to adopt this adducted posture. Flexor hallucis longus, peroneus longus and tibialis posterior are involved and become stretched or hypotonic, with the consequence that they are unable to perform their individual actions of controlling the navicular or depressing the first metatarsal distally as well as controlling the position of the fibula proximally. The ingredients for pes planovalgus are present.

The ankle and talocalcaneal joints are intimately related. The ankle joint, apart from the complications of stabilisation explained above, is relatively simple, but the talocalcaneal system has two components, one anterior and related to the navicular and the cuboid, the other posterior, the subtalar joint.

The ankle-talocalcaneal system amounts to a torsion bar transmitting load from the ankle, which is stable in the coronal plane but mobile sagittally, to the calcaneum, which is stable in the sagittal plane but mobile coronally. The configuration of the talocalcaneal joints results in movements relative to the transverse horizontal plane of pronation and supination, divergence and convergence, and backward and forward displacement. These movements are determined by the position of the talus; dorsiflexion of the talus corresponds to convergence of the longitudinal axis of the calcaneum with that of the talus (supination, adduction, dorsiflexion and forward displacement of the calcaneum, equivalent to pes cavovarus), while plantarflexion of the talus corresponds to divergence of the calcaneum with respect to the axis of the talus (pronation, abduction, flattening or even plantarflexion, and backward displacement, equivalent to pes planovalgus).

In the normal foot, the anterior system of the talocalcaneal complex, at the Chopart joint line, controls and transmits the movements of convergence and divergence of the posterior system and transforms them respectively into supination and pronation of the midtarsus. They are then converted inversely through the torsion bar (Hendrix 1934) into pronation and supination of the forefoot so as to assure final balance of the foot on the ground. In pes planus, there is restriction of these movements and loss of adaptation of the foot to the ground due to alteration of the stability of the mortice and of the talocalcaneal complex and displacement of the midtarsus. The coronal balance of the tarsal and midtarsal systems depends on perfect function of the malleolar mechanism, good axial position of the talus, balance of the calcaneum and muscle and ligamentous tensions. On the variations in position of the talus and the calcaneum depend the orientation and the distribution of pressures. Imbalance of loading and reactions from the ground can be influenced by almost any of the mechanisms postulated by various earlier authors and listed above; general hypotonia, absence of bimalleolar control, instability of the talocalcaneal complex brought about by the tendo Achillis mechanism, or abnormal orientation of the long axis of the calcaneum.

Unbalanced muscle action, ligament laxity and osteoarticular displacements accentuate the forces of pressure and propulsion along the internal longitudinal elements of the foot.

This takes the following forms:

1. The main plantar calcaneocuboidal, calcaneonavicular and above all talonavicular ligaments are stretched and no longer limit the descent of the talar head, with the result that lowering of the plantar arch and internal displacement of the midtarsus occurs.
2. Muscle balance is disturbed on account of pronation and lowering of the talocalcaneal system. The intrinsic plantar muscles and tibialis muscles and the long flexors are insufficient to counteract the falling of the internal arch together with the internal subluxation of the midtarsus; peroneus longus proves insufficient to maintain the angle of declination of the hypermobile first metatarsal and the pronating muscles (peroneus brevis and extensor communis) predominate. These have the tendency to elevate the outer longitudinal arch of the foot, thereby augmenting metatarsal abduction. The pronating action of triceps surae on the calcaneum becomes as exaggerated as the pronated position of the calcaneum (which has considerably diminished its angle of inclination) and its tendency to become horizontal. The augmentation of the calcaneal lever (a result of its horizontal posture) increases the relative power of triceps surae, which is retracted and blocks the talocalcaneal complex in plantarflexion and pronation.

This attitude of plantarflexion and pronation of the midtarsal region becomes self-perpetuating.

The site of angulation along the medial aspect of the pes planus varies according to the degree of muscle control exercised. Thus, if the angulation is at the talonavicular joint or the navicular itself, it is likely that tibialis posterior is most deficient; if at the medial cuneiform, tibialis anterior is likely to be the weakest muscle; if at the Lisfranc joint, the muscle deficiency predominates in peroneus longus. The aspects which have been discussed may be summarised as follows:

1. Two primary tarsal displacements (Figs. 16.1–16.3): (a) talocalcaneal horizontal divergence (adduction of the neck of the talus with pronation and abduction of the calcaneum); (b) divergence of the talus and calcaneum vertically (plantarflexion of the neck of the talus, augmentation of declination of the talar neck, horizontal alignment and backward displacement of the calcaneum). These two divergences combine to result in a valgus calcaneum.
2. Two secondary midtarsal displacements: (a) lowering of the midtarsus, involving the head of the talus, the navicular, and the medial cuneiform and identified by obtuse angulation at the talonaviculocuneiform region open above and by lowering of the head of the talus and of the navicular; (b) medial midtarsal angulation, of which the summit is determined by the internal subluxation of the navicular or that of the medial cuneiform.
3. Two bony deformations: (a) either hypertrophy in length of the talar neck, when it is abducted, or shortness, when it adopts a plantarflexed posture; (b) medial hypertrophy of the navicular, which becomes deformed like a comma, or its dorsal subluxation onto the lowered talar head. These two deformations involve excessive length of the internal border of the foot.
4. Four sources of muscle imbalance: (a) Hypertonia and contracture of triceps surae, (b) hypotonia of peroneus longus, (c) elongation and weakness of tibialis posterior and flexor hallucis longus, and (d) weakness of tibialis anterior.
5. Two metatarsal displacements: (a) pronation and (b) abduction of the antetarsus. True supination of the antetarsus does not exist; supination is relative to calcaneal pronation and only ap-

pears after correction of the pronated calcaneum with the foot unloaded.

6. Various joint disorders seen in the adult, the sites of which relate to maximum deformities, overloading or local pressure.

These aspects of pes idiopathic pes planus apply in varying degrees at all ages of presentation.

16.1.1 Summary of Aims of Treatment

Detailed analysis of management at different ages will be presented later in this account, but it is convenient at this stage to summarise, in the light of the foregoing description, the corrections which must be achieved at any age. Whether conservative or operative, treatment must:

a) Correct the two talocalcaneal divergences by reduction of the pronation and abduction of the calcaneum
b) Remedy the plantarflexed posture of the talus
c) Reduce the midtarsal and tarsometatarsal angulation
d) Establish a normal plantar arch, thereby relieving the plantar tie beam from excessive traction forces
e) Ensure duration of the new stability by preserving muscle balance and restoring an undistorted flat internal border to the foot

Operative measures are directed at the sites of displacement, and the aim is to preserve the mobility of the joints whenever possible.

With regard to the posture of the calcaneum, in the *infant,* release of the subtalar joint may need to be accompanied by ligamentoplasties of the calcaneonavicular region (Pisani 1979b, c) and the talonavicular joint (Regnauld 1974) and by tendinous transpositions of one or both tibialis muscles and sometimes of triceps surae. In the *adult,* elongation or tendo Achillis is necessary if the calcaneum is horizontal in order to release the talocalcaneal complex from the traction which elevates its posterior part and thus re-establish a normal angle of calcaneal inclination. This is followed by replacement of the anterior process under the talar head.

In the case of a plantarflexed talus of which the head plunges inwards and forwards, towards the sole of the foot, bulging the plantar talonavicular ligament, one of two operative procedures may be necessary according to the length of the talar neck: if the talus is *long,* shortening resection ostectomy of the neck allows it to rise; if the talar neck is *short* but *vertical,* resection of a segment of the talonavicular ligament from its plantar and internal aspect permits reduction and support of the talar head.

In both instances, midtarsal internal angulation can be reduced by intranavicular ostectomy continued laterally by osteotomy of the cuboid and associated with transposition of tibialis posterior on to the medial cuneiform bone when the summit of the angulation is at the level of the navicular. Alternatively, when the angulation is at the medial cuneiform, intracuneiform ostectomy and intracuboidal osteotomy are appropriate.

16.1.2 Juvenile Pseudo Pes Planus

When a mother brings her young child for consultation because of apparent flat foot, it is usually pseudo pes planus which is causing the problem. This condition is due to the podginess of the plantar tissues, which yields a completely flat print on the podoscope. The internal border of the foot presents angulation, again on account of soft tissue protuberance, but careful palpation reveals that there is normal horizontal alignment of the bony structures and no midtarsal angulation. At the heel, there is a false appearance of valgus, due in part to the physiological genu valgum in children of this age and to the bulge of the soft tissue of the heel. It is very easy to make the mistake of diagnosing pes planus.

The important indications that there is actually nothing seriously amiss are the absence of any complaint of pain, the appearance of a normal plantar arch when tiptoeing, normal wear of shoes and the straightness of the bony structure along the internal border of the foot, together with a neutral alignment of the calcaneum.

Treatment is unnecessary and correction occurs spontaneously. It is wise only to recommend the use of a pair of shoes with solid stiffeners of the heels and shanks which give adequate support to the arches. These are the hallmarks of suitable shoes for young children.

16.1.3 Juvenile Pes Planus

This condition affects 1% of children (Courriades 1973b; Bensahel 1977). The presenting symptom is usually a gait abnormality; the worried mother notices that the child turns the foot inwards and has a tendency to walk on the outer border. The child falls frequently and deforms his shoes. There is often accompanying genu valgum of varying severity.

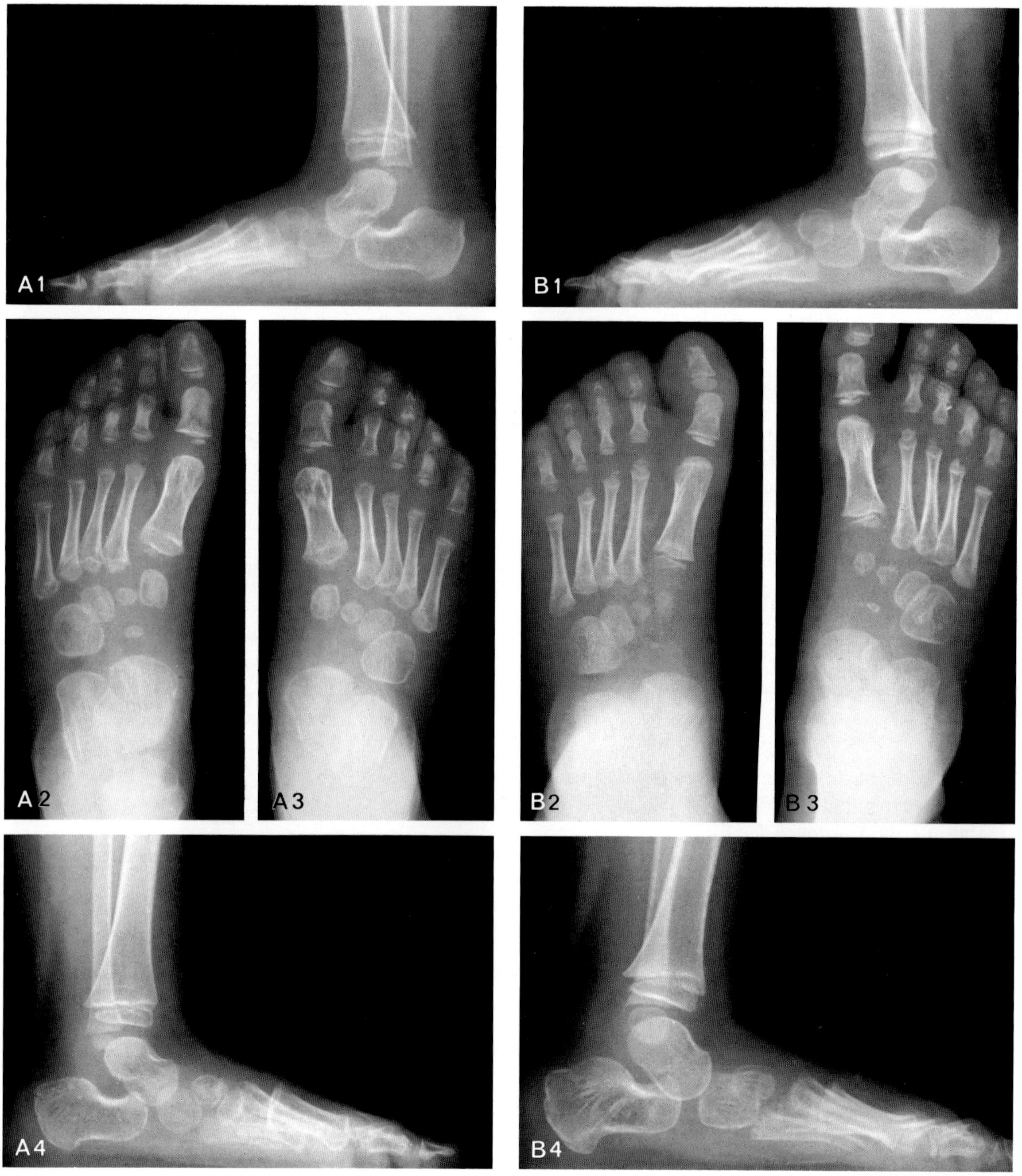

Fig. 16.1 A–D. Idiopathic pes planovalgus in four children aged between 2 and 3½ years. **A** Age 2 years. *1* Left foot, weight-bearing lateral view; *2* both feet, non-weight-bearing dorsoplantar view; *3* right foot, weight-bearing dorsoplantar view: divergence of axes of talus and calcaneum, both vertically and horizontally; *4* right foot weight-bearing lateral view. **B** Age 2½ years. *1* Left foot, weight-bearing lateral view; *2* left foot, weight-bearing dorsoplantar view; *3* right foot, weight-bearing dorsoplantar view; *4* right foot, weight-bearing lateral view: marked equinus of talus. **C** Age 3 years. *1* Left foot, weight-bearing lateral view; *2* left foot, weight-bearing ▷ dorsoplantar view; *3* right foot, weight-bearing dorsoplantar view; *4* right foot, weight-bearing lateral view: marked lowering of midtarsal region, medial angulation of midtarsus. **D** Age 3½ years. *1* Left foot, weight-bearing lateral view; *2* left foot, weight-bearing dorsoplantar view; *3* right foot, weight-bearing dorsoplantar view; *4* right foot, weight-bearing lateral view; *5* left foot, non-weight-bearing lateral view; *6* right foot, non-weight-bearing lateral view: diminution in angle of inclination of calcaneum and metatarsus. **C, D** see p. 179

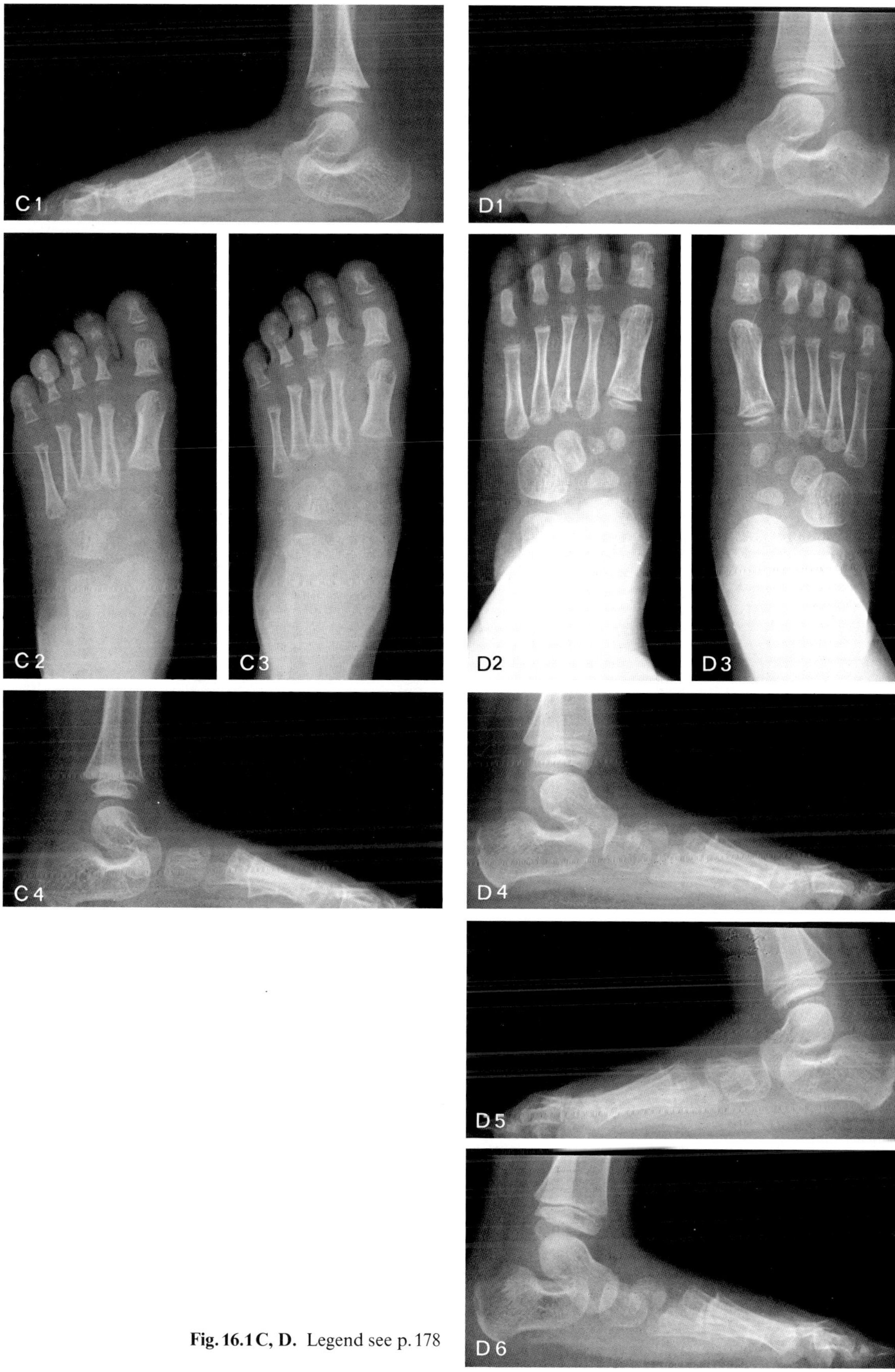

Fig. 16.1 C, D. Legend see p. 178

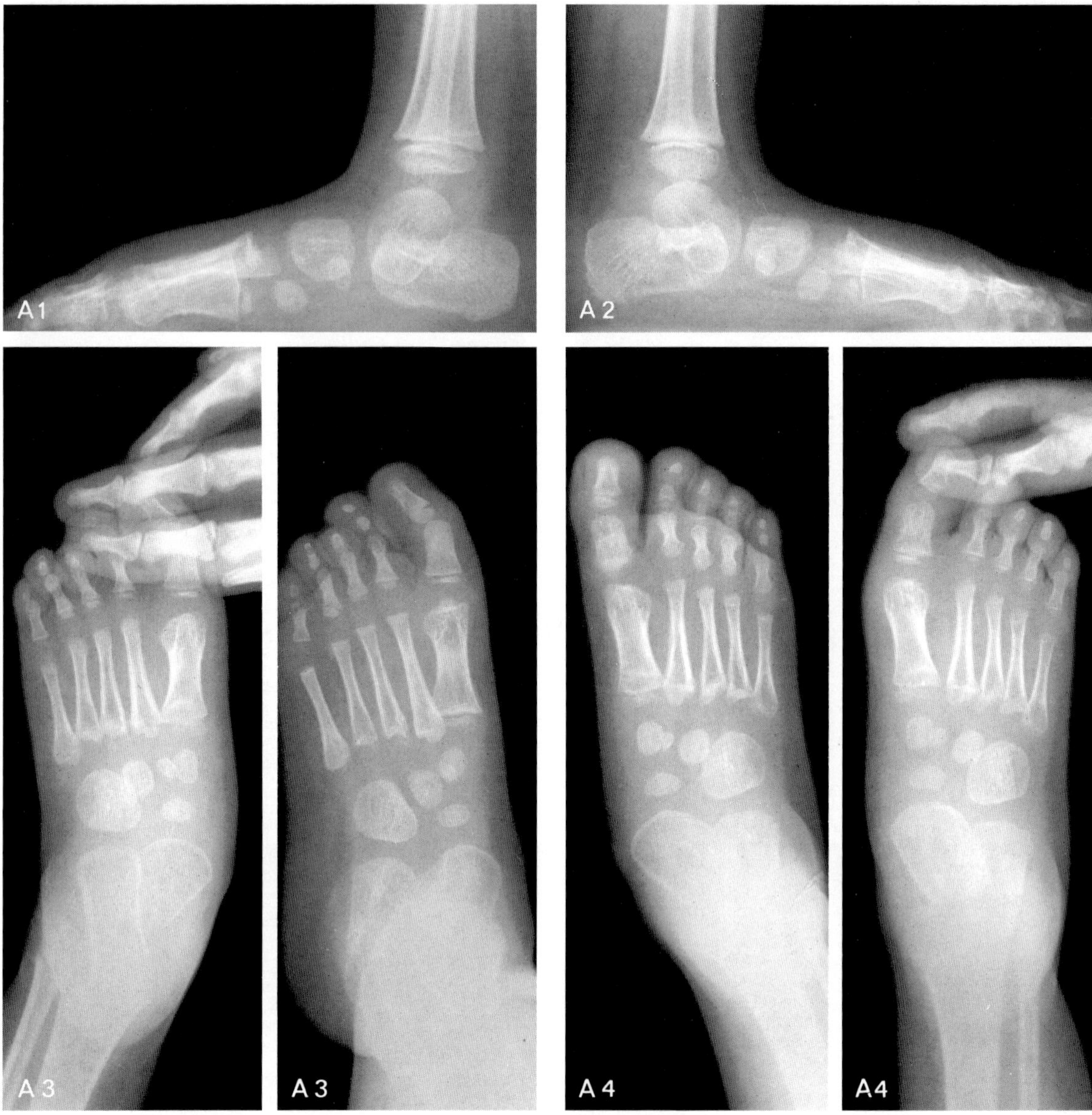

Fig. 16.2 A–C. Second- and third-degree idiopathic pes planovalgus in three children aged between 3 and 5 years. **A** Second degree, age 3 years. *1* Left foot, weight-bearing lateral view; *2* right foot, weight-bearing lateral view: shortness and equinus of talus, marked divergence of axes of talus and calcaneum, lowering of midtarsus; *3* left foot, non-weight-bearing *(left)* and weight-bearing *(right)* dorsoplantar views: divergence of axes of calcaneum and talus, abduction of metatarsus, adduction of talus; *4* right foot, weight-bearing *(left)* and non-weight-bearing *(right)* dorsoplantar views: divergence of axes of talus and calcaneum, adduction of talus. **B** Second degree, age 5 years. *1, 2* Left foot, weight-bearing and non-weight-bearing lateral views: normal length of neck of talus, divergence between axes of talus and calcaneum less ▷ marked, lowering of navicular; *3, 4* left foot, non-weight-bearing and weight-bearing dorsoplantar views: angulation of midtarsal region marked; *5, 6* right foot, weight-bearing and non-weight-bearing lateral views: left foot. **C** Third degree, age 5 years. *1* Left foot, weight-bearing lateral view: shortness and equinus posture of neck of talus, marked lowering of naviculocuneiform region, horizontal alignment of calcaneum; *2* both feet, dorsoplantar views: considerable divergence of axes of talus and calcaneum, abduction of calcaneum; *3* right foot, weight-bearing lateral view: talus normal shape, light equinus of neck of talus, lowering of navicular, horizontal alignment of calcaneum. **B, C** see p. 181

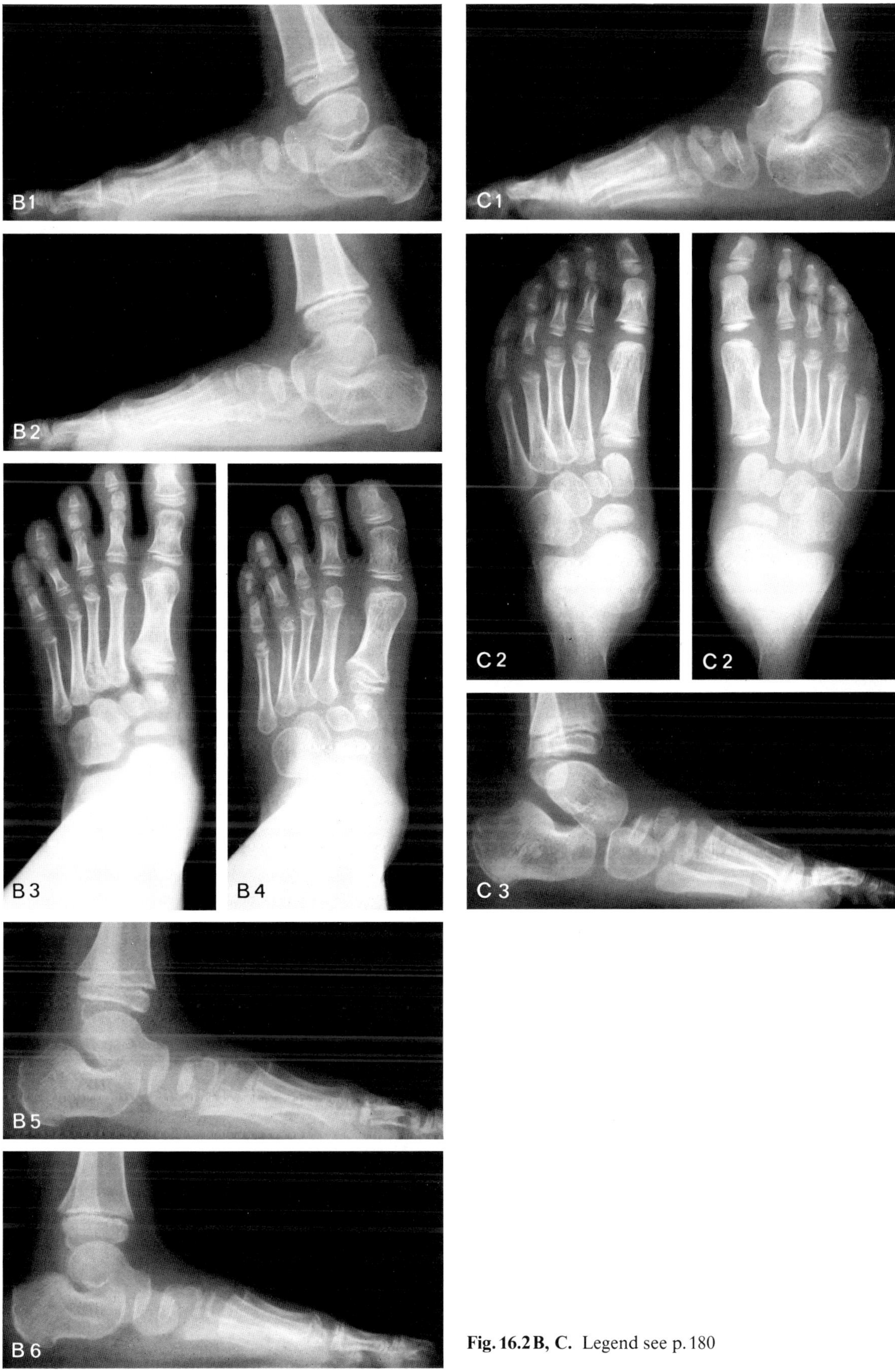

Fig. 16.2 B, C. Legend see p. 180

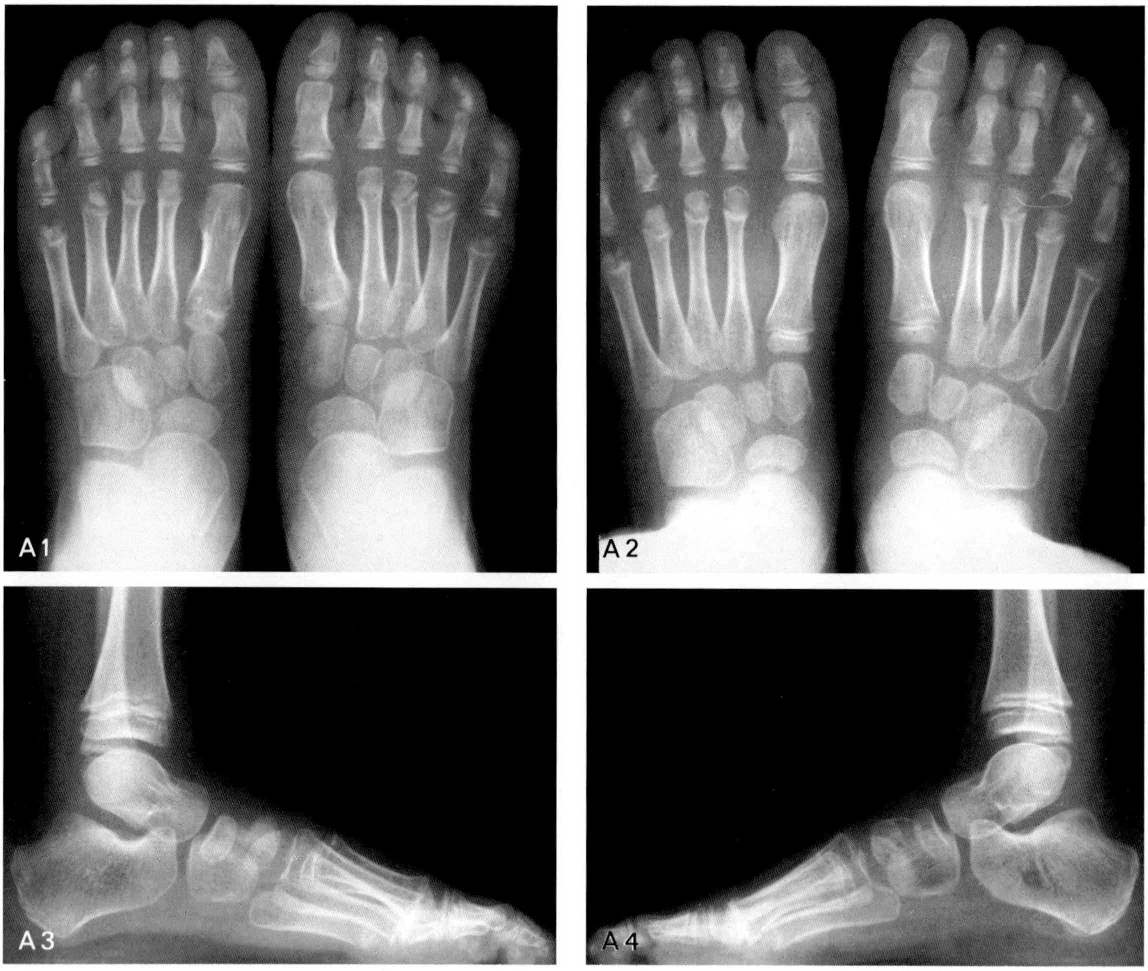

Fig. 16.3 A, B. First- and second-degree pes planovalgus in two children aged 7 and 6 years. **A** First degree, age 7 years. *1, 2* Both feet, non-weight-bearing and weight-bearing dorsoplantar views: convexity of medial border of foot, adduction of neck of talus; *3, 4* right foot and left foot respectively, weight-bearing lateral views: smaller than normal bony outlines, slight lowering of navicular. **B** Second degree, age 6 years. *1* Left foot, weight-bearing lateral view: lowering of midtarsal region, diminution of ▷ angles of inclination of calcaneum and metatarsals; *2* right foot, weight-bearing lateral view: outline of bones smaller than normal; *3, 4* both feet, weight-bearing and non-weight-bearing dorsoplantar views: accentuated angulation of medial border of foot, abduction of cuneiform-cuboidal region, significant adduction of neck of talus. **B** see p. 183

Important features include the condition of the weight-bearing tissues of the sole, the divergence of the toes (most marked in the first interdigital space due to adduction of the great toe) and the general displacement of the bony skeleton of the foot, with complete flattening of the longitudinal arch in the midtarsal region associated with a valgus calcaneum (Figs 16.4, 16.5).

The longitudinal axis of tarsometatarsal alignment shows both vertical and horizontal displacements. The vertical displacement leads to internal projection of the talar head, lowering of the navicular and horizontal alignment of the first metatarsal. Palpation reveals the general valgus of the foot, although this is manually correctable; the calcaneum is neutral or in valgus of up to 15°. The tarsus is adducted with respect to the metatarsus, which is abducted. The essential feature is the angulation of the internal border of the foot associated with a valgus calcaneum, rather than the disappearance of the longitudinal arch itself.

Podoscopic examination shows the common flat foot appearance of a young child, but accompanied by the clinical signs described above. The longitudinal displacement does not correct when the child stands on tiptoe.

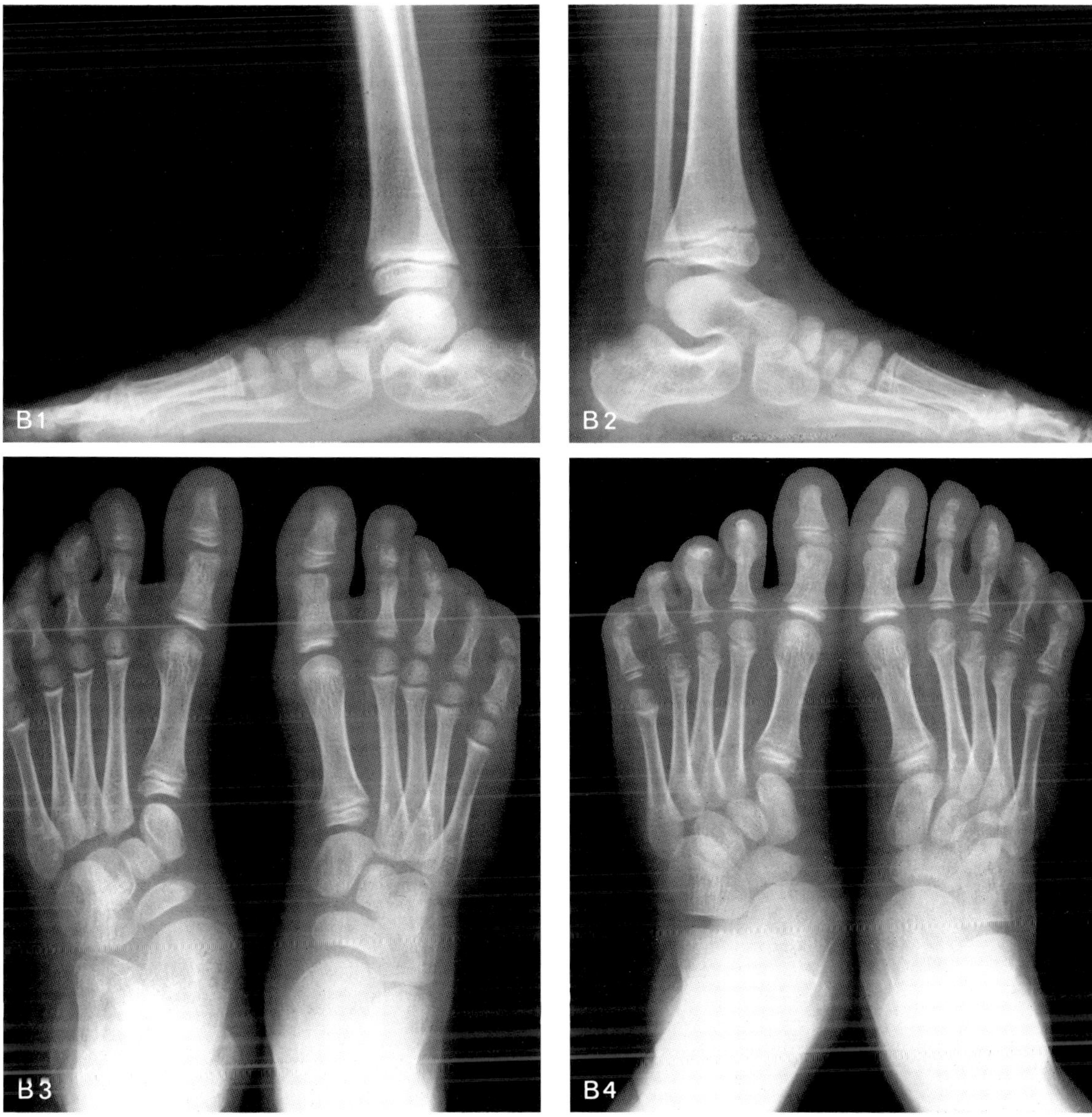

Fig. 16.3 B. Legend see p. 182

Radiographic examination (Fig. 16.6), with views taken under loading and in relaxation, reveals the following:

1. Absence of alteration of normal shape of the bones of the foot.
2. Lowering and subluxation of the navicular.
3. In the lateral view, superimposition of the profiles of the navicular and the cuboid – a most important pathognomonic sign of pes planovalgus, whatever its etiology.
4. Again in the lateral view, horizontal straight alignment of the calcaneum, the head of the talus, the navicular, the medial cuneiform and the first metatarsal. In the vertical view, the internal angulation may be evident.
5. Distortion of the talocalcaneal relationship. In the dorsoplantar view, this divergence is shown by abduction of the calcaneum, forming an angle of 25°–40° with the axis of the talus (normally 10°–20°). In the lateral view the divergence is characterised by horizontal alignment of the calcaneum and plantarflexion of the talus; the axes of the bones form a divergence of 35°–60°, whereas the normal is 20°–30°. The two angles of divergence do not diminish when the foot is loaded, and this persistence is an indication that treatment is necessary.

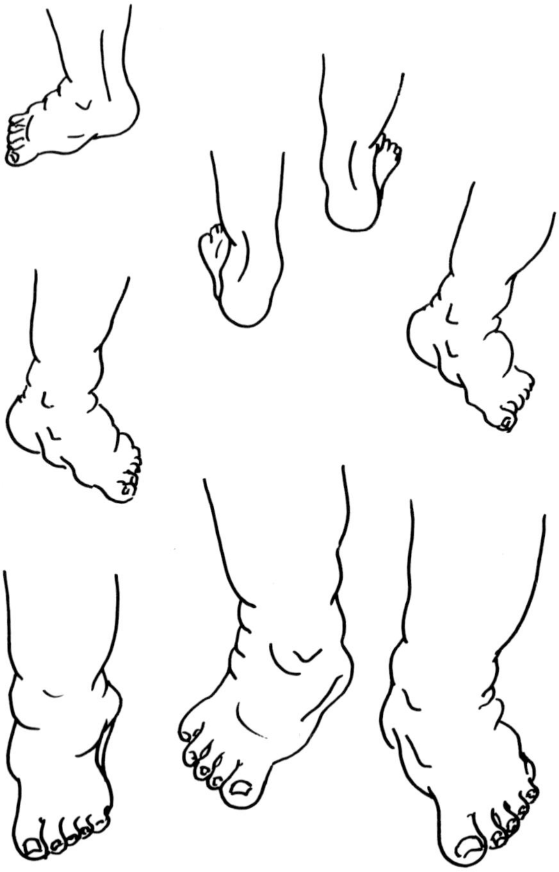

Fig. 16.4. Juvenile pes planus

16.1.3.1 Treatment

The fundamental aim is correction of the distorted relationship between the calcaneum and the talus and of ths displacement of the midtarsus.

16.1.3.1.1 Conservative

In the vast majority of instances the use of an insole suffices, but it is essential that the orthosis is fitted perfectly and that the deformity should be passively correctable (see Chap. 40). Insoles must be worn in properly adapted shoes permanently for some 5–7 years and perhaps intermittently thereafter. The shoes should provide adequate lateral support to the heels and need to be stiffened at the instep, which must be narrow, so that they do not deform. Regular follow-up with careful measurement of the corrective process is essential. In juvenile pes planus, a pronating wedge under the metatarsal region with a supinating wedge under the heel can be well tolerated in first- and second-degree cases (see below) whereas in an adult, a similar insole without a supporting dome under the navicular proves intolerable. The use of an internal dome alone should be avoided in the young child because it produces a cavovalgus foot.

In more detail, the essential features of the insole are as follows: Along the outer border of the foot, a pronating external wedge behind or under the fifth metatarsal head should measure 6–8 mm in height, and the supinating calcaneal wedge along the inner border of the heel should be 7–8 mm high. The two must harmonise, the supinating element always being 1–2 mm higher than the pronating element. An accessory element is an internal dome with summit corresponding to the navicular, which it supports. The height must not exceed that of the normal infantile arch by more than 2–3 mm. An internal support of 13–14 mm may be necessary, but this will be indicated only when the navicular rise has been provoked by the pronating and supinating wedges. When these do not suffice to induce elevation of the internal longitudinal arch, the height of the internal dome must be significantly more than the normal, up to as much as 15–16 mm. It then aids the rise of the navicular, diminishes the vertical disposition of the talar neck and corrects the pronation of the calcaneum by replacing the sustentaculum tali underneath the talar head.

The elements constituting this insole must be calculated in millimetres using the podoscope. The harmonious action of the elements of the insole has been aptly formulated by Delchef and Soeur (1956) and Lelièvre (1952) as: supination of the calcaneum + pronation of the metatarsus = cavus of the longitudinal arch. Every case is individual in terms of these measurements.

It is useless to attempt a complete correction from the outset (Valenti 1977c). After fitting, the insole must be reviewed every year and the prescription for height adapted as correction is achieved. It must be worn continuously until complete restoration of the equilibrium of the heel and reconstitution of a normal plantar arch with a straight internal border have been achieved. This may take from 3 to 15 years, so that in some instances the patient will continue wearing the insole until the age of 18 years. As stated earlier, the shoe must be adequate. The first insole should be of leather and have rigid narrow alignment, while the posterior uppers of the shoes, especially laterally, should be strong enough to prevent the foot sliding towards

Fig. 16.5 A–I. Pes planovalgus with genu valgum in childhood ▷

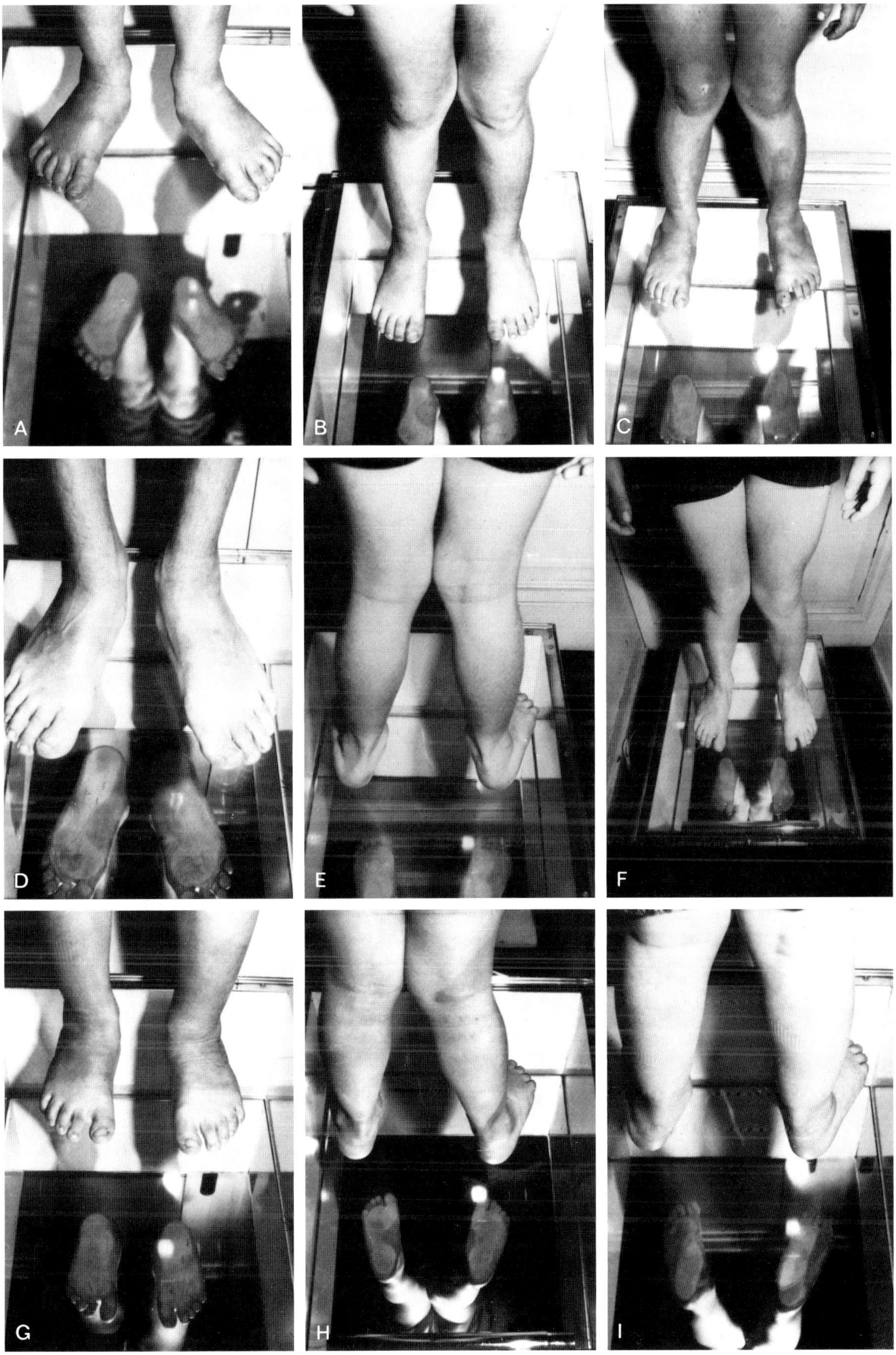
A
B
C
D
E
F
G
H
I

the outer side, bulging the shoe and thereby losing the corrective effect of the insoles. The posterior part of the shoe heel cup should be higher than normal so that the hindfoot is adequately stabilised. The upper of the shoe should be sufficiently capacious to accommodate the insole of the foot without tightness.

16.1.3.1.2 Operative

In 1%–2% of cases, early follow-up will show that correction is not occurring. This may be assessed at the age of 4–5 years and is an indication for possible surgical management. The radiographic estimation of displacements is essential, especially of the failure to correct or improve when standing on tiptoe.

In such instances, any operative intervention must avoid limitation of subtalar movement. Thus the Grice (1952) extra-articular arthrodesis, which has a place in juvenile paralytic flat foot, is inappropriate here; there is evidence that it provokes late arthrosis of the subtalar joint despite its immobility. Comments are appropriate on certain aspects of many operations which have been described for the condition:

Kidner (1929) described a procedure in which the tibialis posterior tendon is passed as a sling under tibialis anterior and re-inserted onto the inferior aspect of the navicular. This corrects the angulation of the midtarsal region fairly well but does nothing to correct pronation of the calcaneum. Stabilisation of the subtalar joint, preferably by means of capsuloligamentoplasties, is essential.

Lelièvre (1965 c) used a stapling procedure in cases of marked aplasia of the sustentaculum tali in young children. The staple cannot be left in place for more than 2 years and must always be supplemented by corrective insoles to prevent the progressive reappearance of the valgus heel. In other words, its effect is temporary.

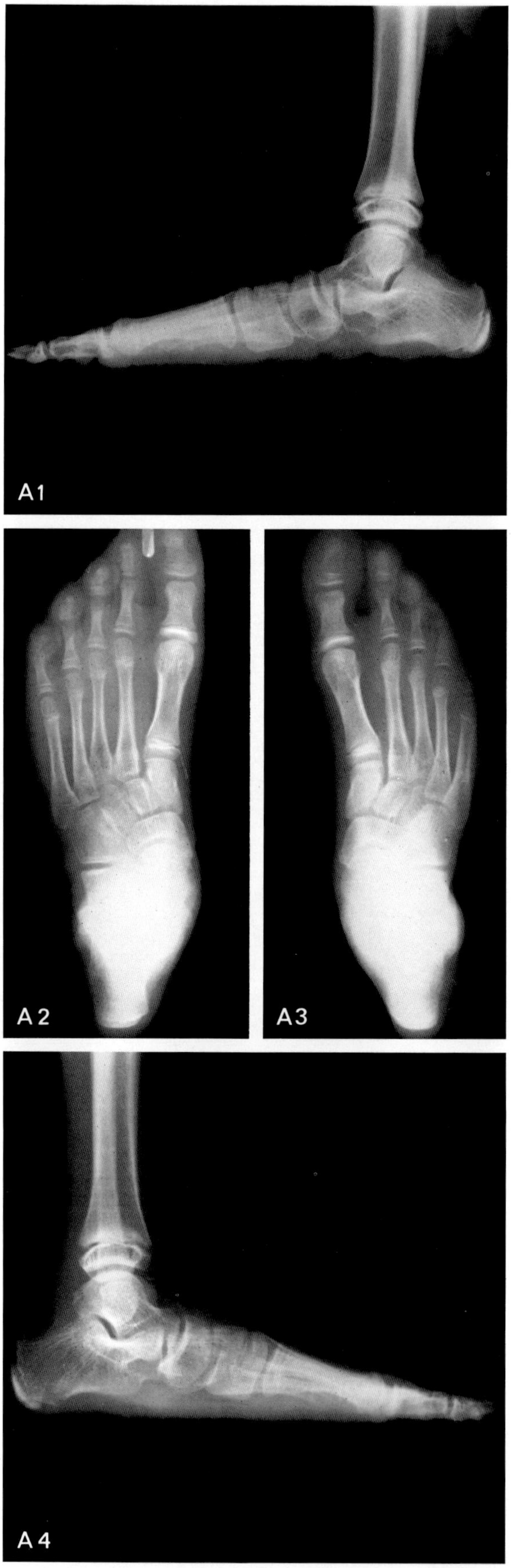

Fig. 16.6 A–C. Second-, third- and fourth degree idiopathic pes planovalgus in three children aged between 5 and 8 years. **A** Third degree, age 5 years. *1* Left foot, weight-bearing lateral view: equinus of talus, divergence of talar and calcaneal axes, lowering of naviculocuneiform region, superimposition of navicular and cuboid, diminution of angles of inclination; *2, 3* left foot and right foot respectively, weight-bearing dorsoplantar views: angulation of tarsomidtarsal region, adduction of neck of talus, divergence of talar and calcaneal axes, abduction of cuneiform-cuboidal region; *4* right foot, weight-bearing lateral view: as left foot. **B, C** see pp. 187, 188

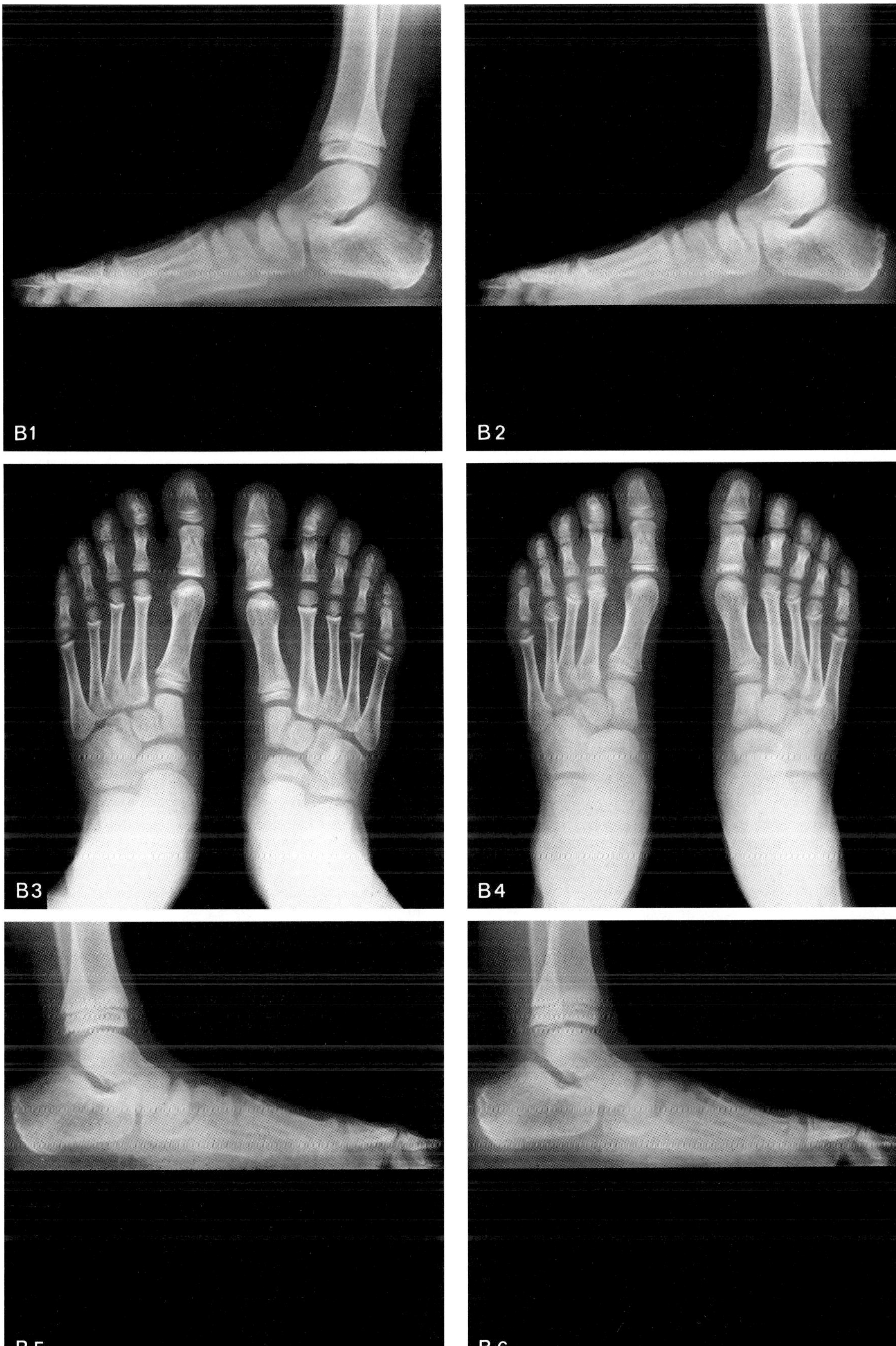
B1
B2
B3
B4
B5
B6

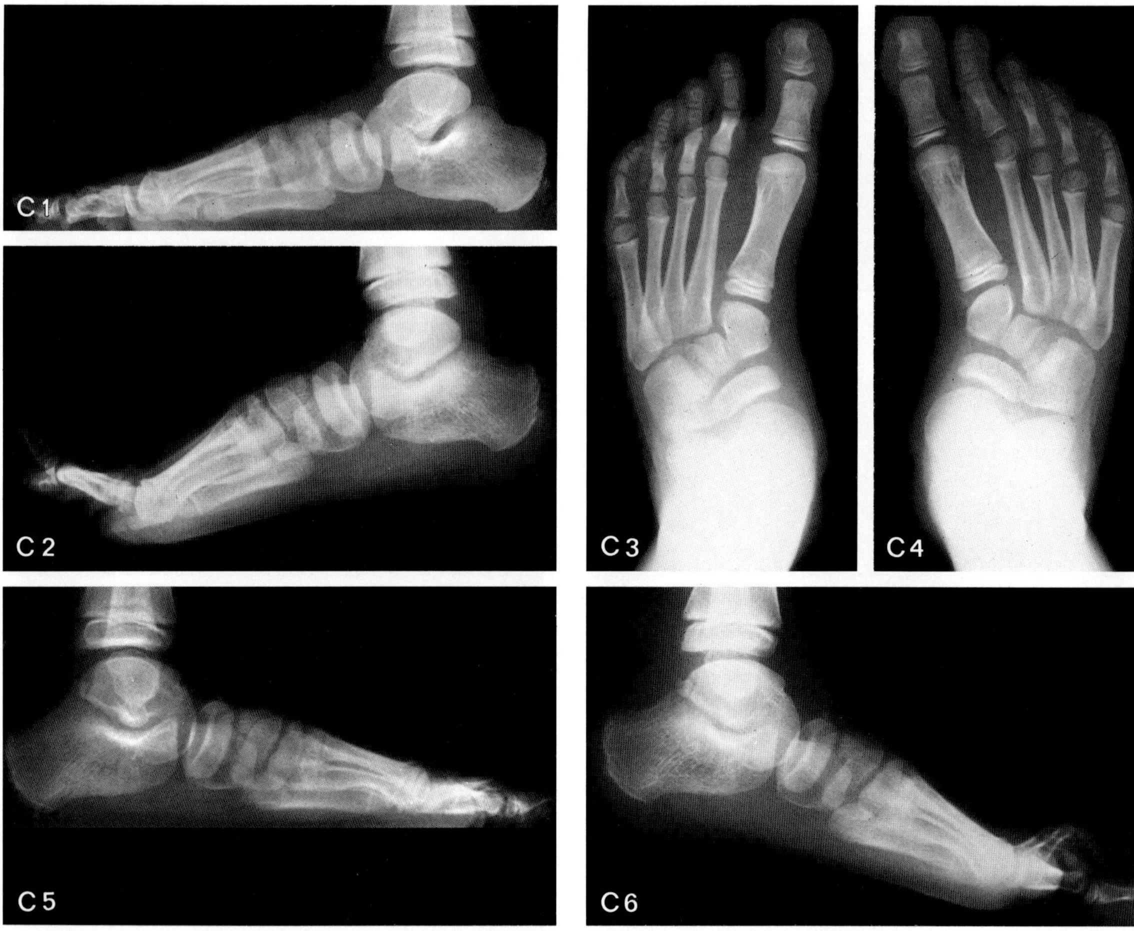

Fig. 16.6 *(continued).* **B** Second degree, age 7 years. *1, 2* Left foot, non-weight-bearing and weight-bearing lateral views: divergence of talocalcaneal axes, lowering of navicular and cuboid, hypertrophy of length of neck of talus, reduced angles of inclination of calcaneum and metatarsus; *3, 4* both feet, weight-bearing and non-weight-bearing dorsoplantar views: angulation of talonaviculocuneiform region, aplasia of navicular, divergence of talar and calcaneal axes; *5, 6* right foot, non-weight-bearing and weight-bearing lateral views: as left foot. **C** Fourth degree, age 8 years. *1* Left foot, weight-bearing lateral view: divergence of talar and calcaneal axes, shortness and equinus of neck of talus; *2* left foot, non-weight-bearing lateral view: collapse of navicular, superimposition of navicular and cuboid; *3, 4* left foot and right foot respectively, weight-bearing dorsoplantar views; extreme divergence of axes of talus and calcaneum, marked adduction of neck of talus, angulation and displacement of midtarsal mass, abduction of naviculocuneiform-cuboidal mass, compensatory varus of metatarsus; *5* right foot, weight-bearing lateral view: shortness and aplasia of neck of talus, equinus of neck of talus, divergence of talar and calcaneal axes; *6* right foot, non-weight-bearing lateral view: collapse of navicular, superimposition of navicular and cuboid, diminution of angles of inclination of calcaneum

Judet (1972) called his procedure "the horseman operation". It seems to have a place in dealing with the difficult problem associated with talocalcaneal divergence of congenital origin leading to valgus foot. It comprises temporary stabilisation with a screw for about 2 years; delaying removal can be dangerous, as it leads to a cavovarus foot due to the blocking of normal physiological valgus play of the tarsus. However, provided delay is not excessive there are advantages compatible with the law of Delpech; the procedure re-establishes the axes of pressure of the normal foot and permits normal alignment of the calcaneum and talus while respecting the articular integrity of the subtalar and midtarsal regions. When the bones are normally aligned, recovery of normal muscle action occurs and contributes to the maintenance of the reduction during growth.

Lelièvre (1965 c), Viladot (1975 c), Voutey (1970 a), Grassin (1977), Valenti (1976 a), Lopez and Zuzuarregui (1963) and Burutaran (1968) have all described techniques of stabilisation of the subtalar joint. The operations are difficult but have in common the concept of extra-articular implantation in the sinus tarsi of a bone graft, a Silastic, metallic or Teflon prosthesis, or a screw. It should be emphasised that these procedures preserve some mobility of the subtalar joint (Fig. 16.7). However, they do not correct either the talonaviculocuneiform angulation which results from contracture of the dorsal ligaments or the hypertrophy which holds the talar head in its low position (Judet). Any stabilising procedure of the talocalcaneal divergence must be accompanied (as confirmed by Judet and Viladot) by excision of this mass of fibrous tissue, so allowing correction of the midtarsus. Further, I have found that subtalar stabilisation causes pain in the region of the sinus tarsi perhaps 8 years after the grafting procedure of Lelièvre. Thys reported on a case of arthrosis of the subtalar joint occurring 10 years after such an operation. I am chary with respect to the implantation of any prosthesis. Rodgvelle (1976) [cited by Pisani (1978b)] eschewed stabilisation or other bony procedures in the infant. They developed a technique, according to demand, of distal transposition of tibialis posterior, transposition of tibialis anterior to the navicular or the tenodesis described by Albanese (1948) (thereby tethering tibialis anterior and tibialis posterior), associated with elongation of triceps surae if necessary. There then follows a capsuloligamentous procedure involving shortening of the glenoid talonavicular ligament by resection of a segment at its plantar internal aspect (Fig. 16.8). The resulting tightening realigns the midtarsal region with respect to the tarsus.

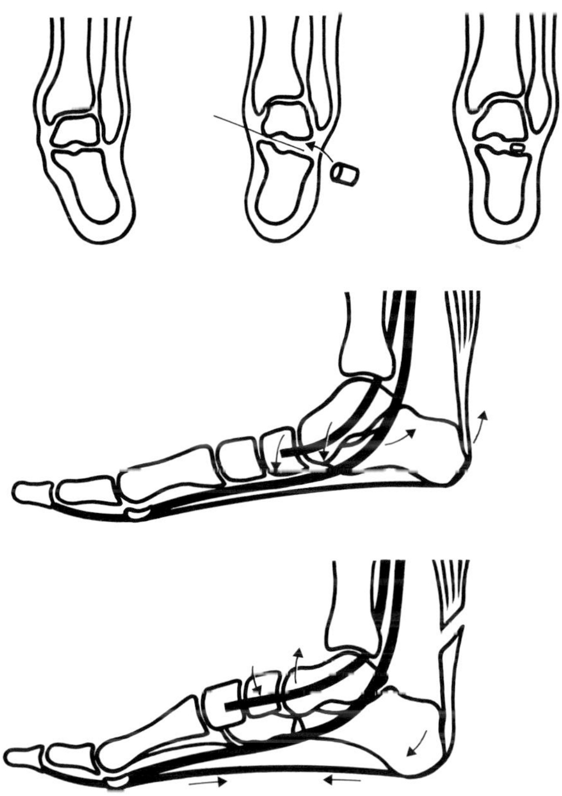

Fig. 16.7. Correction of pes planus by arthrorisis of subtalar joint. (*Arrows* indicate displacements occurring before and as a result of operation)

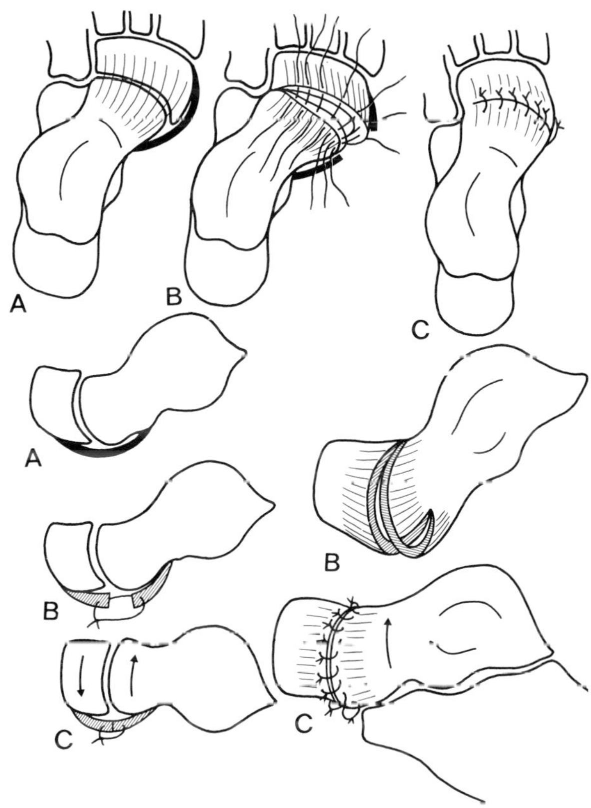

Fig. 16.8 A–C. Semilunar ligamentoplasty in subtalar arthrorisis for pes planus. **A** Talonavicular ligament and spring ligament before operation. **B** Plantar-medial crescentic resection of spring ligament and plantar talonavicular ligament (modified Pisani technique). **C** Suture of the resection and correction of the plantar-medial angulation at the talonavicular joint (modified Pisani technique)

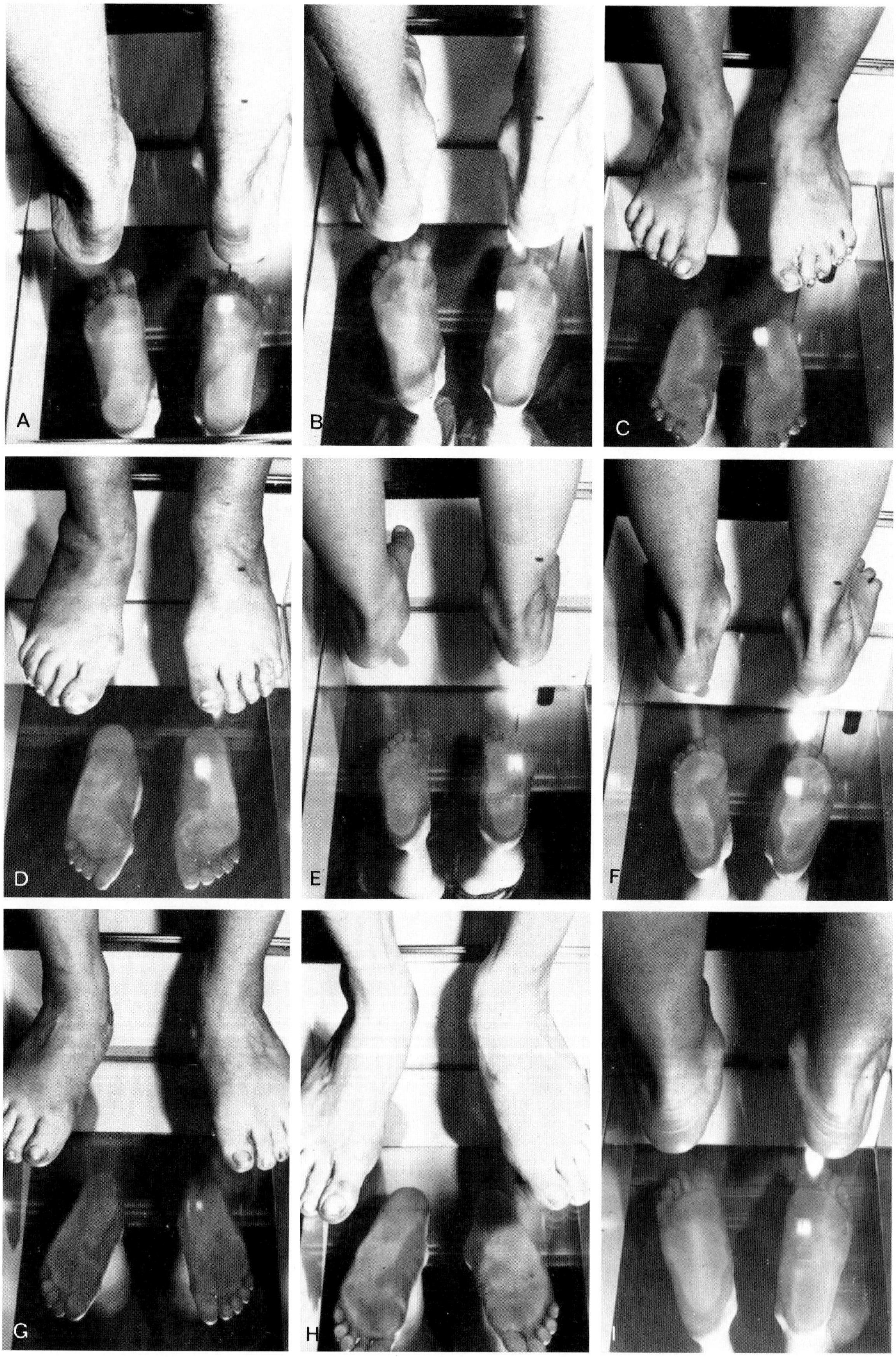
A
B
C
D
E
F
G
H
I

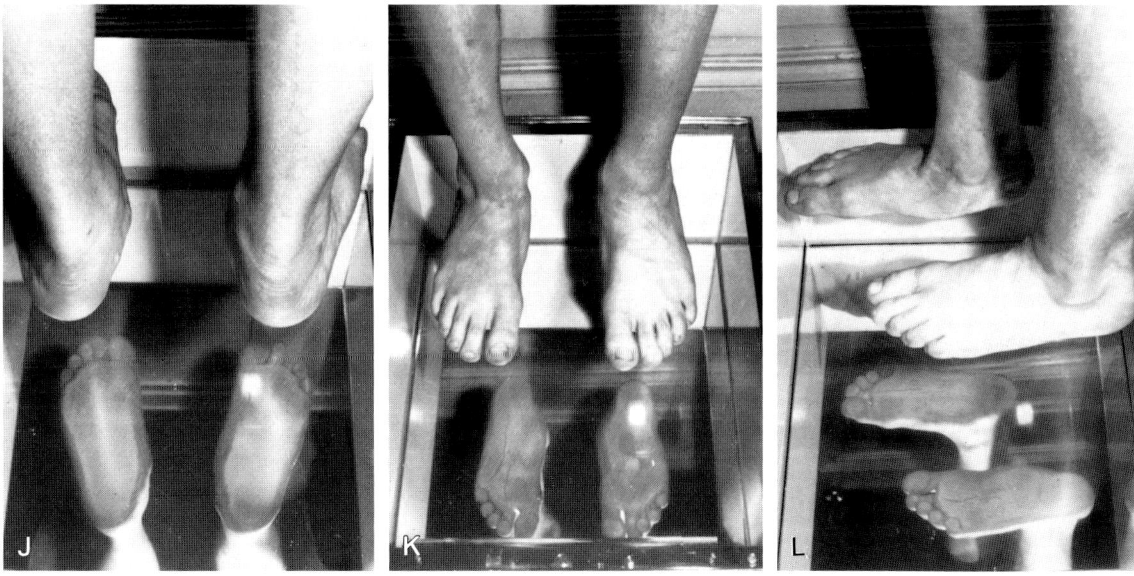

◁ **Fig. 16.9 A–L.** Idiopathic pes planovalgus. **A–D** First degree: obliteration of retrocapital central hollowing, widening of external subcuboidal band, incipient collapse of midtarsal, light valgus posture of tarsus, early abduction of forefoot. **E–H** Second degree: very wide subcuboidal load-bearing band, continuous with axis of the heel print, lowering and medial displacement of midtarsus with longitudinal convexity of internal border of foot, valgus posture of tarsus, abduction of forefoot. **I–L** Third degree: total plantar print with straight or convex medial margin, disappearance of medial longitudinal arch, lowering and medial displacement of midtarsus, pronation and valgus posture of heel. **A–I** see p. 190

I recommend that the only clinical criterion for surgery should be failure to achieve orthotic correction despite 5 years of carefully supervised use of proper insoles. The slightest improvement in the superimposition of images of the navicular and cuboid indicates the need for further conservative efforts; the majority of cases not corrected in early childhood complete their improvement during adolescence.

16.1.4 Adolescent Pes Planovalgus

Presenting between the ages of 10 and 18 years, the findings are basically similar to those in the juvenile variety. The relative diminution in soft tissue padding makes the deformity very obvious, and Lannelongue described three prominent bosses from bony protuberance: the medial malleolus, the head of the talus and the navicular tuberosity (Figs. 16.9–16.11).

16.1.4.1 Treatment

As in juvenile pes planus, the treatment of preference is conservative, with the use of an insole. In the majority of properly treated cases, perfect correction is achieved. However, towards the age of about 14 years, in the presence of persistent displacement, poor gait and pain, especially when the foot abnormality reflects on the limb and trunk above, surgery becomes necessary. It should be performed in such a way as to preserve integrity of articular surfaces. In this age group there is an important difference in that muscle imbalance may be apparent, and will spoil orthopaedic correction unless treated simultaneously. Its components are: hypertonia of triceps surae due to shortening associated with the horizontal and pronated attitude of the calcaneum; hypotonia of tibialis posterior and flexor hallucis longus, which encourages hypertrophy of length of the talar neck and augmentation of volume of the internal part of the navicular; and hypotonia of peroneus longus which is able only to weakly depress the first metatarsal and yet favours abduction of the metatarsus with diminution of the angle of inclination of the metatarsus.

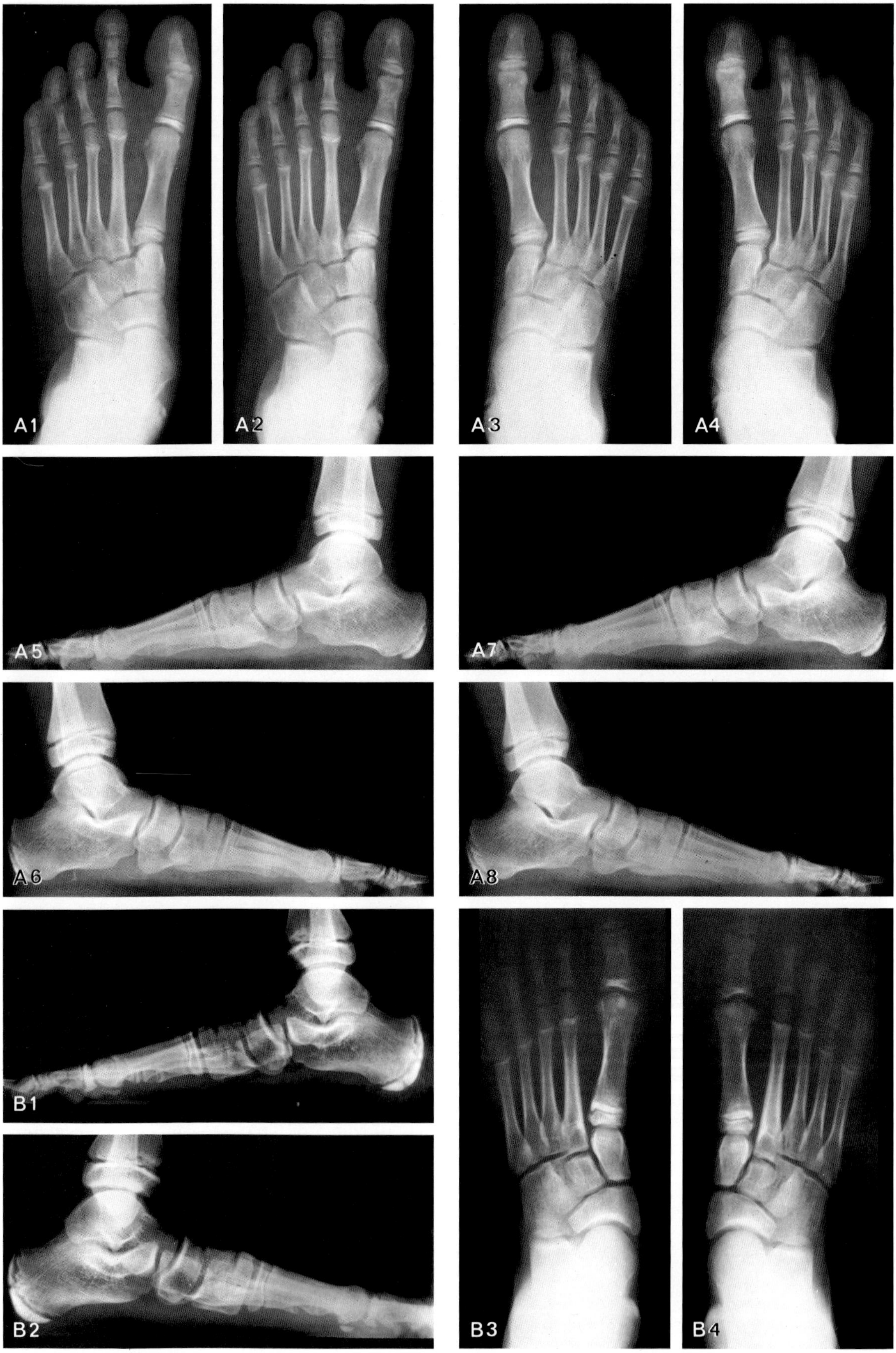
A1
A2
A3
A4
A5
A7
A6
A8
B1
B2
B3
B4

Arthrodesis procedures near epiphyses disturb growth and are likely to have a deleterious effect on later equilibrium of the foot. Stabilising operations of the calcaneum and with respect to the talus, however, will re-establish the normal axis of loading and normal development. The selective bone resections described for the juvenile foot (Regnauld 1974) with particular attention to the length of the neck of the talus and of the navicular are the procedures of choice and must be accompanied by elongation of triceps surae, transplantation of tibialis posterior onto the medial cuneiform and an Albanese tenodesis. The ligamentoplasties associated with the calcaneonavicular and talonavicular joints are most effective. Simple correction of talocalcaneal disalignment is not sufficient.

16.1.5 Adult Pes Planovalgus

In the juvenile form of pes planovalgus it is calcaneal pronation which predominates, and in the adolescent variety pronation of the calcaneum and displacement of the metatarsus are equally significant; in the adult planovalgus foot, the emphasis is shifted to midtarsal displacement, which overshadows the valgus heel. It is rational to distinguish three degrees of planovalgus.

◁ **Fig. 16.10 A, B.** Second- and third-degree idiopathic pes planovalgus in two children aged 10 years. **A** Second degree. *1–4* Weight-bearing (*1* left foot; *3* right foot) and non-weight-bearing (*2* left foot; *4* right foot), dorsoplantar views: angulation of tarsomidtarsal region, marked adduction of neck of talus, abduction of axes of naviculocuneiform-cuboidal complex; *5–8* weight-bearing (*5* left foot; *6* right foot) and non-weight-bearing (*7* left foot; *8* right foot) lateral views: lowering of midtarsal region of second degree, straightness of talonaviculocuneiform axis, two-thirds superimposition of navicular and cuboid, diminution of angles of inclination of calcaneum and metatarsus. **B** Third degree. *1* Left foot, weight-bearing lateral view: marked lowering of midtarsal region, lowering of naviculocuneiform region; *2* right foot, weight-bearing lateral view: superimposition of navicular and cuboid, diminution of angles of inclination of calcaneum and metatarsus; *3, 4* left foot and right foot respectively, weight-bearing dorsoplantar views: angulation of midtarsal region, adduction of neck of talus, medial hypertrophy of navicular

16.1.5.1 First Degree

First-degree planovalgus is characterised by progressive onset of pain, which may present in the midtarsal region and ankle when standing, as a general aching of the instep during prolonged walking, as a sensation of fatigue and tension along the medial border of the instep during standing, or perhaps as metatarsalgia emanating from the second metatarsal head, which may be misdiagnosed as rheumatic or arthritic.

Clinical examination reveals slight calcaneal valgus, internal displacement of the midtarsus accentuated by projection of the navicular tuberosity, and a residual plantar longitudinal arch (of diminished height), but at this stage there is no abduction of the antetarsus.

Podoscopic examination reveals widening of the band of medial midtarsal support, light internal angulation of the print of the heel with respect to the subcuboid band and the disappearance of metatarsal retrocapital concavity (Figs. 16.12, 16.13).

16.1.5.2 Second Degree

The symptoms described above become more intense and lead to true arthralgia, accentuated by standing, walking, and the use of over-supple shoes, in the region of the talonavicular joint. The classic patient presents in the autumn after a holiday during which he or she has worn unaccustomedly soft shoes. Pain on the medial border of the ankle is permanent and irradiates into the calf, where the sensation of heaviness is often attributed to venous circulatory disorder. A sensation of tension at the back of the knees is noticeable on walking after resting. Metatarsalgia under the second metatarsal head is now of a burning character associated with troublesome callus or keratoma formation. This particular feature is aggravated by stair-climbing and sport and impedes normal rolling of the forefoot.

On examination, the valgus of the calcaneum may exceed 15°. Although the medial longitudinal plantar arch is noticeably lower, it still exists, compressing the underlying soft tissue (Fig. 16.13), as evidenced by palpation. Internal angulation remains mild except for the projection of the navicular tuberosity, but there is now undoubted abduction of the antetarsus with evident angulation at the cuboid laterally. The persistent tension on the tibialis posterior tendon may lead to tendinitis at its insertion into the navicular.

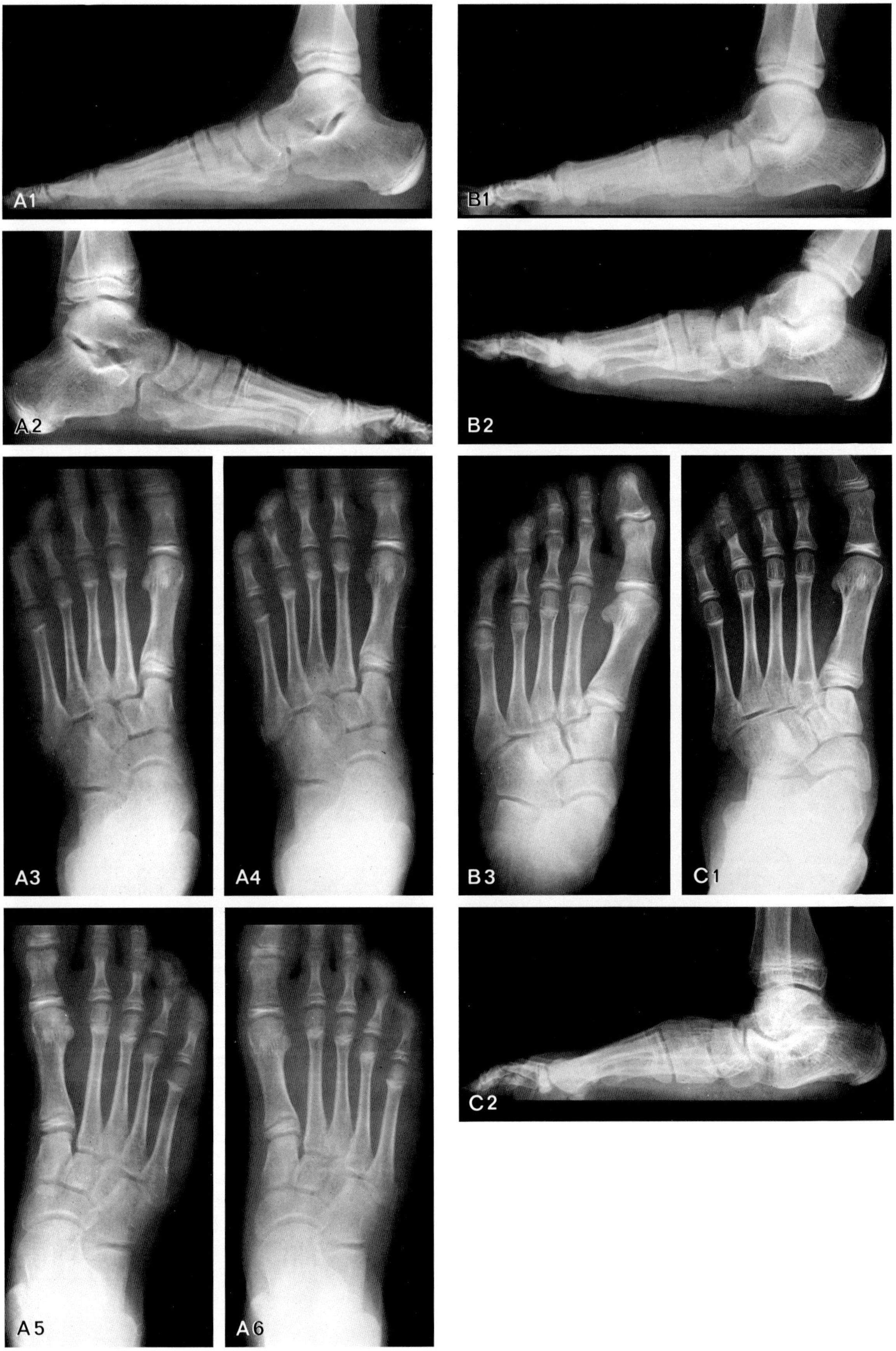
A1
B1
A2
B2
A3
A4
B3
C1
C2
A5
A6

Podoscopy shows a flat print with a straight internal border (evidence of lowering of the medial plantar arch) while the axis of the heel print falls inside the backward-projected axis of the antetarsus print.

Radiography: The lateral view shows lowering of the plantar arch and superimposition of the images of the navicular and the cuboid so that the former shadows the superior two-thirds of the latter bone (Figs. 16.14–16.16). The longitudinal axis of the calcaneum is less than 25° with respect to the floor (the normal is 30°–40°), and the vertical divergence between the axes of the talus and calcaneum is apparent. The surface of the head of the talus is orientated inwards and forwards. The dorsoplantar view shows horizontal divergence of the talus and the calcaneum, diminution in the angle of declination of the neck of the talus to 120°–130° (normally 130°–150°) and hypertrophy in length of the talar neck, especially along its inner margin, while the exaggeration of the posterior concavity of the navicular is accentuated by hypertrophy of the navicular tuberosity. Abduction of the metatarsus is obvious.

The second-degree planovalgus foot in the adult represents a stage in deterioration to the planovalgus contracted foot. Increasing rigidity is accompanied by acute pain in the hindfoot which is rendered violent and sudden by walking, especially on irregular ground. The patient limps because of pain associated with the sinus tarsi due to intolerable tension of the interosseous talocalcaneal ligament, but this pain can still be alleviated by an insole or injection of local anaesthetic and topical steroid. Pain may predominate at the midtarsal joints, being agonising, syncopal and sensitive to shoe pressure, especially when climbing stairs and attempting to stand on the toes. It may be located at the inferior tibiofibular joint, reflecting to either malleoli, or may predominate at the Lisfranc joint line.

◁ **Fig. 16.11 A–C.** Second- and third-degree idiopathic pes planovalgus in three children aged between 13 and 15 years. **A** Second degree, age 13 years. *1* Left foot, weight-bearing lateral view: lowering of midtarsus, two-thirds superimposition of navicular and cuboid, diminution of angles of inclination of calcaneum and metatarsus; *2* right foot, weight-bearing lateral view: lowering of midtarsal region less marked than in left foot, absence of superimposition of navicular and cuboid; *3–6* weight-bearing *(3, 5)* and non-weight-bearing *(4, 6)* dorsoplantar views: medial angulation of midtarsus, convexity of medial border of foot, marked adduction of neck of talus, abduction of axes of cuneiforms. **B** Third degree, age 14 years, left foot. *1* Weight-bearing lateral view: complete collapse of midtarsal region, accentuated lowering of navicular, superimposition of navicular and cuboid; *2* non-weight-bearing lateral view: plantar convexity, inversion of angle of inclination of calcaneum; *3* weight-bearing dorsoplantar view: abnormal shape of head of talus, onset of compensatory varus of first metatarsal. **C** Third degree, age 15 years, left foot. *1* Weight bearing dorsoplantar view: angulation at midtarsal region, marked abduction of longitudinal axes of cuneiforms and cuboid, abnormal shape of head of talus; *2* weight-bearing lateral view: shortness of neck of talus, collapse of midtarsal axis with marked lowering of navicular, superimposition of navicular and cuboid, sinusoidal dorsal angulation of talonaviculocuneiform region, plantar convexity, horizontal alignment of calcaneum

Fig. 16.12 A–F see pp. 196, 197

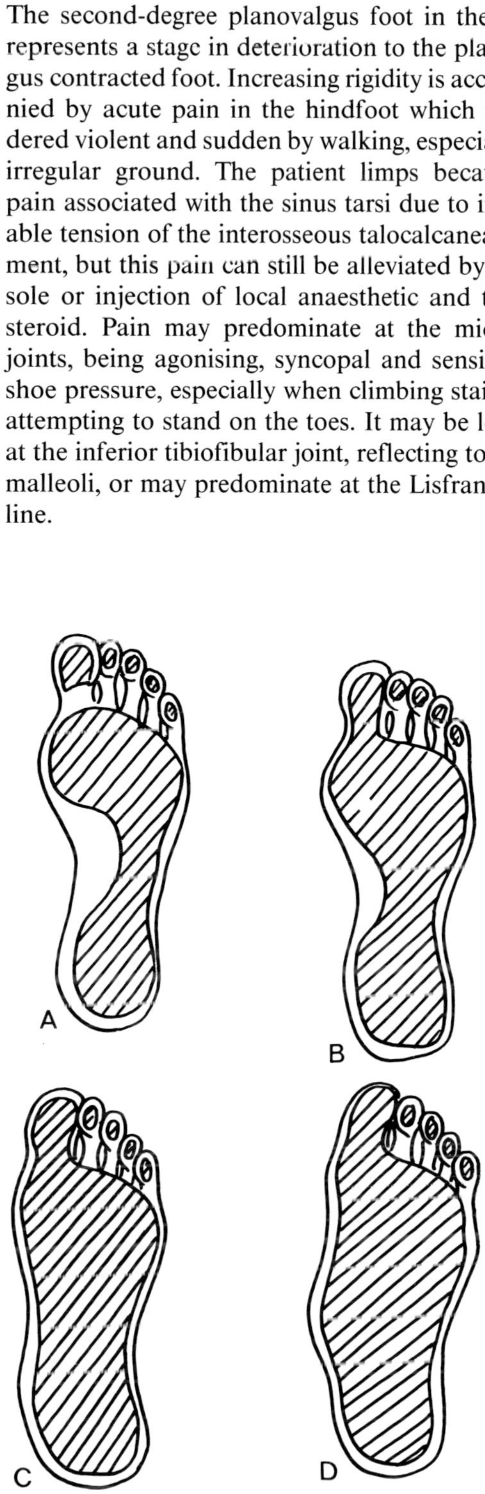

Fig. 16.13 A–D. Patterns of loading in a normal foot and in pes planovalgus. **A** Normal. **B** First-degree planovalgus. **C** Second-degree planovalgus. **D** Third-degree planovalgus

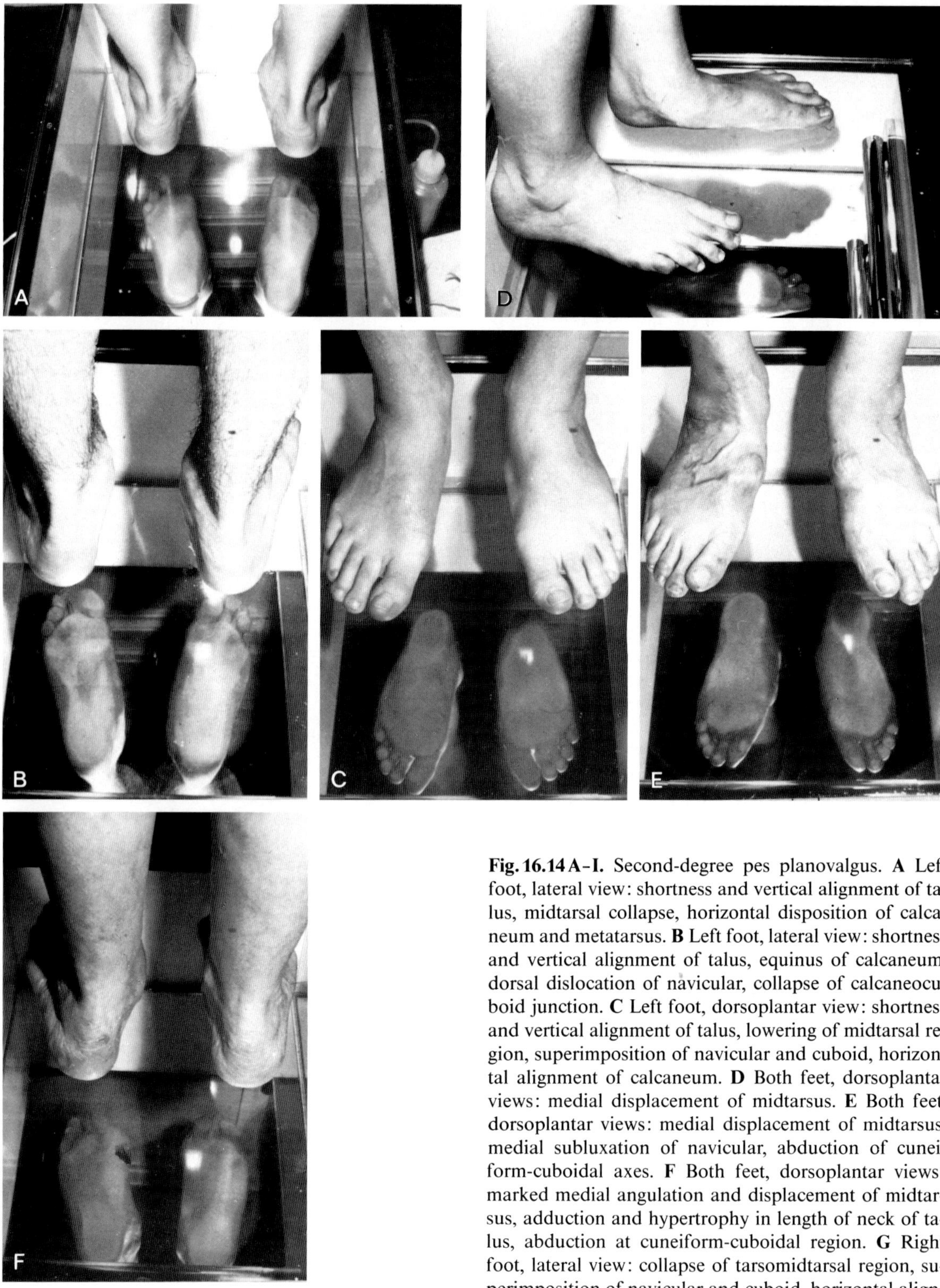

Fig. 16.12 A–F. Third-degree idiopathic pes planovalgus in adulthood: various appearances of the footprint. Note valgus and pronation of tarsus and lowering with medial displacement of midtarsus. **D** Collapse centred on navicular. **E** Collapse centred on medial cuneiform. **F** Right foot corrected by extra-articular osteotomies

Fig. 16.14 A–I. Second-degree pes planovalgus. **A** Left foot, lateral view: shortness and vertical alignment of talus, midtarsal collapse, horizontal disposition of calcaneum and metatarsus. **B** Left foot, lateral view: shortness and vertical alignment of talus, equinus of calcaneum, dorsal dislocation of navicular, collapse of calcaneocuboid junction. **C** Left foot, dorsoplantar view: shortness and vertical alignment of talus, lowering of midtarsal region, superimposition of navicular and cuboid, horizontal alignment of calcaneum. **D** Both feet, dorsoplantar views: medial displacement of midtarsus. **E** Both feet, dorsoplantar views: medial displacement of midtarsus, medial subluxation of navicular, abduction of cuneiform-cuboidal axes. **F** Both feet, dorsoplantar views: marked medial angulation and displacement of midtarsus, adduction and hypertrophy in length of neck of talus, abduction at cuneiform-cuboidal region. **G** Right foot, lateral view: collapse of tarsomidtarsal region, superimposition of navicular and cuboid, horizontal alignment of tarsometatarsal axes. **H** Right foot, lateral view: vertical alignment of neck of talus, horizontal alignment of calcaneocuboidmetatarsal axes, dorsal subluxation of navicular. **I** Right foot, dorsoplantar view: lowering of navicular, equinus attitude of talus, superimposition of navicular and cuboid ▷

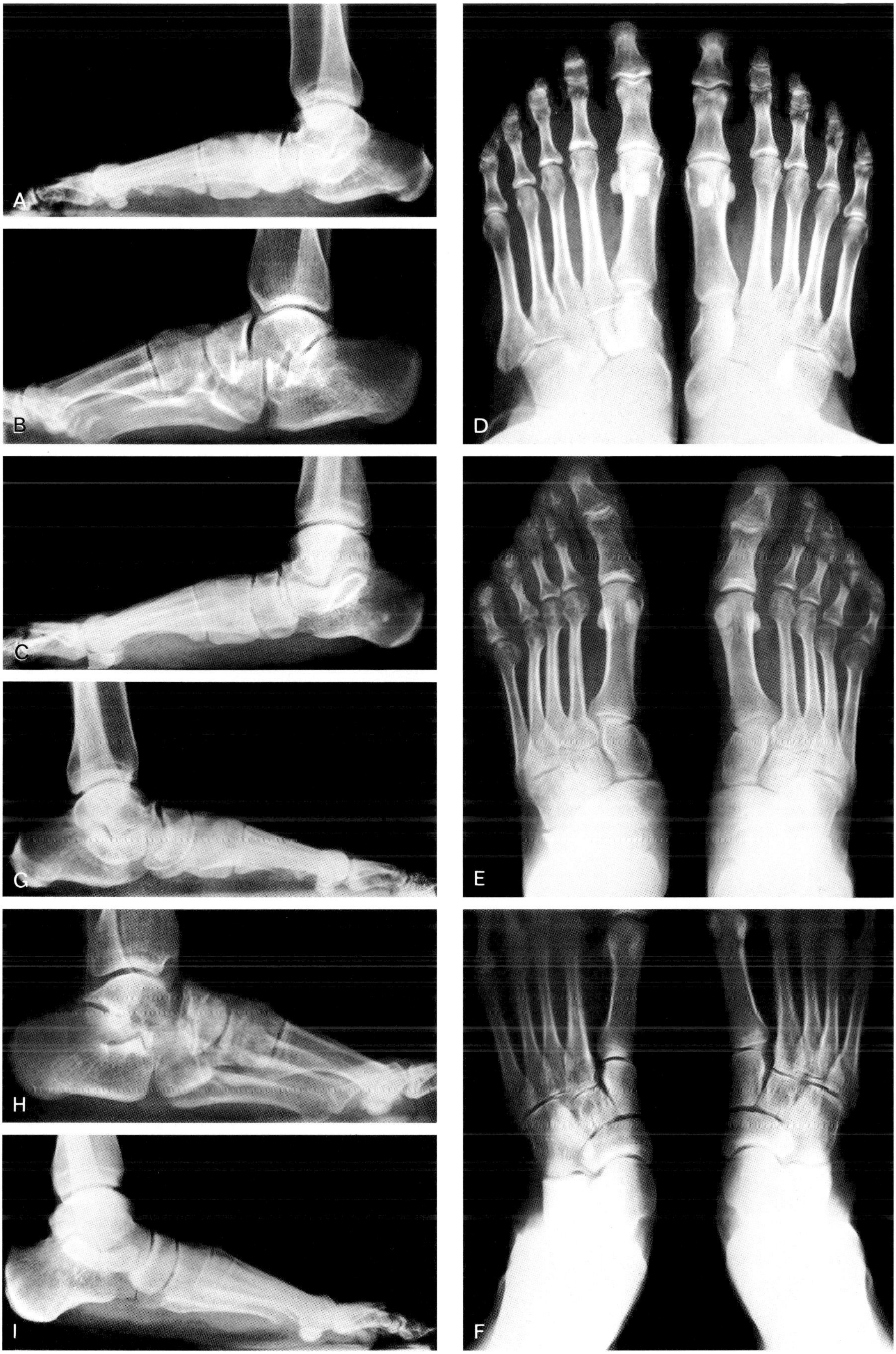
A
B
C
G
H
I
D
E
F

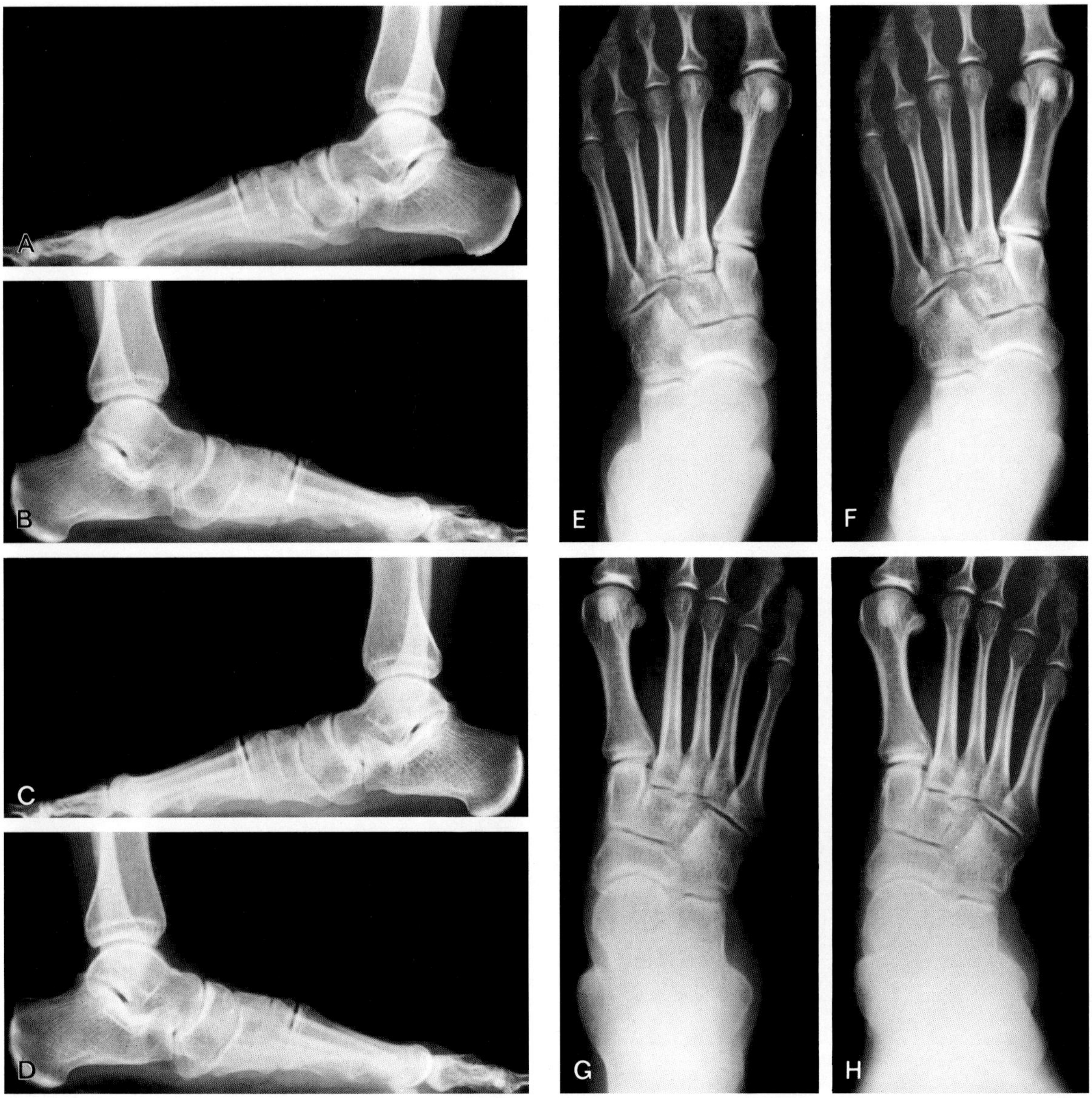

Fig. 16.15 A–H. Second-degree idiopathic pes planovalgus in a patient aged 17 years. **A** Left foot, non-weight-bearing lateral view. **B** Right foot, weight-bearing lateral view: lowering of midtarsal mass, increased equinus of neck of talus in weight-bearing posture. **C** Left foot, weight-bearing lateral view. **D** Right foot, non-weight-bearing lateral view: superimposition of navicular and cuboid, diminution of angles of inclination of calcaneum and midtarsus. **E–G** Weight-bearing (**E** left foot; **G** right foot) and non-weight-bearing (**F** left foot; **H** right foot) dorsoplantar views: light adduction of neck of talus, medial hypertrophy of navicular, abduction of longitudinal axes of cuneiforms

Fig. 16.16 A–C. Second-degree pes planovalgus. **A** *1* Left foot, weight-bearing lateral view: lowering of tarsomidtarsal axis and naviculocuneiform region, superimposition of navicular and cuboid, horizontal alignment of calcaneum and cuboid; *2* left foot, non-weight-bearing lateral view: lowering of midtarsal region with subluxation plantarwards of naviculocuneiform mass, horizontal alignment of calcaneum; *3* left foot, weight-bearing and non-weight-bearing dorsoplantar views: displacement of midtarsal region; *4* left foot, non-weight-bearing and weight-bearing dorsoplantar views (9 years after *3*): displacement of midtarsal region, adduction of neck of talus. **B** *1* Left foot, lateral view: light equinus of talus, straight outline and rigidity of the midtarsal region; *2* both feet, dorsoplantar view: midtarsal displacement associated with medial subluxation and hypertrophy of navicular, abduction of cuneiform-cuboidal mass, compensatory triangular forefoot syndrome. **C** Right foot (different patient), lateral view: shortness of neck of talus, equinus of neck of talus, sinusoidal dorsal angulation of talonavicular-cuneiform mass, midtarsal lowering, superimposition of navicular and cuboid

▷

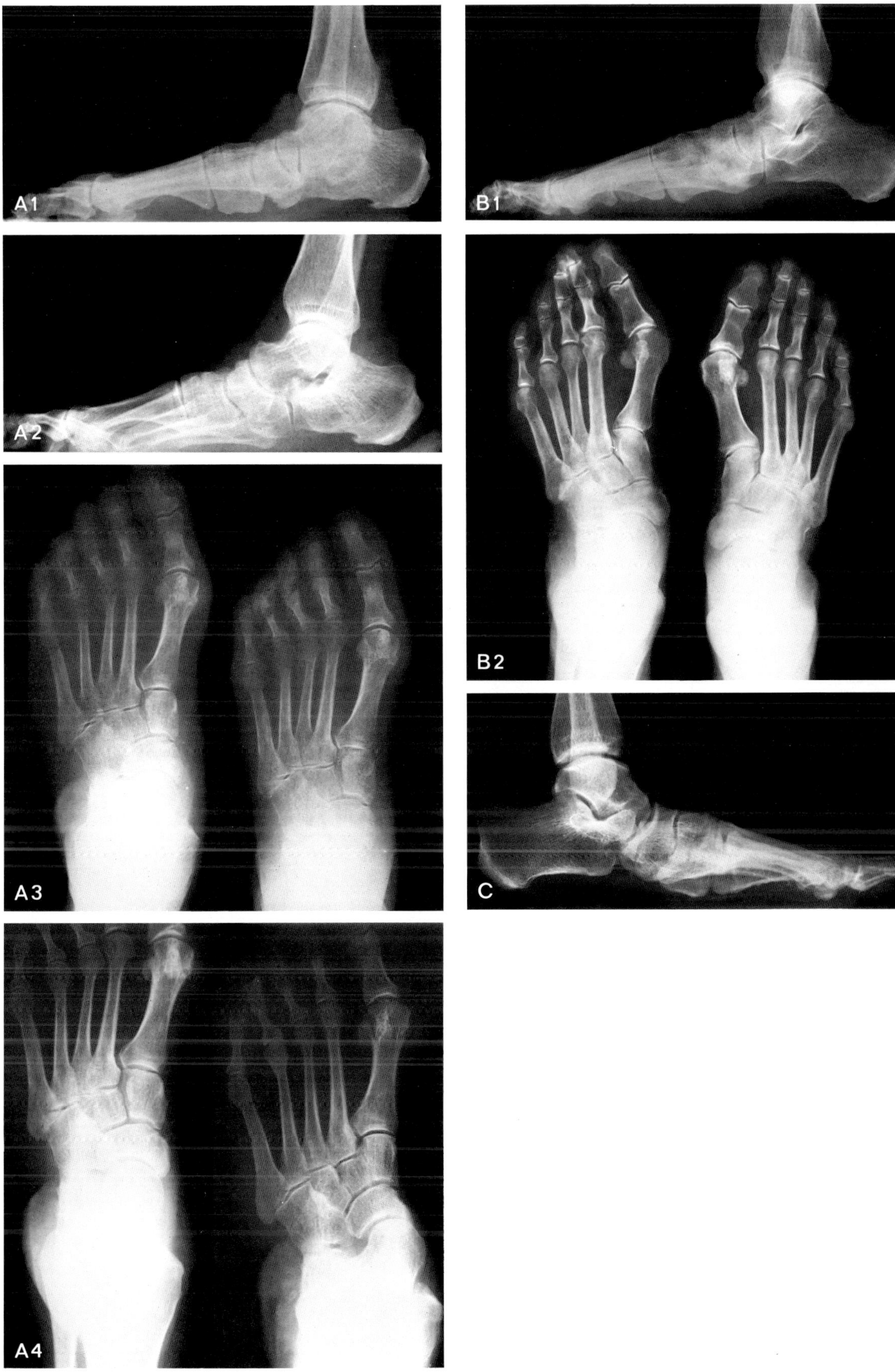
A1
B1
A2
B2
A3
C
A4

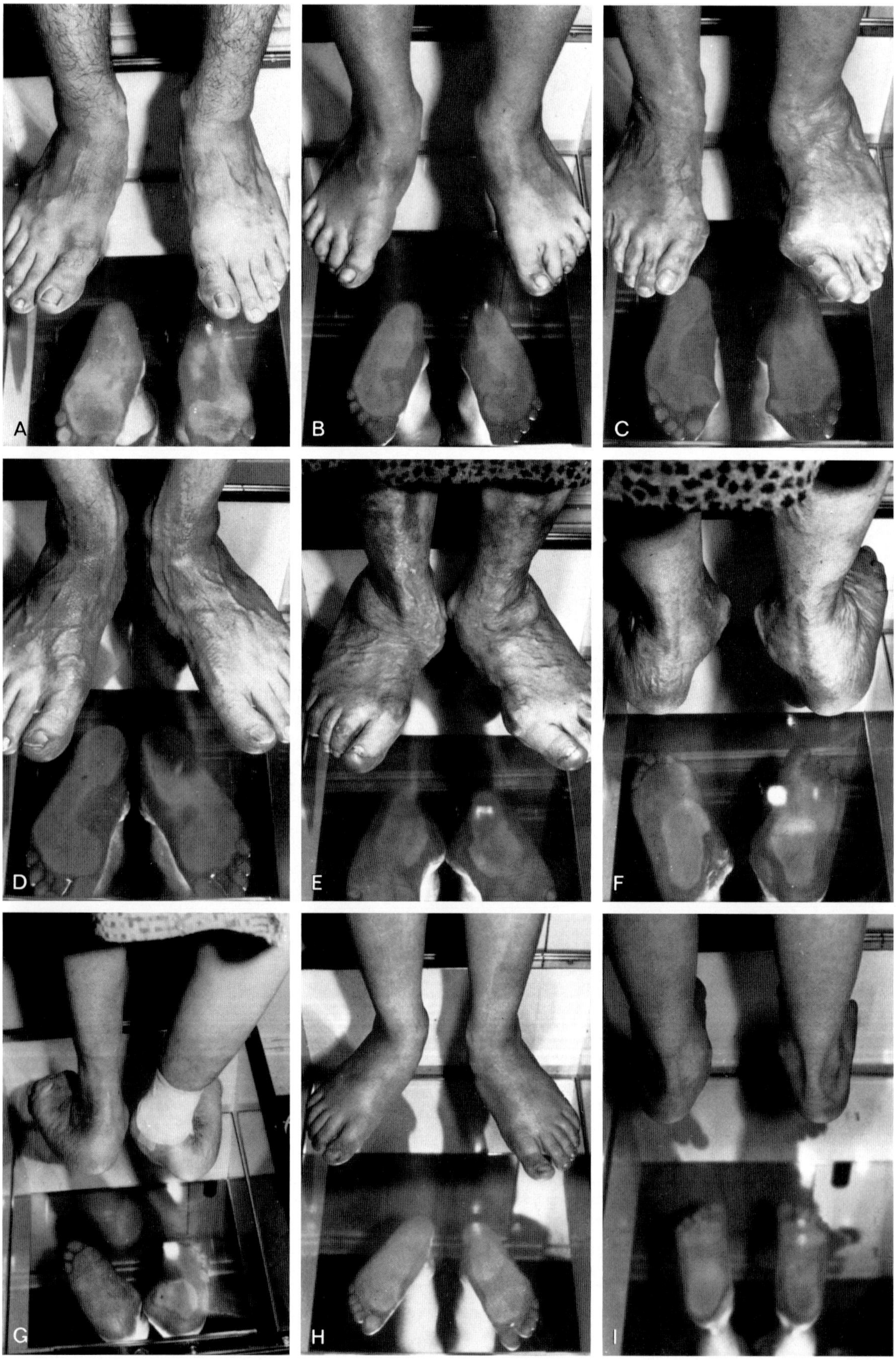
A
B
C
D
E
F
G
H
I

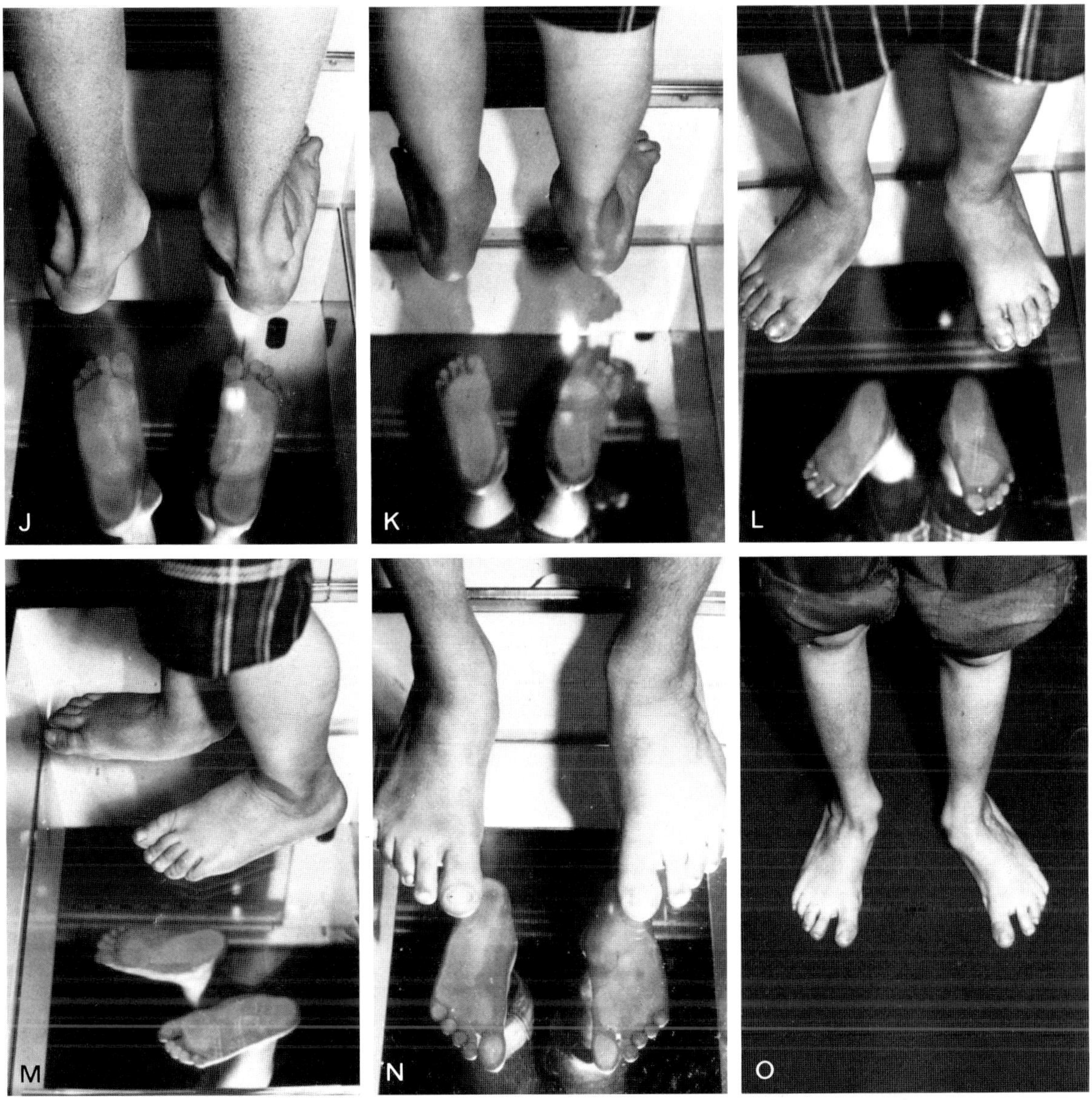

◁ **Fig. 16.17 A–P.** Pes planovalgus. **A–G** In adulthood: **A** Third degree with contracture; **B, C** second and third degree; **D** third degree with contracture of arch; **E–G** fourth degree: collapse and medial displacement of midtarsal mass, significant tarsal pronation, projection of tibial axis medial to internal border of foot. **H–P** In childhood: **H** Second degree: lowering of midtarsus and abduction of foot; **I** first and second degree: axis of heel print disposed externally, lowering of midtarsus with medial displacement, some tarsal valgus; **J** second and third degree: marked tarsal pronation and valgus, lowering of midtarsus with medial displacement; **K–M** third degree with early fourth degree features: collapse and medial displacement of midtarsus, convex medial border of foot, calcaneum pronated, valgus and horizontally aligned, abduction of forefoot; **N** following overcorrection of equinovarus club foot; **O** accompanying pes adductus Dengler; **P** third degree: congenital origin

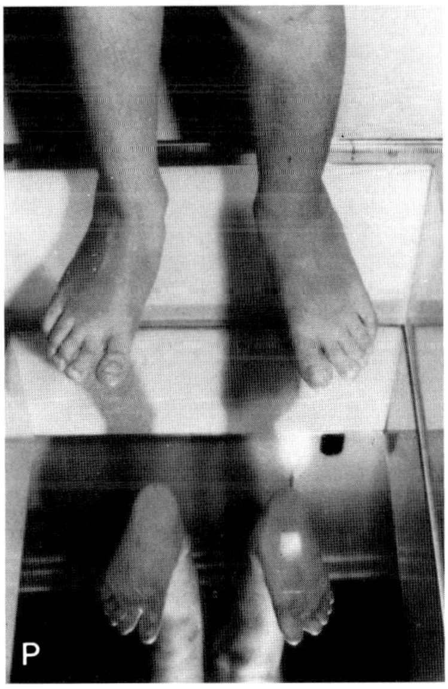

In the contracted foot, Gosselin's sign is positive (pain in midtarsal region produced by passive dorsiflexion of the forefoot), while the test described by Duchenne de Boulogne (1867) demonstrates the weakness of peroneus longus (inability to depress the first metatarsal head actively).

16.1.5.3 Third Degree

In this final stage, pain is permanent and displacements are irreversible. The pain is due to capsuloligamentous tension along the medial border of the foot and affects all joints; it originates in the sinus tarsi and midtarsal joints, and there is associated distortion of the subtalar joint. Pains from tendinitis affecting tibialis posterior and peroneus longus at their insertions are common, while the reverberation of the disorder into the lower limb and trunk causes various muscular pains and also joint pains in the knee, the sacro-iliac and lumbar spine regions or even the neck. Sciatica is frequent. The patient fatigues easily when attempting to walk and is seriously disabled.

On clinical examination the foot is now completely lowered so that the plantar aspect rests totally on the ground with true bony pressure producing bands of thickening in the skin or even causing the development of adventitious bursae (Fig. 16.17). The patient takes to walking in floppy flat shoes which probably serve to aggravate the situation further by their lack of support. The three bosses of Lannelongue (see Sect. 16.1.4) are accompanied by areas of oedema, which is also apparent behind the malleoli.

Podoscopy findings show typically that the heel appears squashed against the ground, with its soft pad protruding externally and backwards, and that the external border is angulated outwards with an apex at the cuboid level. The podoscopic appearance corresponds to the hypertrophy of length of the talar neck with projection of the talar head and the incompetence of tibialis posterior with elongation of its tendon (sometimes associated with painful tension of the tibialis anterior tendon as well); the toes show evidence of contracture due to shortening of the extensor tendons. The antetarsus is abducted under the influence of the peronei. On the medial side of the foot the convexity of the border has its apex at the level of the navicular.

Radiography is essential to guide the choice of treatment. The lateral view shows very severe divergence of the talar and calcaneal axes, horizontal alignment or even plantar obliquity of the calcaneum, and vertical alignment of the neck of the talus, while lowering of the midtarsal mass is proved by total superimposition of the outlines of the navicular and the cuboid (Fig. 16.18). The alignment of the bones on the medial side of the foot may become convex towards the ground, and there is now flattening of the axes of the calcaneum, cuboid and fifth metatarsal, indicating disappearance of any external longitudinal arch. Shortness or hypertrophy in length of the talar neck is evident and there is increased thickness of the image of the navicular. In the dorsoplantar view, the talocalcaneal divergence is constituted by adduction of the talar neck, reduced angle of declination of the talus (120°–130°; normally 105°), subluxation or internal dislocation of the navicular, triangular appearance of the internal base of the navicular, abduction of the anterior process of the calcaneum and abduction of the metatarsus emanating from the Lisfranc joint level.

Adult pes planovalgus is usually a painful sequel of untreated or poorly treated adolescent pes planus. As stated above, only in 1%–2% of such cases can correction not be achieved by the conservative use of properly designed insoles. In other words, in the vast majority of cases, the adult form is avoidable.

16.1.5.4 Treatment

16.1.5.4.1 Conservative

The use of an orthopaedic insole is indicated in first- and second-degree pes planovalgus in all adults and in third-degree cases in elderly patients unfit for surgery. These insoles do not correct all the displacements and it is illusory to expect otherwise. They are designed at this stage to relieve pain, but will do so only if properly measured and accommodated in appropriate shoes. The form and shape is very individual. A stabilising corrective insole bearing a supinating wedge under the heel and a pronating external wedge behind the outer metatarsal heads may be effective for the young adult woman, especially because its small size does not necessitate a bulky shoe (Fig. 16.19). It must be supplemented by an internal dome the height of which is augmented progressively following the corrective rise of the navicular until a good position has been achieved.

In the late second-degree case or in the elderly person this will not be adequate; the insole must be more bulky, with an internal dome adapted exactly in accordance with the patient's tolerance, and requires a larger shoe.

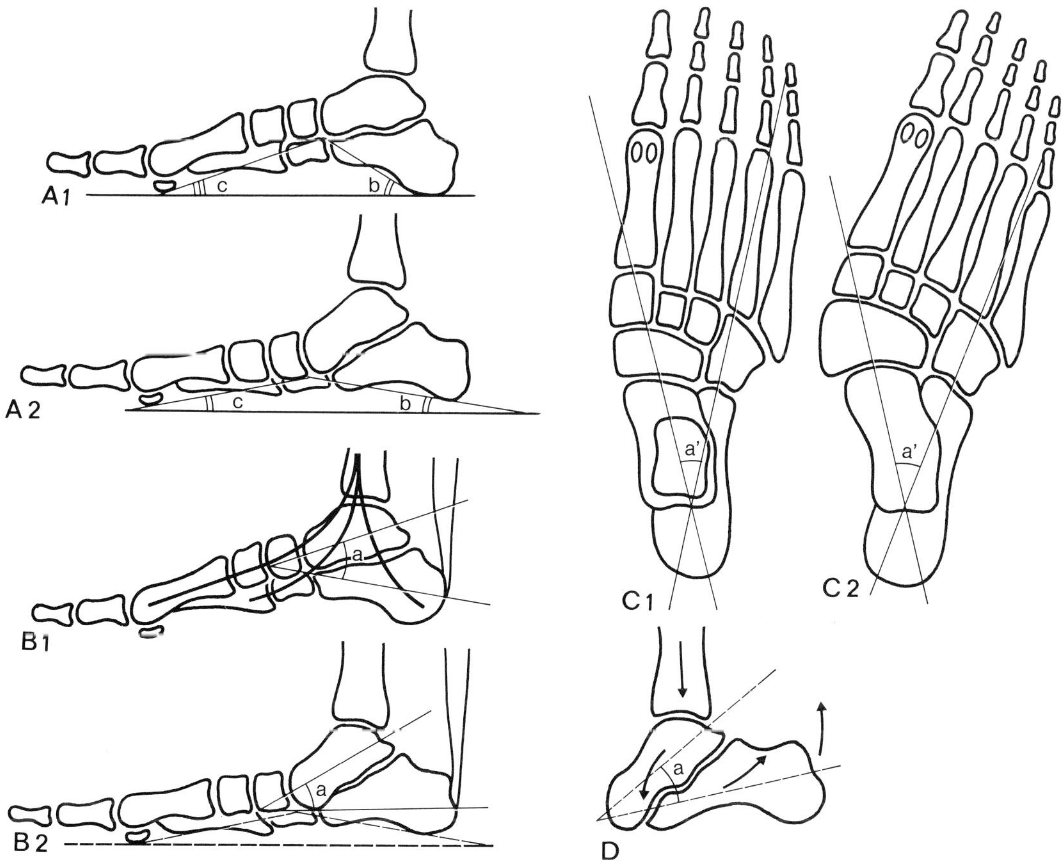

Fig. 16.18 A–D. Comparison of normal foot and planovalgus foot in lateral and dorsoplantar views. **A, B** Lateral view. **A** *1* Calcaneal (*b*) and metatarsal (*c*) angles of inclination in the normal foot; *2* in the planovalgus foot there is reduction of these angles, superimposition of the navicular and cuboid and lowering of the midtarsal mass. **B** *1* In the normal foot the angle of talocalcaneal divergence (*a*) is 15°–30°; *2* in the planovalgus foot the angle is increased to 40°–60°. The talus is displaced downwards, forwards and inwards, the calcaneum upwards, backwards and outwards. **C** *1, 2* Dorsoplantar view. *1* In the normal foot the angle of talocalcaneal divergence (*a'*) is 20°–30°; *2* in the planovalgus foot the angle is increased to 40°–60° and there is plantar and internal displacement of the midtarsus. **D** Relative displacement of talus and calcaneum indicated by *arrows*

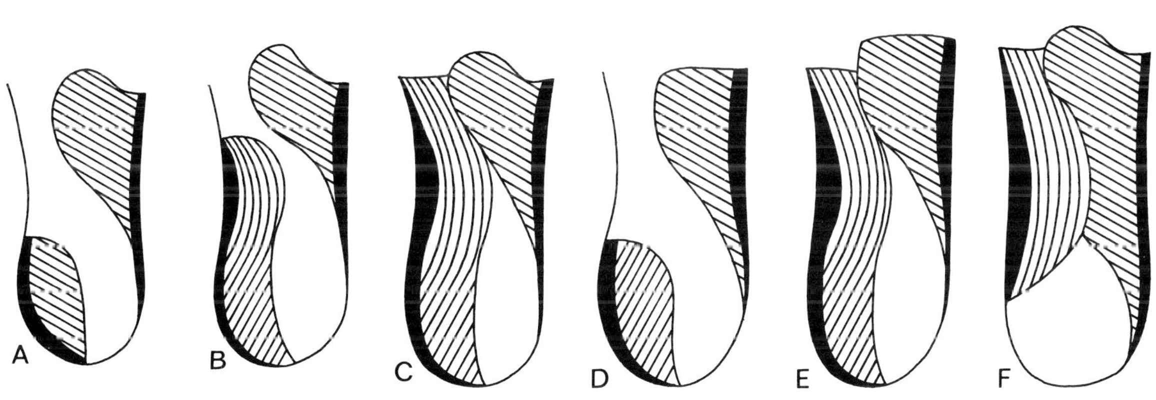

Fig. 16.19 A–F. Insoles for pes planovalgus. **A** Supinating wedge under heel, retrocapital pronating wedge under metatarsus. **B** Navicular support, supinating wedge under heel, pronating wedge behind metatarsal heads. **C** Medial dome support, supinating wedge under heel, retrocapital pronating wedge under metatarsals. **D** Supinating wedge under heel, pronating subcapital metatarsal wedge. **E** Medial dome support, supinating wedge under heel, pronating wedge under metatarsal heads. **F** Physiological supporting monoblock insole

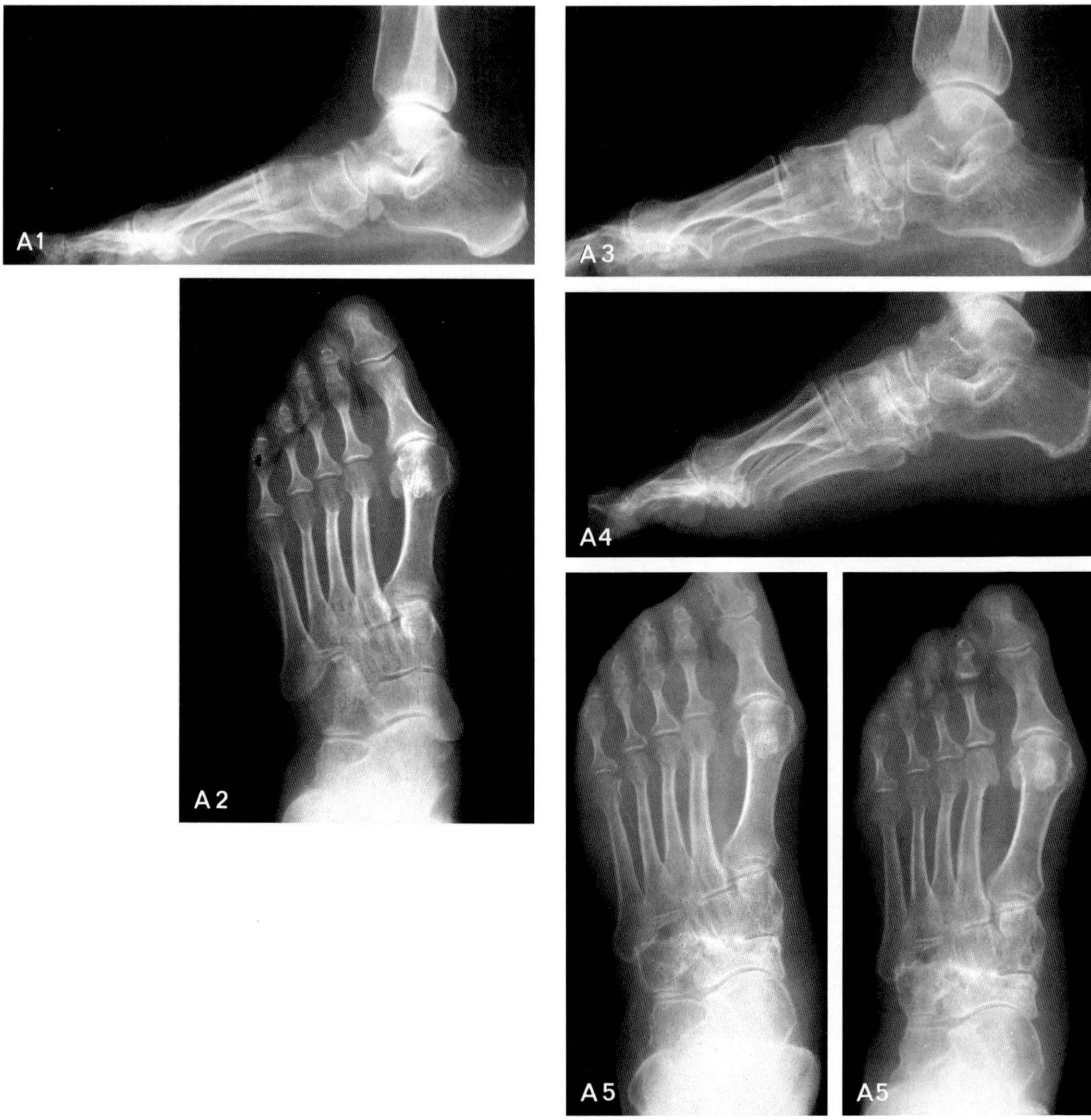

Fig. 16.21 A–C. Adult pes planovalgus before and after treatment. **A** Left foot. *1* Preoperative lateral view: lowering of midtarsal axis relative to navicular, superimposition of navicular and cuboid; *2* preoperative dorsoplantar view: adduction of neck of talus, angulation of talonaviculocuneiform axes; *3, 4* weight-bearing and non-weight-bearing lateral views after osteotomy through naviculocuneiform joint line, transcuboidal osteotomy; *5* non-weight-bearing, dorsoplantar view after osteotomy of navicular medially involving naviculocuneiform joint space, arthrodesis of navicular and intermediate and lateral coneiforms. **B** Left foot. *1* Preoperative lateral view: straightness of talonaviculocuneiform-metatarsal axes, superimposition of navicular and cuboid; *2* weight-bearing lateral view after osteotomy of neck of talus and navicular, reconstitution of longitudinal plantar arch, elevation of navicular; *3* non-weight-bearing lateral view after osteotomy of neck of talus and navicular, augmentation of angles of inclination of calcaneum and metatarsus; *4* non-weight-bearing preoperative dorsoplantar view: pes planus, medial hypertrophy of navicular; *5* weight-bearing preoperative dorsoplantar view: abduction of cuneiforms and cuboid; *6* non-weight-bearing dorsoplantar view after realignment of talonaviculocuneiform axes; *7* weight-bearing dorsoplantar view after osteotomy of neck of talus and navicular, longitudinal reorientation of cuneiform, cuboidal and talonavicular axes. **B, C** see p. 205, 206

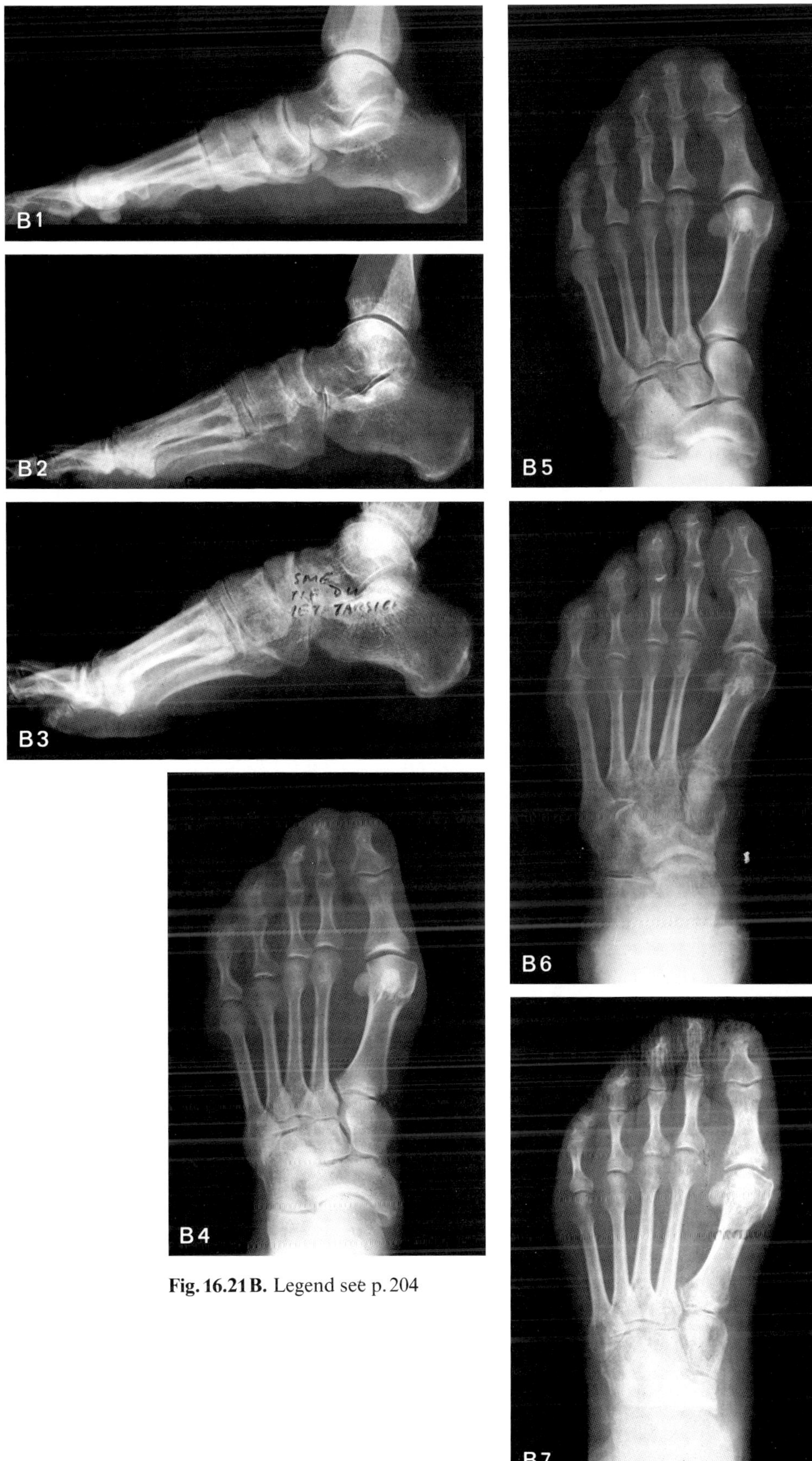

Fig. 16.21 B. Legend see p. 204

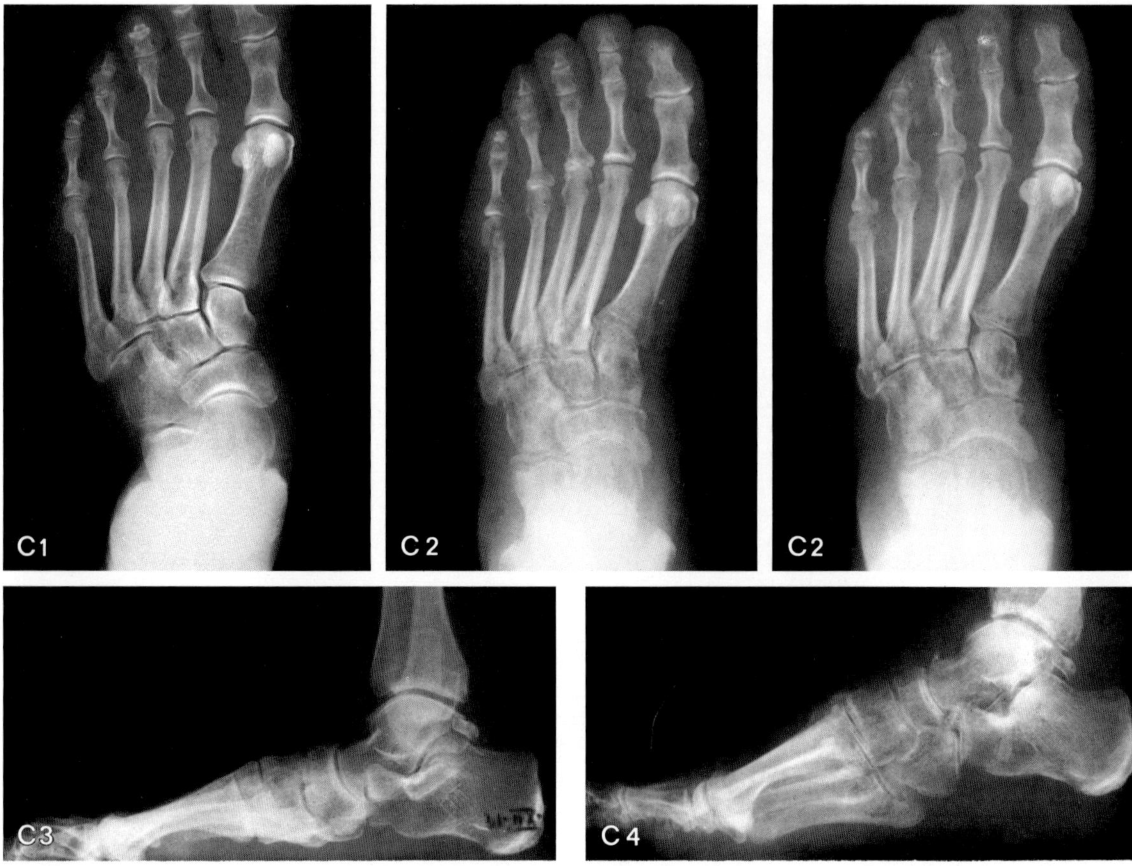

Fig. 16.21 *(continued).* **C** Left foot. Weight-bearing preoperative dorsoplantar view: *1* medial angulation of midtarsus, adduction of neck of talus, metatarsus varus; *2* weight-bearing and non-weight-bearing dorsoplantar views after extra-articular osteotomy of neck of talus and of navicular, correction of midtarsal angulation, correction of adduction of neck of talus; *3* weight-bearing preoperative lateral view: lowering of naviculocuneiform region, superimposition of navicular and cuboid; *4* non-weight-bearing lateral view after correction of lowering of midtarsal region, repositioning of navicular: no superimposition of navicular and cuboid

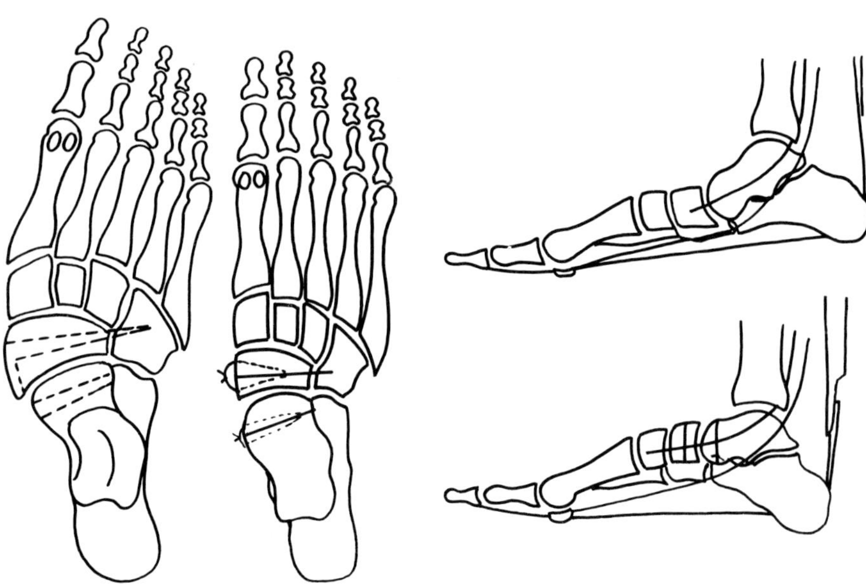

Fig. 16.20. Extra-articular corrective wedge osteotomies of navicular and neck of talus (Regnauld)

The internal dome may amount to 13–18 mm in height or even more, the supinating wedge to 7–8 mm [this should not be exceeded (Valenti 1977c)], and the pronating corner will be some 6–7 mm high. The difference between the heights of the wedges is interesting; some authorities state that it should be considerable, but in my opinion it should be only 1–2 mm, the supinating calcaneal wedge being the higher.

This classic insole may be unsuccessful when it attempts corrective action which cannot be tolerated by irritable arthrosic joints. In these cases, the insole must be relegated to a role of pure support for the midtarsal region and, in effect, immobilise especially the tarsomidtarsal joints. A physiological monoblock insole, perfectly fitted, may afford great relief and allow comfortable walking.

Additional measures include regular changing of the insoles in hot weather, anti-inflammatory agents and local massage.

16.1.5.4.2 Operative

Surgery is indicated in advanced second-degree and third-degree pes planovalgus in otherwise fit patients. It must be stated from the outset that isolated correction by stabilisation of the talocalcaneal joint will not be successful, because this does not correct the osteoarticular displacements of the midtarsal region which are a predominant source of discomfort. In general, the choice of surgery depends upon the state of the joints, arthrosic or non-arthrosic.

Without Arthrosis. Joint fusion procedures are not indicated and should be avoided whenever possible, as they limit movements of the foot especially those necessary for sport or the wearing of elegant shoes by young women. The procedures chosen should stabilise the tarsal displacement and correct the midtarsal disalignment. Particular attention should be paid to the presence of hypertrophy of the talar neck and of the navicular, which together with the vertical alignment of the talus and internal hypertrophy of the body of the navicular opposes any stable reduction of the angulation at the tarsometatarsal region (Fig. 16.20).

The procedure I have used since 1969 has achieved uniformly satisfactory results in terms of pain relief and permanent correction. There has been excellent restoration of function, particularly in young adults. The approach is as follows:

1. Correction of the horizontal posture of the calcaneum by elongation of triceps surae.
2. Correction of the vertical and horizontal divergence of the calcaneum and talus by osteotomies of the talar neck and of the navicular; one or both may be necessary, according to the case.
3. Preservation of the corrected posture of the calcaneal pronation by stabilisation of the subtalar joint or by varus calcaneal osteotomy (Dwyer 1959), accompanied as indicated by osteotomies in the midtarsal region.
4. Preservation of the correction of the longitudinal plantar arch and the medial border of the foot by transplantation of tibialis posterior onto the medial cuneiform and/or of tibialis anterior onto the navicular if thought necessary.

These measures are adequate; as stated above, fusions are not necessary, serving only to distort the action of neighbouring joints and produce other problems.

The principles of this operative programme can be amplified according to the individual case:

a) If the angle of inclination of the calcaneum is normal or below normal, simple elongation of triceps surae suffices, but if there is pronation with horizontal alignment, elongation by the technique of Vulpius (1920) or a Z-elongation preserving the inner part of the tendinous insertion is employed so as to obtain a varising supplementary action.
b) Resection of bone from the comma-shaped hypertrophied navicular or the elongated talar neck together with transplantation of tibialis posterior onto the medial cuneiform (Figs. 16.21, 16.22) may suffice to produce overall correction, but if valgus of the calcaneum persists despite these resections and elongation of triceps surae, stabilisation arthrorisis of the sinus tarsi may be necessary, perhaps with capsuloligamentoplasties of the plantar aspect [shortening of the calcaneonavicular ligament (Pisani 1979b)] and of the talonavicular ligament (Regnauld 1979) (Figs. 16.23, 16.24).
c) In cases where the maximum angulation of the internal border is at the midtarsal joints, the talar neck is vertical and of normal length and there is dorso-internal subluxation of the hypertrophied navicular, the most effective treatment may be plantarwards and internally based segmental (like a quarter of an orange) resection of the glenoid talonavicular ligament, repaired using nylon, together with either triangular bony resection of the plantar internal base of the

navicular or extra-articular resection across the body of the navicular extended onto the cuboid (Fig. 25). This may have to be accompanied by elongation of triceps surae, transplantation of tibialis posterior and Albanese tenodesis (1948) solidifying tibialis anterior and tibialis posterior.

d) If the maximum angulation of the internal border is at the navicular, navicular osteotomy or transverse curvilinear transnaviculocuboidal bone resection with a base directed plantarwards and internally may be chosen in addition to the tendinous transplants (Fig. 16.26).
e) If the maximum angulation in the midtarsal region is at the medial cuneiform, extra-articular transverse curvilinear resection passing through the cuneiform bones to the cuboid with the base plantarwards and internally is selected to accompany the tendon procedures (Regnauld 1978 b) (Figs. 16.27, 16.28).
f) If the summit of medial angulation is at the Lisfranc joint line, an exception is made in that bone resection with arthrodesis of the tarsometatarsal joints is performed together with the tendon procedures.
g) The presence of significant abduction in the metatarsus may indicate the need for elongation of the peroneus brevis tendon together with extra-articular bone resections.
h) Finally, if the tarsus is in general valgus despite the midtarsal correction, the transcalcaneal osteotomy of Dwyer (1959) complemented by the implantation of a cuneiform graft with its base externally at the site of the osteotomy will correct the posture of the calcaneum (J. Judet 1972).

With Arthrosis. Early arthrosis, for example first- or second-degree hallux rigidus, comprises osteophytosis with peripheral eburnation but preservation of the central articular cartilage. Whenever possible, this central preservation should be exploited, and in accordance with the teaching of Pauwels, extra-articular procedures with correction of alignment can in early cases provoke some recovery of the joint condition. It is only when the arthrosis is irreversible, as evidenced by central erosion visible on radiographs and total disappearance of the joint spaces associated with subchondral condensation, that this concept has to be regretfully abandoned. Conservative treatment with insoles can only be antalgic but retains a role in the elderly or unfit patient. Fusions may be performed as follows according to the sites of the destroyed joints:

Midtarsal, intertarsal and subtalar arthrosis occurring together are relieved by arthrodesis of the affected joints, provided that the resections allow correction of the tarsal displacements and recreate a plantar arch. If the subtalar joint is supple but painful, the section of the talocalcaneonavicular joint extended into the body of the cuboid suffices to correct the foot (Figs. 16.29, 16.30). If the arthrosic lesions of the subtalar and naviculocuneiform joints are accompanied by valgus displacement of the calcaneum, the triple arthrodesis as modified by Viladot (1971) affords excellent correction in the midtarsal and subtalar regions. This operation comprises double arthrodesis of the talonavicular and navicular-medial cuneiform joint lines associated with extra-articular arthrodesis of the subtalar joint by means of insertion of cylindrical bone grafts in a hole bored along the sinus tarsi, completed by reinsertion of tibialis posterior (Fig. 16.31).

Midtarsal lesions confined to the intertarsal joints are best managed by wedge resection with the base internally and plantarwards, as described by Ombredanne (1949) and Cauchoix (Fig. 16.32). With this procedure, however, there is the risk of development of progressive arthrosis of the subtalar joint as a result of distorted movement of the anterior part of the talocalcaneal complex.

Arthrosis limited to one or two joints can be treated by local arthrodesis in the inner part of the midtarsus. Thus, in talonavicular arthrosis, trapezoidal resection arthrodesis of the joint based internally and plantarwards limits the painful movement and corrects the midtarsal displacement (Ogston-Cauchoix). At the naviculocuneiform joint, Hohmann (1951) arthrodesis resects the joint line together with an internally based wedge from the medial cuneiform (Fig. 16.33). The Müller arthrodesis finds its true indication in arthrosis associated with marked lowering at the naviculocuneiform joint. After resection of a fibroperiosteous tongue of tibialis posterior, a double arthrodesis is performed, modelling the naviculocuneiform joint and the medial cuneiform-first metatarsal joint by raising a trapezoidal bony block with its base plantarwards. The procedure is completed by transplantation of the fibroperiosteous tongue of tibialis posterior to the base of the first metatarsal. These localised arthrodeses give excellent results in the adult aged over 50 years provided the indications for their choice are present.

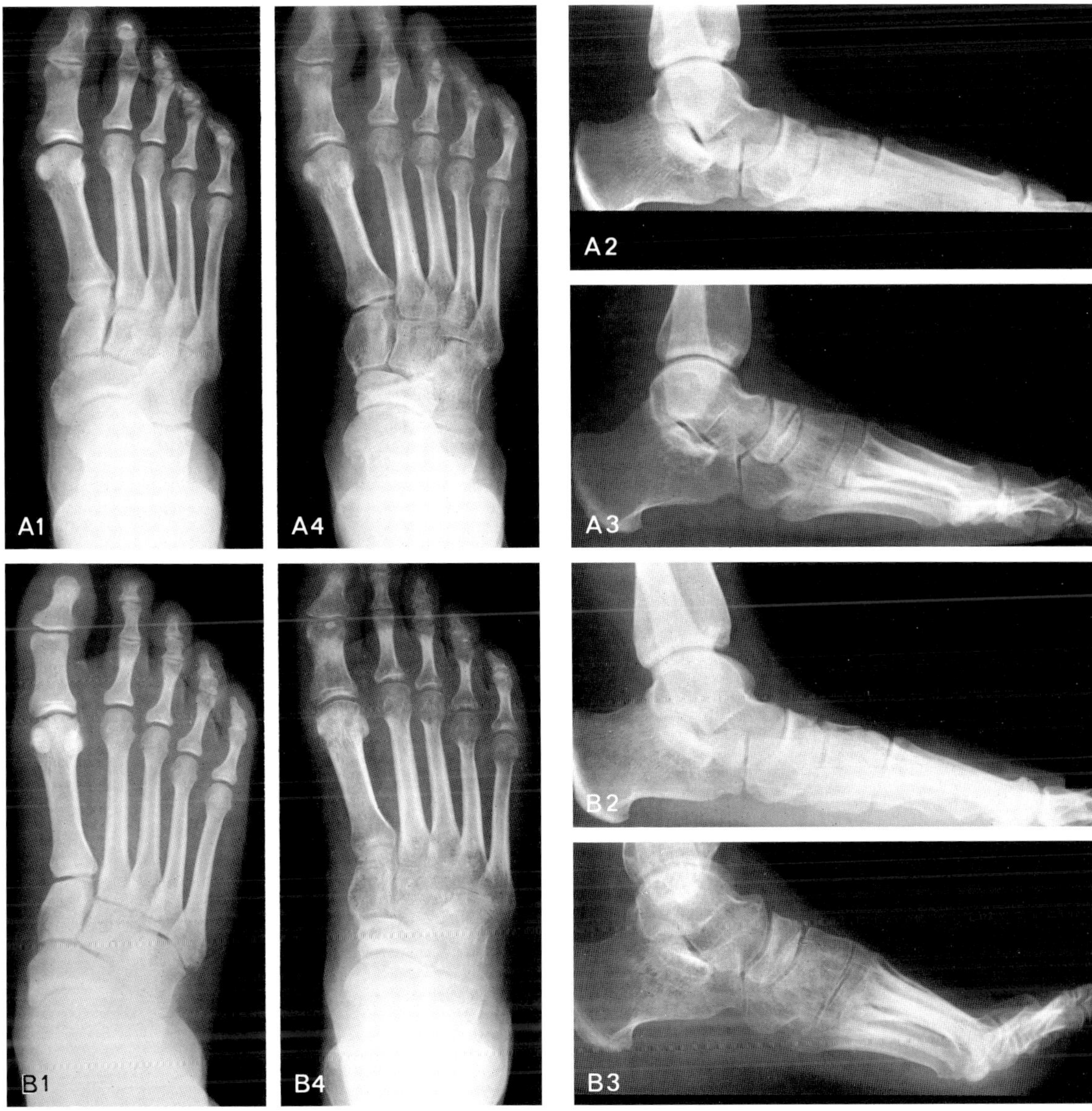

Fig. 16.22 A, B. Third-degree pes planovalgus. **A** Right foot. *1* Preoperative dorsoplantar view: midtarsal angulation, adduction of talus; *2* preoperative lateral view: complete lowering of plantar longitudinal arch, horizontal disposition of calcaneum, superimposition of navicular and cuboid; *3* lateral view after osteotomy of neck of talus and navicular, reconstitution of medial longitudinal plantar arch, elevation of navicular and cuneiform, inclination of calcaneum and metatarsus; *4* dorsoplantar view after osteotomy of neck of talus and of navicular with good longitudinal realignment of midtarsus. **B** Right foot. *1* Preoperative dorsoplantar view: angulation of midtarsal region, adduction of neck of talus, abduction of cuneiform-cuboidal mass; *2* preoperative lateral view: lowering of naviculocuneiform region, equinus of neck of talus, superimposition of navicular and cuboid; *3* lateral view after osteotomy of neck of talus and navicular, re-establishment of medial plantar arch (disappearance of superimposition of the navicular and cuboid), elevation of naviculocuneiform region; *4* dorsoplantar view after osteotomy of neck of talus and navicular, longitudinal realignment of midtarsus and cuneiforms

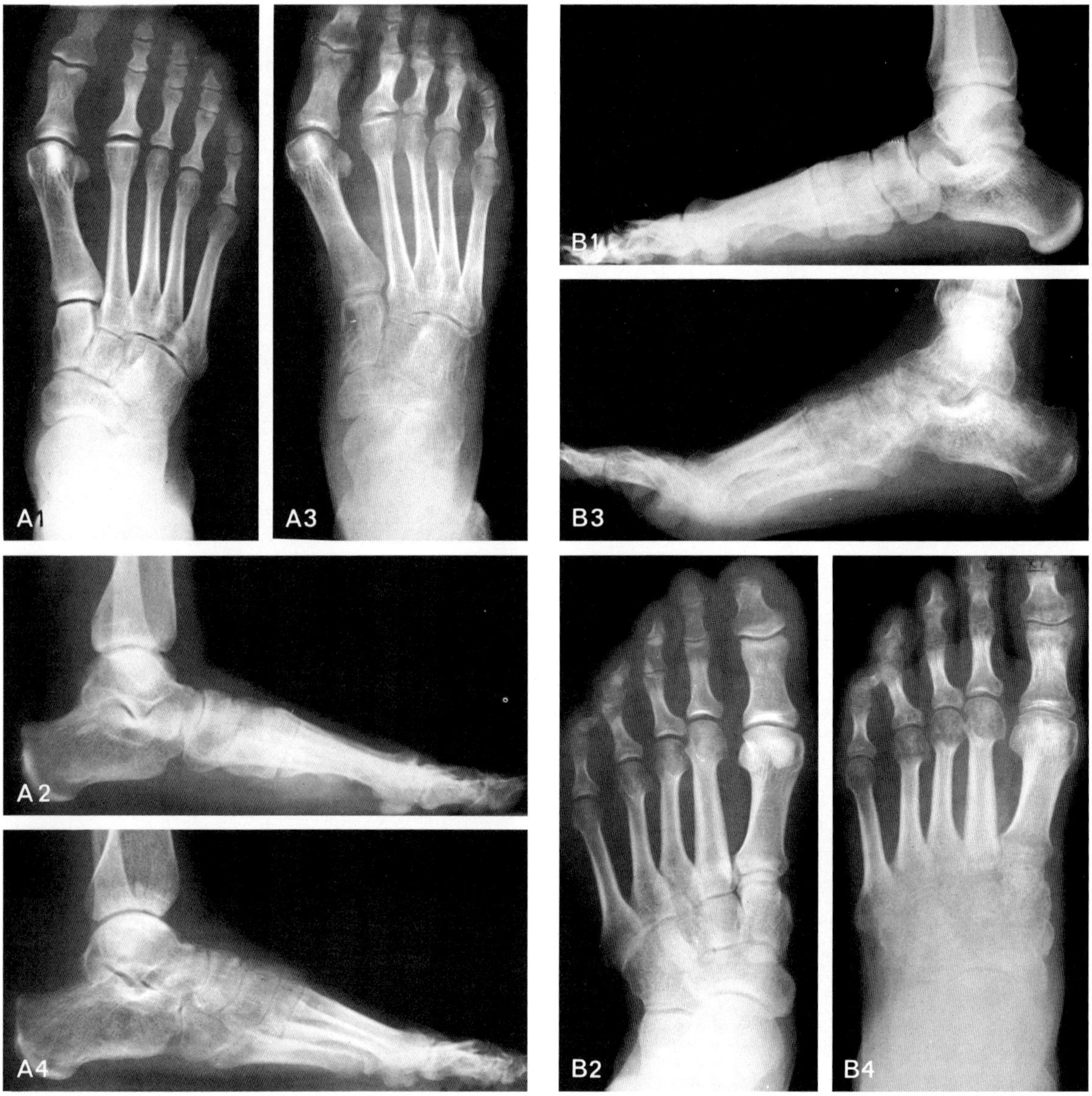

Fig. 16.23 A–D. Second- and third-degree pes planovalgus before and after treatment. **A** Third degree, right foot. *1* Preoperative dorsoplantar view: angulation of midtarsal region; *2* preoperative lateral view: lowering of naviculocuneiform region, superimposition of navicular and cuboid; *3* dorsoplantar view after extra-articular osteotomies of neck of talus and navicular; *4* lateral view after re-establishment of plantar arch, elevation of naviculocuneiform mass. **B** Third degree, left foot. *1* Preoperative lateral view: lowering of midtarsal region, superimposition of navicular and cuboid; *2* preoperative dorsoplantar view: adduction of talus, angulation of midtarsal region, hypertrophy of navicular; *3* lateral view after extra-articular osteotomy of neck of talus and of navicular; *4* dorsoplantar view after reconstitution of medial plantar longitudinal arch, realignment of midtarsus. **C, D** see p. 211 ▷

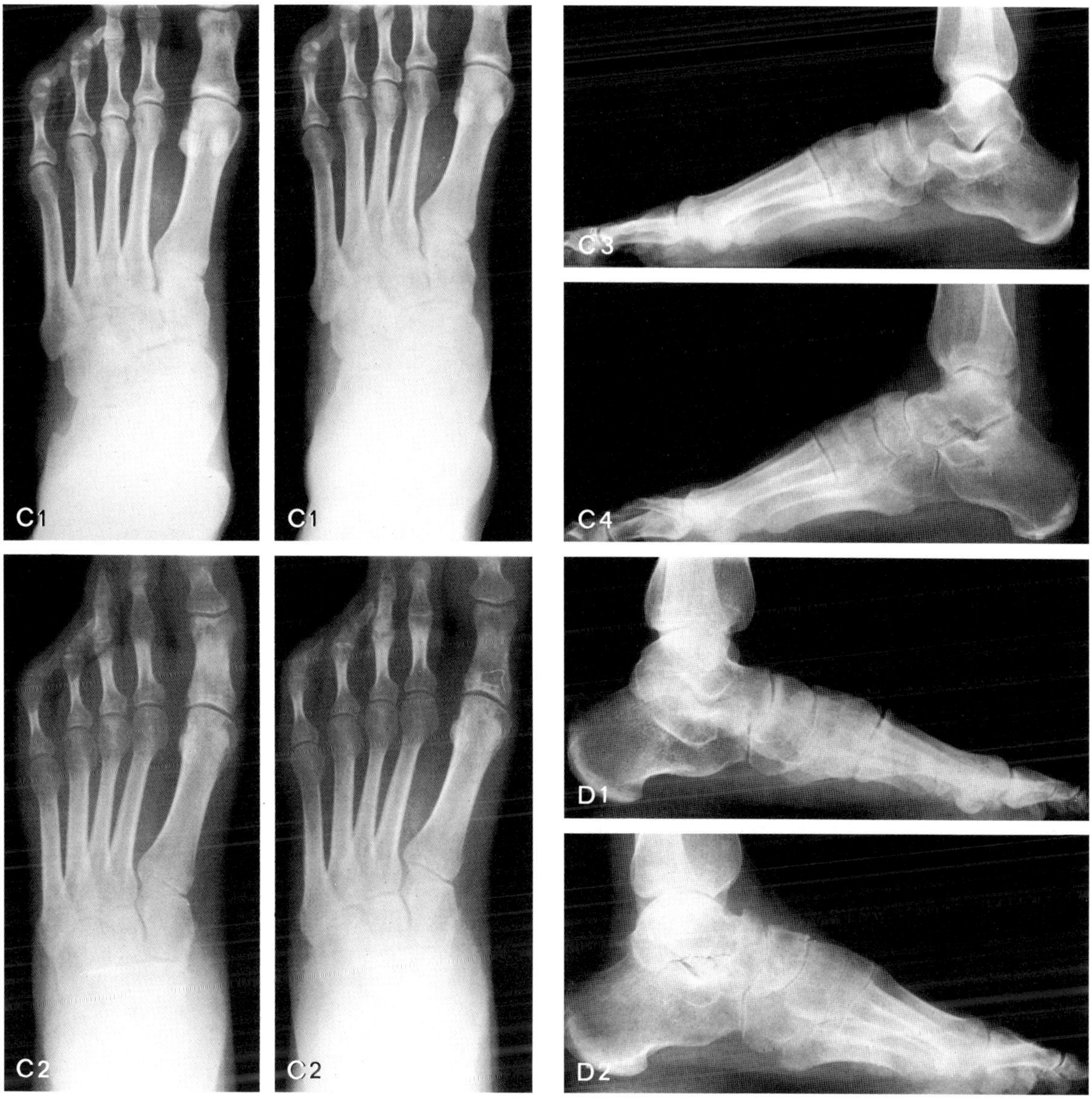

Fig. 16.23 *(continued)*. **C** Second degree, left foot. *1* Weight-bearing and non-weight-bearing preoperative dorsoplantar views: angulation of midtarsal region, adduction of neck of talus, medial hypertrophy of navicular; *2* weight-bearing and non-weight-bearing dorsoplantar views after osteotomy of neck of talus and of navicular, straightening of medial border of foot, realignment of midtarsus; *3* weight-bearing preoperative lateral view: lowering of midtarsal region; *4* weight-bearing lateral view after extra-articular osteotomy of neck of talus and of navicular. **D** Second degree, right foot. *1* Weight-bearing preoperative dorsoplantar view: lowering of naviculocuneiform; *2* weight-bearing lateral view after extra-articular osteotomies of neck of talus and of navicular, reconstitution of longitudinal arch, elevation of naviculocuneiform mass

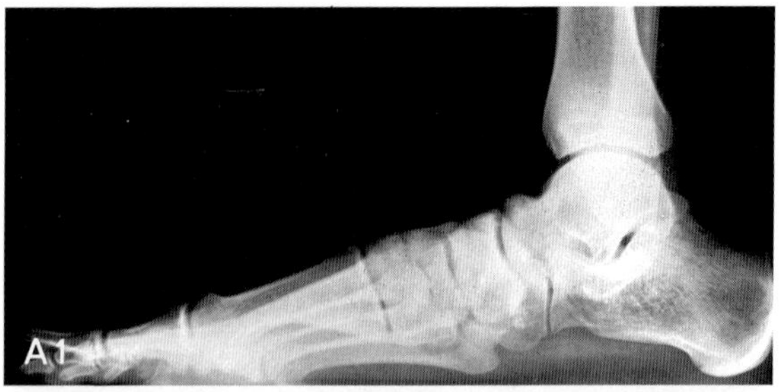

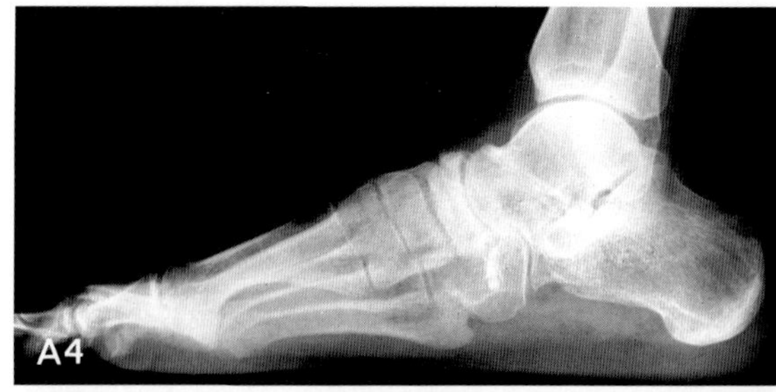

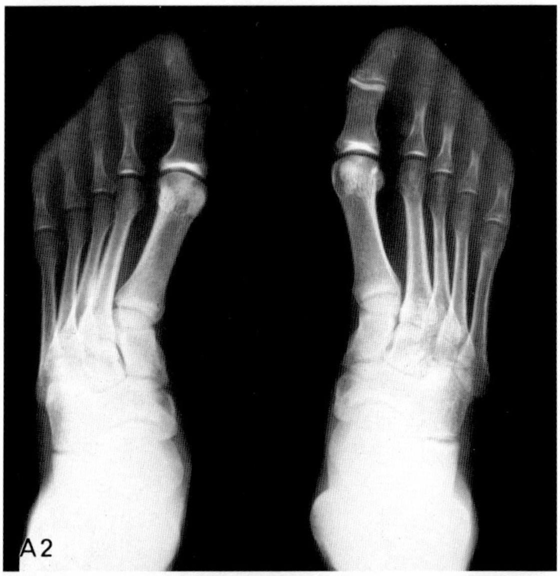

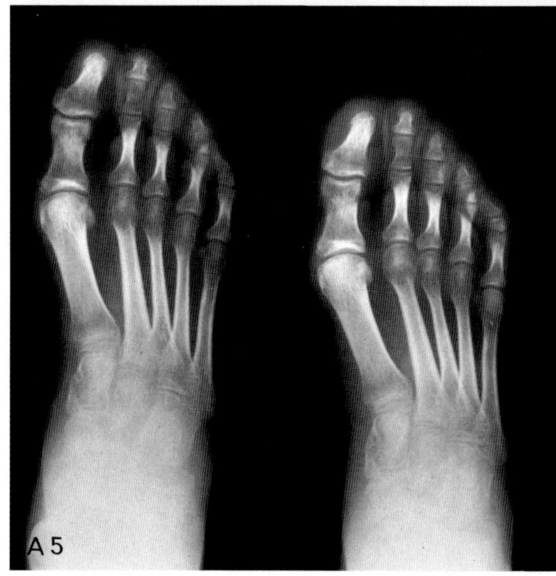

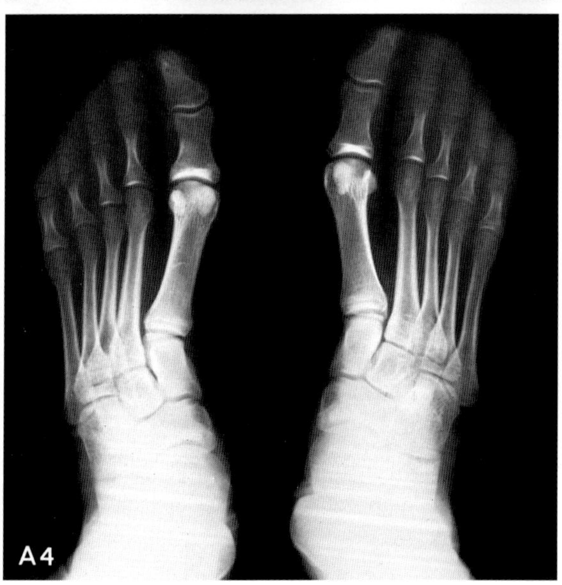

Fig. 16.24 A, B. Pes planovalgus: treatment by extra-articular osteotomies of neck of talus and navicular with transposition of tibialis posterior onto medial cuneiform. **A** *1* Left foot, preoperative weight-bearing lateral view; *2, 3* both feet, preoperative non-weight-bearing and weight-bearing dorsoplantar views: note medial displacement of midtarsus; *4* left foot, weight-bearing lateral view 12 months postoperatively; *5* right foot, weight-bearing and non-weight-bearing dorsoplantar views 6 months postoperatively. **B** *1-5* Right foot, lateral views: *1* Preoperative weight bearing; *2* weight bearing 6 months after navicular osteotomy, transposition of tibialis posterior to medial cuneiform; *3, 4* non-weight bearing and weight bearing 6 months postoperatively; *5* non-weight bearing 13 months postoperatively; *6, 7* both feet, weight-bearing and non-weight-bearing dorsoplantar views 13 months postoperatively. **B** see p. 213 ▷

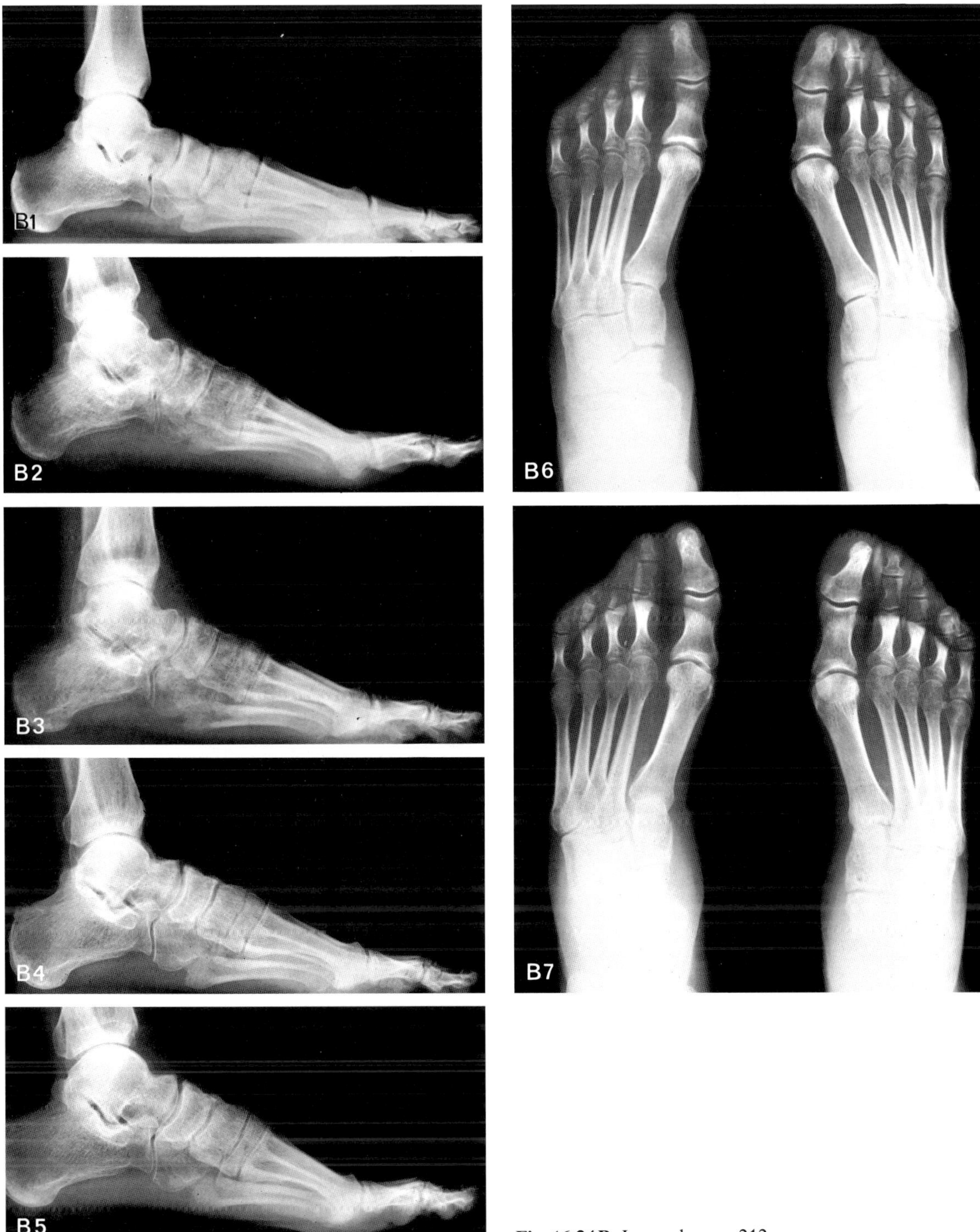

Fig. 16.24 B. Legend see p. 212

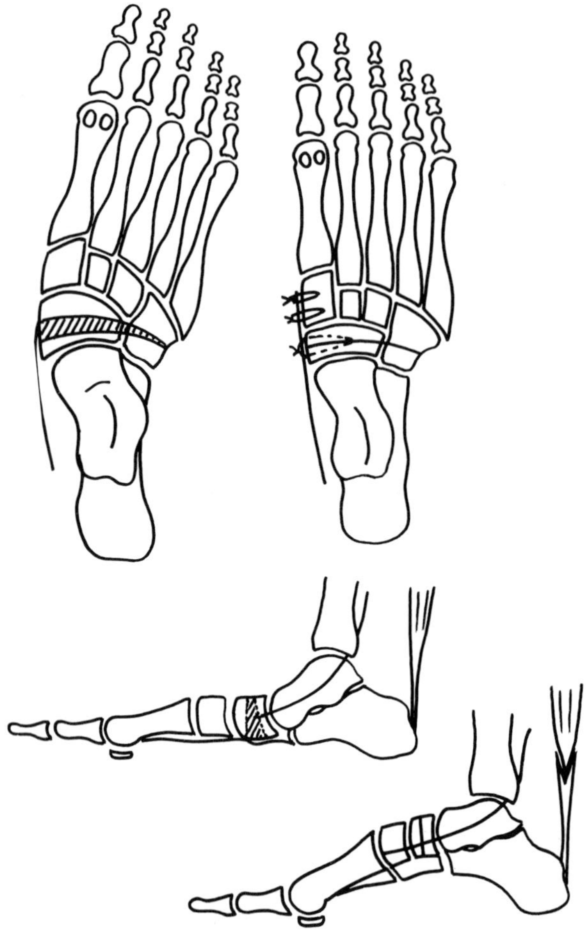

Fig. 16.25. Extra-articular plain or curved wedge osteotomies of navicular and cuboid (Regnauld)

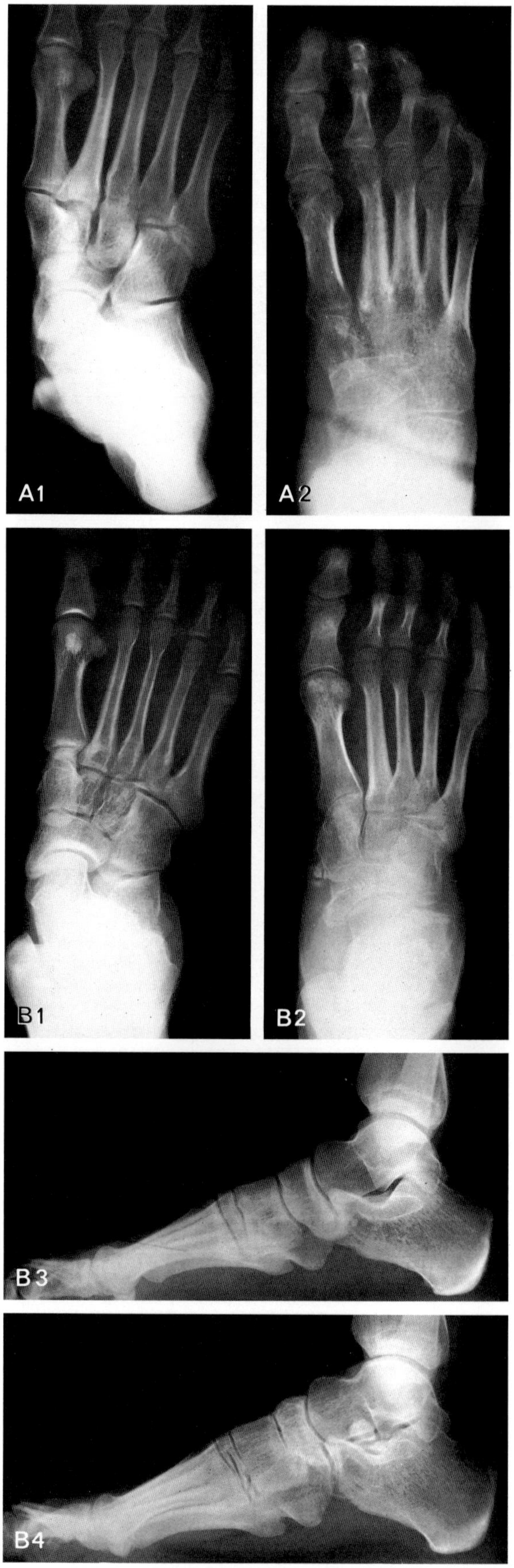

Fig. 16.26 A, B. Adult pes planovalgus before and after ▷ treatment. **A** *1, 2* Right foot, weight-bearing dorsoplantar views; *1* Preoperative: medial displacement of midtarsus, adduction of neck of talus, abduction of cuneiform-cuboidal region, abduction of metatarsus; *2* after osteotomy-arthrodesis of naviculocuneiform complex extending to cuboid, correction of midtarsal medial angulation, realignment of talonaviculocuneiform metatarsal axis. **B** Right foot. *1* Preoperative weight-bearing dorsoplantar view: lowering of axis of tarsus, abduction of naviculocuneiform-cuboidal region, metatarsal pronation, medial hypertrophy of navicular; *2* after extra-articular transnaviculocuboidal osteotomy, longitudinal realignment of tarsometatarsal axis; *3* preoperative weight-bearing lateral view: lowering of naviculocuneiform region, partial superimposition of navicular and cuneiforms on cuboid; *4* weight-bearing lateral view after reconstitution of medial longitudinal arch, elevation of naviculocuneiform mass, sagittal realignment of tarsus, transnaviculocuboidal osteotomy, subtalar arthrorisis (Lelièvre) with free bone graft in sinus tarsi, transposition of tibialis posterior onto medial cuneiform

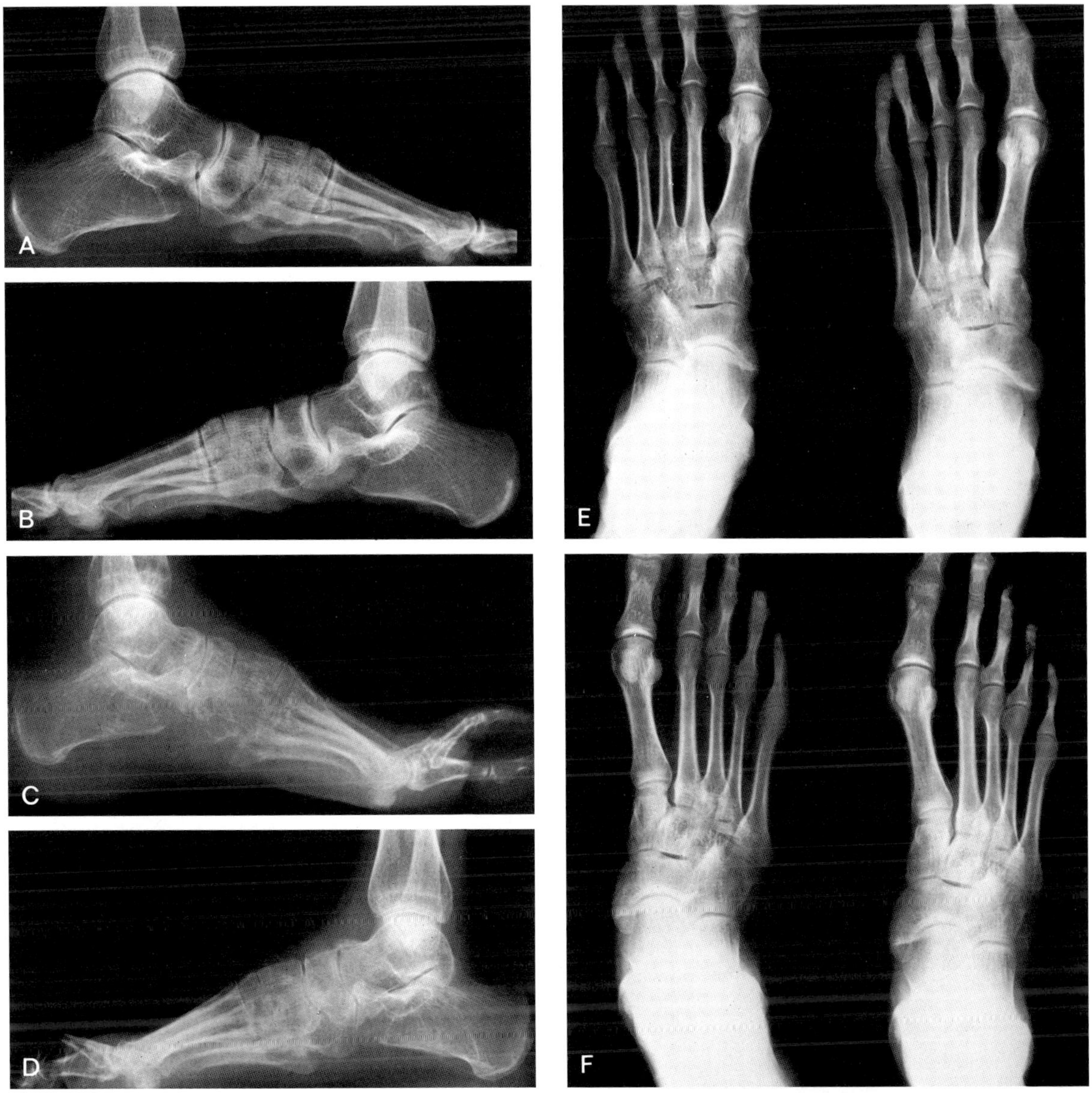

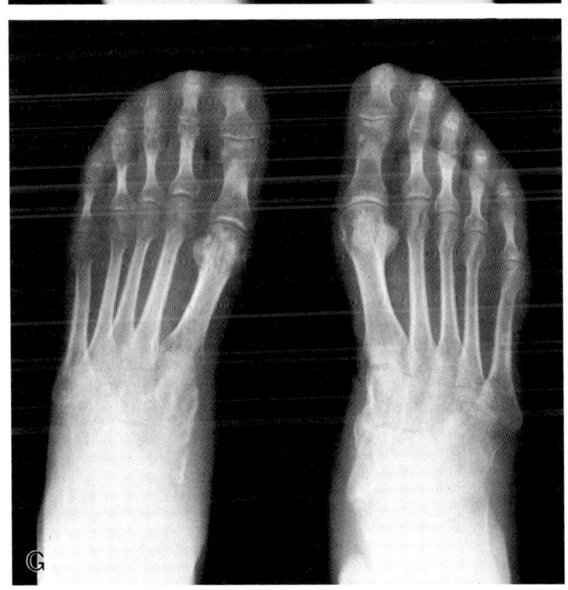

Fig. 16.28 A–G. Adult pes planovalgus before and after treatment. **A, B** Left and right foot, preoperative weight-bearing lateral views: lowering of navicular, superimposition of navicular and cuboid. **C, D** Left and right foot, weight bearing lateral views after correction of lowered position of navicular, osteotomy of navicular, transposition of tibialis posterior onto medial cuneiform. **E, F** Left foot (**E**) and right foot (**F**), weight-bearing *(left)* and non-weight-bearing *(right)* dorsoplantar views: medial midtarsal displacement, adduction of talus. **G** Both feet, non-weight-bearing dorsoplantar views after extra-articular osteotomies of neck of talus and navicular, transposition of tibialis posterior onto medial cuneiform

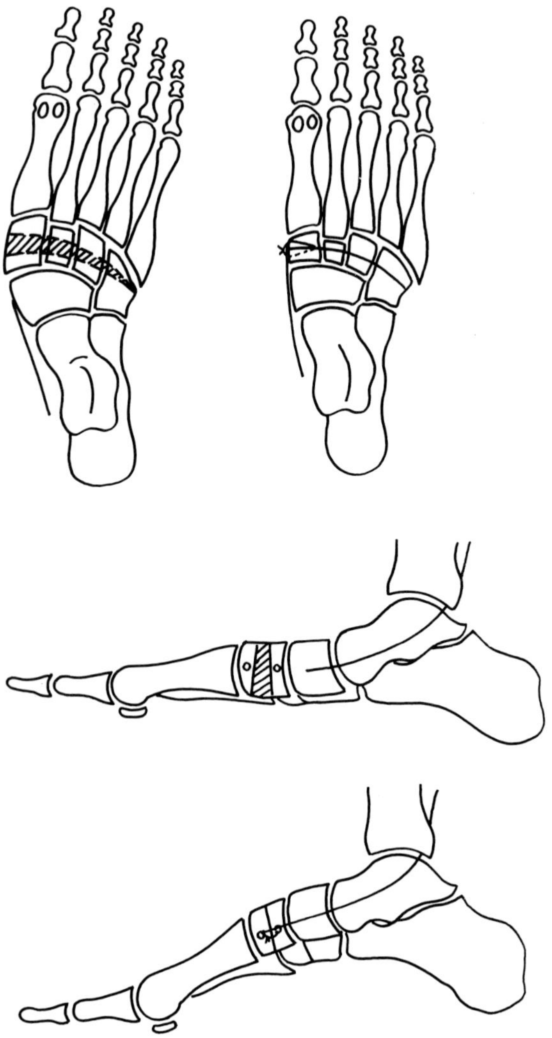

Fig. 16.27. Extra-articular transcuneiform-cuboidal wedge resections (Regnauld)

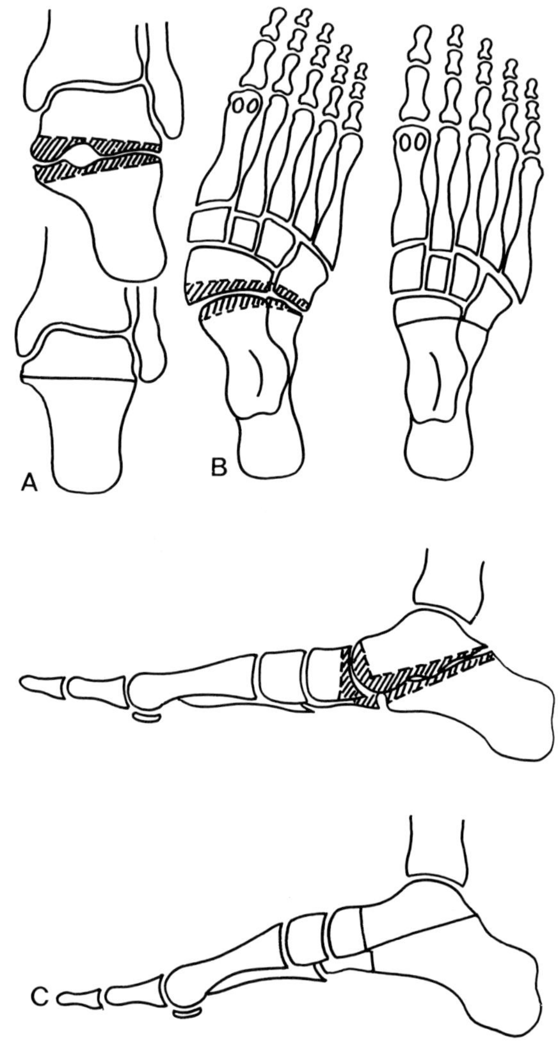

Fig. 16.29 A–C. Combined arthrodesis. **A** subtalar joint (wedge resection based medially). **B** Midtarsal joint (wedge resection based plantar-medially). **C** End result

Fig. 16.28 A–G see p. 215

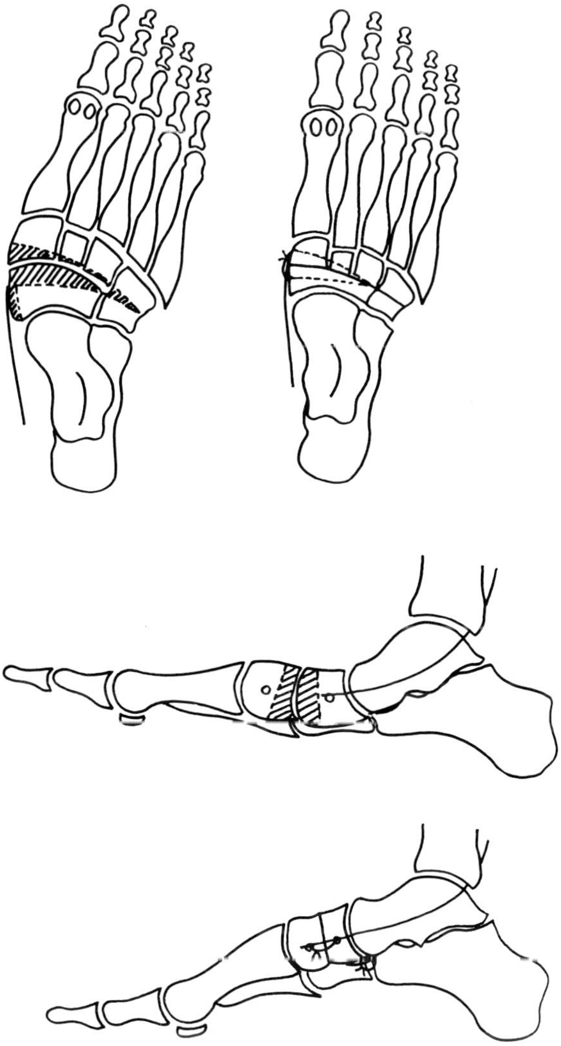

Fig. 16.30. Curvilinear resection arthrodesis of naviculo-cuneiform joints and body of cuboid with the wedge based plantar-medially (Regnauld)

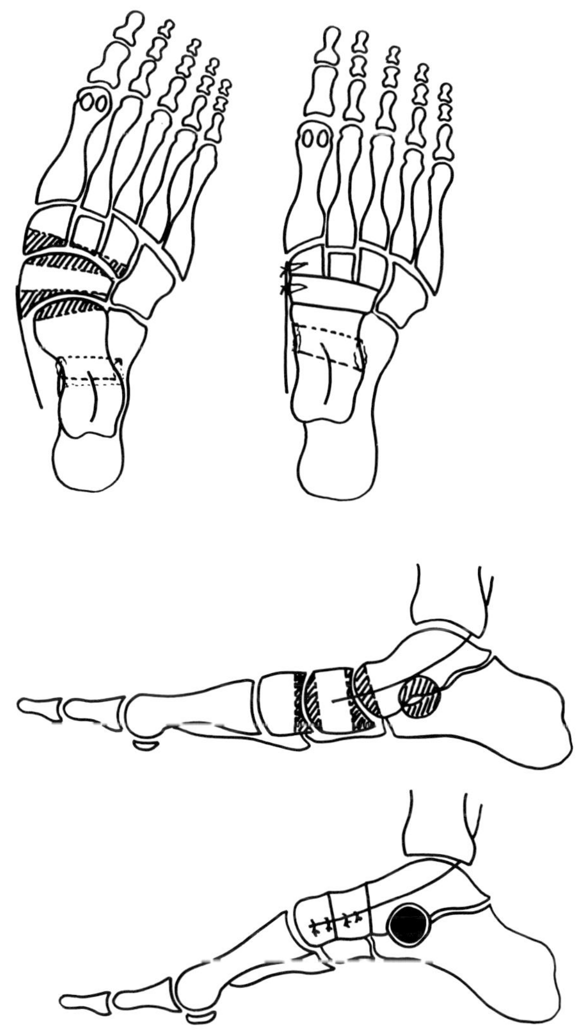

Fig. 16.31. Combined arthrodeses of naviculocuneiform joints, talonavicular joint and subtalar joint (by cylindrical bone graft in sinus tarsi). Wedge resections as appropriate (Viladot-Torner)

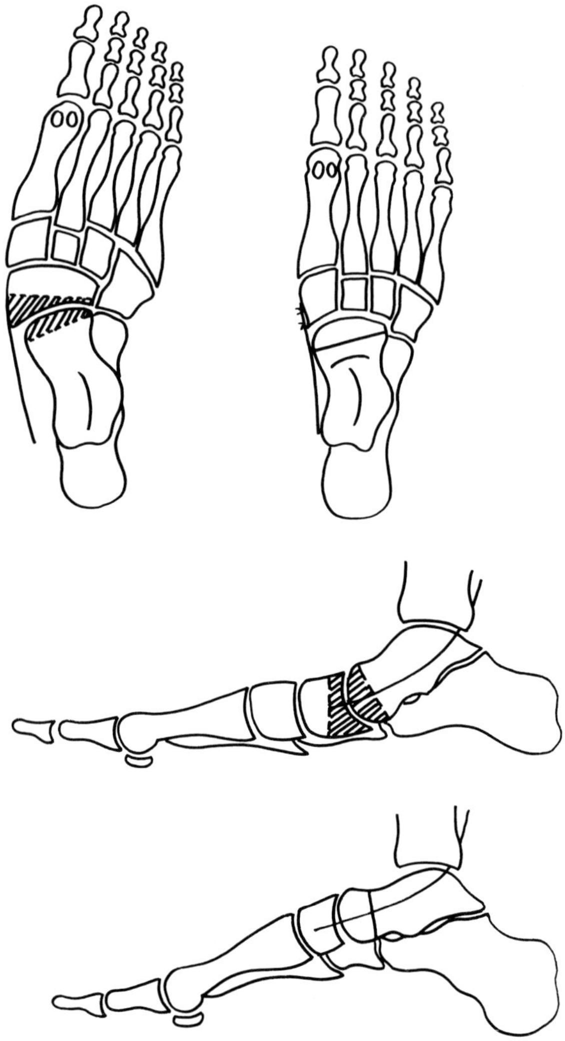

Fig. 16.32. Wedge resection arthrodesis (based plantar-medially) of talonavicular joint (Ogston-Cauchoix)

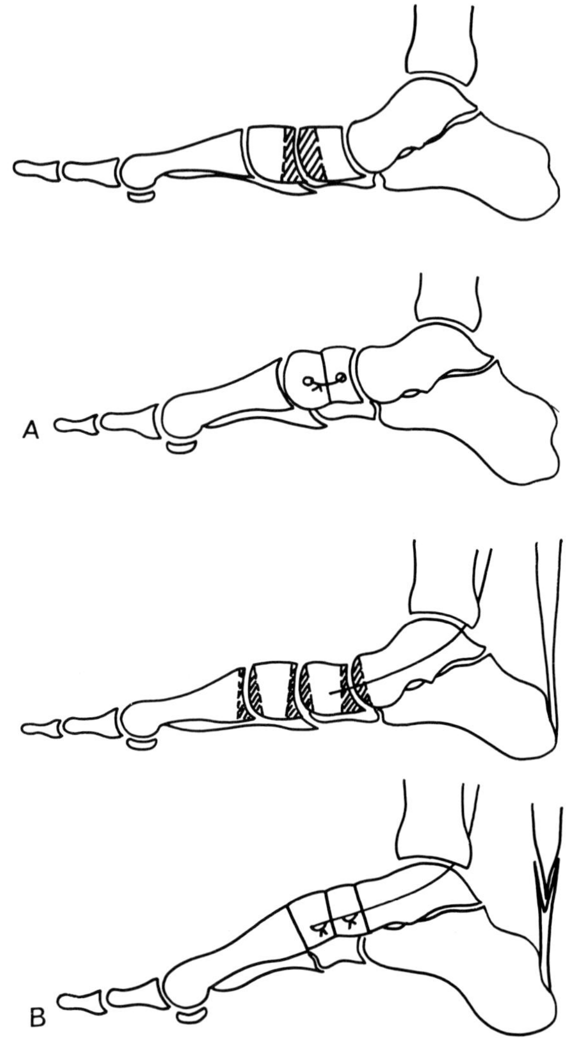

Fig. 16.33. A Wedge resection arthrodesis (based plantar-medially) of naviculocuneiform joints (Hohmann). **B** Combined wedge resection arthrodeses of talonavicular, naviculocuneiform and cuneiform-metatarsal joints (Müller)

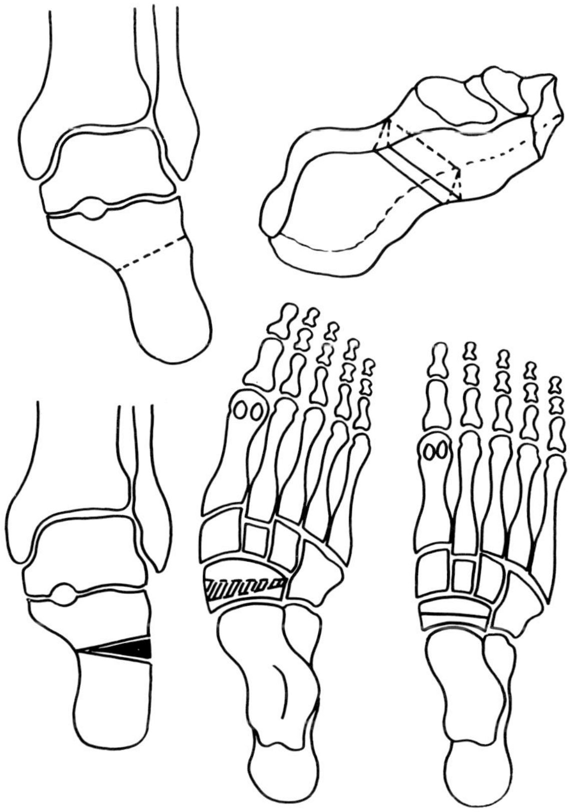

Fig. 16.34. Calcaneal osteotomy (Dwyer) with bone graft opening wedge (Judet)

Arthrosis of the subtalar joint is especially significant in advanced arthrosic pes planus by virtue of its frequency and intensity of pain. The extra-articular arthrodesis described by Grice (1952) is most valuable, while the subtalar arthrodesis of J. Judet (1972) will also correct the valgus heel by implantation of a cuneiform graft based externally (Fig. 16.34).

As stated earlier, these procedures do not correct the midtarsal displacement. When the latter is accompanied by advanced arthrosis in the medial joints, there is no problem in choice of treatment in that arthrodeses are necessary, but in the instances where arthrosis is less advanced and it is desirable to preserve joint movement, the greatest care is required in selection of other local fusions.

16.2 Congenital Pes Planovalgus

Pes planovalgus arising from congenital causes comprises two main groups: congenital conditions and those associated with synostosis.

16.2.1 Congenital Convex Pes Planovalgus (Vertical Talus)

This condition should be regarded as a club foot in which there is aplasia of the navicular analagous to that of the equinovarus club foot but differing in the inverted position of the talus. In the planovalgus variety, the foot is displaced superior and lateral to the talar head, whereas in the equinovarus foot, the foot is above and medial to the talar head. Examination of the neonate may reveal a simple protrusion of the head of the talus, although the foot, while presenting a convex flat appearance, may appear as pes adductus with talovalgus. The important sign is that the planovalgus convex foot is rarely isolated. It is frequently accompanied by other congenital deformities, perhaps in the opposite foot (varus club foot or pes adductus) or in the hips, the spine or the hands (cf. Chap. 26).

16.2.2 Planovalgus with Tarsal Coalition

The main tarsal coalitions associated with planovalgus foot are the talocalcaneal and calcaneonavicular types (see Figs. 27.10, 27.11). Treatment has been classified by Meary and Robert (1969). Harris advocates arthrodeses of the immediately associated joints, namely talonavicular arthrodesis for the calcaneal bar and talonavicular and subtalar arthrodesis for the calcaneonavicular.

Treatment. Conservative management is usually ineffective or at best affords temporary relief of pain and spasm. I favour local resection of the bony bars, associated when necessary with osteotomy-arthrodesis of the related joints or extra-articular midtarsal osteotomy. Thus, for calcaneocuboid or talonavicular synostosis, the procedure comprises transverse osteotomy across the synostosis with arthrodesis of the talonavicular joint fashioned by removal of a wedge with its base on the plantar and internal aspects, thereby correcting the lowering of the arch and the valgus posture. In calcaneonavicular synostosis, if the calcaneocuboid and talonavicular joints are normal, arthrodesis here should be avoided and wide resection of the synostosis should be performed together with midtarsal, extra-articular transnaviculocuboidal osteotomy with a wedge based plantarwards and medially. Arthrodeses are indicated only if it is impossible to preserve the integrity of the associated joints during the resection of the synostosis.

16.3 Post-Traumatic Pes Planovalgus

Pes planovalgus can result from fracture of the calcaneum when the angle of Böhler (1944) is so modified that the calcaneum is horizontally aligned, from diastasis of the inferior tibiofibular joint or from other bimalleolar fractures which are poorly reduced and become consolidated in abduction and pronation. Severe sprains of the foot with rupture of the inferior tibiofibular ligaments or the medial ligament of the ankle can also lead to pes planovalgus. In the midtarsal region, the commonest traumatic causes are fracture subluxation of the navicular, external dislocation at the Lisfranc joint line associated with diastasis, and poorly reduced intercuneiform-metatarsal joints.

Mention should be made of iatrogenic pes planovalgus following midtarsal arthrodesis and subtalar fusion (Fig. 16.35) (see Chap. 22).

16.4 Myopathic Pes Planovalgus

Myopathy, according to the distribution of muscles involved, can lead to pes cavovarus or pes planovalgus (Erb-Goldflam 1878). The condition is usually hereditary, familial and bilateral. When the resulting muscular hypotonia involves both tibialis muscles, it leads to irreversible pes planovalgus of second or third degree.

The foot is amenable to *conservative* management with orthopaedic insoles comprising arch supports, which re-establish lateral equilibrium and relieve the pains at the midtarsal region.

16.5 Paralytic Pes Planovalgus

Flaccid paralysis of various origins produces muscle imbalances and elongation of the associated muscles, leading to corresponding deformities of the foot. These follow the expected patterns, which are the converses of the predominant actions of various muscle groups. They may be summarised thus:

1. Simultaneous action of tibialis anterior and tibialis posterior produces a varus adducted attitude.
2. Triceps surae produces equinovarus posture, especially when acting together with the tibialis muscles and the long flexors and long extensors of the toes.
3. Peroneus brevis and extensor digitorum longus produce a valgus posture with abduction, while peroneus longus, the long and short flexors of the toes and tibialis posterior and anterior contribute to the maintenance of the longitudinal arch of the foot.

It follows from these summaries that diminution or absence of function of muscles producing varus cavus or equinus will lead to the formation of a pes planus (with the exception of triceps surae).

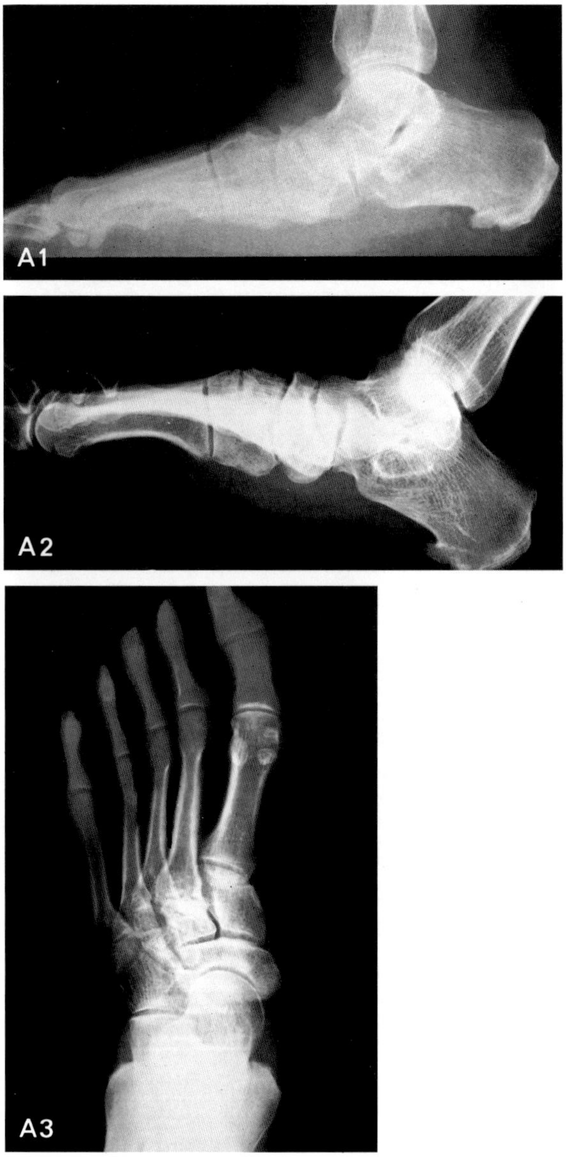

Fig. 16.35 A–D. A case of iatrogenic pes planovalgus in ▷ the left foot before and after treatment. **A** *1* Weight-bearing lateral view: third-degree pes planovalgus with horizontal position of calcaneum, equinus of talus, collapse of midtarsus; *2* non-weight-bearing lateral view; *3* dorsoplantar view: medial displacement of midtarsus, hypertrophy in length of neck of talus. **B–D** see p. 221

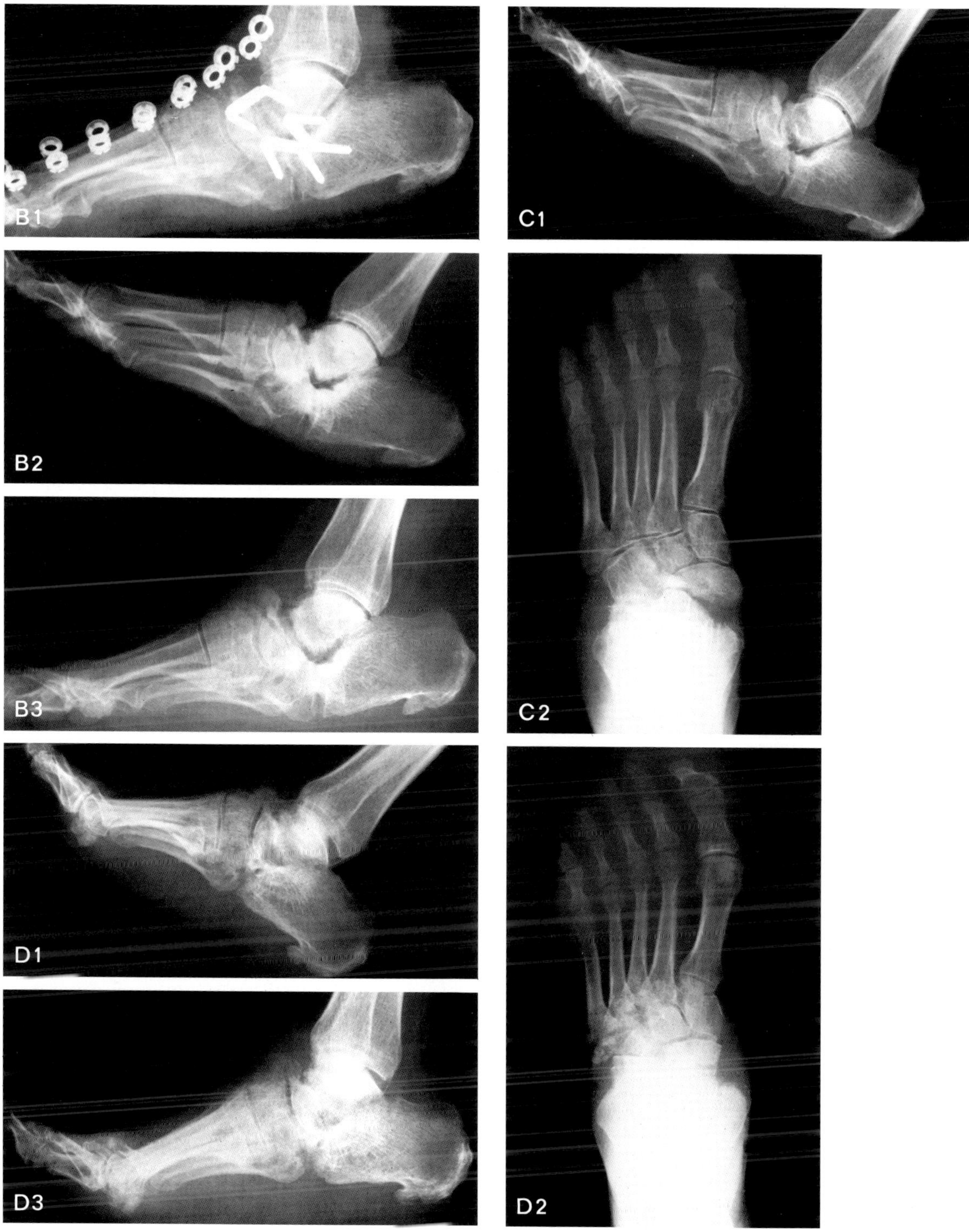

Fig. 16.35 *(continued)*. **B** *1–3* Results of ill-chosen operation: osteotomy-arthrodesis of midtarsal region and of subtalar joint. Severe pes planovalgus with pain, inability to walk, and difficulty in wearing shoes. **C** *1* Lateral view: pseudarthrosis at attempted arthrodesis sites in midtarsal and subtalar regions, convexity of calcaneocuboid joint; *2* dorsoplantar view: displacement at Chopart joint line. **D** *1, 2* After osteotomy of midtarsal region with excision of a wedge based medially and plantarwards together with osteotomy of talocalcaneal joint with removal of a wedge based medially and frontally; *3* weight-bearing lateral views 6 months later: good balance in restored foot, gait normal

The main etiologies of flaccid paralysis (poliomyelitis, medial popliteal nerve palsy, flaccid hemiplegia and spina bifida) confer somewhat different appearances and present different prognoses. Each will be described separately.

16.5.1 Poliomyelitis

The distributions of paralysis leading to planovalgus deformity are typically:

a) Complete paralysis of the sciatic nerve, especially of its medial popliteal component. This type of foot is flail; the subject walks with a high stepping gait, and when the foot is unloaded it falls into equinus, looking like a third-degree valgus foot. Sensory involvement may lead to plantar anaesthesia with trophic changes of ulceration, which can make therapy difficult.
b) Isolated paralysis of tibialis anterior or of both tibialis muscles.
c) Associated paralysis of triceps surae and the two tibialis muscles.
d) Associated paralysis of peroneus longus and flexor digitorum longus.

16.5.1.1 Clinical Features

There is usually atrophy of the postero-internal muscles involved and overaction of the extensors and peronei. The plantar longitudinal arch lowers very rapidly, the foot resting totally on its plantar surface. Along the internal border there is a tarsometatarsal convexity, the angular summit of which is situated according to the muscles involved: when it is located at the medial cuneiform, there is involvement of tibialis anterior and peroneus longus; when at the navicular, there is paralysis of both tibialis muscles; when at the head of the talus, there is usually paralysis of peroneus longus and flexor digitorum longus. The hindfoot appears to be significantly pronated, with the posterior process of the calcaneum deviated into valgus, and a horizontal groove presenting on the outer aspect of the tarsal region accompanies this displacement. The general alignment of the calcaneum is horizontal and valgus, or even equinus and abduction, when triceps surae is not involved. The midtarsal region is severely everted; the navicular and cuboid are in the same horizontal plane due to elevation and abduction of the latter. In the metatarsus, there is pronation and abduction due to unrestrained action of peroneus brevis and extensor digitorum longus.

The areas of overloading along the medial side of the foot are evidenced by callosities under the navicular and the head of the talus. The prominence of the three bony protrusions described by Lannelongue (Sect. 16.1.4) may be very marked. The deformity is exaggerated by active dorsiflexion of the foot, which causes the long extensor tendons and peroneus brevis to tent the overlying skin.
Pain arises from capsuloligamentous strain, this relating especially to the ankle and subtalar joints and the midtarsus, and from calluses under the first metatarsal head and those mentioned above. The pain may be progressive.
Podoscopic examination shows the typical print of severe third-degree pes planovalgus, marked by uniformity of plantar loading. The tarsometatarsal angulation with convexity at the internal border and concavity of the external border is clear.
Radiography: In the anteroposterior view, divergence of the talocalcaneal axes, midtarsal adduction, metatarsal abduction and, in advanced cases, medial subluxation of the navicular are usually clear. The site of angular distortion at the medial border can be located. The lateral view shows disappearance of the longitudinal arch, horizontal alignment of the calcaneum and the metatarsus and superimposition of the images of the navicular and the cuboid. The neck of the talus is in equinus.

16.5.1.2 Treatment

Appropriate support from insoles and adapted shoes may control the progression of the condition for a significant and useful period of time, but in general, these feet are best treated by surgery. Capsuloligamentous, tendon, and bony procedures are chosen according to the distribution and stage of the deformity.

16.5.1.2.1 Capsuloligamentous Procedures

These procedures comprise resection of segments like quarters of an orange from the plantar and internal aspects of the talonavicular capsule. Repair is with nylon sutures (Regnauld 1974).

16.5.1.2.2 Tendon Procedures

One of the following procedures is chosen according to the indications:

- V-shaped elongation of triceps surae by the Vulpius technique (1920) for simple liberation of a horizontally aligned calcaneum.
- Elongation of tendo Achillis, preserving its internal half so as to relax the calcaneal position and encourage varus action.
- Haglund tenodesis (1923), which unifies the actions of tibialis anterior, extensor hallucis longus and extensor digitorum longus. All or part of extensor hallucis longus is tenodesed, and at the same time peroneus brevis is elongated and a modified tenodesis of tibialis posterior according to Delitala (1921) is performed. The last-named technique consists of fashioning a loop of the paralysed tibialis posterior and anchoring this by several thick nylon stitches to the distal end of the tibialis anterior tendon. It is then sutured to itself after passage under tension through a tunnel in the medial malleolus. Transplantation of all or half of the peroneus brevis tendon can be performed together with part of extensor hallucis longus onto the navicular or medial cuneiform or onto the distal insertion of tibialis anterior.

These tendinous operations will be complemented as necessary by the correction of claw toes and subluxation or dorso-external dislocation of the metatarsophalangeal joints.

16.5.1.2.3 Bony Procedures

Bony operations vary according to the site of the paralysis.

Isolated Paralysis of Tibialis Anterior. The procedure of choice comprises osteotomy of the neck of the talus and of the navicular (Regnauld 1974) associated with stabilisation of the subtalar joint by arthrodesis through the sinus tarsi or the Grice procedure (1952) augmented by anterior transplantation of tibialis posterior. The osteotomy across the naviculocuboidal region includes a wedge resection with the base directed internally and plantarwards, as well as a shortening segmental resection of the talonavicular ligament.

Combined Paralysis of Tibialis Anterior and Tibialis Posterior. A variety of procedures are effective: (a) Arthrodesis of the midtarsal and subtalar joint and cuneiforms as described by Ombredanne (1949) or by Ducroquet and Launay (1909). These procedures correct the planovalgus and re-establish a medial plantar arch. A Haglund tenodesis is associated with these operations. (b) In the paralytic flail foot, pantalar arthrodesis may be indicated. (c) Stabilisation by the arthrodesis described by Torner (1984), in which a cylindrical subtalar graft is inserted into the sinus tarsi (really a modified Grice procedure) and associated with double arthrodesis by cuneiform resection of the plantar aspect of the talonavicular joints and the naviculocuneiform joint lines, thereby remodelling the plantar arch. This must be complemented by reinsertion of the shortened tibialis posterior. (d) Extra-articular resection osteotomy of the talar neck or of the navicular (Regnauld 1974) is effective and must be accompanied by multiple tendinous procedures, including Haglund tenodesis, anterior transplantation of tibialis posterior (Delitala 1950) and hemitransplantation of extensor hallucis longus on to the stump of tibialis anterior.

16.5.2 Pes Planovalgus from Medial Popliteal Nerve Lesions

Traumatic medial popliteal nerve paralysis creates pes planovalgus accompanied by trophic disorders, ulceration or perforating ulcer associated with the sensory impairment.

Treatment is simultaneously orthotic and surgical. The use of orthopaedic shoes and supporting insoles cushions the pressure points and supports the longitudinal arch, while surgery comprises triple arthrodesis accompanied by tendon transplants (partial or total transfer of peroneus brevis onto tendo Achillis compensates slightly for the paralysis of triceps surae). Midtarsal arthrodesis and subtalar arthrodesis with wedge resections of bone based plantarwards and internally can correct the position of the midtarsus and may be accompanied by an anterior transfer of tibialis posterior (Delitala 1950) and also by transplantation of tibialis anterior onto the navicular in an effort to support the plantar arch.

16.5.3 Flaccid Hemiplegia

This syndrome of encephalitic origin with the development of a planovalgus foot should be treated conservatively with supporting insoles. The central origin of the weakness is likely to render any surgical intervention worthless, with the possible exception of pantalar arthrodesis.

16.5.4 Paralytic Pes Planovalgus from Spina Bifida

This condition appears when the myelomeningoceles are located at the L5-S1 level. The imbalance between the active extensors and the paralysed flexors leads at the outset to a club foot and then to a planovalgus foot due to paralysis of the posterior muscles: tibialis posterior and the long flexors.

16.6 Spastic Flat Foot

Niederecker (1959), Giannestras (1973) and Barouk (1981) have made important contributions to our understanding of spastic flat foot, described originally by Little (1861) as spasmodic hemiplegia in infants. There is generalised spasticity of the whole lower limb during the first months of life and frequently a history of difficult delivery.

The planovalgus posture is accompanied by equinus of the foot, flexion contracture of the knee and internal rotation at the hip. The presence of a peroneus tertius, shortening of peroneus brevis and a more distal insertion of tibialis anterior onto the first metatarsal (Niederecker 1959) are further features in the foot itself.

The foot posture is characterised by valgus displacement under loading, generalised external rotation and the constant clawing of the toes, which appear to "grasp" the ground. The plantar print exhibits lowering of the internal border and absence of loading externally, together with the grasping effect of the pulps of the toes. The foot is valgus internally and cavus externally.

16.6.1 Treatment

Treatment is surgical and complex, and directed at correction of the imbalance at the knee and hip as well as at the foot itself. Management of the foot in isolation is bound to fail.

Barouk (1983) recommends the following measures:

Hip: Adductor longus and brevis tenotomies, and if necessary rotation osteotomy of the femur.

Knee: Division of semitendinosus and oblique elongation of the aponeurosis of semimembranosus and biceps femoris as described by Coste; less frequently, retensioning of the quadriceps apparatus (Hurmich, Vima and Grenier) with detachment of rectus femoris.

Foot: In the *child or adolescent,* early correction of the equinus and grasping toes can be secured by gastrocnemius release and elongation of the triceps surae tendon as described by Green. In this method, section is performed intero-internally and supero-externally, so that elongation is achieved by sliding of the spiral fibres. The flexors of the toes are elongated or tenotomised. An above-knee plaster cast maintains correction of the foot in 10° of equinus with the toes in dorsiflexion and the knee extended; walking is encouraged at 2 weeks. After removal of the cast, splints must be worn at night and re-educative exercises pursued regularly for many months. Subsequent measures which may be indicated include tenotomy of peroneus tertius or transposition of its insertion to the lateral cuneiform, elongation of peroneus longus, Grice (1952) arthrodesis, the use of an insole with a corrective supinating wedge under the heel, and transposition of the insertion of tibialis anterior looped under tibialis posterior (Niederecker 1959) so as to depress the first metatarsal and elevate the navicular.

In the *adult,* bony procedures are required. These comprise corrective arthrodesis of the subtalar complex and midtarsus from the medial aspect associated as necessary with Niederecker (1959) and Albanese (1948) tenodeses, corrective semicircular osteotomy of the first metatarsal, thereby depressing it, interphalangeal arthrodeses for the clawed toes and corrective arthroplasties for hallux valgus or hallux flexus.

17 Disorders of the Toes

Painful conditions of the toes are significant because of their frequency and the common failure of practitioners to recognise their part in the overall context of a foot disorder. It is easy to miss the fact that more serious problems underlie an apparently simple toe disorder. Inconvenience, pain and troublesome infection bring the patient to the doctor, but treatment is likely to be ineffectual if directed only at the site of the symptom rather than the basic source of the disease.

17.1 Nail Plate

17.1.1 Ingrown Toenail

This common lesion most frequently affects the great toe but can involve others (Fig. 17.1). It is due to mechanical, multidirectional compression of the fleshy prominence in the para-ungual region. In order of frequency, the abnormalities of the nail are: rigidity of the plate and its lateral vertical borders; a spatulate configuration; the longitudinal wavy Provence deformity (so named from its similarity to the roofing tile used in Provence); and onychogryphosis. Extrinsic causes are shoe pressure, pressure from adjacent toes and other pathological affectations.

Sustained pressure exerted by the lateral border of the nail in the depths of the nail fold produces a pressure ulcer. This becomes infected, and irritation leads to a permanent overgrowth of granulation tissue. The inflammatory state presents with a violaceous red appearance in the ingrown area, with oedematous tissue underlying the stretched skin. Local heat and tenderness may be marked. There is permanent maceration, whitish at the ingrown area, and the pain on weight bearing is aggravated by the slightest contact of the shoe or sock when walking and especially in sport. When the ingrown condition becomes chronic due to cracking of the nail and suppuration, pain may become less severe, assuming a pricking character and relieved by rest and avoidance of compression. Diagnosis is usually easy.

17.1.1.1 Treatment

Chiropody or surgery may be appropriate. The following measures should be *avoided:*

1. Total removal of the nail. This does not obliterate the cause. Regrowth of the nail usually results in a repetition of the same condition, and the trauma may lead to abnormalities of parts of the nail bed which would otherwise have remained normal; the surface of the bed may become dry and then irregular, often impeding adherence of the new nail when it grows.
2. Excision of the nail and its bed which is disproportionate to the gravity of the lesion. This removes the protection afforded by the nail and produces long-term discomfort. It is an unaesthetic procedure.
3. Cauterisation of the granulation tissue with silver nitrate. This again does not suppress the cause. Local applications of antiseptic and antibiotic will also prove ineffectual.

Chiropody may be curative, especially if instituted early. It comprises implantation of a small plate of silver or springy metal onto the dorsum of the nail as described by Voelcker [cited by Klages (1933)]. The extremities of the Voelcker plate are curved so as to grasp the lateral borders of the nail, and as a result of its compliance they progressively diminish the vertical disposition of the borders and the transverse convexity of the plate. This may provoke a definitive cure by modifying the shape of the nail.

The efficacy of the plate may be augmented by creating a small longitudinal groove in the central longitudinal axis of the nail in order to weaken it. During an infective episode, the technique described by Wallet (1942) can be used.

The lateral portion of the incarcerated nail is lifted and a spur removed through a small, obliquely disposed, anterior to posterior incision close to the nail fold. Chiropody must be accompanied by the administration of tetanus prophylaxis if the subject has not been immunised and by the application of antiseptic cream for 3 weeks in preparation for sur-

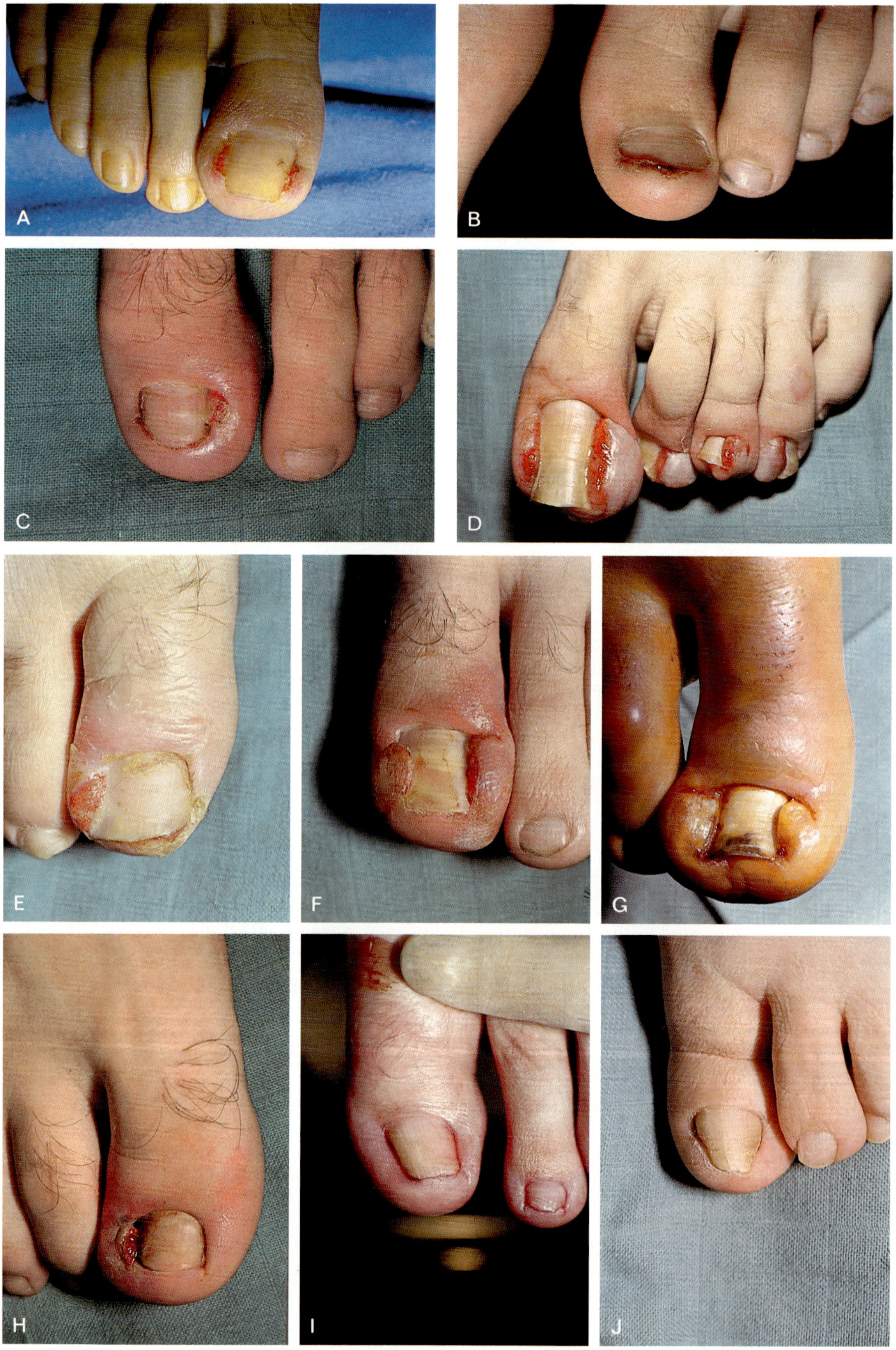
A
B
C
D
E
F
G
H
I
J

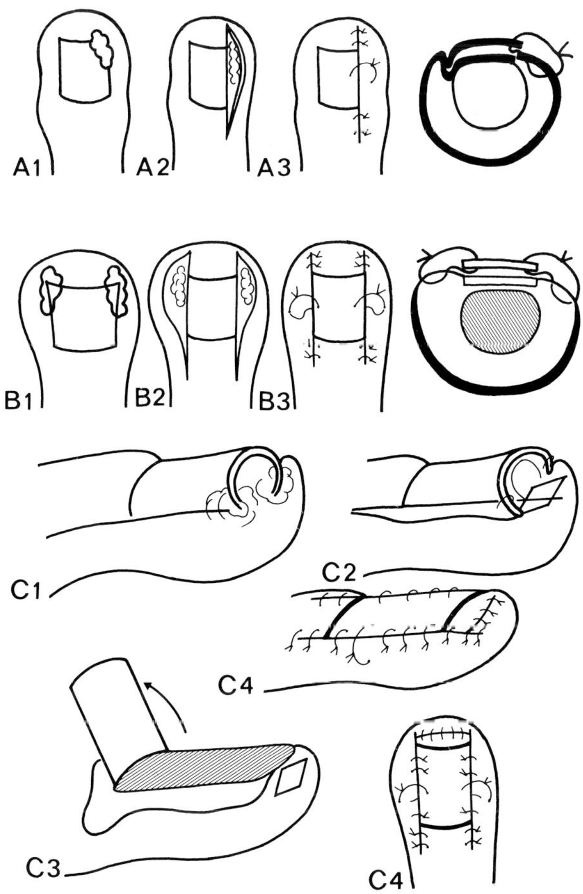

Fig. 17.2. A Ingrown toenail. *1* Before treatment; *2* wedge resection of nail matrix corresponding to ingrown portion; *3* method of suture whereby skin margin is maintained deep to nail margin, so avoiding recurrence. **B** Spatulate deformity of nail resulting in ingrown condition. *1* Before treatment; *2* resection of lateral margins of distal phalanx; *3* method of suture similar to that for ingrown toenail *(above)*. **C** Provence tile deformity. *1* Before treatment; *2* bilateral resection of vertical margins of nail and removal of a lozenge-shaped portion distally; *3* elevation of nail bed and flattening of dorsal surface of terminal phalanx and its tuft; *4* method of suture of skin margins to nail bed

◁ **Fig. 17.1 A–J.** Ingrown toenail. **A** Ingrown medial and lateral nail folds. **B** Distal incarceration with a flat nail. **C, D** Medial and lateral ingrown nail folds. **E** Flat nail with lateral incarceration of nail fold. **F, G** Medial and lateral nail fold incarceration. **H, I** Horseshoe incarceration of whole nail fold. **J** Cone-shaped nail with chronic medial and lateral nail fold incarceration at distal ends

gical intervention should conservative measures not prove successful.
Operation should be undertaken during an uninfected phase, and the technique of O'Donoghue (1940) and Sibley (1945) is recommended (Fig. 17.2). This curative procedure has the advantage of being aesthetic and reconstitutes the normal morphology of the toe.

Operative Technique. Operation can be performed under local ring-block anaesthesia with a small tourniquet around the base of the toe. A longitudinal strip of the vertical border of the nail is removed with narrow scissors. The central part of the nail plate should not be disturbed. A wedge-shaped band of nail bed and adjacent matrix is then removed together with the nail fold and hypertrophied tissue. With small rongeurs, hypertrophied bone from the distal phalanx is trimmed and a suture coapting the cutaneous lip beneath the lateral border of the nail is placed meticulously. A dressing of tulle gras with gauze soaked in physiological saline is applied. The dressing is changed on the following day, leaving the tulle gras in situ until removal of the sutures at about the 10th day.

In addition to the classical ingrown toenail described above, in which the nail is of normal shape, the condition being due to extrinsic pressure, two anomalies of the nail plate itself may occur.

17.1.2 Provence Nail

This characteristic deformity of the nail is due to a growth abnormality affecting the distal phalanx (Figs. 17.1 H–J, 17.3 A–C, G, H). The great toe is affected most frequently, but the lesser ones can also be involved, and it is then usual for all nails to be affected. There appears to be an absence of the dorsal cortex of the distal phalanx, so that a marked transverse convexity at the base of the phalanx presents where the nail root is situated. This continues towards the extremity and a longitudinal crest presenting a reversed V-shape on the dorsal face terminates in a narrow tuft. The nail corresponds to the configuration of the underlying bone on which it rests and assumes an aspect like a Provence roof tile, being cone-shaped and diminishing in size towards the distal extremity. It separates gradually from its bed, and in the space so created, fungal infection is likely to develop and skin debris to accumulate, while the two collateral borders have a tendency to incurve more and more towards the distal aspect until they almost meet, thereby

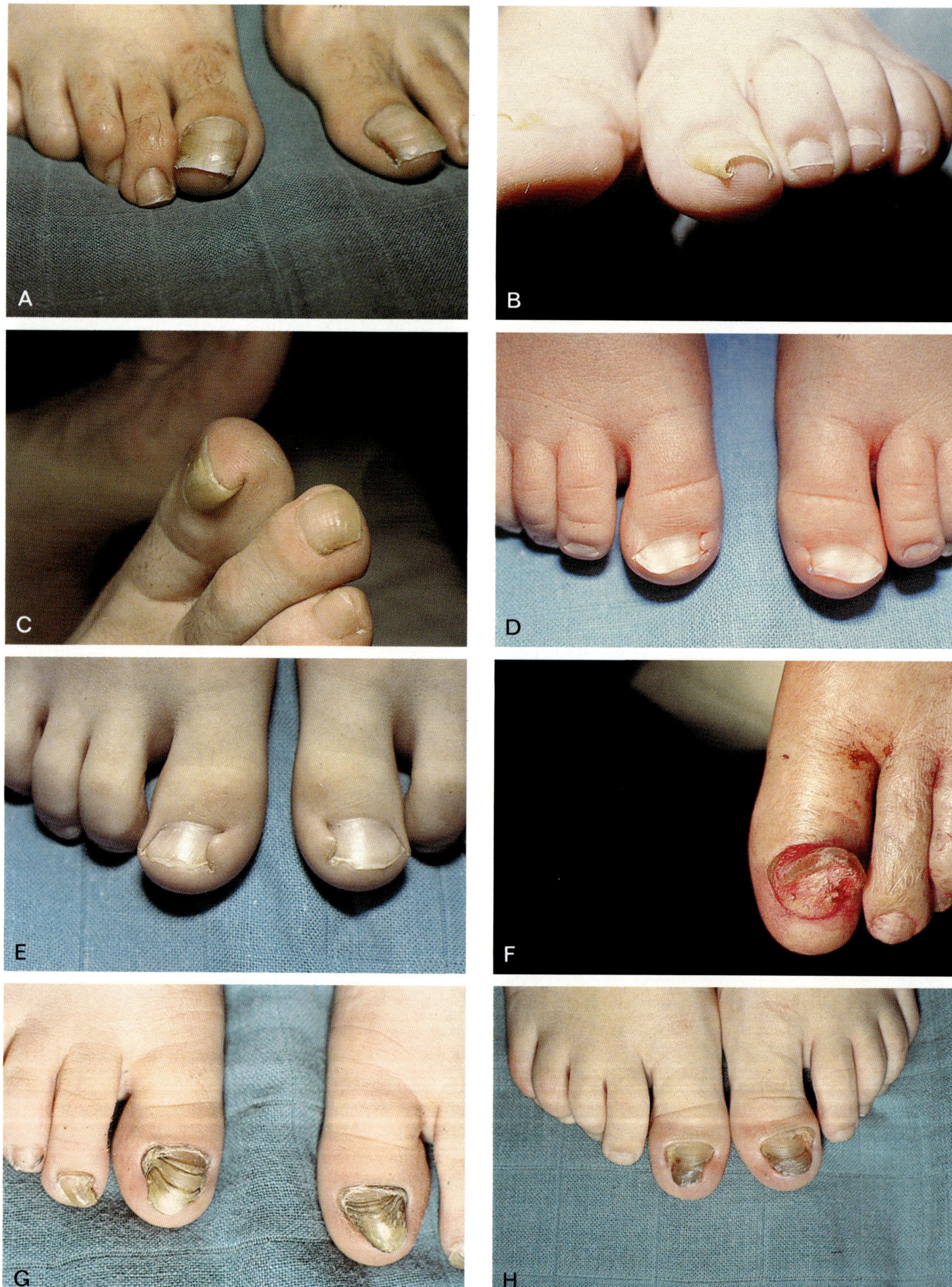

Fig. 17.3 A–N. Onychodystrophy. **A–C** Provence tile deformity. **D, E** Spatulate nail. **F** Onychorrhexis. **G, H** Cone-shaped nail. **I–N** Onychauxis, onychogryphosis and onychomycosis. **I–J** Onychomycosis. **I–N** see ▷ p. 229

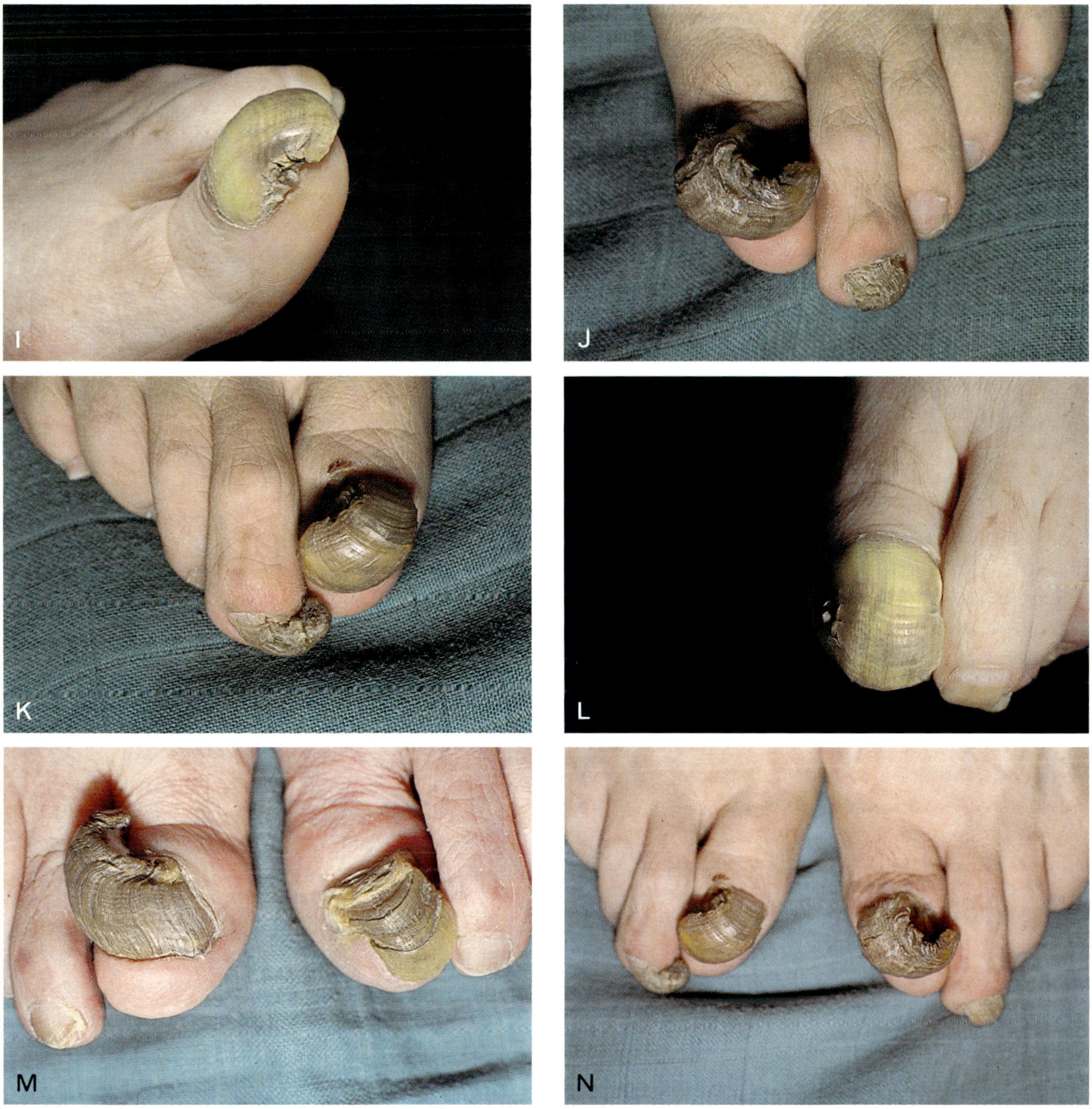

Fig. 17.3 I–N. Legend see p. 228

producing pressure symptoms and inflammation. These may persist for a long time without infection, but sooner or later overgrowth of soft tissue and abscess formation occur and symptoms increase in severity.

17.1.2.1 *Treatment*

Conservative treatment, which has some chance of success, comprises removal of the soft tissue debris and horny skin in the nail folds, separation and division of the free borders of the nail and protection of the nail folds by splintage. Conservative measures commonly fail, and operation is then required (Regnauld 1974).

Operative Technique. Performed under local anaesthesia and with tourniquet at the base of the toe, the following steps have proved successful (Fig. 17.2). A minimal amount of the two vertical borders of the nail plate is removed, together with the related nail bed, but the nail folds are preserved. A transverse lozenge-shaped incision is made distally with removal of the area of skin enclosed. At the level of the bone, the mucous part of the nail bed and nail folds is separated cleanly as far as the base of the phalanx.

The bed, plate and folds are hinged backwards so as to permit horizontal resection of the bone, removing the crest and the convex swelling near the epiphysis and thus rendering the dorsal aspect of the phalanx flat. The nail and its bed are repositioned, involving further cutaneous resection distally, in such a way that the alignment of the nail folds is restored. A compressive dressing with tulle gras and gauze soaked in physiological saline is left in position for 10 days, changing the gauze alone after the first day.

17.1.3 Spatulate Deformity

This condition, in which an infection leads to exaggeration in the size of the nail plate, results, especially in the adult, in the appearance of a classical ingrown toenail, while in the infant it may constitute the cause of nail incarceration (Fig. 17.3 D, E). Predominantly the great toe is affected, but the lesser toes may also be involved in the adult. There is a further relationship with claw toe and hammer toe, affecting predominantly the second, third and fourth digits. The enlarged nail is flat and lacking in the normal suppleness, and may develop a transverse concave configuration, thin, translucent and supple, sometimes crossed by transverse striae in the newborn infant. Despite careful attention to hygiene, the infant may suffer from episodes of inflammation of the soft tissues at the side of the nail, painful due to incarceration of the end of the nail plate, or repeated episodes of cellulitis around the nail edge leading to paronychial abscess formation. In time, the infections result in irreversible changes to the point that there is hypertrophy of the nail folds, which tend to cover the lateral portions of the nail plate. The nail, while thin and supple at birth, hardens progressively and develops its typical spatulate appearance, wider than it is long. Eventually, the mother brings her child for consultation because of the ingrown toenail. This may affect both sides of the nail as well as its distal end, so that the enlarged plate appears encased within three pads of tissue.
Treatment of the spatulate deformity is surgical.

Operative Technique. The operation is performed with an elastic tourniquet under general anaesthesia in the baby, local anaesthesia in the adult. The skin, bone and nail bed on the outer and inner aspects of the spatulate nail are resected so as to reduce the nail to a normal size with respect to the surrounding soft tissues. If there is distal thickening of the free border, resection of a wedge-shaped transversely disposed piece of tissue should be performed in the region of the distal nail bed. The soft tissues distal to the nail are shortened down to the level of the tuft of the terminal phalanx from which the dorsal border is resected so as to restore bony alignment. Careful suturing distally obliterates the soft tissue fold in the hyponychium which before surgery hindered growth of the nail by obstructing its free border.

17.1.4 Onychodystrophy

This group of conditions includes onychogryphosis, onychophosis and onychauxis.
Onychogryphosis entails a longitudinal claw-like thickening of the nail while onychauxis looks like a paving stone hypertrophy (Figs. 17.3 I, K, M, N, 17.4 A–C). Both, according to Achten (1964), are due to thickening of the hyponychial keratin (onychophosis) and of the bed of the nail, which constitute a homogeneous mass one upon the other. The thickening of keratin at the junction of the hyponychium and the nail root creates a soft tissue pad against which the free border of the nail abuts. The nail, stopped in its growth by this obstacle, thickens and separates. In onychogryphosis, the thickening and separation result in the curvature of the nail into its claw shape and separation from all or part of the nail bed. It is as if the nail abutting distally against the keratinised soft tissue pad, which is thickened by transverse striae, is attempting to separate and raise itself in order to get over the obstacle. The nail plate thickens with the development of transverse striae, separates as described, and there is accumulation of waxy debris of more or less infected tissue, which becomes odorous. There is opaque (greyish or dirty-yellow) discoloration of the nail (Fig. 17.3 I, J). A tendency to ingrowth proximally in the region of the root results in permanent discomfort, and difficulty of shoe fitting arises from the sheer bulk of the nail together with aggravation of the painful disturbance of its bed. It may be several years or even decades before onychogryphosis becomes complicated by infection.
In contrast to the progressive narrowing of the nail towards its distal end in onychogryphosis, the thickening in *onychauxis* is more regular, variously described as plate-like or paving-stone-like in type. Occasionally as much as 1 cm of thickening results, provoking the same inflammatory reactions of the nail bed and difficulty in shoe fitting together with accumulations of debris underneath the nail and

sometimes purulent separation of nail from bed (Figs. 17.3 E, F, 17.4 A–C).

Treatment of onychodystrophy is by chiropody or surgery. Chiropody may be successful for a considerable period but does not result in a curve. It comprises cutting, drilling or filing of the nail plate so as to reduce its stiffness and allow it to remain coapted to the nail bed. The debris under the paraungual regions must also be removed. Surgery may be necessary.

Operative Technique. Under local anaesthesia with an elastic tourniquet, the aim is to oblate the nail, excise the soft tissue margins of the nail fold in the distally keratinised and hypertrophied part of the tuft of the terminal phalanx and resect the cornified hypertrophied proximal nail root and protuberant basal apophyses. The nail bed is reconstituted by flattening the surface of the phalanx distally and laterally to the nail bed so as to enlarge the distal extremity of the toe. Surgery must be followed by regular chiropody to control and guide the reposition of the nail. Oil must be applied in order to lubricate the bed of the reconstituted nail until complete repositioning has been achieved.

17.1.5 Onychomycosis

The nail tissue is invaded by dermatophytes or yeasts (Fig. 17.3 I, L).

According to Achten (1964), infection by *Trichophyton rubrum* is three times as frequent as that by other agents, e.g. *Trichophyton mentagrophytes* and *Candida albicans*. Children are much less frequently affected than adults. The condition may be a complication of fungal infection between the toes which may have been present for several years. Transmission is rarely direct, usually via the ground, and is favoured by warmth, alkaline conditions and above all, dampness from sweat. Several nails may be involved, and the multiplicity of attacks makes the condition difficult to cure (see Chap. 4).

There is usually no pain or discomfort in the early stages.

An attack begins on any nail, the most frequent site being along the free border or a lateral border. The lesion is characterised by the appearance of little opaque stains, at first whitish but then becoming yellowish and irregular, which rapidly provoke separation of the nail and accumulation of subungual debris. Yellowish stripes may appear parallel or perpendicular to the longitudinal axis of the nail. Sometimes the infection totally involves the nail bed, which thickens, deforms, and separates at the site of the yellowish stains with accumulation of cornified debris under these separated areas. The condition develops very slowly but progressively until finally the whole of the nail, its bed and the surrounding soft tissues are involved and there is variable superinfection. The nail eventually disappears, leaving a mass of waxy keratinised debris.

Treatment. Medicinal treatment comprises oral administration of nystatin or amphotericin in the case of yeast infections, griseofulvin in dermatophyte infections. Chiropody includes filing of the nail and excision of the loose parts separated by debris, together with the application of local fungicides (dimethylsulphoxide and others). Surgery comprises excision of the nail and curettage of the nail and is followed by local application of fungicides until complete regrowth of the nail, aided by chiropody, has been achieved. This treatment may have to continue for several years, being complemented by general treatment when the mycosis is due to

Candida albicans. A mycogram is indispensable in determination of the most useful antibiotic treatment.

17.2 Nail Bed

17.2.1 Subungual Exostosis

This condition is seen most frequently in the adolescent, less frequently in the infant and only exceptionally in the adult (Fig. 17.5 I, M). Most cases are due to trauma, usually a crush injury, although microtrauma provoked by shoe pressure can be responsible. The great toe is affected most frequently, followed by the fourth, third, second and (rarely) fifth toes. Two sorts of exostosis occur:

17.2.1.1 Diaphyseal Exostosis

This small, benign tumour can be osteocartilaginous, chondromatous or bony and arises in the middle part of the dorsal face of the terminal phalanx, or occasionally to one side. In the latter instance it may provoke soft tissue granulations which confuse the diagnosis. It presents as a small, roundish swelling, always very hard, which produces pain on walking or at rest, especially from shoe pressure. Its size usually corresponds to that of the toe. When it is central, it elevates the whole nail plate, which bulges.

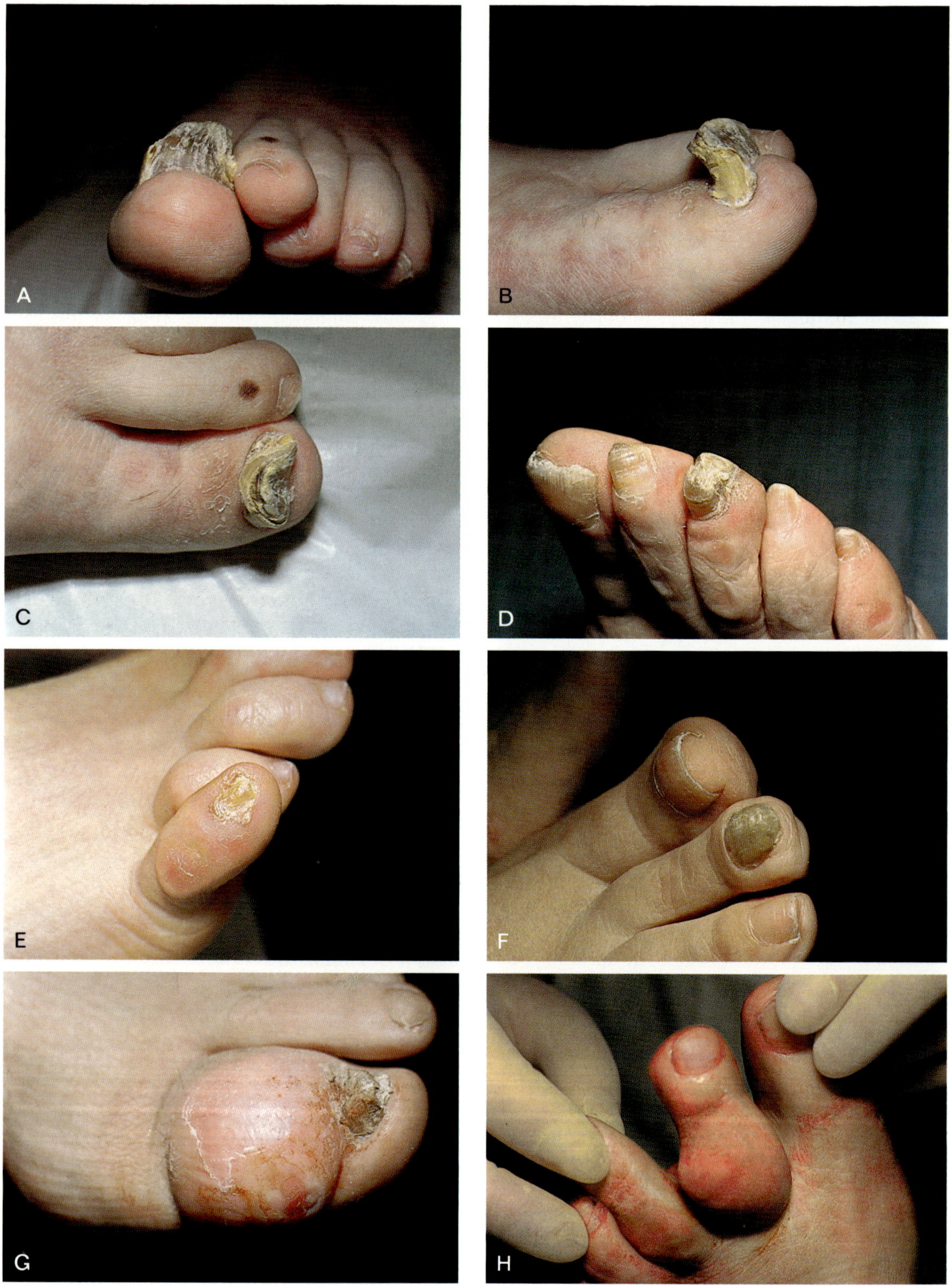

Fig. 17.4 A–K. Onychodystrophy and claw toes. **A–C** Onychauxis, onychorrhexis. **D–F** Traumatic onychodystrophy. **E** Onychodystrophy due to rubbing and pressure. **G–I** Tophaceous gout. **J, K** Quintus varus with ▷ supraductus. **I–K** see p. 233

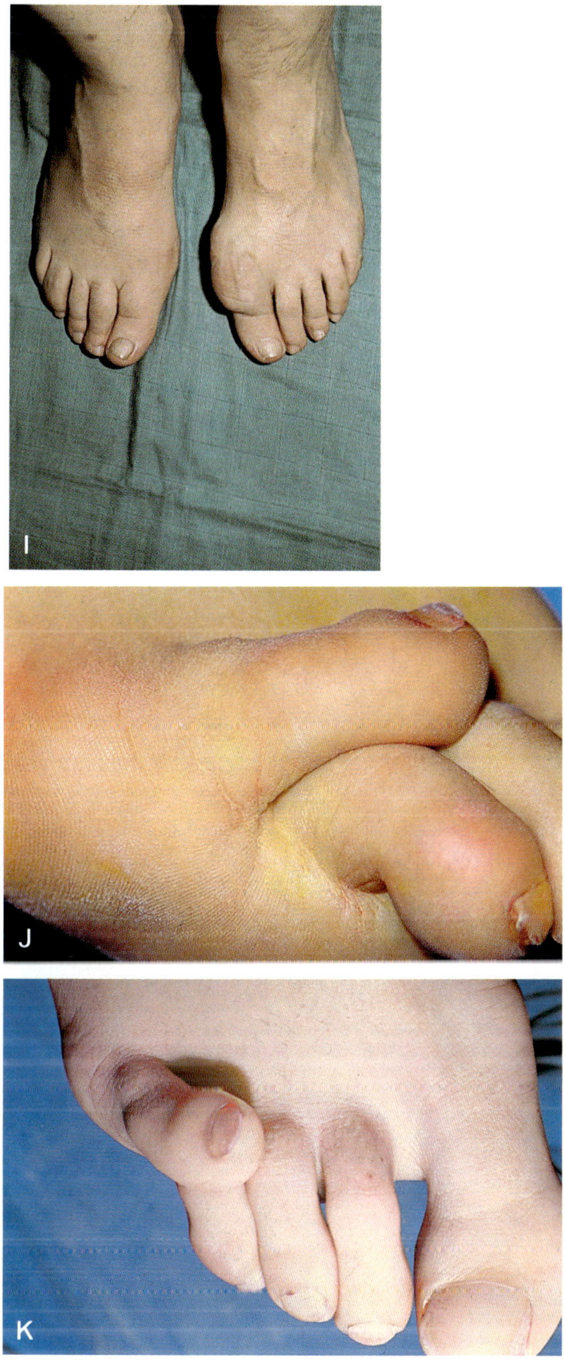

Fig. 17.4 I–K. Legend see p. 232

When situated more proximally, it may elevate the free border of the nail and the hyponychial skin. On the lateral borders of the nail, the fold becomes obliterated by the development of granulation tissue. The skin in the hyponychial area may become thin, whitish due to epidermal reaction and perhaps cornified, thereby producing further confusion with a diagnosis of distal corn or verruca. The skin is usually thin, red and ulcerated. The small hard tumour can be palpated.

Radiography (Fig. 17.6) may show the exostosis as (a) a tuft with a wide base, (b) more flattened with a zone of posterior attachment, or (e) spiculate, usually lateral, developing at the junction of the lateral and dorsal surfaces of the bone.

Treatment comprises removal under local anaesthesia with a tourniquet. In the case of a central exostosis, a shark-mouth incision across the hyponychium on the terminal aspect of the toenail allows development of the dorsal plane on the bone at the level of the stratum germinativum of the nail bed. The exostosis is resected using cutting forceps, and after careful curettage and cleaning, the skin is sutured. In a lateral exostosis, the first step is longitudinal resection of the lateral overlying portion of the nail, followed by complete ablation of the exostosis, curettage of its base, and closure of the skin as in the operation for ingrown toenail, suturing it to the mucosa of the nail bed below the lateral border of the nail (Duries 1959).

17.2.1.2 Distal Epiphyseal Exostosis

Usually seen on the dorsal extremity of the distal phalanx of the great toe, under the free border of the nail, this lesion develops at the expense of the lateral border of the tuft. It is a small, heaped-up, bony tumour characterised by extreme pressure pain from the upper of a hard shoe and often not detected. Elevation of the nail does not occur, and there is no obvious change in the surface except for the presence of a small, brownish stain indicating traumatic haematoma provoked by the wound in the nail bed. The skin under the free border of the nail is acutely tender on palpation.

Radiography shows the small, heaped-up spicule from the tuft and indicates its true nature.

Treatment is by surgical removal under local anaesthesia, using a tourniquet. Distal transverse incision of the hyponychium allows resection with nibblers and levelling of the tuft of the phalanx.

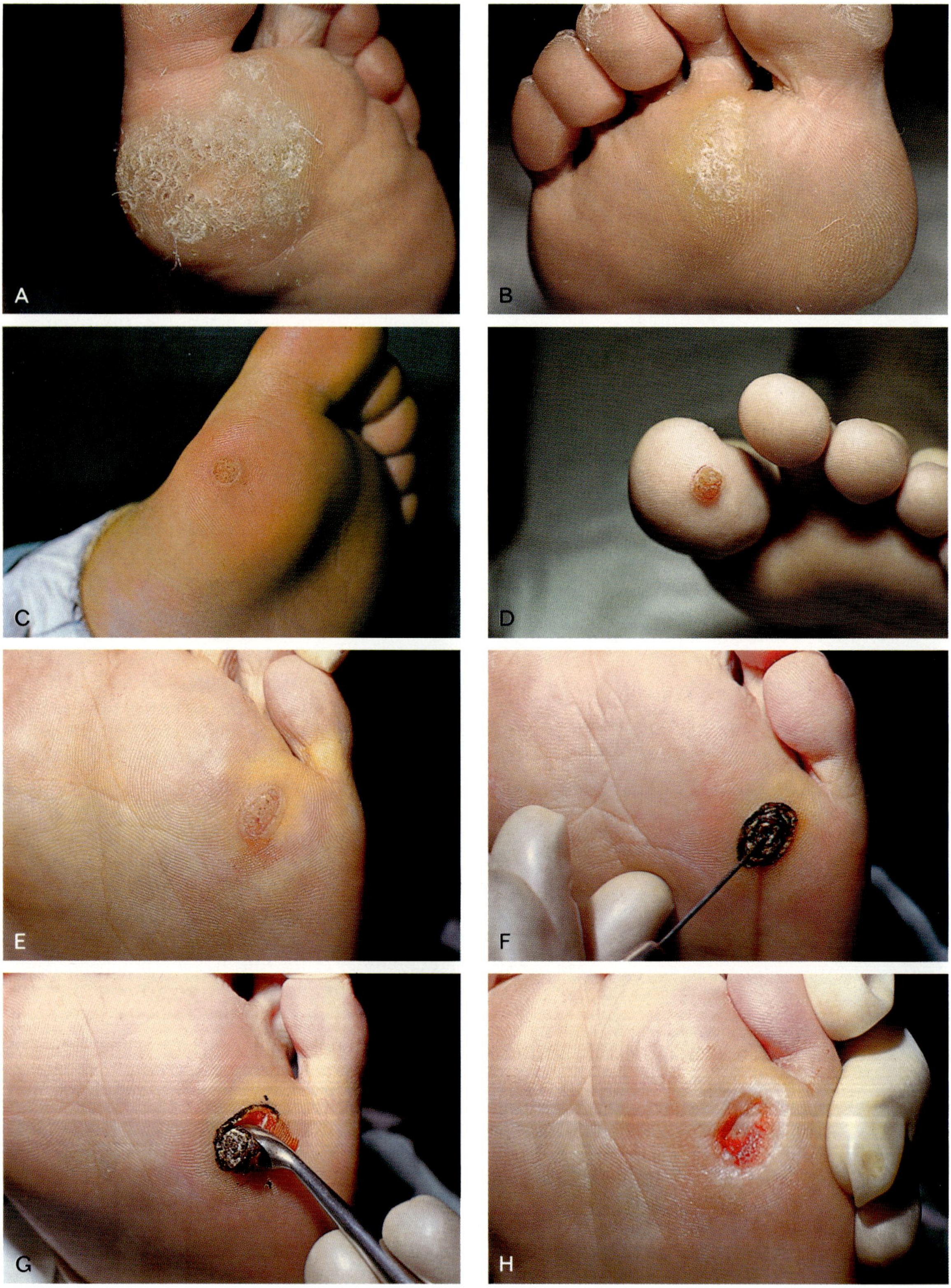

Fig. 17.5 A–M. Verruca. **A–E** Plantar verruca. **F** Electrocoagulation. **G** Curettage with care to protect underlying dermis. **H** Trimming of hypertrophied epidermal borders. **I** Subungual osteochondroma. **J** Verruca hidden by massive callus formation. **K, L** Koenen tumour. **M** External subungual exostosis. **I–M** see p. 235 ▷

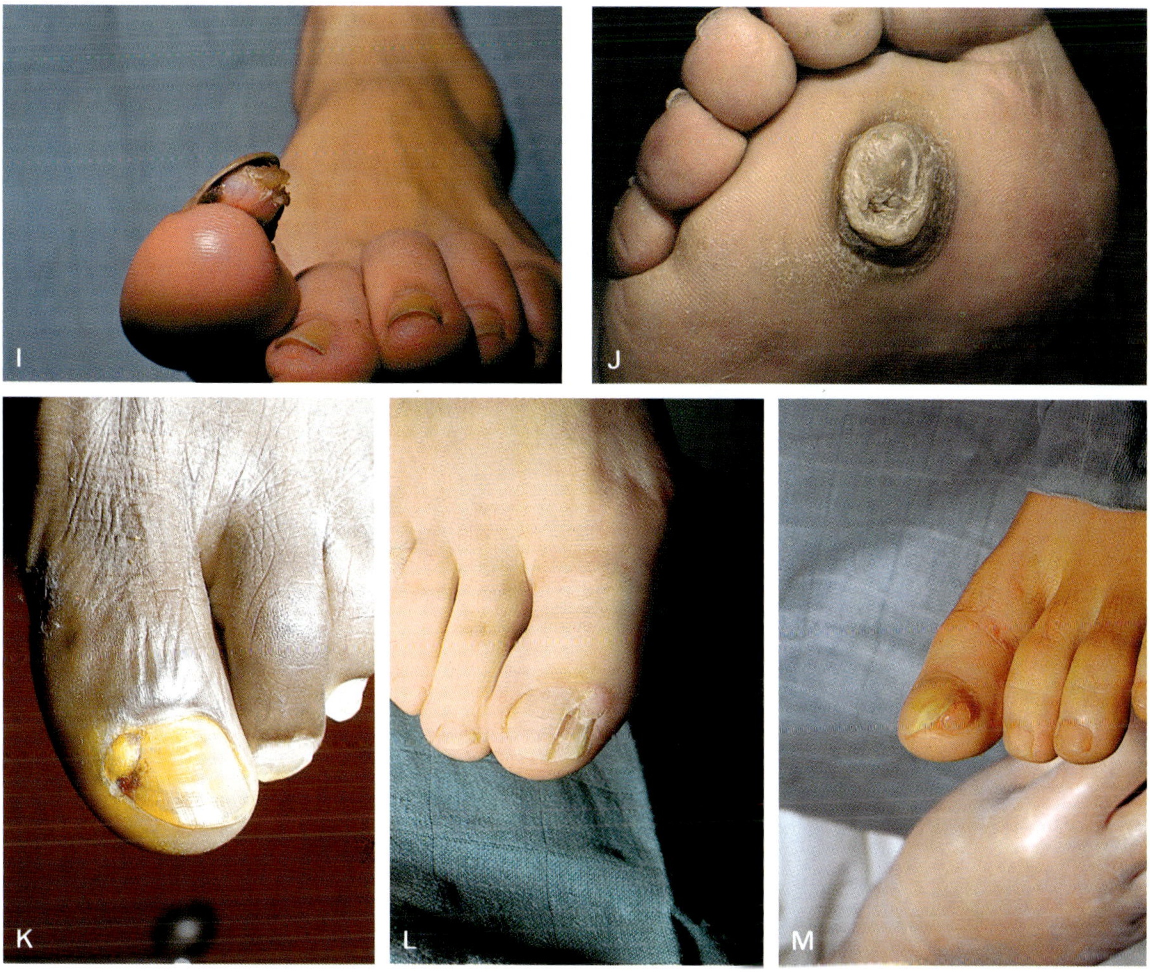

Fig. 17.5 I–M. Legend see p. 234

17.2.2 Subungual Chondroma

Subungual chondroma is similar in presentation to dorsal diaphyseal exostosis. Only its smooth, rounded, regular form distinguishes it clinically, and its chondromatous nature is confirmed histologically.
Treatment is the same as for dorsal exostosis but it is necessary to curette the base of the tumour with even greater care so as to prevent recurrence, which is otherwise common.

17.2.3 Angioneuromyoma

Described by Masson (1924), this lesion is also known as glomus tumour and has in addition been called perithelioma (Müller 1901), haemangiopericytoma and subcutaneous painful nodule (Wood 1812) [cited by Pierre (1978)]. It develops from arteriovenous glomus, such glomi being very numerous in the nail bed - 10–20 cm^2 according to H. Bureau [in Pierre (1978)]. It is very rare, presenting as a single tumour ranging in size from a pinhead to a grain of rice, rarely larger, and being multilobulate, regular, encapsulated, and benign. It can be seen as a red, violaceous or blue spot under the nail bed and is characterised by exquisite pain, which is sometimes spontaneous but is provoked by the least pressure, cold or heat. Occasionally it can be confused with a subungual corn, but it is distinguished by the severe pain and the reddish colour.
Treatment is by surgery under local anaesthesia. The nail is separated from its bed, and complete excision of the tumour should be verified by magnification in case lobular prolongations should be present. The nail is replaced on its bed and held in place by a compressive dressing or by two transverse sutures.

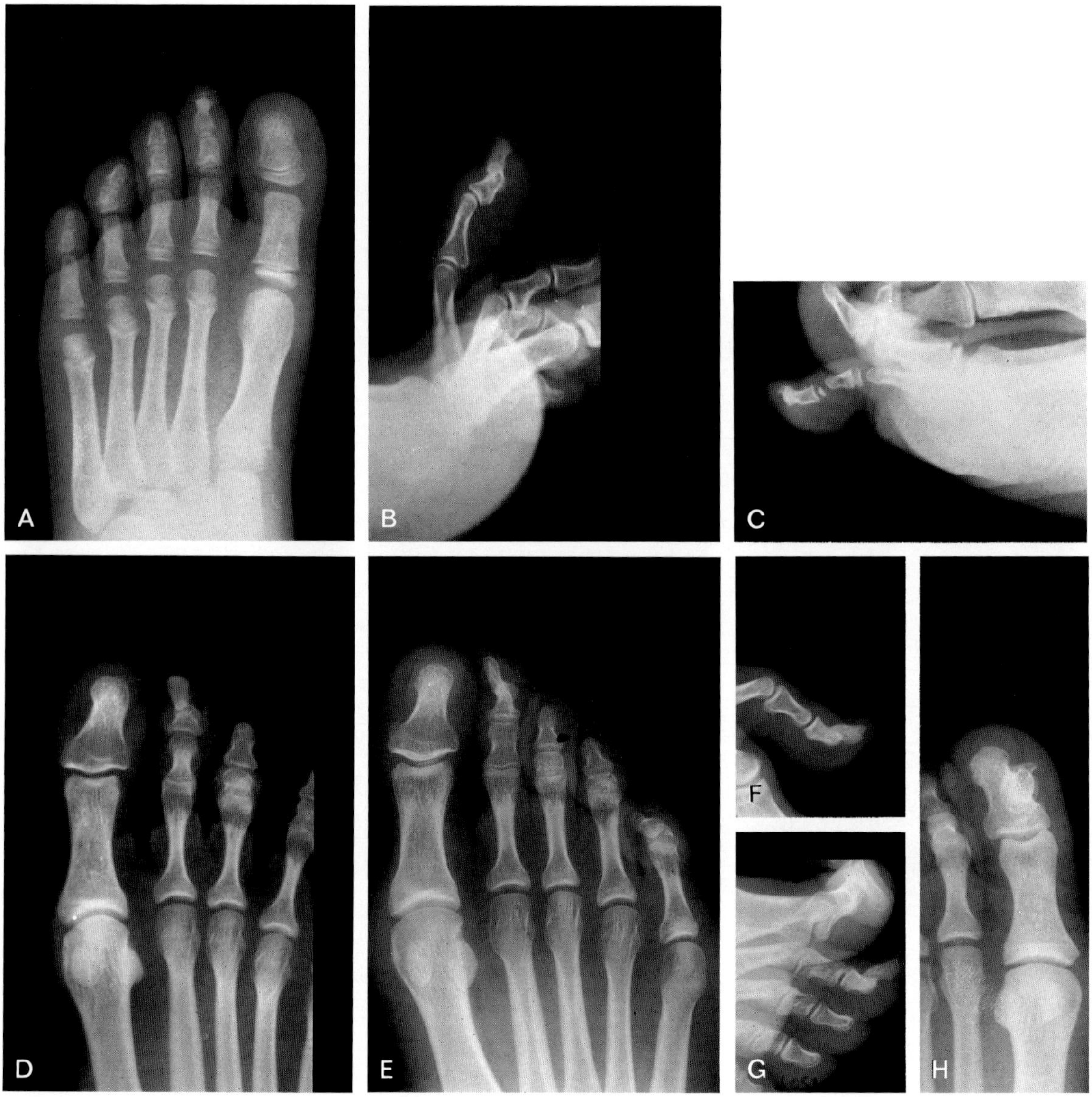

Fig. 17.6 A. B. Subungual exstosis of distal phalanx of second toe. **C** Exostosis of distal phalanx of third toe. **D, E** Exostosis of distal phalanx of second toe. **F, G** Subungual exostosis. **H** Dorsolateral exostosis of distal phalanx of great toe. **I** Plantar exostosis of distal phalanx of great toe. **J** Spiculate subungual exostosis of tuft of distal phalanx of great toe. **K** Lateral plantar exostosis of distal phalanx of third toe. **L, M** Dorsolateral subungual exostosis of terminal phalanx of great toe. **N** Subungual osteochondroma of distal phalanx of great toe. **O, P** Dorsal ▷ subungual exostosis of great toe. **Q** Dorsomedial subungual exostosis of great toe. **R** Dorsal subungual exostosis of great toe. **S** Dorsal exostosis of distal phalanx of great toe. **T** Dorsal subungual exostosis of great toe. **U** Medial subungual exostosis of distal phalanx of great toe. **V, W** Subungual chondroma of great toe. **I-QQ** see pp. 237-239

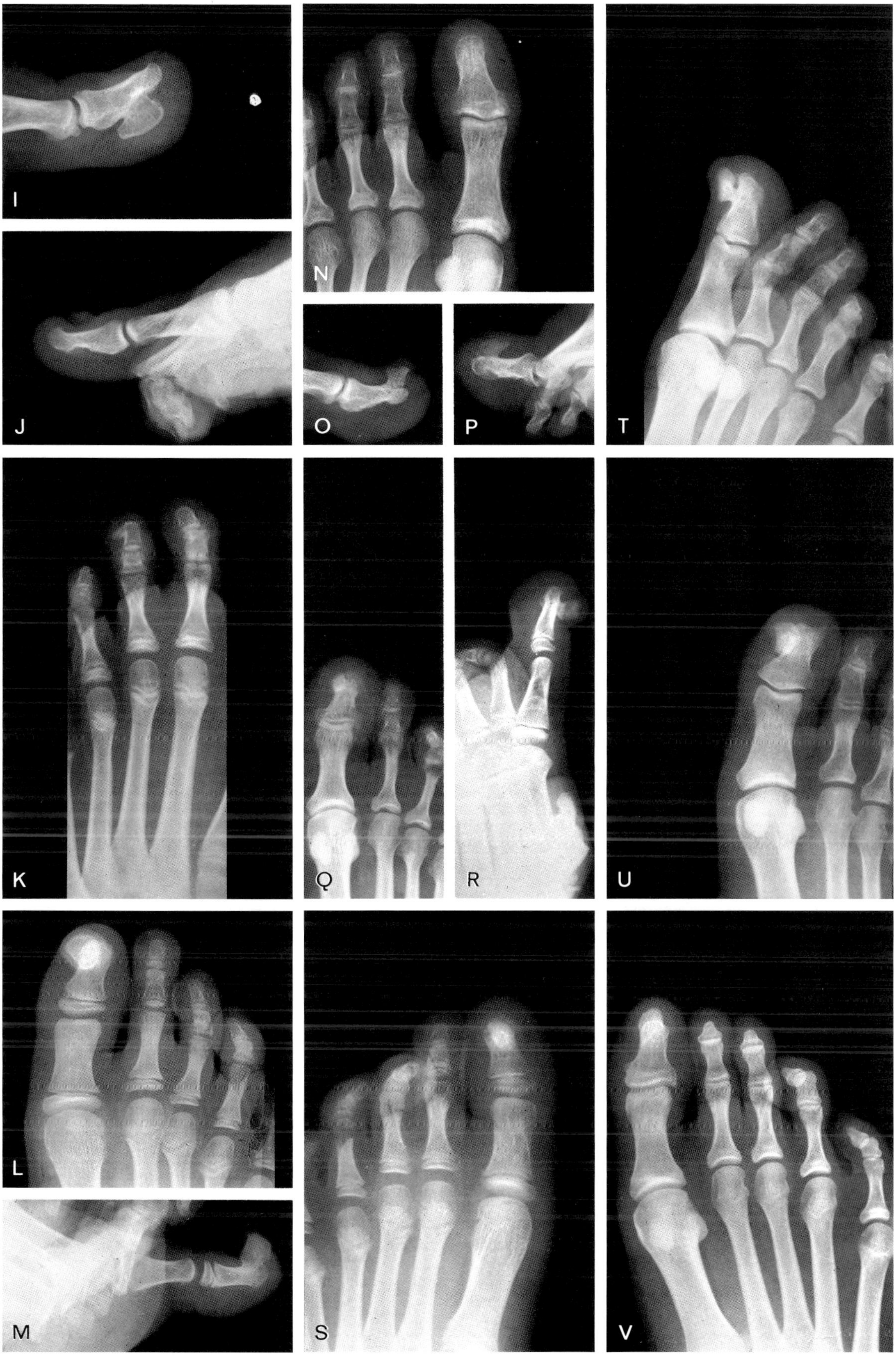
I
J
N
O
P
T
K
Q
R
U
L
M
S
V

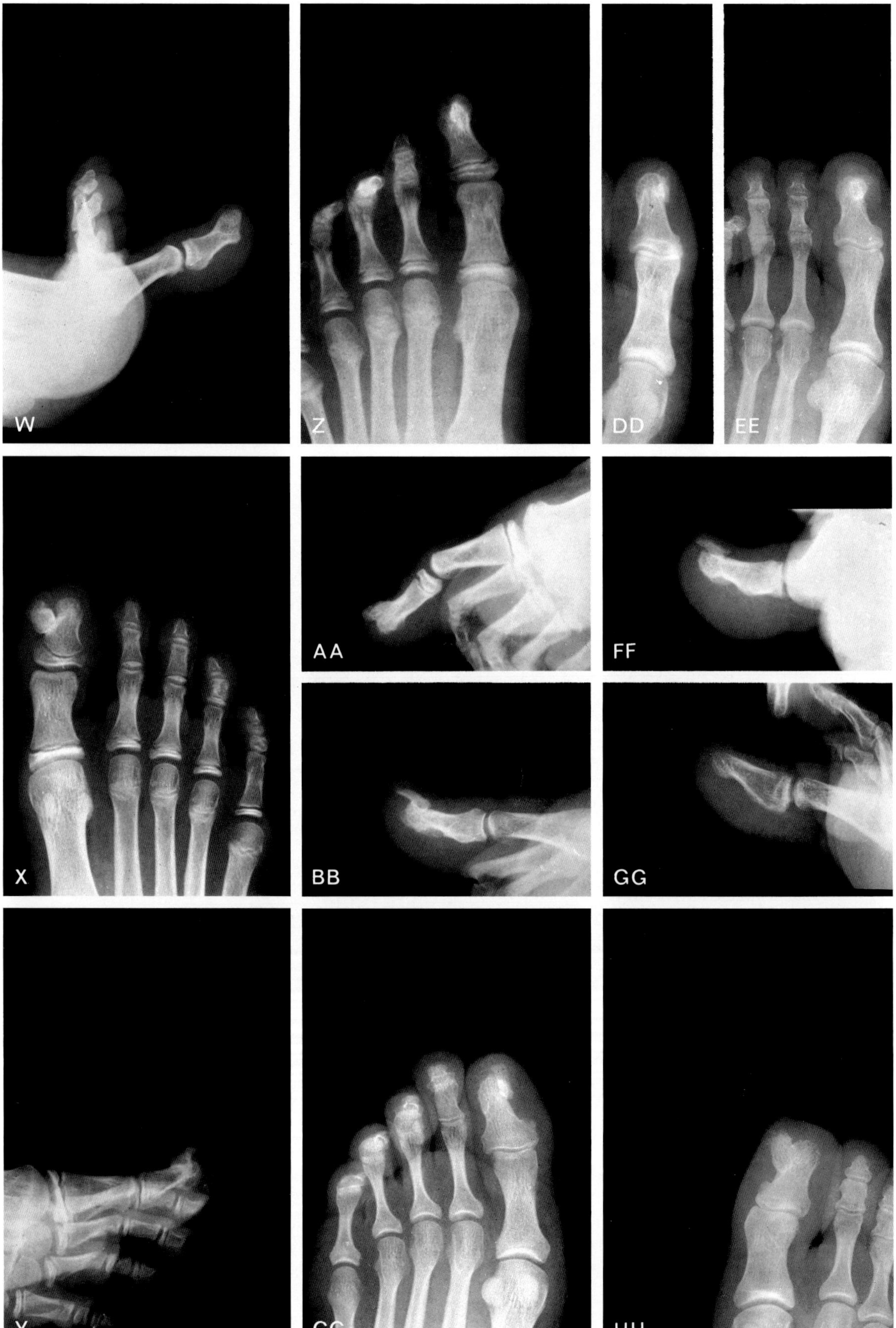
W
Z
DD
EE
X
AA
FF
BB
GG
Y
CC
HH

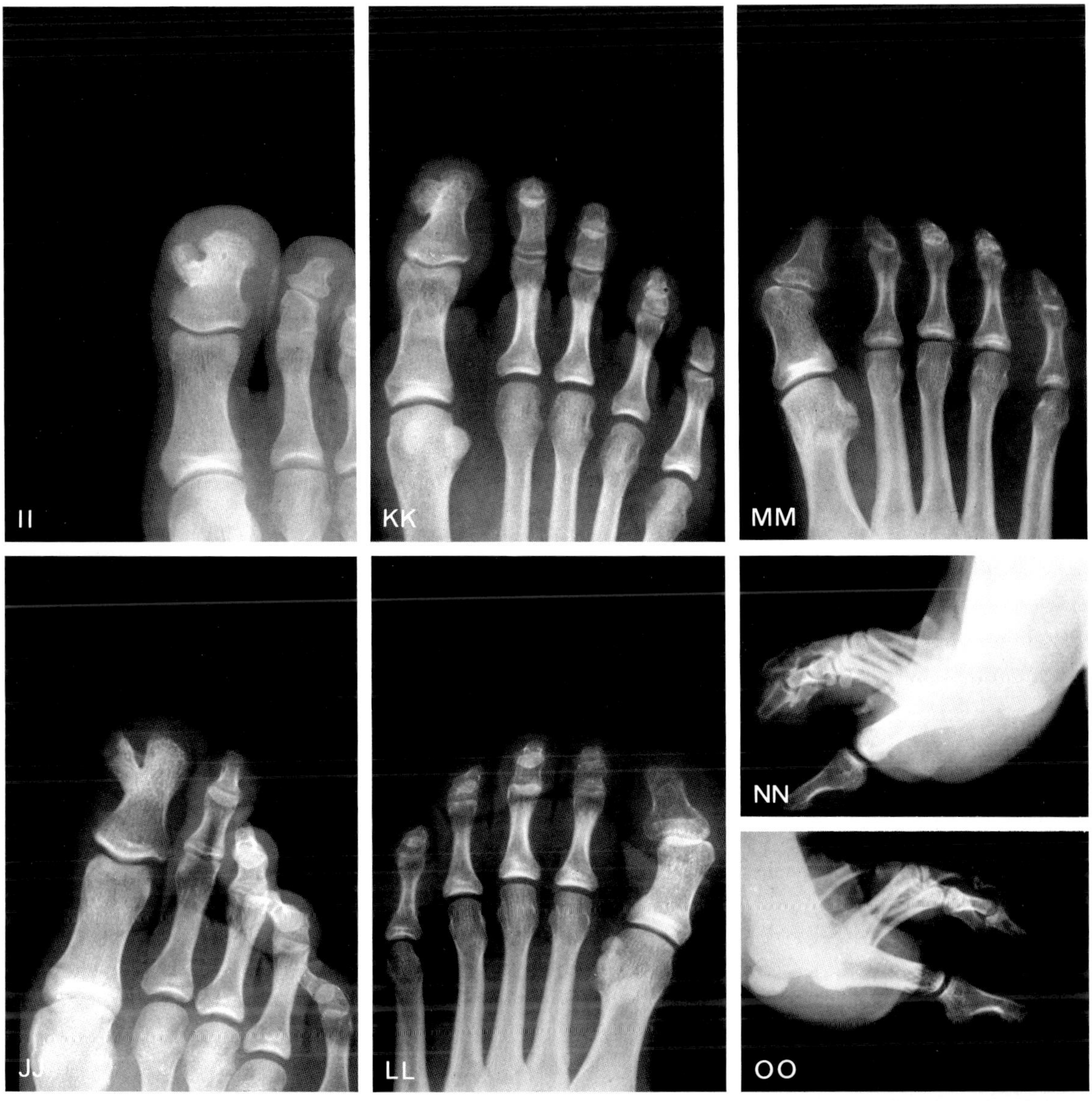

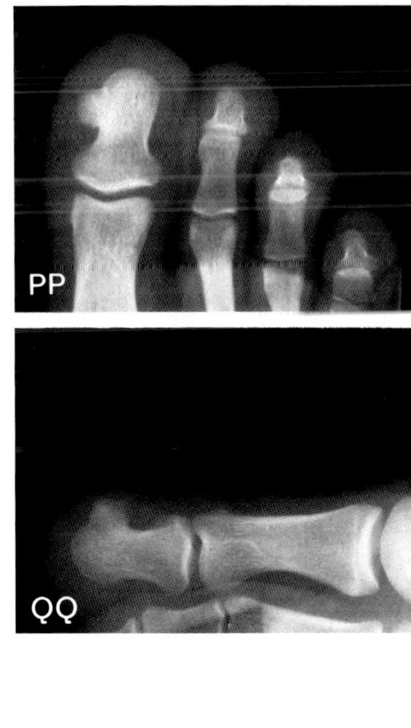

◁ **Fig. 17.6** *(continued)*. **X** Medial subungual exostosis of great toe. **Y** Dorsal subungual exostosis of great toe. **Z** Subungual osteochondroma of great toe. **AA, BB** Subungual exostosis of great toe. **CC** Medial subungual exostosis of great toe. **DD, EE** Medial subungual exostosis of great toe, pre- and postoperative. **FF, GG** Dorsal subungual exostosis, pre- and postoperative. Various forms of medial subungual exostosis. **LL, MM** Transverse deformity of third toe. **OO, PP** Enostosis on plantar aspect of base of proximal phalanx of great toe

17.2.4 Subungual Corn

A subungual corn consists of a small mass of avascular keratinised tissue, developing most frequently a few millimetres behind the free border of the nail. It may be provoked by a tiny spiculate exostosis on the tuft of the phalanx, and appears as a white area under the nail plate. Excision of the cornified tissue and the related exostosis cures the condition.

17.2.5 Subungual Haematoma

Chronic or acute trauma may lead to the development of subungual haematomas of varying size, ranging from a small speck to one so large that it may cause separation of the whole nail from its bed. In sportsmen, "tennis toe" may extend to the subungual region. Microtrauma from shoe pressure or from wearing an excessively high heel may also be the cause. The condition may be painless, the patient noticing only the red or purplish staining which gradually darkens to black, and advances progressively towards the end of the nail with growth, eventually disappearing and leaving a normal plate. Alternatively, the lesion may be painful, with yellow or dirty-white discoloration due to suppuration, and may therefore present as an apical infection with all the signs and symptoms of inflammation.
Treatment must include tetanus prophylaxis. Surgical intervention is a minor procedure (Wallet 1933), comprising the drilling of two holes into the nail plate and evacuation of the haematoma. The cavity should be cleansed using alcohol or physiological saline and irrigation of antiseptic solution through the holes. In the case of a dessicated haematoma, which may be very painful, resection of the separated part of the nail should be performed under local anaesthesia. The cavity is then cleansed as above.

17.3 Nail Fold

Conditions of the nail fold not produced by disorders of the nail plate include the following.

17.3.1 Nail Fold Corn

Commonest on the great and fifth toes, this corn can cocur in any. On the great toe it presents as a mass of keratinous, white or greyish punctiform tissue in the depths of the fold and is produced by pressure from the side of the nail. In the fifth toe it is softer on the outer aspect, flattened, yellowish and tends to widen the nail plate at its site near the root; here it is very painful and permanent.
Treatment by chiropody involves removal of the cornified mass of tissue and resection of the lateral border of the nail, which usually allows it to settle. Fashioning of a longitudinal furrow in the centre of the nail plate reduces the pressure exercised by the borders of the nail. When chiropody fails, resection of a narrow vertical band along the margin of the nail, similar to that for ingrown toenail, produces cure.

17.3.2 Koenen Tumour

This lesion, a variety of tuberous sclerosis, was described by Bourneville (1880, 1900), Koenen (1932) and more recently by Galmiche (1983) and Martin (1981) (Fig. 17.5 K, L). It is a subungual tumour developing at the level of the nail root and presenting on the inner or outer aspect. It is lozenge-shaped, about the size of a rice grain, possibly lobulated, of soft consistency and usually lies in the gutter of the nail fold. It is very frequently found in the fifth toe, but may occur elsewhere.
Treatment comprises excision and resection of the part of the nail root involved.

17.3.3 Para-Ungual Verruca

This lesion presents with all the characteristics of a papillomatous verruca: rounded appearance, yellowish colour, surface punctate with little brown or black points, soft consistency. Lying in one of the nail folds or under the free border of the nail, it is tender on pressure or collateral compression. It has a tendency to bleed.
Treatment is by electrocoagulation and curettage, should chiropody fail.

17.4 Skin

17.4.1 Digital Corn

Digital corns may be classified according to site (cf. Figs. 18.2, 18.7).

Dorsal Corn. This variety comprises a small regular mass in the epidermis developing between the skin and the subjacent bone. The lesion is rounded, ses-

sile and tends to spread over a bed of cornified tissue subjacent to a serous bursa. It is situated on the dorsal face of the proximal or distal interphalangeal joints over the heads of the proximal or middle phalanges. It is induced by claw toe deformity affecting these parts and results in pain or inflammation which may lead to ulceration.
Treatment is by arthroplasty or arthrodesis of the proximal or interphalangeal joints.

Lateral or Interdigital Corn. This lesion develops on the lateral faces of the proximal or distal interphalangeal joints or in the interdigital commissure. It may present as a keratinous mass or as a "partridge eye" characterised by a nucleus in the centre of a whitish zone. One particular example of the "partridge eye" appearance occurs in the commissure of the fourth interdigital space where there is a white or dirty-grey flattened mass in the epidermis, without precise limits, which may be either hard and cornified or soft, and can be confused with interdigital mycosis. The most frequent site is on the inner aspect of the base of the fifth toe where the corn is painful on pressure on the outer side of the toe. Palpation detects a bony protuberance which provokes the condition, most often located on the external aspect of the apophysis of the base of the proximal phalanx of the fifth toe.
Treatment may be conservative, involving ablation of the epidermis bed and protection of the area with felt in front of the corn. Failure necessitates surgery, which comprises simple removal of the underlying bony prominence or perhaps resection arthroplasty of the nearby joint.

Distal or Pulp Corn. In this condition the cornified mass, presenting as a conical or flattened callosity, is a true callus provoked by compression of the pulp against the ground over the distal extremity of the terminal phalanx. It is associated with claw or hammer deformity of the proximal and distal interphalangeal joints, which results either from swan-neck deformity or from excessive length of a toe with respect to its neighbours, and is markedly painful. Inflammation occurs gradually and eventually results in ulceration, and persistence leads to hypertrophy of the end of the toe associated with a seropurulent discharge which ceases only after relief of compression.
Treatment is by chiropody, comprising excision of the protective keratinous mass and subsequent protection from pressure. When this fails, the claw deformity must be corrected by surgery, namely arthrodesis of either the distal or the proximal interphalangeal joint or of both.

Plantar Digital Corn. This cornified yellowish or whitish mass, rounded in contour, develops in relation to a bony projection. It is rarely keratinous. Frequently, an inverted claw deformity - mostly affecting the middle phalanx, more rarely the proximal phalanx - has resulted in a prominence on the plantar aspect.
Treatment is chosen according to whether there is claw deformity of the proximal phalanx. If so, mobilisation of the metatarsophalangeal joints should be associated with arthrodesis of the proximal interphalangeal joint or arthroplasty of this and the distal interphalangeal joint. If not, arthrodesis of the distal interphalangeal joint alone may be adequate.

*17.4.2 **Digital Verruca***

Digital verrucas, which can arise in any portion of the toe, have the same characteristics as plantar verrucas (see Chap. 14.5.2) (Fig. 17.5 C, D).

*17.4.3 **Chilblain***

Girls, young women and elderly people are most commonly affected by chilblains, the appearance of which on one or several toes during autumn and winter is favoured by humidity and the wearing of waterproof shoes. There may be a limited cutaneous lesion in the pulp, similar to chilblains of the plantar aspect of the forefoot, or the whole toe may be involved. The lesion is characterised by swelling, a violaceous appearance, smarting, pricking or burning pain which varies in intensity and is aggravated by compression, shoes or damp cold weather. Rarely, an ischaemic condition leads the patient to consult his doctor at an early stage because of the marked pain involved.
Treatment comprises measures to improve the circulation. These include administration of oligosols, vitamin C and D supplements and flavonides; application of anti-inflammatory and vasodilatory creams; improvement of shoe fitting, eliminating wrinkles; morning massage with alcohol; and careful drying with talc.

17.5 Joints

Painful conditions of the toe joints are due to local compression which results in inflammation and relates to deformities which produce bony prominences and associated corns, callosities, hygromata

and subcutaneous bursitis. The joints themselves may be painful if dislocated or subluxed, and trauma may have produced fractures involving the joint surfaces. The latter can be associated with epiphyseal detachment.
It is convenient to divide these painful disorders into five categories (Fig. 17.7): clawing of the great toe; clawing of the lesser toe (clinodactyly); transverse deformations of the toes (camptodactyly); digital subluxation or dislocation; articular fractures.

17.5.1 Clawing of Great Toe

Longitudinal cavus deformity of the whole foot, with or without dropped forefoot, is commonly associated with clawing of the great toe (cf. Fig. 18.7 E). Whether this is correctable or fixed, the posture leads to static problems of overloading. Bursitis or callosity develops under the first metatarsal head, although this may be a consequence of the supinated position of the forefoot associated with a varus reaction. On the dorsal aspect, blistering from shoe pressure or corn formation may occur at the summit of the claw deformity, while compression of the extensor hallucis longus tendon, which tends to bowstring, may produce marked discomfort, especially in females.
Two subvarieties exist. In the first, the great toe develops a hammer deformity with a hygroma over the dorsal aspect of the interphalangeal joint. The metatarsophalangeal joint remains supple, and despite slight contracture of the long extensor tendon, full plantarflexion at the metacarpophalangeal joint remains possible. *Treatment* comprises arthrodesis of the interphalangeal joint associated if necessary with capsulotomy of the dorsal aspect of the metatarsophalangeal joint. Interphalangeal arthroplasty is not advised because of the risk of recurrence of the deformity (cf. Fig. 17.7).
The second variety is the Z-deformity involving contracture of the dorsal capsular tissue of the metatarsophalangeal joint. When of short duration, this does not produce any distortion of the base of the proximal phalanx; the plane of the articular surface remains perpendicular to the longitudinal axis of the bone. Realignment can be achieved by elongation of the extensor tendons and dorsal capsulotomy on either side. However, when the Z-deformity of the toe has been present for several years, the base of the proximal phalanx undergoes hypertrophy on its plantar aspect, producing an exostosis. There is, as a result, obliquity of the surface of the base of the proximal phalanx, a feature which prejudices stability and correction. *Treatment* must be more extensive, including elongation of the extensor tendons, capsulotomies, and arthroplasty of the metatarsophalangeal joint by means of osteotomy of the base of the phalanx and incorporation of an osteocartilaginous graft, thereby restoring correct alignment and stability. It is often necessary to maintain the toe in line with the metatarsus by temporary insertion of a pin through the phalanges until consolidation of arthrodesis of the interphalangeal joint has been achieved.

17.5.2 Clawing of Lesser Toe

Claw deformities of the lesser toes may be divided into four categories:

Flexion Contracture of Proximal Interphalangeal Joint. Commonly there is a callosity over the prominent proximal interphalangeal joint, the toe adopting a claw deformity with the proximal phalanx dorsiflexed at the metatarsophalangeal joint and the distal interphalangeal joint remaining properly aligned. The deformity may be fixed or correctable, and may be associated with subluxation of the metatarsophalangeal joint. Capsular contracture on the dorsal aspect of the metatarsophalangeal joint with shortening of the long tendons is aggravated by contracture of the lumbricales, the interossei and the skin on the dorsal aspect of the metatarsophalangeal joints and the plantar aspects of the interphalangeal joints. *Treatment,* when the condition is correctable, comprises relatively simple operative measures: arthroplasty of the proximal interphalangeal joint and arthrodesis of the distal interphalangeal joint. In the case of a fixed contracture, arthrotomy of the metatarsophalangeal joint with collateral releases and elongation of the tendons by VY-plasty of the dorsal skin is necessary. The extensor tendons must also be elongated. Finally, arthroplasty of the proximal interphalangeal joint – or preferably arthrodesis in the case of the great and second toes – is performed. The long and short flexor tendons must be detached.

Flexion Contracture of Distal Interphalangeal Joint. In this condition the metatarsophalangeal and proximal interphalangeal joints are mobile, although at the latter there may be a correctable flexion posture. *Treatment* is by arthrodesis, performed from the dorsal aspect. An ellipse of skin, tendon and capsule is excised, and after resection of the joint surfaces the resulting new surfaces are coapted by a U-shaped wire loop.

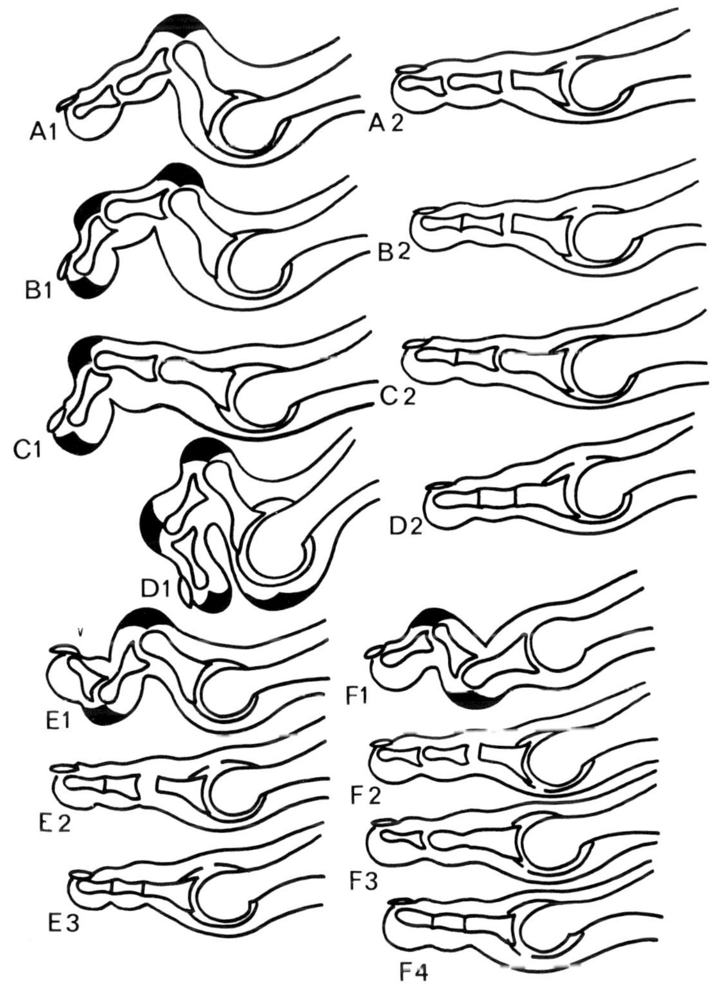

Fig. 17.7. **A** Simple clawing of proximal interphalangeal joint: *1* Before treatment; *2* after arthroplasty. **B** Clawing of proximal and distal interphalangeal joints: *1* Before treatment; *2* after arthroplasty of proximal interphalangeal joint and arthrodesis of distal interphalangeal joint. **C** Clawing of distal interphalangeal joint (hammer toe): *1* Before treatment; *2* after arthrodesis. **D** Combined flexion contracture of proximal and distal interphalangeal joints: *1* Before treatment; *2* after arthrodesis of both joints. **E** Reversed claw deformities of toe with dorsal callosity over proximal interphalangeal joint and plantar callosity under distal interphalangeal joint: *1* Before treatment; *2* after arthroplasty of proximal interphalangeal joint and arthrodesis of distal interphalangeal joint; *3* after arthrodesis of both joints. (Both procedures accompanied by dorsal capsulotomy of the metatarsophalangeal joint.) **F** Reversed claw deformities of toe with plantar callosity under proximal interphalangeal joint and dorsal callosity over distal interphalangeal joint: *1* Before treatment; *2* after arthroplasty of proximal interphalangeal joint; *3* after arthrodesis of proximal interphalangeal joint; *4* after arthrodesis of both joints. (All procedures accompanied by plantar capsulotomy of metatarsophalangeal joint)

Flexion Contracture of Both Proximal and Distal Interphalangeal Joints. Callus forms over the prominent dorsal aspects, perhaps associated with a third callosity on the tip of the toe from compression against the ground. As well as painful pressure over the prominent joints, nail deformities, thickenings and inflammations can develop. The toe becomes very clawed and fixed, with hyperextension at the metatarsophalangeal joint due to capsular contraction associated with shortening of the flexor tendons and contracture of the plantar skin. The skin over the dorsal aspect of the metatarsophalangeal joint is contracted, and the extensor tendons are shortened. *Treatment* comprises arthrotomy of the metatarsophalangeal joint, release of the collateral ligaments and the overlying skin, elongation of the extensor tendons and arthrodesis of the proximal and distal interphalangeal joints.

Inverted Claw Deformity Due to Plantarflexion at the Proximal Interphalangeal Joint and Dorsiflexion of the Distal Interphalangeal Joint. In this condition, pain arises from pressure over the proximal joint dorsally and from the corns or callosities which develop on the plantar aspect of the distal interphalangeal joint. The metatarsophalangeal joint remains in a normal position. A reverse situation can exist in which the proximal interphalangeal joint is dorsiflexed while the distal interphalangeal joint is plantarflexed, (i.e. a swan-neck deformity). There is always contracture of the short flexor tendon. *Treatment* comprises division of the short flexor tendon from the middle phalanx, arthrodesis of the proximal interphalangeal joint with removal of a bone wedge based dorsally and arthrodesis of the distal phalangeal joint with removal of a wedge based inferiorly. Alternatively, arthroplasty of the proximal interphalangeal joint with arthrodesis of the distal phalangeal joint may be successful.

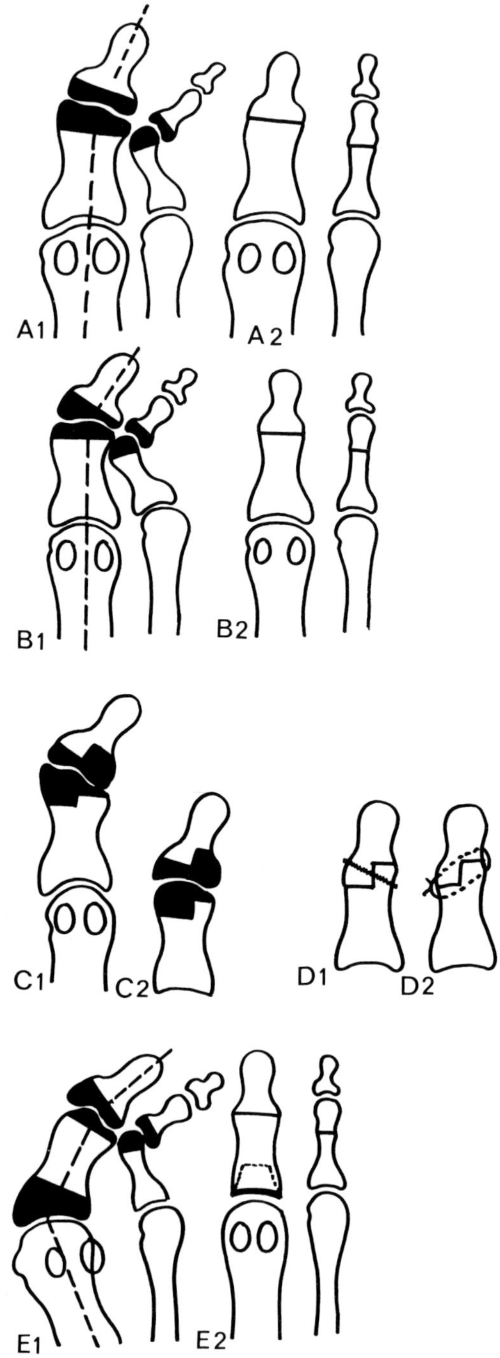

Fig. 17.8. A Transverse clinodactyly of interphalangeal joint of great toe, affecting principally head of proximal phalanx, and swan-neck deformity of second toe: *1* Before treatment; *2* after interphalangeal arthrodeses. **B** Transverse clinodactyly of same joint, affecting principally base of distal phalanx, again with swan-neck deformity of second toe: *1* Before treatment; *2* after interphalangeal arthrodeses. **C** *1, 2* My technique of interphalangeal arthrodesis. **D** Fixation: *1* Screw or pin; *2* nylon suture. **E** Interphalangeal arthrodesis of great and second toes for hallux valgus: *1* Before treatment; *2* after treatment

17.5.3 Transverse Deformities: Clinodactyly

It is convenient to subdivide transverse deformities into two well-defined clinical entities: (a) valgus deformity of the distal phalanx of the great toe associated with swan-neck deformity of the second toe (Fig. 17.8) and (b) transverse deformity of the middle three toes (Fig. 17.9).

17.5.3.1 Transverse Deformity of Great Toe

There is valgus deviation of the distal phalanx which may be associated with some general degree of hallux valgus. The deformity most often arises in the head of the proximal phalanx, as can be confirmed on X-ray, and treatment must be related to this part. Less frequently, it arises at the base of the distal phalanx, near the junction of the proximal and middle thirds.

Valgus deviation of the great toe is commonly associated with swan-neck deformity of the second toe. The two must be studied together and treatment directed at both. The swan-neck deformity may be congenital in origin or may be acquired when shoe pressure produces collapse of the toe. The proximal phalanx is dorsiflexed, and subluxation of the metatarsophalangeal joint tends to occur. Depression of the second metatarsal head breaks the normal concavity of the anterior transverse arch and encourages callus formation underneath. The middle phalanx is plantarflexed and is deviated lateral-

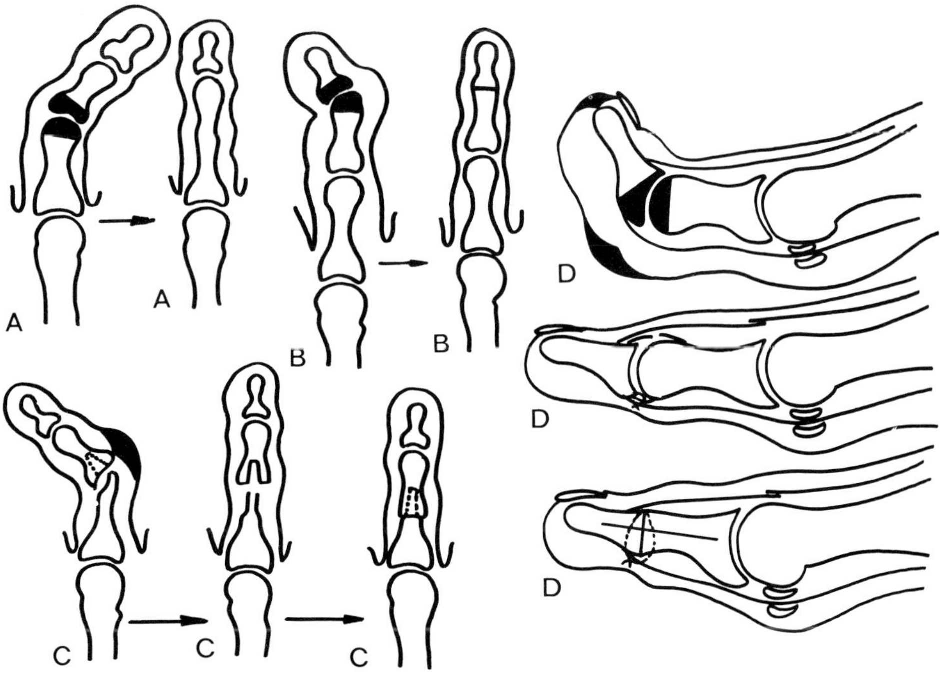

Fig. 17.9. **A** Transverse clinodactyly of proximal interphalangeal joint: *1* Before treatment; *2* after arthrodesis. **B** Transverse clinodactyly of distal interphalangeal joint: *1* Before treatment; *2* after cuneiform arthrodesis. **C** Iatrogenic transverse clinodactyly of proximal interphalangeal joint: *1* Before treatment; *2, 3* enclavement arthrodesis of proximal interphalangeal joint (my own technique). **D** Dorsiflexion contracture of interphalangeal joint of great toe: *1* Before treatment; *2* after treatment by interphalangeal arthroplasty with elongation of extensor hallucis longus; *3* after interphalangeal arthrodesis with cuneiform resection of interphalangeal joint. Fixation is with a nylon suture through the resected bone ends and a Kirschner wire under or inside the phalanges

ly by pressure from the great toe. Secondary pressure on the outer aspect of the joint produces narrowing like an hourglass. The dorsal surface is painful from shoe pressure and presents with a callus. The distal phalanx is spared all pressure from both sides and tends to swell like a club. There may be callus formation on the extremity of the pulp, on account of the continuous pressure from the hard sole of the shoe, and there is secondary deformity of the nail, which becomes widened, thickened and striated.

While tendon contracture may be the original cause of the swan-neck deformity, there is little doubt that it can be aggravated or precipitated from abnormal position of the toe in the shoe. Ankylosis of the joints occurs progressively. Shortening of the long extensor tendon produces the dorsiflexion deformity of the metatarsophalangeal joint, while more distally, its two slips of insertion dislocate plantarwards, thereby flexing the interphalangeal joints, reversing their normal extensor action, maintaining fixed flexion. The condition tends to be progressive. The lumbricales normally balance this tendency, but their action becomes distorted by the sagging of the transverse arch and reversal occurs, contributing to the fixed flexion contracture.

A congenital predisposition to the condition is evident from the fact that hammer toe can be seen in a small child or in a person who has never worn shoes. Molière [cited by Regnauld (1956)] suggests that an initial laxity of the intermetatarsal ligaments provokes collapse of the anterior arch and allows the proximal phalanx to develop a dorsiflexion posture. Kirmission (1908) and Ombredanne (1949) consider that abnormal valgus deviation of the proximal epiphysis of the phalanx, affecting its basal, plantar segment, forms an enostosis which leads to hyperextension of the proximal phalanx and secondary flexion contracture of the middle phalanx. There is no proof that hyperlaxity of the ligaments is the cause, but it is reasonable to suppose that swan-neck deformity is related to other etiological factors, including the following:

1. Cavus deformity of the foot in which the unbalanced arch stretches the extensor mechanism and encourages the claw position of the toe.

2. Injudicious choice of footwear for a child, resulting in cramping of the foot and compression of the toes, affecting predominantly the second toe because of its length.
3. The wearing of high heels tends to drive the forefoot into a wedge-shaped shoe, perhaps elegant but altogether disastrous.
4. Other shoes may exert similar combined pressure on the great and fifth toes, producing a tendency towards hammer deformity in all of the lesser toes. This is most marked in the second toe, which adopts passive swan-neck deformity as a result of pressure from the neighbouring toes, i.e. varus in the lateral three toes and valgus in the distal phalanx of the great toe.

Observations during operations for valgus deviation of the great toe show that the insertion of the extensor hallucis longus on the distal phalanx tends to lie more laterally than normal, thereby encouraging a valgus posture of the distal phalanx of the toe. Pressure is exercised on the outer side by the shoe, and a bony deformity develops in the interphalangeal joint due to loss of normal compression on the internal half of the joint, according to the law described by Delpech stating that bony hypertrophy is likely to occur in such unloaded circumstances. Enostosis, once developed, will fix the valgus posture permanently. There is little doubt that the wearing of shoes aggravates any pre-existing congenital tendency to the deformity. The frequent association of valgus of the great toe with the swan-neck deformity raises the question of which is the primary condition; if the valgus deformity of the great toe is primary, it probably originates in the abnormal external insertion of extensor hallucis longus, but if the swan-neck deformity is primary, the valgus of the great toe is due to loss of the prop normally afforded by the second toe. The latter is seen also in cases of aplasia or amputation of the second toe.

Clinically, after one of these two deformities has been diagnosed and the pressure signs of callus formation have been noted, it may be useful to inspect the general shape of the foot for possible cavus deformity, pes planus, and Egyptian toe configuration, such factors influencing the choice of treatment. It should be noted whether the deformities of the great and second toes are reducible. The swan-neck configuration may be classified as follows:

First degree: The swan-neck deformity is slight and manually reducible in extension and there is no associated dorsal callus formation over the proximal interphalangeal joint or in the pulp, apart perhaps from a small area of congestion corresponding to a point of friction from the shoe, the site of a future corn.

Second degree: The swan-neck deformity is obvious and irreducible. There is an associated small dorsal callus, but the whole length of the toe is visible from above.

Third degree: Typical swan-neck deformity is fixed by tendinous and fibrous retraction and cannot be reduced. Calluses over the dorsal aspect and the tip of the toe are present and painful, and the extremity of the toe cannot be seen from above because it is tucked under. The middle portion of the toe is swollen due to pressure, and occasionally there is vascular insufficiency.

Radiographic examination must include dorsoplantar and lateral views, which will confirm the presence of any bony swelling at the medial side of the base of the distal phalanx of the great toe, the site of the transverse deviation (i.e. base of distal phalanx or head proximal phalanx) and the degrees of angulation.

The severity of the valgus deformity may be graded as follows:

1. Slight valgus of the distal phalanx. This may be treated by chiropody and shoe adjustment.
2. Angulation of the distal phalanx on the proximal not exceeding 5°. Treatment may be by soft tissue release.
3. Valgus deviation of between 10° and 20°. This is the most frequent state and necessitates a bony procedure.

General assessment includes oscillometry of the lower limbs, and operation should be conducted after antitetanus vaccination.

Operative treatment is directed at both the great toe and the commonly associated swan-neck deformed second toe. In the great toe, if the valgus stems from the head of the proximal phalanx and is not accompanied by contracture of the extensor hallucis longus tendon, interphalangeal arthroplasty can be performed but may result in discomfort on motion. Especially in the presence of contracture of the long extensor tendon, arthrodesis of the interphalangeal joint is preferable. Another possibility is cuneiform resection at the neck of the proximal phalanx with the base of the wedge lying medially. If the valgus stems from the base of the distal phalanx, arthrodesis of the interphalangeal joint is indicated, accompanied by resection of an appropriate bony wedge together with elongation of extensor hallucis longus. Either intervention must be associated with elongation of the long extensor tendons.

The swan-neck deformity of the second toe may be corrected by simple tenotomy of the flexor tendons together with plantar capsulotomy extended on either side of the proximal interphalangeal joint. If the structures on the plantar layer are too contracted, however, arthroplasty or arthrodesis of the proximal interphalangeal joint is required. During arthroplasty, it may be necessary to excise the head of the proximal phalanx in order to relax the soft tissues and reduce the length of the toe, which will continue to buckle if cramped in the shoe.

17.5.3.2 *Clinodactyly of the Lesser Toes*

Occasionally this deformity affects the proximal interphalangeal joints, in which case resection of the head of the proximal phalanx or, better, arthrodesis of the joint corrects the deformity and maintains stability. In a majority of cases, however, the transverse deviation arises in the distal interphalangeal joint, the terminal phalanx then displaying valgus or varus. This posture is usually accompanied with some degree of plantarflexion contracture, and is associated with under- or overriding of a neighbouring toe. Discomfort is produced by compression at the summit of the angulation, where callus or even an ulcer forms, and occasionally there is painful para-ungual corn formation. *Treatment* then comprises either cuneiform arthrodesis directed at correcting the valgus or varus posture or arthrodesis by a peg and socket technique. A particular cause of deformity is unsuccessful phalangeal arthroplasty. Scarring and bone hypertrophy contribute, and the apposed ends of the bone become eburnated and irregular. Fresh attempts at arthroplasty by further resection may realign the long axis of the toe but encourage further instability; relapse is almost inevitable. For this reason, *treatment* by peg-and-socket arthrodesis is advised. The peg is driven into the base of the middle or distal phalanx and fixed by a small pin until consolidation is assured.

17.5.4 **Dislocation**

Dislocation can affect any of the joints of the toes, and may be provoked by microtrauma from shoe pressure, in which case it is seen most commonly at the metatarsophalangeal joint with dorsal and lateral displacement of the proximal phalanx. Other possible causes are direct trauma or failure of interphalangeal arthroplasty. Capsular contracture maintains the malposition, and lateral clawing of the toe may occur, especially after failed arthroplasty. Symptoms are produced from pressure over the most prominent aspect of the toe. *Treatment* varies according to the site.

Dislocation of a metatarsophalangeal joint necessitates elongation of the contracted overlying dorsal skin by VY-plasty, elongation of the extensor tendons, lateral and dorsal capsulotomy, mobilisation of the joint if adhesions have occurred and subsequent correction of any fixed displacement of the related interphalangeal joints.

Interphalangeal dislocations, when plantarwards, require correction of the irreducible claw deformity by arthroplasty or arthrodesis accompanied by any necessary tendinous elongations. Failed arthroplasty can present greater difficulties, due to scarring and fragmentation of the distal end of the proximal phalanx. As above, a fresh attempt at arthroplasty should be avoided and the peg-and-socket technique of arthrodesis employed.

Dorsiflexion deformity at the interphalangeal joint of the great toe may accompany hallux rigidus, but in this instance mobilisation of the metatarsophalangeal joint will correct the deformity. It is not necessary to do anything other than occasional capsulorrhaphy on the plantar aspect of the interphalangeal joint. This deformity often exists in the Egyptian foot configuration and may be associated with hyperlaxity of the ligaments.

Dorsiflexion contracture of the distal segment of the toe may be associated with permanent shortening of the extensor hallucis longus tendon and the development of painful onychogryphosis, subungual exostosis, or a plantar callosity under the interphalangeal joint. *Treatment* of the latter conditions includes Z-elongation of the extensor hallucis longus tendon through a longitudinal incision or alternatively transverse wedge excision of skin and tendon through the capsule of the joint from the dorsal aspect. In the latter operation, care must be taken that the incisions are rigorously perpendicular to the longitudinally running structures, and correction is maintained by non-absorbable sutures passed through two small vertical holes through the base of the distal phalanx. During healing, correction is maintained by a pin inserted axially, close to the plantar face of the two phalanges. Skin, tendon and capsule are sutured in one block. Healing is achieved after 6 weeks and walking without rolling onto the toes is permitted after 1 month.

17.5.5 Osteochondral Fractures

Osteochondral fractures result from direct trauma, hyperflexion or torsion. One particular type involves damage to the articular surface of the proximal phalanx of the fifth toe and is seen in dancers. The following forms may be considered:

Fracture of distal end of phalanx. When there is no significant displacement, treatment is usually by a simple elastic dressing. Otherwise, arthroplasty by resection of the head of the phalanx or arthrodesis of the interphalangeal joint is necessary.

Comminuted fracture of end of a phalanx. This should be treated by resection of the damaged part. Conservative treatment by immobilisation nearly always leads to bony hypertrophy and stiffness, the deformity from the hypertrophy producing pressure symptoms.

Avulsion fracture of articular surface of an interphalangeal joint. This again necessitates removal of the fragment. Further resection to restore alignment may be necessary. Arthrodesis may be safer than arthroplasty.

17.6 Summary of Operative Procedures

At the proximal interphalangeal joint, arthroplasty, arthrodesis or articular reconstruction by head-shaft enclavement of the proximal phalanx may be considered. At the distal interphalangeal joint, arthrodesis is always preferred because it ensures permanence of corrections with stability in a part subject to lateral pressure from the shoe and perhaps under strain from the wearing of high-heeled shoes.

Arthroplasty. Whenever an arthroplasty is performed, it is essential that muscle balance is restored by tendinous elongation and alignment of the proximal phalanx, secured appropriately by capsulotomy of the metatarsophalangeal joint. The procedure may be one part of the general management of a foot in which weight-bearing properties have been altered as a result of subluxation of the bases of the phalanges and contracture of the long and short extensor tendons and the flexor tendons. Arthroplastic resections of the toes must be fashioned so as to re-establish the parabola of normal digital propulsion and alignment of the metatarsal heads (Lelièvre 1952). Frequent reference to the toes is made in other chapters. When arthroplasty involves only one toe, phalangeal resection must be limited so as not to produce too much shortening. Failure to observe this rule results in claw deformity or hammer toe deformity of the then relatively overlong adjacent toes. Arthroplasty does not assure long-term stability of a toe. When in doubt, it is preferable to resort to resection arthrodesis.

Arthrodesis of Interphalangeal Joints. As stated, arthrodesis of the proximal interphalangeal joint is safer when severe tendinous contractures are present, e.g. in swan-neck deformity of the second toe or claw deformities of the third and fourth toes, especially when there is axial torsion or lateral deformity. An even stronger rule is that arthrodesis must be chosen at the distal interphalangeal joint; the likelihood of failure from other techniques is too great.

Enclavement. This, my own technique (Regnauld 1968), is indicated in claw toes in the young subject or the sportsman, for after adequate elongation of the tendons it allows full amplitude of interphalangeal movement (see Chap. 42).

18 Disorders of the Great Toe

18.1 Hallux Valgus

18.1.1 Description

The term hallux valgus is incomplete, for the condition is overall a clinodactyly of the first ray. Nevertheless, the more usual name will be used in this account.

Hallux valgus is a deformity of the forefoot which is seen more frequently in women than in men. It will be emphasised repeatedly that surgical correction depends totally on an exact understanding of the genesis of the deformity of the first ray and the complex interdependent abnormalities involving tendon, capsule and bone. The neglect of one element risks failure of treatment. The outward deviation of the great toe is associated with a varus posture of the metatarsal and it is the latter which is the more primitive factor, becoming irreversible as a result of subluxation of the underlying sesamoid bones. The angulation at the metatarsophalangeal joint results in the formation of an exostosis on the medial aspect of the head of the first metatarsal adjacent to the oblique base of the phalanx and, secondarily, various deformities of the adjacent lesser toes, including varus, clawing and valgus. Stretching of the abductor muscle of the great toe and the medial capsule of the metatarsophalangeal joint, contracture of the lateral aspect of the capsular ligament, contracture and lateral displacement of extensor hallucis longus and outward displacement of the sesamoids all contribute to the permanence of the condition (Fig. 18.1).

In its early stage, the valgus posture of the great toe is influenced largely by the long extensor and flexor muscles. Their tension maintains the displacement, bowstringing the metatarsophalangeal joint and aggravating the beginnings of the valgus. Contraction of the short flexors and of the transverse and oblique heads of the adductor muscle drags the sesamoid bones outwards and posteriorly. The load from the weight of the body accentuates the varus of the first metatarsal, the lateral subluxation of the base of the proximal phalanx and the medial displacement of the metatarsal head; abductor hallucis subluxes towards the plantar aspect and causes pronation of the great toe.

This involvement of the first ray of the foot leads to changes in the posture of the lesser toes (Fig. 18.2). The great toe presses against the next three toes, sometimes resulting in valgus angulation of the metatarsophalangeal joints or dorsiflexion leading to clawing; mixed deformities can occur. The long extensor and short extensor tendons to all of the toes bowstring laterally, accentuating the deformity. External and dorsal subluxation of the phalangeal bases inevitably follows. Finally, the deformities become fixed by capsular and tendinous contractures. Occasionally, the great toe underrides the second toe, and in this instance clawing and varus deformity of the latter can develop. The adjacent third and fourth toes follow suit. The involvement of the three central rays results in lowering of their metatarsal heads and contractures of the long extensor and short extensor tendons. Arthralgia relating specifically to one or more metatarsophalangeal joints may be associated with callus formation underneath affected metatarsal heads. In a more advanced stage, inflammatory arthritis and osteophytic arthrosis of the joints develop. In general, the forefoot takes on a flat triangular or convex triangular form.

The complex interrelations of hallux valgus with disordered weight bearing have been demonstrated by Chiappara and Berardi (1976), who drew attention to the displacement of the line of load bearing progressively towards the medial side of the foot. A general lowering of the longitudinal arch to second or third degree pes planovalgus occurs (see Chap. 16.1.5), and it is essential to appreciate that a real cause of hallux valgus lies in this abnormality: the *flat* valgus foot. This must be corrected at the outset, realigning the normal line of loading in the axis of the *second* metatarsal before any attempt is made to correct the more obvious forefoot deformity.

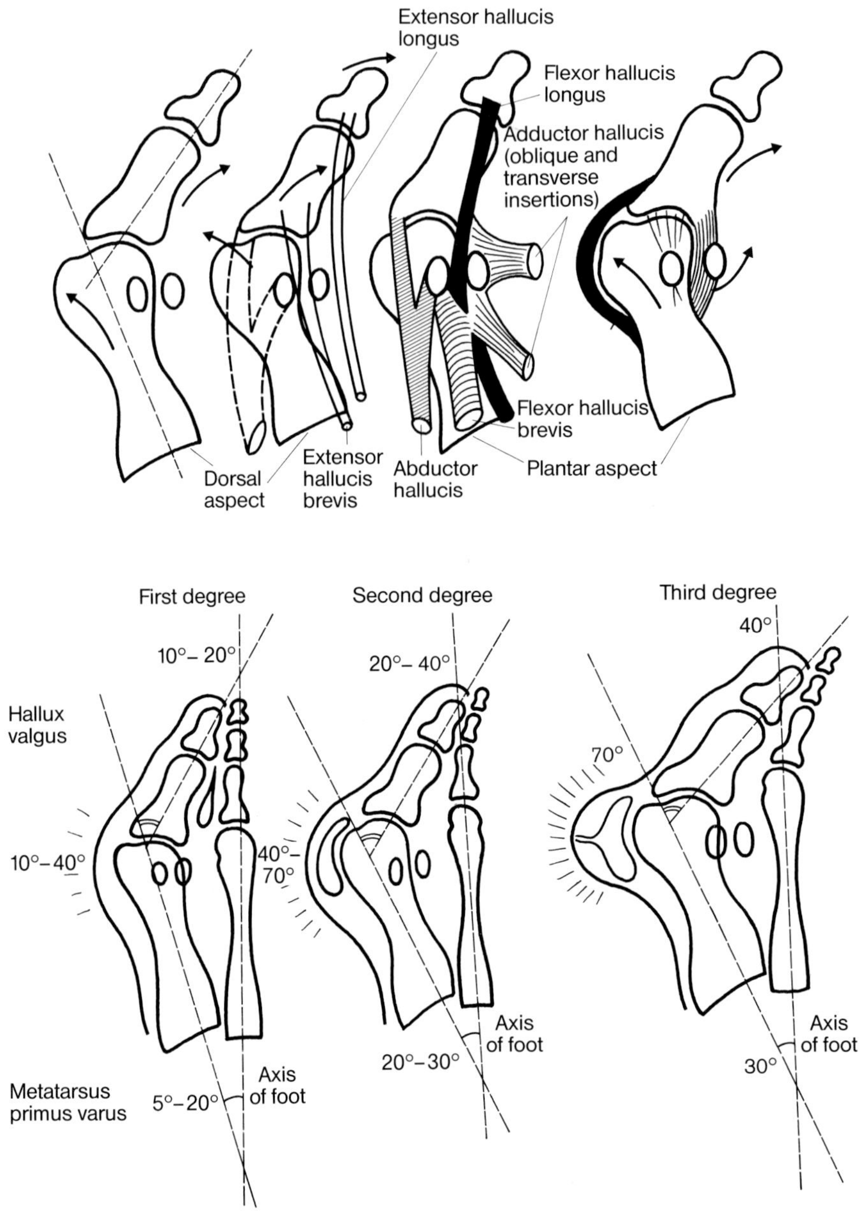

Fig. 18.1. Hallux valgus and metatarsus primus varus (*arrows* indicate displacement)

Fig. 18.2 A–G. Claw toes. **A** Third-degree hallux valgus with second toe clawed and in varus with supraductus. **B** Egyptian forefoot: first-degree hallux valgus, second toe supraductus, third toe infraductus, irreducible clawing of fourth and fifth toes. **C** Third-degree hallux valgus with supraductus of second and third toes and supple clawing of fourth and fifth toes. **D** Third-degree hallux valgus with valgus and clawing of outer toes. **E** Irreducible clawing of fifth toe in pes cavus. **F** Hallux valgus with erectus from failed previous operation accompanied by dorsal dislocation of metatarsophalangeal joints of outer toes with clawing. **G** Third-degree hallux valgus with irreducible clawing of second toe in varus and supraductus and dorsal corns on third and fourth toes ▷

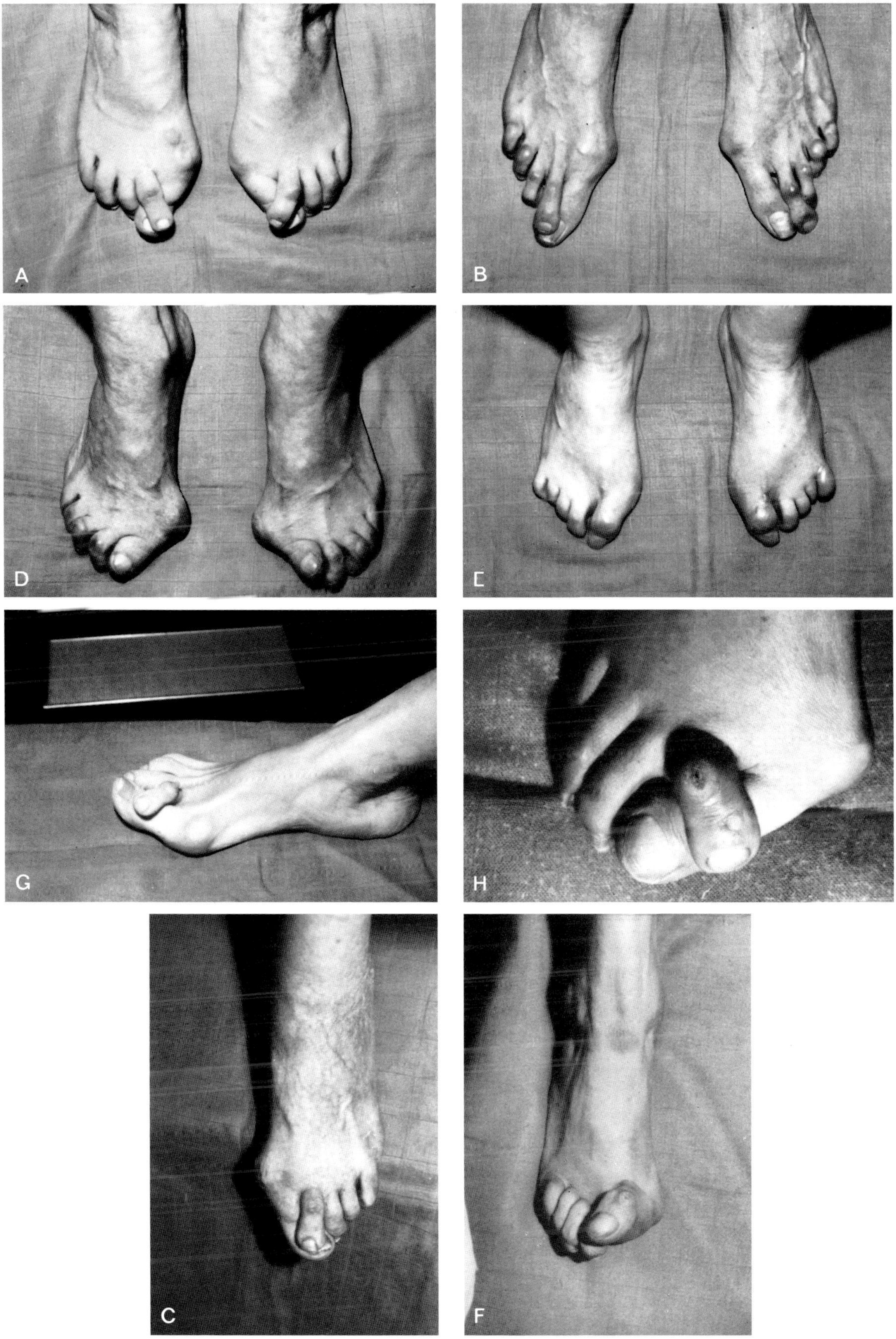
A
B
D
E
G
H
C
F

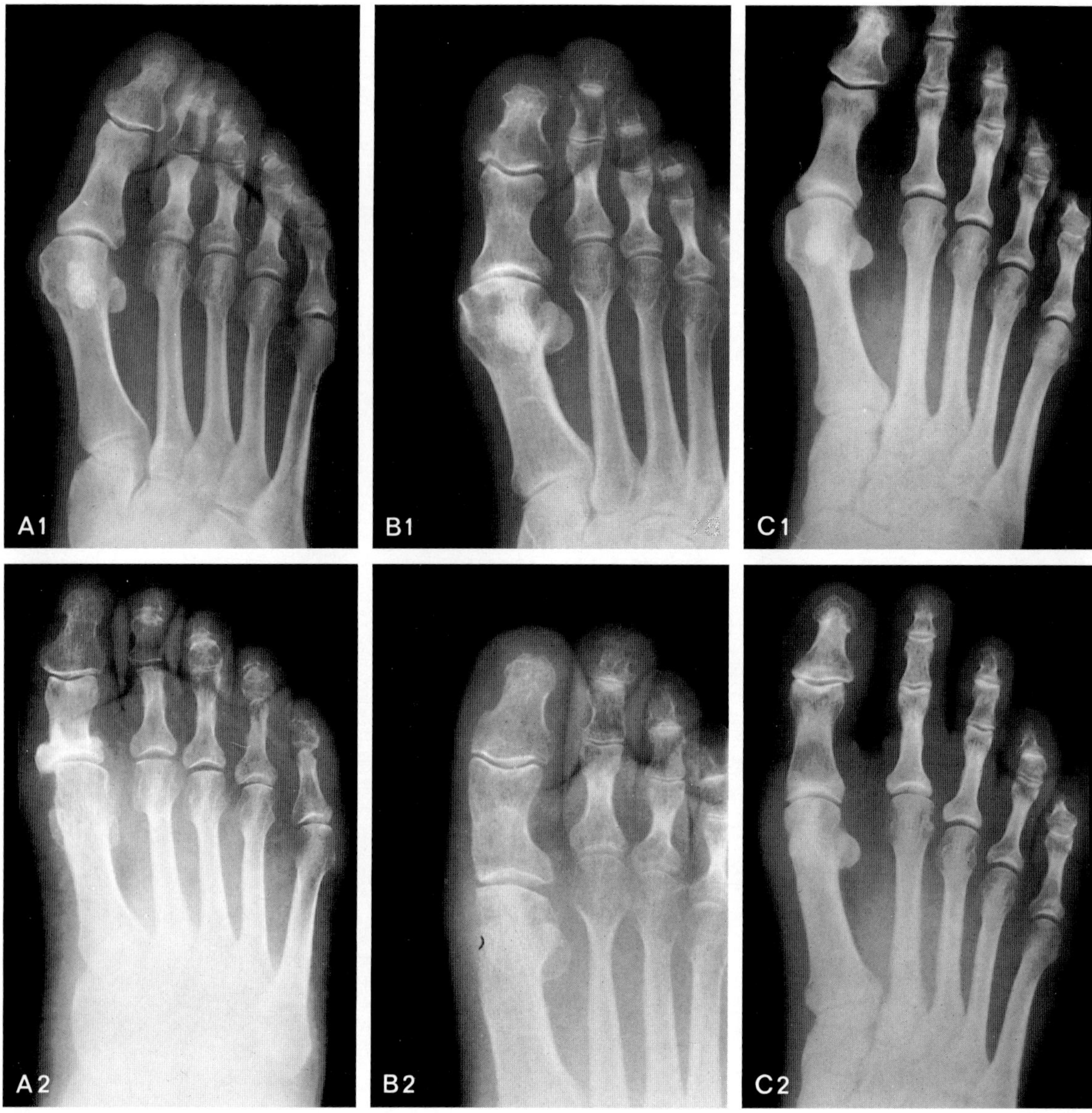

Fig. 18.3 A–J. Operative treatment of first- and second-degree hallux valgus. **A-1** First degree. **A** *1* Preoperative; *2* after hat-shaped graft. **B–D** *1* Preoperative; *2* after modified Schède operation. **E** *1* Preoperative; *2* after hat-shaped graft. **F** *1* Preoperative; *2, 3* a year after ▷ cork-shaped graft; *4* 2 years after operation. **G–J** see pp. 253–255

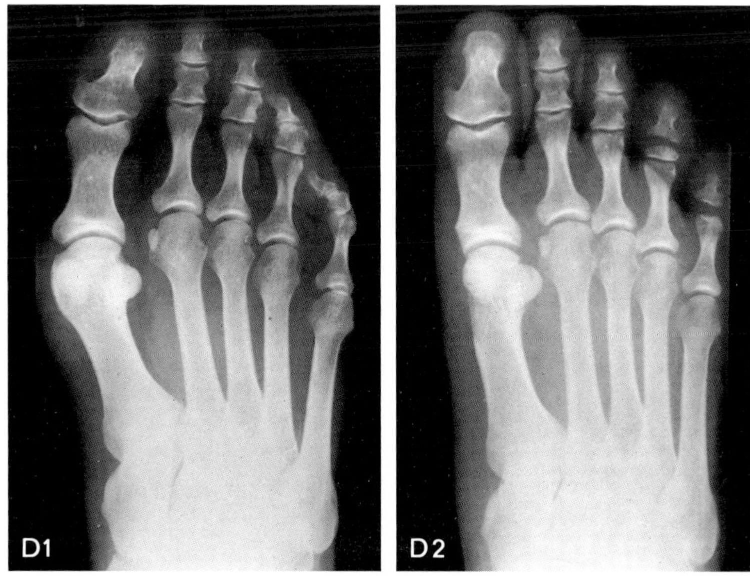

Fig. 18.3 D–F. Legend see p. 252

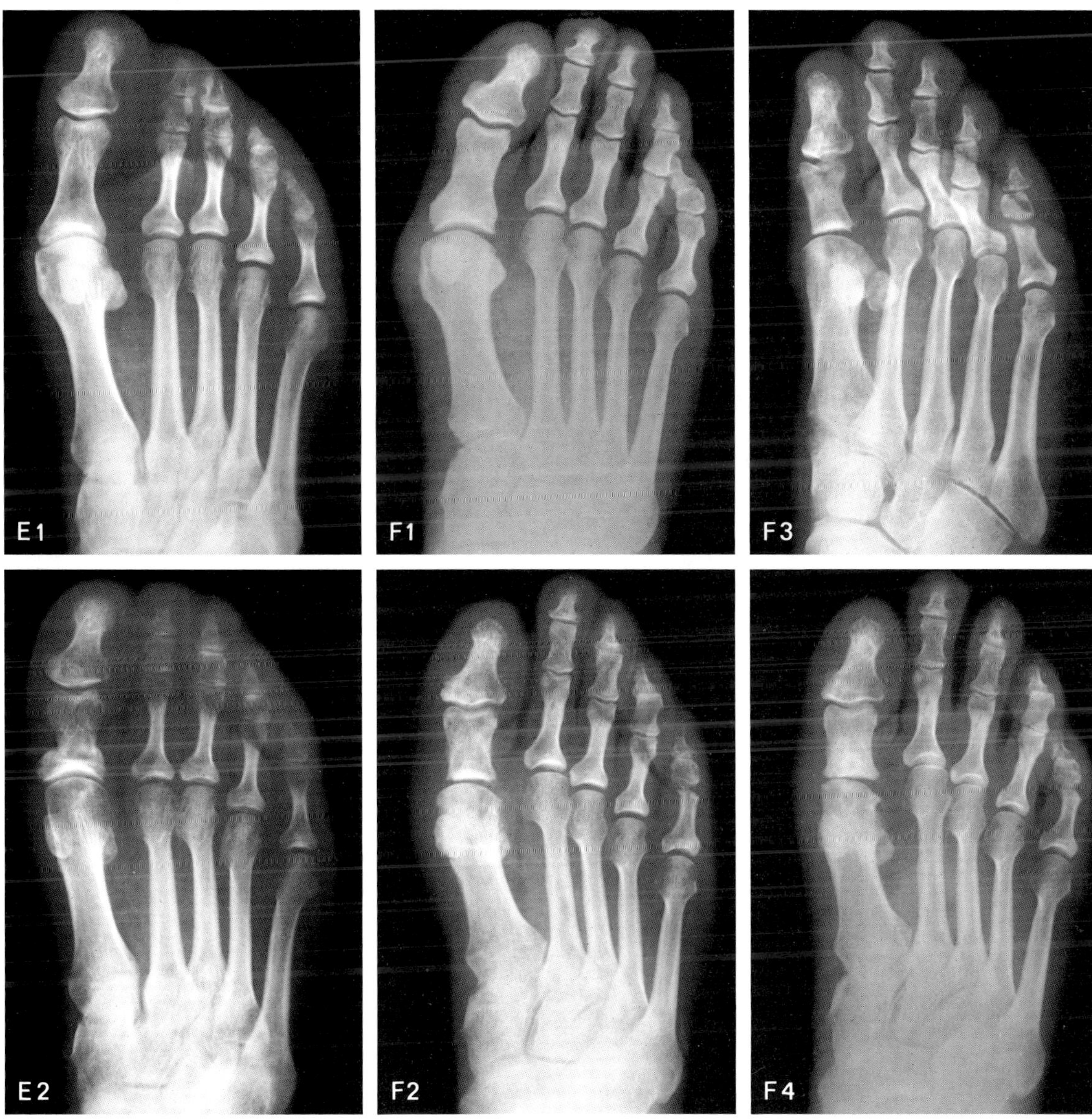

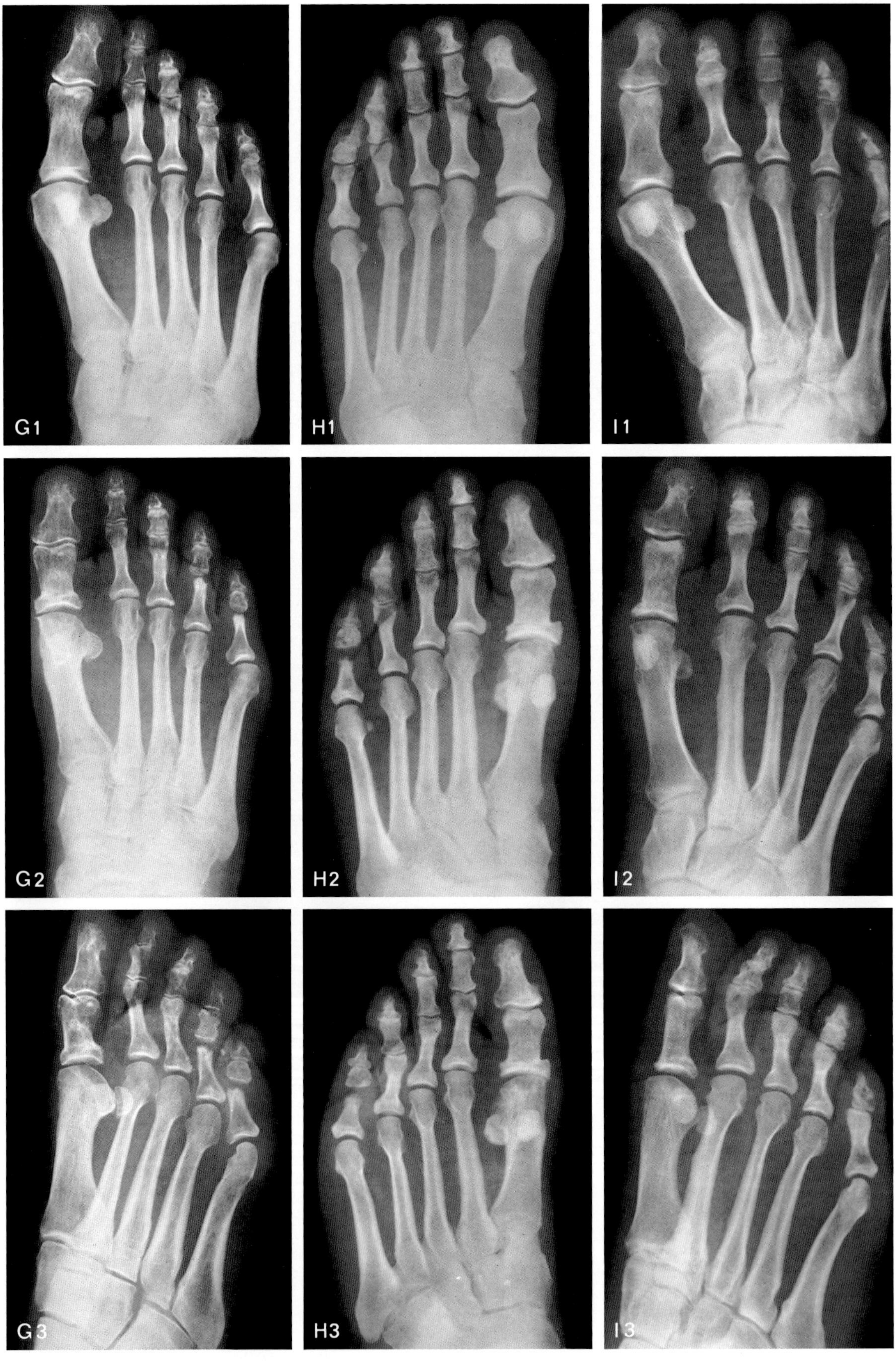
G1
H1
I1
G2
H2
I2
G3
H3
I3

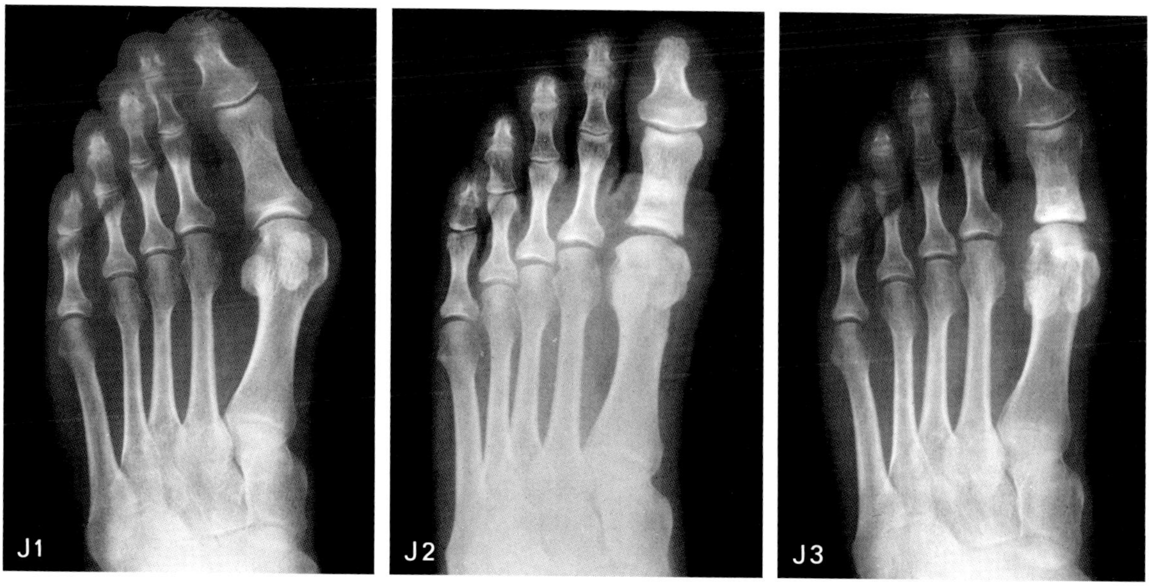

◁ **Fig. 18.3** *(continued)*. **G** *1* Preoperative; *2* a year after hat-shaped graft. **H, I** *1* Preoperative; *2, 3* dorsoplantar and oblique views 10 months after hat-shaped graft. **J** Second degree. *1* Preoperative; *2* 3 months after cork-shaped graft; *3* a year after operation

In first-degree planovalgus deformity, there is a tendency for the load-bearing area to be along the inner border of the foot, while the forces of muscular contraction during propulsion may produce general abnormalities of pressure over the whole of the forefoot; the condition may respond satisfactorily to isolated correction of the hallux valgus. Restoration of the normal alignment of the first ray restores the arch of the forefoot and enables the intrinsic muscles and peroneus longus to establish the cavus of a normal arch. In both the planovalgus and cavovalgus varieties can occur the valgus deformities of the lesser toes, associated much later with dorsal angulation, which were described above.

Cavovarus deformity of the foot can lead to a tendency of the forefoot to pronate in order to restore equilibrium. A tendency to equinus of the metatarsal increases progressively, and associated hypertonia of the extensor muscles accentuates not only hallux valgus, but also dorsal angulation of the metatarsophalangeal joint with clawing. In this case, hallux valgus is a consequence of dynamic derotation of the forefoot combined with overaction of the extensors.

Accentuated equinus of the first metatarsal, and secondarily of the other metatarsals, becomes accompanied by sesamoid hypertrophy and the tendinous contracture mentioned above. The hallux valgus is also associated with a permanent dorsiflexion component in all the toes, often concentrated at the fourth ray, which leads to a convex or cavus forefoot. Again, it must be emphasised that in these complex displacements, no one element can be neglected and premature intervention without a general planned overall programme will prove inadequate.

The severity of the hallux valgus deformity can be measured objectively with reference to the axis of the second metatarsal, comparing this with the degree of varus of the first metatarsal. The valgus of the great toe may be measured against the same line of reference or against that of the first metatarsal (Figs. 18.3–18.6).

- Varus of the first metatarsal (Fig. 18.7)
  First degree: 5°–20°
  Second degree: 20°–25°
  Third degree: > 25°
- Valgus of the great toe (Fig. 18.1):
  First degree: 10°–20° in relation to the long axis of the foot; 10°–40° in relation to the metatarsal
  Second degree: 20°–40° in relation to the long axis of the foot; 40°–60° in relation to the metatarsal
  Third degree: > 40° in relation to the longitudinal axis of the foot; > 60° in relation to the base of the metatarsal

The severity may also be graded according to the degree of soft tissue involvement (Fig. 18.8).

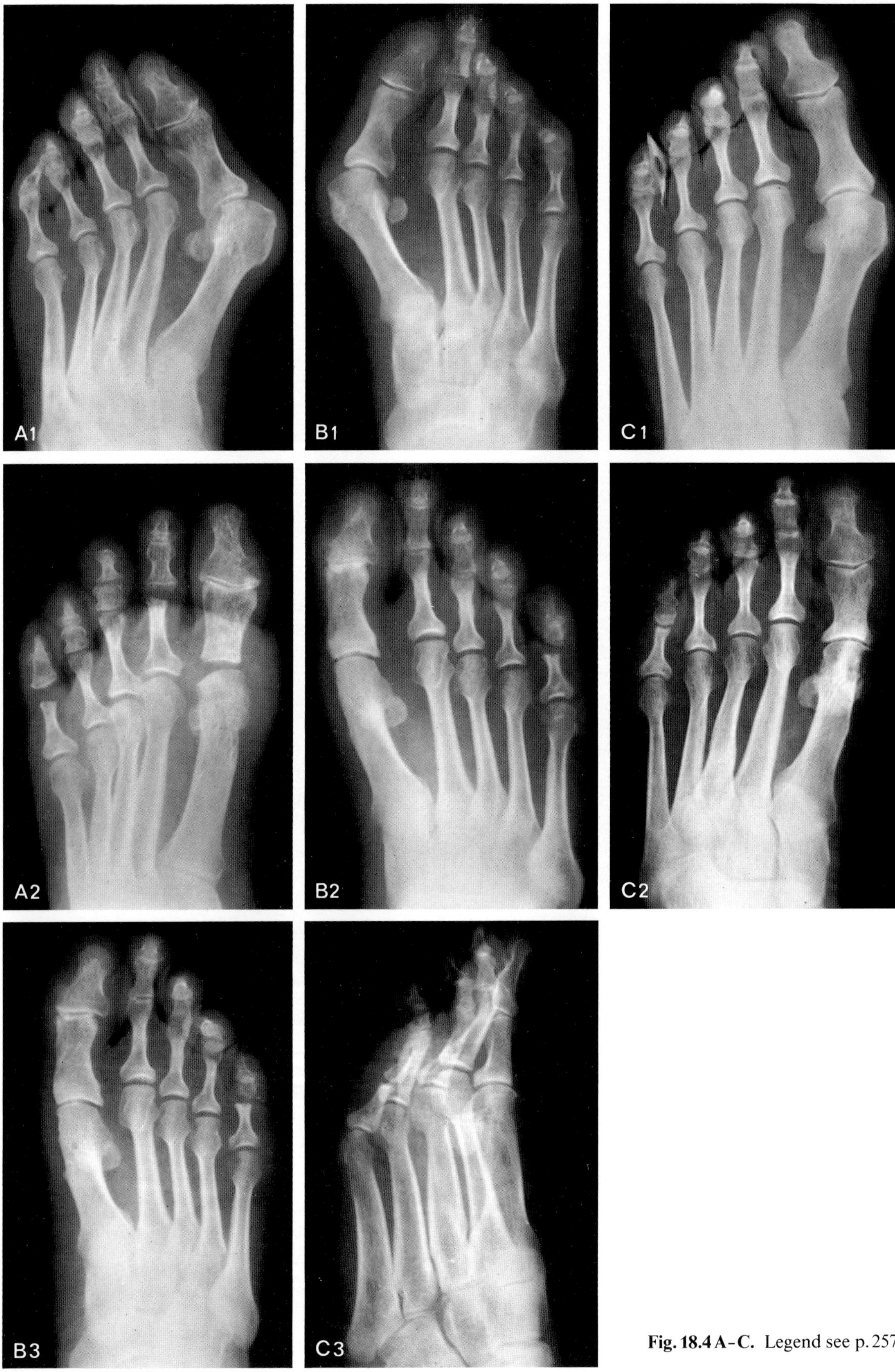

Fig. 18.4 A-C. Legend see p. 257

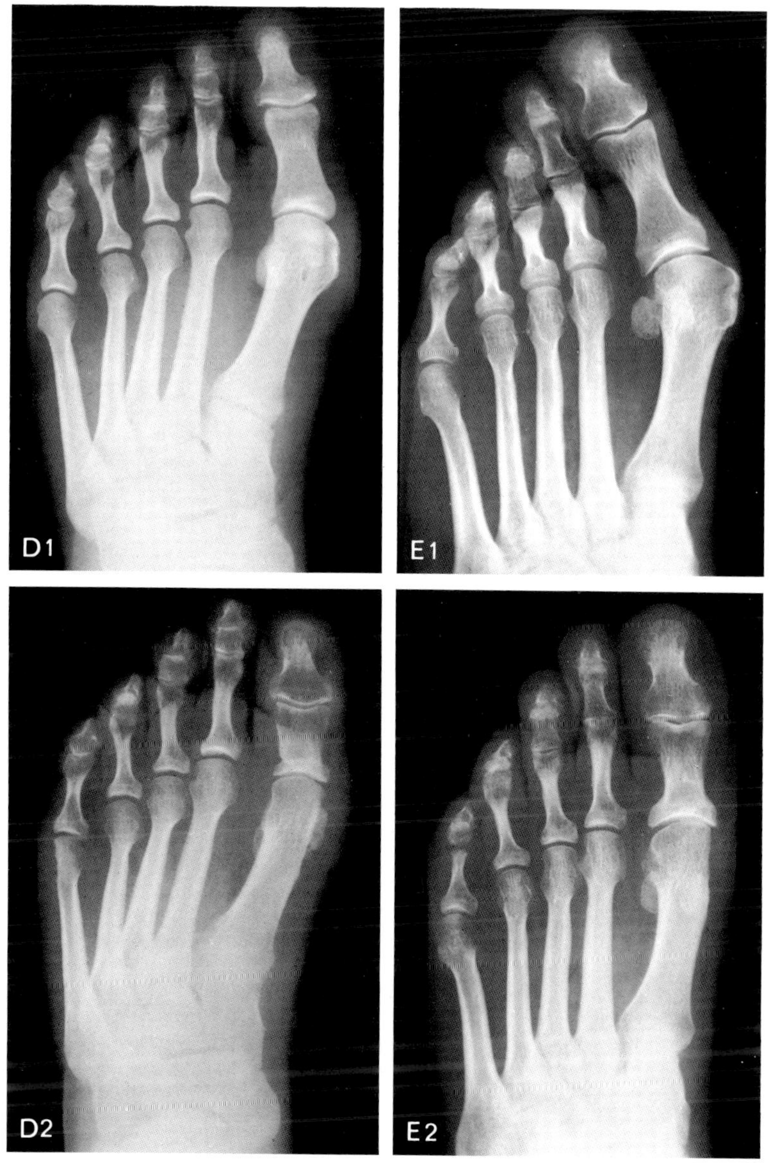

◁ **Fig. 18.4 A–H.** Operative treatment of hallux valgus. **A** Third degree: *1* Preoperative; *2* after metatarsophalangeal arthroplasty with cork-shaped graft. **B** Second degree: *1* Preoperative; *2* 6 months after modified Schède operation; *3* a year after operation. **C** Second degree: *1* Preoperative; *2, 3* a year after hat-shaped graft. **D, E** Second degree: *1* Preoperative; *2* a year after metatarsophalangeal arthroplasty with hat-shaped graft. **F** Second degree: *1* Preoperative; *2* 6 months after hat-shaped graft; *3* a year after operation; *4* 3 years after operation. **G** Second degree: *1* Preoperative; *2, 3* 6 months after metatarsophalangeal arthroplasty with hat-shaped graft; *4, 5* 18 months after operation; *6, 7* 3 years after operation. **H** First degree: *1, 2* Preoperative dorsoplantar and oblique views; *3, 4* 5 months after metatarsophalangeal arthroplasty with hat-shaped graft; *5, 6* 2 years after operation. **F–H** see pp. 258, 259

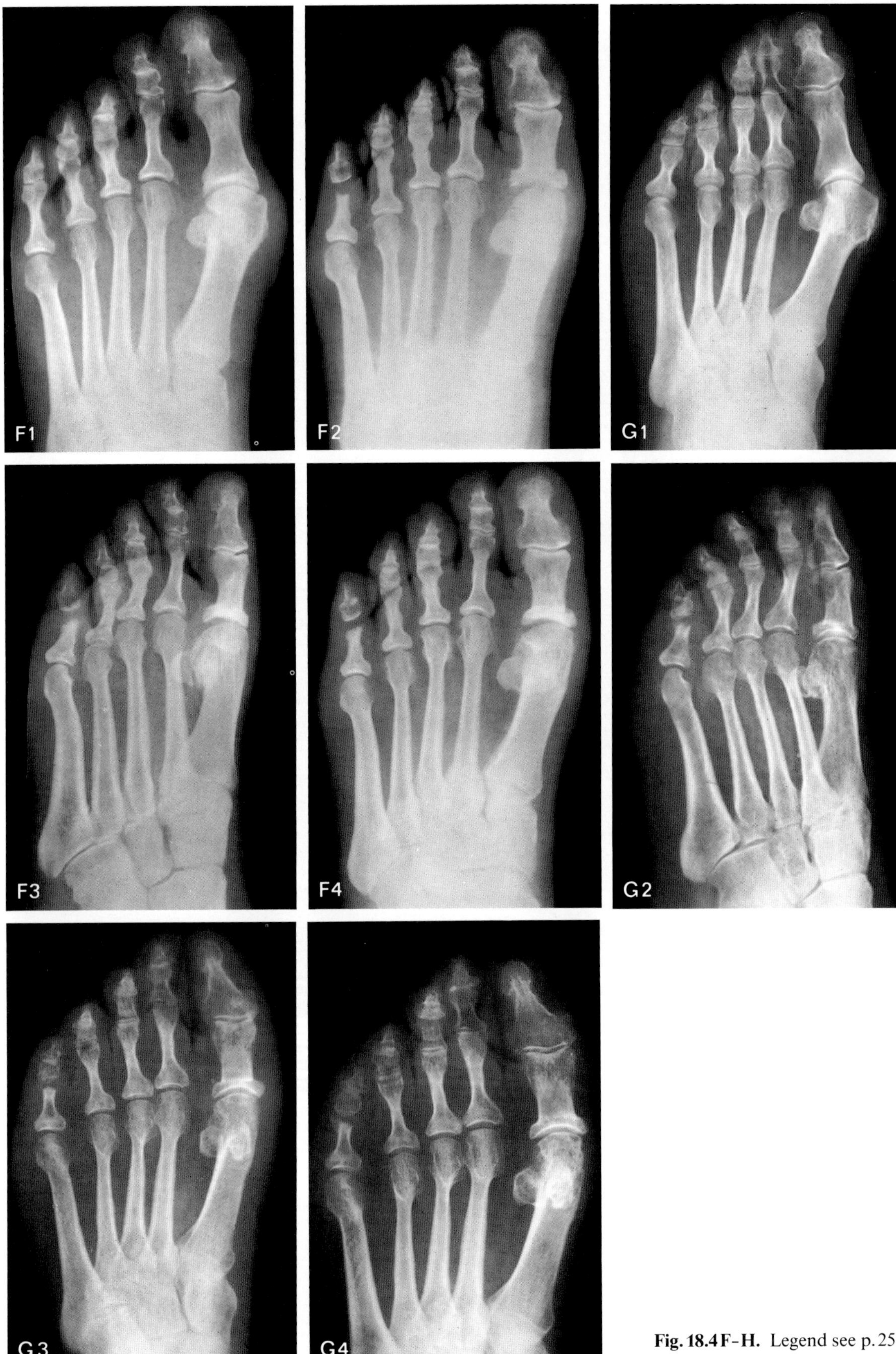

Fig. 18.4 F–H. Legend see p. 257

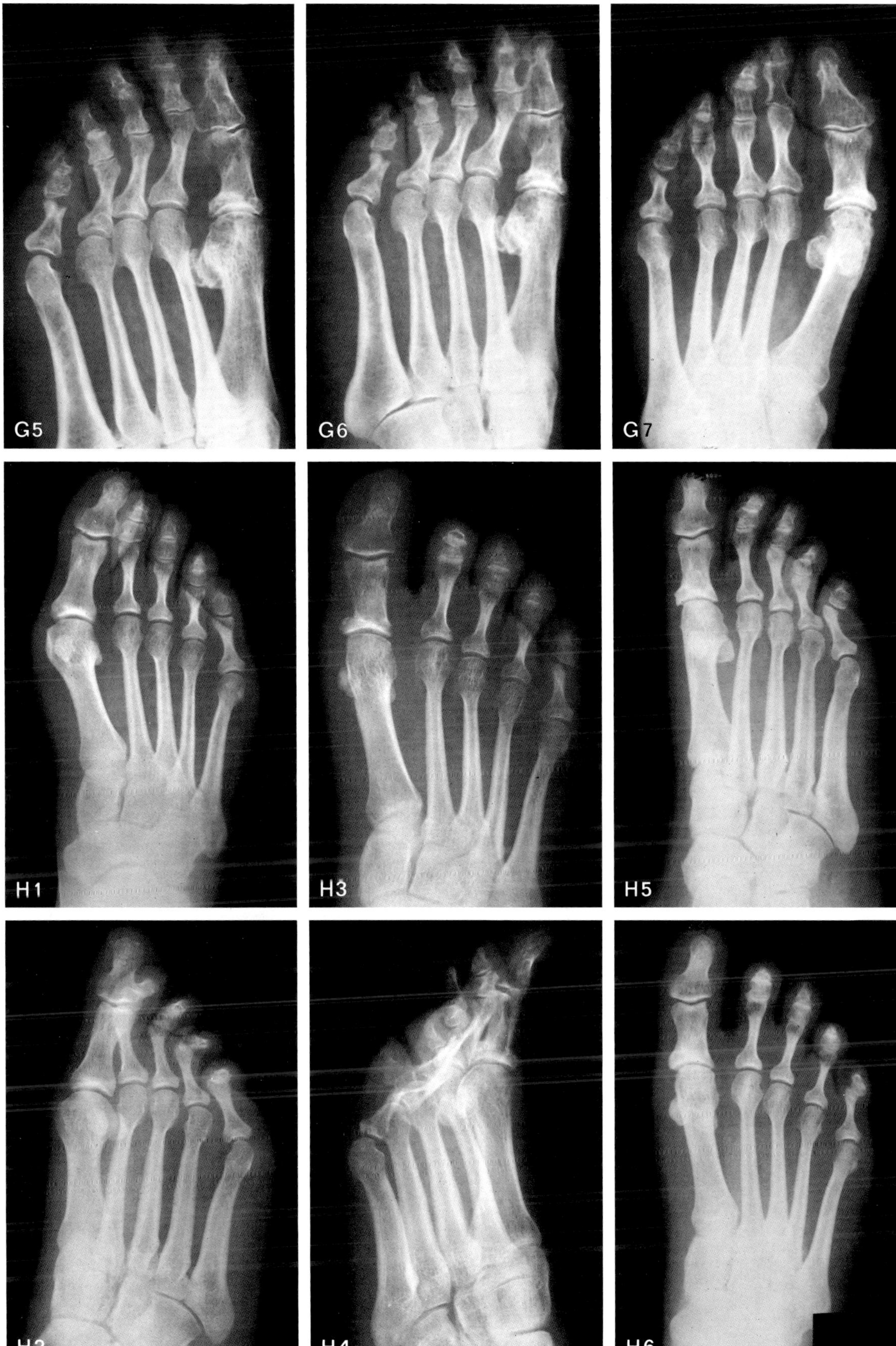
G5
G6
G7
H1
H3
H5
H2
H4
H6

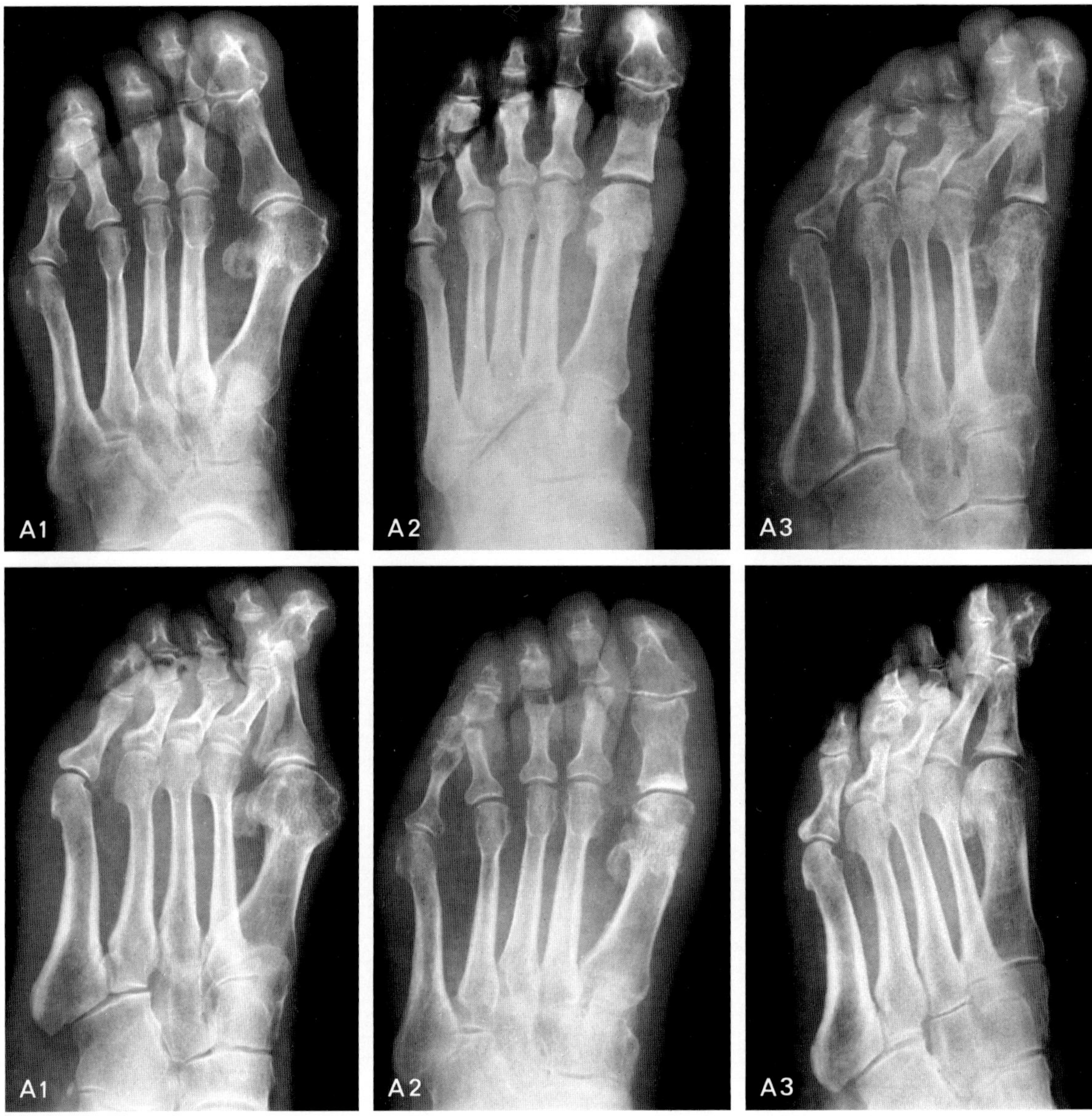

Fig. 18.5 A–D. Treatment of second- and third-degree hallux valgus by arthroplasty with osteocartilaginous graft (Regnauld). **A** Second degree: *1* Preoperative; *2, 3* after metatarsophalangeal arthroplasty with cork-shaped graft. **B** Third degree: *1* Preoperative; *2* a year after metatarsophalangeal arthroplasty with hat-shaped graft; *3* 2 years after operation. **C** Third degree: *1* Preoperative; *2* after metatarsophalangeal arthroplasty by enclavement of phalangeal base onto resected end of proximal phalanx. **D** Third degree, following forefoot trauma and malconsolidation of fractures of metatarsal necks: *1* Preoperative; *2* after metatarsophalangeal arthroplasties with hat-shaped graft, reduction of lateral angulation of toes. **B–D** see p. 261 ▷

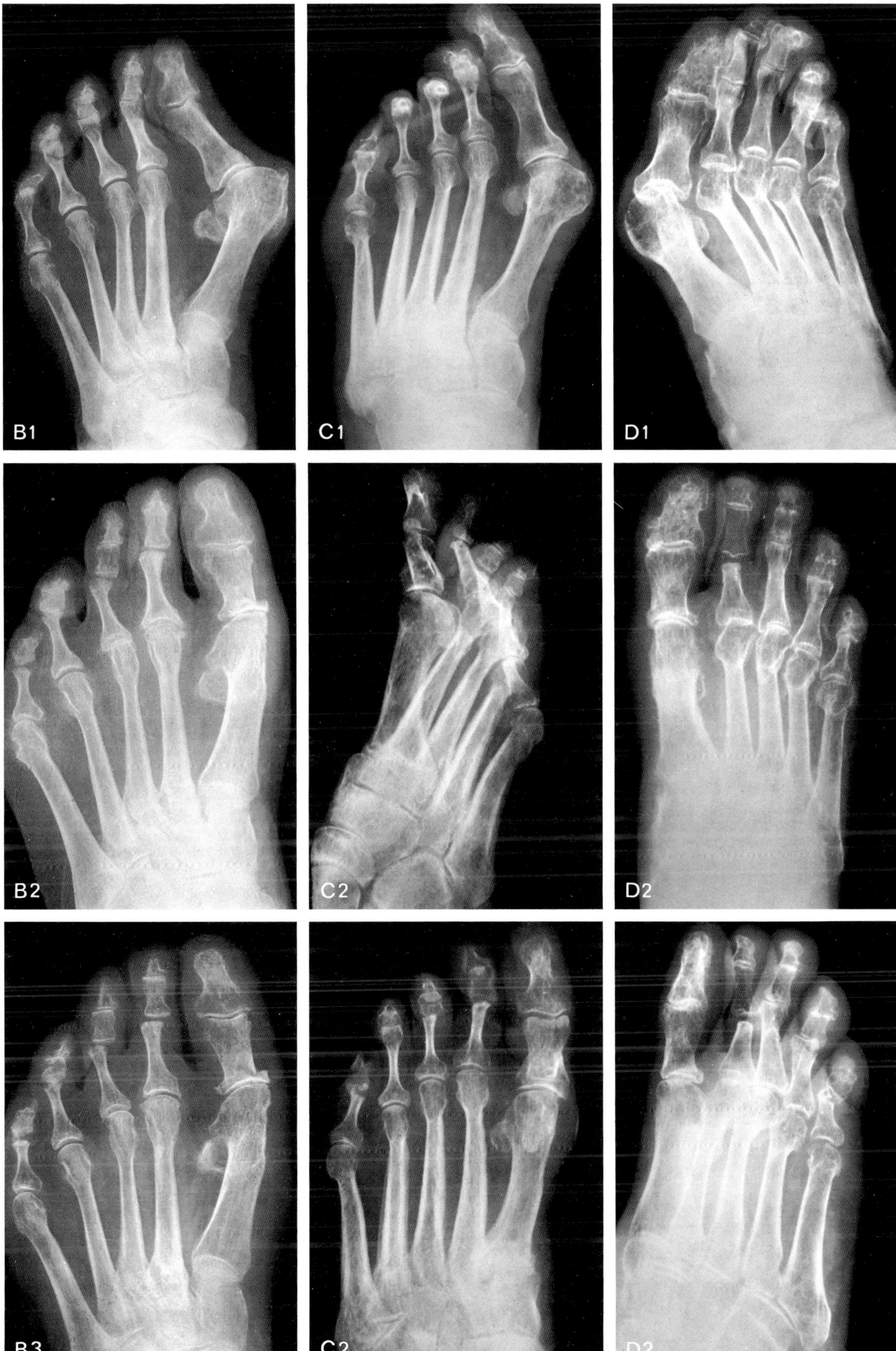
B1
C1
D1
B2
C2
D2
B3
C2
D2

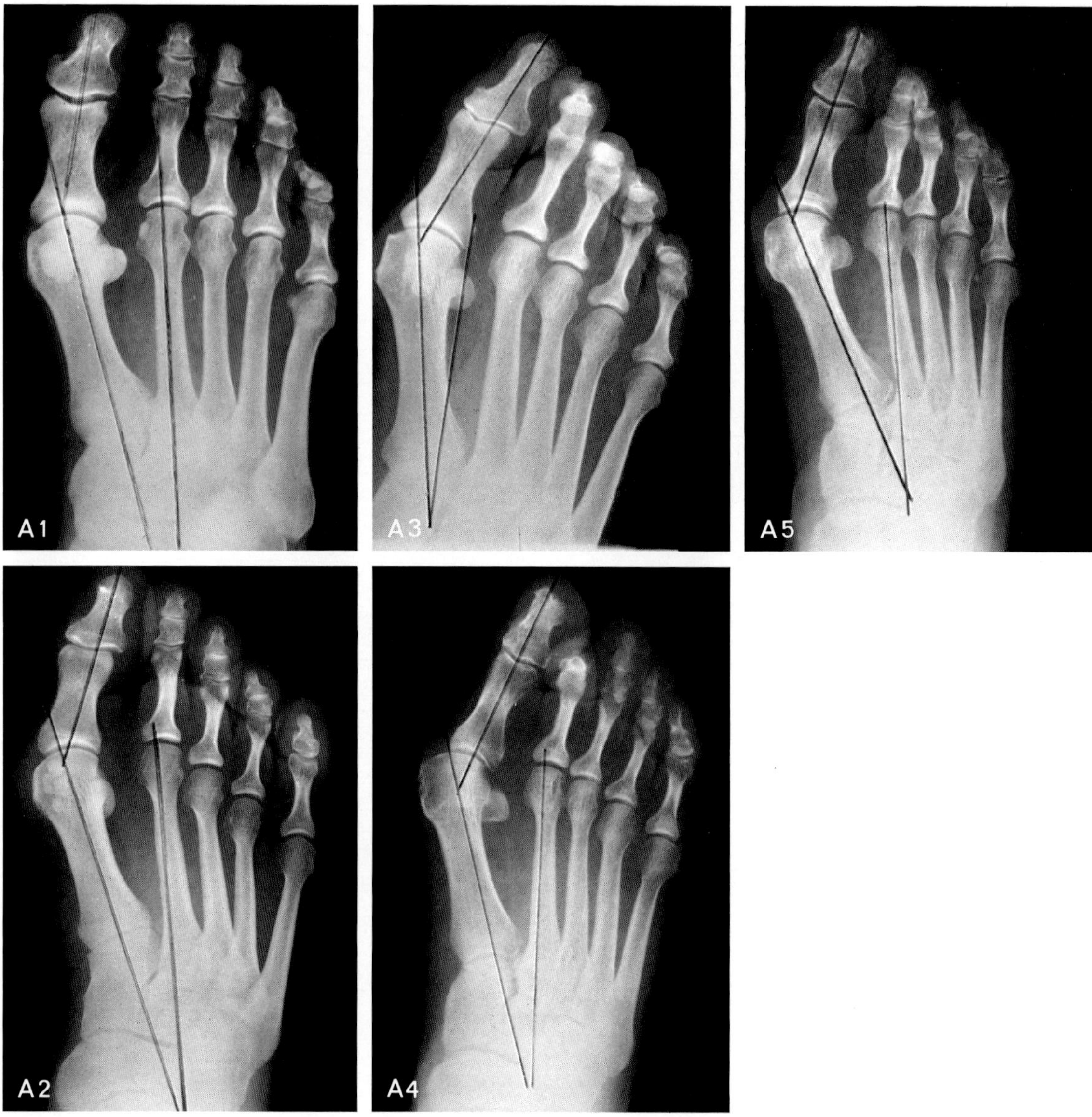

Fig. 18.6 A–C. Examples of hallux valgus. **A** *1* Normal forefoot but with onset of pain due to commencement of subluxation of external sesamoid. Metatarsus primus varus (M) = 15°; hallux valgus (H) = 24°; *2* third degree: slight metatarsus primus varus and hallux valgus, widening of first intercapital space. M = 16°; H = 36°; *3* fifth degree: slight clinodactyly of metatarsophalangeal joint, subluxation of sesamoid, lateral sesamoid appears within ▷ first intercapital space. M = 13°; H = 37°; *4* second degree: clinodactyly, lateral sesamoid appears in first intercapital space. M = 18°; H = 43°; *5* second degree: clinodactyly, lateral sesamoid appears in first intercapital space. M = 21°; H = 49°. **B, C** see pp. 263, 264

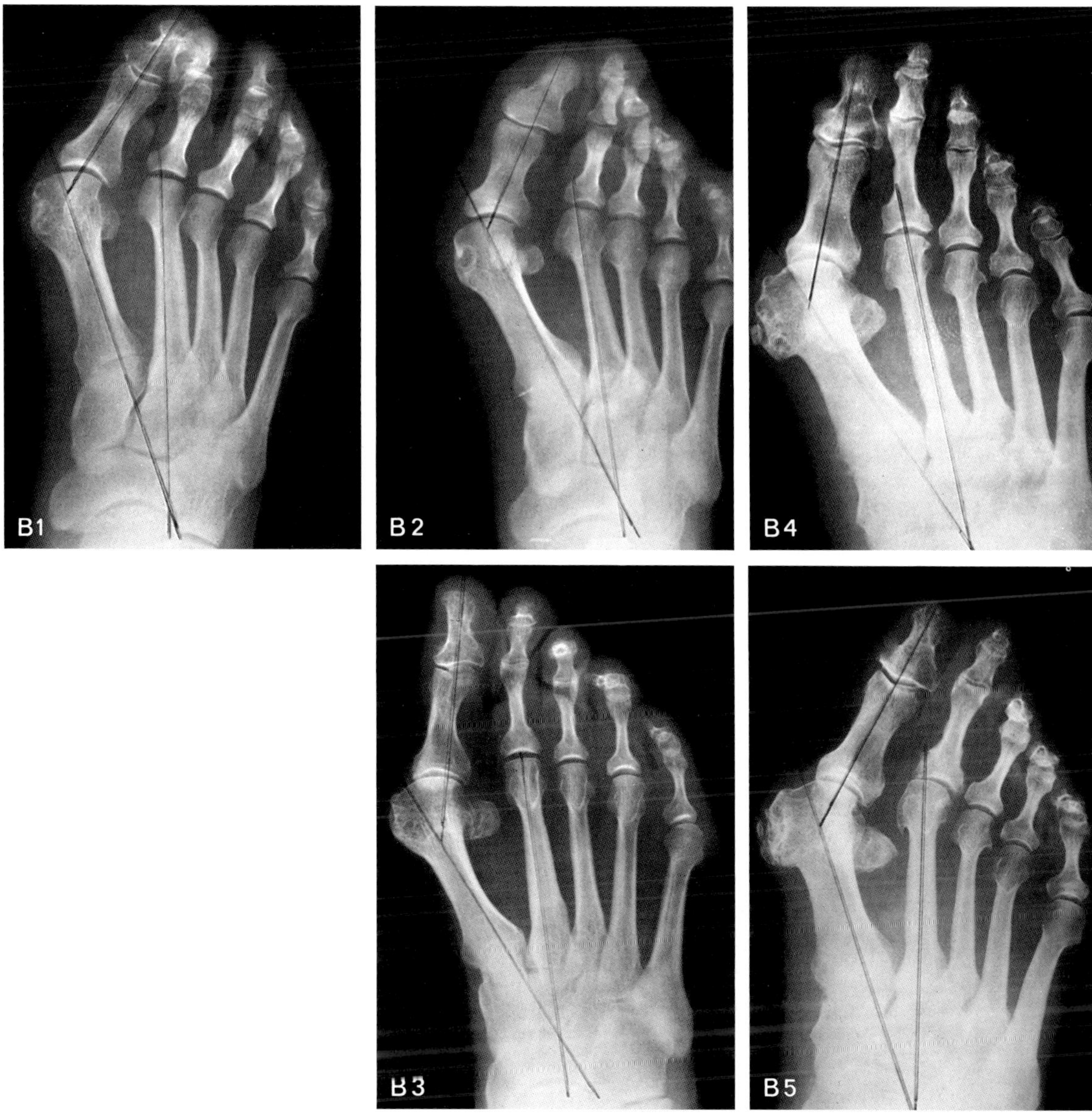

Fig. 18.6 *(continued)*. **B** Second degree. *1* Metatarsus primus varus slight but obvious, hallux valgus more marked, slight subluxation of lateral sesamoid, metatarsal exostosis. M = 19°; H = 56°; *2* clinodactyly more significant, lateral sesamoid entirely within first intercapital space. M = 21°; H – 55°; *3* clinodactyly slight, appearance of lateral sesamoid in first intercapital space. M = 22°; H = 41°; *4* large metatarsal exostosis, lateral sesamoid in first intercapital space. M = 25°; H = 52°; *5* large metatarsal exostosis, lateral sesamoid in first intercapital space, one-third of outline of medial sesamoid also seen in first intercapital space, clinodactyly accentuated. M = 25°, H = 54°

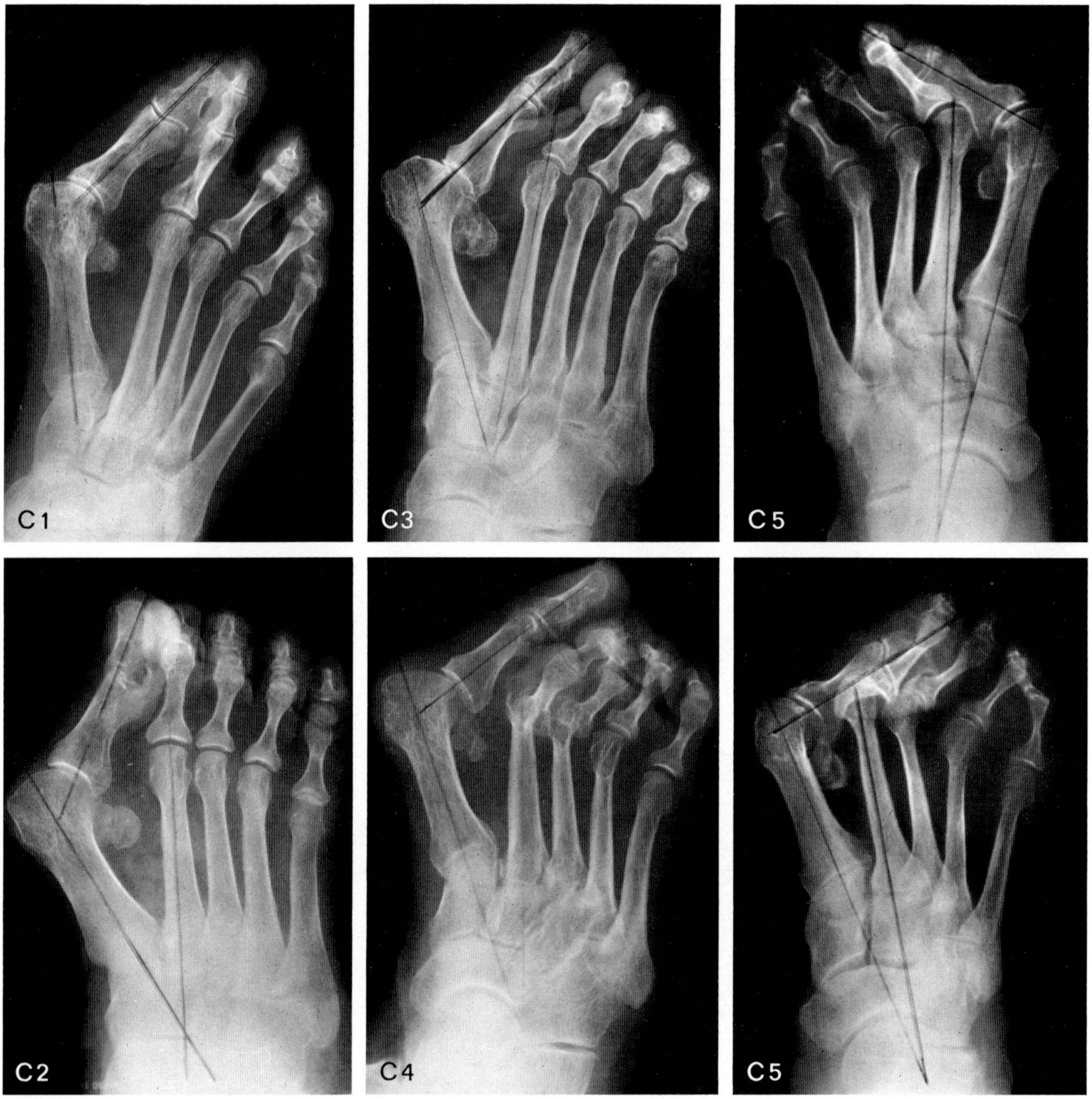

Fig. 18.6 *(continued).* **C** *1* Third degree: clinodactyly, severe hallux valgus, lateral sesamoid in first intercapital space. M = 27°, H = 58°; *2* third degree: marked metatarsus primus varus, severe hallux valgus, torsional deformity of great toe, both sesamoids in first intercapital space. M = 34°; H = 60°; *3* third degree: very severe hallux valgus, marked metatarsus primus varus, exostosis of metatarsal head, both sesamoids in intercapital space, torsional deformity of great toe, two-thirds of head of first metatarsal now extra-articular, lateral dislocation of toes. M = 31°, H = 70°; *4* fourth degree: both metatarsus primus varus and hallux valgus very severe, both sesamoids in first intercapital space, torsional deformity of great toe, lateral dislocation of toes. M = 22°, H = 80°; *5* fourth degree: severe clinodactyly, lateral dislocation and retropulsion of both sesamoids in first intercapital space, lateral dislocation of toes. The condition here is more than isolated hallux valgus, including general outward dislocation of forefoot. M = 15°; H = 78°

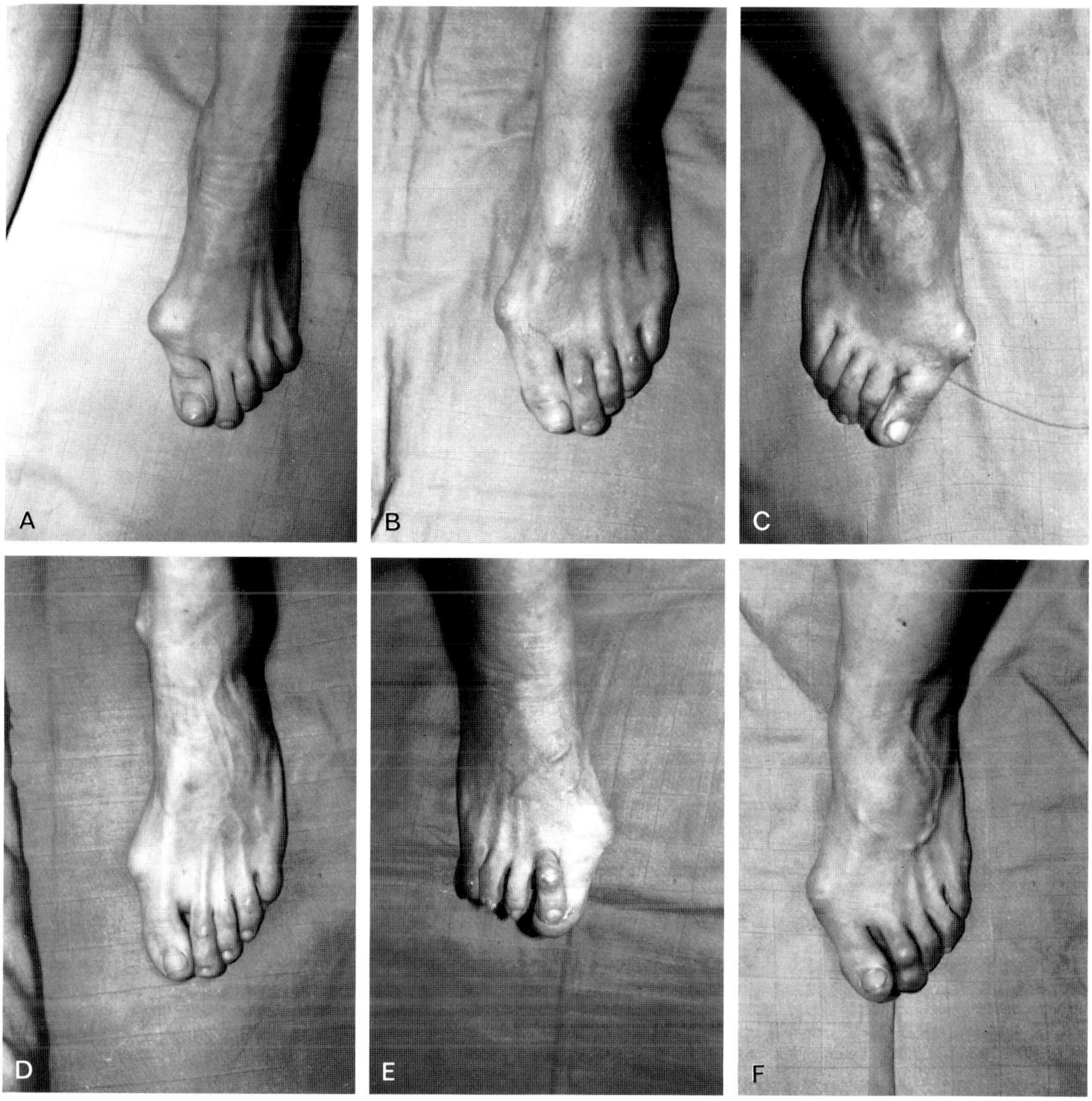

Fig. 18.7 A–L. Claw toes associated with hallux valgus. **A** Second-degree hallux valgus with onset of supple clawing of toes. **B** Second-degree hallux valgus with supple clawing of toes and evidence of dorsal pressure. **C** Second-degree hallux valgus with irreducible clawing of all toes except second. **D** First-degree hallux valgus with correctable tendinous contracture. **E** Second-degree hallux valgus with fixed clawing of second toe in supraductus and commencement of digital clawing and tendinous contracture of other toes. **F** Second-degree hallux valgus with irreducible clawing of second and third toes and supple clawing of fourth and fifth toes. **G–L** see p. 266

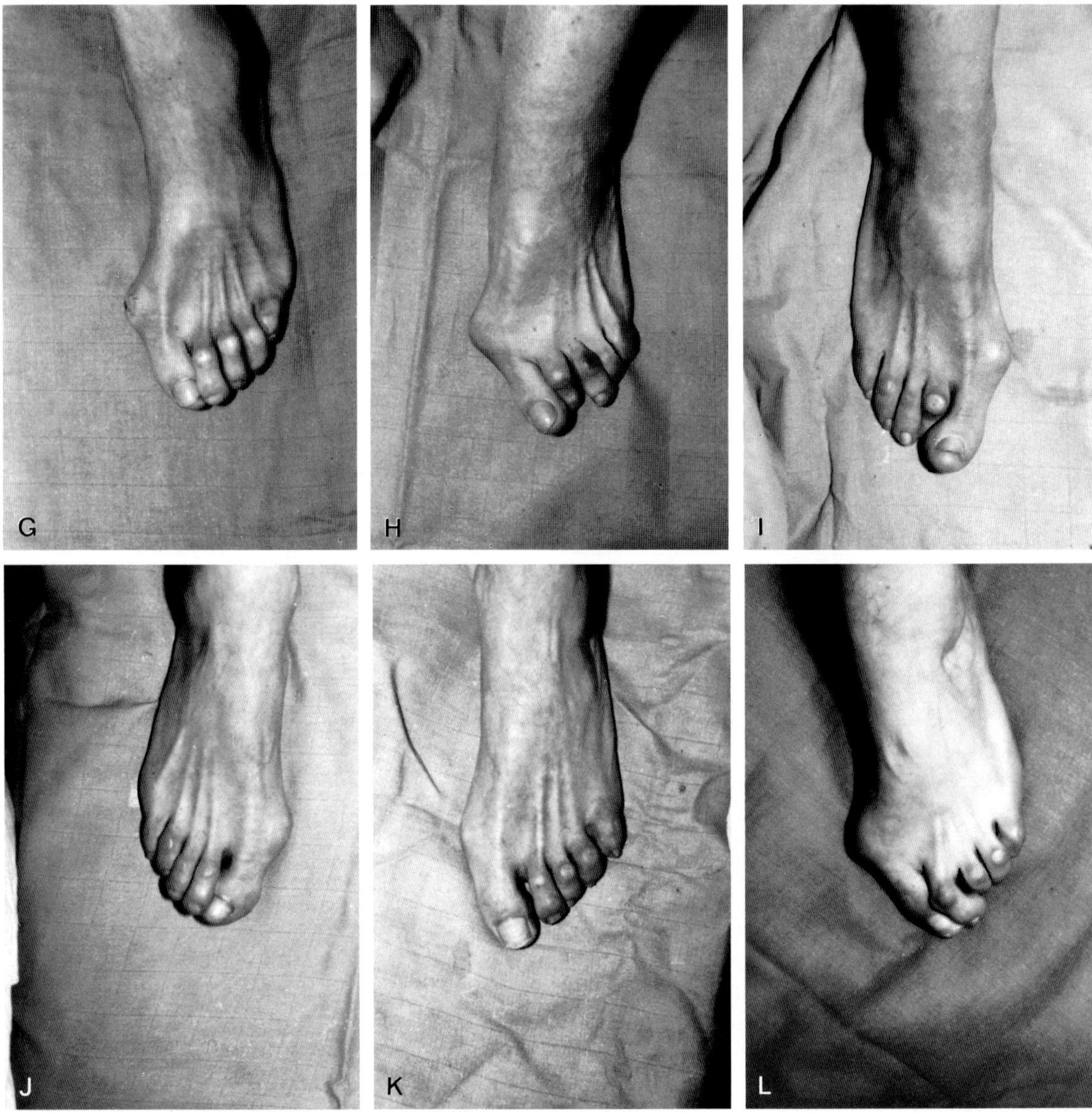

Fig. 18.7 *(continued)*. **G** Second-degree hallux valgus with irreducible clawing and tendinous contracture. **H** Third-degree hallux valgus with fixed clawing, valgus of toes and tendinous contracture. **I** Second-degree hallux valgus with swan-neck deformity of the second toe and supple clawing of the other toes. **J, K** First-degree hallux valgus with tendinous contracture and clawing of toes with dorsal corns. **L** Third-degree hallux valgus with clawing and transverse deformities of middle and distal phalanges of the second toe, and fixed clawing of other toes

Fig. 18.8 A–I. Inflammation in hallux valgus. **A, B** Inflammation from local pressure and rubbing. **C, D** Inflammatory bursitis. **E–I** Ulceration of serous bursa ▷

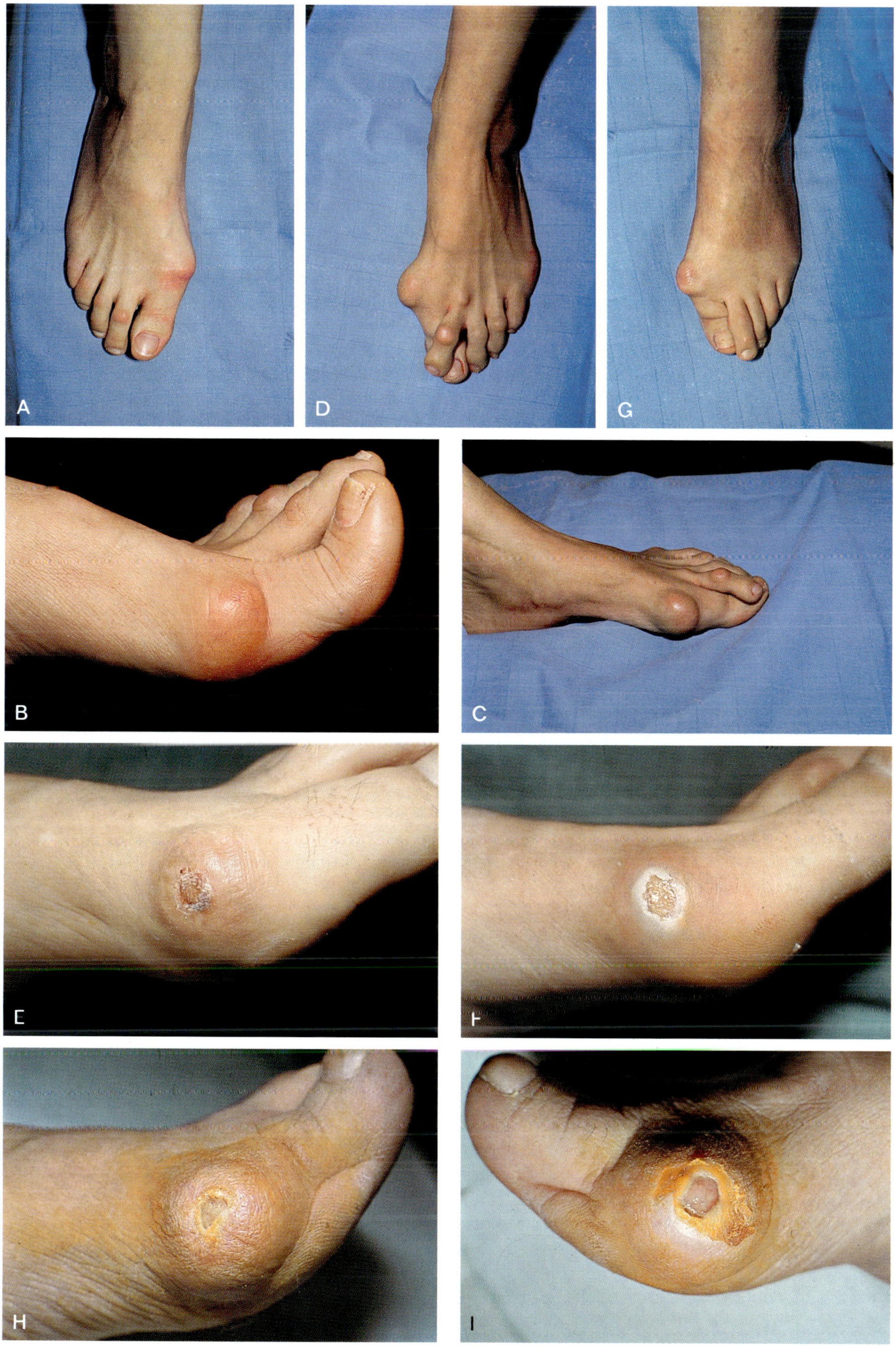
A
D
G
B
C
E
F
H
I

- Soft tissue deformity:
  First degree: painful inflammation
  Second degree: serous bursa, serous bursitis
  Third degree: ulceration

18.1.2 Clinical Features

Related pathology must be sought; arthrosis, polyarthritis or dislocation of one or both hips can be of great relevance. The last-mentioned will be associated with shortening and this will influence the posture of the foot into equinus. The ankle must be evaluated in case of loss of dorsiflexion from some mechanical cause. The degree of cavus in the midtarsal region should be assessed together with its suppleness or rigidity, this again being influenced by any instability of the hip. Valgus or varus posture of the heel should be noted. Any specific equinus of the first metatarsal demands careful neurological examination; poliomyelitis, encephalitis or hemiplegia may be revealed in this way, and their existence renders the cure of hallux valgus much more difficult, even minor degrees possibly constituting a source of therapeutic error. Other etiological factors include poor footwear and a tendency to familial inheritance. The general examination of the foot must include assessment of the circulation. While the normal foot or well balanced precavus foot does not present any problem, the association of a valgus heel with a dropped arch or a cavovalgus deformity is common. Pronation of the tarsus with displacement of the midtarsal joints towards the inner and plantar aspects leads to a forefoot abduction, and it is apparent that abnormalities of loading operate in both static and dynamic actions of the foot. There is a useful test which makes it possible to decide with certainty how much correction can be achieved in some cases of calcaneal pronation or midtarsal displacement: the patient is asked to stand on tiptoe, and as pressure on the forefoot increases, the abnormal posture of the heel can be seen to correct. In such instances, isolated treatment of the hallux valgus is perfectly safe on the condition that the patient subsequently uses an arch support and avoids shoes with high heels. If the calcaneal displacement persists during this test, it is necessary from the outset to envisage correction of the hindfoot before going on to management of the forefoot. The presence or absence of an exostosis and overlying serous bursitis, the reducibility of rigidity of the varus first metatarsal and the valgus of the great toe, the amplitude of dorsiflexion and plantarflexion at the metatarsophalangeal joint, the exact position of the sesamoids, the mobility of the first metatarsal head and any degree of axial rotation of the great toe should all be noted. The history of pain should be related to the deformity, and discomfort may be extremely variable; shoe pressure may be due to friction or simple compression of the forefoot, while inflammatory pains with repeated exacerbations, eventually becoming continuous, are related to the joints and to the inflammatory bursitis. The joint pains will be aggravated by shoe-wearing, walking or sport and can be localised by selective manipulation of the joints. Continuous pain with joint effusion is usually relieved by rest. An additional source of pain is compression of nerves in the first metatarsal head interspace, aggravated markedly by wearing an overtight shoe, especially when the foot swells. The patient may describe forefoot pain in a poorly defined fashion as a sense of engorgement, tingling, or "drawing" of the forefoot. A more lancing type of pain comes from infection and inflammation or even ulceration of the serous bursa.

Lelièvre (1952) distinguished two sorts of clinical hallux valgus: In the *young* woman it is supple and reducible and the foot is mobile. There is little obvious deformity but a great deal of pain. The condition is frequently accompanied by joint effusions. In the *older* woman there is irreducible deformity rendered painful by serous bursitis. This is related more to discomfort from shoe pressure than to true arthralgia.

The tightness of the tendons of extensor hallucis longus and extensor hallucis brevis, the degree of exostosis formation and the varus of the metatarsals should all be assessed by inspection and by palpation. The positions of the metatarsal heads with respect to each other should be observed, and it is in this respect that *podoscopy* and *podometry* are most valuable. The following may be established:

1. The degree of irregularity of metatarsal load bearing, measured according to Lelièvre (1952).
2. Possible protrusion of the central metatarsal heads without any depression into the plantar aspect. In such cases there may be no callus formation, no metatarsalgia from overloading and no tendinous retraction, and the forefoot is normal and supple with the exception of the hallux valgus deformity.
3. Possible depression or protrusion of one or more of the central metatarsal heads. This will be associated with:
   a) Early claw deformity of the second toe alone or of several toes, which may be supple and

reducible but persists on account of slight overactivity of the extensor longus and extensor brevis tendons (Fig. 18.9). Alternatively, the deformity may be irreducible due to more severe tendinous contractures and subluxation of the metatarsophalangeal joints into dorsiflexion.

b) Mechanical metatarsalgia related to the depression of the metatarsal heads, usually of a burning or tingling type. Initially the pain is worse in the evenings, but it starts progressively earlier in the day and eventually becomes permanent.
c) Localised callus formation under one of the middle metatarsal heads, proving that loading is excessive and indicating that correction is necessary at the time of the hallux valgus operation.
d) A large diffuse callosity centred under the central three metatarsal heads and associated with serous bursitis and a convex forefoot.
e) Specific equinus of one or more central metatarsal heads with thick skin or keratoma on the plantar aspect, usually associated with fixed clawing of the toe and tendinous contracture of the extensors and flexors.

Attention should be directed towards the fifth ray, which may be normal or in valgus posture with or without plantar callus formation or an external bursa over the head of the metatarsal. The fifth toe may be displaced into varus, and frequently this coincides with overlength of the toe relative to its neighbour.

Any abnormality in the metatarsophalangeal components of the other toes should be recorded. For example, epiphysitis of the Freiberg-Köhler type may occur. Mobility, rigidity, dorsal subluxation and osteophytosis of long standing should all be noted. Any angulation at a metatarsophalangeal joint should be registered as valgus or varus, supple or fixed, and painful or not painful.

The interphalangeal joints may present slight supple claw deformity, perhaps with an area of inflammation of the dorsum of the proximal interphalangeal joint and with tendinous contracture. There may be a corn on the pulp tip associated with shortening of the long extensor and flexor tendons.

18.1.3 Treatment

The surgical treatment plan must encompass correction of the lesser metatarsophalangeal joints by elongation of the extensor tendons, tenotomy of the short extensors, capsulotomy of the deformed metatarsophalangeal joints, especially towards the dorsum, and detachment of the lumbricales and interossei. Clawing of the toes should be corrected by (a) arthroplasty of the proximal interphalangeal joint or (b) arthrodesis of the distal interphalangeal joint associated with tenotomy or release of the contracted long flexor tendon and especially of the short flexor. Basal osteotomy of one or more metatarsals which are in equinus, producing specific symptoms under the corresponding metatarsal heads, will result in the disappearance of the plantar callus formation. The reduction of valgus of the fifth metatarsal and of varus deformity of the fifth toe by capsulorrhaphy of both fourth and fifth metatarsophalangeal joints may be necessary.

It is sometimes possible to re-establish the transverse alignment of the forefoot in one operative procedure by correcting the hallux valgus, repositioning the five metatarsal heads in the same horizontal plane, establishing correct parallel alignment of the five toes and rectifying the multiple dislocations of the tendons and associated soft tissues. The exact combination of procedures can be determined only by careful clinical examination.

The chosen operation must relate to the genesis of the hallux valgus and embody the following corrections:

1. The first metatarsal varus, the sesamoid subluxation and the hallux valgus must be reduced simultaneously.
2. The medial capsulotendinous layer of the metatarsophalangeal joint must be restored. Elongation of extensor hallucis longus becomes less necessary as soon as the capsular plantar tissue of the sesamoid-phalangeal zone is corrected.
3. Any resection of the base of the proximal phalanx must be calculated to respect the proper length of the first metatarsophalangeal ray relative to the adjacent second ray. In a Greek forefoot, for example, it is useless to resect the base of the phalanx.
4. Shortening of the first metatarsal which results in irregularity of the line of weight bearing in the zone of the metatarsal heads must be avoided, e.g. there must be no total or partial amputation of the metatarsal head or implantation of any prosthesis into the metatarsophalangeal joint which would result in shortening. Even the insertion of a temporary prosthesis is justified only by significant destruction of the cartilaginous surfaces.
5. The outward displacement of the sesamoids must be corrected by replacing them accurately

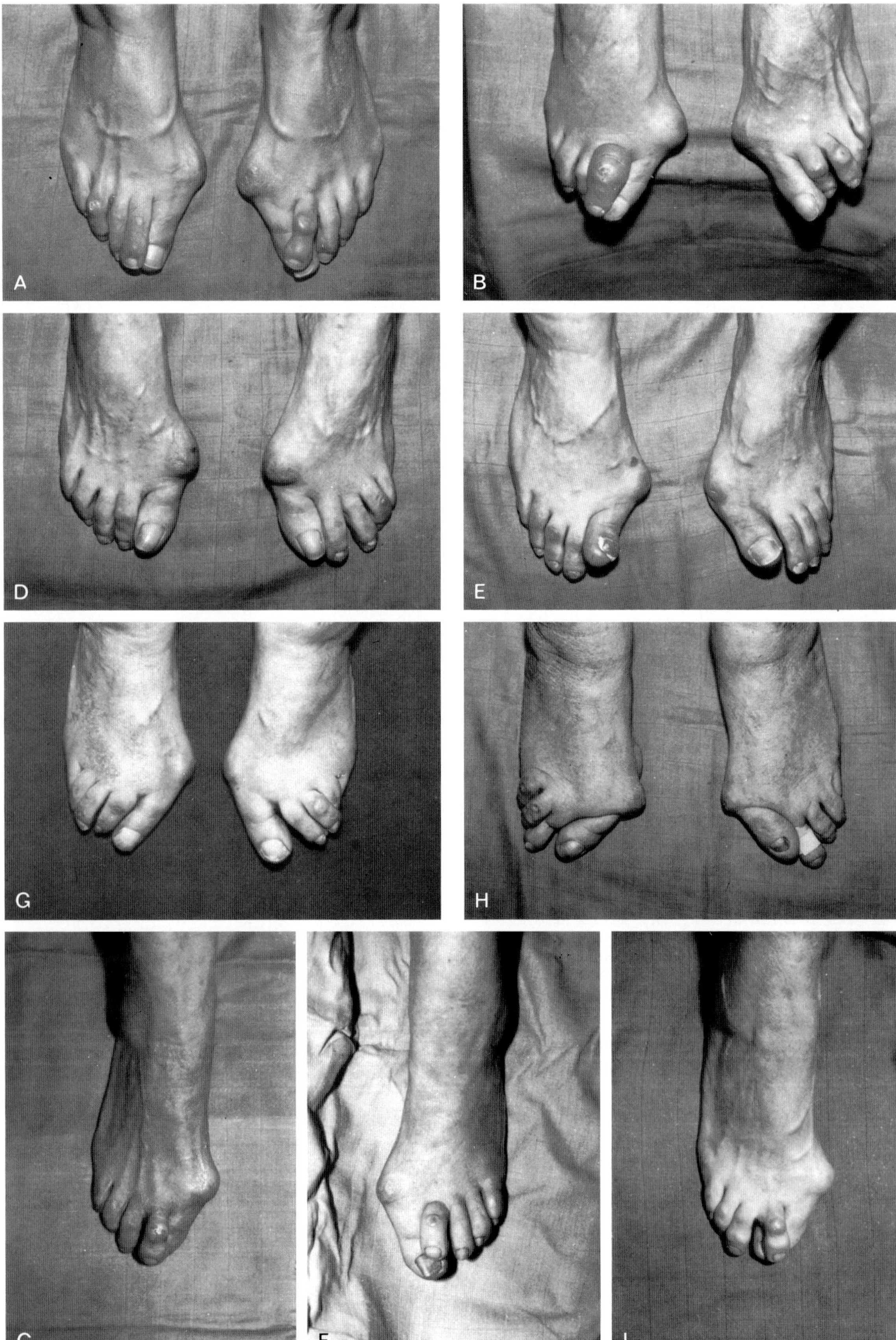
A
B
D
E
G
H
C
F
I

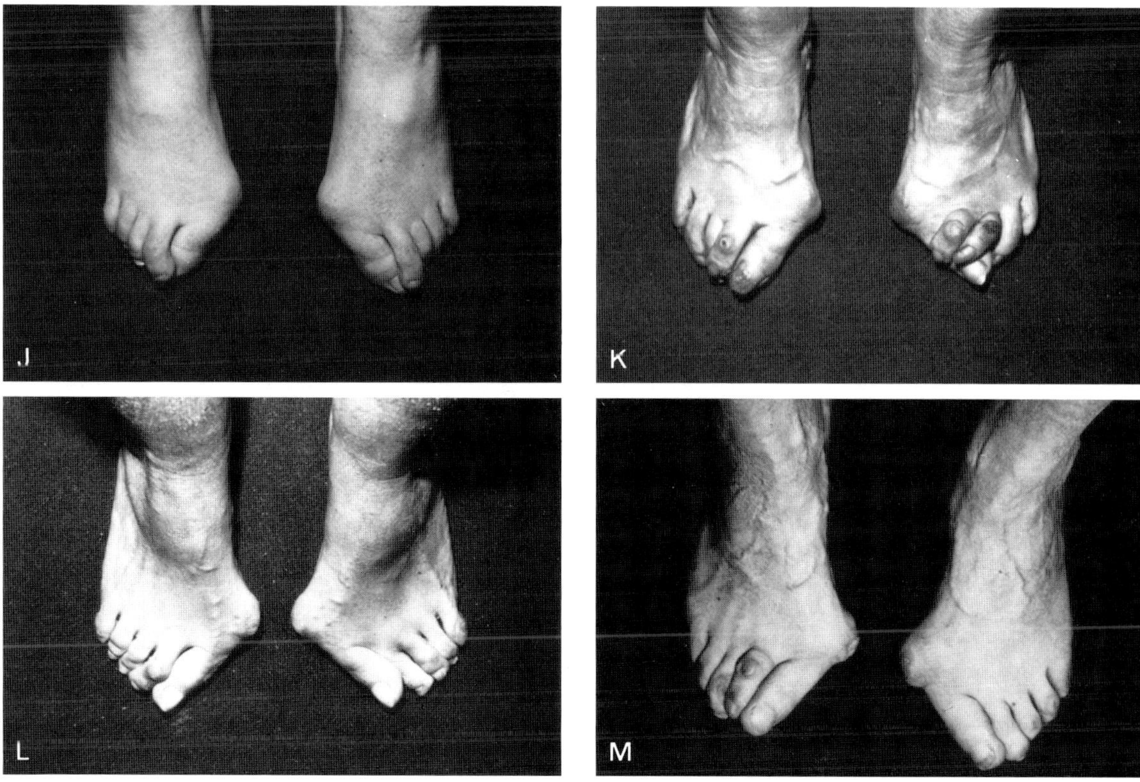

◁ **Fig. 18.9 A–M.** Deformities of forefoot. **A, B, G, H, K–M** Simple triangular forefoot. **C, F, I** Second-degree hallux valgus with extensor tendon contractures. **D, E, J, K** Convex triangular forefoot

under the first metatarsal head, avoiding retro position, which would impede the normal slightly dorsiflexed position of the proximal phalanx.
6. The final aim must be restoration of the normal anatomy and dynamic physiology of *all* the met atarsophalangeal joints. A range of 90° dorsiflexion and 40° plantarflexion should be maintained.

Of the numerous operations which have been described for the correction of hallux valgus, some are ineffective because they do not take into account the global function of the forefoot. While some produce temporary benefit and control of pain, this is not permanent. The classical studies by Lelièvre (1952) and Viladot et al. (1956) show the necessity of correcting adduction of the metatarsal and valgus of the great toe while preserving the overall length of the first ray, as well as the indispensability of correcting the sesamoid subluxation. Together with Viladot (1973a) and Burutaran (1973), I have emphasised the importance of positioning the sesamoid under the metatarsal head and adopting measures to avoid subsequent backward displacement.

Simple arthroplasty by resection of the base of the phalanx leads frequently to articular contracture as a result of the absence of normal phalangeal articular surface, and long painful rehabilitation is necessary if the formation of osteophytes is to be avoided.

Since 1968, with these considerations in mind, I have practised an operation in which the metatarsophalangeal joint is reconstituted by implantation of an osteocartilaginous graft tailored to fit the resected base of the phalanx and fitted into a mortice gouged into the phalanx. The graft articulates with the head of the metatarsal, which rests on sesamoid bones relocated to their proper place, thereby recreating normal function at both metatarsophalangeal and metatarsosesamoid joints and dispensing with long painful rehabilitation (Figs. 18.10, 18.11).

Operative Technique. The cutaneous incision is longitudinal on the inner aspect of the joint, exposing the subcutaneous tissue, in which lies a lace-like configuration of superficial vessels. As many as possible of these are preserved during development of the incision. An area of only some 2–4 mm

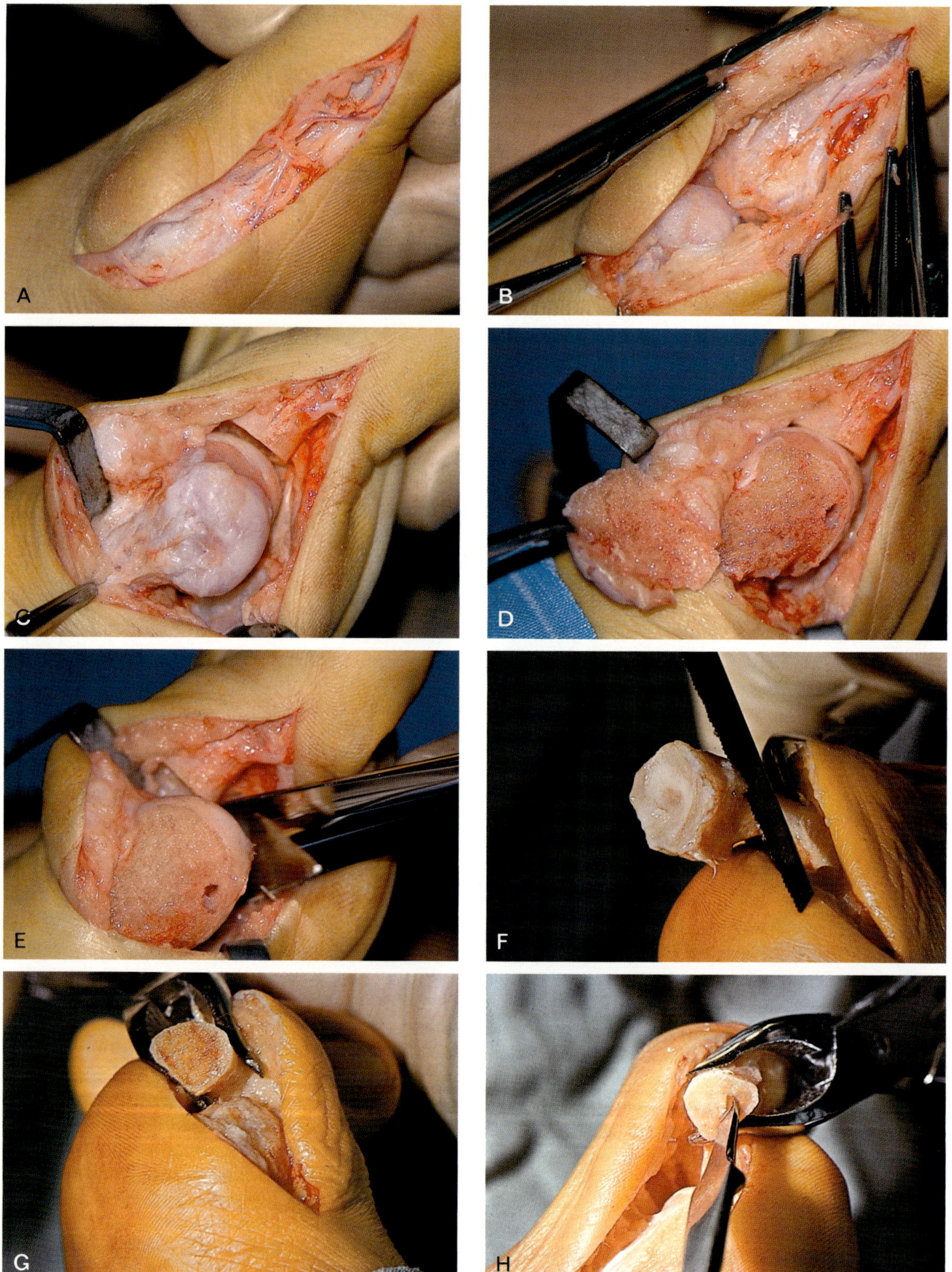

Fig. 18.10 A–J. Correction of hallux valgus by arthroplasty with implantation of a cork-shaped osteocartilaginous graft. **A** Medial longitudinal incision. **B, C** Haemostasis, detachment of capsule around base of phalanx and head of metatarsal. **D** Minimal resection of medial metatarsal exostosis. **E** Freeing of sesamoids. **F, G** Division of base of proximal phalanx. **H** Fashioning of mortice in cut surface of proximal phalanx. **I, J** see p. 273

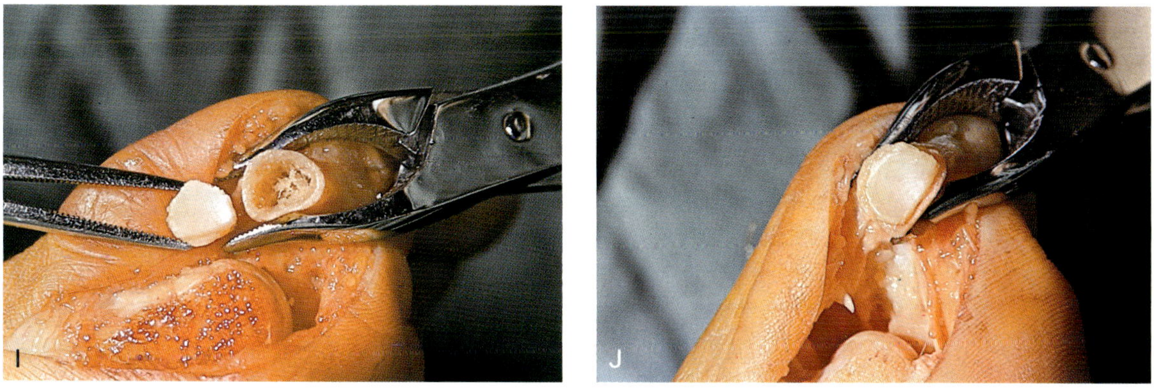

Fig. 18.10 *(continued)*. **I, J** Preparation of cork-shaped graft and implantation into mortice in proximal phalanx

breadth should be exposed. It is necessary to limit the subcutaneous exposure in order to obtain better closure of the skin at the end of the operation, without the puckering which appears if the cutaneous plane adheres to the capsular plane and is the source of necrosis, minor wound dehiscences and keloid formation.

During incision of the capsule of the metatarsophalangeal joint, great care must be taken to preserve the arterial supply to the metatarsal head and the phalanx.

The incision is made longitudinally on the medial aspect, carefully dividing some of the anastomotic venous branches which are seen superficially. The capsuloperiosteal incision must stop at the posterior limit of the exostosis without encroaching upon the medial nutrient artery of the metatarsal head, which penetrates the bone at this level. Capsular detachment ensures separation of the capsuloperiosteum in one layer and is achieved by sharp dissection, maintaining careful contact with the cortex of the phalanx. The plantar aspect of the diaphysis of the phalanx should not be disturbed, for here the artery to the phalanx enters the bone. The use of a rugine which is traumatic and imprecise should be avoided.

Sharp dissection separates the capsuloperiosteal layer over the medial aspect of the exostosis while preserving its dorsal attachment and its posteromedial attachment behind the exostosis (where the nutrient artery is located). Vascular damage will result in postoperative necrosis of the first metatarsal head. Preservation of the plantar artery of the phalangeal diaphysis aims at avoiding necrosis of the graft at the base of the phalanx.

By means of a bone forceps, the first metatarsal head is displaced inwardly and the insertion of the oblique head of the adductor at the base of the outer aspect of the phalanx is divided. The base of the proximal phalanx is amputated at an appropriate level so that after putting in a graft, the length of the first toe is restored, giving a Greek forefoot configuration. Using a fine rugine, a mortice is foraged into the base of the phalanx. The exostosis on the medial aspect of the metatarsal head is resected as atraumatically as possible without damaging the medial diaphyseal cortex. The blade of a scissors is insinuated between the lateral and plantar surfaces of the head of the metatarsal, thereby freeing the sesamoid and reducing any external subluxation by dividing the medial sesamoid capsule. This allows reduction of a varus metatarsal and repositions the sesamoids under the first metatarsal head. The posterior insertion of the plantar capsular plane does not usually limit reposition of the sesamoid and resists any tendency for the sesamoid to luxate posteriorly.

The osteocartilaginous graft[1] is fashioned after inspection of the base of the phalanx. The configuration of the graft (Fig. 18.12) may be:

"Hat-shaped": A central spongy bone tissue of healthy quality is fashioned according to the shape of the phalangeal base.

"Cork-shaped": This is necessary when the base of the phalanx presents with bone of poor, friable quality, likely to collapse easily and accompanied by osteophyte formation around the base of the phalanx.

"Inverted": The shaft of the phalanx is inserted into an excavation made in the base of the graft.

1 Editor's footnote: the author uses the term "graft" because the base of the proximal phalanx is detached completely and then replaced in the manner described

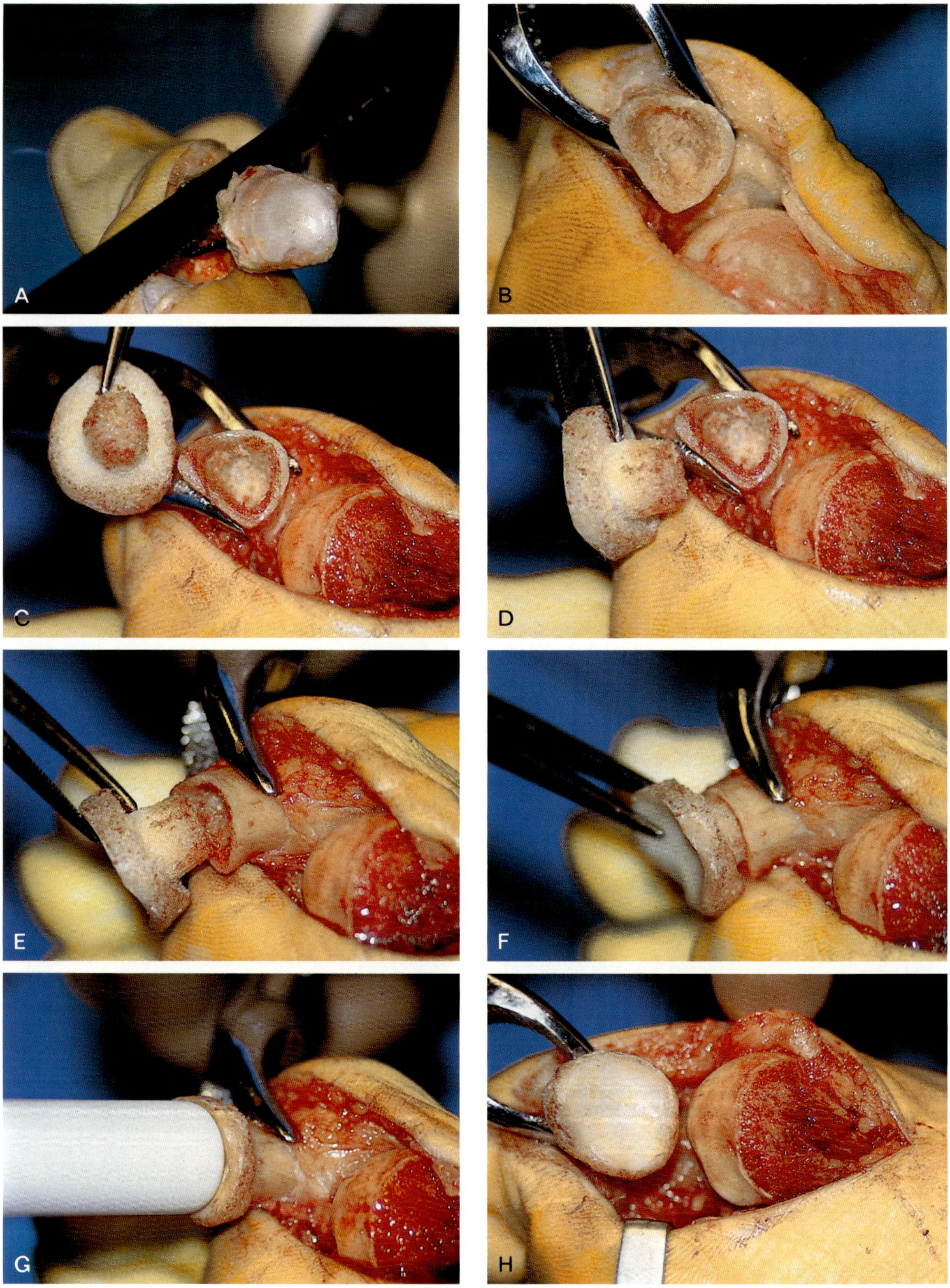

Fig. 18.11 A–H. Correction of hallux valgus by arthroplasty with implantation of a hat-shaped osteocartilaginous graft. **A** Section of base of proximal phalanx after exposure. **B** Fashioning of phalangeal mortice. **C–G** Implantation of graft in mortice. **H** Positioning of graft on metatarsal condyle

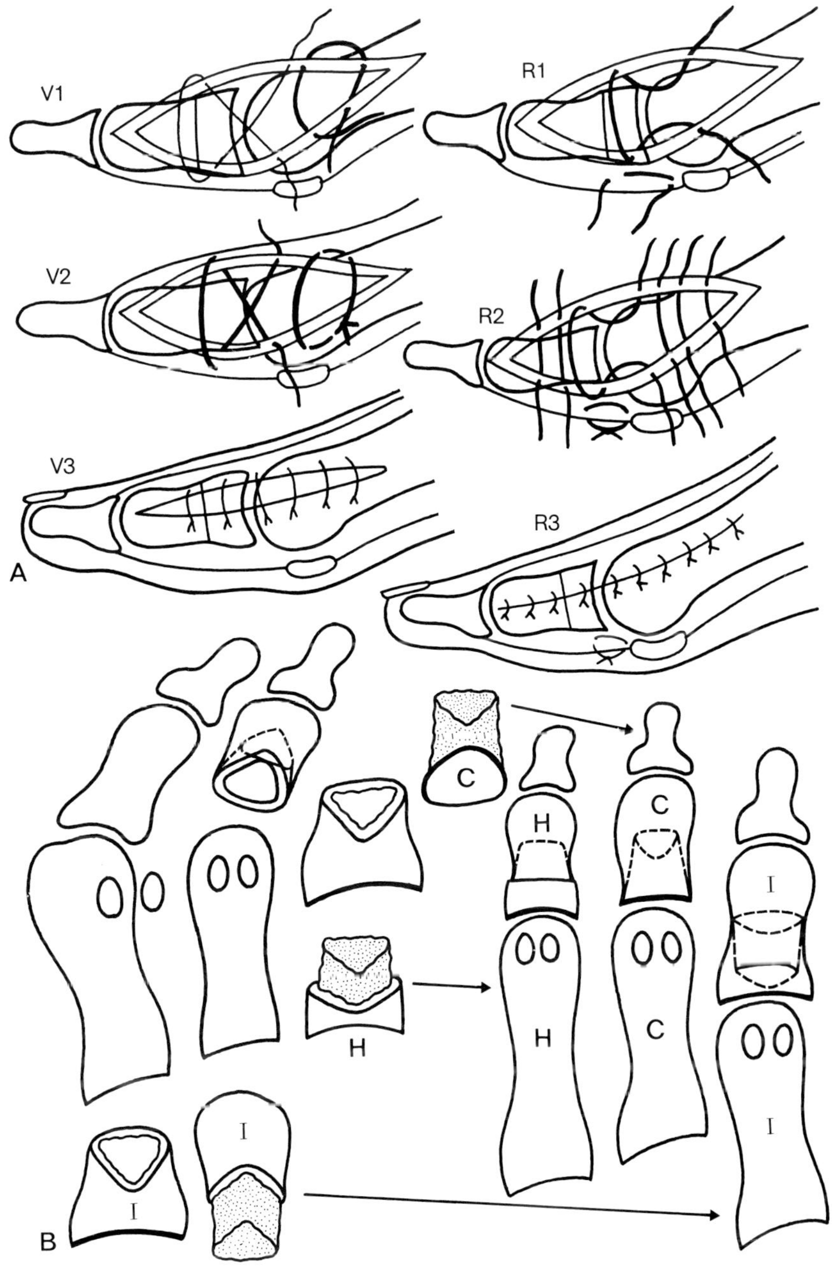

Fig. 18.12 A, B. Operative techniques for hallux valgus. **A** *V1–V3* Stages of Valenti procedure. *R1 R3* Stages of Regnauld procedure: *1* Suture from sesamoid to metatarsal; *2* capsule closure. **B** Forms of graft for base of phalanx: *H* Hat-shaped; *C* cork-shaped; *I* inverted

The *hat-shaped* graft is fashioned using a saw, shaping a peg by resecting bone some 6–8 mm from the cartilaginous margin, which is carefully preserved so as not to provoke osteophyte formation. The graft must fit firmly into the medullary canal of the phalangeal diaphysis, which is suitably excavated.

The *cork-shaped* graft is fashioned so that the peg surfaces slope to form a cone which fits the internal dimension of the phalangeal diaphysis, its margins approaching the edges of the cartilaginous surface. The hat-shaped graft confers excellent stability, while the cork-shaped graft may necessitate some removal of the margins of the joint surface of the phalanx and is thus smaller and less stable. The *inverted* graft is least satisfactory.

During impaction of the graft, great care must be taken to avoid damage to the cartilaginous surface. The capsule of the joint is repaired by two relaxed catgut sutures. A third suture of nylon or slowly resorbable material is used to repair the zone between the sesamoid and the phalanx.

Capsulorrhaphy to reduce the hallux valgus may comprise a U-suture spanning the metatarsophalangeal joint in mattress form. Tightening this suture reduces the hallux valgus and restores alignment of the great toe on the metatarsal. Alternatively, the suture in alignment may be used (Valenti 1980a). It presents the advantage of providing a thick cover by plication of the capsular ligament.

The varus of the first metatarsal is corrected by approximating the capsuloperiosteal tissue on the metatarsal head to the tissue overlying the medial sesamoid bone. This suture replaces the sesamoid under the metatarsal head as well as correcting the varus. While correcting varus, it is important to preserve the vertical amplitude of movement of the first metatarsal by allowing sufficient freedom between the first and second metatarsal heads. If they are bound together too tightly, hallux rigidus, necrosis of the first metatarsal head or degenerative changes from overloading of the metatarsophalangeal joint may result. Once this suture has been tied, the superficial capsular plane can be restored and reinforced. Valenti (1980a) uses a U-suture doublebreasting the capsuloperiosteal tissue, reinforcing it with separate stitches.

Posterior subluxation of the sesamoid is resisted by a third suture of slowly resorbable material or nylon which approximates the plantar capsular plane in the sesamoid-phalangeal zone. This suture passes backwards in the substance of the capsule between the two sesamoids and the remaining capsuloperiosteal tissue of the phalanx. It is desirable not to insert this stitch so as to involve the flexor tendon, otherwise irritation from tendinous adhesion will be inevitable.

Burutaran (1973) employs a capsulosesamoid plantar suture which reconstitutes the plantar capsule very adequately. Final repair of the capsule is with simple gauge 0 catgut interrupted sutures over the resected exostosis, which has the advantage of preventing postoperative bleeding. The skin is closed using interrupted sutures, and a dressing of tulle gras and compresses of cotton bandage soaked in physiological saline are applied. The dressing extends to the knee and is lightly compressive, impeding the appearance of oedema.

As well as correcting alignment, this operation preserves the metatarsophalangeal and metatarsosesamoid joints and makes postoperative rehabilitation easy (Fig. 18.13). Protection from loading is necessary for 30 days, after which active mobilisation is pursued. Only *active* exercises are allowed; no passive attempts at mobilisation should be made. The use of a heel-shoe (Barouk 1984) allows occasional partial weight bearing from the 4th postoperative day.

Consideration of the osteocartilaginous graft and its survival is important. Follow-up since 1968 of some 8000 operations practised according to the above technique by myself and other surgeons confirms that long-term stability with good function can be expected. Valenti (1976) studied the osteocartilaginous graft radiographically and histologically; among the 102 operations performed in 1975, in 96% of cases the reconstruction proved morphologically and functionally perfect and in 87% there was complete restoration of articular mobility. Valenti has subsequently performed some 2000 operations with the same quality of results. He states that "the studies of transplantation of cartilage in the hip and in the hand made by Tuffier (1901), Judet (1906), Dalla Vedova (1911) and MacKeever (1952) were pessimistic, and these authors abandoned osteocartilaginous grafts because of a significant occurrence of cartilage necrosis. They believed that the cartilage would die if it was not transplanted with its capsule and synovium. In contrast, Herndon and Chase (1954), Graham and Riordan (1948) and Stringa and Vigliani (1958), performing osteocartilaginous grafts in the hand, obtained favourable results, but there was uncertainty with regard to the heavy loading which would be experienced in the foot".

I have carefully considered the nutrition of the osteocartilaginous graft, concluding that this is achieved by interstitial fluid and articular synovial fluid and assured by compression of the graft by muscular action, tightness of the capsule, and perfect coaptation of the spike within the wall of the phalanx, as well as by a snug fit of the osteoarticular collar. The fringe of capsular insertion around the margins of the graft facilitates the rapid penetration of new vessels.

Valenti (1976) remarks that the load across the metatarsal head is distributed largely on the sesamoids, the only forces acting on the implant being due to isometric contraction of the flexor and extensor muscles of the great toe, which tend to reinforce the stability of the mortice and tenon; during walking the metatarsophalangeal angle distributes force into three components, one passing through the sesamoids, one passing through the centre of the phalanx tending to impact the implant, and a very minor shearing component, probably of no significance, operating through the margins of the graft.

Judet, Lexer, Axhausen and Vigliani, as well as Valenti, conclude that the incorporation of the graft develops in four phases:

1. Fibroblastic phase: during the 1st–4th days, the osseous part of the graft necroses completely and, with the exception of a few islands of tissue, the cartilaginous surface also dies. Tissue fluid and new cells invade the graft around its periphery and new vessels begin to penetrate it.
2. Healing phase: this lasts from the 20th to the 40th day and is associated with proliferation of capillary tufts in all directions, modifying the structure of the implant. Mesenchymal cells undergo metaplasia to form osteoblasts in the tissue and at the same time, around the islands of remaining articular cartilage, fibrous tissue undergoes metaplasia to form fibrocartilage with numerous cells which continue to function well.
3. Consolidative phase: the biological graft becomes reintegrated, forming definitive bone around the margins, largely from periosteum.
4. Phase of functional reconstitution: from the 60th to the 80th day, the mechanical and histological architecture of the graft reforms according to the forces exerted upon the area.

These phases are not distinct, but overlap. The articular cartilage, in part replaced by fibrocartilage, is functionally satisfactory.

Clinically, healing is shown by the resorption of oedema, but care must be taken for some 6 months after the operation in order to prevent recurrence of oedema. Usually, half to two-thirds of the normal range of motion is restored by the 15th–20th day. Contracture is unusual (Valenti 1976). Any attempt at passive re-education is likely to provoke oedema of the tissues generally and lead to contracture. Only *active* re-education should be employed, the patient using his own muscles.

Many other techniques have been described (Fig. 18.14). Those directed towards the first metatarsal head alone should never be employed, for they result in shortening and encourage the development of insufficiency of the great ray with its consequent complications of overloading of the middle phalangeal heads, intolerable metatarsalgia after a few months and complete alteration of articular function of the great metatarsophalangeal joint, perhaps with ankylosis. Thus, the operations described by Mayo (1908), and Ombredanne (1937), which diminish the length of the first metatarsal, disrupt the normal line of loading of the great metatarsal and lead to a syndrome of insufficiency.

The operation of Bilboquet [described by Lance (1936)] shortens the great metatarsal to a lesser extent and does not reduce its loading so much. However, bony consolidation of the metatarsal head necessitates a long period of plaster cast immobilisation; painful sequelae and capsular contraction are encouraged, and recurrence is likely because the great toe is not shortened, an Egyptian foot configuration remaining.

The operation of Keller-Brandes (1904) and the hourglass resection of Wallet (1942) do not correct a varus metatarsal, but do result in a very shortened toe which is functionless, unaesthetic and constitutes an insufficiency syndrome of the first ray by misalignment of its line of propulsion.

Lelièvre (1952) and Viladot et al. (1956) have advocated correction of the varus metatarsal together with shortening of the great toe by resection of the base of the phalanx. However, ankylosis may occur even after a long period of painful re-education.

The operation advocated above is appropriate because in most instances the hallux valgus has occurred in the Egyptian type of forefoot. It is equally appropriate in the square forefoot and in the presence of metatarsophalangeal angulation, osteophytes at the base of the phalanx or obliquity of the articular surface of the phalanx. With the same intention of creating a Greek forefoot as opposed to the Egyptian or square configuration, Burutaran (1977) has described another technique designed to preserve the integrity of the phalangeal base and the metatarsal head while shortening the great toe in the region of the proximal phalanx diaphysis (Fig. 18.15). A Z-form phalangeal osteotomy, shaped in two half cylinders of equal dimensions, one lateral and one medial, allows general shortening by sliding of the two segments after removal of some bone. Coaptation is maintained by a screw.

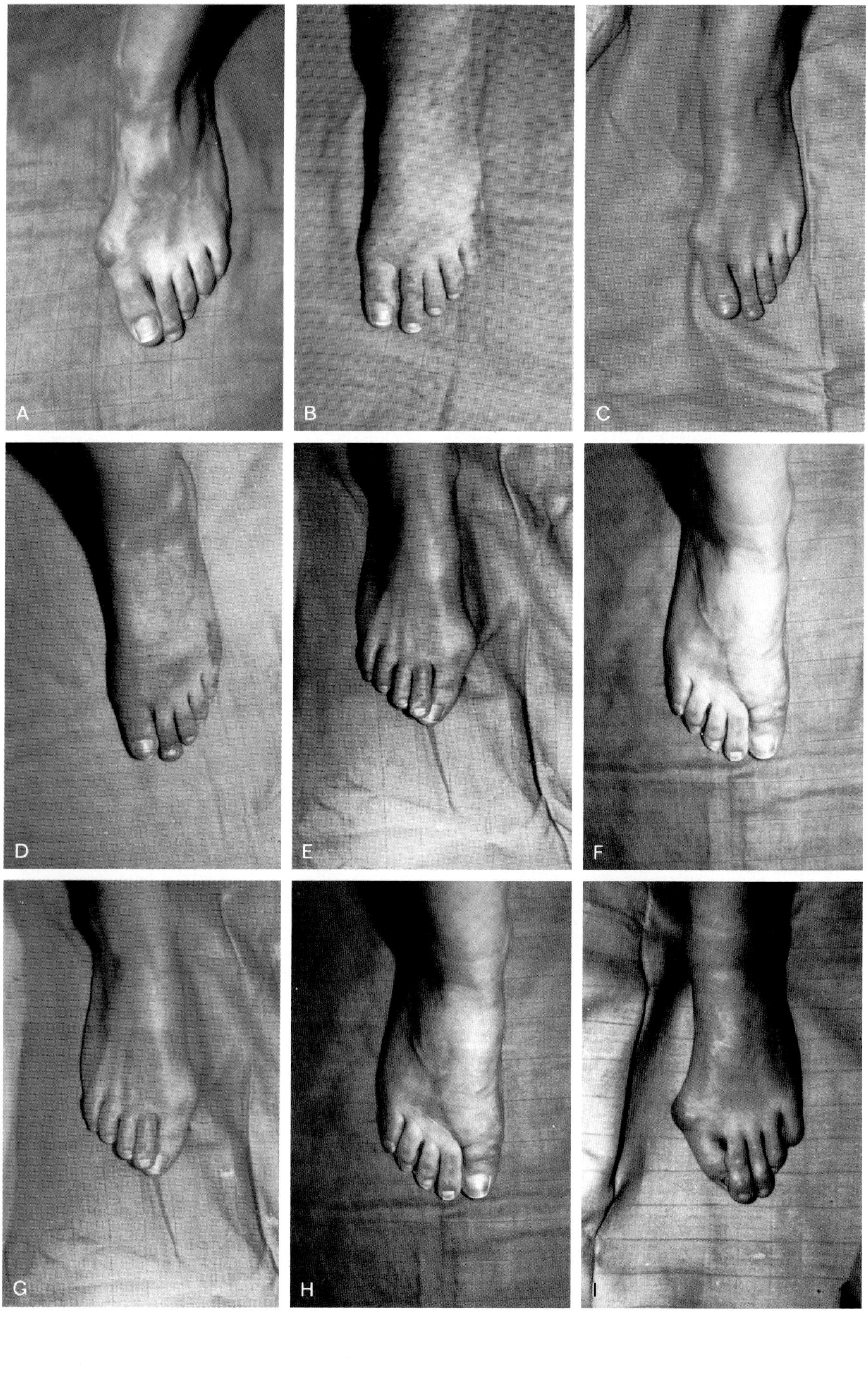
A
B
C
D
E
F
G
H
I

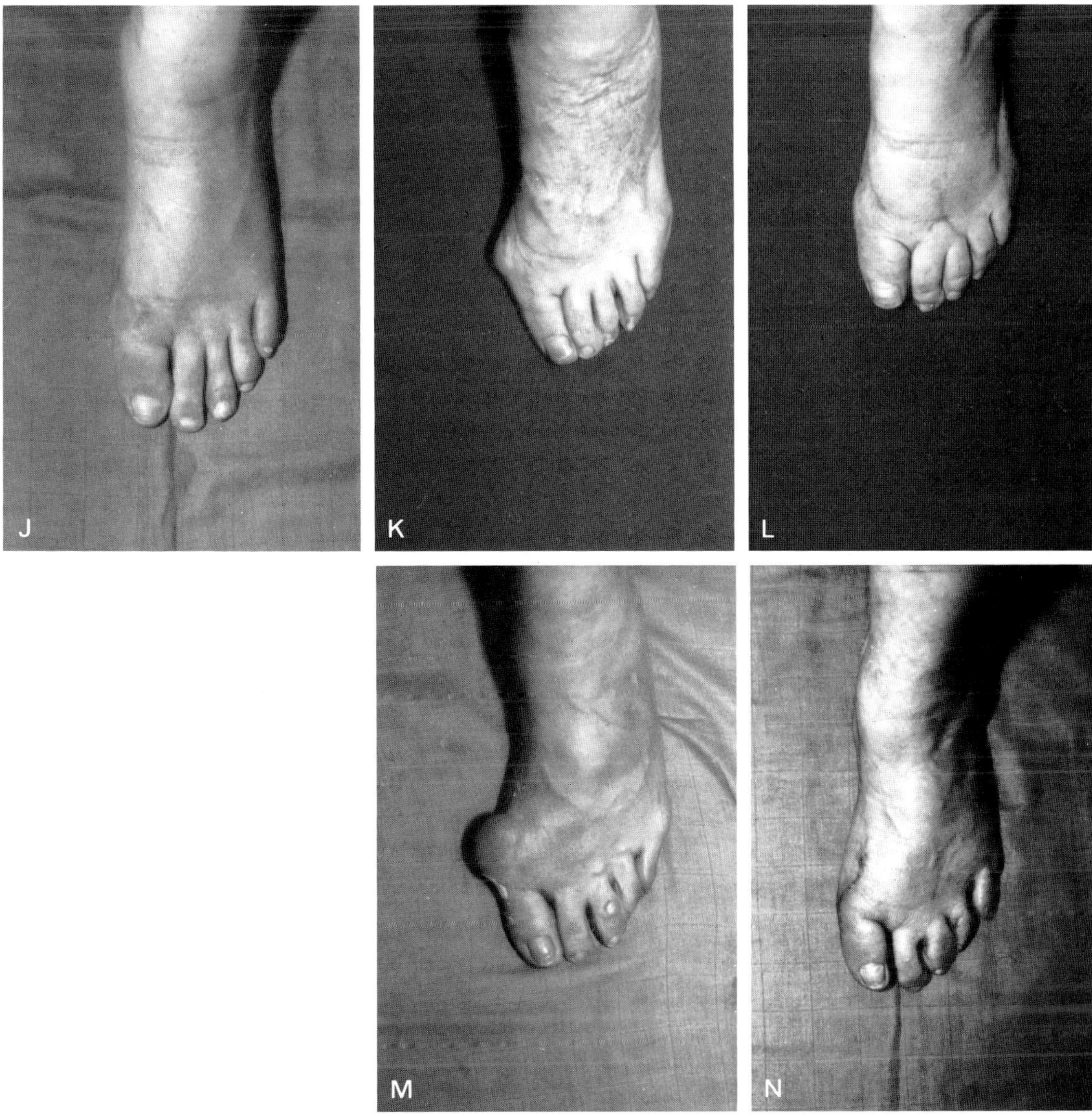

◁ **Fig. 18.13 A–N.** Results of correction of hallux valgus using Regnauld technique. **A–D** First degree: pre- and postoperative appearance in two cases. **E–H** Second degree: pre- and postoperative appearance in two cases. **I–N** Third degree: pre- and postoperative appearance in three cases

At the same time, the metatarsus varus is reduced by resection of the exostosis and a capsular suture. This operation gives excellent aesthetic and functional results, but the screw fixation of the phalanx is difficult and there is a danger of injury to the nutrient artery of the phalanx.

In the case of the Greek forefoot, when there is metatarsophalangeal angulation of first or second degree without obliquity of the phalangeal base and without osteophyte formation, three other operations can be employed. These have the advantage of preserving the metatarsophalangeal joint, but only when there is no need for shortening.

Schede Operation (Fig. 18.3 A–D). This operation (Schede 1955) comprises simple excision of the medial exostosis which if performed in isolation will result in recurrence in most instances (Fig. 18.3 A–D). It must be complemented by

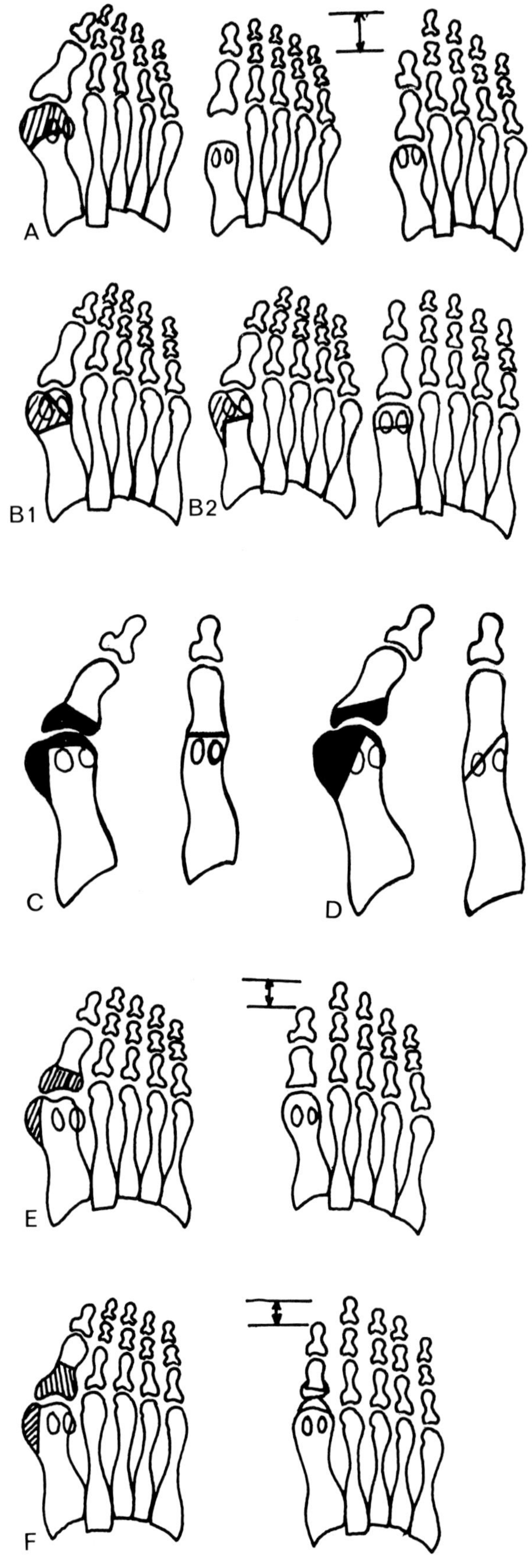

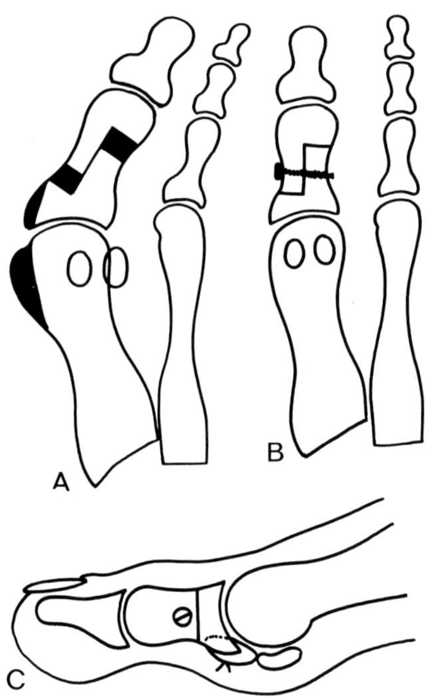

△ **Fig. 18.15 A–C.** Correction of hallux valgus (Burutaran technique). **A** Sliding corrective osteotomy of proximal phalanx. **B** Shortening of proximal phalanx with screw fixation. **C** Reposition of sesamoid bone by capsulorrhaphy and intra-osseous suture

◁ **Fig. 18.14 A–F.** Operative procedures for hallux valgus. **A** Hueter-Mayo amputation of condyle of metatarsal. **B** *1* Reverdin procedure; *2* Ombredanne procedure. **C** Simple arthrodesis. **D** Mauclaire arthroplasty. **E** Keller-Brandes arthroplasty. **F** Wallet arthroplasty detachment of the metatarsophalangeal capsule, while preserving the nutrient arteries of the phalanx of the metatarsal, by means of capsulorrhaphy of the sesamoid bone as described by Lelièvre (1952), which corrects varus of the great metatarsal, and by reduction of the hallux valgus (Fig. 18.16). Probably this procedure has a place in first- and second-degree hallux valgus in the Greek forefoot, in both the young and the older patient. In such cases it gives excellent functional and aesthetic results, provided that, at the end of the procedure, the great toe does not exceed the second toe in length.

McBride-Joplin Operation. The adductor tendon of the great toe is transplanted from its normal insertion onto the head of the first metatarsal. McBride (1928) cautioned against removal of the lateral sesamoid, which prejudices the stability of the plantar strap, and against transplantation of the tendon under the neck of the great metatarsal. The results are good functionally and aesthetically if performed in the Greek forefoot where the hallux valgus is of first or second degree and in the presence of a good quality metatarsophalangeal joint in which the base of the phalanx is perpendicular to the longitudinal axis of the bone. However, it is important not to perform too tight a reduction of the varus. This operation is contra-indicated in hallux valgus in the Egyptian type of foot, in third-degree hallux valgus, in which the adductor muscle has become stretched and incompetent, and when there is arthrosis of the metatarsophalangeal joint or obliquity of the basal surface of the phalanx. Its main complications are too tight a reduction of the varus of the metatarsal, pain due to tension, hallux varus and postoperative arthrosis of the rigid type. Courriades, de Doncker and Kowalski, Regnauld and Valenti have all stressed the importance of preservation of vertical motion of the great metatarsal against the neighbouring second metatarsal; this movement is essential if normal configuration of the metatarsal heads on an irregular ground surface is to be achieved.

Operative Technique. Through a dorsal longitudinal incision in the region of the first interspace, the two heads of the adductor are detached from the base of the proximal phalanx on the outer aspect of the sesamoids and secured by a nylon or slowly resorbable suture. Through a second, medial longitudinal incision, the metatarsophalangeal joint is exposed and the exostosis on the metatarsal head resected. The dislocation of the sesamoids is reduced, a hole is bored through the metatarsal head as described by Joplin (1928) and the adductor tendon is passed through this transverse canal by means of the stay suture, which is secured under tension to the capsular layer of the metatarsal.

Recaredo-Alvarez Operation. This operation (Recaredo-Alvarez 1969) comprises removal of the medial exostosis from the metatarsal head and preserves the integrity of the proximal phalanx. The lateral subluxation of the sesamoid is corrected by the capsulorrhaphy of Lelièvre (1952) and the varus of the first metatarsal is corrected by means of a YV-plasty of the inner capsular layer. Recaredo-Alvarez performs a Y-shaped longitudinal internal incision in the capsulo-aponeurotic tissue with the two branches of the Y distally. After separation of the intervening triangular tongue of tissue and reduction of the sesamoid dislocation and the metatarsus varus, the tongue is drawn proximally under tension and sutured to the capsular layer sufficiently far proximally to maintain correction of the valgus of the great toe. The operation is useful for first- and second-degree hallux valgus but is not effective for third-degree cases or when there is obliquity of the articular surface of the phalanx which will resist long-term correction of the hallux valgus. It has the advantage of conserving the articular surfaces and should be confined to the Greek type of forefoot.
It is definitely contra-indicated for hallux valgus of the square or Egyptian foot, as the long great toe, the basic origin of hallux valgus in these cases, is preserved.

18.1.4 Metatarsal Osteotomy

Complementary osteotomy of the base of the metatarsal may be useful in those rare cases where varus of the metatarsal has been irreducible by transverse capsulorrhaphy of the sesamoids alone. Trethowan (1923) and Garelli (1976) independently described osteotomies in which, after division of the bone transversely and correction of the varus, a bone graft is inserted into the medial aspect to maintain ing reduction. A semicircular transverse osteotomy is preferable, with an anterior concavity, which is very easy to regulate.
The indications for metatarsal osteotomy should be carefully assessed, because there is the danger of impaired physiological abduction of the first metatarsal and this can create the conditions for the development of hallux rigidus, phalangeal necrosis or metatarsal epiphyseal necrosis due to increased joint pressure. The normal physiological

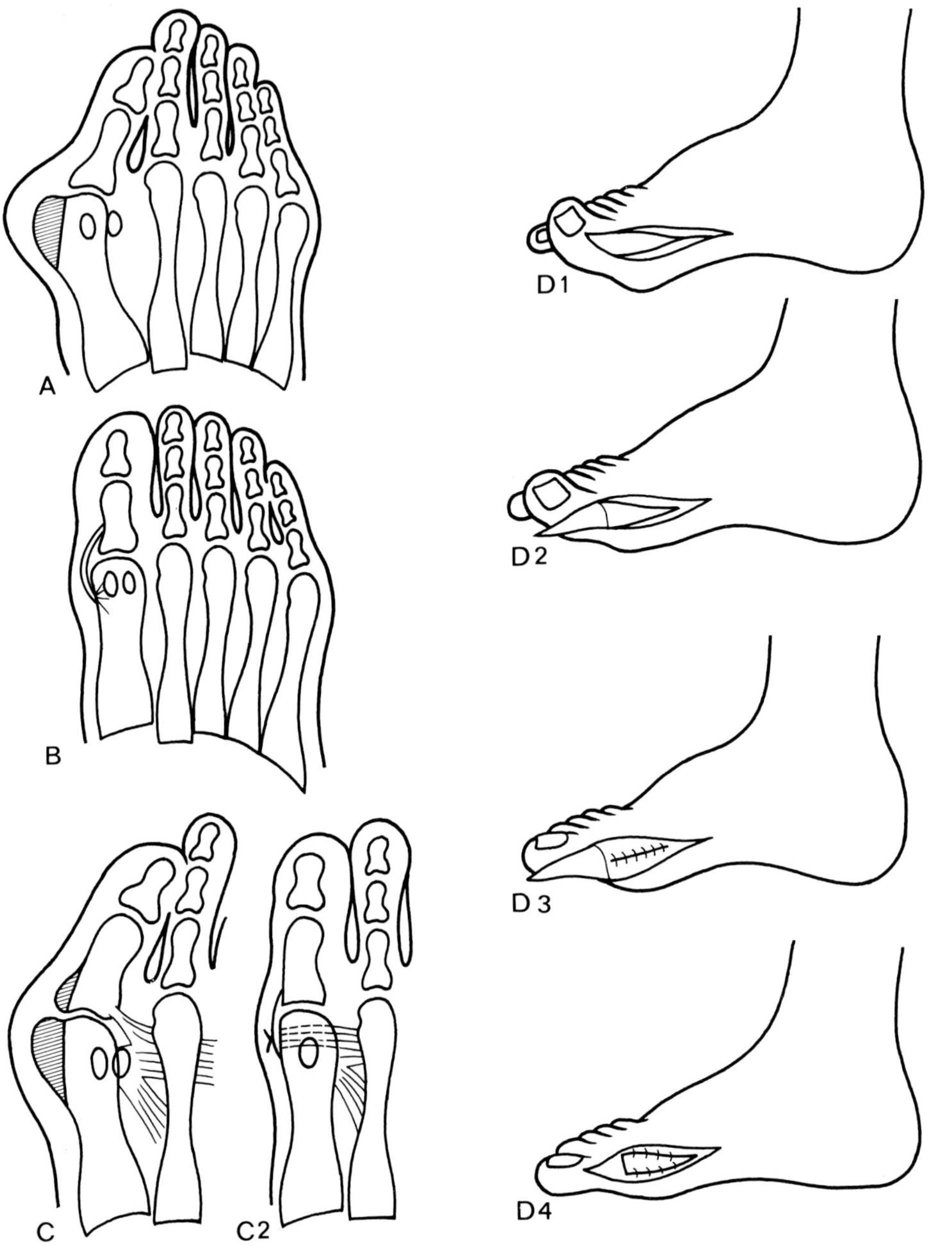

Fig. 18.16 A–D. Operative procedures for hallux valgus. **A** Schède procedure. **B** Modified Schède procedure with sesamoid capsulorrhaphy (Lelièvre). **C** *1, 2* Stages of MacBride-Joplin procedure. **D** *1–4* Stages of Recaredo Alvarez-Rodriguez procedure

movement of the first metatarsal must be preserved.

In summary, success demands the following (Figs. 18.3–18.5):

1. Reconstitution of a forefoot in which metatarsal loading is conserved or restored so as to assure painless propulsion
2. Correction of hallux valgus in relationship to the wearing of a normal shoe
3. Preservation of amplitude of movement at the joints and of the metatarsals
4. A great toe equal to or slightly (2–3 mm) shorter than the second toe (except in the Greek forefoot configuration)
5. Avoidance of overcorrection of varus of the first metatarsal
6. Protection of the nutrient arteries of the first metatarsal head and the proximal phalanx in all operative procedures
7. Correction of the plantar capsule maintaining the position of the sesamoids, but never involving the long flexor tendon otherwise postoperative clawing of the great toe will occur
8. Active re-education, never passive mobilisation
9. Restoration of normal walking action as soon as possible allowing for postoperative discomfort and the resolution of postoperative oedema

18.2 Hallux Varus

18.2.1 Description

The term hallux varus is self-explanatory and relates to an adduction of the great toe which brings about difficulty with footwear, callus formation and sometimes the development of ingrown toenail involving the medial nail fold. It may be acquired, as in trauma involving the joint, or iatrogenic, the result of unsuccessful operative treatment for another condition. Congenital causes include syndactyly.

18.2.2 Clinical Features

There is adduction of the great toe with respect to the axis of the first metatarsal, the latter being correctly orientated with respect to the second metatarsal (cf. Fig. 25.1 G, I–K, O). Contracture of the abductor tendon of the great toe and of extensor hallucis longus, which tends to bowstring across the dorsal border of the foot, is an associated feature, and while the great metatarsal preserves its normal vertical range of motion, it loses the property of lateral movement. The first interdigital space becomes widened distally.

The varus posture of the great toe may be reducible or fixed, depending on the degree of tension in the skin, the abductor tendon and the extensor hallucis longus and brevis tendons. Correction may be resisted by hypertrophy of the soft tissues of the first interdigital commissure. The quality of joint movement is usually normal, especially when the cause has been congenital, in which case the hallux varus may be hypermobile.

In the various forms of iatrogenic hallux varus, the amplitude of movement varies from flail mobility to ankylosis. Thus, in osteolytic hallux varus due to excessive removal of bone in resection arthroplasty, the great toe is short, varus and hypermobile. In contrast, ankylosis can occur in this shortened condition; it may result when poor re-education after arthroplasty has led to excessive scarring. There will be significant loss of function during walking due to supination.

Varus deformities of the lesser toes may be apparent due to contracture of the extensor communis and brevis tendons and of the capsular layers of the dorsal and medial aspects of the joints. Standard *radiographs* reveal the angulation developed at the metatarsophalangeal joints and the alignment of the five metatarsals; any arthrosis or osteophyte formation around the joint is apparent, together with any mishaps of previous surgery such as overresection of bone and loss of joint space. In the varus congenital foot, the absence of signs of arthrosis or other irritative features should be noted. At the base of the proximal phalanx, it may be that only the internal two-thirds is articulating with the metatarsal head.

18.2.3 Treatment

Various forms of surgical management are appropriate for congenital hallux varus in the child and sometimes in the adult, and for those forms secondary to previous surgery or trauma.

Child. If hallux varus is associated with a bifid phalanx, ablation of the supernumerary digit is indicated, the less-developed component usually being chosen (Fig. 18.17). Plastic resection of the soft parts and the nail can allow restoration of normal appearance and good function. Metatarsophalangeal arthrotomy with elongation of contracted tendons (extensor hallucis longus, extensor brevis and the abductor of the toe) may be necessary. If the

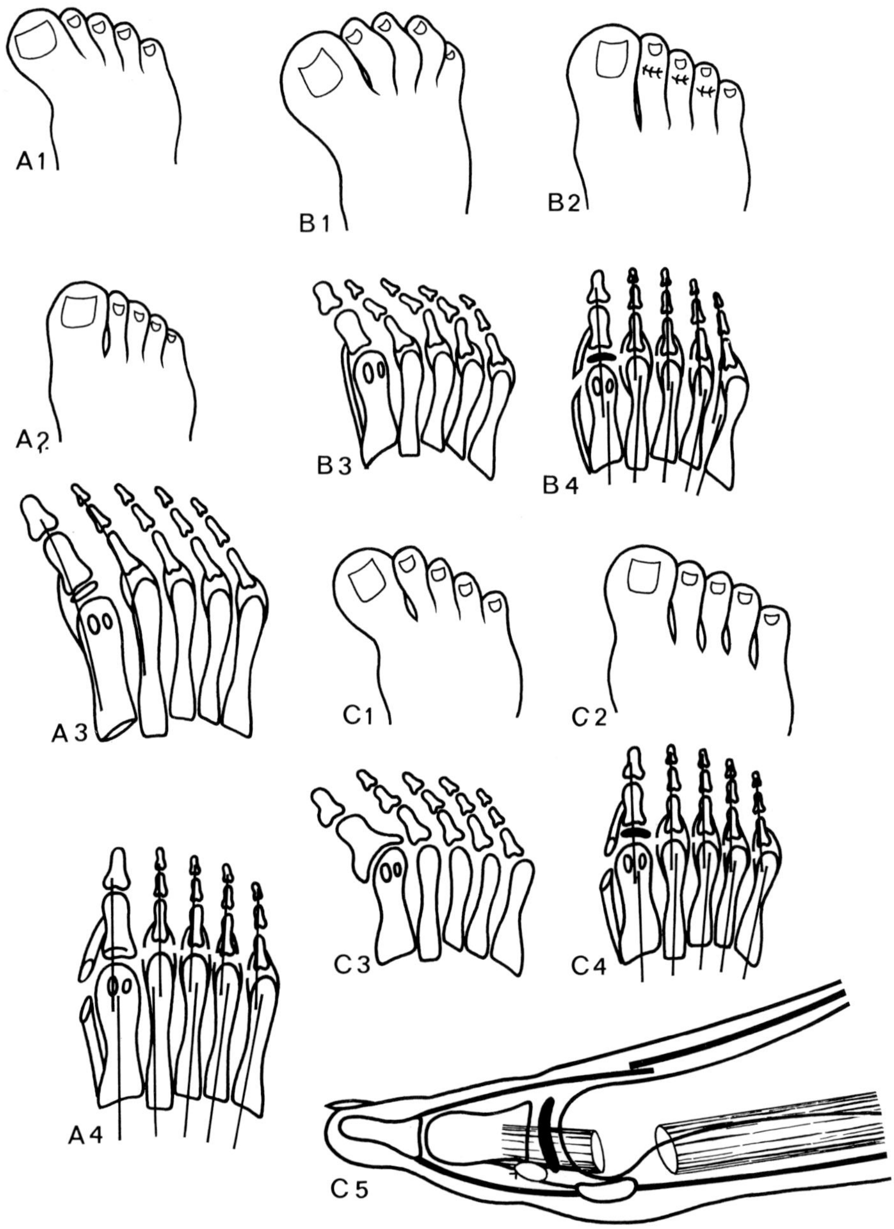

Fig. 18.17 A–C. Treatment of hallux varus. **A** Congenital: *1, 3* Before operation; *2, 4* after metatarsophalangeal arthrolysis, capsulotomy, elongation of extensor tendons and tenotomy of adductor tendon of great toe. **B** Iatrogenic hypermobile: *1, 3* Before operation; *2, 4* after metatarsophalangeal arthroplasty with cup prosthesis if necessary, metatarsophalangeal arthrolysis, internal capsulotomy, elongation of extensor tendons and tenotomy of adductor tendon of great toe. **C** Iatrogenic rigid: *1, 3* Before operation; *2, 4, 5* after tenotomy of adductor tendon of great toe, metatarsophalangeal arthroplasty with cup prosthesis, metatarsophalangeal arthrolysis and internal capsulotomy

hallux varus is a component of overall pes adductus, correction of the abducted metatarsal associated with arthrolysis of the metatarsophalangeal joint may be indicated.

Adult. The hallux varus has usually become irreducible on account of skin and tendon contractures together with consequent displacement of the metatarsophalangeal joint. Shortening of the proximal phalanx of the great toe is essential for correction of the angulation and the repositioning of the toe into a normal axis with respect to the metatarsal. This can be achieved by reconstitution of the articular surface of the phalanx by means of application of an osteocartilaginous graft onto the base of the resected phalanx, as described above in the operative treatment of hallux valgus, and constitutes the first stage of the operative management. Elongation of the extensor hallucis longus and brevis tendons is required, sometimes together with elongation of the flexor hallucis longus tendon. Next, the abductor tendon is divided, passed under the neck of the first metatarsal and reinserted on the lateral aspect of the base of the proximal phalanx (Lelièvre 1952). The detachment, or perhaps Z-elongation, of this tendon suffices in many instances to allow long-term correction. Finally, the soft tissues in the interdigital space between the first and second metatarsal heads may require resection in order to allow the metatarsal heads to come together, and the commissural gap may have to be sutured to allow approximation of the great toe towards the second toe. This preserves the axis of the first metatarsal. Rehabilitation is similar to that for hallux valgus, but during the first 3 months after treatment the position of the great toe should be maintained by an elastic bandage, ensuring its longitudinal axis as long as any postoperative oedema remains.

Post-traumatic. Permanent malunion of a comminuted fracture of the proximal phalanx, provoking varus of the great toe, demands resection of the base of the phalanx and – if the contiguous metatarsal surface is normal – insertion of an osteocartilaginous graft. Otherwise, a cup prosthesis should be interposed.

Iatrogenic. As stated earlier, iatrogenic hallux varus may be hypermobile or rigid. In the *hypermobile* variety, adduction of the great toe supervenes in the weeks following the operation performed most commonly for hallux valgus. In this case, simple tenotomy of the abductor tendon and corrective bandaging may re-establish proper alignment before the situation gets out of control. In other instances, osteolysis of the base of the phalanx may be progressive a few months after the operation for hallux valgus, causing the great toe to become misaligned in varus and dorsiflexion. Medial and dorsal cutaneous contracture and shortening of extensor hallucis longus, the medial insertion of the short extensor and the abductor tendon may be involved. This condition can be satisfactorily rectified by the interposition of fibrous tissue between the metatarsal head and the base of the phalangeal remnant.

The *rigid* variety relates to insufficiency of resection of the base of the phalanx and failure to ensure corrective re-education after operation. Peripheral osteophytes develop, and a poor gait encourages progressive varus displacement and ankylosis. Mobility of the great toe must be achieved by interpositional cup arthroplasty (Regnauld and Grassin 1975) or by the cutaneous interpositional arthroplasty described by de Wulf (1978). This is complemented by excision of the fibrous scarring in the intermetatarsophalangeal area and repositioning of the sesamoids under the first metatarsal heads, accompanied by elongation of extensor hallucis longus and extensor brevis, tenotomy of the abductor tendon, and closure of the capsular layer and skin. Establishment of correct alignment with stability inhibits any osteolytic process. The management of hallux varus of the rigid type is the same as that for hallux rigidus in general.

Should a varus posture of the lesser toes accompany the main hallux varus, arthrotomy of the appropriate metatarsophalangeal joints with elongation of the long and short extensors and capsulotomy of the internal and dorsal planes of the capsules will allow re-establishment of their normal longitudinal axis.

18.3 Hallux Flexus

18.3.1 Description

The abnormality comprises a displacement of the metatarsophalangeal joint as a result of varying degrees of dorsiflexion of the great metatarsal and flexion deformity of the interphalangeal joint. (cf. Fig. 23.3 D, E). This may result in the distal phalanx being relatively in the same axis as the metatarsal or in a plantarflexed posture. There is associated muscular imbalance due to atonia or paralysis of extensor hallucis longus with hypertonia or contracture of the long flexor tendon. The configuration of the metatarsophalangeal joint is altered in that the articular curvature is flattened and narrowed dorsally, accompanied by protuberance of the cartilaginous margin of the metatarsal head. There is osteophytosis of the base of the proximal phalanx, and in this respect the condition is analogous to first-degree hallux rigidus. Kingreen (1933) regarded hallux flexus as being provoked by osteochondritis or epiphyseal necrosis of the base of the proximal phalanx in the young adolescent, but the condition becomes painful only in later life, after closure of the epiphyseal line, thus leaving no evidence of the pregrowth etiology.

The etiology varies: Primary hallux valgus may appear without any obvious cause, associated with some degree of rigidus, or an associated plantar keratoma under the first or second metatarsal head may lead to a protective attitude of plantarflexion of the great toe. Sometimes the origin is congenital, secondary to varus club foot or to pes adductus in the adult. A paralytic origin relates to the peroneal muscles or extensor hallucis longus. Inflammatory causes are seen in ankylosing spondylitis. Following trauma, ischaemic contracture may lead to foot deformity due to contracture of the long flexor tendon; initially, there is no deformity of the metatarsophalangeal joint.

18.3.2 Clinical Features

The patient complains of discomfort during walking because of difficulty in performing the normal rolling action of the foot. He tends to supinate during toe-off.

Examination reveals a cavus supinated foot which rests predominantly on the heel, the outer border and the extremity of the toes. There is longitudinal internal cavus, associated with an irreducible dorsiflexed posture of the first metatarsal. The condyle does not reach the ground, failing by some 5–15 mm. The plantarflexed posture of the proximal phalanx of the great toe, with the distal phalanx in the same axis or even more plantarflexed, amounts to a claw deformity or occasionally an interphalangeal dorsiflexion deformity. In such instances, there may be a plantar keratoma on the distal pulp, or painful thickening of the skin under the interphalangeal joint of the great toe can result from a hyperextended distal phalanx. The dorsal prominence of the metatarsophalangeal joint may result in formation of a serous bursa or callus on the dorsal aspect, associated perhaps with a bony exostosis of the cartilaginous margin of the joint. Contracture of the short and long flexors of the great toe is present, together with atrophy, elongation or even paralysis of extensor hallucis longus. During walking, the impossibility of plantarflexion of the metatarsal and dorsiflexion of the great toe becomes apparent. This is due to the distortion and flattening of the articular curvature of the metatarsophalangeal joint and abutment of the base of the proximal phalanx against a metatarsal dorsal osteophyte. Extensor hallucis longus and brevis insufficiencies preclude dorsiflexion of the proximal phalanx.

The exact cause of loss of motion at the metatarsophalangeal joint can be ascertained by examination of the foot in acute plantarflexion of the ankle; relaxation of the long flexor tendon is allowed, and if the impediment to dorsiflexion is mechanical in the joint itself, this will become quickly apparent. There may be passive reduced amplitude or even complete loss of movement. Displacement at the joint may be associated with capsular contraction on the plantar aspect and adhesions of the sesamoid underneath (Figs. 18.18, 18.19).

Radiography: The loaded lateral view shows the orientation of the metatarsophalangeal joint, any flattening or hypertrophy of the dorsal cartilaginous margin of the great metatarsal head, and the orientation of the base of the proximal phalanx with respect to the longitudinal axis of the metatarsal. Loss of joint space indicates the development of hallux flexus rigidus.

18.3.3 Treatment

Operative treatment must re-establish the normal purchase of the metatarsal head on the ground by lowering the first metatarsal to its normal degree of inclination.

The primary cause must be sought, and operative technique must vary according to the cause. For instance, hallux flexus due to Volkmann ischaemic contracture demands simple elongation of the long flexor tendons and there is no indication for disturbing the metatarsophalangeal joint. In talipes equinovarus in which there is persistent metatarsal supination together with the hallux flexus deformity, the main condition must be corrected first; in a congenital planovalgus foot, the same principle applies. Poliomyelitis leading to muscle imbalance demands correction of equilibrium between the flexors and extensors by shortening or elongation of tendons, by tenodesis or by transposition procedures. If there should be associated hallux rigidus or misalignment from ankylosing spondylitis, pri-

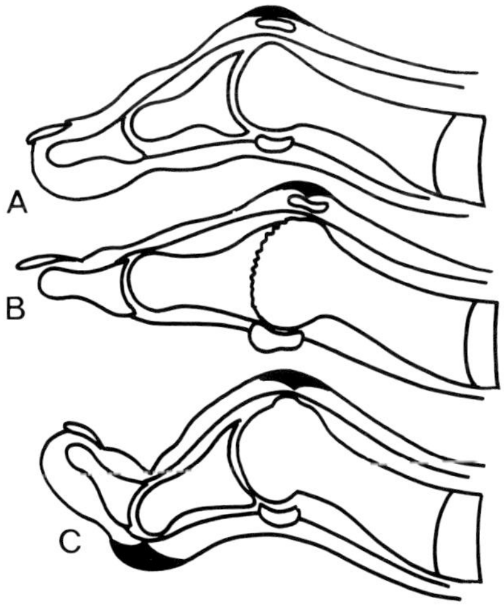

Fig. 18.18. A Hallux flexus with normal articular cartilage. **B** Rigid hallux flexus: articular cartilage destroyed. **C** Hallux flexus with reverse clawing of great toe

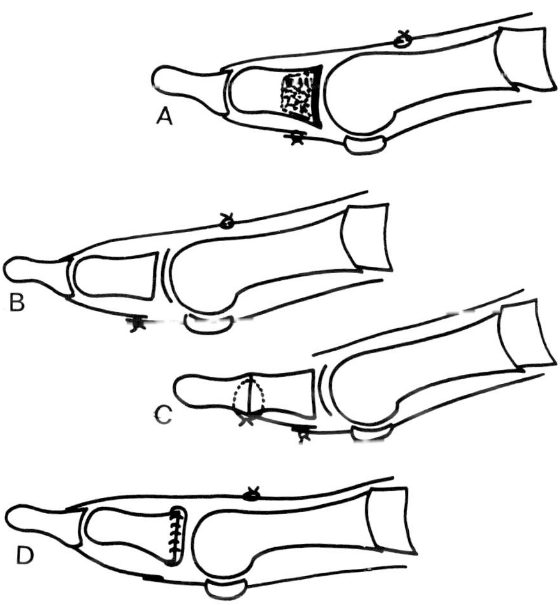

Fig. 18.19 A–D. Correction of hallux flexus by curvilinear basal osteotomy of the first metatarsal, thereby lowering the metatarsal heads, accompanied by elongation of the flexor tendons and shortening of the extensor tendons. The metatarsophalangeal joint is corrected by one of the following procedures. **A** Metatarsophalangeal arthroplasty using a cork-shaped graft (in hallus flexus with preservation of articular cartilage) (Regnauld). **B** Metatarsophalangeal cup arthroplasty (in hallux flexus with damage to articular cartilage) (Regnauld). **C** Metarsophalangeal arthroplasty with interposition cup prosthesis and arthrodesis of interphalangeal joint (in rigid hallux flexus with reverse clawing of the great toe) (Regnauld). **D** Metatarsophalangeal arthroplasty by skin interposition (de Wulf)

mary treatment must be directed towards the cartilaginous structure of the joint itself.
After correction of any primitive displacement underlying the hallux flexus, final treatment comprises, in this order:

1. Metatarsophalangeal arthroplasty, effected by resection of the base of the proximal phalanx and implantation of an osteocartilaginous "graft" (see Fig. 18.12) to restore the integrity of the joint surface. Alternatively, a cup prosthesis can be interposed if the articular surfaces are too damaged or distorted. De Wulf (1978) has described an interposition skin graft procedure.
2. Correction of the interphalangeal angulation by arthrodesis.
3. Basal osteotomy of the great metatarsal, necessary to correct its dorsiflexed posture (Fig. 18.20). Either the technique of Lelièvre (1952), in which a cuneiform resection with a wedge based on the plantar aspect is performed, or the technique of Hammond (1943), in which a wedge resection at the base is stabilised by an osseous triangular corner, may be used. I have described a comma-shaped ostectomy with a plantar base and a simple curvilinear osteotomy with a posterior concavity; this allows controlled reorientation of the first metatarsal, and coaptation is assured by insertion of a transosseous wire or a staple.
4. Balancing of the joint by restoration of the lengths of the flexor tendons (elongated) and extensor tendons (shortened).

Immobilisation with relief of weight bearing is necessary for 6 weeks postoperatively. Progressive weight bearing is allowed only after radiography confirms bony union of the various osteotomies concerned.

18.4 Hallux Extensus and Hallux Erectus

This deformity comprises a permanent dorsiflexion of the great toe; two types should be distinguished (Fig. 18.21).

18.4.1 Idiopathic Hallux Extensus

Primary hallux extensus occurs most frequently in the heavy woman who has persisted in wearing high heels, and is associated with a mobile cavus foot. Exceptionally, it occurs in the heavily built man with a cavus foot, but here an irreducible claw deformity of the great toe is more common. Lacer-

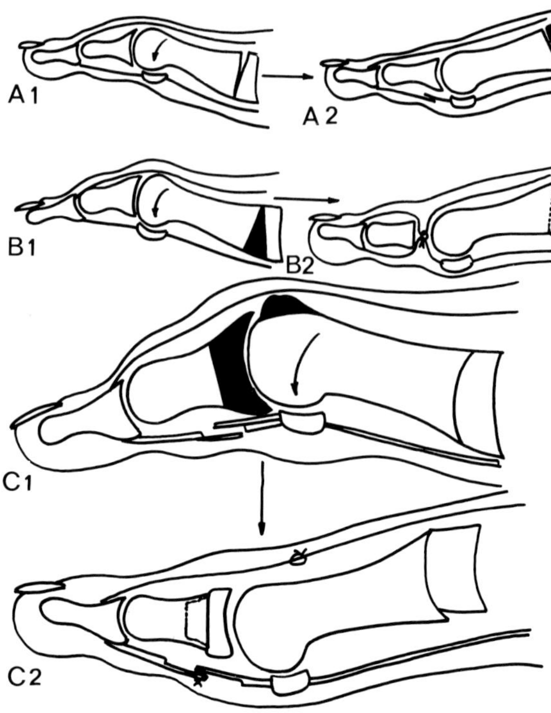

Fig. 18.20 A–C. Operation techniques for hallux flexus. **A** *1* Hammond metatarsal osteotomy; *2* metatarsophalangeal arthroplasty and insertion of triangular bone graft. **B** *1* Lelièvre wedge resection metatarsal osteotomy; *2* metatarsophalangeal arthroplasty. **C** *1* Regnauld curvilinear basal metatarsal osteotomy; *2* metatarsophalangeal arthroplasty, autograft, elongation of flexor hallucis longus and shortening of extensor hallucis longus (Regnauld)

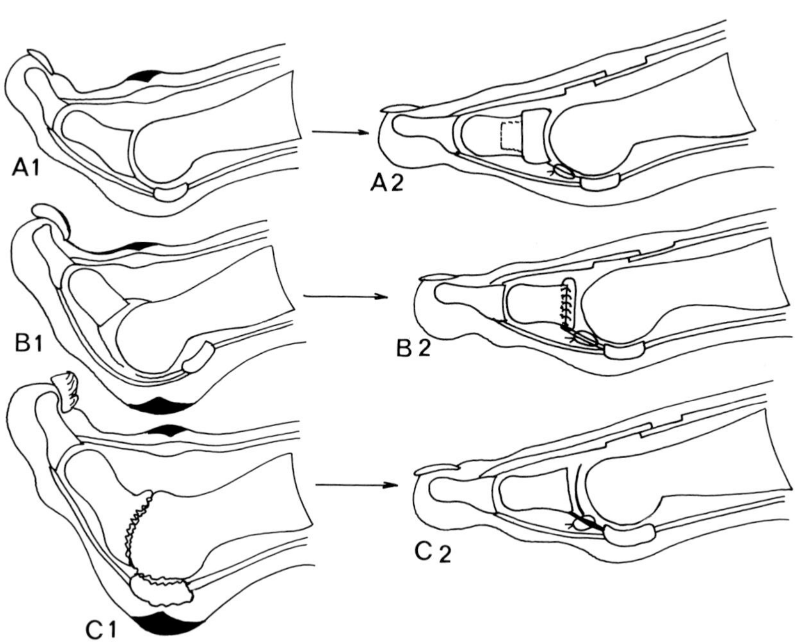

Fig. 18.21 A–C. Operation techniques for hallux erectus. **A** Idiopathic: *1* Before treatment; *2* after metatarsophalangeal arthroplasty with autograft (Regnauld). **B** Iatrogenic mobile: *1* Before treatment; *2* after metatarsophalangeal arthroplasty by skin interposition (de Wulf). **C** Iatrogenic fixed: *1* Before treatment; *2* after metatarsophalangeal cup arthroplasty (Regnauld)

ation of the long flexor tendon or paralysis of flexor hallucis longus can lead to the condition. Permanent dorsiflexion of the great toe develops at the metatarsophalangeal joints, and the two phalanges remain aligned. Contracture of the short extensor and long extensor tendons is associated with bowstringing across the dorsal aspect of the metatarsophalangeal joint and troublesome thickening of the overlying skin associated with repeated episodes of inflammation and infection. This thickening of the skin results from compression of the tendon against the free border of the upper of the shoe, especially when there is a high heel, and it is the resulting symptoms which bring the patient to consultation.

Limitation of plantarflexion leads to failure of the prehensile action of the great toe and development of a convex forefoot. Dorsal capsular contracture renders the condition irreversible.

Secondarily, a subungual corn of the nail bed is provoked by constant friction against the toecap of the shoe, and serous bursitis with or without skin thickening and plantar keratoma can occur under the first metatarsal head.

Radiography shows angulation at the metatarsophalangeal joint associated with straight alignment of the toe. The metatarsophalangeal articular surfaces are congruent, there being no displacement of the sesamoids. After many years, plantar hypertrophy of the base of the proximal phalanx develops together with obliquity of the proximal surface of the proximal phalanx, and this contributes to the irreducibility of the displacement. The sesamoids hypertrophy. A small exostosis in the subungual region is the result of localised pressure from the shoe upper

18.4.1.1 Treatment

Initially, when the hallux extensus is supple, *orthotic* treatment may be successful. An insole with a bar behind the heads of the metatarsals can completely restore equilibrium if high-heeled shoes are no longer worn.

In irreducible cases, *operative* treatment is necessary. The short extensor and extensor hallucis longus tendons should be elongated after excision of any dorsal callus due to bowstringing. Mobilisation of the metatarsophalangeal joint by dorsolateral capsulotomy and shortening of the flexor tendon can re-establish joint balance, but subsequent careful rehabilitation and avoidance of precipitating factors are essential. In more advanced cases, arthroplasty of the metatarsophalangeal joint by resection of the base of the phalanx and implantation of an osteocartilaginous graft is recommended, as for hallux valgus. This is the only way to realign the transverse plane of the base of the phalanx correctly.

Obviously, any rupture or shortening of the long flexor tendon has to be corrected.

In the presence of paralysis of flexor hallucis longus, transplantation of the abductor tendon to the long or short flexor tendon superficial to the attachment of the sesamoid bones can stabilise the metatarsophalangeal joint, provided rehabilitation is careful.

18.4.2 Iatrogenic Hallux Erectus

Hallux erectus can follow unsuccessful arthroplasty in which the stability of the sesamoids has not been taken into account, so that they have subluxed posteriorly. Osteolysis of a resected proximal phalanx or an osteocartilaginous graft can occur if the reduction has been too tight due to persisting varus of the great metatarsal, which produces overloading of its lateral margin. The overloading results in osteonecrosis which may in some instances result in mobile hallux erectus, while in others, due to osteophyte formation, the deformity may be rigid. In either case, the incorrect siting of the plantar sesamoid assembly in relation to the capsule is the basic problem.

If the sesamoids are not stable under the metatarsal head, posterior subluxation can occur together with laxity of the plantar capsule and mobile hallux erectus. If operation has led to scarring, the deformity becomes rigid due to peripheral osteophyte formation and the destruction of the articular surface.

Clinically, iatrogenic hallux erectus presents as permanent dorsiflexion of the great toe with loss of active plantarflexion and failure of prehensile action. There is contracture of both long and short extensor tendons, but the development of a pressure callus where these bowstring is less common in the iatrogenic form than in the primary variety. The sesamoids become displaced posteriorly, as can be demonstrated on palpation, so that the condyles of the metatarsal heads are prominent. The failure of action of the first ray results in insufficiency which leads secondarily to overloading of the second metatarsal head, under which a serous bursa or painful corn may form, or the development of a convex forefoot with central pressure signs and claw deformities of the second, third and fourth toes.

Broadly, two forms of iatrogenic hallux erectus are seen:

1. *Mobile* hallux erectus follows excessive resection of the base of the proximal phalanx, subsequent lysis of the remaining bone of the proximal phalanx and instability of the sesamoids. The great toe is shortened, erect and sometimes flail and becomes displaced dorsally and occasionally laterally, being maintained in its subluxed position dorsomedially by contracture of extensor hallucis longus. These features are apparent clinically and on radiography
2. *Rigid* hallux erectus occurs following excessively conservative resection of the base of a phalanx during arthroplasty and over tight reduction due to varus of the great metatarsal, and is associated with fixity of the sesamoids. The great toe is fixed in dorsiflexion with contracture of the long and short extensor tendons; ankylosis of the metatarsophalangeal joint with hypertrophy of the bony margin is clearly palpable, and the sesamoids can hypertrophy, becoming fixed under the metatarsal condyles. Secondary nail complications may occur (onychogryphosis, onychosis, ingrown toenail).

Radiography, shows that the deformity of the metatarsal joint is accompanied by arthrosis in the rigid type of hallux erectus. Osteophytes may be seen, together with narrowing of the joint space. Osteophytes may also present around the margin of the sesamoid bones, where loss of joint space may be apparent as well.

18.4.2.1 Treatment

Iatrogenic hallux erectus always requires surgical measures. Of prime importance is correction of the plantar sesamoid displacement and the instability, following which balancing of the extensors and flexors by appropriate elongations or shortenings should correct the posture at the metatarsophalangeal joint.

In *mobile* hallux erectus, stability can be achieved after excision of intra-articular fibrous tissue by the implantation of a skin graft over the remaining margin of the phalanx (de Wulf 1978). In *rigid* hallux erectus, further resection of the base of the arthrosic phalanx, removal of osteophytes, proper modelling of the head of the first metatarsal and interposition of a cup prosthesis is the procedure of choice (Regnauld and Grassin 1975).

Operative Technique. Through a dorsal incision, extensor hallucis longus and brevis are elongated. Through a medial incision, the capsular ligament is detached from around the dorsal and plantar aspects of the metatarsal head. The sesamoid bones are freed from their fibrous adhesions, and at the same time the flexor hallucis longus tendon is mobilised in its sesamoid gutter as far distally as the joint space. Here, fibrous tissue between the metatarsal head and the remainder of the phalanx is removed carefully and the surfaces trimmed so as to allow the interposition of the cup prosthesis. The plantar capsule is sutured, ensuring that the sesamoid bones remain in their proper place under the metatarsal head. The capsule is closed without tension, and after careful haemostasis the skin is sutured. The cup prosthesis must be removed after a year.

If the great toe shortening is gross, it may prove necessary to shorten the adjacent toes in order to re-establish, as nearly as possible, the proper line of digital propulsion.

If the hallux erectus is accompanied by insufficiency of weight bearing of the great metatarsal head, further procedures may be necessary. Osteotomy or basal ostectomy (Mau 1940 or Thys 1974b) of the second metatarsal will correct overloading of its condyle. In the presence of a convex forefoot with tendinous contractures and metatarsophalangeal joint displacements enclavement procedures of the second, third and fourth metatarsals are indicated, accompanied by basal osteotomies of the second and fourth metatarsals (Mau 1940; Thys 1974b). The bone resections from these ostectomies must be precisely calculated and performed so as to avoid development of a cavus forefoot.

19 Quintus Varus

19.1 Description

Clinodactyly of the fifth ray is usually of congenital origin, sometimes becoming progressive during adolescence. It is less common than comparable deformities of the other toes. When it occurs in infancy the concerned parent notices supraductus (dorsal overlapping) of the little toe. The condition is easily correctable, and the fifth metatarsal is not in a valgus posture; there is no cutaneous contracture, but the extensor tendon is tight.

From the age of about 12 years, metatarsus quintus varus begins to be responsible for shoe discomfort, and lateral prominence of the metatarsophalangeal joint and obtuse angulation between the metatarsal and the toe are responsible for friction and pressure. A tailor's bunion becomes apparent on the dorsolateral surface of the proximal interphalangeal joint, and the local pressure on the nail can also be troublesome. The deformity is analogous to that of hallux valgus, with which it may be associated in the adult. The two displacements ultimately constitute a triangular forefoot.

19.2 Clinical Features

In its more developed permanent state, the most characteristic sign of quintus varus is the valgus posture of the fifth metatarsal (cf. Fig. 17.4 J, K), which varies in degree, amounting to some 10°–20° relative to the neighbouring fourth metatarsal. It can usually be reduced by lateral compression, but recurs immediately when this is released. Occasionally, the abduction posture is associated with inward distal curvature of the metatarsal, which produces an abnormal projection towards the end of the bone. The valgus posture of the fifth toe stems from the metatarsophalangeal joint, and the base of the proximal phalanx articulates with the inner two-thirds of the metatarsal condyle. The general alignment of the phalanges of the little toe remains normal in most instances, but the varus at the distal interphalangeal joint can be augmented. The digit may come to rest under the fourth toe (infraductus) or over it (supraductus), the latter being the more frequent. Pressure leads to spatulate deformity and hypertrophy of the nail.

In the *infraductus* position, a dorsal corn of the first phalanx with a partridge eye on the plantar external aspect of the fourth toe will be associated with the quintus varus. In the *supraductus* posture, a dorsal corn develops on the proximal phalanx, and a partridge eye on the plantar aspect of the proximal phalanx corresponds to a similar partridge eye on the dorsal aspect of the first phalanx of the fourth toe.

Significant contracture of the extensor tendons results in their subluxing medially to overlie the fourth interspace and form a tie beam which maintains the deformity. Some contracture of the dorsal skin is common, and exceptionally the syndrome may be associated with relative lengthening of the fifth toe.

On *radiographs*, the varus deformity of the metatarsophalangeal joint is clearly seen, associated with the valgus posture of the fifth metatarsal and perhaps distal curvature of the metatarsal with its concavity external (Fig. 19.1). Medial subluxation of the proximal phalanx may relate to the external exostosis and some hypertrophy of the condyle.

19.3 Treatment

In the infant treatment is rarely necessary. In children aged 12 years upwards, only if the situation is deteriorating, tenotomy and elongation of the extensor tendon may be indicated, accompanied exceptionally by VY-plasty of the contracted skin on the dorsal aspect (Wilson 1953). These procedures may be followed by recurrence of the angulation, but this may be acceptable.

Bony operations should not be performed before closure of the epiphyseal line, at the age of about 18, unless there is gross discomfort. All *operative* treatment must be designed to correct the longitudinal alignment of the metatarsal and phalanx (Fig. 19.2). Various operations have been advised (Fig. 19.3):

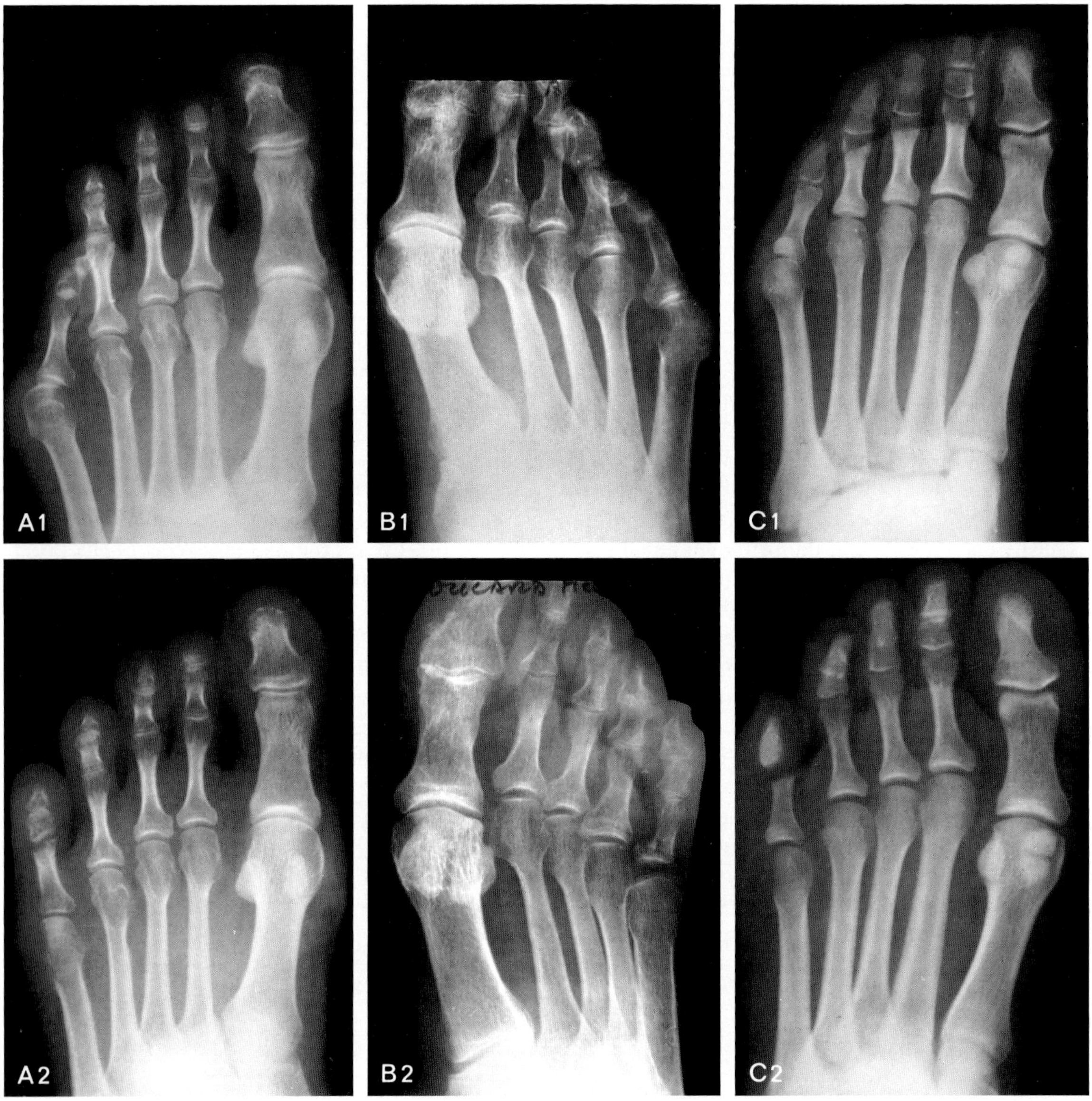

Fig. 19.1 A–H. Treatment of clinodactyly of fifth ray: quintus varus, metatarsus valgus. **A** Early clinodactyly: slight metatarsus valgus and quintus varus. *1* Preoperative; *2* after capsulorrhaphy of fourth and fifth metatarsophalangeal joints, flattening of lateral aspect of fifth metatarsal condyle, interphalangeal arthroplasty of fifth toe. **B** Quintus varus with infraductus, hypertrophy of fifth metatarsal head. *1* Preoperative; *2* after flattening of lateral aspect of fifth metatarsal head, arthroplasty of metatarsophalangeal joint with hat-shaped graft. **C** Clinodactyly with slight quintus varus and slight deformity of fifth metatarsophalangeal joint. *1* Preoperative; *2* after arthrolysis of fifth metatarsophalangeal joint, interphalangeal arthroplasty of fifth toe. **D–H** see pp. 293, 294 ▷

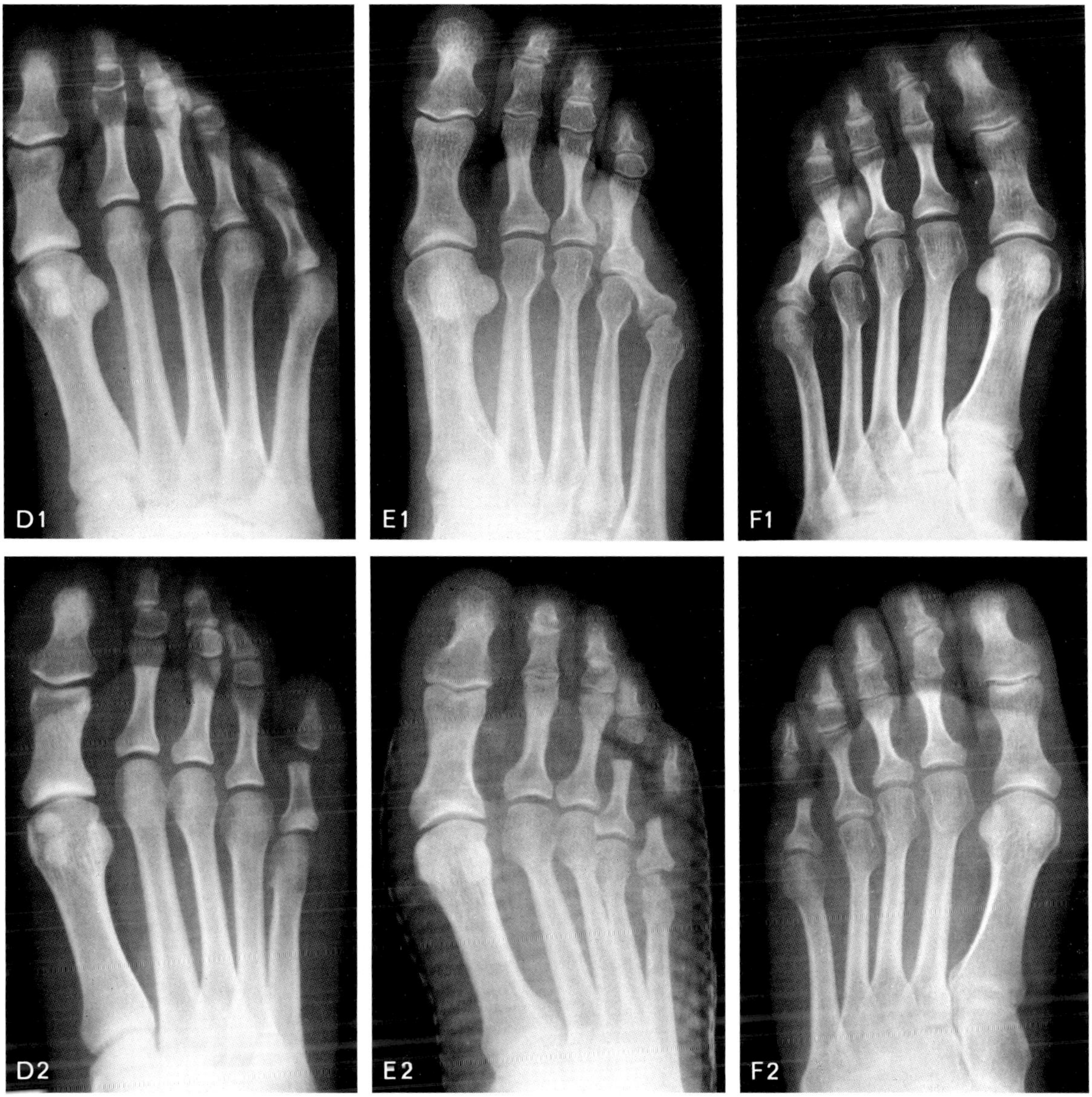

Fig. 19.1 *(continued)*. **D** Marked clinodactyly with lateral displacement of fifth metatarsal and quintus varus. *1* Preoperative; *2* after basal osteotomy of fourth and fifth metatarsals, capsulorrhaphy of fourth and fifth metatarsophalangeal joints, arthroplasty of fifth toe. **E** Rheumatoid quintus varus with involvement of fifth metatarsal head. *1* Preoperative; *2* after arthrolysis of fifth metatarsophalangeal joint, interphalangeal arthroplasty of fourth and fifth toes. **F** Clinodactyly of fifth ray, external deviation of fifth metatarsal, quintus varus with infraductus. *1* Preoperative; *2* after basal osteotomy of fourth and fifth metatarsals, metatarsophalangeal arthrolysis, arthroplasty of fifth toe, dorsolateral dermoplasty

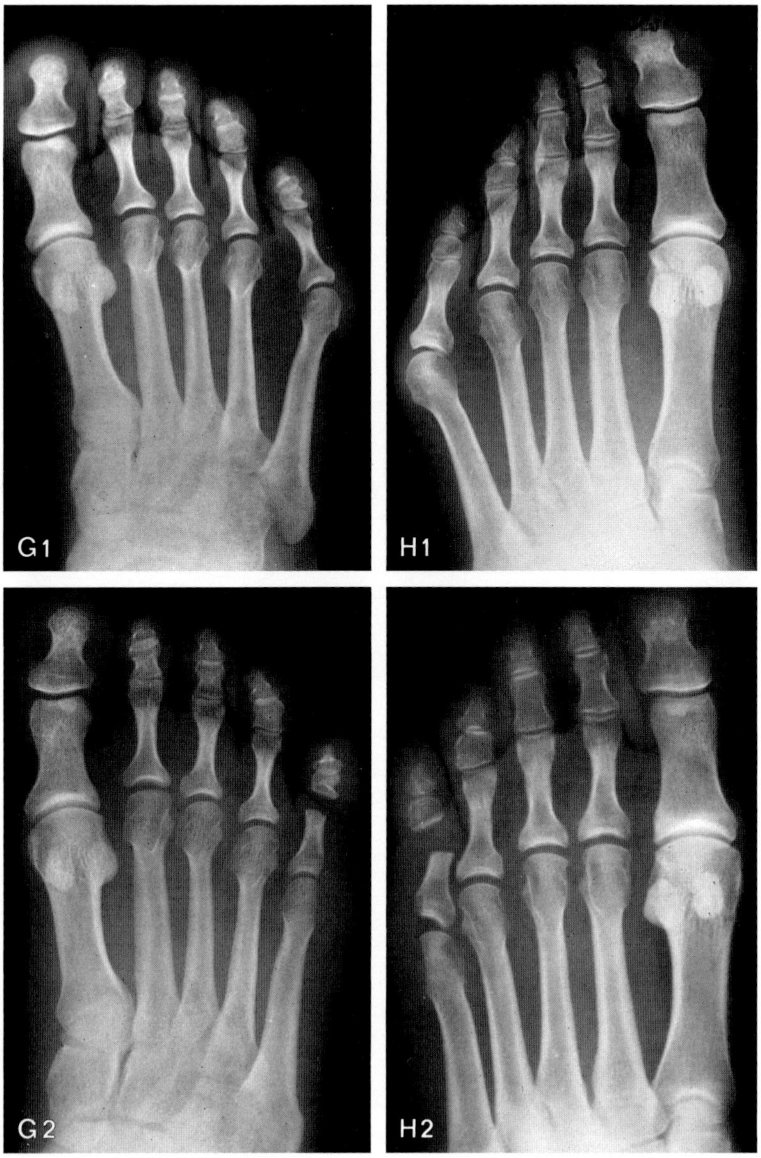

Fig. 19.1 *(continued)*. **G, H** Clinodactyly of fifth ray with valgus and lateral displacement of fifth metatarsal, quintus varus. *1* Preoperative; *2* after basal osteotomy of fourth and fifth metatarsals, capsulorrhaphy of fourth and fifth metatarsophalangeal joints, flattening of lateral aspect of fifth metatarsal head, metatarsophalangeal arthrolysis, interphalangeal arthroplasty of fifth toe

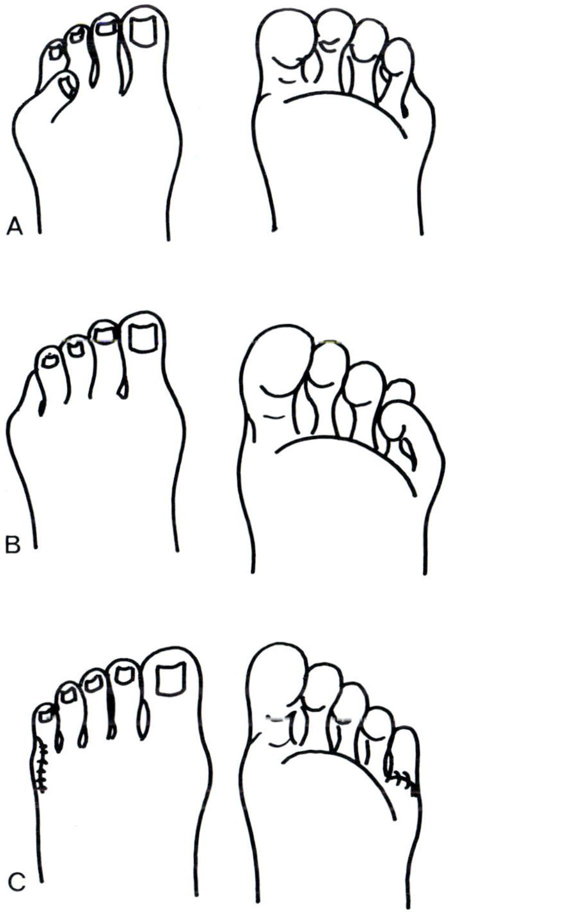

Fig. 19.2 A–C. Adult quintus varus. **A** Supraductus. **B** Infraductus. **C** After correction

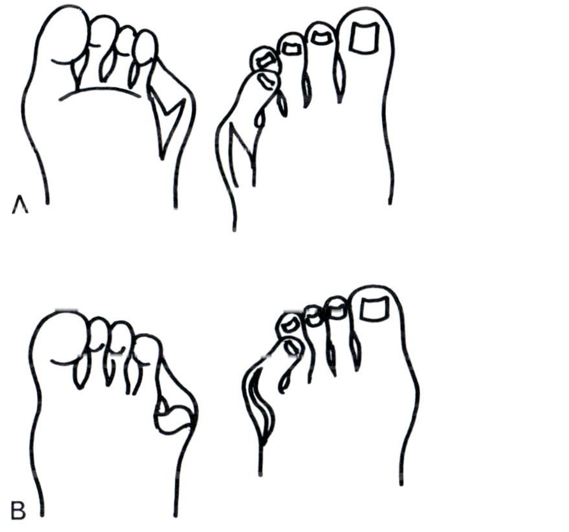

Fig. 19.3 A, B. Overlapping varus of fifth toe. **A** *Left,* plastic plantar incision (Butler); *right,* dorsal incision. **B** Lazy S incision: *left,* plantar; *right,* dorsal

Butler described a Y-plasty on both dorsal and plantar surfaces accompanying elongation of the extensor tendons. Lapidus (1942) divided the extensor longus tendon and transposed the distal end to the tendon of the abductor digiti minimi. Du Vries (1978) recommended division of the extensor tendon and the capsule of the metatarsophalangeal joint with a plastic skin procedure similar to Z-plasty on the dorsal surface. Finally, mention should be made of the repair technique of Lelièvre (1961).

Arthroplastic shortening of the toe is the best measure for long-term correction, and on no account should the head of the fifth metatarsal be amputated. I advise a method of my own for definitive care (Regnauld 1974).

Surgical Technique. The site of the cutaneous incision depends upon whether the toe is in supraductus or infraductus. For supraductus, it extends laterally and transversely across the plantar aspect of the base of the toe and curves proximally on the dorsolateral surface to end longitudinally – an ellipse of skin is excised along this configuration. For infraductus, a longitudinal incision over the dorsal aspect suffices. The metatarsophalangeal joint is opened longitudinally and detached from the outer half of the metatarsal head and completely from the base of the proximal phalanx, protecting the underlying flexor tendons. The medial aspect of the capsule is stripped carefully from the head of the metatarsal with a fine curved rugine.

If complete correction is possible, interphalangeal arthroplasty which shortens the toe suffices to maintain it. Otherwise, a grafting procedure is necessary: The base of the proximal phalanx is exposed, and the shaft divided and the base removed. Boring of a hole in the remaining shaft allows insertion of a spike fashioned on the base, thereby shortening the phalanx. The corrected position is maintained in a relaxed state. A mattress stitch doubles the outer capsular repair, and the extensor tendon is elongated Z-fashion. The remainder of the capsule is repaired with tiny stitches. The valgus of the fifth metatarsal is held corrected by a loop suture around the adjacent fourth metatarsal neck. Skin closure consolidates the corrected position. Weight bearing is avoided for at least a month.

20 Tarsalgia

Pain relating to the tarsal region generally can be conveniently called tarsalgia. It may be classified according to origin or, for practical purposes, according to site. In this account, the causes of tarsalgia will be described first, and then summarised for diagnostic purposes.

20.1 Integument

20.1.1 Skin

Fissures. Skin fissures in the weight-bearing zone of the heel are associated with horny proliferation of the skin, which becomes yellowish, hard and of varying thickness. They are usually located towards the junction of the weight-bearing zone and the sides of the heel. They produce a burning, pricking or sharp pain on loading, and in the absence of treatment, the symptoms become more severe as separation of the lips of the fissure is provoked and the crevice becomes deeper. There is a hereditary familial tendency, but the lesions are sometimes acquired, being related to psoriasis or eczema or simply resulting from improper hygiene. *Treatment* is directed first at any associated skin complaint. The thickened area is then pared repeatedly by a chiropodist, and later, pumice stone is used regularly in the bath. Antiseptic greasy lotions should be applied if there is an infective element or an underlying dermal inflammation. The closure of a fissure can be encouraged by the application of an aerated mud plaster after disinfection, and treatment is usually quick to take effect.

Plantar Verruca. See Chap. 14.5.2.

Radiodermatitis. See Chap. 14.5.5.

Plantar Keratoma. This small conical corn under the heel is very painful on compression on loading. It develops insidiously and becomes noticeable and painful only when it is compressed into the richly innervated dermis.

Sclerokeratoma. This is a sequel of a plantar scar following electrocoagulation, application of silver nitrate or carbon dioxide snow, or surgery for a papilloma, miliary corn or keratoma. A cornified sclerotic lesion which is hard, whitish, painful and persistent develops in the scar. *Treatment* is by chiropody and involves paring, flattening and extirpation of the keratoma; excision or plastic surgical procedures should not be necessary.

Heel Ulcer. This lesion (Fig. 20.1 A) may arise from osteitis of the calcaneum after a fracture, from infection or from pressure from immobilisation in bed or a tight plaster cast. The ulcerated area is cornified, thickened and projecting, irregularly roundish in shape, and some 10–15 mm in diameter. It produces constant discomfort, impeding wearing of shoes. Soon, a moist discharging perforation develops relating to a small area of osteitis. The margin becomes violaceous, and there are repeated cycles of drying, scab formation and further discharge. *Radiography* may show an area of osteosclerosis of the calcaneal surface with tiny osteophytes relating to the ulcer due to areas of erosion around its margins at the bone junction. The pain from shoe pressure can be controlled only by operation: crescent-shaped excision of the skin, curettage of the ulcer, trimming of the underlying bone, suture (Fig. 20.2). Thereafter the foot must be kept in full plantarflexion for 2 weeks, during which period a painless scar of good quality can be achieved (Fig. 20.1 A) (Regnauld 1965).

20.1.2 Subcutaneous Tissue

Granuloma, angioma, myeloid tumour, lipoma and epidermoid cyst all lead inevitably to pain on loading, often detected as a sensation of a foreign body in the tissues with tension and internal compression. On examination, the tumour may not be obvious, having become buried in the connective tissue, but it is usually palpable. All these lesions are small and mobile, except for angioma, which may reach a considerable size. Local excision should be followed by regular inspection, as there is a tendency towards recurrence. Occasional malignant tumours may present a serious problem of excision.

20.1.3 Aponeurosis

20.1.3.1 Juvenile Aponeurotic Fibroma

Originally described by Keasbey (1953) and later discussed by Lempereur (1962), this is a rare lesion; I have seen only two examples, presenting bilaterally in children of 7 and 12 years. Lempereur described it as a plantar swelling on the inner aspect of the heel, producing a protrusion visible through the skin and situated in the plantar aponeurosis in front of the calcaneal apophysis. The fibroma is ovoid or rounded and easily palpable, being fixed to the underlying aponeurosis. There are variable degrees of spontaneous pain, but no particular tenderness on palpation or during standing. The discomfort is strictly localised to the area of swelling, without significant irradiation or inflammatory features. Local excision is curative.

20.1.3.2 Plantar Spur

This common lesion (Fig. 20.1) comprises a painful subcalcaneal exostosis at the insertion of the plantar aponeurosis into the inner tubercle. There is inflammatory myotendinitis at the origin of flexor digitorum brevis. The essential lesion seems to be a degenerative osteophytosis. It may be a consequence of repeated microtrauma related to the lack of elasticity of the musculo-aponeurotic system on the plantar aspect of the foot. It is more frequently unilateral than bilateral, typically affecting a 50-year-old woman whose weight has been increasing who presents with a several-year history of pain. It can appear in any type of foot, but is more frequent in the presence of other imbalances. The patient complains of localised pain, most frequently sharp and confined to the inner aspect of the heel, burning, pricking or lancinating in nature and of sudden onset. Its neuralgic character gives the sensation of a nail or thorn penetrating the heel. The pain appears in the morning as soon as the patient bears weight, but may be relieved at first by the use of heel-less slippers. It is initially intermittent, exaggerated by standing, but becomes increasingly constant, and may eventually persist even at rest during the night, although it is usually relieved by elevation. Occasionally, the pain is more to the centre of the heel, in front of the tubercles, related to the serous bursa of Lenoir, it then often presents symptoms similar to those of inflammatory rheumatic disease.

Inspection of the two heels reveals swelling of the affected side on the inner aspect, with filling of the normal hollow in front of the heel. Palpation may detect thickening due to tension of the overlying subcutaneous tissue, while local pressure reproduces the sharp pain which is aggravated by dorsiflexion of the foot and the toes.

Radiography (Fig. 20.1 F) may show no abnormality or only slight reactive periostitis. In other cases, the classical subcalcaneal spur, varying in size from a few millimetres to as much as 1 cm, may be obvious in the lateral view. Most important is the fact that there is no relationship between the intensity of the tarsalgia and the size, or even the presence, of osteophytosis or a spur; this leads to the view that the spur may be of little significance in the genesis of this pain.

Treatment. It may require 6 months for therapy to be effective. Localised radiotherapy and the use of an insole constitute the treatment of choice. The insole comprises a soft rubber heel or a compliant physiological felt or elastic support. If there is any imbalance, correction of pes planus or pes cavus may be indicated. Local infiltration with topical steroids is not effective and is sometimes poorly tolerated. Local anaesthesia of the calcaneal nerve in the retromalleolar gutter may be helpful, and occasionally, in some intensely painful cases, a period of bed rest is necessary. Systemic and local anti-inflammatory agents and local massage may be useful in the absence of gastric contra-indication. Surgery is only exceptionally indicated, but in occasional cases, the operation described by Benassy (1975) is effective; it involves the implantation of two screws into the calcaneum.

20.2 Tendons and Tendon Sheaths

Clearly, there is a close relationship between tendons and their sheaths.

20.2.1 Partial Rupture

Partial rupture of tendons may lead to lengthening.

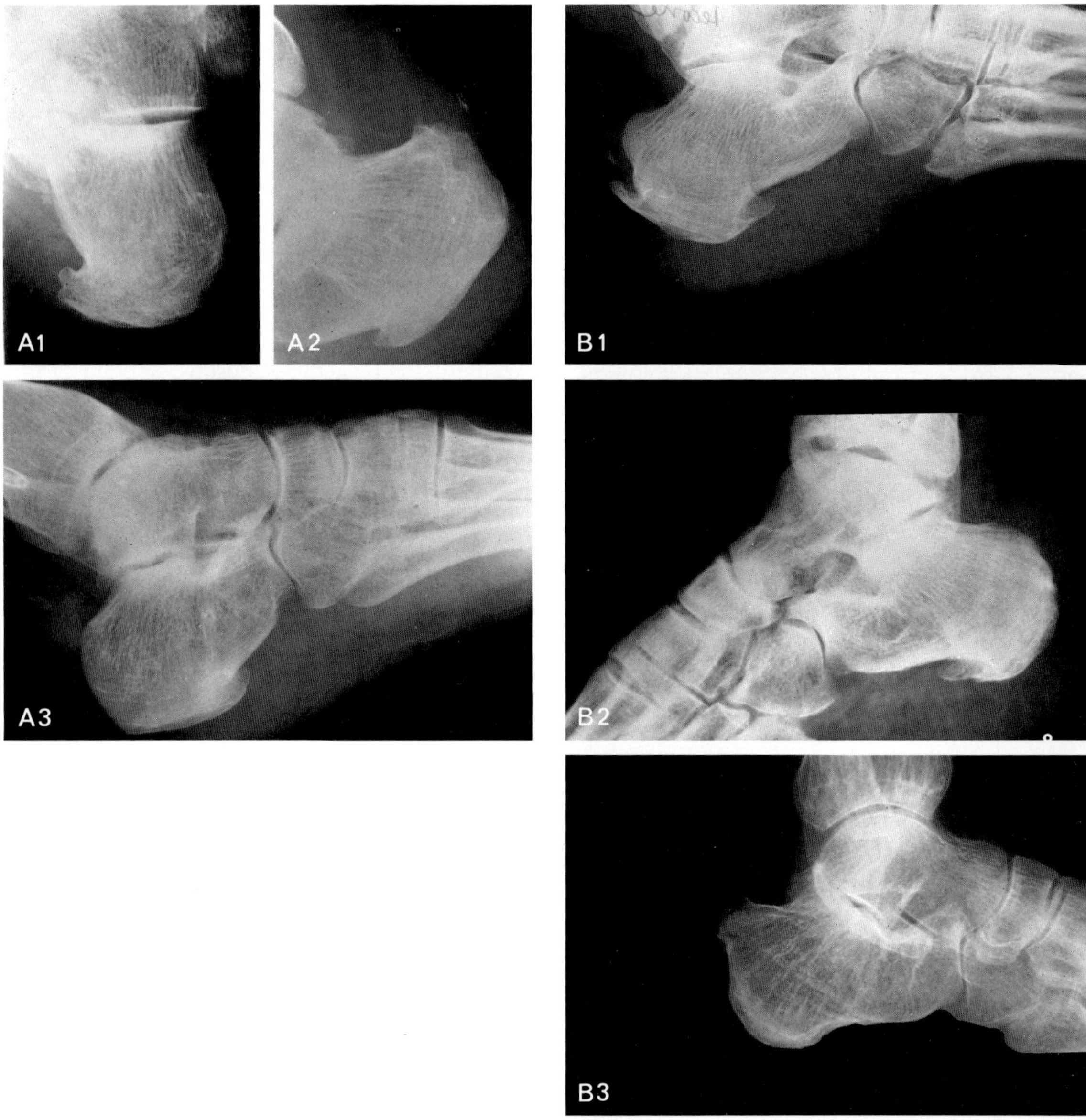

Fig. 20.1 A–H. Calcaneal exostoses, cuneiform-metatarsal exostoses calcaneal spur. **A** Posterior calcaneal sinus: *1, 2* Preoperative; *3* after resection and trimming of calcaneum, posterior dermoplasty. **B** *1, 2* Spiculate exostosis of posterior calcaneum: *1* preoperative; *2* after resection and trimming. *3* Posterosuperior exostosis of calcaneum. **C** Posterior calcaneal exostosis: *1* Preoperative; *2* after ▷ resection. **D** Posterosuperior exostosis of calcaneum: *1* Preoperative; *2* after posterosuperior resection. **E** *1,2* Osteophytes associated with arthrosis of cuneiform-metatarsal joints. **F** *1–3* Examples of calcaneal spur. **C–H** see pp. 299–301

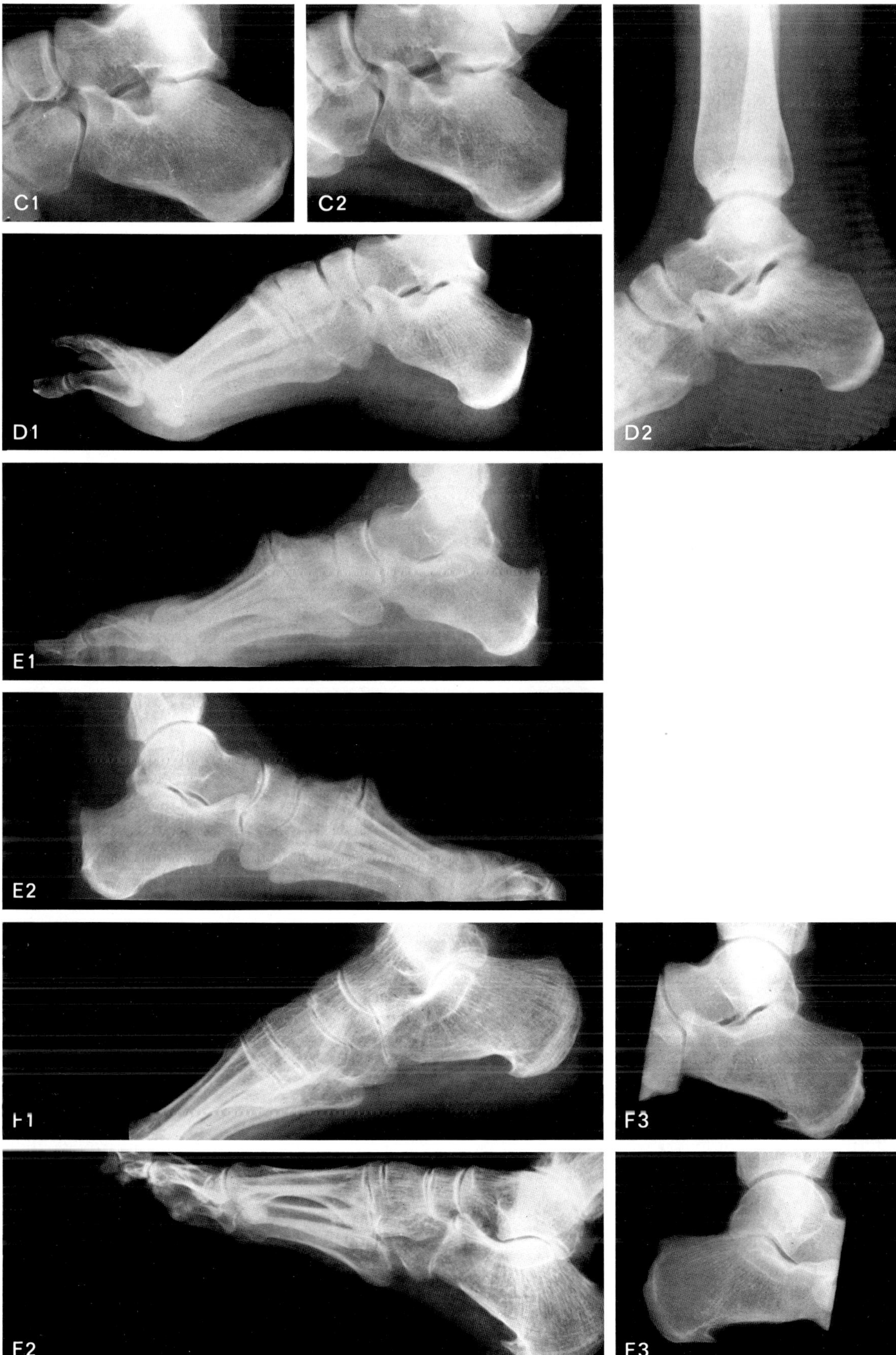
C1
C2
D1
D2
E1
E2
F1
F3
F2
F3

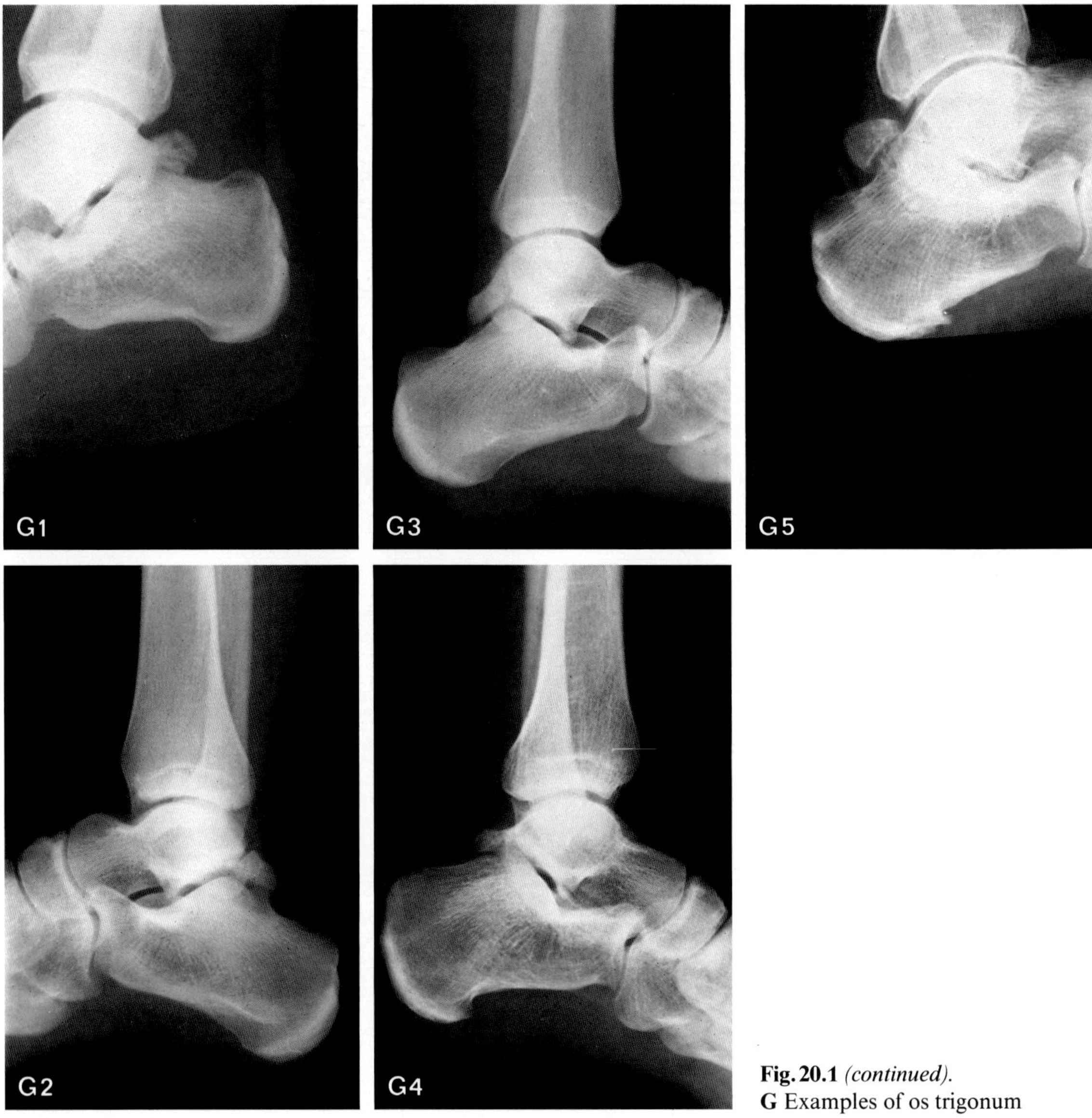

Fig. 20.1 *(continued).*
G Examples of os trigonum

Tibialis Anterior and Extensor Hallucis Longus. Partial rupture is usually the result of injury, typically incurred when kicking a ball and catching the toe on some irregularity in the ground. The tendons are severely stretched, leading to pain and limitation of movement with weakness. On examination, some bridging of the overlying subcutaneous tissue during contraction may be obvious. *Treatment* to restore normal function comprises tenoplasty with shortening of the stretched tendon followed by appropriate re-educative physiotherapy.

Tendo Achillis. Partial rupture may be produced by forced dorsiflexion, which is common in skiing and can also occur on commencement of exercise, during gymnastics, or on faulty landing from a jump. In the majority of cases, there is a snapping sound and a relatively brief stab of pain. Inspection and palpation rarely detect the true dehiscence of the tendon, more often revealing only a soft peritendinous swelling. Discomfort rather than pain is accompanied by inability to stand on tiptoe and loss of plantarflexion strength. Discomfort may be produced when the foot adopts a fully dorsiflexed position. The patient may attend as a result of hearing the rupture occurring. *Treatment* comprises immediate surgical repair, or in late cases a plastic procedure, followed by adequate physiotherapy.

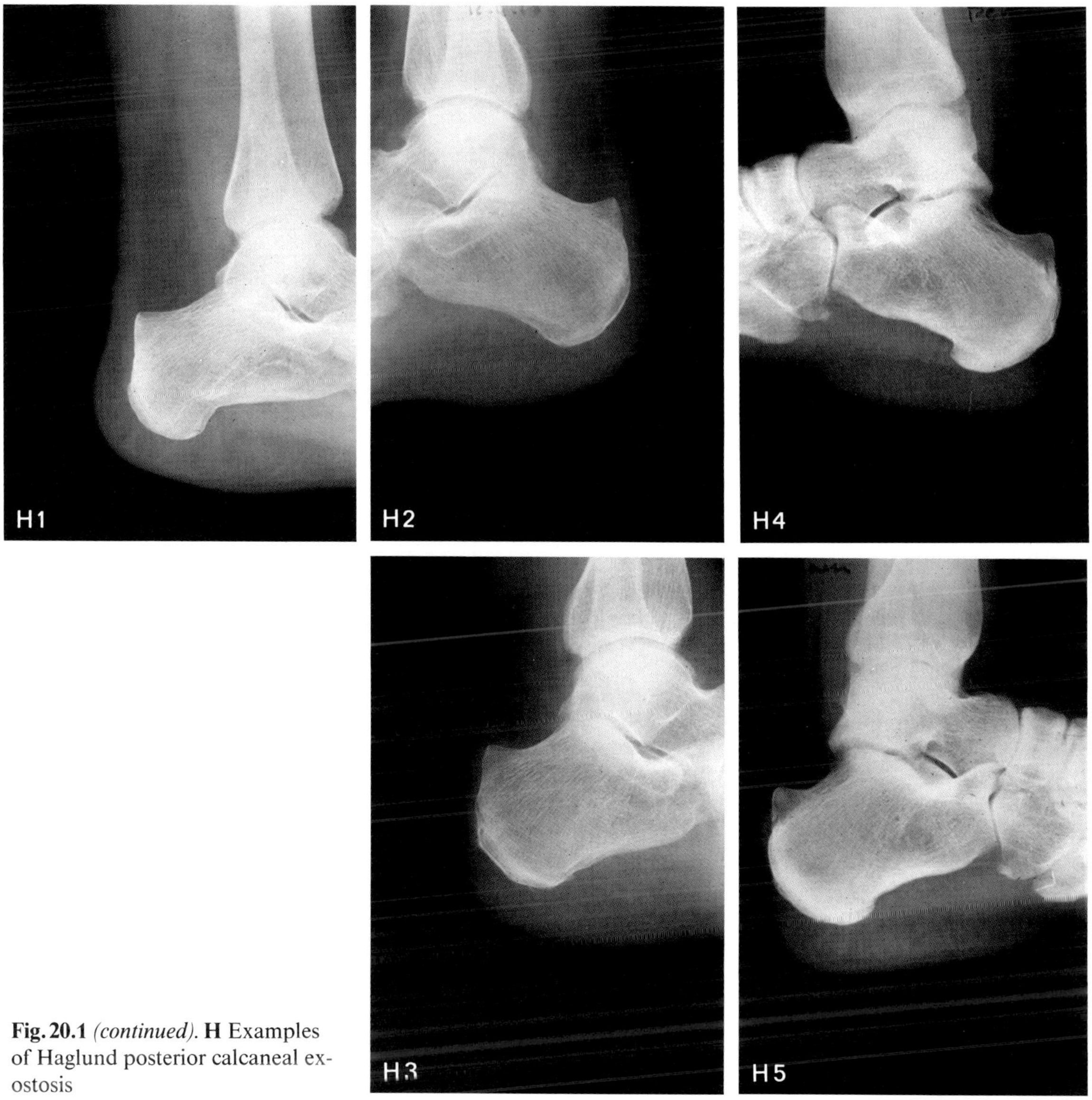

Fig. 20.1 *(continued)*. **H** Examples of Haglund posterior calcaneal exostosis

Tibialis Posterior. Partial rupture is a sequel to sprain in eversion associated with marked abduction stress and is manifested by pain along the course of the tendon in the medial retromalleolar gutter after the trauma. It is aggravated by standing and walking and frequently complicated by typical tenosynovitis. Untreated, it leads to displacement of the midtarsus with lowering of the medial longitudinal arch. *Treatment* with insoles is not effective, but tenoplasty with shortening of the tendon and synovectomy of the tendon sheath usually are.

20.2.2 Tendinitis at Insertions

Tendo Achillis and Tibialis Posterior. Tendinitis here may be associated with some fixed deformity of the foot. In the majority of cases, there is either pes planus or pes cavus accompanied by a significant degree of pronation of the calcaneum and internal and plantar displacement of the midtarsal region. The tendinitis may also be traumatic in origin, associated with poor choice of footwear, a stumble, an unaccustomedly long walk, or a sports injury, perhaps involving an eversion strain (affecting tibialis posterior) or severe dorsiflexion of the foot (leading to damage of tendo Achillis). Tendinitis at the insertion of tibialis posterior manifests itself by

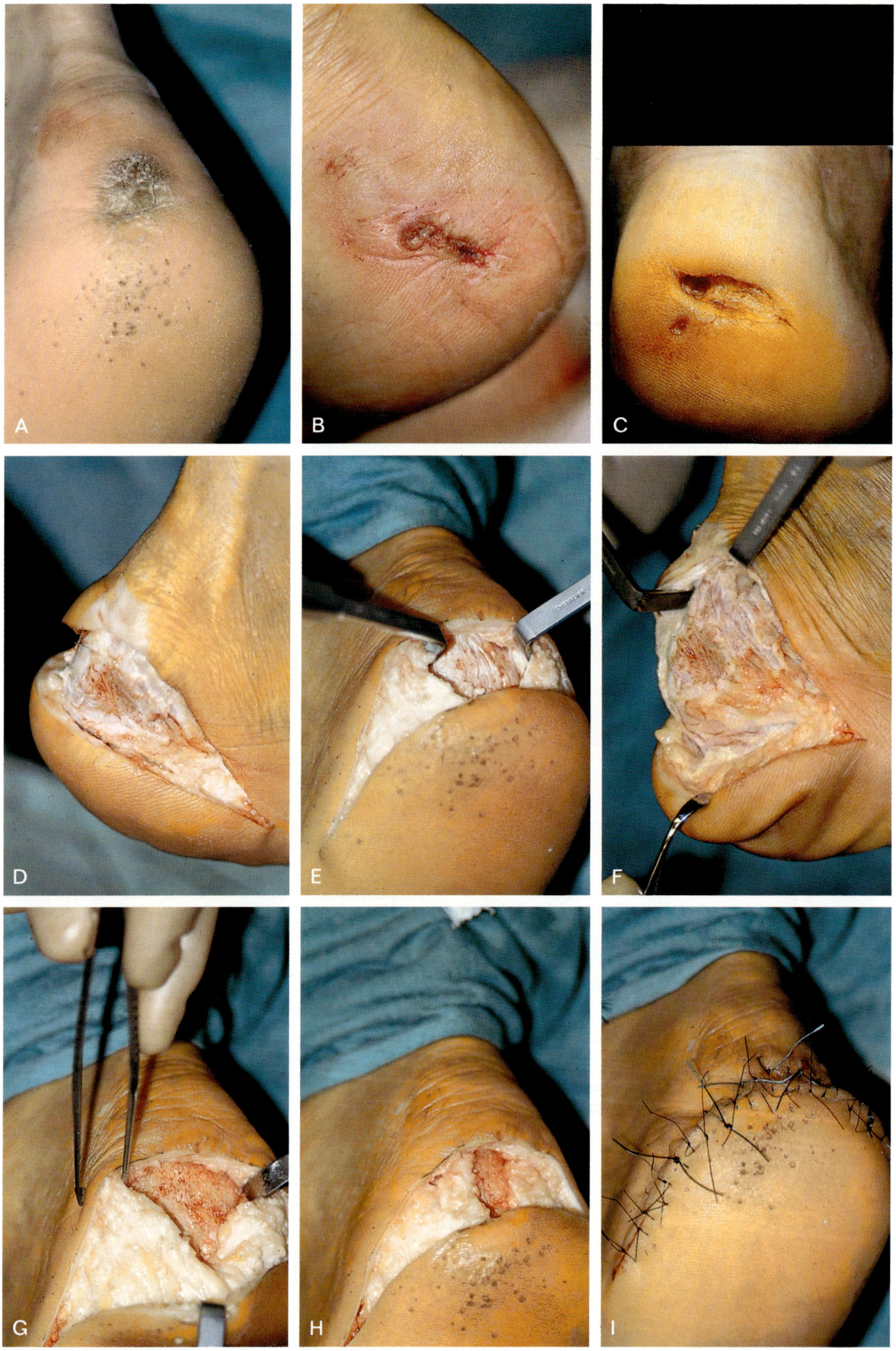
A
B
C
D
E
F
G
H
I

pain and tenderness over the navicular tuberosity, where, in an adolescent, there may be a supernumerary ossicle. Tendinitis of tendo Achillis can occur in the 12-year-old, but seems to occur more frequently in the young adult sportsman. There is no gross swelling but sometimes a slight thickening may be palpable. Local tenderness of tendo Achillis and any tension during activity or examination indicate the site. *Treatment* comprises corrective insoles for imbalance, local and general anti-inflammatory agents (with medication-free intervals), massage, physiotherapy and sometimes radiotherapy.

Peroneal Tendons. In 7- to 12-year-old children, tarsalgia on the outer side of the foot may arise from tendinitis at the insertions of the peroneal tendons, and seems to relate to a congenital lack of development of the retromalleolar gutter for the tendons. In later cases, in adults, there is usually a traumatic origin involving severe sprain into inversion. There is diffuse discomfort in the region of the instep together with chronic instability of the ankle, which feels weak. Repeated episodes of instability aggravate the condition, and anterior subluxation of the tendons may occur. This picture of instability accompanied by swelling of the ankle with thickening in the retromalleolar gutter is typical. *Treatment* is surgical, comprising the Lannelongue periosteal plastic operation (Ombredanne 1932).

Rupture. All ruptures of the insertions of tendo Achillis, tibialis posterior, tibialis anterior, or the peroneal tendons are traumatic in origin, and if left untreated they cause inconvenience due to the loss of function of the tendon concerned. Pain is produced by the displacements which follow this loss of function: equinovalgus pes planus from tibialis anterior, valgus pes planus from tibialis posterior, pes varus from peroneal origins and pes talus (calcaneus) from tendo Achillis. If there is not much pain at the time of rupture, the condition can go almost unnoticed but lead later to the functional disability from displacement. *Treatment* is surgical, comprising reattachment of the tendon concerned.

◁ **Fig. 20.2 A–I.** Retrocalcaneal sinus. **A, B** Keratotic appearance of sinus. **C** Cutaneous necrosis and sinus formation. **D, E** Transverse elliptical excision. **F, G** Curettage of bony cavity. **H** Closure, especially of tendinoperiosteum. **I** Skin suture

20.2.3 Stenosing Tenosynovitis

This may affect the peroneal tendons, tendo Achillis or, less frequently, tibialis posterior and extensor hallucis longus. The tenosynovitis causes sharp pain along the course of the tendon concerned, aggravated by action or palpation. There may be a burning sensation or one of tension with aching. The swelling of the tendon sheath may be accompanied by oedema of the surrounding tissues.

Peroneal Tendons. Machacek 1940 and Denis (1962) have both described the typical form of this lesion. I have twice seen a dry hypertrophic variety, once in a woman of 30 accustomed to wearing inordinately high heels and once in a man of 42 in which the late development followed an inversion strain of the ankle. The tarsalgia is limited to diffuse functional discomfort during walking or standing on tiptoe. It is related to a fusiform swelling some 10–15 cm long around the peroneal tendons. The swelling in the distal third of the leg is of irregular sausage shape, hard, crepitant and partially blocks the range of movement of the involved muscles; the skin overlying the gutter behind and underneath the lateral malleolus is stretched. According to Lelièvre, Machacek and Denis, the pain sometimes irradiates to the peroneal tubercles but I have not seen this in my patients. *Treatment* is surgical, comprising total synovectomy and tenolysis of the involved peroneal tendons.

Tendo Achillis. Stenosing tenosynovitis of tendo Achillis is an exceptional condition which I have seen on only one occasion, when the clinical presentation was analogous to that in the peroneal tendons. The subject was a tennis player in whom the condition had developed gradually, without any specific precipitating event. The pain was limited to the tendo Achillis region and associated with painful synovial thickening some 15 cm in length, filling the normal paratendinous hollows. The pain was of a lancing, burning, tense nature, and was exacerbated by contraction of the muscle, standing or walking. It progressively prevented all sporting activities. *Treatment* is surgical, comprising synovectomy associated with anti-inflammatory agents, physiotherapy and the transverse type of massage described by Cyrriax.

Tibialis Posterior Tendons. The tenosynovitis presents in one of two forms, serous or hypertrophic. The *serous* form is more frequent and may be simultaneously postural and traumatic in origin. It seems to follow a simple stumble caused by the imbalance of a pre-existing valgus foot. The tarsalgia is at the outset sharp, persistent and aggravated by standing or walking, and is localised to the course of the tendon below and behind the medial malleolus. There is local thickening and oedema, and fluctuation indicates the serous nature of the lesion. The intensity and persistence of discomfort soon leads the patient to consult, and early *treatment* comprising rest, anti-inflammatory agents, massage, physiotherapy and appropriate insoles will allow rapid settling of the lesion. It is rare that this tenosynovitis requires surgical management. The *hypertrophic* form with chronic stenosis may be dry and frequently follows the serous form. It is provoked by violent trauma such as sprain, eversion injury or a direct blow from the foot against an irregularity in the ground, leading to abduction. Lapidus, Powler, Roblins and Denis talk of a chronic hypertrophic form leading to persistent irregular distension along the course of the synovial sheath, sausage-like under the medial malleolus. The *treatment* of choice is synovectomy and tenolysis.

Extensor Hallucis Longus Tendons. Tenosynovitis here is rare, but when it occurs it is analgous to that of tibialis posterior and the peronei. In one case which I treated, at synovectomy the swelling was bossilated, irregular and confined to the dorsal aspect of the foot.

20.3 Capsules and Ligaments

Capsuloligamentous tarsalgia is related to sprains of the tarsal region, which are dealt with in Chap. 21.

20.4 Joints

20.4.1 Arthrosis

Arthrosis of the ankle, the subtalar joint or the Chopart joint line may be secondary to trauma, may be primarily associated with fixed deformities of the foot or may be seen in rheumatoid arthritis or idiopathic arthrosis.

Post-traumatic. Arthrosis, usually related to a fracture involving one of the joint surfaces or to a dislocation, however minor, can affect any of the joints of the tarsus. It may also arise from sprains or from microtrauma associated with sport, for example the impingement exostosis described by O'Donoghue (1957) which is due to repeated hyperplantarflexion in football. Cabot and Moragas described an exquisitely painful lesion located at the back of the malleoli during plantarflexion associated with radiographically evident fragmentation of an os trigonum or enlargement of the postero-external tubercle of the talus (Fig. 20.1 G). The trigonal synostosis described by Outland and Shands is associated with tarsalgia which is either of an arthralgic nature and comes from the subtalar joint, or has a neuralgic quality, is sudden and intensely lancing in character and radiates into the retromalleolar gutters towards the heel. This pain is aggravated by loading and cured by excision of the os trigonum or resection of a tubercle. Finally post-traumatic arthrosis may be a sequel of a fracture of the malleoli, the distal tibia, the calcaneum or the waist of the foot. Post-traumatic arthrosis occurs, in ascending order of frequency, in the ankle joint alone, the inferior tibiofibular joint, the talonavicular joint or the subtalar joint.

Postural Deformities. Typically, pes planus and pes cavus do not involve the ankle joint but cause symptoms from disorder of the joints more distally. They may, however, eventually lead to arthrosis of the Chopart joint line, the subtalar joint or in some instances the knee joint.

Rheumatic Disease. Rheumatoid arthritis or metabolic disorders of bone of long standing may lead to panarthrosis of the tarsal region with osteophyte formation. Gout may be especially significant, leading to enormous exostosis formation associated more with the calcaneum.

Dysmorphic Conditions. This term refers to certain deformities affecting the shape or size of individual bones which can result in incongruity between the talus and the calcaneum. This is manifested by the long or short talar neck or by abnormalities in the shape of the talar head. Pes cavus is provoked by tarsomidtarsal biomechanical disharmony. According to Voutey (1978) the arthralgias resulting from dysmorphic conditions are associated with involvement of the midtarsus and subtalar joint and lead to rapid evolutive destruction of the cartilaginous joint surface together with severe osteophytosis of the ankle joint and the talocalcaneal joints. The problem is at first confined to one joint, but progressively other tarsal joints become involved. At first the pains occur only on first getting up in the morning, but progressively they become continuous, lancinating and diffuse, involving the whole tarsus, with the maximum intensity at the level of the joint most affected. They are associated with sensations of constriction and tension, crepitus and progressive loss of range of movement. Often there is swelling, which may become generalised. *Radiography* shows osteophytosis of varying degrees, usually around the joint, with a spicular appearance and with condensations around the joint borders. The narrowing of the joint spaces is variable, depending on the area concerned, but is seen most constantly and markedly in the subtalar joint. Sometimes, particularly in metabolic disorders, there are signs of panarthrosis affecting the tarsus, the arthrosic areas showing a bristled appearance (Weissenbach and Francon). *Treatment* is conservative by means of insoles, corticotherapy, the use of carefully fitted shoes. Surgery may be necessary if this fails, and is dealt with in Chap. 22.

20.4.2 Specific Arthritides

Specific arthritides may be rheumatic or infective (especially tuberculous and gonococcal), although the latter are relatively uncommon at the present time. Systemic signs, local heat, swelling filling the retromalleolar gutters, and evidence of joint effusions suggest these etiologies when symptoms are of sudden origin. *Radiography* shows, according to the state of development, narrowing or irregularity of the joint line with erosions and later frank destruction with secondary sclerosis. Subchondral osteoporosis with localised necrosis appears only at a late stage and may be detected in only about 25% of cases by objective densitometry (Collard and Wullaert 1976).
Acute septic arthritis leads to very severe tarsalgia with nocturnal recrudescence. Positive bacteriological tests are pathognomonic.
Tuberculous arthritis predominantly involves the ankle joint, leading to diffuse tarsalgia with the appearances of subacute arthritis. Synovial biopsy and a check for the typical biological signs are the essential steps in diagnosis.

20.5 Bones

20.5.1 Post-Traumatic Tarsalgia

While any bone in the tarsal region may be fractured, the ones which most commonly present post-traumatic pains are the calcaneum, the talus and the navicular.

Calcaneum. The pain usually relates to the subtalar joint, the function of which is disturbed by anatomical distortion and incongruence associated with modification of the angle of Böhler (1944), and is especially marked on walking on irregular ground. There is usually localised diffuse swelling in both retromalleolar gutters. *Treatment* in the first instance is conservative, by physiotherapy and an insole. If this fails, double arthrodesis of the subtalar joint and the Chopart joint line is necessary, correcting any pes planus or lateral imbalance of the calcaneum.

Talus and Navicular. Fractures of these bones lead to disturbance of the inner part of the Chopart joint line, which results in poor transverse adaptation of the foot to irregularities in the ground. The tarsalgias relate to the joint involved but tend to be diffuse, are aggravated by loading and walking and lead to very severe loss of function. *Radiography* may show osteophytosis of the midtarsal joint and post-traumatic lowering of the plantar arch. *Treatment* comprises arthrodesis of the subtalar joint and the midtarsal joint with grafting of the talonavicular joint. This re-establishes balance and restores comfort, although there is limitation of function of the foot.

20.5.2 Aseptic Necrosis of Talus

See Chap. 22.

20.5.3 Solitary Cyst of Calcaneum

This benign tumour included in the Mikulicz group (1906) is rarely met in the calcaneum. It develops in the spongy bone under the subtalar joint posteriorly and does not invade the joint cartilage. When small, it may exist unperceived for a long time and eventually be discovered only on radiographic examination, perhaps for some other cause. It may, however, result in permanent localised pain without significant radiation, invariably of a tension or lancing type, and local heat, which can be detected by comparing the two feet.
Large examples may result from pathological fracture of the calcaneum due to weakening of the bone. *Radiography* shows a cyst with an intact or fractured outline, ovoid or rounded, clear, homogeneous or speckled, marked by circumscribed thin lines and never involving the articular cartilage. The cortex may show some periosteal reaction, which leads to patchy condensation or ero-

sions as described by Ombredanne and Mathieu (1937). *Treatment* is surgical, with reduction of the fracture if any, curettage, and filling with bone graft.

20.5.4 Retrocalcaneal Tarsalgia

There are four origins of retrocalcaneal tarsalgia.

Rheumatoid or Psoriatic Arthritis or Metabolic Disturbance. Gout and chondrocalcinosis are the two main examples.

Growth. Associated with growth, tarsalgia may be due to the apophysitis of the posterior calcaneum which occurs in childhood and was described by Sever (1930) between the ages of 7 and 12 years. It develops insidiously, beginning with slight discomfort in the heel which may be precipitated by minor trauma and may produce a limp. Gradually, the pain increases and becomes more localised to the postero-inferior aspect of the heel. There may be a localised inflammatory response with local tenderness and this kind of tarsalgia frequently occurs in the precavus balanced or valgus foot. *Radiography* shows absence of fusion of the metaphyseal line and increased condensation and fragmentation of the posterior epiphysis. The epiphyseal line may appear irregular. *Treatment* by conservative means suffices in the majority of cases, and consists of periods of rest, avoidance of athletics and prolonged walking, calcium supplements associated with ultraviolet light and poultices, and the use of supporting insoles with soft material for the heel. If after 3–6 months this is unsuccessful, surgery may be required, comprising multiple perforation of the epiphyseal line with a Kirschner wire, which accelerates the process of ossification. This is, however, only exceptionally necessary.

Retrocalcaneal Bursa. This lesion (Fig. 20.3) occurs more often in young women than in men, being provoked by shoe pressure associated with an overhigh heel or a poorly shaped heel cup. A growth disturbance can lead to the heel being rather large and this can be the origin of the exostosis. The patient presents with inflammatory bursitis of varying extent on the posterior aspect of the heel. There are two serous bursae, one in front of and one behind the insertion of tendo Achillis, which may become inflamed alternately. The retrotendinous bursitis is the more significant and is accompanied during the cold seasons by cutaneous conditions such as erythema pernio which are aggravated by the mechanical aspects of the bone configuration. Examination detects that although tendo Achillis itself is not painful, there is a persistent swelling of varying size giving the heel a rounded projecting aspect, perhaps with evidence of acute inflammation. Infection is rare. The severity of symptoms relates very much to the type of shoe worn. *Radiography* (Fig. 20.1 B–D, H) reveals abnormal projection of the posterosuperior corner of the apophysis of the calcaneum, sometimes with spiculate exostoses or the classical image of the pointed high calcaneum described by Haglund (1928), the verticality of the posterior aspect contrasting with its normal convexity and obliquity.

Treatment should be conservative initially, especially if the condition has presented in winter, comprising local and general anti-inflammatory agents and medication against erythema pernio. A hollowed heel cup can be fitted to the shoe to protect the inflamed bursa. Surgical treatment is necessary in the event of failure and should be confined to the months between May and September so as to allow the wearing of shoes without heels after resection of the posterosuperior protuberance of the calcaneum.

Retrocalcaneal Ulcer. See Sect. 20.1.1 above and Chap. 31.

20.6 Postural Tarsalgia

Postural tarsalgia can be due to extrinsic factors, arising usually in the knee, or to intrinsic conditions involving the balance of the foot itself. The treatment differs according to the age of the subject (see Chap. 3).

20.6.1 Extrinsic Causes

Genu valgum and genu varum result in abnormal loading of the foot inside or outside its median axis in relation to the talus.

Genu valgum in the child induces a valgus foot which may become cavus or flat. In the adult, there is a tendency for the medial longitudinal arch to fall with age, leading to a pes planovalgus.

Genu varum in the child leads to a cavovarus foot, but paradoxically, adult genu varum leads gradually and irreversibly to a pes planus, not only on account of the external convexity of the lower limb, but also because of an axial deformity which leads to a shift of loading to the medial side of the foot.

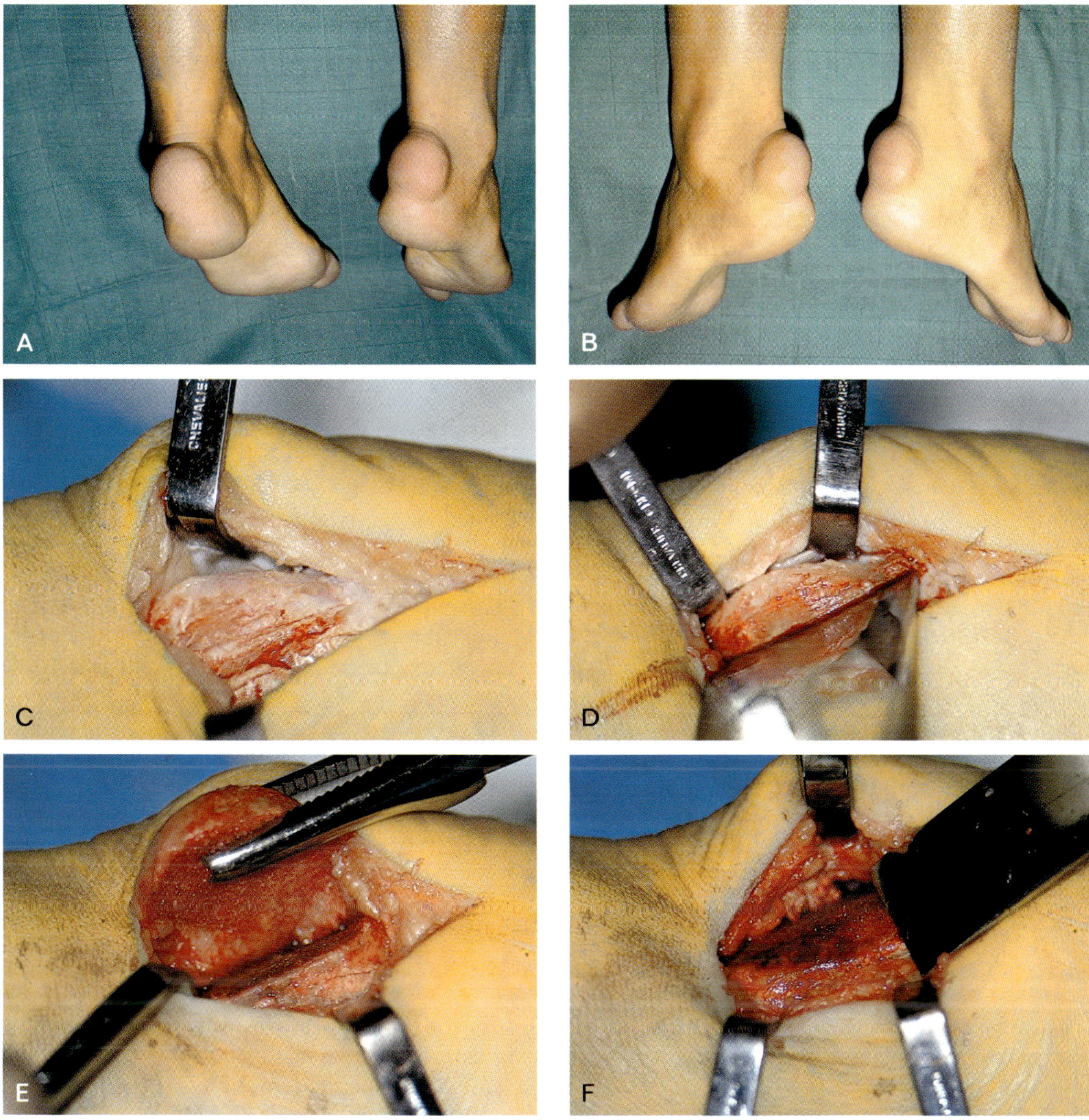

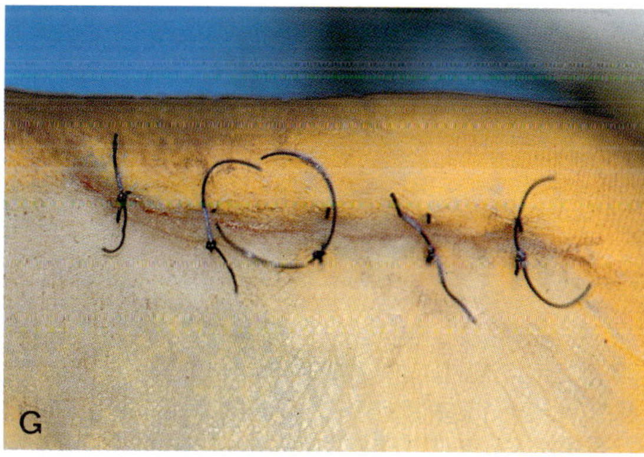

Fig. 20.3 A–G. Retrocalcaneal exostosis. **A, B** Exostosis and retrocalcaneal bursitis. **C** Detachment of tendinoperiosteum. **D** Resection of posterosuperior margin of calcaneal apophysis. **E** Removal of exostosis. **F** Trimming of margins of resected area. **G** Skin suture

In both displacements, in the child and especially in the adult, one sees tarsalgias of a tension, stretching type affecting the internal aspect of the tarsus, localised pain at tendinous insertions and tenosynovitis of tibialis posterior. In the adult there is frequently joint pain from the internal midtarsus and pain from distortion of the sinus tarsi, particularly on the outer side of the subtalar joint in genu varum.

Treatment. In the *child,* treatment with an insole gives favourable results in the majority of cases but if this fails, surgical treatment by stabilisation of the subtalar joint as described by Blunt is appropriate. In the *adult,* insoles are usually successful but the persistence of the knee deformity leads eventually to joint damage. The only solution is correction of the basic deformity by tibial osteotomy bearing in mind the additional need to correct any axial torsional deformity thereby recreating normal physiological balance of the foot and the knee. Finally, it is necessary to mention tarsalgia of dynamic origin associated with neurological disease, syndromes due to pyramidal, extrapyramidal or medullary disorders leading to pes planovalgus or flaccid hemiplegia, pes equinovarus in spastic hemiplegia and Parkinson's disease and pes cavovarus associated with Friedreich's ataxia and Roussy-Lévy's syndrome. Poliomyelitis and its effects are described in Chap. 16.5.1.

20.6.2 Intrinsic Conditions

The tarsalgia can relate to congenital conditions such as club foot, planovalgus foot, and tarsal coalition (see Chap. 26) or to acquired cavovalgus, planovalgus or cavus (described in Chaps. 15 and 16).

20.7 Sites of Tarsalgia

For diagnostic purposes it is useful to provide the reader with an *aide-mémoire* of the conditions likely to produce symptoms localised to various sites:

1. *Dorsal:* Tenosynovitis or tendinitis of toe extensors and tibialis anterior at the ankle region
   Capsular calcification, cartilaginous loose bodies in the joint, post-traumatic osteoarthrosis and impingement of dorsal osteophytes (O'Donoghue 1957)
   Dorsal spur formation at Chopart joint line, static pain from pes cavus
   Avascular necrosis (Köhler; Müller-Weiss) of navicular (usually tends to cause metatarsalgia)
2. *Posterior:* Apophysitis of calcaneum during growth and development
   Bursitis of tendo Achillis due to prominence of calcaneum
   Static deformities of foot leading to transverse imbalance of heel into valgus or varus
   Post-traumatic rupture or partial rupture of tendo
   Achillis, fracture of talar apophysis or os trigonum, ulceration, or traumatic synovitis of tendo Achillis sheath
   Arthrosis of subtalar joint
3. *Plantar:* Cutaneous conditions including fissures, scars from previous trauma or operation, and epithelioma
   Subcutaneous tumours
   Radiodermatitis: necrosis or sclerosis
   Plantar sclerokeratoma
   Periostitis and fibrositis of plantar aponeurosis associated with calcaneal spur
   Post-traumatic conditions including fracture of calcaneum
   Arthritic conditions
4. *Medial:* Vascular conditions, especially varicose veins and varicose ulcer
   Tarsal canal syndrome
   Postural deformities: genu valgum, genu varum and tibia varum
   Post-traumatic conditions such as sprain, rupture or elongation of tibialis posterior, tenosynovitis of tibialis posterior and extensor hallucis longus
   Fracture of calcaneum
   Fracture of medial malleolus
5. *Lateral:* Postural deformities: congenital or acquired pes cavus or cavovarus
   Neurological conditions leading to pes varus, e.g. spastic hemiplegia, Parkinson's cavovarus, Friedreich's ataxia, poliomyelitis
   Peroneal tendon conditions, including subluxation, peroneal tubercle irritation and tenosynovitis
   Sinus tarsi syndrome
   Fracture of calcaneum
6. *Diffuse:* Many causes, including sprains of any joints, algodystrophy, arthrosis, aseptic necrosis of talus, rheumatic conditions, metabolic disorders (e.g. gout, chondrocalcinosis) and neurological disease associated with sciatica or polyneuritis

III Trauma and Arthrosis

21 Ligamentous Injuries of Ankle and Hindfoot

Stability of the ankle and hindfoot is assured by muscles and ligaments, which must be considered together. Normal synergic control is through the proprioceptive Golgi organs in the tendons, which control the associated reflex muscle contraction. The mechanism is complex. It seems clear, however, that when the mechanical force is too sudden for reflex protective stimulation of the muscles, ligaments are likely to be stretched or torn.

21.1 Classification

Ligamentous injuries can be classified either according to the mechanism which produces them (eversion, inversion, pure abduction, pure adduction, plantar hyperflexion, dorsiflexion, or shearing) or in terms of the severity of the injury; thus, a minor sprain may be classified as one producing loss of function and involving swelling or tenderness at the insertions but displaying no radiographical abnormality, whereas major sprains lead to severe pain, loss of articular motion, oedema and bruising, and instability is manifested on X-ray by tilting, forward displacement and bony involvement of the malleoli or talus.

21.1.1 Eversion Injuries

Forced abduction, pronation and some degree of dorsiflexion lead to injury of the inferior tibiofibular joint and the medial ligament of the ankle, most commonly involving both structures. If both fasciculae of the medial ligament are ruptured, this is equivalent to a fracture of the medial malleolus as far as treatment is concerned and the possibility of extension of the injury to the talonavicular ligament must be borne in mind.

Clinically, there is pain and tenderness along the whole length of the medial ligament, especially at its insertion into the medial malleolus extending distally to the talonavicular joint. There may be local tenderness at the insertion of tibialis posterior into the navicular.

Radiography may show an avulsion fracture of the medial malleolus, and if there is instability of the talus in its mortice on valgus stressing, both fasciculae of the medial ligament must have been ruptured.

21.1.2 Inversion Injuries

When the foot has been stressed into adduction and supination, the complex of ligamentous injuries depends on whether it was in plantarflexion or dorsiflexion at the time of injury. If in plantarflexion, there is likely to be damage to the anterior talofibular ligament; if in a neutral position, the calcaneofibular ligament can be primarily involved, the injury usually extending to the anterior talofibular ligament; if in dorsiflexion, there is often a lesion of the posterior talofibular ligament, almost always of the calcaneofibular and anterior talofibular ligaments as well. According to Judet et al. (1972), there cannot be injury of the posterior components without involvement of the anterior talofibular ligament. When the whole lateral ligament complex is ruptured, there is often damage to the interosseous ligament of the subtalar joint and to the inferior tibiofibular ligament.

Radiography may show avulsion fractures of the lateral malleolus and the styloid of the fifth metatarsal and tilting of the talus; according to Judet, tilting of more than 10° demands early operative treatment.

21.1.3 Pure Abduction Injuries

These are essentially subtalar injuries occurring when the foot is in a neutral position with respect to the axis of the leg. The superficial fasciculus of the medial ligament of the ankle, the interosseous ligament of the sinus tarsi, the internal talonavicular ligament and, exceptionally, the plantar calcaneonavicular ligament are ruptured. Local pain and tenderness extends from the medial ligament of the ankle joint to the talonavicular ligament.

21.1.4 Pure Adduction Injuries

Such injuries are exceptional, for in most instances there is an inversion component. They can occur, however, and lead to lateral ligament damage, particularly of the calcaneofibular and anterior talofibular components.
Pain and tenderness relate to the lateral malleolus, the outer aspect of the calcaneum, the outer aspect of the head of the talus and the talonavicular joint, and the anterior fasciculae of the anterior talofibular ligament.

21.1.5 Plantarflexion Injuries

These injuries occur most commonly in football, due to a forward slip, or on the stairs, on catching the heel on the edge of a step when falling. The lateral and anterior components of the anterior talofibular ligament, and perhaps the peroneal tendons, sustain most of the force, but the dorsal ligaments of the talonavicular joint may also be involved.
Tenderness relates either to the lateral ligament at its malleolar insertions or to both medial and lateral tarsal attachments. It may extend from the dorsal aspect of the talar head near the talonavicular joint, or exceptionally more distally, to the naviculocuneiform line.

21.1.6 Dorsiflexion Injuries

These injuries result when landing awkwardly from a jump is associated with backward slipping of the foot; the posture leads to forced separation of the ankle mortice by engagement of the wider anterior mass of the talar articular surface between the malleoli. Primarily, there is damage to the inferior tibiofibular ligament, but with progression on the injury, the talonavicular plantar ligaments, the calcaneocuboid ligament, the Y-shaped ligament (Testut) and the calcaneonavicular ligaments become involved, perhaps with detachment of a beak of bone from the anterior process of the calcaneum. The interosseous ligament of the sinus tarsi and the posterior part of the lateral ligament of the ankle are always associated, according to Judet, with a lesion of the calcaneofibular ligament. A more significant degree of trauma can provoke fracture of the neck of the talus or of the navicular. The injury complex leads to tibiofibular diastasis and instability of the talus with lateral shifting, a positive anteroposterior draw sign, and damage to the articular surface of the talus. Later complications may be seen, e.g. the formation of exostoses at the anterior or posterior margins of the tibial articular surface and the anterior border of the talar surface (impingement exostosis of O'Donoghue). Calcification of the damaged collateral ligaments of the ankle may occur.
Ultimate recovery from any of these injuries depends largely upon subsequent muscle control, the presence of disadvantageous foot postures (as occur in the cavovalgus or cavovarus foot), and the inclinations of the subject with respect to physical activity, quality of footwear, and the sort of terrain on which he chooses to walk. Frequently, seemingly minor trauma, consequently undertreated, may lead to complications.

21.2 Clinical Features

21.2.1 Severity

Efforts should be made to assess the severity of the injury clinically. The following aspects should be considered:

1. The presence of predisposing abnormalities in the foot: cavovarus makes lateral injuries most likely, cavovalgus tends to lead to either external or internal injuries
2. The history of the mechanism of trauma and its intensity
3. The rapidity of onset of particular signs after the trauma, and the occurrence of a cracking or grating sound at the time of injury
4. The site and severity of pain occurring at the time of injury or afterwards, and the extent and site of any swelling, oedema and ecchymosis
5. Loss of movement and its cause – pain or mechanical blockage
6. The exact points of tenderness and the presence of crepitus
7. The clinical evidence of tilting of the talus or a positive drawer sign, which may be difficult to appreciate
8. The muscular state and sporting activities of the subject

21.2.2 Pain

Pain of immediate onset is of variable duration. An initial improvement may provide reassurance but obscure the presence of a serious injury. Sometimes, pain is progressive, involving the whole of the region, or recurrent, precipitated by the slightest movement. The presence of a cracking sensation is no guide to the severity of the injury.

21.2.3 Swelling

The most common sites of swelling are (a) below and in front of the lateral malleolus and (b) beneath the medial malleolus. In either case, there is filling of the retromalleolar gutter according to the side of the lesion. Early swelling may be localised; it reaches its maximum at the end of the 2nd day, and is then resorbed under the influence of an elastic support and immobilisation. It may be accompanied by ecchymosis of early onset, but this can disappear very rapidly, depending on the severity of the injury. The ecchymosis may be diffuse. Generalised oedema occurring some 5–8 h after injury and accompanied by local heat and loss of function is more a manifestation of vasomotor disorder.

21.2.4 Loss of Function

Characteristically, the foot adopts a light equinovarus posture, with loss of function, perhaps lasting for a few minutes, perhaps for a few days. The subject cannot load the foot due to pain with complete loss of active and passive movement.

This may sometimes give the impression of a mechanical blockage of motion. There are cases where loss of movement seems to be associated with capsular or synovial entrapment, but this can disappear during gentle conservative management, which seems to liberate the synovium.

Loss of function can be analysed in terms of impaired range of dorsiflexion and plantarflexion and of inversion and eversion and related to points of local tenderness. Careful stressing of limits of motion induces pain, which may occur in areas of bony detachment and tendon or tendon sheath damage, as well as in the injured ligaments themselves.

21.2.5 Talar Instability

Clinical assessment is rendered difficult by the pain and local swelling, but in the anteroposterior direction, abnormal mobility anteriorly always indicates involvement of the collateral ligaments, while in the coronal plane, rocking of the talus indicates widening of the mortice due to diastasis or rupture of one or other collateral ligament. A sudden movement of the talus when it is put back into a neutral position from varus stress indicates a lesion of the anterior talofibular ligament (Voutey 1971 a).

21.3 Radiography

Standard anteroposterior, dorsoplantar and lateral views are essential. If this involves much pain, the examinations may be conducted under general anaesthesia. Gentle stressing will reveal instabilities, but any forceful manipulation may extend the lesions or even give a false impression of their severity.

In the dorsoplantar and anteroposterior views, bony injuries involving the malleoli or the base of the fifth metatarsal, the navicular and the neck of the talus may be evident, together with avulsion flake fractures of ligamentous insertions. Diastasis of the inferior tibiofibular joint will be seen if present.

With the foot in dorsiflexion and plantarflexion, anteroposterior displacement of the ankle may be seen on the lateral view. When this amounts to less than 10 mm anteriorly, it indicates a lesion confined to the anterior fasciculae of the collateral ligaments, but in excess of 10 mm, there is an anterior lesion with rupture of the outer ligament of the ankle. Varus or valgus stressing of the foot may show instability of the talus in its mortice. When this is less than 20°, a lesion of the anterior fasciculus of the middle part of the lateral ligament is indicated, but more than 30° betrays rupture of the entire lateral ligament.

Special views include the 45° external oblique view with the foot in plantarflexion, which shows the inferior tibiofibular joint and the sinus tarsi (Voutey 1971 a), and the views described by Harris and Beath (1948), which demonstrate the integrity of the talocalcaneal joint line.

In late lesions, tomography is valuable in locating an area of avascular necrosis of the talus or a lesion of the sinus tarsi or the subtalar joint (Voutey). Arthrography, advocated by Motta (1966) and Wolkas and Mondo (1966) is needed only in exceptional cases.

21.4 Treatment

21.4.1 Minor Injuries

Treatment is *conservative*, comprising elevation, ice therapy, alternating hot and cold bathing, and elastic support for 4 weeks; alternatively, a brief period of immobilisation in a plaster cast if the lesion is very painful. Anti-inflammatory agents, analgesics and relaxants are valuable. In some instances, infiltration with local anaesthetic, limited to small volumes (less than 10 ml), is useful. Light massage and gentle passive and active mobilisation with strengthening exercises for the stabilising muscles of the ankle are valuable.

Irritability arising from old injuries requires prolonged elastic support and proprioceptive re-education. Slight postural displacement may occur in these cases, but will respond to the wearing of a supporting insole correcting the transverse imbalance; pronating or supinating wedges should be fitted as appropriate if there is any varus or valgus posture of the tarsus.

In more severe cases, a longer period of plaster immobilisation is valuable, using a walking plaster which can be removed. Proprioceptive re-educative exercises in a figure-of-eight supporting bandage are well worthwhile, beginning a month after injury. If there is evidence of tibiofibular diastasis, the plaster cast should be carefully moulded so as to control possible separation of the malleoli and to maintain the foot in equinus for 6 weeks.

21.4.2 *Major Injuries*

In terms of treatment, severe injuries should be regarded as seriously as fractures.

21.4.2.1 Recent

In general, a plaster cast boot should be worn for 1 month followed by appropriate kinesitherapy, proprioceptive re-education and soft dressing support for about a further month. Acupuncture associated with the treatment has been found to alleviate pain, but is clearly a specialised procedure.

Surgical Management. Judet, Glorion, Witvoet, Legré, and Voutey (1971 a) have all emphasised that surgical management is necessary in the subject less than 30 years old, but after the age of 40 years, the accent should be on conservative management. Suture of the damaged ligament should be performed within 3 days of injury if surgery is intended. Complete rupture of a collateral ligament of the ankle with more than 20° tilt on stress radiography is an absolute indication for immediate repair by edge-to-edge suture of the ligament with fine simple stitches or, when necessary, reinsertion of the ruptured ligament onto the surface of the bone. Immobilisation for 1–2 months, according to the severity of the lesion, should be followed by massage and proprioceptive re-education (Freeman et al. 1965).

21.4.2.2 Older

In older cases where no treatment was undertaken immediately, if persistent instability is moderate, support with an elastic bandage and proprioceptive re-education may be all that is necessary. Persistent instability with pain is an indication for surgical management in the young subject. Repair of an old injury is, however, ineffective when the ligament has been lacerated and stretched and has become atrophied or shredded; correction must then be achieved by a ligamentoplasty such as those described by Watson-Jones (1943), Castaing (1968 a) and Schnepp (1979) which use peroneus brevis tenoplasty for the lateral ligament of the ankle. These tendon transfers function passively, in contrast with the procedure described by Bousquet in which peroneus brevis is shortened and actively supports the joint. I have described a technique (Regnauld 1974) in which a strip of the peroneus longus tendon is doubled back on itself, as shown in Fig. 21.1; this has proved effective.

Judet (1975) and Francillon (1961) advocated dermoplastic procedures, Storen (1959) used a tongue from tendo Achillis, and d'Aubigne (1949 b) suggested bolting together the components of the inferior tibiofibular joint; as the latter prevents normal rotation of the lateral malleolus, it should never be performed unless there is a severe diastasis or total disruption of the lateral ligament. All of these operations necessitate postoperative immobilisation and subsequent re-education.

21.5 Late Complications

Renewed or persistent symptoms several months or even years after trauma do not seem to relate to the intensity of the original trauma. They are usually functional impairments, comprising pain of varying degrees which particularly interferes with sporting activities. Other examples, however, clearly relate to obvious mechanical derangements.

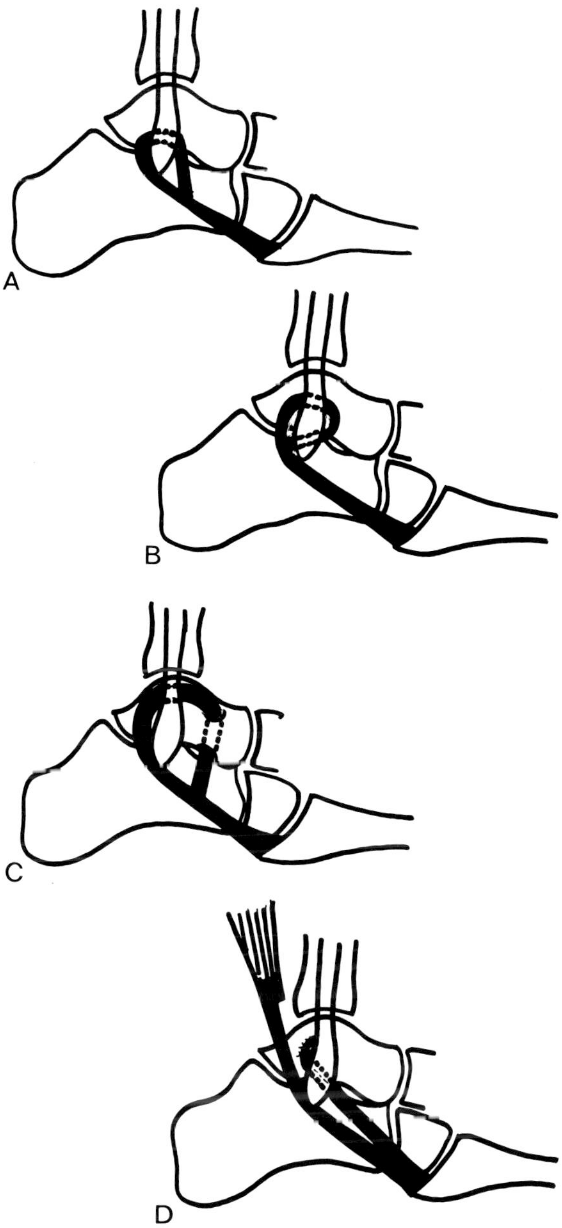

Fig. 21.1 A–D. Tenodesis of lateral peroneus brevis. **A** Castaing technique. **B** Watson-Jones technique. **C** Schnepp technique. **D** Regnauld technique

21.5.1 Functional Sequelae

Functional sequelae may comprise simple limitation without any obvious ligamentous abnormality, ligamentous laxity with instability of the foot and tilting of the talus, or vasomotor sequelae classified as reflex algodystrophy, sinus tarsi syndrome, contracted foot, diffuse oedema, tarsal tunnel compression syndrome (described fully in Chap. 33).

Complications due to joint involvement include the impingement of exostoses as described by O'Donoghue (1957), osteophytosis of the neck of the talus, avascular necrosis of the articular surface of the talus, arthrosis of the ankle joint, and loose bodies in the ankle joint. Pain can begin as soon as the patient resumes walking after a ligament injury which has apparently been successfully treated. It is commoner in subjects aged 50 or over and seems to be due to persistence of capsular oedema or hypertrophy of the articular synovial membrane. The patient complains of a feeling of stiffness accompanied by rather diffuse tenderness. Simple or diffuse swelling may be palpable in the various articular recesses, but radiography reveals no abnormality. *Treatment* comprises supportive bandage, massage, active re-education and proprioceptive rehabilitation accompanied by anti-inflammatory agents, and is usually successful.

21.5.2 Ligamentous Laxity with Subluxation of Talus

The lateral, anterior and medial ligaments can all be the predominant site of instability.

21.5.2.1 Lateral Instability

Lateral instability occurs most frequently after a neglected sprain, and questioning usually confirms the presence of haematoma immediately after the injury. There is often an associated postural abnormality, most frequently cavus but sometimes cavovarus, which is more obvious when the foot is not loaded (Voutey 1971 a).

Examination detects hypermobility of the ankle with instability, as described by Grant and Bonnin (1944), or true looseness of the talus in the mortice (Voutey 1971 a). Sometimes no obvious mechanical instability will be present despite the clinical symptoms of lowering into inversion; this must be ascribed to functional instability leading to a sensation of giving way due to incoordination of the ankle, especially in sport and in walking on irregular ground.

There is usually pain at the region of the anterior talofibular ligament or over the sinus tarsi when the outer subtalar region is involved. The ankle may have an effusion with oedema outside the capsule, and Voutey (1978) has described an irregularity of quality of motion during manipulation indicative of malleolar incongruence.

Radiographic examination usually shows increased varus of the talus of about 20° on gentle stressing.

Comparison with the opposite side shows a difference of some 15° if rupture is confined to the anterior talofibular ligament (second degree), while opening of 20°–50° (Bosse 1957) indicates additional rupture of the calcaneofibular component (third degree). Varus of between 10° and 20° is indicative of a "weak ankle" (first degree) (Voutey 1978).

21.5.2.2 Anterior Instability

The subject experiences a sensation of longitudinal instability when he puts his foot down in either dorsiflexion or plantarflexion. Examination reveals a drawer sign which is confirmed in lateral view X-rays under anterior or posterior stress – there is incongruence of the two curvatures of the tibial and talar articular surfaces. When the drawer sign is 10 mm, rupture of the anterior fasciculae can be expected, but in excess of 15 mm the three components of the lateral ligament must be involved.

21.5.2.3 Medial Instability

Occurring after eversion injuries, medial instability is nevertheless uncommon. Usually, a precavus valgus foot or a cavovalgus foot predisposes to isolated rupture of the medial ligament, perhaps associated with diastasis of the inferior tibiofibular joint, proved by radiography. Occasionally, interposition of soft tissue between the medial malleolus and the talus apposes reduction of the diastasis (Trillat et al. 1965).

Treatment of minor ankle instability from whatever cause comprises a supporting bandage, good shoes, proprioceptive re-education and exercises for the leg muscles. Frank recurrent subluxation in first-degree cases should again be treated conservatively but in the event of failure, or in second- and third-degree cases, surgery is usually indicated. Any of the following procedures may be appropriate:

- Suture of ligaments to their osseous attachment using transosseous stitches, after any necessary retensioning or shortening
- Plication of the extensor retinaculum, especially if instability is medial or anterior
- Stabilisation of the sinus tarsi with respect to the interosseous ligament injury
- Various tenoplasties and other procedures described above (Sect. 21.4.2.2)

21.5.3 Vasomotor Conditions

Alteration of vasomotor response leads to a painful dystrophic state (algodystrophy) which may manifest as a contracted foot, an oedematous foot or articular neuralgia.

Thus, a severe sprain of either of the ankle ligaments (more frequently the lateral) or of the interosseous ligament of the sinus tarsi may lead to painful restriction of both ankle and subtalar joints with severe spasm in eversion due to contraction of the peronei and the long extensor tendons (spasmodic flat foot). This responds to treatment comprising rest in a plaster cast for 6 weeks, injections of topical steroids and local anaesthetic into the sinus tarsi and re-educative physiotherapy.

Ligamentous lesions can result in diffuse oedema around the whole circumference of the ankle region, filling the retromalleolar gutters. The oedema may or may not be painful, and may occur months or even years after the injury. Small calcified plaques may be observed in the substance of the ligaments. Effective treatments include massage, anti-inflammatory drugs, physiotherapy and radiotherapy.

Other causes include the tarsal tunnel syndrome (cf. Chap. 33), while neuralgic articular pains can be produced by capsulosynovial herniations into the joint, which may require operative exploration and excision of an intra-articular synovial fringe.

21.5.4 Joint Complications

Osteophytosis of Anterior Margins of Ankle Joint. The osteophytosis can involve both tibia and talus, and is characterised by spiculate exostoses, sometimes with impingement (O'Donoghue 1957). The osteophytes follow hyperdorsiflexion strains and are seen in the lateral radiograph. Painful limitation of movement necessitates surgical resection of both tibial and talar osteophytes.

Avascular Necrosis of Talar Articular Surface. Several authors have described these lesions which are more frequent than perhaps thought (Berndt and Harty; Soeur; Delahaye; Besson; Wellinger; Voutey; Axhausen; Kessel). Axhausen and Kessel ascribe the condition to obliteration of the nutrient artery of the talus or to traumatic shock. Clinical signs are few, usually comprising pain in the ankle joint associated perhaps with crepitus and, exceptionally, loss of movement. *Radiography,* especially tomography, makes the diagnosis obvious, possibly revealing a classical "egg in a nest", sometimes a small notch with an opaque sequestrum, perhaps flattening of the superior border of the talus in the region of a niche visible in the anteroposterior view and slight widening of the joint space, also in the anteroposterior view (Besson). *Treatment* by conservative means is often ineffective, even after prolonged immobilisation, in which case operative removal of the sequestrum is indicated.

Osteoarthrosis of Ankle Joint. This is commoner when injury is associated with a varus posture of the foot. *Treatment* is conservative in the first instance, involving the use of an insole bearing an external pronating wedge under the heel. Surgical management is relatively rarely indicated.

Intra-articular Loose Body. A joint mouse leads to intermittent loss of motion with sudden catching and pain. *Radiography* shows the offending lesion and the *treatment* of choice is surgical excision.

22 Post-Traumatic Osteoarthrosis

It is often difficult to define the boundary between idiopathic arthrosis and trauma. Thus, hallux rigidus and Freiberg-Köhler osteochondritis may be related to microtrauma, and considering the strenuous use to which the foot is put, it is perhaps surprising that osteoarthrosis is not more common. The wearing of poorly adapted shoes and the performing of unsuitable surgical procedures are examples of the abuse to which the evidently robust structures can be subjected. Arthroses are frequent in occurrence, and the failure of one particular component reverberates throughout the organ. Every plan for surgical management of arthrosis must embody a clear appreciation of any overall disturbance.

The concept of microtrauma applies in a variety of diverse situations. Thus, in the Egyptian configuration there is an absence of lateral physiological mobility of the first metatarsal, predisposing to a trophic stiffness of the metatarsophalangeal joint with some degree of aseptic necrosis of the head. Unnatural immobilisation of the foot following a fracture can have similar consequences. The postural deformity embodied in pes planus leads to diminution of the angle of inclination of the great metatarsal and to medial and plantar displacements of the midtarsus; these mechanical conditions can provoke, at one or several metatarsal joints, arthrosis consequent upon microtrauma from the twisting or the compression which operate at the site. In this way the arthroses of the midtarsus which affect the talonavicular and naviculocuneiform joints in pes planus can appear. Microtrauma from an everted posture of the foot leads to painful dysfunction of the midtarsal region, mostly affecting the outer side, and is associated with a varus tarsus comparable to that seen after the more severe trauma of talar dislocation and after reduction of an ankle fracture, a tarsal fracture or, especially, comminuted fractures of the waist of the foot (Fig. 22.1).

Painful syndromes, such as the algodystrophy of Sudeck-Leriche and the cavo-equinus foot seen in Volkman's syndrome, are dealt with in other chapters.

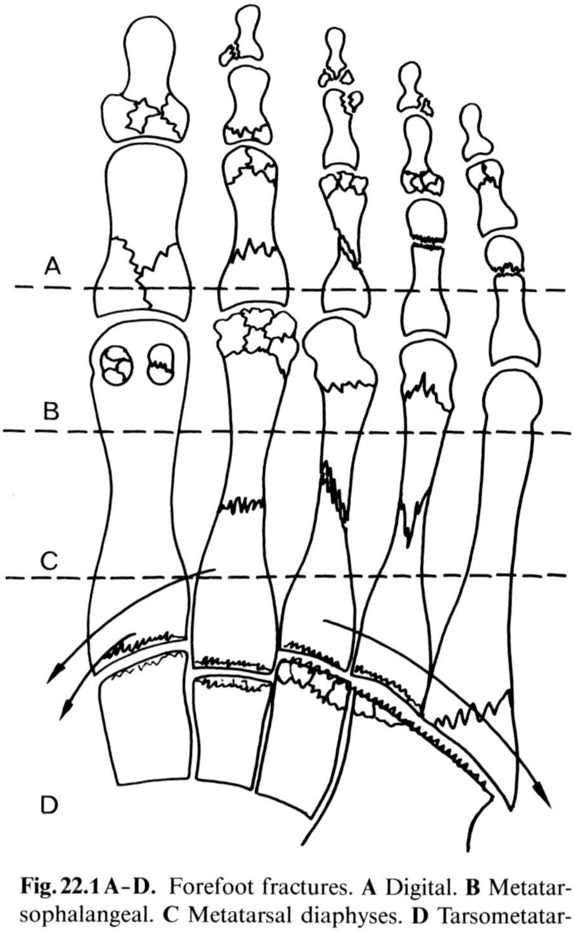

Fig. 22.1 A–D. Forefoot fractures. **A** Digital. **B** Metatarsophalangeal. **C** Metatarsal diaphyses. **D** Tarsometatarsal

22.1 Toes

22.1.1 Etiology

Arthrosic complications may supervene some months or years after compressive injury or crushing directly affecting the articular surfaces of the interphalangeal joints (Fig. 22.2).

Compressive injury may be due to direct axial force producing severe plantarflexion stresses or less commonly dorsiflexion stresses, in the small joints. This may result in fracture of the diaphysis of the proximal phalanx, which in turn leads to an-

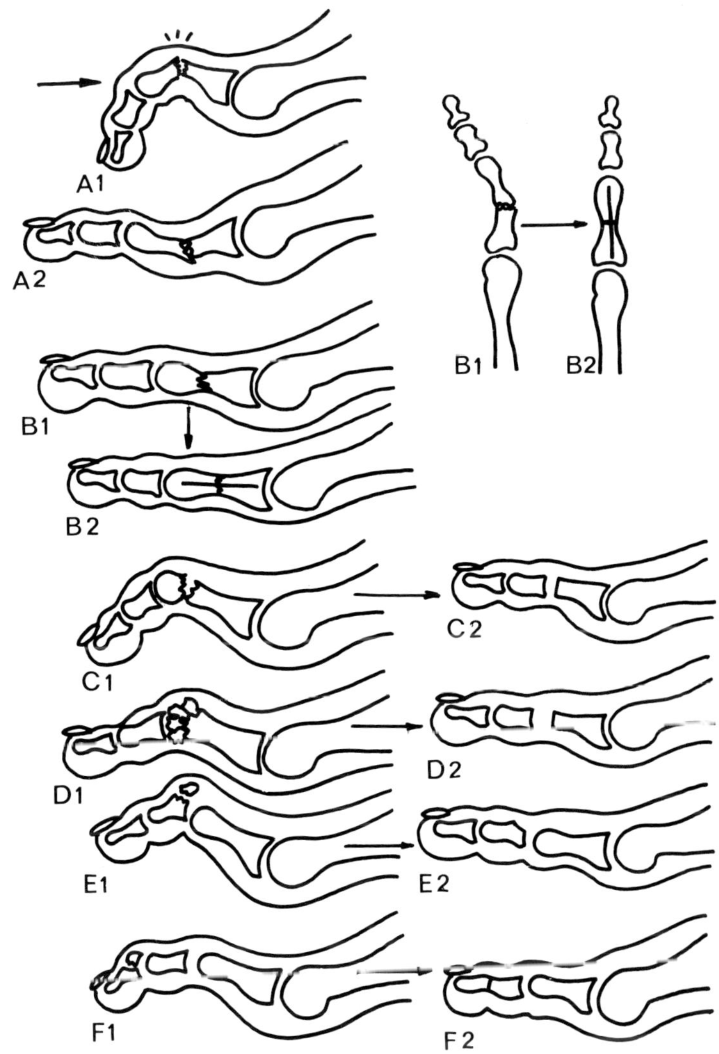

Fig. 22.2 A–F. Fractures of phalanges. **A** Diaphyseal fracture: *1* Displacement in plantar flexion (*arrow* indicates direction of force); *2* displacement in dorsiflexion. **B** Diaphyseal fracture: *1* Before treatment; *2* after fixation by secret intramedullary pin. **C** Fracture of neck: *1* Before treatment; *2* after resection arthroplasty. **D** Comminuted fracture of head: *1* Before treatment; *2* after resection arthroplasty. **E** Avulsion fracture of base of middle phalanx: *1* Before treatment; *2* after excision of avulsed fragment. **F** Avulsion fracture of base of distal phalanx: *1* Before treatment; *2* after interphalangeal arthrodesis

gulation of the toe and to abnormal pressure over a joint, manifested by a partridge-eye cutaneous lesion or, more distally, a pulp corn. Occasionally, comminuted fracture of the joint surface may occur. Direct application of force can produce lateral displacement of the toe with sprain or dislocation of the interphalangeal joints, sometimes associated with fracture involving the joint surface or fracture of the shafts of the bones. These injuries predominate in the first and fifth toes; the latter, because of its exposed external position, especially in an open shoe, is likely to be stubbed against an object on the ground, sprained during activities like dancing or sport, or crushed by some falling object.

22.1.2 Clinical Features

The sequelae of injuries to the toes are likely to include trophic changes from vascular or autonomic sources – sweating, hypothermia, painful swelling and red violaceous discoloration, general podginess of the digit involved, and pain and loss of function – in addition to the direct effects of ar-

throsis or deformity. Pain is aggravated by wearing shoes, walking and manipulation.
Radiography confirms the deformity or damage of the bones and joints.

22.1.3 Treatment

Mild deformities are compensated in many cases without treatment, while others respond to a judicious choice of foot wear. The presence of pressure symptoms such as a distal corn necessitates surgery.
In general, interphalangeal deformities should be corrected by arthrodesis, while malunited diaphyseal fractures with lateral angulation which will affect neighbouring toes and be accompanied by reflex contracture of tendons can be corrected by open operation at which the normal axis of the phalanx is corrected and fixed by the hidden pin technique (Regnauld 1974) (see Chap. 14).
It must be emphasised that in the immediate post-traumatic period, however severe the accompanying soft tissue involvement, the temptation to amputate should be resisted. Under the cover of antitetanus and antibiotic therapy, minute excision of toe injuries, realignment by splintage in tulle gras and a compress and protection with a plantar plaster of Paris insole extending beyond the ends of the toes is nearly always successful in salvaging the digit. Disability from amputation of a toe is frequently underestimated. Fractures of the neck of a phalanx (Fig. 22.3) involving the joint surface can, however, be treated by primary local excision, perhaps followed later by arthrodesis, especially in the case of the second proximal interphalangeal joint, where the pressure produced by the adjacent normal great toe risks valgus displacement of the second toe, which is always poorly tolerated.

22.2 Metatarsophalangeal Joints

22.2.1 Etiology

Post-traumatic metatarsophalangeal arthrosis can result from indirect injury by compression, torsion or crushing and lead to a general disturbance, not only in the forefoot but reverberating back to other elements. Very frequently, the lesions of the tarsus or midtarsus appear more important and those of the forefoot relatively minor, and it is as a result of this neglect that painful disturbances of the forefoot later predominate.
Arthrosis may be a consequence of dislocation or subluxation of a metatarsophalangeal joint, perhaps accompanied by an articular fracture of the head of a metatarsal or the base of a phalanx, or

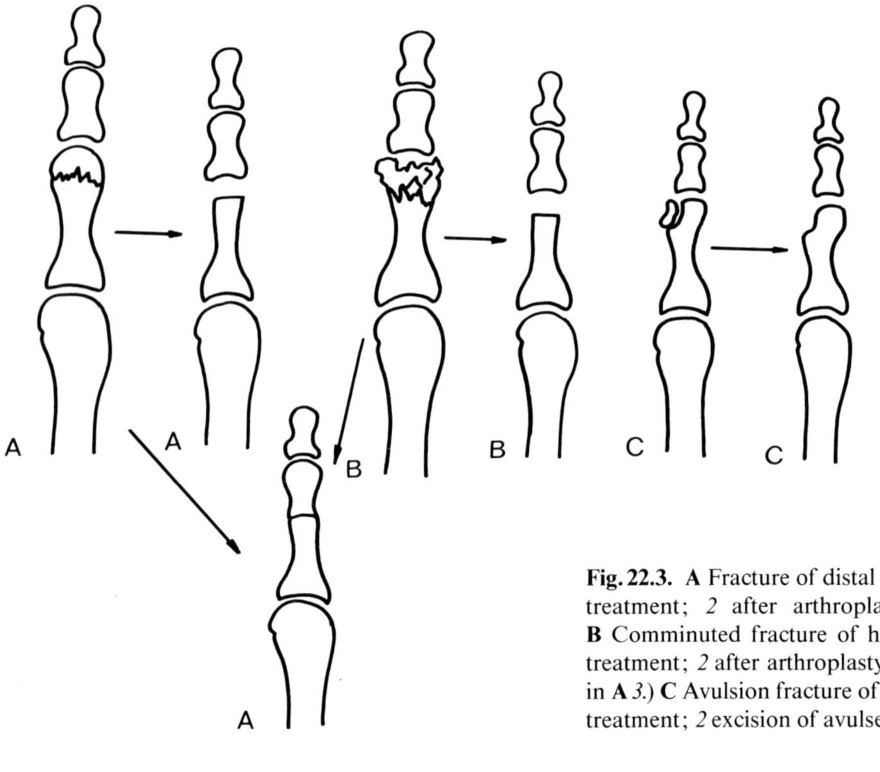

Fig. 22.3. **A** Fracture of distal shaft of phalanx: *1* Before treatment; *2* after arthroplasty; *3* after arthrodesis. **B** Comminuted fracture of head of phalanx: *1* Before treatment; *2* after arthroplasty. (Result of arthrodesis as in **A** *3*.) **C** Avulsion fracture of head of phalanx: *1* Before treatment; *2* excision of avulsed fragment

may occur after displacement of a metatarsal head stemming from a fracture of the neck of a metatarsal. Limitation of articular motion is accompanied by local pain, and there is frequently generalised metatarsalgia due to disturbed loading of the metatarsal heads; overloading of the neighbouring heads accompanies insufficiency of loading of the affected head. Symptoms may reflect proximally at the Lisfranc joint line and tarsal segments, following distortion secondary to protective postures adopted to relieve the painful forefoot. One or more joints may be involved but the disruption of loading and the individual sources of pain need to be analysed. Soft tissue injuries with scars and contractures and an impaired vascular state are features requiring very careful assessment, especially before surgery.

Treatment planning requires assessment of the distortions of anatomy, with special attention to loss of uniform load bearing of the metatarsal heads due to elevation, depression or backward displacement, as well as of the physiological aspects of incoordination of loading consequent upon individual joint involvement and protective reflexes.

22.2.2 *Clinical Features*

Careful establishment of the date of the accident, the nature of the trauma and its early treatment and the subsequent development of post-traumatic symptoms is essential.

Analysis of symptoms may immediately yield evidence of overloading of one or two metatarsal heads due to malalignment. A syndrome of insufficiency of loading, perhaps associated with pseudarthrosis of a diaphyseal fracture or consolidation of the fracture with the affected metatarsal head in a poorly elevated position may be accompanied by lateral or medial displacement.

Overloading will be accompanied by callus or keratoma formation which recurs despite chiropody or the wearing of an insole while in later cases an antalgic posture of the foot may lead to similar formations under the fourth or fifth metatarsal heads. Localised pain of the affected metatarsophalangeal joint relates to articular displacement.

In cases of underloading, palpation may reveal a simple depression between the two adjacent metatarsal heads or a plantar longitudinal skin fold more commonly associated with pseudarthrosis of the diaphysis or neck of the metatarsal. One or both of the adjacent metatarsal heads may display underlying corns or keratomata.

Associated contractures may involve the long and short extensors or sometimes a flexor; contractures are always accompanied by metatarsophalangeal subluxation and displacement of the associated toe. Inverse action of the lumbricales and interossei help to fix articular displacement. The general imbalance of the forefoot, partly engendered by pain, may lead to supination of the forefoot and malposition of the hindfoot into varus and consequent tarsometatarsal, midtarsal or subtalar joint pains.

Podoscopy identifies the pattern of the footprint and the position of the painful calluses, together with retraction or contracture of the forefoot and of the toes and any transverse imbalance into inversion or eversion. The configuration of the longitudinal arch may be cavus or planus.

Podometry allows exact identification of the disordered pressure of the forefoot, identifying each metatarsal head in this respect.

Radiography: Features of importance are pseudarthrosis, malignment of fractures of metatarsals, the state of the articular surfaces, subluxation or dislocation, particularly at the metatarsophalangeal joints, osteoporosis or lytic areas, osteophyte formation and the absence or significance of digital displacements. The dorsoplantar view reveals the degree of forward or backward displacement of metatarsal heads, and depression or elevation can be assessed in the anteroposterior load-bearing view of the metatarsal heads.

Referring to the state of the joint surfaces, flattening and marginal osteophytosis of the peripheral areas may be accompanied by conservation of a central cartilage area on either phalanx or metatarsal head. This will influence the possibility of recovery of joint function after reposition of a metatarsal head in its proper position, the behaviour of a homograft or prosthetic replacement of a metatarsal head or, if the cartilage of both head and phalanx has been destroyed, the need for a cup prosthesis. Osteophytes can be removed, thereby relieving ankylosis, and central preservation of articular cartilage can be used to advantage.

Of paramount importance in the radiological examination is the assessment of the positions of the metatarsal heads with respect to under- or overloading. As stated repeatedly, this can be produced by horizontal or vertical displacement from any cause. Displacements of the joints should be related to elongation or shortening of the flexor and extensor tendons.

22.2.3 *Treatment*

Whenever possible, surgical treatment is indicated, for it is the only means of anatomical correction likely to cure the condition whether there is localised arthrosis responsible for local symptoms or disordered weight bearing under the metatarsal heads with respect to the metatarsophalangeal joints. The interphalangeal joints, which are nearly always involved, have been dealt with in Chap. 17. The principles of surgical treatment will depend upon assessment of displacement and the state of the joint surface.

22.2.3.1 *Metatarsophalangeal Arthralgia with Preservation of Metatarsal Head*

The postural arthralgic syndrome is due to malposition of the metatarsal head consecutive to fracture of the neck of the bone rather than due to the development of true arthrosis. Operative treatment contrives to replace the metatarsal head in a good position (Fig. 22.4). When possible, osteoclasis is performed, and correct malalignment of the fracture site and subsequent fixation is achieved with an axial intramedullary pin. If this repositioning is too difficult, perhaps due to the impossibility of adequate fixation, a realignment head-shaft enclavement constitutes the only solution. This will diminish the length of the metatarsal concerned in comparison with its neighbours and perhaps lead to a syndrome of insufficiency. Accordingly, in such an event it is necessary to realign and enclave adjacent metatarsal heads, thereby restoring frontal and horizontal alignment.

22.2.3.2 *Metatarsophalangeal Arthrosis with Destruction of One or Both Articular Surfaces*

In some cases the metatarsal head is predominantly involved and the base of the phalanx is intact. Complete destruction of the former demands replacement of the metatarsal condyle, either by homograft or with a metatarsal prosthesis (Fig. 22.5). When there is peripheral eburnation with flattening of the metatarsal condyle but with preservation of a central zone of cartilage, the margins can be trimmed of osteophytes peripherally and further mobilisation can be achieved by capsulotomy and adequate elongation of the associated tendons. The joint surface can be improved by temporary insertion of a cup prosthesis. Realignment head-shaft enclavement of adjacent metatarsal heads may be necessary. Finally, attention must be devoted to any accompanying interphalangeal deformities.

When the arthrosis involves the corresponding phalangeal base, reconstitution of the joint has to be achieved by either (a) homograft of the metatarsal head associated with trimming of the circumference of the base of the phalanx and perhaps temporary interposition of a cup prosthesis, although in some instances this may not be necessary (Fig. 22.6), or (b) implantation of a metatarsal prosthesis together with trimming of the proximal end of the phalanx, which may be adequate in gross cases.

22.2.3.3 *Multiple Metatarsophalangeal Joint Involvement*

Clearly, every case will be individual, but in general, attention must be paid to the integument, the joint capsules, involvement of neighbouring tendons, the articular surfaces and accompanying digital involvement (Figs. 22.7, 22.8). Thus, there may be atrophy of the skin with local corns and contractures, erythrocyanosis, excessive sweating, alterations of the nail bed and peripheral vascular problems of an algodystrophic type. Capsular involvement will lead to contracture aggravated by shortening of the tendons and inverse action of the interossei and lumbricales, while ankylosis of the metatarsophalangeal joints accompanies and aggravates the destruction of their surfaces. Clawing of the interphalangeal joints leads to painful pressure symptoms.

However bad the general state, amputation of metatarsal heads should be avoided rigorously, and as stated earlier, amputation of the toes will lead to loss of protection of the associated metatarsal heads. The aim has to be the reconstitution of forefoot metatarsal loading in a uniform line with preservation of both plantar flexion and dorsiflexion. Accordingly, the operation of choice should be realignment as described by Lelièvre (1952) (see Chap. 40) associated with interposition cup prostheses or head-shaft enclavement of metatarsal heads which are otherwise intact although displaced (Fig. 22.9). In each metatarsophalangeal joint the two bones should be restored to proper alignment after restoration of position by means of capsulotomy and appropriate tendinous elongations.

To recapitulate, the rather complex indications for the various procedures available for damaged metatarsal heads are as follows:

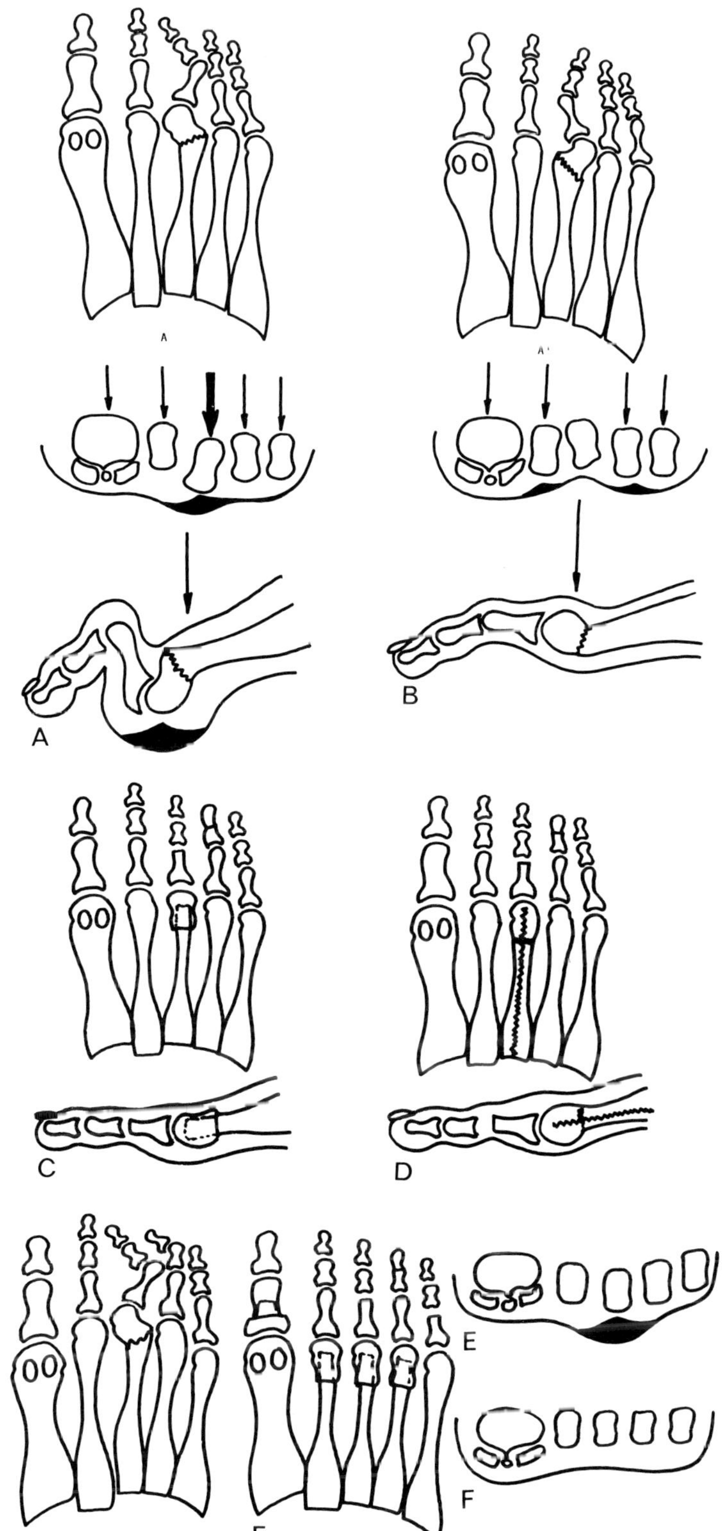

Fig. 22.4 A–F. A Localised post-traumatic metatarsal overloading. **B** Post-tramatic deficient loading of single metatarsal head. **C** Realignment by enclavement of malunited metatarsal head. **D** Realignment of malunion of metatarsal condyle by secret pin technique. **E** Isolated post-traumatic overloading in convex forefoot. **F** Realignment by enclavement of central three metatarsal heads, metatarsophalangeal arthroplasty if necessary, arthroplasty or arthrodesis of interphalangeal joints

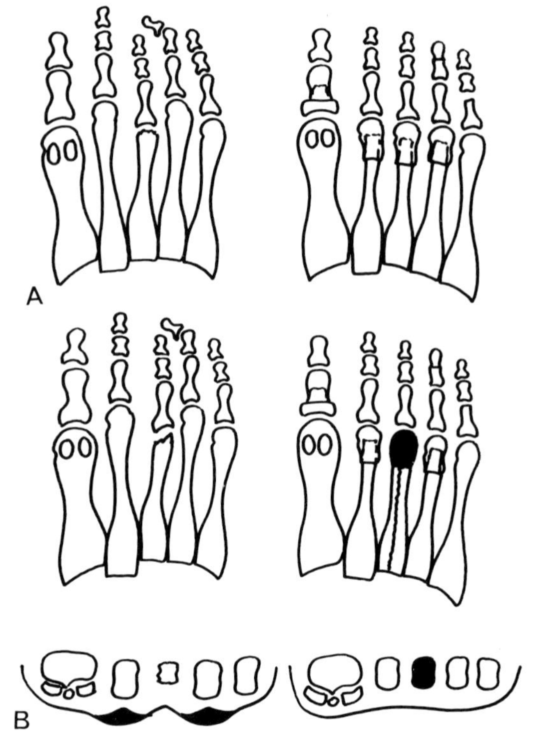

◁ **Fig. 22.5 A, B.** Isolated post-traumatic osteonecrosis in convex forefoot. Treatment: arthroplasty of first ray if necessary, realignment by enclavement of the adjacent metatarsal heads, and, for the osteonecrotic metatarsal, either **A** enclavement of metatarsal head by homograft (Regnauld) or **B** implantation of a metatarsal prosthesis with stem into the stump of the resorbed metatarsal

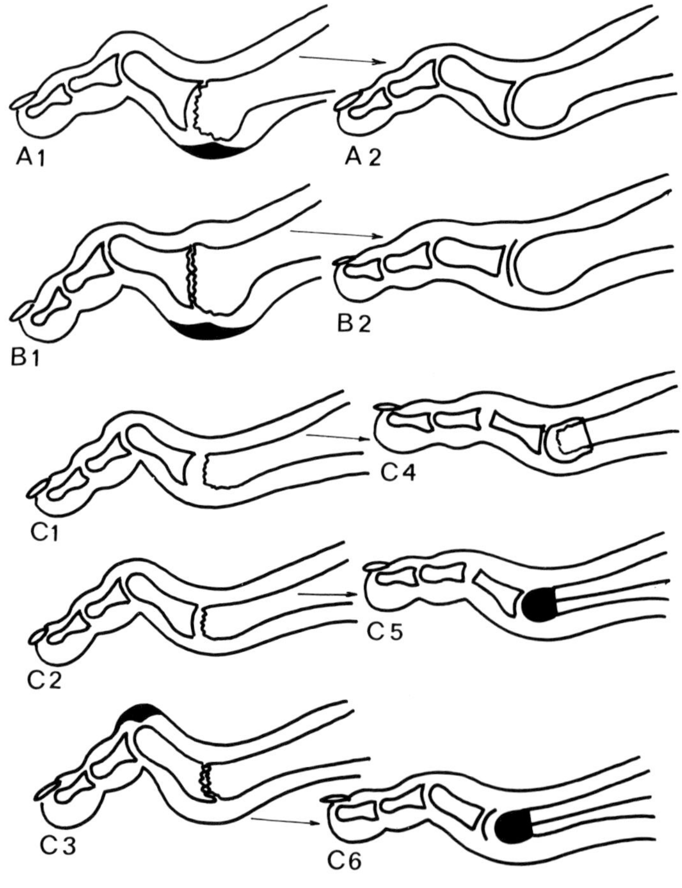

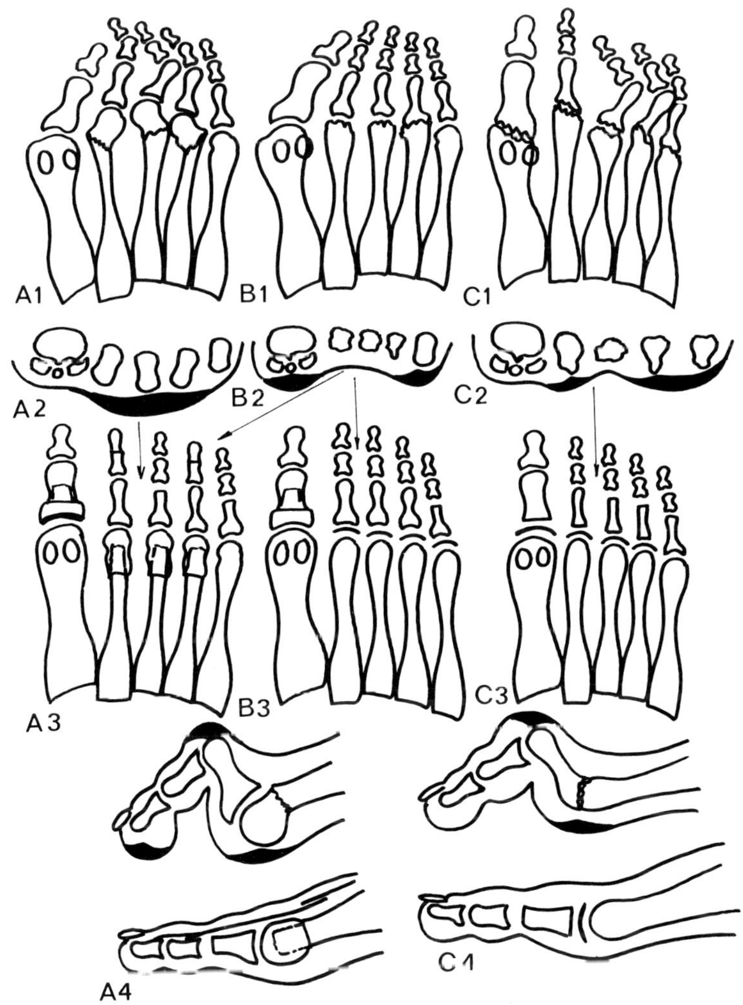

Fig. 22.7. A *1* Malunion of fractures of central metatarsal condyles; *2* overloading of central metatarsal heads; *3* realignment of central metatarsal heads by enclavement of autografts or homografts (Regnauld); *4* old and new profiles. **B** *1* Fracture of metatarsal condyles: post-traumatic osteoarthrosis with bone resorption leading to forefoot cavus but with preservation of the phalangeal bases; *2* forefoot cavus leading to overloading of first and fifth metatarsal heads; *3* metatarsal realignment (Lelièvre) with interposition of cup prostheses and arthroplasty or arthrodesis of interphalangeal joints (Regnauld). **C** *1* Multiple post-traumatic osteoarthrosis with loss of articular cartilage affecting metatarsals and phalanges; *2* irregular disorder of loading; *3* metatarsal and phalangeal realignment (Clayton) and interposition of cup prostheses and arthroplasty or arthrodesis of interphalangeal joints (Regnauld); *4* old and new profiles

◁ **Fig. 22.6 A–C.** Post-traumatic arthrosis of metatarsophalangeal joint. **A** Isolated metatarsal involvement: *1* Before treatment; *2* after remodelling of metatarsal head. **B** Arthrosis and ankylosis of metatarsophalangeal joint: *1* Before treatment; *2* after remodelling, conservative resection of the base of the proximal phalanx and cup arthroplasty. **C** Osteonecrosis of metatarsal head; *1–3* Before treatment; *4* after condyle homograft enclavement (Regnauld); *5* after prosthetic replacement of metatarsal head (Regnauld); *6* after prosthetic replacement of metatarsal head, conservative resection of base of proximal phalanx and cup arthroplasty (Regnauld)

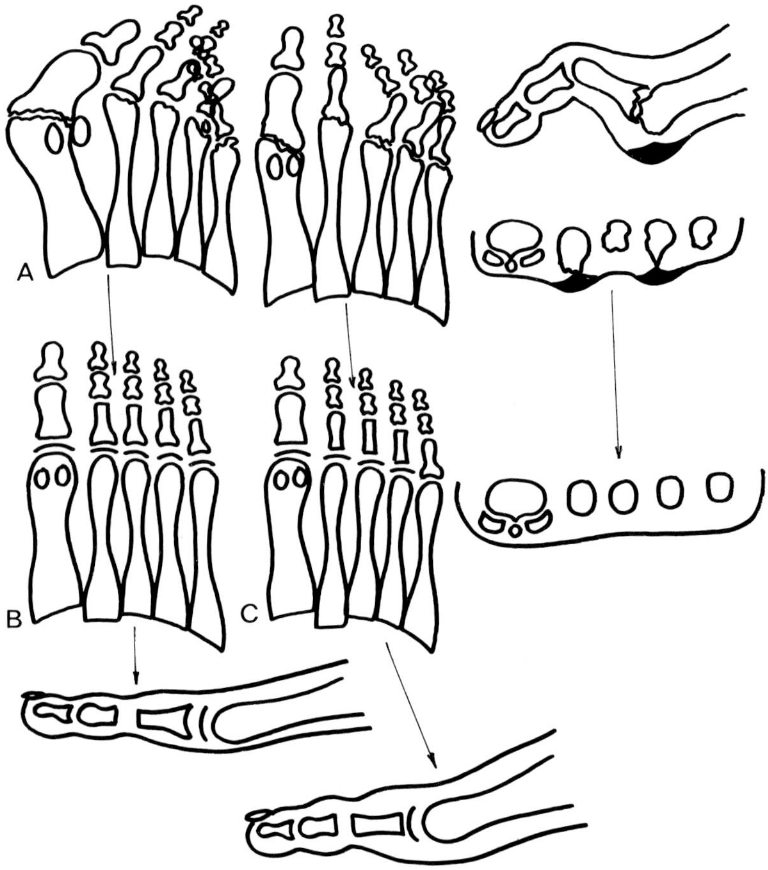

Fig. 22.8 A–C. Post-traumatic metatarsophalangeal osteoarthrosis. **A** Before treatment. **B** After metatarsal realignment (Lelièvre) with interposition of cup prostheses (Regnauld). **C** After metatarsal realignment (Clayton) with interposition of cup prostheses (Regnauld)

1. When the metatarsal head is consolidated in a poor position, realignment head-shaft enclavement is the most useful solution.
2. When the metatarsal head is partly or totally destroyed, enclavement using a metatarsal head homograft is the treatment of choice.
3. When all of a metatarsal head or one large part of it is destroyed, whether or not the bases of the corresponding phalanges are involved, the realignment modelling described by Lelièvre (1952) - digital arthroplasty and tendinous elongations together with the interposition of a cup prosthesis - will reconstitute a forefoot compatible with normal loading.

22.3 Complications of Metatarsal Fracture

Fractures of the diaphysis or neck of a metatarsal leading to disturbance of loading of the metatarsal heads has just been dealt with above; the definitive treatment is likely to be surgical correction of malunion or pseudarthrosis involving internal fixation with a secret intramedullary pin (Regnauld 1974) (Fig. 22.10) or with miniature plates.

Fractures of the bases of the middle three metatarsals do not generally produce serious complications. They consolidate well, apart from occasional hypertrophic callus with local pressure symptoms, and do not require treatment. Fracture of the base of the first and fifth metatarsals, on the other hand, may lead to pain if an arthrosis develops, because of the greater mobility expected from these rays. De Wulf (and Robyns) (1962b) described a technique of coaptation and screwing of the fragments of a pseudarthrosis in the fifth metatarsal, while in the first metatarsal, reduction and fixation by staple, wire or plate re-establishes proper orientation.

22.4 Lisfranc Joint Line

The injury most likely to produce late symptoms is fracture dislocation of the tarsometatarsal joint

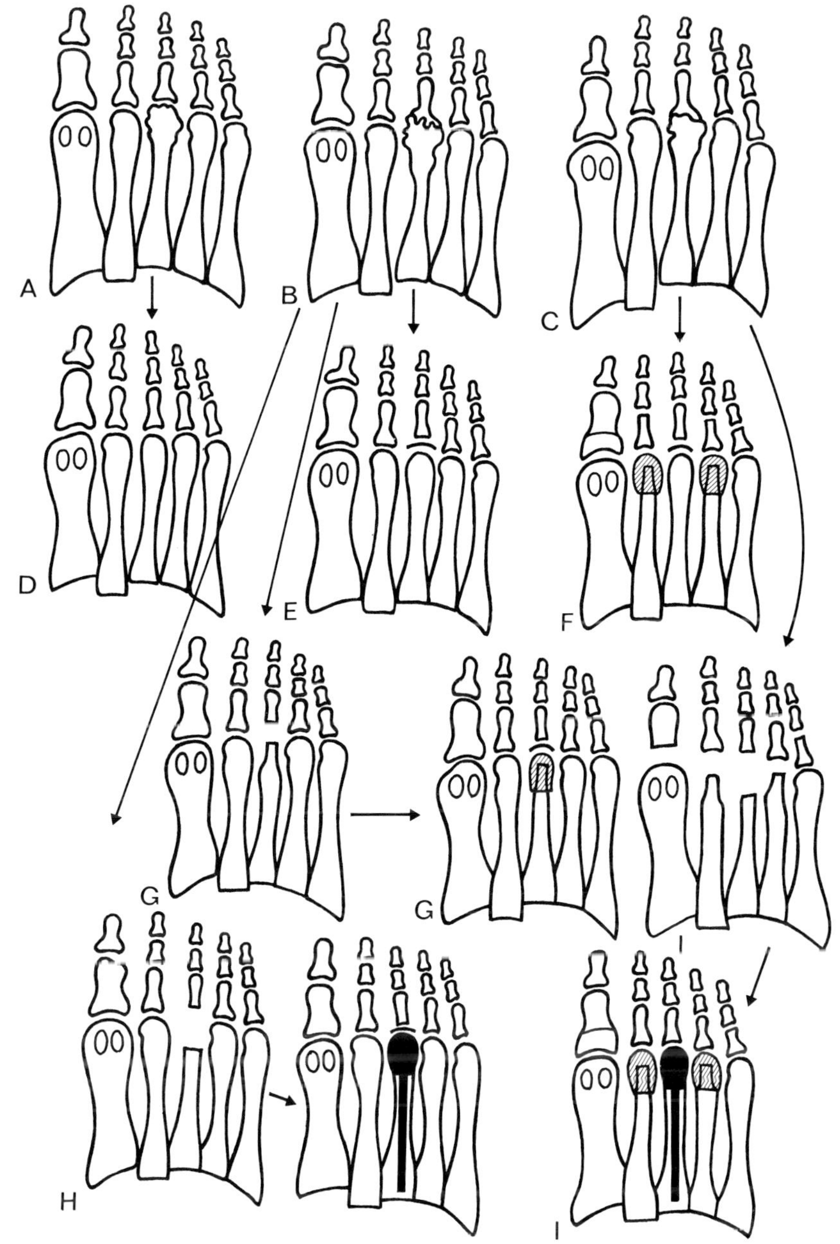

Fig. 22.9 A–I. Post-traumatic osteophyte formation. **A** In post-traumatic arthrosis. **B** In post-traumatic osteoarthrosis with ankylosis. **C** In post-traumatic arthrosis with ankylosis in a convex forefoot. **D** Metatarsophalangeal arthrolysis and remodelling of metatarsal head (Regnauld). **E** Clayton procedure completed by interposition of cup prosthesis (Regnauld). **F** Metatarsophalangeal arthroplasty with graft for first ray, realignment enclavement of adjacent metatarsal heads, Clayton procedure limited to remodelling of the metatarsal condyle and completed by implantation of cup prosthesis (Regnauld). **G** Enclavement of metatarsal head with homograft, limited resection of the phalangeal base, implantation of cup prosthesis (Regnauld). **H** Implantation of metatarsal prosthesis, interposition of cup prosthesis (Regnauld). **I** Metatarsophalangeal arthroplasty of first ray, realignment enclavement of neighbouring metatarsal heads, implantation of metatarsal prosthesis (Regnauld)

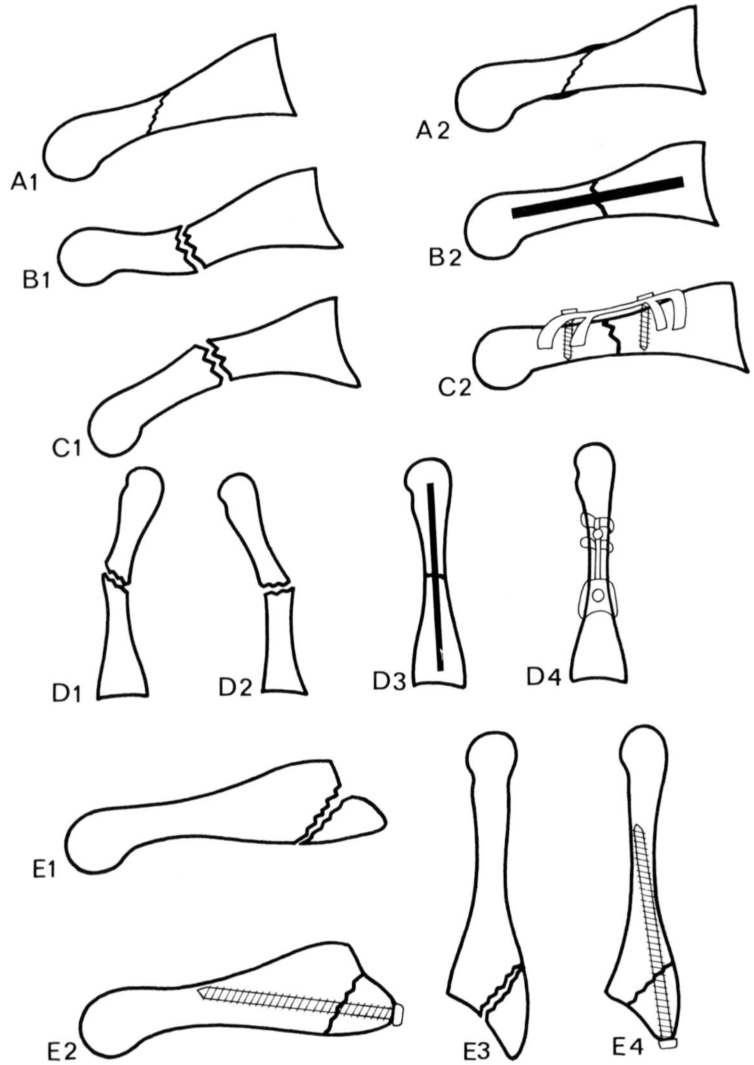

Fig. 22.10 A–E. Fractures of shaft of metatarsal. **A** Without displacement: *1* Before treatment; *2* after immobilisation. **B** With dorsal displacement: *1* Before treatment; *2* after reduction and fixation using secret pin technique. **C** With plantar displacement: *1* Before treatment; *2* after fixation with a Müller staple. **D** With lateral displacement: *1, 2* Before treatment; *3* secret pin technique; *4* Müller staple. **E** Base of fifth metatarsal: *1, 3* Before treatment; *2, 4* after screw fixation (de Wulf)

line, which can happen in trauma of direct impact, a fall onto the point of the foot, severe twisting during running, or road traffic accidents, accompanied by forceful abduction or adduction. The tarsus is wedged or fixed at the time of injury (Fig. 22.11). Quenu and Kuss (1909) classified these injuries for practical purposes as:

1. Valgus angular displacement of all metatarsals *en bloc*
2. Divergent angular displacement with medial deviation of the first metatarsal and lateral deviation of the outer four
3. Localised dislocation of one or more metatarsals

Although these injuries are relatively rare, a number of authors have described them.

Months after an unsuccessfully treated injury, there may be persistent swelling on the dorsal aspect accompanied by obvious bony projections from the bases of the metatarsals which have not been reduced. Pain is variable, but usually of a twisting, tension, burning, constrictive or grinding character and is exaggerated by standing and walking, especially on uneven ground, by mobilisation of the foot into pronation and plantar flexion and by abduction or adduction of the metatarsus. Often there coexists a pes planus with variable diastasis

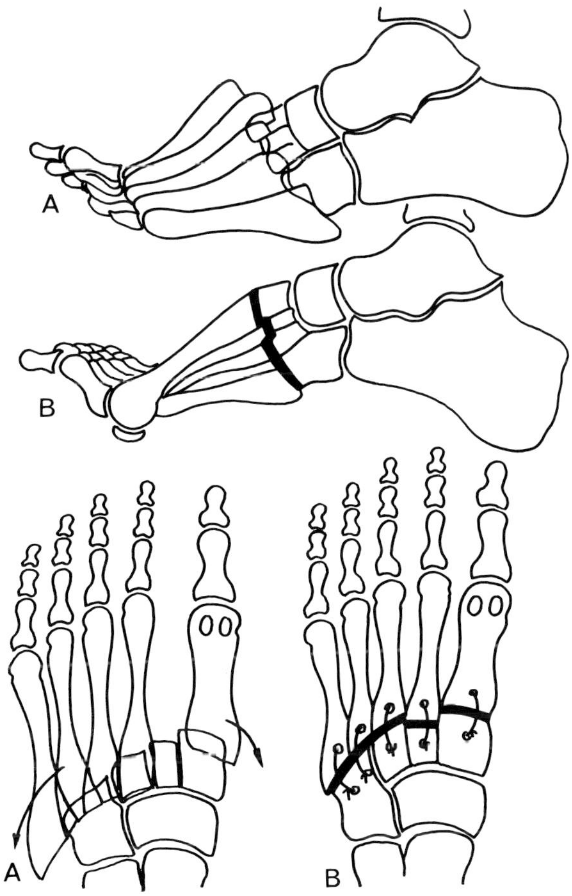

Fig. 22.11. A Lisfranc joint dislocation. **B** After reduction, arthrodesis and fixation by resorbable suture

between the outer and inner cuneiform-metatarsal joints.

Radiography (Fig. 22.12): The lateral view shows no abnormality, or perhaps some dorsal projection of the base of the first and second metatarsals. In the dorsoplantar view, basal diastases of the intermetatarsal spaces of the first and second rays are apparent, with evidence of comminuted fractures of the bases of the metatarsals and the cuneiforms. Special views may show subluxation upwards or outwards of the five metatarsals, possibly accompanied by divergence of dislocation with respect to each other; the first metatarsal base may be dislocated inwards and downwards, the other metatarsal bases subluxed in one mass upwards and outwards.

Treatment: Conservative management is usually unsuccessful. Surgery is indicated, and comprises arthrodesis of the cuneiform-metatarsal joints, which corrects any planus deformity and preserves the congruity of the antetarsus with respect to the long axis of the foot. It is important to re-establish the proper angle of declination of the metatarsus, identical to that of the opposite foot. Maintenance of the reduction is achieved by splintage, or better by transosseous nylon sutures at the level of each cuneiform-metatarsal and cuboidometatarsal joint after careful coaptation of the cut surfaces of the bones. A plaster cast for 2 months followed by suitable physiotherapy restores function.

22.5 Midtarsal Region

Etiology. Microtrauma from pes planovalgus or cavovarus is the commonest cause of arthrosis of the midtarsal joints, followed by fracture of one or several of the bones. Most frequently affected is the navicular, followed by the cuneiforms and then the cuboid. Fractures of the cuneiforms or the cuboid do not usually disturb the balance of the midtarsal complex, whereas fracture of the navicular leads to subsidence or arthrosis of the talonavicular, naviculocuneiform or naviculocuboidal joints. Paradoxically, it may induce painful pes cavovarus due to contracture of the intrinsic muscles. Dislocation of one of the perinavicular joints may have similar results.

Clinical Features. The persistent pain in the midtarsal region is exaggerated by standing, is of a burning, tight character and is experienced both during the day and at night. It is little relieved by anti-inflammatory or analgesic agents. The *radiographs* show the severity of any bony lesion and of the associated joints. Osteophytic proliferation may be marked, while overall appreciation of the foot clinically and radiologically may exhibit flattening or cavus deformities.

Treatment. Conservative management may be successful if there is no alteration in size of the navicular and no accompanying arthrosis. A monoblock insole is used to correct any transverse displacement as gently as necessary, and together with anti-inflammatory agents can relieve pain. Irreversible arthrosis of one or more joint spaces without crushing of the navicular bone itself can best be treated by arthrodesis of the joints affected, accompanied by arthrodesis of the subtalar joint if necessary. If the navicular is reduced in volume, arthrodesis should be accompanied by the interposition of a bone graft so as to restore the volume of the foot and the longitudinal arch. Fractures of the cuneiforms and cuboid do not usually lead to late painful sequelae, and surgical indications are exceptional.

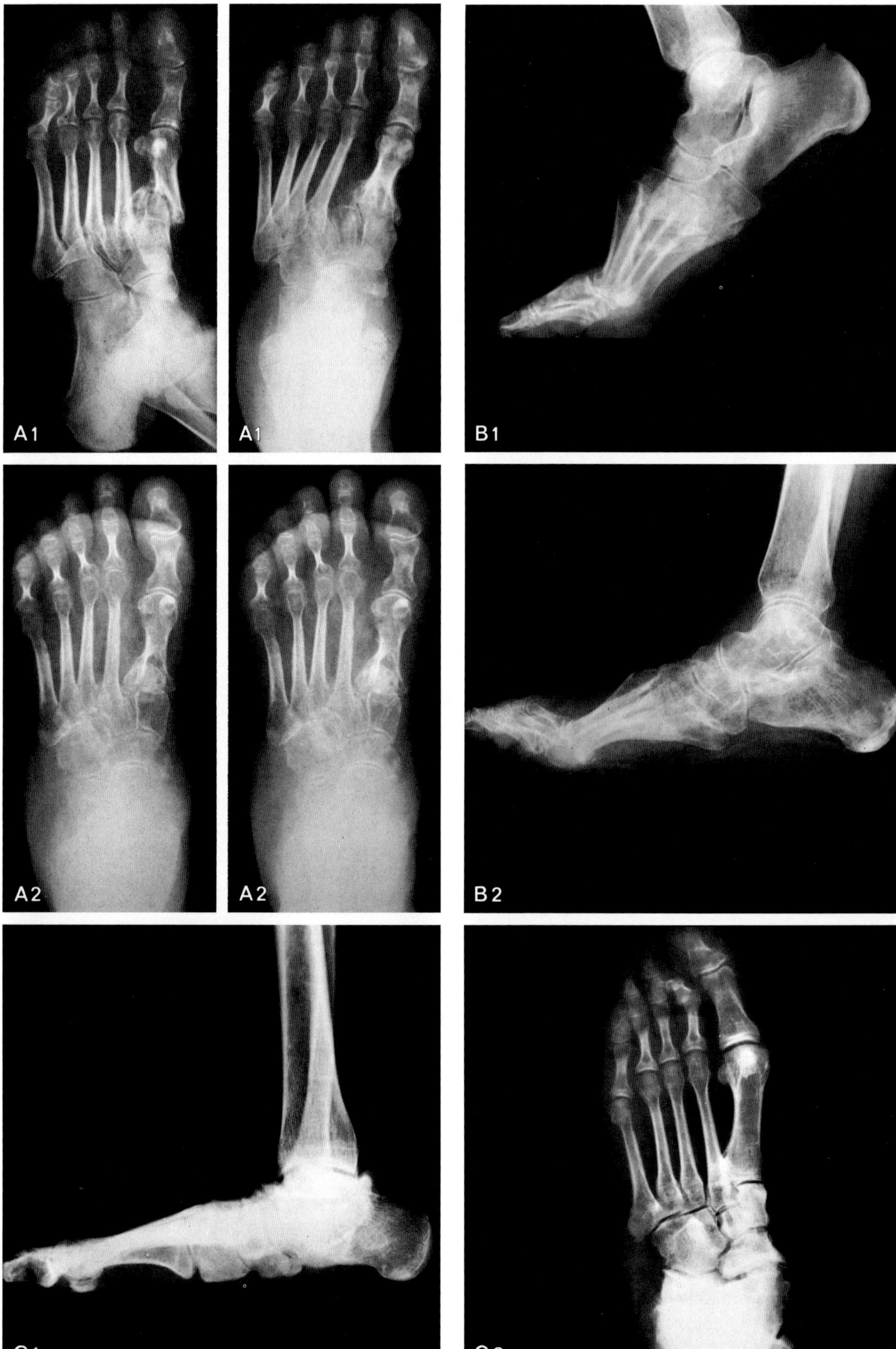
A1
A1
B1
A2
A2
B2
C1
C2

22.6 Tarsus

Etiology. Post-traumatic sequelae of tarsal injuries commonly relate to fractures of the calcaneum or talus and the development of subtalar arthrosis. Isolated or associated fractures of the calcaneum or talus may, despite apparent excellence of the initial reduction, be followed by the appearance of progressive pain and disability from arthrosis of the subtalar joint due to incongruity of the joint surfaces, varus or valgus posture of the calcaneum or sinking of the arch of the foot. Arthrosic lesions of the subtalar joint can occur after arthrodesis of the ankle joint. When the latter has been fixed in an excessively equinus position, the demands for compensation at the subtalar joint are too severe; the midtarsal joint cannot compensate for this posture, and it is the subtalar joint which suffers.

Clinical Features. The onset of pain progressively months or years after trauma or arthrodesis of the ankle joint is accompanied by diffuse swelling in the tarsal region. The pain is of a pricking or grinding character, sometimes with a sensation of pinching at the level of the subtalar joint. Intermittent to begin with, it becomes permanent, even at night, and is exacerbated by loading, walking on an irregular surface and climbing up and down stairs. It becomes resistant to conservative measures, including insoles.

Treatment. The only solution to the painful subtalar joint is arthrodesis. If it is only the subtalar joint which is to be fused, prerequisites are a normal axis of the foot with respect to the leg and the absence of other more anterior injury. The muscles of the foot must be balanced. At operation, valgus or varus must be corrected, although a light valgus posture of about 5°–7° is advantageous. It must be checked that the longitudinal axis of the foot is less than 10° equinus. Any involvement of the ankle joint or talonavicular joint indicates extending the arthrodesis to these parts.

◁ **Fig. 22.12 A C.** Post traumatic foot: fracture dislocation of Lisfranc joint line. **A** Fracture of base of first metatarsal, dorsolateral dislocation of outer four metatarsals, disruption of first intercapital space. *1* Preoperative; *2* after reduction of dislocation, re-establishment of alignment, arthrodesis of Lisfranc joint. **B** Post-traumatic pes planus, dorsal dislocation of bases of metatarsals. *1* Preoperative; *2* after reduction of metatarsal dislocations, re-establishment of alignment in sagittal plane, arthrodesis of Lisfranc joint line. **C** Post-traumatic flat foot: 70-year-old patient had fractured navicular and talus at age of 12 years

22.7 The Ankle

The ankle joint is unique in its role of transmission of forces from the leg to the foot in that it is the only joint involved and there is no neighbouring joint which can compensate if its range of movement is impaired.

22.7.1 Ligamentous Injuries

Early injuries have been dealt with in Chap. 21, while late complications may be associated with intracapsular or intraligamentous calcification. In general, these do not produce severe symptoms, and only exceptionally do they constitute an indication for surgery.

22.7.2 Dorsiflexion Injuries

O'Donoghue (1957) named the late sequela of these injuries "impinging exostosis". The condition appears very frequently in sportsmen after jumping or sliding with the foot in acute dorsiflexion, and the development of the exostoses lead to impingement and pain. They are clearly shown in the lateral radiograph as blunt or sometimes spiculate protuberances of bone on the margin of the joint anteriorly (Fig. 22.13). When symptoms are significant, surgical excision is curative.

22.7.3 Contracture of Ankle Joint Without Joint Surface Involvement

22.7.3.1 Etiology

Intrinsic Causes. Impaired range of movement may supervene after a prolonged period of immobilisation in a plaster cast (H. Judet 1976) or be associated with synostosis or fibrous contracture of the inferior tibiofibular joint as described by Lecoeur (1938, 1976). In the latter cases, I have noted persistent equinovarus displacement of the talus with antero-external subluxation. Because the antero-external portion of the articular surface of the talus is constantly unloaded, it tends to hypertrophy (law of Delpech), impeding re-entry of the front part of the talus into the tibia mortice and blocking the foot in equinovarus. An equivalent phenomenon is seen in the incompletely corrected equinovarus congenital club foot.

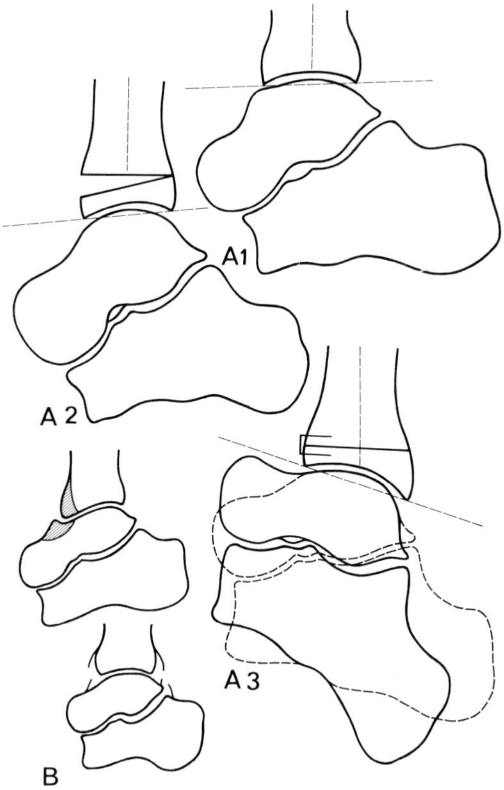

Fig. 22.13. **A** *1–3* Stages of tibial osteotomy for correction of ankle malposition (Judet). **B** Arthrolysis of ankle joint

Extrinsic Causes. These include joint stiffness from ligamentous fibrosis or tendinous adhesions posteriorly or laterally following long immobilisation (Judet 1978).

22.7.3.2 Clinical Features

A history of trauma is usual, and symptomatology comprises difficulty in standing and walking due to the stiffness at the outer aspect of the ankle joint and midtarsal joints which is caused by the varus attitude stemming from the ankle joint. The posture leads to the development of calluses under the metatarsal heads in an atrophic-looking cavus foot. It is often the calluses which lead the patient to consultation. Examination should include a search for evidence of peroneal and flexor tendon adhesions.
Radiography, including special tangential views, will confirm the intact state of the articular surfaces and the presence of any talar subluxation, usually into varus but occasionally into valgus. A synostosis of the inferior talofibular ligament may be evident (Lecoeur 1938); the antero-external hypertrophy of the talus can be identified.

22.7.3.3 Treatment

In conditions of persistent symptoms of stiffness, a restricted range of movement reflecting onto the rest of the foot, but intact articular surfaces, surgical treatment is indicated. This entails arthrolysis of the ankle joint, which must be directed to all aspects and include release of the inferior tibiofibular joint by resection of fibrous or osseous tissue (Lecoeur 1938). The antero-external hypertrophied part of the talus should be excised and the talus allowed to revert to its normal position within the ankle mortice (Regnauld and Saudreau 1978) (Fig. 22.14).
When necessary, elongation of triceps surae should be performed in conjunction with synovectomy of the adhering tendons of tibialis posterior, the long flexor tendons of the toes and, postero-externally, the peronei. Occasionally these tendons must be elongated. Operation must be succeeded by assiduous physiotherapy. If the orientation of the axis of the tibia is disturbed, H. Judet (1976) advises osteotomy of the cuneiform region resecting a wedge of bone with its base anteriorly, so establishing the horizontal alignment of the sagittal plane of the foot and effectively augmenting the amplitude of dorsiflexion of the ankle joint (Fig. 22.13).

22.7.4 Fractures of Malleoli

In the absence of arthrosis of the ankle joint, symptoms may be produced by shortening of the lateral malleolus, and the roof of the mortice can be lowered in some tibial fractures. Scholler (1976) has drawn attention to these two conditions, which provoke diminution of containment by the bimalleolar forceps and cartilaginous incongruity. Para-articular lesions develop, and yet the articular cartilage is preserved. Instability and stiffness predominate. The arthralgia indicates a need for surgical management by osteotomy and elongation of the shortened fibular malleolus, accompanied by arthrolysis of the ankle (Scholler 1976).
In the presence of traumatic osteoarthrosis, which is usually associated with distortion of the tibial articular surface, instability and deviation of the talus can occur into varus or valgus according to the site of the damaged surface. Blaimont et al. (1976) recommend arthrolysis, intra-articular osteotomy to align the malleoli correctly and filling of any de-

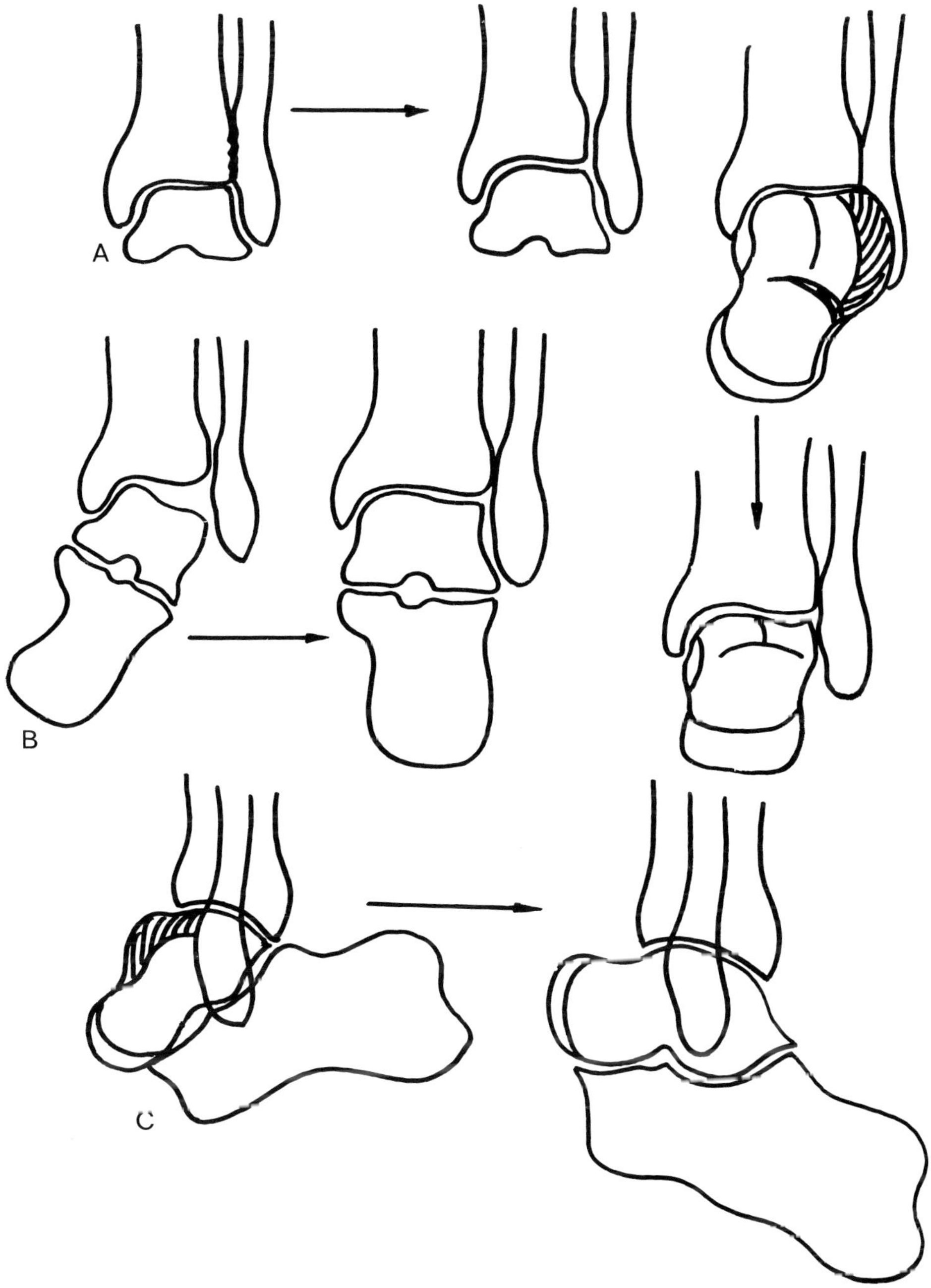

Fig. 22.14. A Release of inferior tibiofibular joint (Lecoeur). **B** Reduction of talar subluxation. **C** Remodelling of anterolateral hypertrophy of talus (Regnauld)

ficiencies by grafting, thereby restoring the mortice in all planes (Fig. 22.15).

Merle d'Aubigné and Judet have emphasised the potential success of osteotomy and arthrolysis of the ankle joint especially when there is no arthrosic lesion in the central part of the load-bearing roof of the mortice. Osteotomies of one or both malleolar fracture sites, if malunited, safely re-establish a normal configuration.

These reconstructive procedures are much more appropriate in the young subject in order to avoid the final solution of arthrodesis. If arthrodesis is thought necessary, however, its orientation is of great importance (Schnepp 1976).

1. In the sagittal plane, if the subtalar and midtarsal joints are ankylosed, the foot should be at 90° with respect to the leg, the procedure perhaps including arthrodesis of the subtalar and midtarsal joints. When the subtalar joint is stiff but the midtarsal joints remain supple, the foot should be in slight equinus but less than 10° plantarflexed. However, if both subtalar and midtarsal joints are mobile, 5°–10° equinus in the male and 10° in the female are permissible.
2. In the transverse plane, arthrodesis should be fashioned to allow a light valgus of 5°–8°, never exceeding 10°; this posture is more appropriate for the tarsal mechanism than a vertical heel. Varus should never be permitted.
3. The end result should be transverse horizontal alignment of the five metatarsal heads rigorously at 90° to the long axis of the tibia.

There are many techniques of arthrodesis of the ankle designed to achieve the same end, but the surgeon should choose one procedure and remain with it.

With reference to arthroplasty of the ankle, ankle replacement prostheses still yield very uncertain results and cannot be recommended.

22.7.5 Avascular Necrosis of Talus and Osteochondritis Dissecans

Ischaemic necrosis localised to the talar articular surface in the ankle can occur without apparent cause or can follow trauma, most usually a sprain. It may be located in any of several places, notably on the supero-internal border or externally. Alternatively, the subtalar joint can be involved, or occasionally the head of the talus (Cayla 1972; Denis 1968).

Whichever joint is involved, symptomatology is clear cut. There is chronic tarsalgia, subsequent perhaps to injury and noticed mostly on prolonged walking on irregular surfaces. It amounts to subacute arthritis with pain at the level of the joint involved, perhaps localised to the outer orifice of the sinus tarsi, perhaps radiating diffusely throughout the tarsus. Usually there is localised swelling of the peri-articular tissues and limitation of joint movement, occasionally acute, if a loose body separates.

Radiography shows the site of the lesion, which begins with a small eggshell-like depression at the superior corner of the talar surface (Denis 1968) associated with local rarefaction of bone texture. Later, a cup-shaped zone of sinking is associated with a geode of bony condensation, in the interior of which is a small sequestrum with regular, clearly delineated contours. Finally, the zone of necrosis becomes more extensive, with collapse of the surface and obvious signs of arthrosis.

Treatment: Conservative management has little to offer, and only excision of the sequestrum gives any possibility of improvement. Subsequent extensive arthrosis will necessitate arthrodesis of the joint affected.

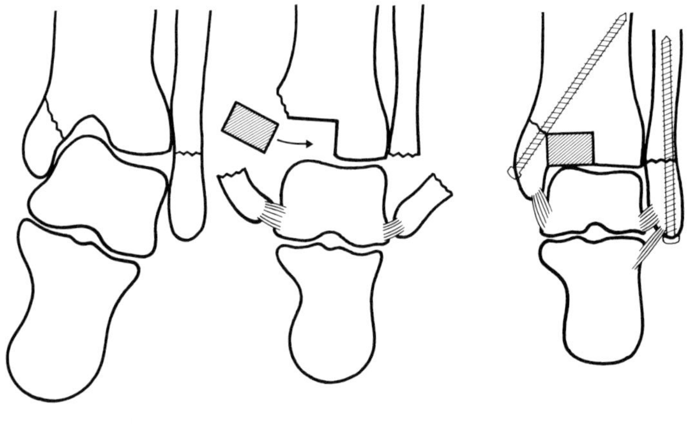

Fig. 22.15. Arthrolysis and osteotomy for realignment of the ankle after grafting of joint surface (Blaimont)

23 Hallux Rigidus

23.1 Description

Hallux rigidus should be regarded as comprising two arthrosic components, one affecting the metatarsophalangeal joint of the great toe, the other the associated metatarsosesamoidal joints. Osteophyte formation and progressive ankylosis involve both sites. The whole foot becomes affected, including integument, muscles and ligaments. The skin loses its normal suppleness and thickness, and there is a reduced amount of local subcutaneous fat. The atrophic capsule becomes greyish in colour and rigid, and is closely moulded to the underlying distorted bone configuration. The capsule rarely hypertrophies, but occasionally some thickened fibres with yellowish concretions are formed within it. Marked atrophy of abductor hallucis and flexor hallucis longus is seen.

The articular cartilage loses its brilliant pearly appearance becoming flattened, eroded and destroyed in plaque-like areas as if struck by a hammer. Osteophytosis around the margins of the joints is irregular, and the osteophytes which form adhere to and distend the capsule.

Leroux (Regnauld and Leroux 1965) has stressed the comprehensive involvement of the joint components and associated tissues.

23.1.1 *Bone*

Osteoporosis is a dominant early feature; diffuse rarefaction of the trabeculae predisposes them to microfractures. The associated medullary spaces are enlarged relatively, and the marrow becomes atrophied, sometimes fatty or fibroblastic. Osteoporosis can have any of a number of causes, and may be aggravated by immobilisation, ischaemia, or pain. Within the substance of the bone, eyelets of repair are apparent. This process may be linear, associated with fibrosis of the medullary spaces with thickening of several local bony trabeculae, on which cement lines with osteoid seams bordered by fusiform osteoblasts are visible. Sometimes, a nodular configuration along the lines of enchondral ossification indicates bony repair associated with the cartilage lesions. Lines of concentric cementation with the inclusion of multiple osteophytes occur in the newly formed nodules of bone.

23.1.2 *Cartilage*

Probably a result of microtrauma, the development of lesions of the articular cartilage associated with osteoporotic deformity of the underlying bone is a determining element of hallux rigidus. Erosion of the surface is associated with areas of enchondral ossification which further distort and disrupt the overlying cartilage. Elsewhere, there is a disturbance of the normal histology in which the groups of cells lose their axial or spheroidal disposition and disperse generally into the chondroid substance, becoming heterogeneous with variable staining properties. Fibres of Sharpey are found in these altered zones.

23.1.3 *Periosteum*

Dystrophic lesions in the form of multiple osteophytic formations are numerous where the cambium has a cartilaginous appearance. The nuclei of the cells are pyknotic. In the sesamoids, there are similar osteophytic lesions associated with osteoporosis and cartilaginous erosion.

23.1.4 *Capsule*

The dystrophic and inflammatory process leads to increased vascularity throughout the dense fibrous tissue and to fibroblastic proliferation. The fibroblasts are compressed by the general oedema of the area, and this causes them to develop wing-like prolongations. The adjoining capsular tissue contains inflammatory granulocytes. The local lesions resembling gouty tophi which occasionally appear are due to central calcific degeneration surrounded by areas of macrophages and giant cell reaction (Regnauld and Leroux 1965).

23.2 Etiology

As stated above, hallux rigidus may originate in osteoporosis supervening after immobilisation for any reason.

A traumatic basis is likely. The primary damage can be elsewhere, perhaps even in the ankle joint, or associated with some sort of direct toe trauma with subluxation or dislocation. In the same way that a fracture of the lower limb with plaster cast immobilisation can lead to an acquired cavus foot, it can also produce hallux rigidus secondary to post-traumatic algodystrophy of Sudeck.

Microtrauma may be due to ill-fitting shoes, most frequently in the Egyptian or square toe configuration. Lelièvre (1967) observed that in 90% of cases of hallux rigidus there was significant lengthening of the first ray with respect to the neighbouring second ray and parallel alignment of the two first metatarsals. Often, there is an absence of transverse mobility of the first metatarsal, and the shock of loading on the end of the toe is transmitted directly to the metatarsophalangeal joint, which becomes a little deviated; when lateral mobility is impaired, the joint is subjected to repeated higher loading and cartilaginous degeneration follows. Disturbance of the longitudinal axis of the foot may result in overloading of the first metatarsophalangeal joint, particularly affecting the sesamoids, which are subjected to repeated trauma. The cavus forefoot and the natural valgus foot, seen frequently in the adolescent, may lead secondarily to adult hallux rigidus. The overloading of the inner ray of the foot affects predominantly the metatarsosesamoidal articulation.

Sometimes there is generalised arthrosis affecting the tarsometatarsal, intertarsal and subtalar joints, as well as several of the metatarsophalangeal joints. Hallux rigidus appears in these instances as part of a generalised disorder. It may also be consecutive to rheumatoid inflammation, gout, ankylosing spondylitis (this often provokes hallux rigidus with flexion contracture), psoriatic arthropathy, acute septic arthritis or gonococcal arthritis.

Apart from these specific causes, I am of the opinion that flattening or cavus deformities of the longitudinal arch lead to abnormal axial compression of the articular cartilage of the great metatarsophalangeal joint especially when accompanied by absence of lateral play (or less significantly, vertical play), of the first metatarsal, which then does not function properly as a shock absorber during walking. In support of this opinion is the development of hallux rigidus after overtight reduction of a varus first metatarsal in hallux valgus (cf. Chap. 18) in which the movements of the first metatarsal are suppressed. This typically happens in McBride's procedure and Petersen's operation.

23.3 Clinical Features

Hallux rigidus rarely presents during adolescence, but usually in adulthood between the ages of 30 and 50 years. There are three stages of development (Figs. 23.1–23.3).

23.3.1 First Degree

This is the period of development of arthrosis, characterised by acute or subacute pain during the phase of rolling onto the forefoot in walking. There is painful limitation of amplitude of movement, normally 40° of dorsiflexion and 20° of plantarflexion.

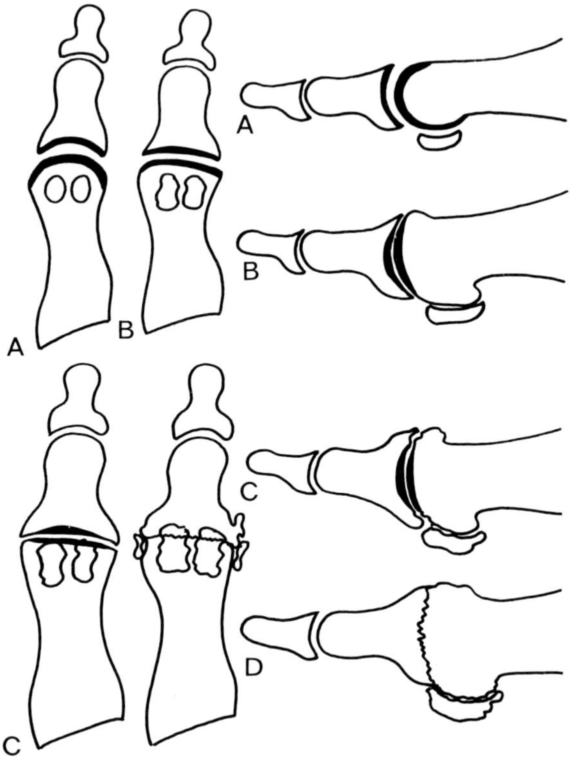

Fig. 23.1 A–D. Hallux rigidus. **A** Normal articulation. **B** First degree. **C** Second degree. **D** Third degree

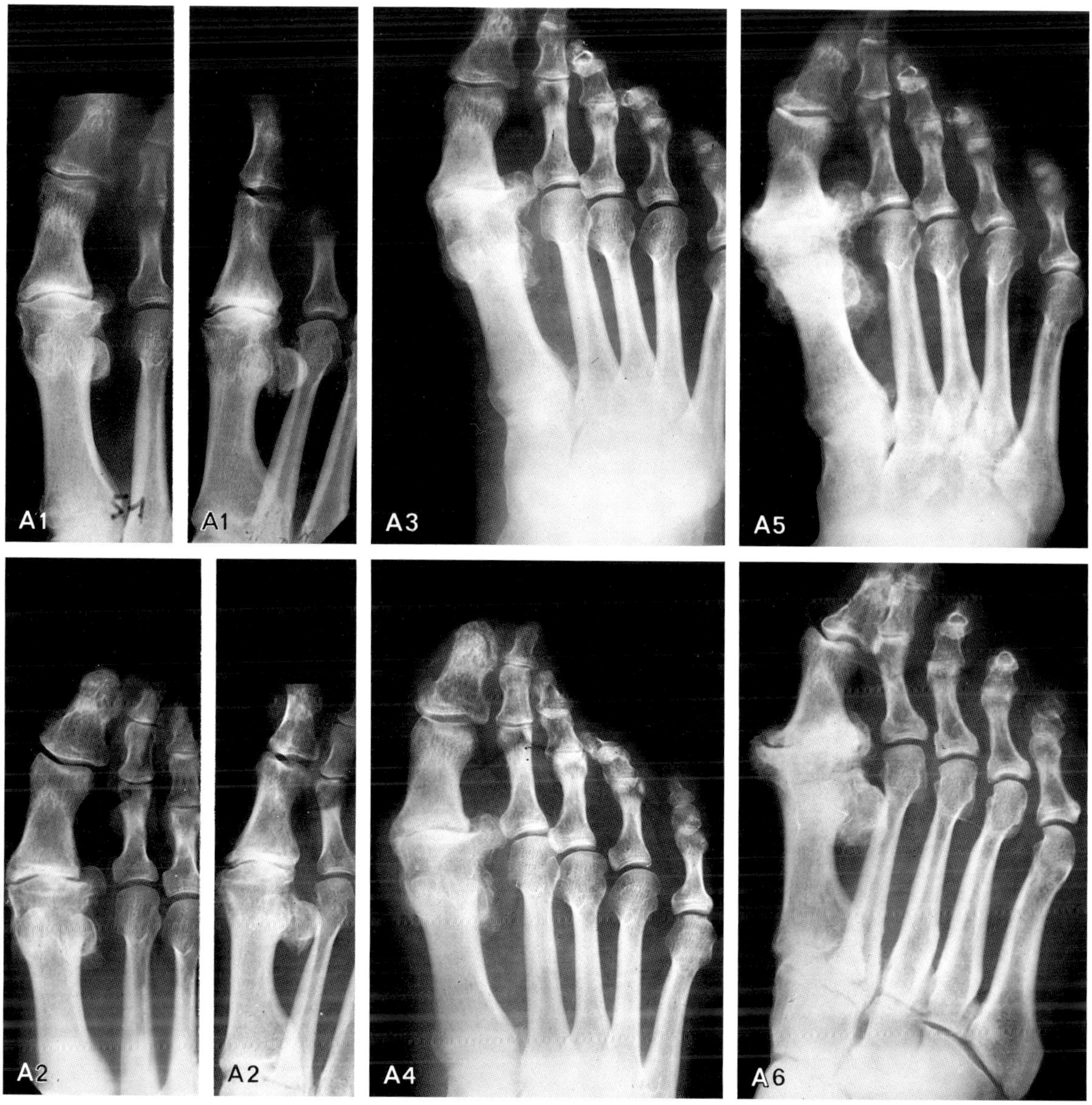

Fig. 23.2 A–N. First- to third-degree hallux rigidus. **A** Development of hallux rigidus between 1951 and 1970. *1, 2* First degree (1951–1952): flattening of articular surfaces, broadening and thinning of joint space, peripheral osteophytosis, preservation of central articular cartilage, limited range of motion; *3, 4* second degree (1953–1954): similar radiological characteristics but with addition of disappearance of central articular cartilage, proliferation and enlargement of peripheral osteophytes, ankylosis; *5, 6* third degree (1970): almost complete disappearance of joint space, ankylosis involving metatarsophalangeal, metatarsosesamoid and sesamoidophalangeal components, significant hypertrophy of joint generally, irregular hypertrophic osteophytosis and peripheral condensation. **B–N** see pp. 338–341

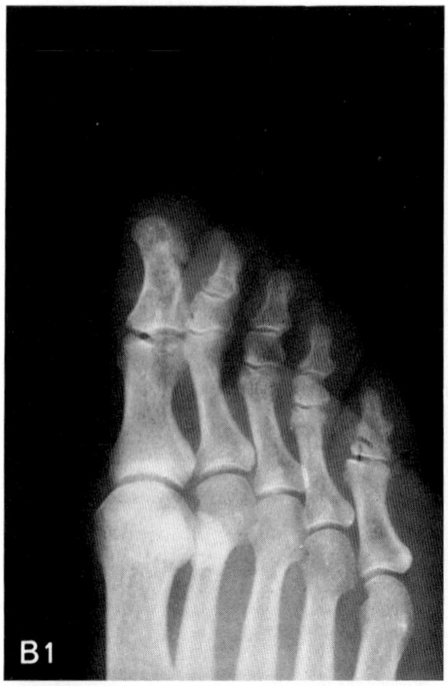

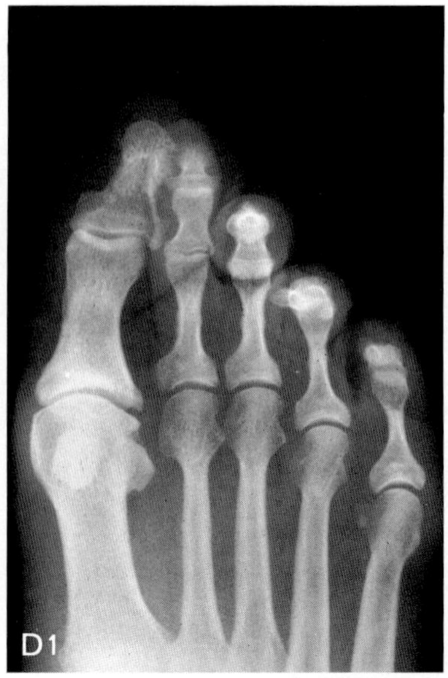

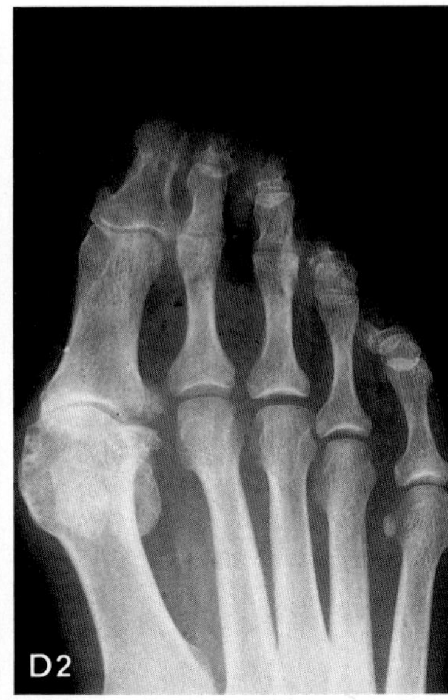

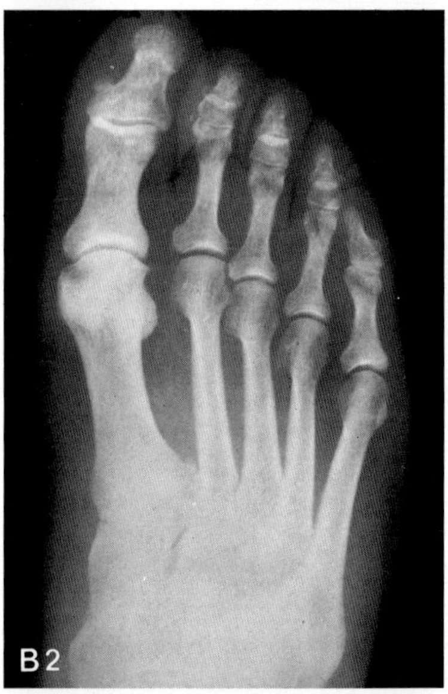

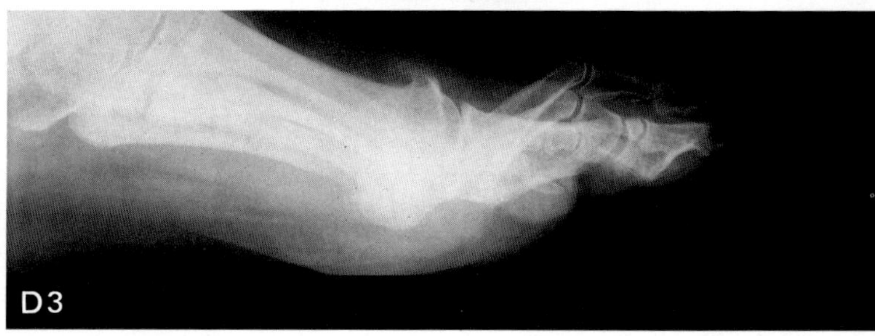

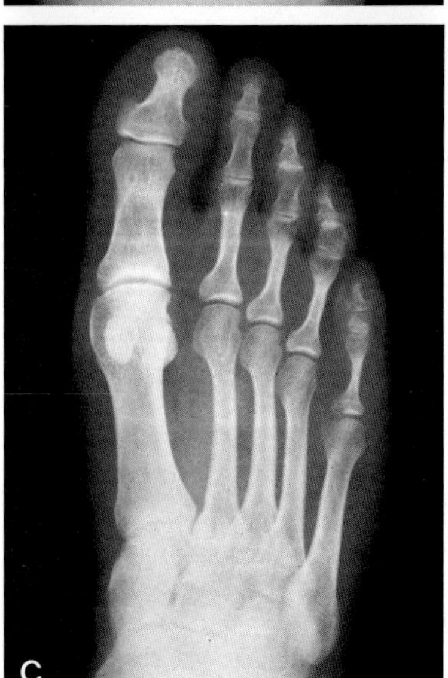

Fig. 23.2 *(continued)*. **B–D** First-degree hallux rigidus with progressive ▷ diminution in range of motion. **B** Early stage: preservation of curved joint outline, presence of first metatarsal head. **C** Early stage: preservation of concavity of phalangeal articular surface, flattening and enlargement of articular surface of metatarsal, commencement of lateral eburnation involving metatarsophalangeal joint. **D** *1–3* Irregularity and thinning of joint space, widening and peripheral eburnation of articular surfaces, moderate hypertrophy and fragmentation of lateral osteophytes, hypertrophy and irregularity of sesamoids, dorsolateral exostosis of head of metatarsal (different patients). **E–G** Second degree. **E** Loss of articular curvatures with flattening and irregular thinning of joint space, peripheral osteophytosis, especially medial, lateral and dorsal, irregular hypertrophy of sesamoids, partial or complete loss of range of motion, compensatory dorsification of distal phalanx. **F** Hallux rigidus flexus, otherwise same characteristics as above. **G** *1, 2* Second-degree hallux rigidus, first-degree rigidus in second ray; *3* after metatarsophalangeal arthroplasty with interposition cup prosthesis for first and second metatarsophalangeal joints; *4, 5* a year after operation

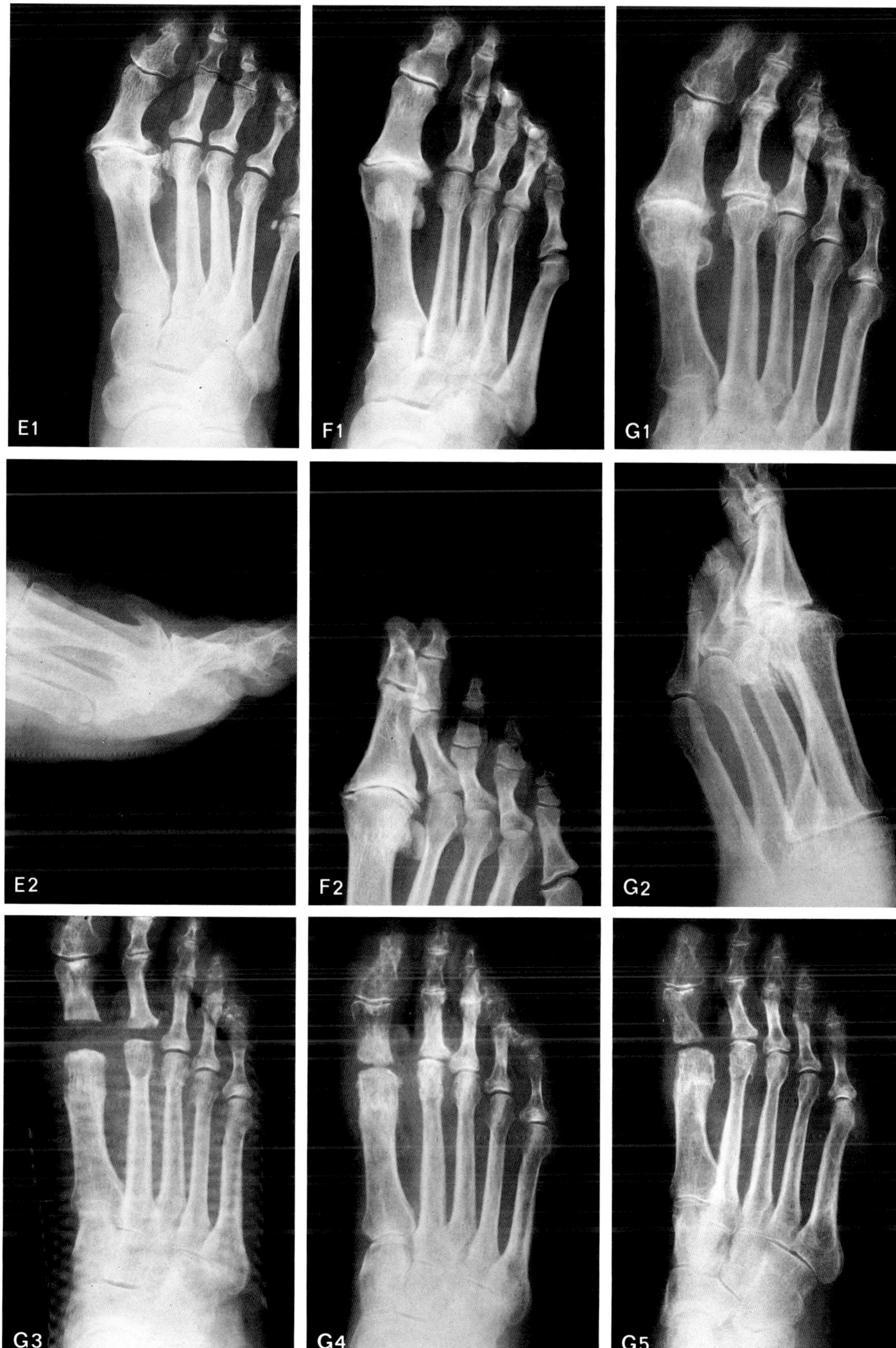
E1
F1
G1
E2
F2
G2
G3
G4
G5

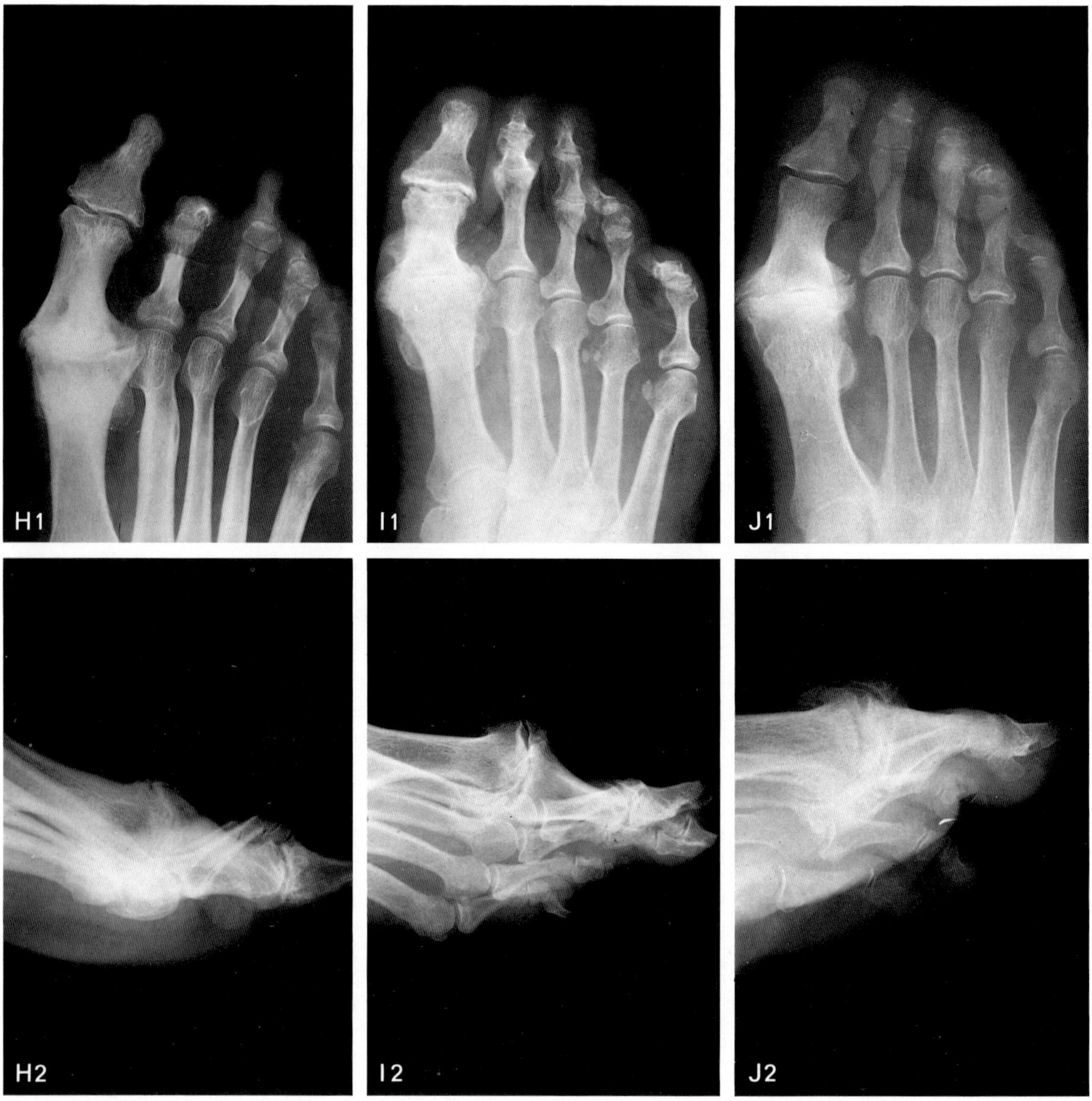

Fig. 23.2 *(continued)*. **H–M** Third degree: complete ankylosis of metatarsosesamoidophalangeal components, irregular hypertrophy of joint, massive irregular osteophytosis ▷

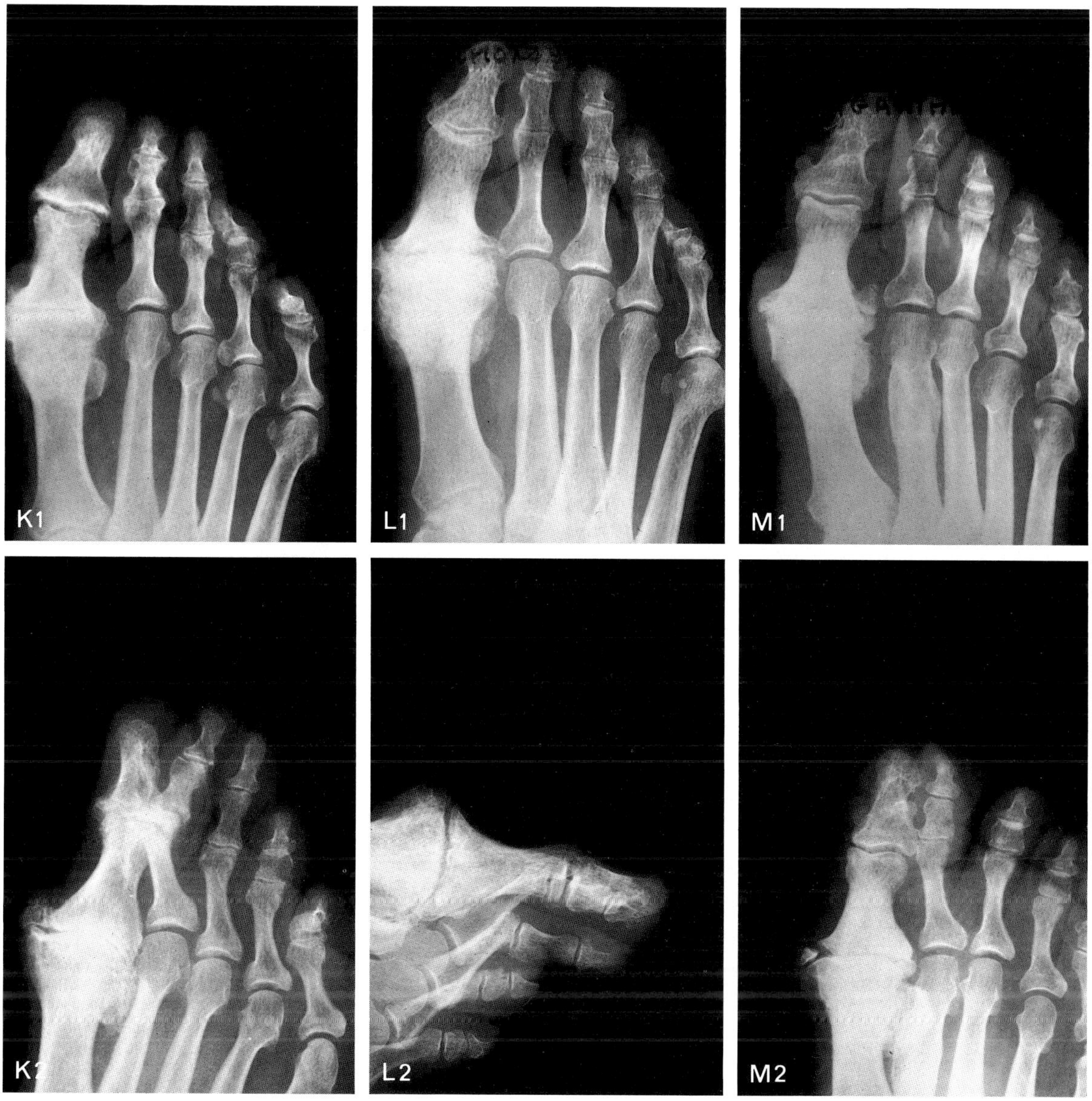

Fig. 23.2 K–M. Legend see p. 340

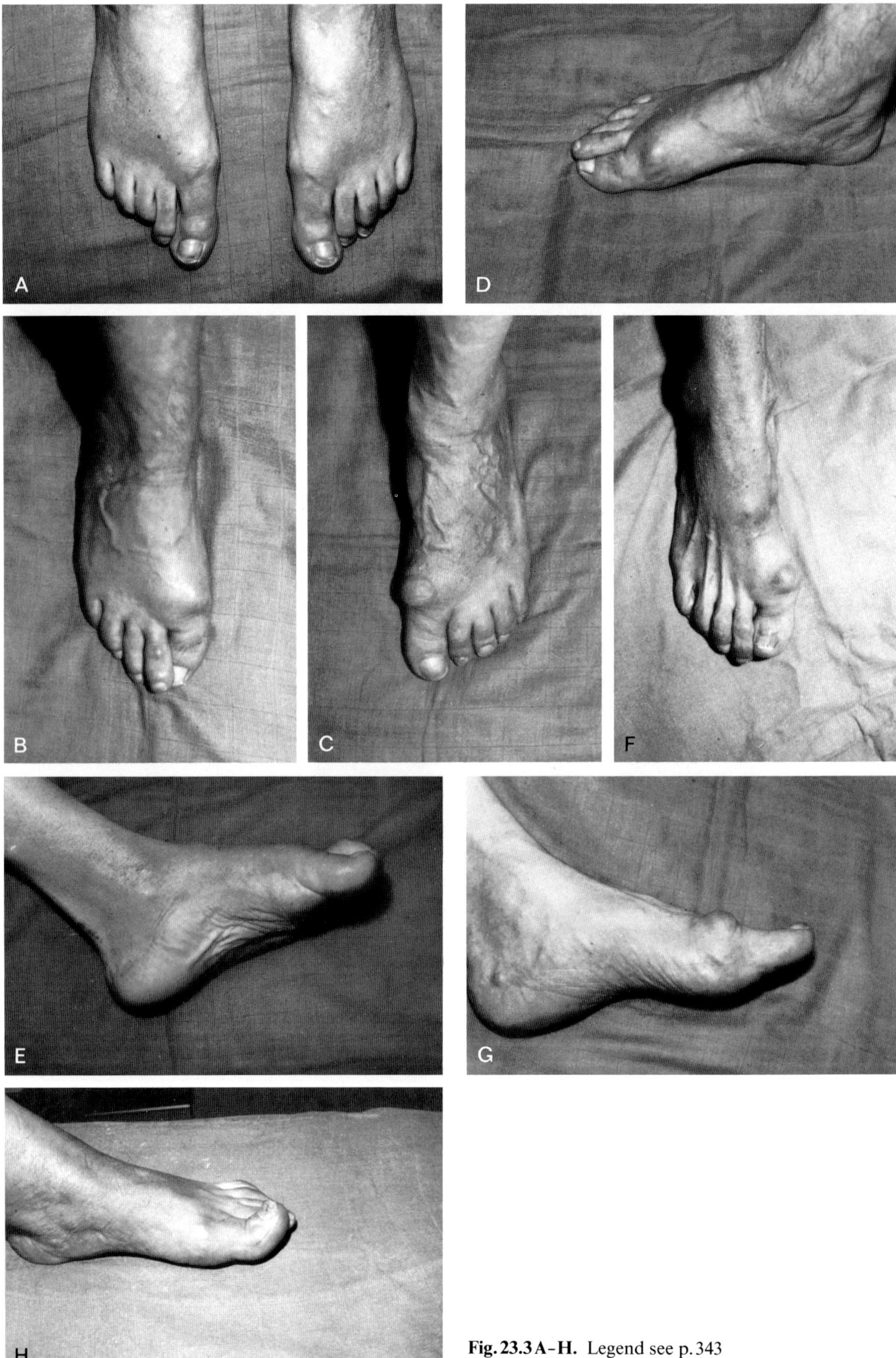

Fig. 23.3 A–H. Legend see p. 343

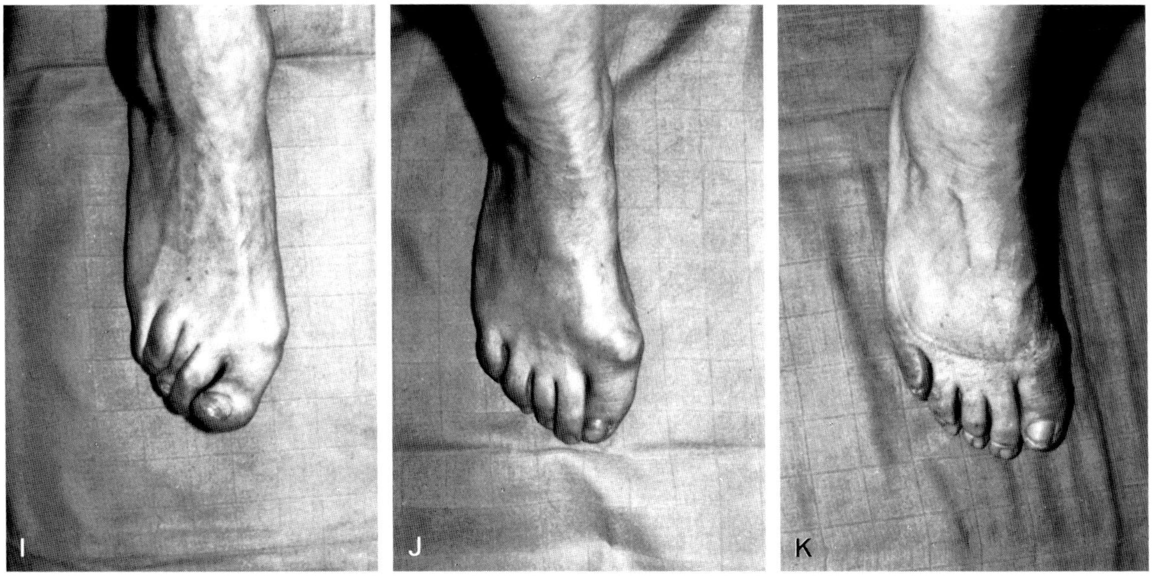

◁ **Fig. 23.3 A–K.** Hallux rigidus. **A** First degree. **B, D, E** With flexus. **E, F, G** Third degree with dorsal exostosis. **H, I** With compensatory dorsiflexion of distal phalanx. **J** With valgus. **K** Correction of hallux rigidus with valgus by arthroplasty and interposition of cup endoprosthesis

The joint is generally somewhat enlarged, and *radiographic examination* displays condensation of bone around the periphery, slight narrowing of the joint space and diminution in the convexity of the metatarsal head mirrored by the opposing phalanx. The sesamoids are regular but slightly enlarged compared with normal. Sometimes there is generalised rarefaction of bone texture throughout the forefoot.

23.3.2 *Second Degree*

The phase of established arthrosis is characterised by variable intermittent pain, tingling at rest, more severe during movement of the part and always during walking when the toe is dorsiflexed. There is limitation of movement to about three-quarters of the normal range and general loss of suppleness of the tissues. A thickening on the weight-bearing plantar surface of the joint is due to a hygroma.

Metatarsalgia develops, associated with the other joints, and postural arthralgia of the tarsometatarsal and intertarsal joints is due to the general distortion imposed during walking as a result of pain at the primary lesion. General hypertrophy of the margins of the joint occurs, producing the prominent border protruding under the skin dorsally.

Radiography shows general narrowing of the joint space with peripheral condensation and an irregular flattened configuration of the joint shape. Hypertrophy of the subarticular bone with eburnation is present, and there is irregular hypertrophy of the sesamoids.

23.3.3 *Third Degree*

This is the phase of ankylosis, in which very little movement is present. As a result, the joint itself is not painful, but discomfort may result from shoe pressure on the margins of articular hypertrophy, inflammation or ulceration of the hygroma on the dorsal face of the first metatarsal, postural pains affecting other joints or neuralgia from compression in the first interspace by osteophytes or articular hypertrophy. The margins are irregular, bristling with bony bosses, and the overlying skin becomes thin and cyanotic. Contracture of flexor hallucis longus and associated soft tissues produces pressure under the interphalangeal joint of the great toe, leading to callus formation. The foot develops a general varus posture.

Radiography shows complete disappearance of the joint space with hypertrophy of bony elements – metatarsal, phalanx and sesamoids. In particular, osteophytes from the sesamoid may bridge the undersurface, reaching the base of the phalanx and enhancing the rigidity.

23.4 Treatment

The aims of treatment are (a) to reduce articular compression by shortening the proximal phalanx, more significantly than necessary for the treatment of hallux valgus (see Chap. 18), (b) to release the cuneiform metatarsal joint in order to allow greater mobility of the metatarsal, and (c) to re-establish normal articular amplitude of movement.

23.4.1 Conservative

In general, conservative treatment will not stop the progress of the condition, but it does have a place in the early treatment of infected hygroma, following which operation should be delayed for at least 3 months. If there is any contra-indication to operative treatment, an insole comprising a pad raising the great metatarsal head may give some symptomatic relief, as the elevation of the head relieves the great toe from dorsiflexion loading during the toe-off phase in walking. The use of a pronating wedge to the outer border of the foot in an effort to reduce wear of the shoe here seems illogical, for by correcting the supinated posture of the forefoot it increases loading on the great toe, accelerates the inflammatory development of the condition and may enhance callus formation on the plantar aspect.

23.4.2 Operative

Minor surgery - removal of a protruding osteophyte from the dorsum of the foot - is occasionally a useful palliative procedure in the elderly.
Operations which should be *avoided* are excision of the proximal phalanx of the toe and resection of the great metatarsal head, which will produce insufficiency of loading of the first ray. Arthrodesis of the metatarsophalangeal joint is a poor operation.
The choice of operation depends on the degree of hallux rigidus (Fig. 23.4).

First Degree (Fig. 23.5 A-D). Revitalisation of an osteocartilaginous graft after transplantation works in hallux valgus and also in first-degree hallux rigidus provided there are still islands of healthy cartilage. There is usually a zone of cartilage in the centre of the joint which remains relatively healthy compared with the peripheral degenerate part. It is a valuable osteocartilaginous element, and after appropriate shaping and reimplantation will reconstitute the joint morphologi-

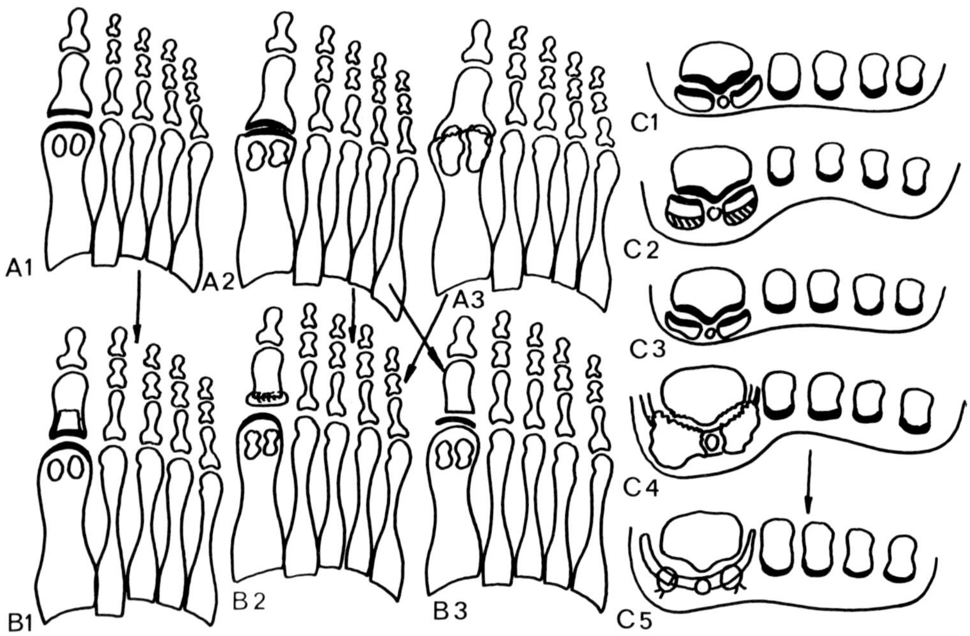

Fig. 23.4 A-C. Operative techniques for hallux rigidus. **A** Stages: *1* First degree; *2* second degree; *3* third degree. **B** Treatment: *1* Arthroplasty using cork-shaped graft (Regnauld); *2* cutaneous arthroplasty (de Wulf); *3* cup arthroplasty (Regnauld). **C** Sesamoids: *1* Normal; *2* hypertrophic; *3* partially excised; *4* arthrosic hypertrophy of sesamoids in forefoot cavus; *5* excision of sesamoids and essential reconstitution of plantar capsule

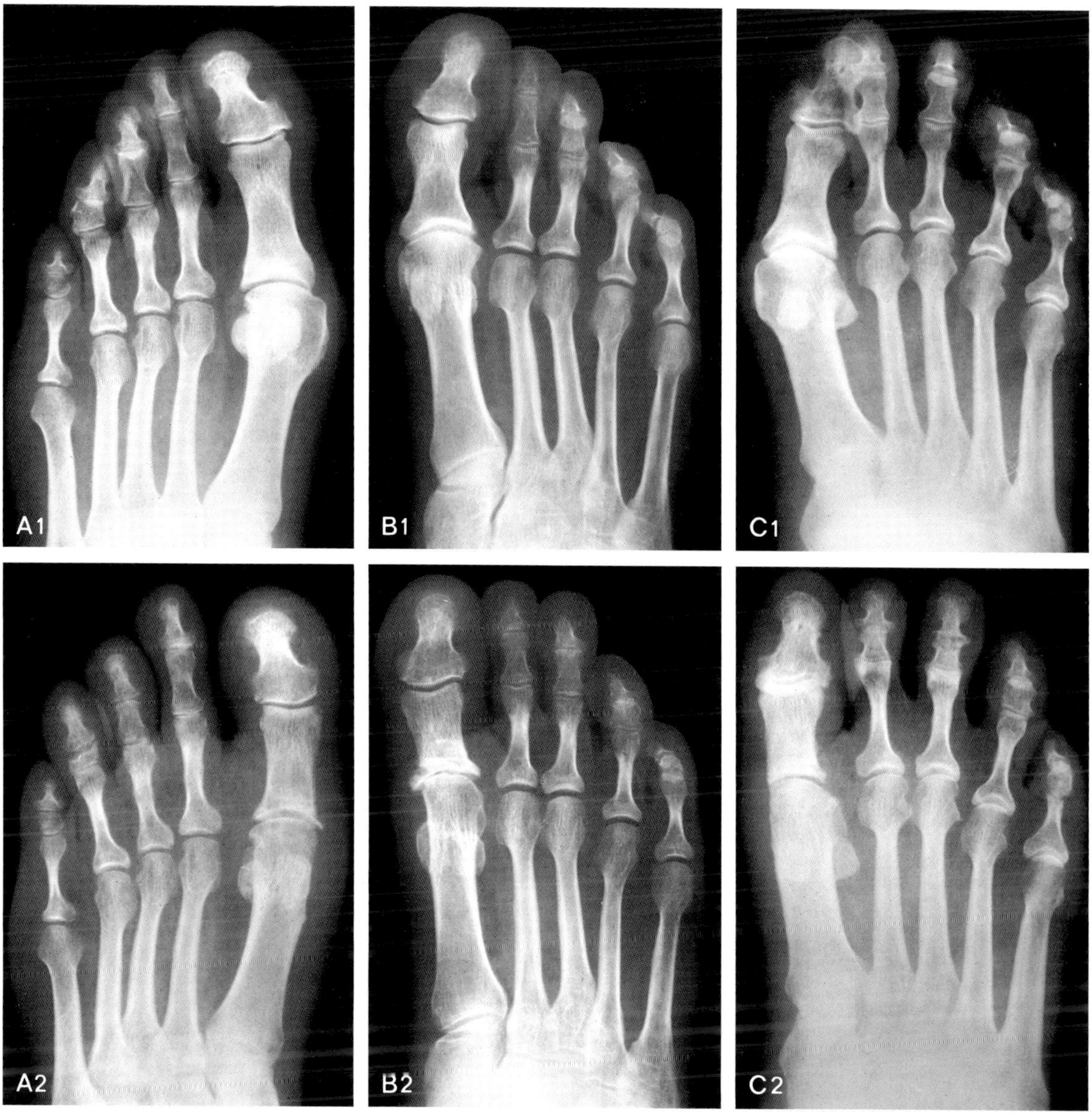

Fig. 23.5 A–G. First- and second-degree hallux rigidus: treatment by metatarsophalangeal arthroplasty. **A–E** First degree, arthroplasty with hat-shaped graft: *1* Preoperative; *2* postoperative. **A, C** With valgus. **B, E** Rigidus alone. **D–G** see pp. 346, 347

cally and functionally. Thus, first-degree hallux rigidus should be operated upon as early as possible, the procedure being similar to that used in hallux valgus, with the exception that tightening of the capsular ligament must be avoided so as to permit restoration of a physiological range of transverse motion.

Operative Technique. During operation great care should be taken not to traumatise the thin skin, which is frequently atrophied and poorly vascularised. A medial longitudinal incision exposes the joint, and the capsule is detached from the base of the phalanx and the head of the metatarsal as far as the lateral aspect of the joint, where it is preserved. The adductor insertion into the base of the proximal phalanx is divided. The base of the proximal phalanx is divided exactly perpendicular to its long axis at a site carefully calculated to avoid too much shortening of the great toe, which would lead to insufficiency of loading. The metatarsal head is trimmed by resection of protruding osteophytes, especially where these intrude into the margins of the articular area. The head must present a

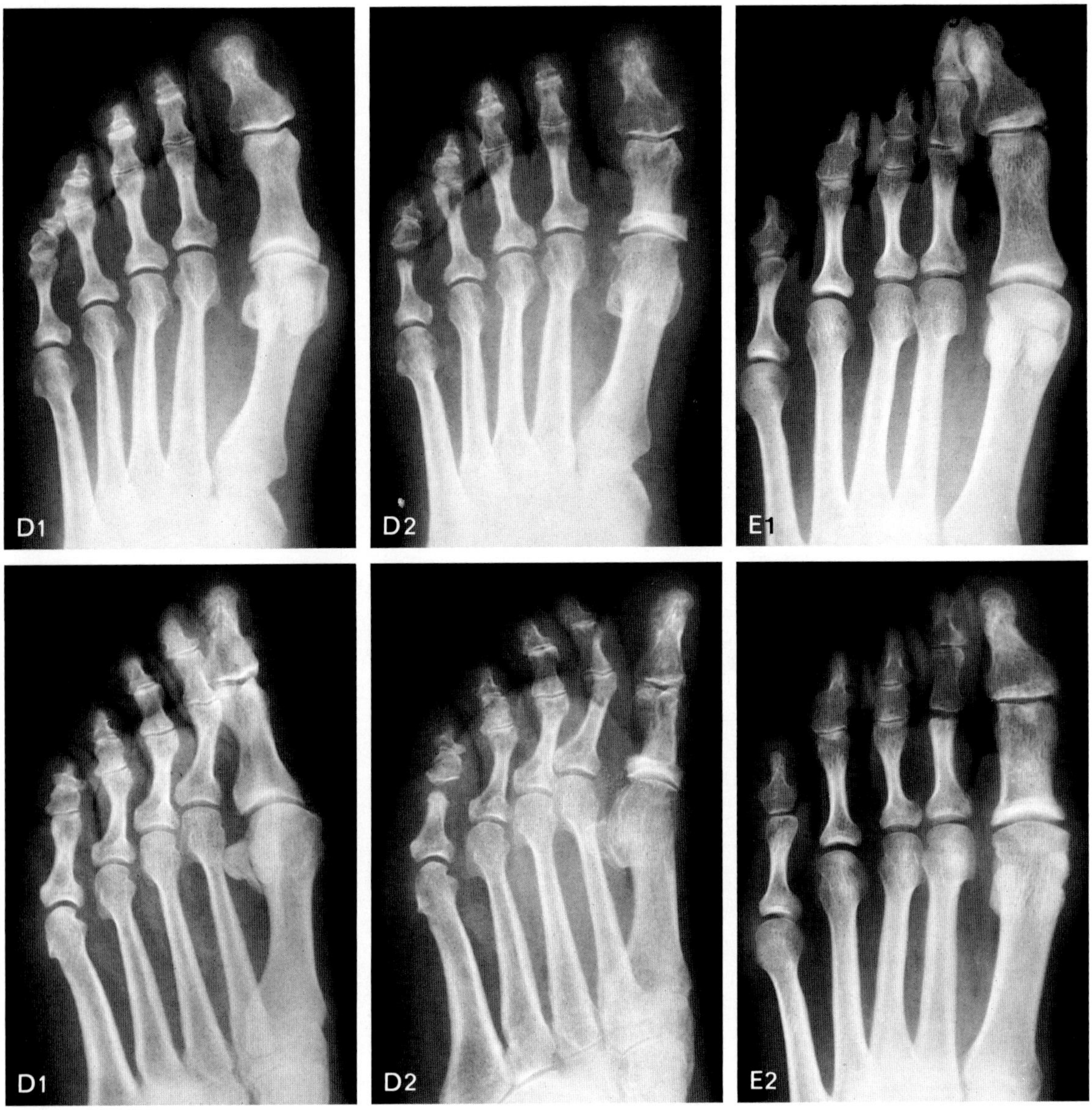

Fig. 23.5 *(continued)*. **D** with flexus. **F, G** Second degree, arthroplasty with interposition of high-density polyethylene ▷ cup prosthesis: *1* Preoperative; *2, 3* postoperative

rounded shape. If cavus forefoot is present, the plantar projection of the hypertrophied sesamoids augments the transverse concavity of the forefoot. Removal of the sesamoids releases the ankylosis of the metatarsosesamoid component and restores the transverse alignment of the forefoot. Removal does not result in insufficiency of flexion, but must be completed by careful closure of the plantar capsule, the scar forming a pad of fibrous tissue which replaces the sesamoids. If the transverse configuration of the metatarsal heads is level or convex, excision of the sesamoids is contra-indicated, because it will produce an insufficiency of the first ray. If the articular surface of the heads is intact, postoperative ankylosis is unlikely, but when involved by the arthrosic process the surface can be nibbled flat, so that with appropriate re-educative measures, a new fibrocartilage layer will form and motion will be preserved. If the heads are hypertrophied, the projecting plantar surface can be trimmed as necessary. The reimplanted osteocartilaginous graft must be of the cork-shaped configuration, the often-present arthrosic osteophytes precluding the hat-shaped variety (see Chap. 18).

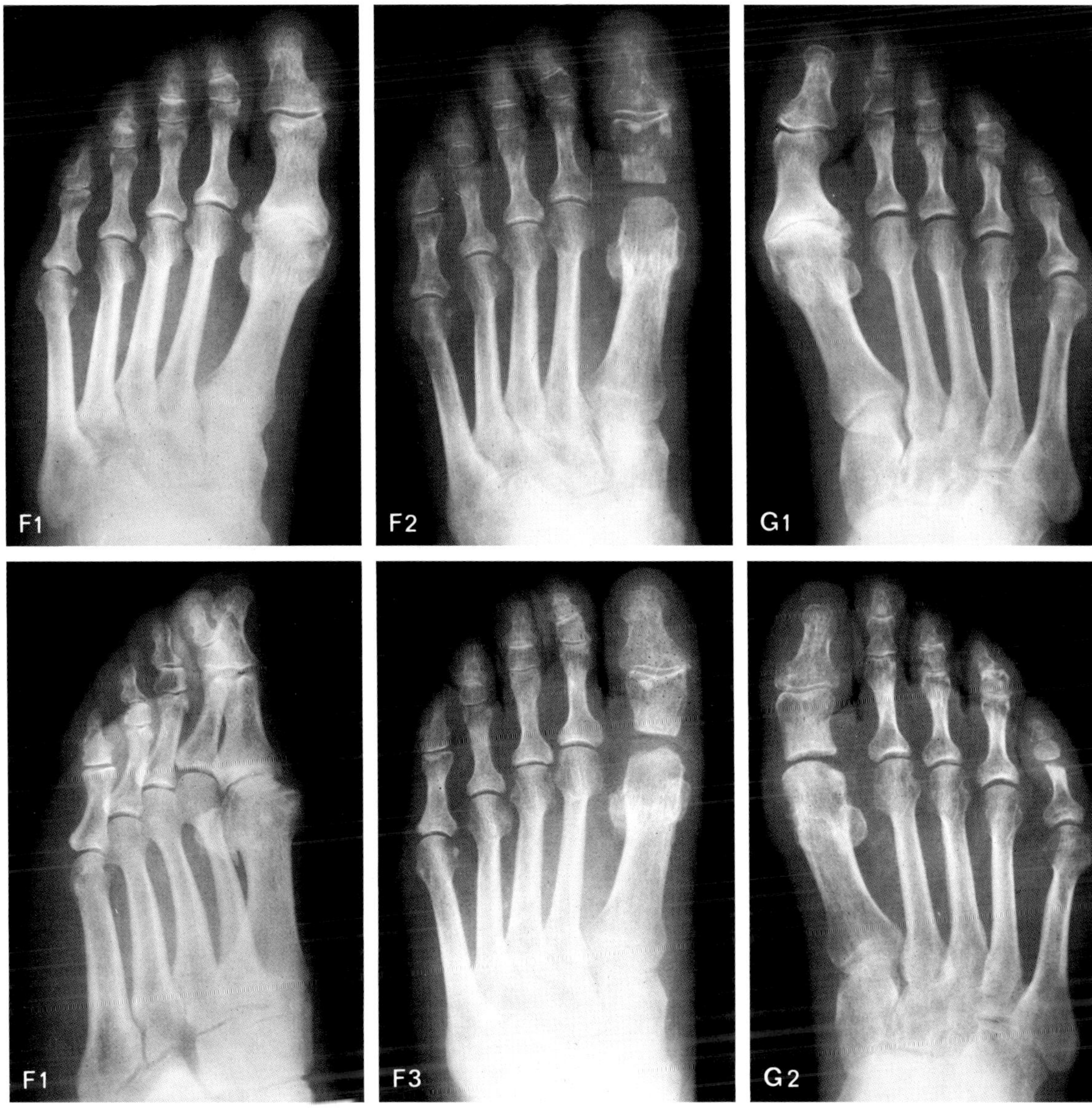

Fig. 23.5 F–G. Legend see p. 346

Capsular repair should be by meticulous edge-to-edge suturing ensuring adequate transverse play of the toe. Postoperatively, the toe should be immobilised and the legs kept strictly elevated for 3 weeks; this favours healing and avoids swelling. Early active exercises are then encouraged, including the normal rolling action of the forefoot on the ground. Passive mobilisation should be avoided rigorously. The patient should be warned that marked stiffness is likely during the first month.

Second and Third Degree (Fig. 23.5 F, G, 23.6). The dystrophic lesions of the articular cartilage in second-degree hallux rigidus are irreversible, and in third-degree cases the complete ankylosis with total loss of articular cartilage necessitates cup prosthesis arthroplasty (Regnauld and Grassin 1975) or implantation of a skin graft as described by de Wulf (1978).

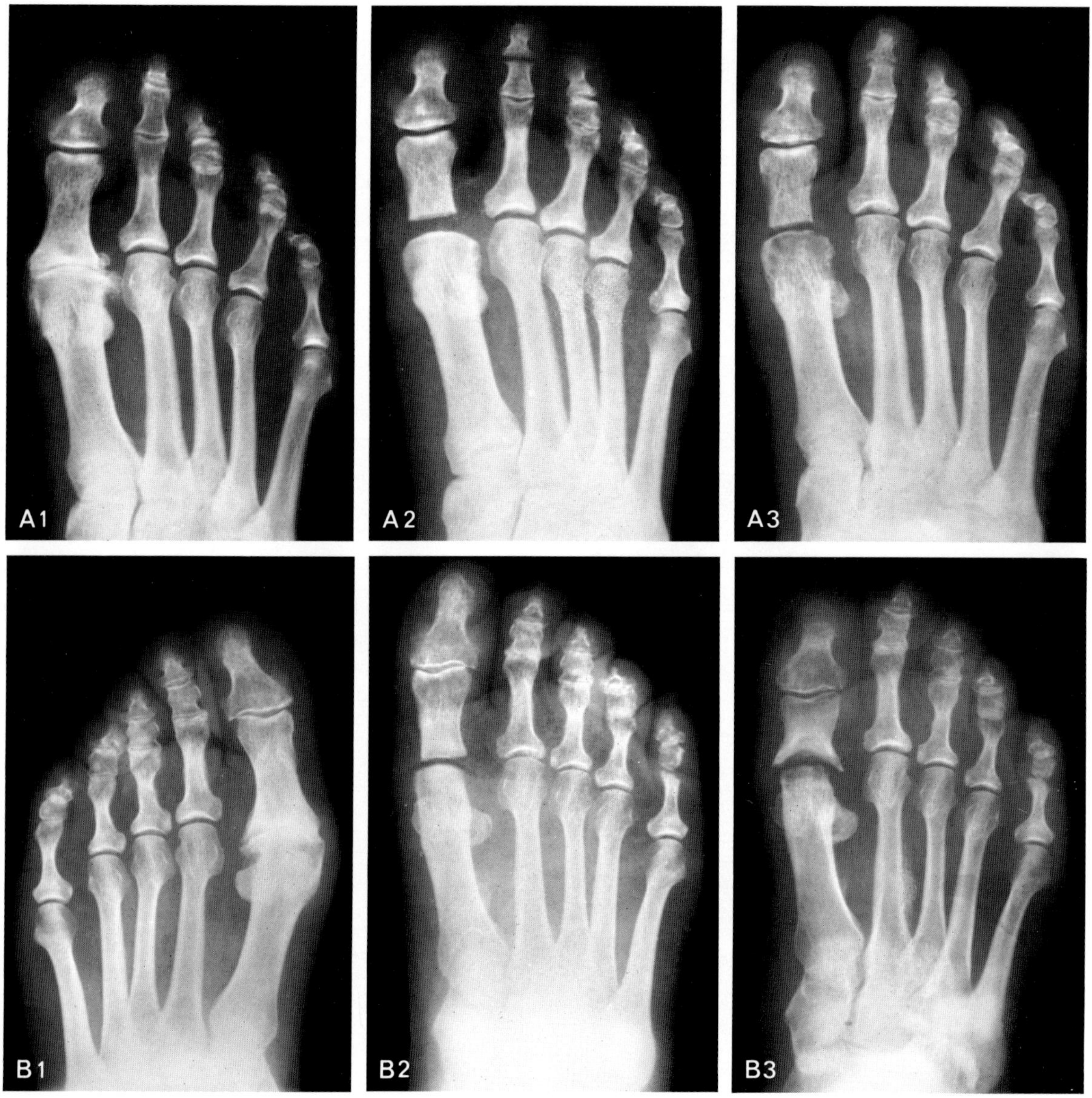

Fig. 23.6 A–E. Second- and third-degree hallux rigidus: treatment by metatarsophalangeal arthroplasty with interposition of a cup prosthesis. **A** Second degree: *1* Preoperative; *2* postoperative; *3* after removal of prosthesis 18 months after operation. **B** Third degree: *1* Preoperative; *2* 6 months after operation; *3* result 33 months after operation after overlate removal of prosthesis (at 2 years) ▷ which led to erosion of base of phalanx – mobility nevertheless good. **C** Second degree: *1* Preoperative; *2* a year after operation. **D** Second degree: *1* Preoperative; *2* a year after operation, the time at which the prosthesis should be removed. **C–E** see pp. 349, 350

Operative Technique. The exposure is similar to that in the osteocartilaginous graft procedure (Regnauld 1968). After modelling of the opposing joint surfaces, a high-density polyethylene cup is inserted into the metatarsophalangeal space and the degree of resection of the base of the phalanx confirmed as adequate. The cup is fixed in place by four sutures, one each on the internal, dorsal, plantar and external aspects. The capsule is repaired by a plantar stitch which coapts the capsulosesamoidal junction, thereby impeding posterior subluxation of the sesamoids, and by multiple circumferential stitches, always without undue pressure. It may be useful to accompany this arthroplasty with arthrotomy of the first cuneiform metatarsal joint in order to restore mobility. Fibrocartilage forms on either side of the cup, which can then be removed after about a year (it is always necessary to inform the patient of this further intervention). The development of the fibrocartilage can be as-

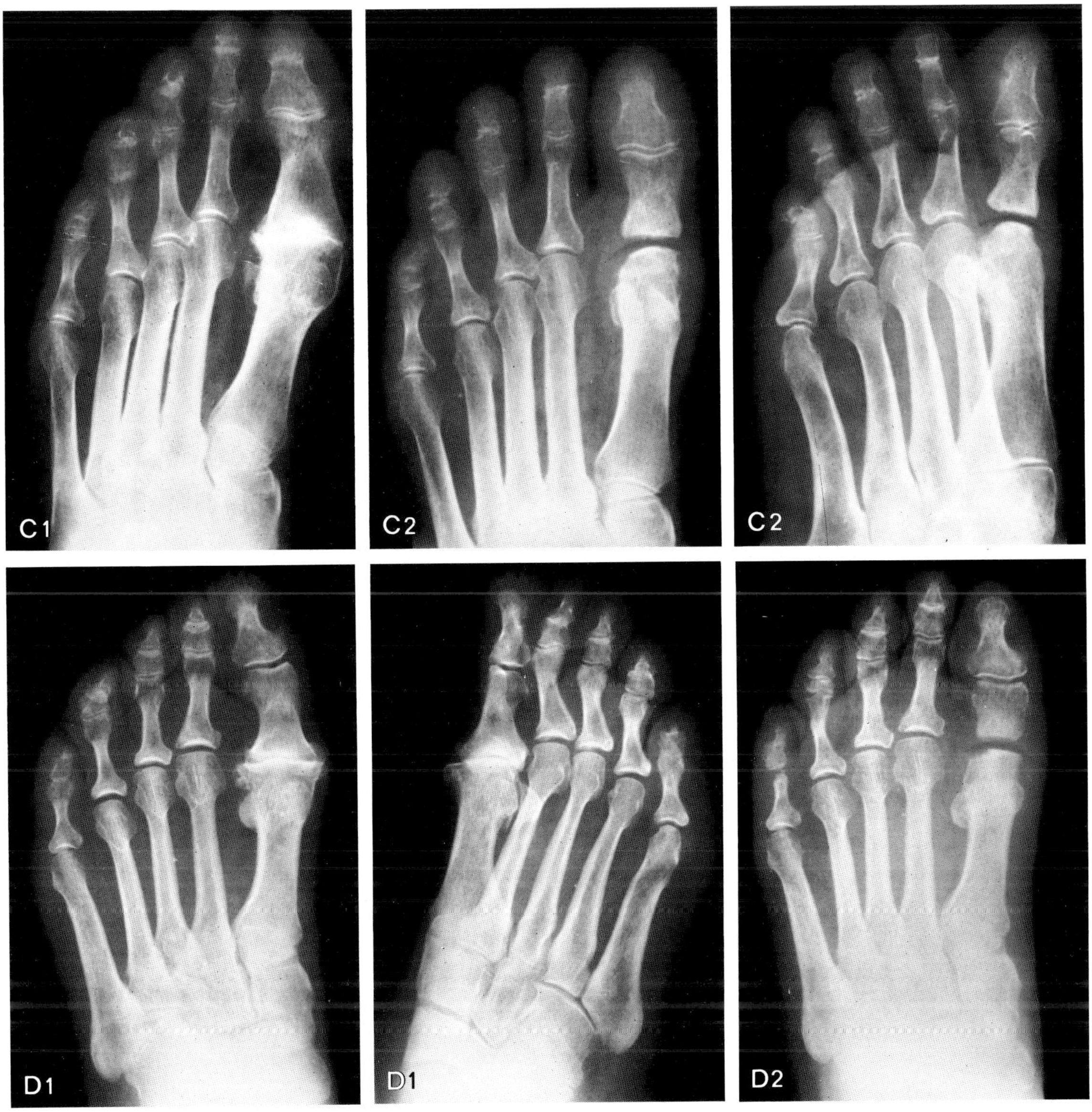

Fig. 23.6 C, D. Legend see p. 348

sessed radiographically every 3 months so as to choose the best time for removal of the cup. The end result is a mobile supple joint.

Alternatively, perhaps avoiding the need for two operations, the skin graft interposition technique described by de Wulf (1978) can be employed. Fat and hair are excised from the graft taken from the donor site on the thigh. The layer of skin is stretched over the metatarsal head and anchored by separate sutures passed through little holes in the margins of the bone. The graft adapts to an articular function with the development of fibrocartilage. It is very important that careful functional re-education is commenced early and continued for 2-3 months.

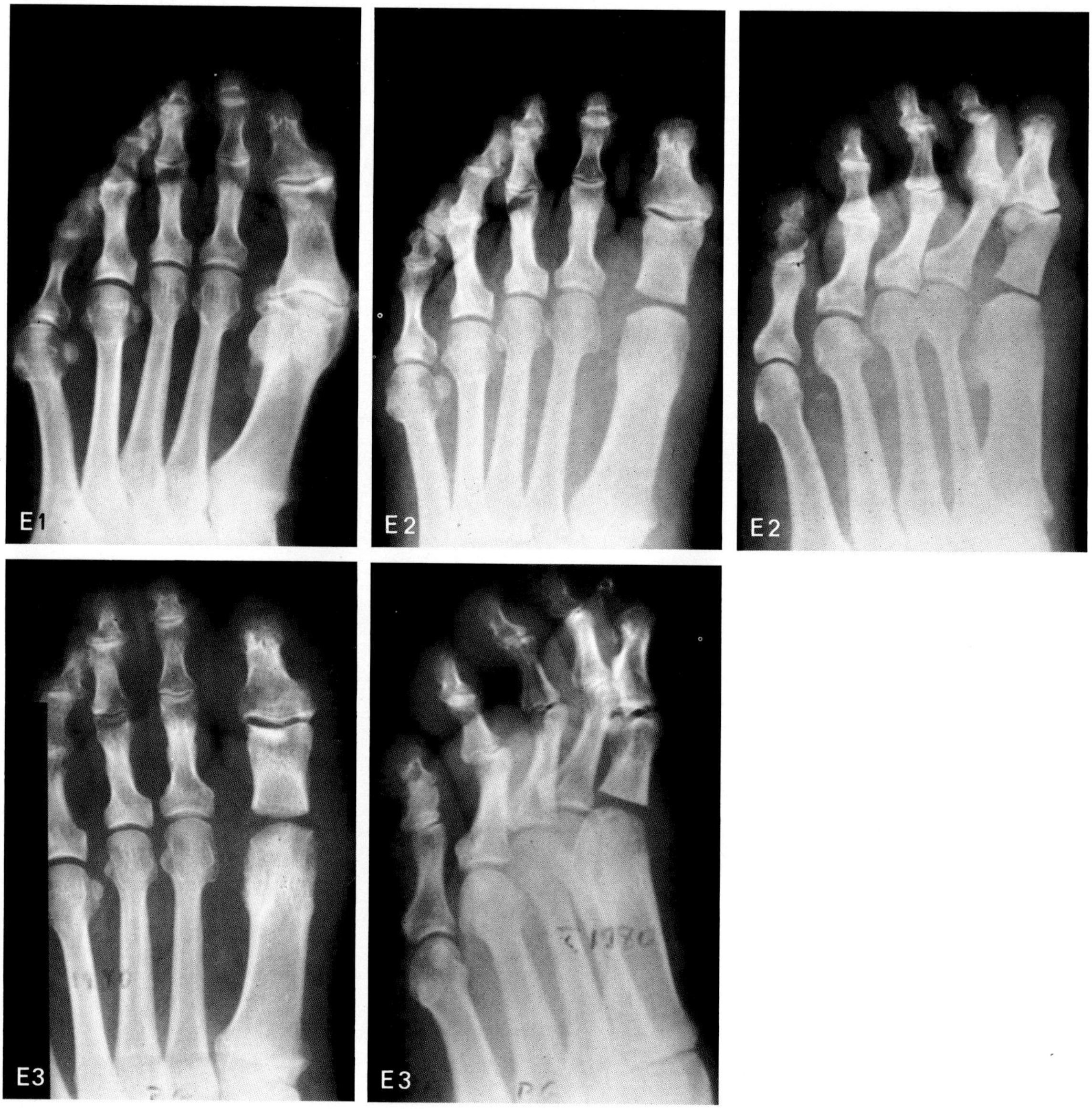

Fig. 23.6 *(continued).* **E** Second degree: *1* Preoperative; *2, 3* 3 and 6 months after interposition of high-density polyethylene cup prosthesis

24 Freiberg-Köhler Avascular Necrosis

This condition was described successively by Freiberg (1914), Köhler (1920) and Pannier (1921). Anatomopathological studies were published by Axhausen (1923), Welfing (1951) and Buchet et al. (1961).

24.1 Etiology

Ombredanne and Mathieu (1937) regarded the condition as an attenuated osteomyelitis, Lelièvre (1952) associated epiphysitis with growth and Denis (1975 c) thought it was an ischaemic necrosis of the head of a metatarsal analogous to Perthes' disease. Hansen and a majority of modern authors regard the condition as a traumatic epiphysitis. Arandes and Viladot (1956) described the condition as occurring in two phases: in phase 1 there is mechanical compression of the arteries nourishing the diaphysis, and in phase 2 arterial spasm leads to ischaemia of the epiphysis succeeded by a period of reconstruction.

Whatever the basic cause, it should be emphasised that the epiphysitis almost always supervenes in a metatarsal subjected to overloading. It is analogous to the microtrauma responsible for hallux rigidus which provokes arterial spasm and epiphyseal ischaemia.

Buchet et al. (1961) regarded Freiberg-Köhler epiphysitis as an exaggerated consequence of the natural sequence of aseptic bone necrosis supervening during normal bone turnover in which necrosis-resorption of cells and rebuilding of new bone lamellae occurs. This is at a microscopic level, and it is not until blood supply is suddenly interfered with that the necrosing element of the process predominates.

Axhausen (1923) defined four stages of evolution:

1. While the gross shape of the epiphysis is preserved, fissuring takes place in the metaphyseal cortex; this process begins at the adjacent periosteum and is due to resorption of bone trabeculae and cartilage. In the latter, tiny marginal erosions appear on radiography.
2. Subchondral fissures extend to separate the osteocartilaginous cap from the main body of the epiphysis. Radiography shows flattening, with atrophy of the spongy bone of the metaphyseal region.
3. The subchondral spongy bone, separated from fragments of the osteocartilaginous cap, resorbs and is replaced by granulation tissue. Radiography shows a cystic appearance, due to erosion, and the formation of osteophytes round the margin of the area.
4. The end result is a deformed hypertrophied condyle, the articular cartilage of which is pitted by deep erosions; there is osteolysis of the spongy subchondral bone. The radiograph shows the classical appearance of hypertrophic arthrosis and osteophytes, and there is ankylosis.

24.2 Clinical Features

The condition begins in adolescence, between 12 and 18 years of age, and affects girls more often than boys. It is usually unilateral, but is frequently seen in both feet. Occasionally it passes unperceived, only becoming apparent in adulthood (Fig. 24.1).

The second, third and fourth metatarsals are involved in descending order of frequency; the great metatarsal head is very rarely affected, although Denis (1975 c) cites several examples.

Symptomatically, there is metatarsalgia in the affected joint on walking, accompanied by slight limitation of movement. As the pain increases, there may be swelling and, on the dorsal aspect, painful hypertrophy of the capsule. At this stage, the condition may appear to resolve and remain quiescent for some years. *Radiography* may show no abnormality or a slight narrowing of the joint space with discrete marginal erosions and blurring of the outline of the epiphysis.

In some instances, discomfort and oedema are much more significant, with local heat, articular contracture and extreme pain on movement. The appearance is one of true inflammatory arthritis. *Radiogra-*

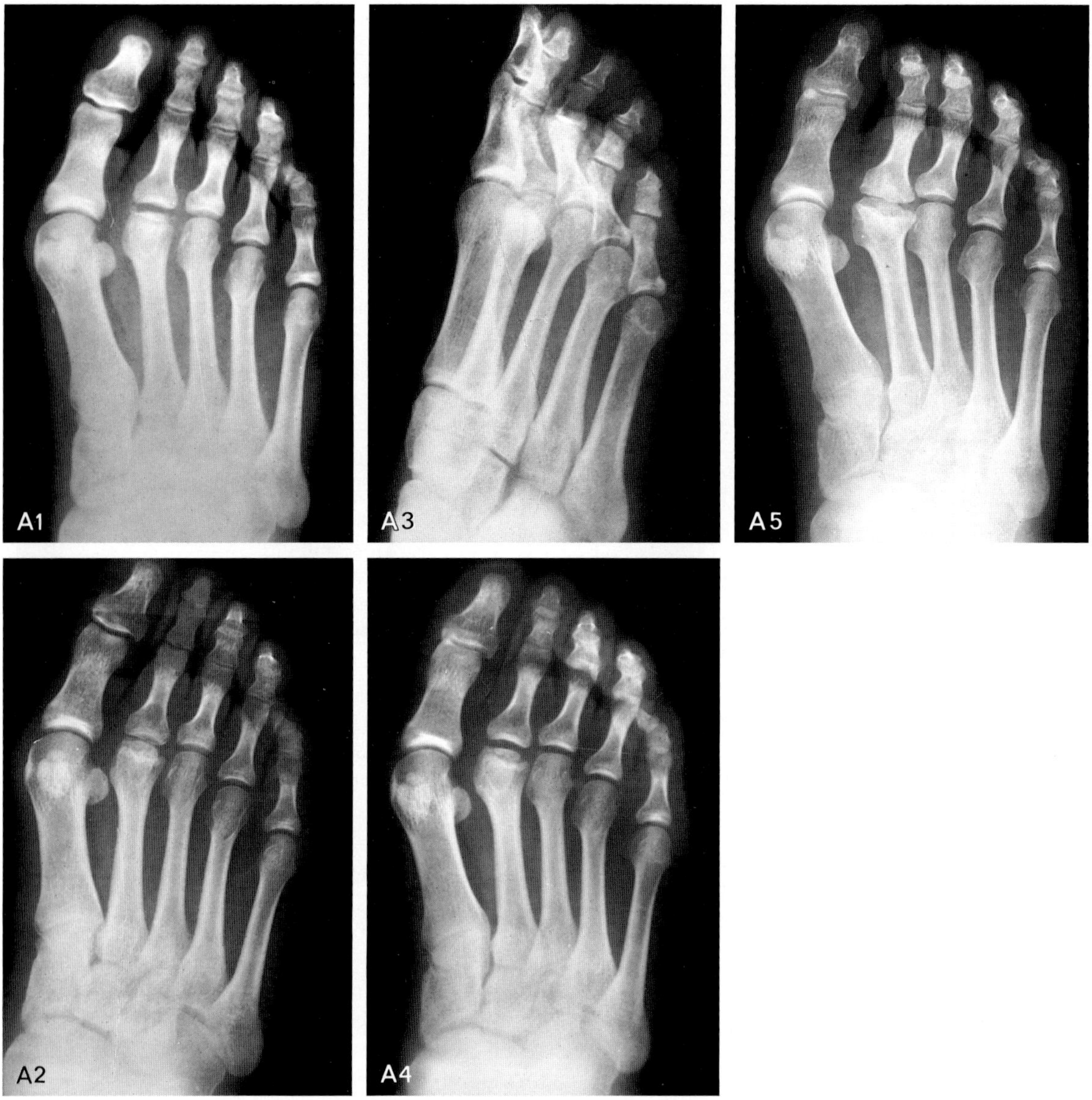

Fig. 24.1 A–D Freiberg-Köhler and Köhler-Mouchet osteochondritis. **A** Osteochondritis of second metatarsal head: *1, 2* Dorsoplantar views in 1964 and 1965; *3–5* lateral views in 1965, 1966 and 1979. **B** Osteochondritis of second metatarsal head. *1, 2* 1975; *3, 4* 1976; *5* 1978; ▷ *6–8* Appearance of intracapital geodes with onset of surrounding changes: *5, 6* 1979; *7, 8* 1980. **B–D** see pp. 353–355

phy shows narrowing of the joint interspace, widening and flattening of the articular surfaces, diminution in the density of the bone trabeculae and, in the centre of the epiphysis, irregular peripheral condensation of bone around the margins, conferring a flecked appearance on the condyle.

In late cases, presenting perhaps in adulthood, arthrosis is accompanied by painful limitation of amplitude of articular movement, fibrous contracture, and pain during walking or mobilisation of the toe. The irregular hypertrophy affects the phalanx and the metatarsal epiphyses. There is hypertrophy, flattening, and perhaps widening of the articular joint space. It may become concave with respect to the metatarsal, fairly often presenting a zone of central sequestration or clearly defined lacunae of resorption. There is sometimes thickening of the diaphyseal cortex and formation of osteophytes inside and around the joint. The latter are usually dorsal and lateral, only exceptionally plantar.

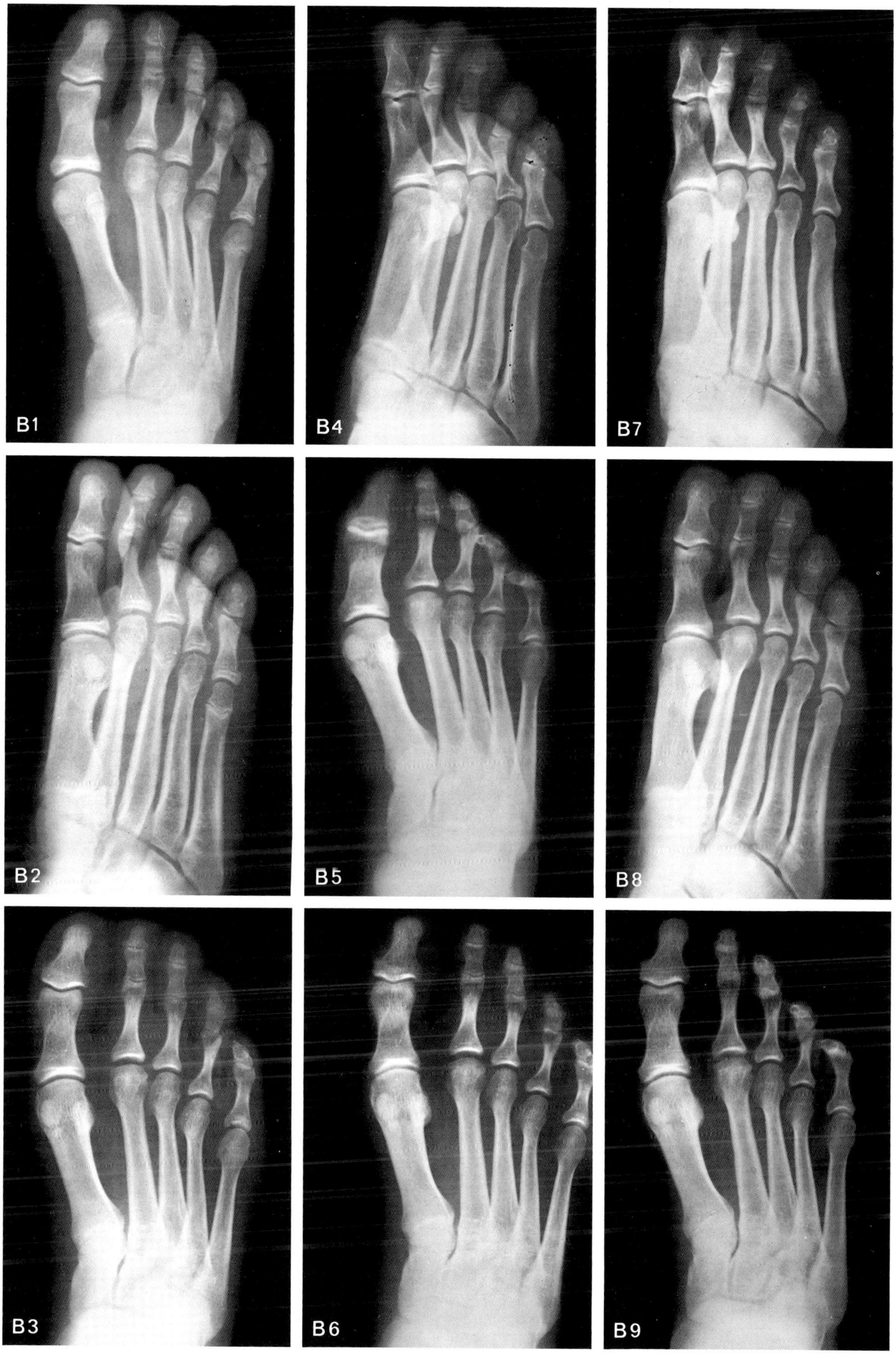
B1
B4
B7
B2
B5
B8
B3
B6
B9

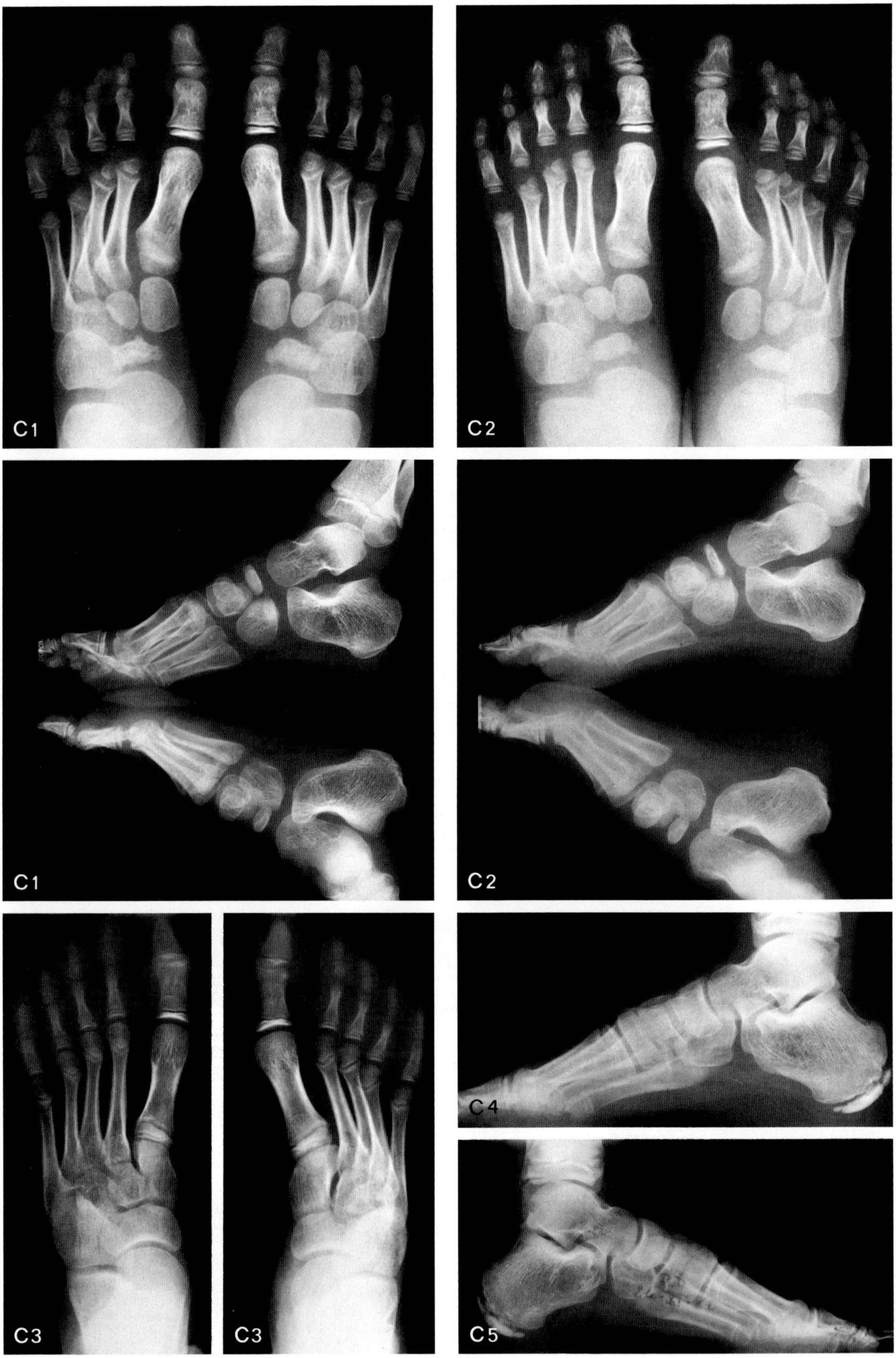
C1
C2
C1
C2
C3
C3
C4
C5

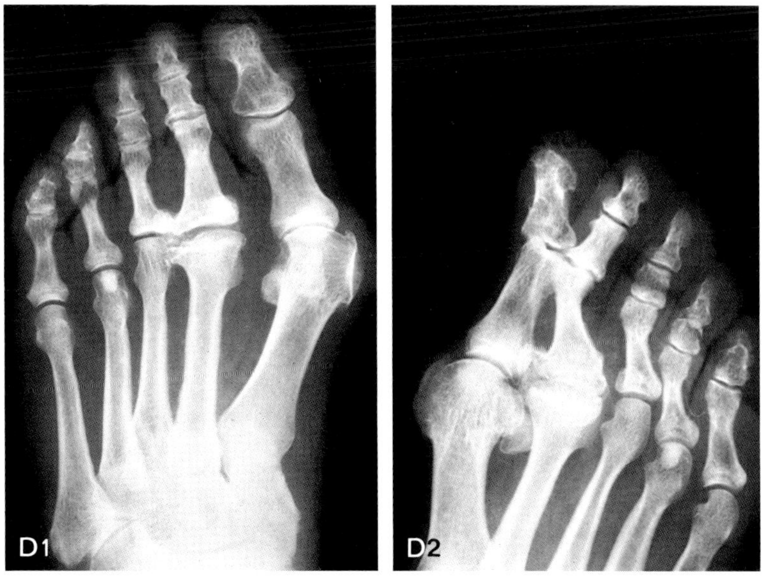

◁ **Fig. 24.1** *(continued).* **C** *1* 1974: avascular changes in navicular of right foot (Köhler-Mouchet); *2* 1974: flattening, irregularity of outline of navicular; *3* 1980: perfect reconstitution of navicular outline; *4, 5* 1980: lateral views showing normal navicular in both feet. **D** *1* Osteochondritis of second metatarsal head; *2* involvement of metatarsophalangeal joint

24.3 Treatment

24.3.1 Conservative

In the early stages, an insole may be prescribed to spare loading underneath the affected metatarsal head, comprising a physiological monoblock insole with an internal dome associated with a retrocapital bar or an excavation under the affected area. Antirheumatic medication may be used as an adjunct.

24.3.2 Surgical

The choice of operation depends on the preservation of articular cartilage, which can best be assessed at operation. As with hallux rigidus, the condition can be classified into three degrees depending upon the state of the cartilage (Fig. 24.2).

First Degree. The cartilage is well preserved, and trimming of the expanded margins of the metatarsal head and the base of the phalanx should avoid further damage and reconstitute normal pathology with mobility. A joint treated by excision of the peripheral eburnation, osteophytes and altered synovium can recover completely. Active re-education is essential.

Operative Technique. A longitudinal incision is made on the dorsal aspect, spanning the metatarsophalangeal joint, and after careful haemostasis the tendons of the long and short extensors are retracted and sometimes lengthened. The capsule is detached at the phalangeal base and from the head of the metatarsal, exposing the joint and the congested synovium, which is excised meticulously. The collateral and dorsal exostoses of the metatarsal heads are trimmed with rongeurs so that they are flush with the margins of the cartilaginous surface. The base of the phalanx is excised and replaced in proper alignment with the metatarsal head. The capsule is sutured, and after closure of the skin a padded dressing is applied, maintaining the toe in a normal position. Re-education must be gentle, progressive and prolonged so as to restore satisfactory amplitude of movement after disappearance of the capsular oedema.

Second Degree. Movement is painful and there is partial damage to the articular cartilage. When there is loss of articular cartilage, the metatarsal head and base of the phalanx should be trimmed of marginal osteophytes and the altered cartilage on their surfaces should be removed. A cup prosthesis must be inserted between the joint surfaces or a cutaneous graft implanted. The long and short extensor tendons should be elongated.

Third Degree. Complete destruction of the metatarsophalangeal cartilage is accompanied by gross distortion of a metatarsal head. Resection of the metatarsal head is required, followed by implantation of a homograft if loss of bone is so extensive that this is necessary. The homograph must be coapted to a properly trimmed phalangeal base. Use of a homograft demands careful attention to alignment of the adjacent metatarsal heads, which may require shortening to preserve a proper line of loading. If there is extensive involvement of the base of the phalanx in addition to the metatarsal head damage, cup arthroplasty may be combined with the metatarsal head homograft. In some instances the surfaces of the joint are very pitted, leading to a central sequestrum. It may be possible to excise this and then apply a cup prosthesis to the remaining healthy bone. The technique of cup arthroplasty is similar to that described for hallux rigidus (Chap. 23) and has given excellent results (Regnauld and Grassin 1975).

Silastic implants, like Teflon and metal, are poor and tend to provoke lysis of the bone after several years, and have to be removed. At the present time, I prefer the use of a homograft for the metatarsal head or the curettage of cysts followed by interposition of a cup prosthesis for a year (Fig. 24.3).

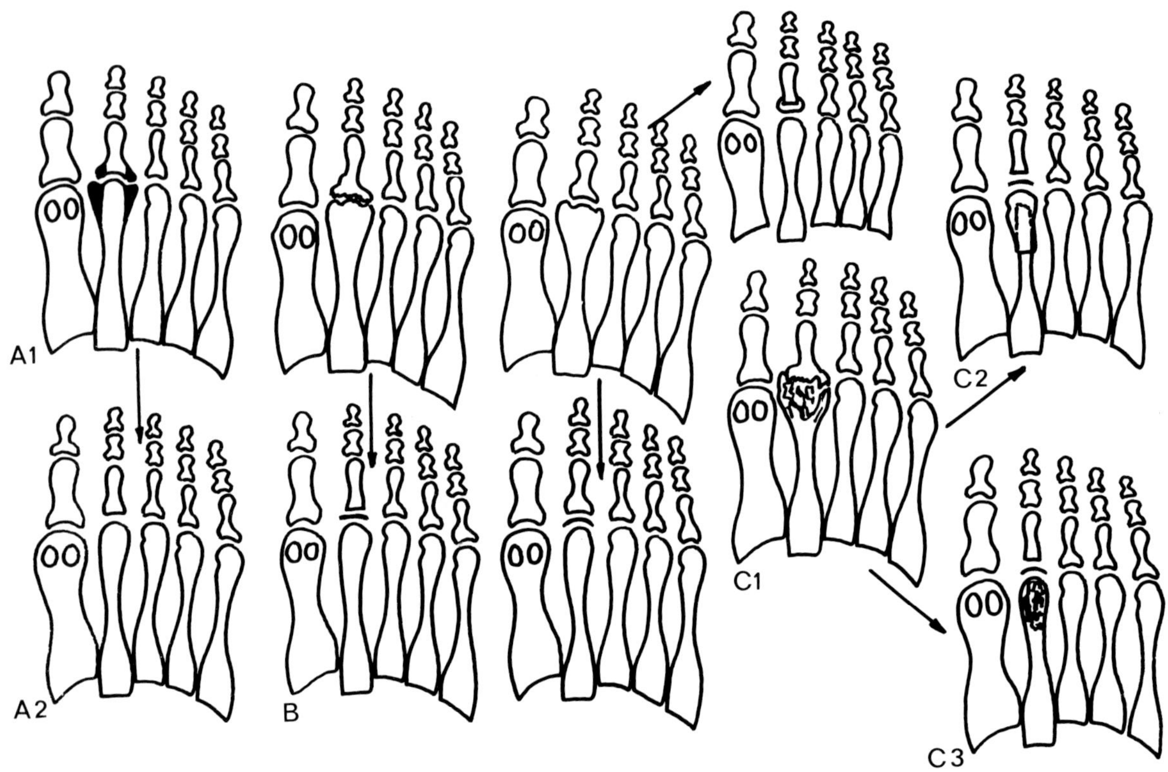

Fig. 24.2 A–C. Freiberg-Köhler avascular necrosis. **A** First degree: *1* Before treatment; *2* after articular remodelling. **B** Second degree: The choice is between metatarsophalangeal arthroplasty with interposition cup prosthesis (Regnauld) and metatarsophalangeal arthroplasty with skin interposition (de Wulf). **C** Third degree: *1* Before treatment; *2* after insertion of metatarsal head homograft and cup prosthesis (Regnauld); *3* after insertion of cancellous bone graft and cup prosthesis

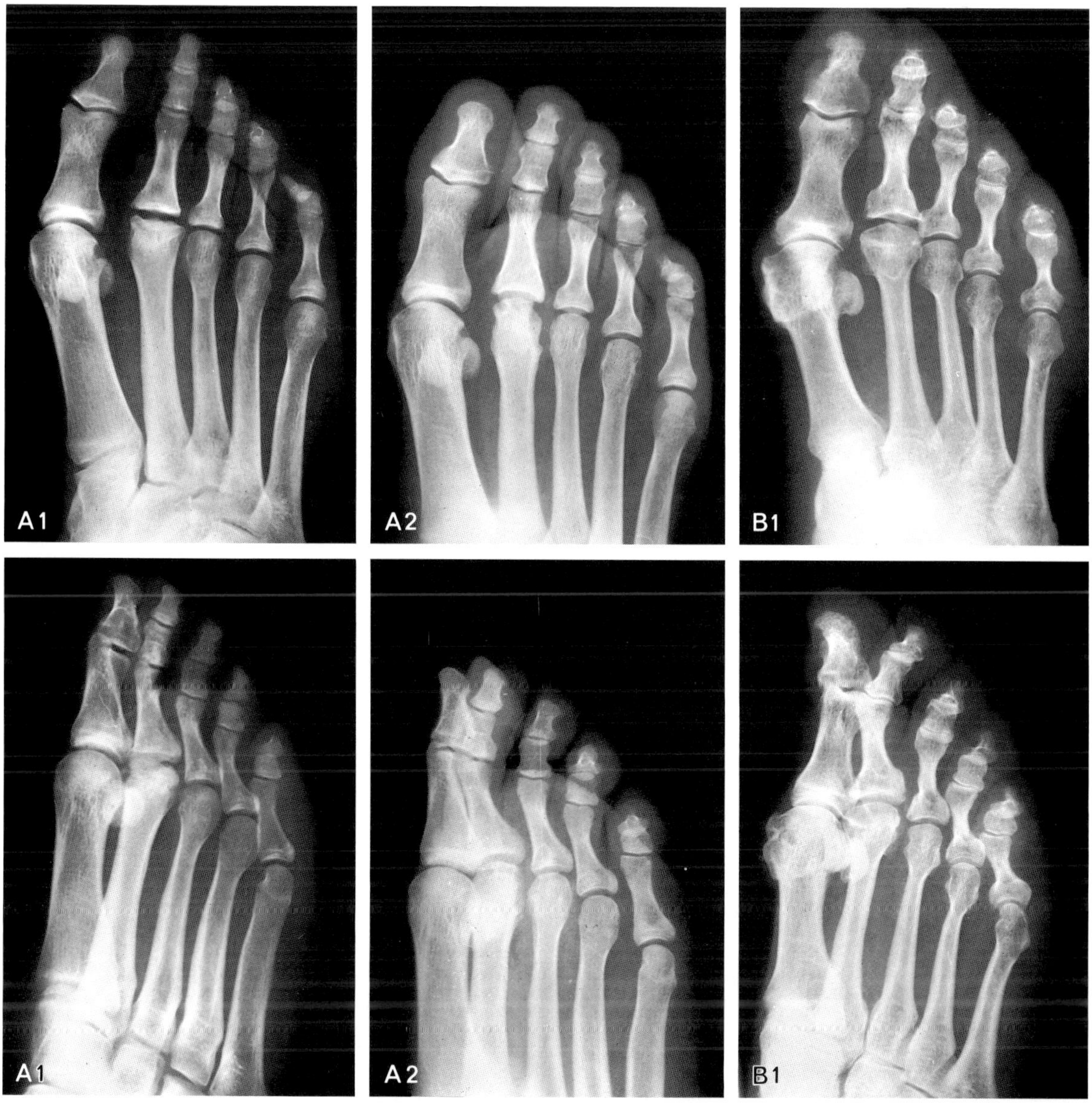

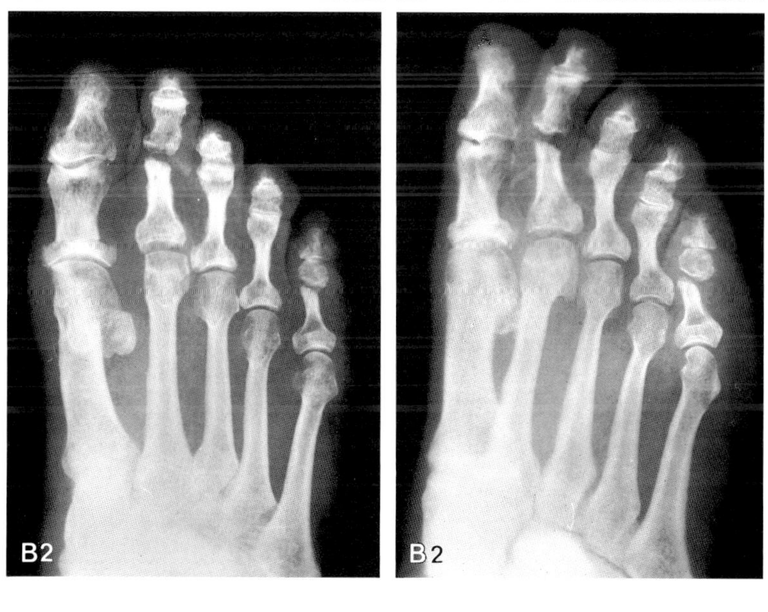

Fig. 24.2 A, B. Legend see p. 358

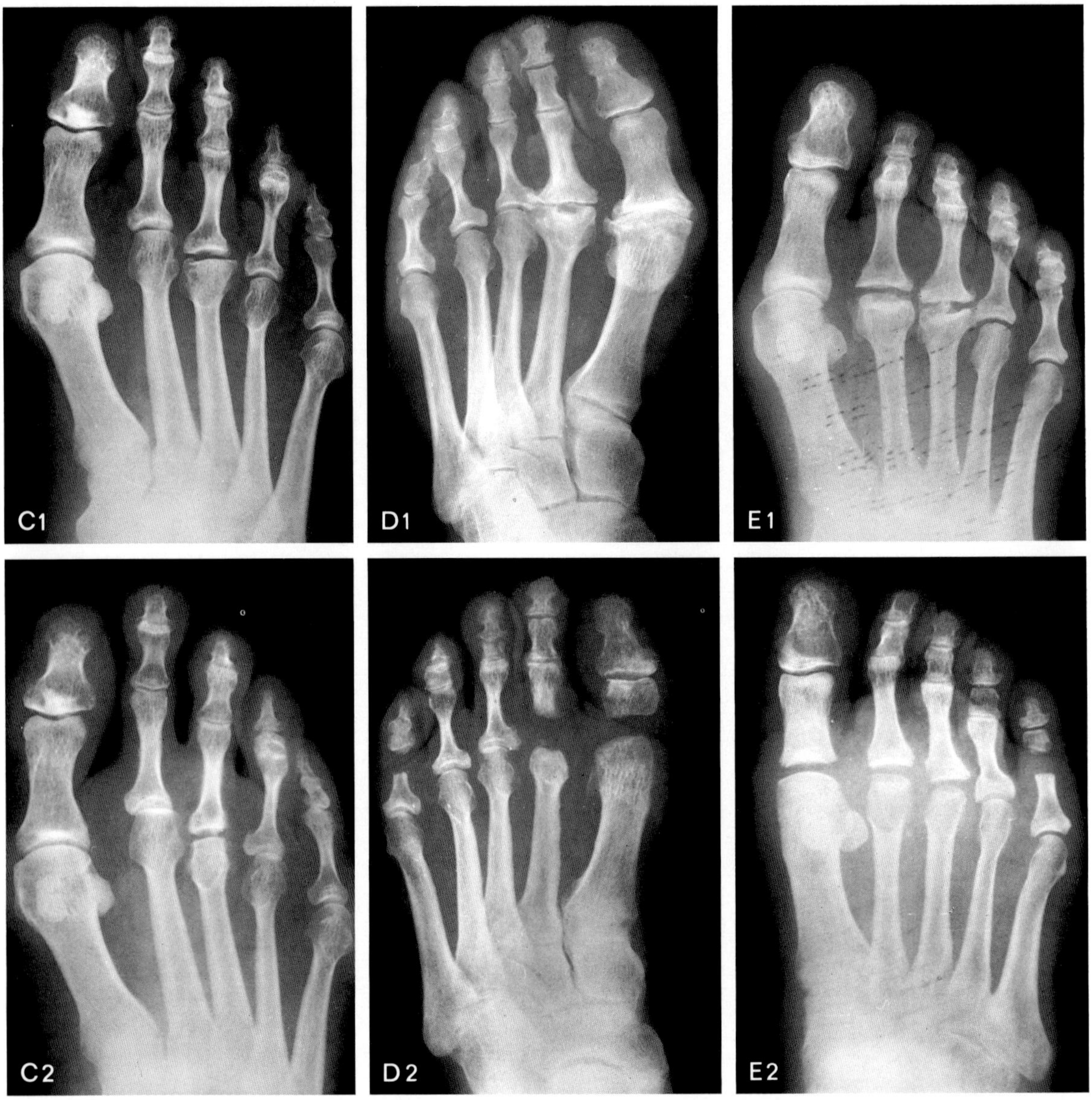

Fig. 24.3 A–G. Treatment of Freiberg-Köhler osteochondritis. **A** Second metatarsal head. *1* Preoperative; *2* after trimming of metatarsal head. **B** First-degree hallux valgus, results of old Freiberg-Köhler disease of second metatarsal head. *1* Preoperative; *2* after correction of hallux valgus with hat-shaped graft in phalanx, trimming of second metatarsal head and metatarsophalangeal joint. **C** Third metatarsal head. *1* Preoperative; *2* after trimming. **D** Hallux rigidus, osteochondritis of second and third metatarsal heads. *1* Preoperative; *2* after trimming. **E** Second and third metatarsal heads. *1* Preoperative; ▷ *2* after trimming. **F** Second metatarsal head. *1* Preoperative; *2* after trimming. **G** Osteochondritis of third metatarsal head, relative frontal protrusion of central three metatarsal heads, hallux valgus. *1* Preoperative; *2* after correction of hallux valgus with cork-shaped graft, realignment of metatarsal heads by head-shaft enclavement; *3, 4* 2 weeks after operation; *5* a year after operation. **F, G** see p. 359

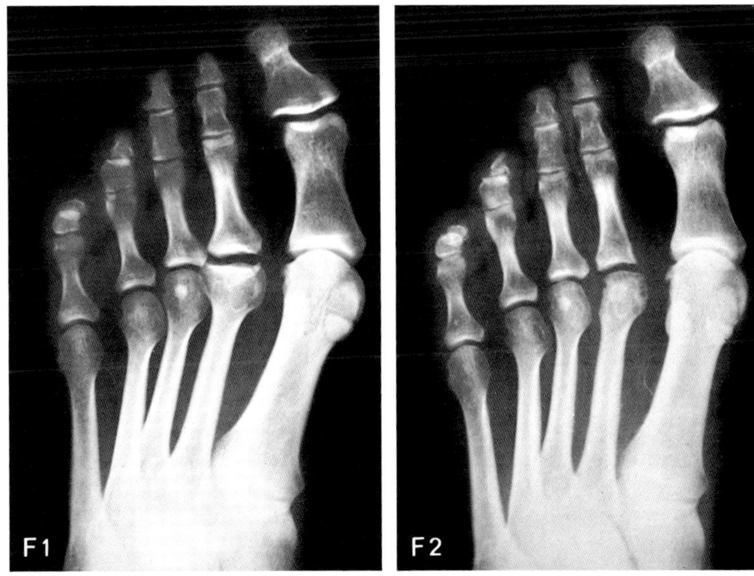

Fig. 24.3 F, G. Legend see p. 358

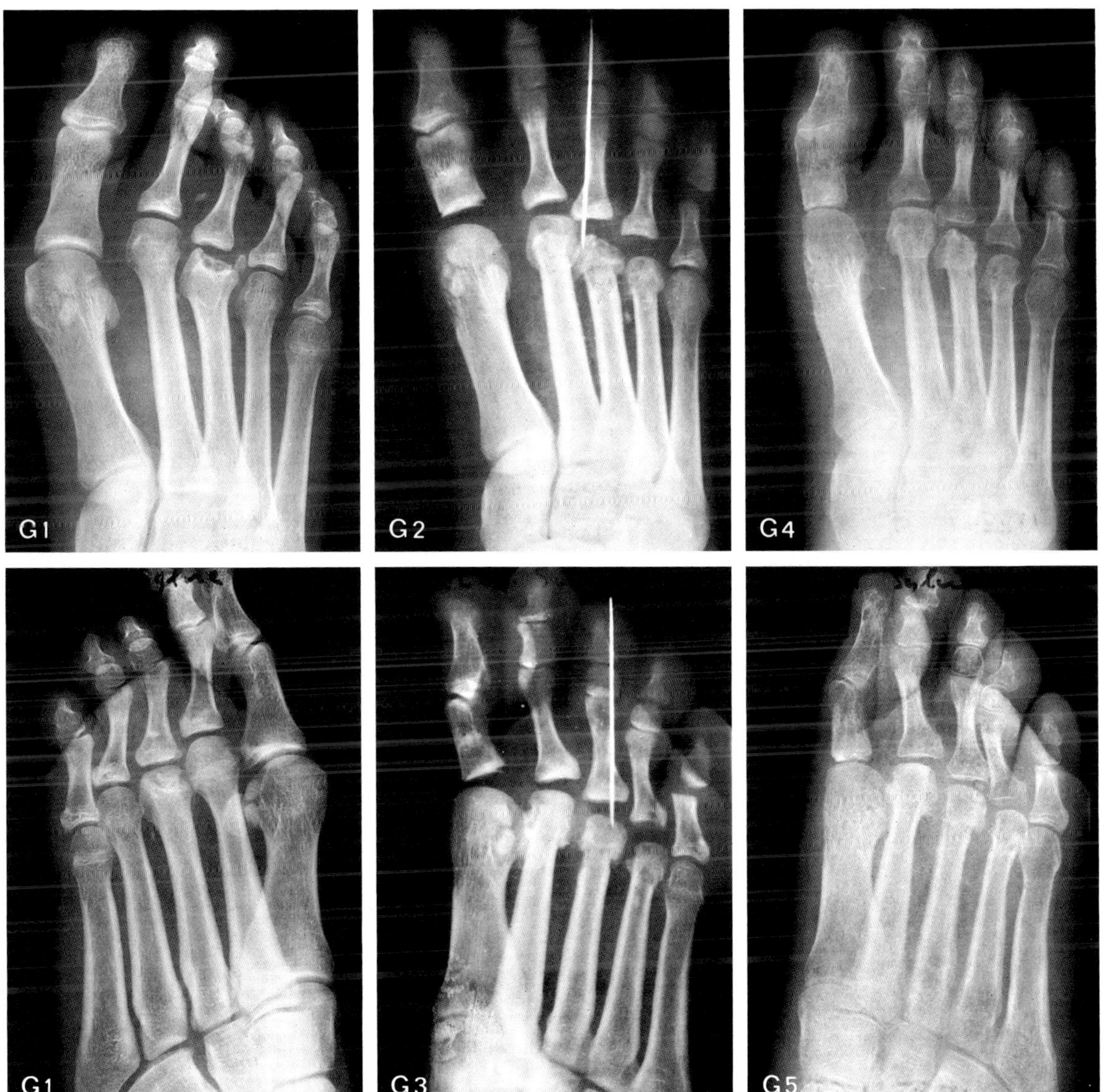

25 Consequences of Failed Operative Treatment in the Antetarsus

The surgeon is frequently faced with the results of failure of previous operative treatment. Sometimes the procedures have been performed well, in other cases they have been poorly conceived or executed or rehabilitation has not been good. It is now realised that certain operative procedures should be avoided because they lead predictably to development of an iatrogenic condition. In this chapter, some guidance is offered on the solution of such problems in the antetarsus (Fig. 25.1).

Whatever the initial condition for which the operation was performed, the poor results have many features in common. Local arthralgia, usually affecting the metatarsophalangeal joints, is accompanied by limitation of movement, crepitus or occasionally total ankylosis. The forefoot tends to roll into supination, while occasionally there is a compensatory varus deformity of the foot as a whole; this antalgic attitude is adopted due to pain when walking, particularly when it emanates from the first metatarsophalangeal joint. Contracture of the extensor tendons commonly produces dorsiflexion contracture. *Radiographic* appearance depends on the nature of the previous surgical intervention, and often the apparent extent of resection procedures becomes exaggerated over the years because of progressive postoperative lysis of bone stock.

One of the main causes of arthrosis following metatarsophalangeal joint procedures is failure to meticulously preserve the blood supply of the metatarsal head and the phalanx. Damage leads to osteolysis. Too tight a correction of any deformity causes atrophy of the cartilage of the joint surfaces, this being seen particularly in procedures like the McBride (1928) operation in which the loss of normal transverse play of the first metatarsal is suppressed, thereby creating a syndrome of overloading in the associated metatarsophalangeal joint. One learns from mistakes, and the aim should always be to recreate a Greek configuration with preservation of proper mobility of the first and fifth metatarsals. *Radiography* will, in addition to revealing the state of the joint or remaining bone stock, show the position of the sesamoids, which can exhibit hypertrophy or lysis as well as subluxation.

Most of these failures of treatment require surgical revision and the following examples are those which I have seen most frequently; the lessons learned are indicated.

25.1 Keller-Brandes and Lelièvre Arthroplasties

Failure of these operations (Keller-Brandes 1904; Lelièvre 1952) (Figs. 25.2, 25.5 B, D, G) may be due to the plantar sesamoid bones not having been anchored into position with respect to the excised phalangeal base, or may occur when phalangeal resection has been insufficient and re-education poorly effected; in other cases, an excess of passive mobilisation has led to persistent postoperative capsular oedema. The patient may have experienced pain, and there may have been infection or cutaneous necrosis. Destructive osteitis can follow oedema, haematoma, cutaneous necrosis or infection. Any of these can impede re-educative measures and mobilisation of the joint.

Similar results may be seen after implantation of an osteochondral phalangeal hat-shaped graft (Regnauld 1968) associated with fracture of the cartilaginous margins of the graft (see Chap. 18.1.3). Progressive osteolysis and osteonecrosis have occurred. These may have been associated with lack of care to protect the site of entry of the nutrient artery of the proximal phalanx during liberation of the plantar aspect of the capsule. In other instances there is a proliferation of the margins of a hat-shaped graft, possibly associated with excessive trimming of the osteocartilaginous crown which has encouraged the development of osteophytes. The osteophytes can almost completely surround the metatarsal head, producing an iatrogenic hallux rigidus. A cork-shaped graft is always preferred when possible.

Treatment comprises elongation of the long and short extensor tendons, trimming of the metatarsal head to a normal shape and conservation or remodelling of the convexity of the condyle. The posteriorly displaced sesamoids should be reduced and their fixation to the base of the phalanx ensured, and after appropriate shaping, the interposition of a high-density polyethylene cup prosthesis is probably the procedure of choice.

When the shortening of the great toe due to osteolysis or resection has ruptured the general line of load bearing, shortening of the neighbouring toes by enclavement may be indicated. If this is not done, callosities will appear under the three central metatarsal heads. In cases where a callosity forms only under the second metatarsal head, basal osteotomy or wedge resection [Mau (1940) and Thys (1976b) procedures] may be adequate.

In the ankylosing type of arthrosis, in which there is involvement of the metatarsophalangeal and metatarsosesamoidophalangeal components, treatment has to be more extensive, with excision of the base of the phalanx, mobilisation of the sesamoids, reconstitution of the capsuloplantar plane, anchoring this to the base of the resected phalanx, and arthroplasty using an interpositional cup. If the residual condition is osteolytic, refashioning of the base of the phalanx is necessary, again accompanied by proper attachment of the sesamoids and a cup prosthesis. The prosthesis must be removed after a few months when mobility and the stability of the joint has been restored.

25.2 Peg Implant Arthroplasties

Metatarsophalangeal lysis may occur months or years after insertion of prostheses such as the Swanson device (Fig. 25.3).

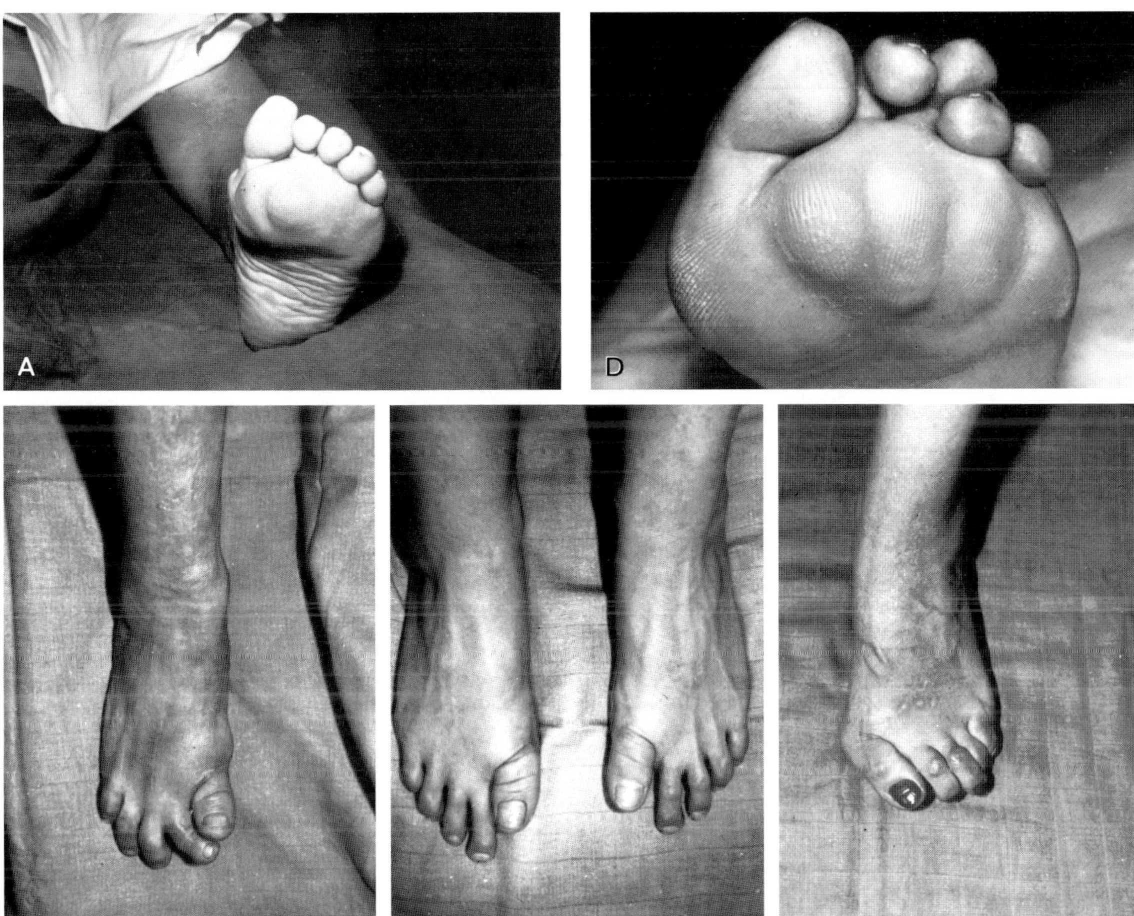

Fig. 25.1 A–R. Forefoot deformities produced by previous operative intervention. **A–H** Following amputation of first metatarsal head for hallux valgus: convex forefoot (**A, D, F, H**) shortness of first ray (**H, C**) valgus displacement (**D–F**) varus displacement (**G, H**) irregular displacements (**H**). **F–R** see pp. 362, 363

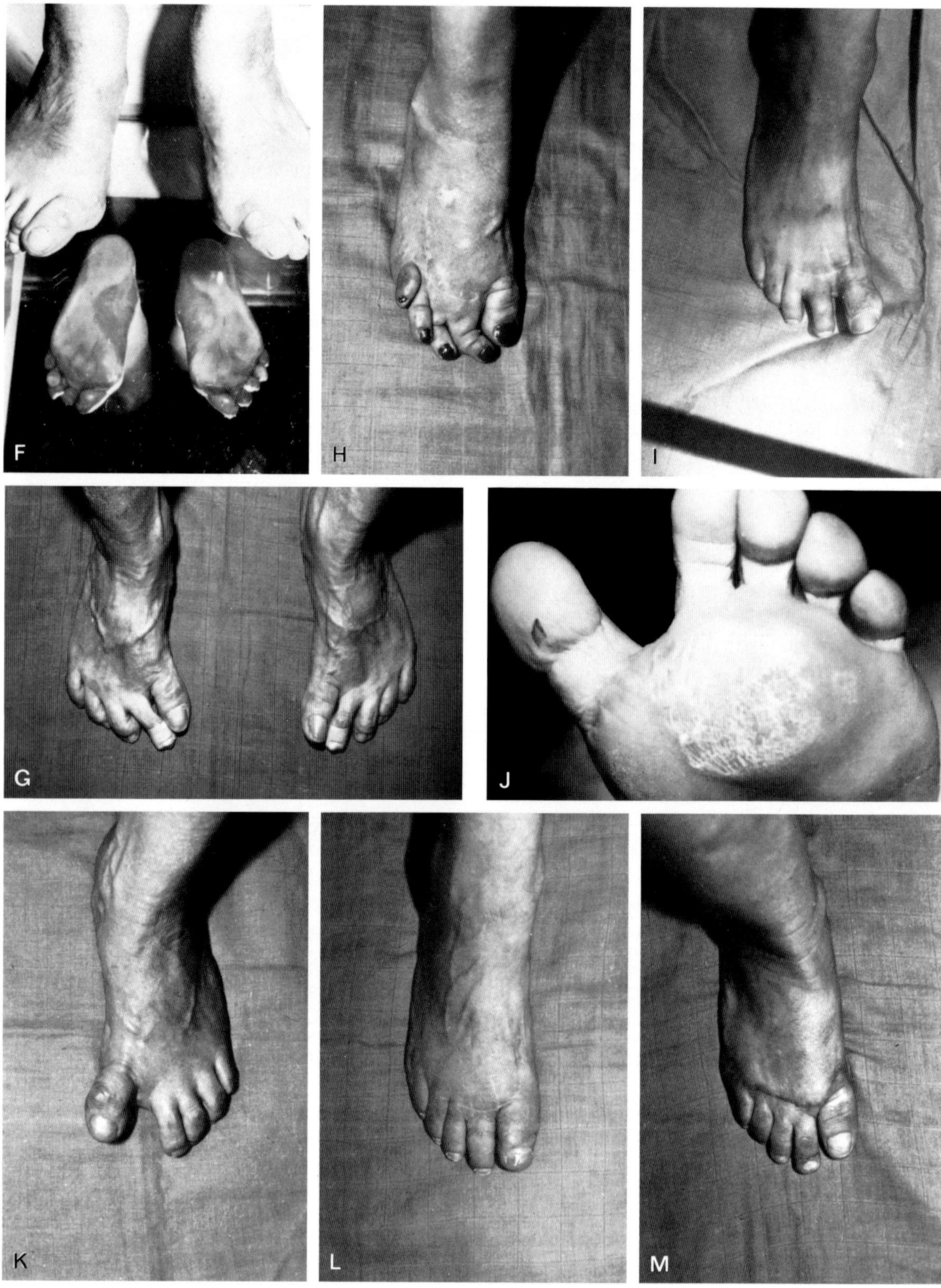

Fig. 25.1 F–M. Legend see p. 363

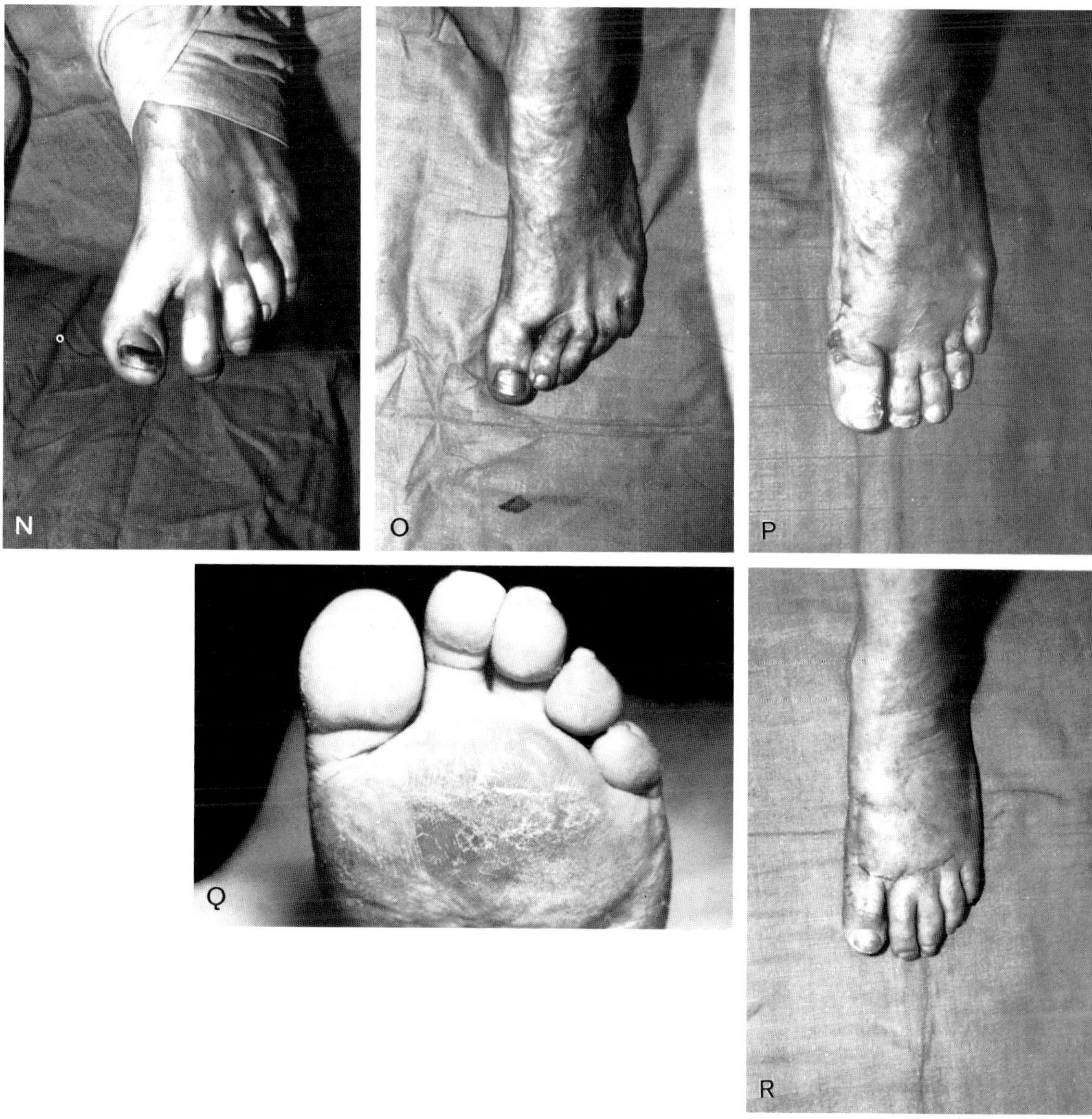

◁ **Fig. 25.1** *(continued)*. **J-K, N** Following operation for hallux valgus leading to hallux varus. **G** Hallux varus with flexion after operation for hallux valgus. **J** Hallux varus with flexion after metatarsophalangeal arthroplasty. **L** Correction of condition in **J** by arthroplasty of metatarsophalangeal joint using cup prosthesis and enclavement of second, third and fourth metatarsal heads. **M** Correction of **C** by enclavement of second, third and fourth metatarsal heads. **O** Hallux rigidus with varus and flexion following metatarsophalangeal arthroplasty. **P** Correction of **O** by arthroplasty using interposition cup prosthesis. **Q, R** Correction of foot shown in **J** and **K** by arthroplasty of metatarsophalangeal joint of great toe and realignment enclavement of second, third and fourth metatarsal heads

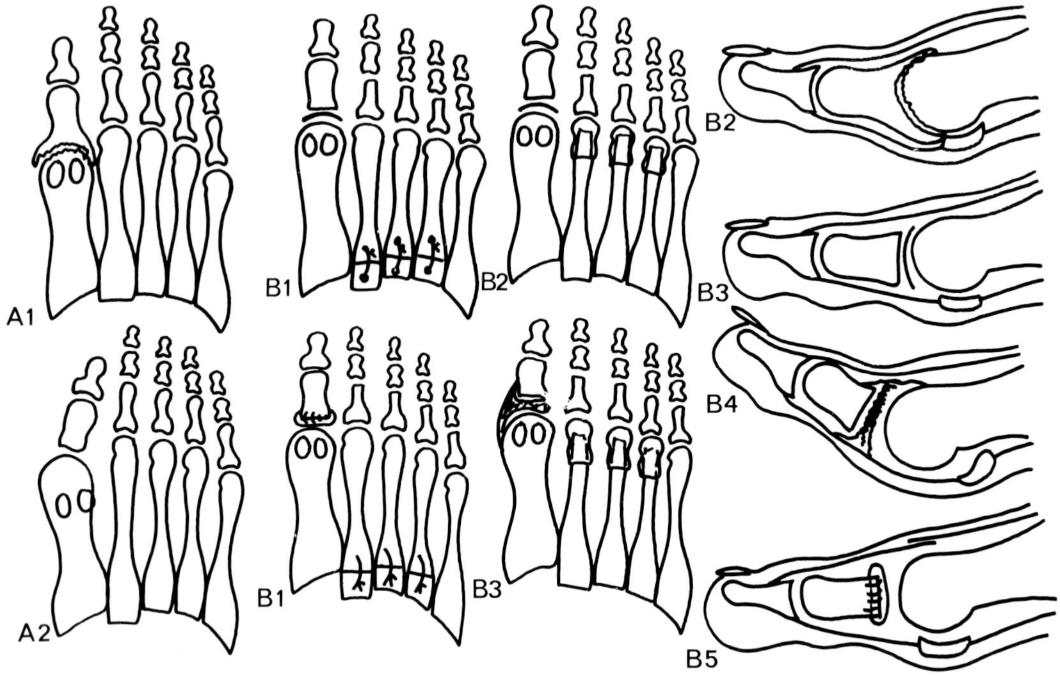

Fig. 25.2. **A** Sequels of arthroplasty of great metatarsophalangeal joint: *1* Ankylosing arthrosis; *2* mobile arthrosis. **B** Treatment. The choice is between *1* metatarsal osteotomies and *2* enclavement of metatarsal heads, accompanied by *3* cup arthroplasty (Regnauld), *4* capsular interposition or *5* cutaneous arthroplasty (de Wulf)

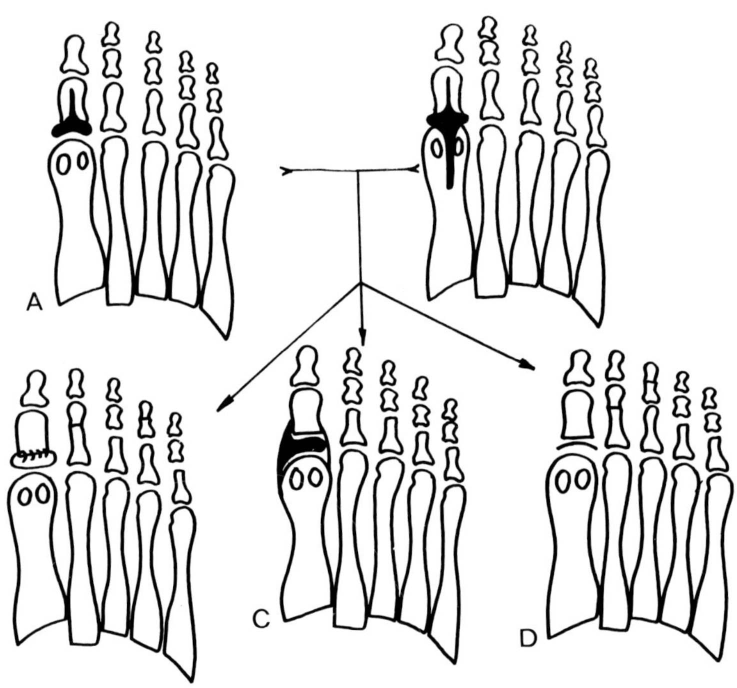

Fig. 25.3 A–D. Operative treatment of the sequelae of metatarsophalangeal arthroplasty using a peg prosthesis. **A** Two types of peg prosthesis. **B** Arthroplasty with skin interposition (de Wulf). **C** Capsular interposition. **D** Cup arthroplasty

The lysis occurs predominantly in the phalanx, at areas of contact with the prosthesis, and progressively diminishes the length of, usually, the great toe. Metatarsal lysis appears less frequently. The condition is associated with an exudative serous inflammation rather than a true arthrosis. Hypertrophy of the periarticular tissues, articular swelling and infiltration with serous fluid all indicate intolerance by the tissues of the prosthesis. The condition is painful most of the time, with crises of greater severity. I used the peg prosthesis in the past, but have abandoned it in favour of the cup prosthesis, especially for hallux rigidus.

Treatment comprises removal of the prosthesis and the interposition of a layer of capsular tissue interwoven with a no. 3 nylon filament, which encourages and allows reconstitution of the metatarsophalangeal arthroplasty rendering the joint stable and comfortable. Alternatively, de Wulf (1978) implantation of a skin graft on the base of the phalanx can be used.

25.3 McBride and Schède Procedures

Failure is likely in two circumstances: when the operation has been performed in an Egyptian foot and when the reduction of the varus of the great metatarsal has been too tight. The result, over months or years, is metatarsophalangeal arthrosis which leads to ankylosis like hallux rigidus (Figs. 25.4, 25.5 A, C, E, F). *Treatment* is analogous to that for hallux rigidus comprising a metatarsophalangeal arthroplasty by resection of the phalangeal base and the interposition of a cup prosthesis.

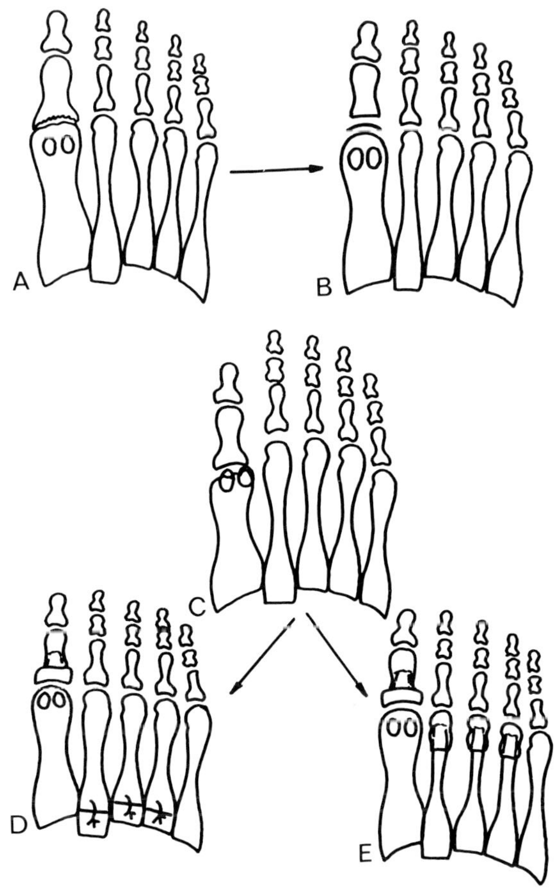

Fig. 25.4. A Arthrosis following McBride's procedure. **B** Remodelling of metatarsal head and phalangeal base and cup arthroplasty (Regnauld). **C** Sequel of Hueter-Mayo operation with healthy cartilage at base of phalanx. **D** Osteocartilaginous graft arthroplasty and realignment of metatarsals by Thys-Martorell procedure. **E** Autograft of arthroplasty and realignment enclavements of central three metatarsal heads (Regnauld)

25.4 Hueter-Mayo Amputation of First Metatarsal Head

This operation (Hueter 1876; Mayo 1908) leads inevitably to overloading of the second metatarsal head with keratoma formation. There may also be a median callosity under the central three metatarsal heads, the condition then presenting as iatrogenic convex forefoot. *Radiography* displays the extent of the metatarsal head resection and the degree of protrusion of the central metatarsal heads. *Treatment* will vary according to the state of the residual phalangeal base and the degree of excision of the metatarsal (Fig. 25.8).

25.4.1 Intact Phalangeal Base with Normal Articular Cartilage

Operation consists of trimming of the extremity of the first metatarsal and arthroplasty by insertion of an osteocartilaginous homograft tailored into the base of the phalanx (Regnauld 1968). Osteotomy to elevate the second metatarsal head is required if the transverse zone of metatarsal weight bearing is only locally disturbed (the Lipstein V-osteotomy is appropriate); realignment head-shaft enclavement of the central three metatarsal heads (Regnauld 1968) or wedge ostectomies of the central three metatarsal bases (Thys 1974b) is indicated if there is a convex forefoot.

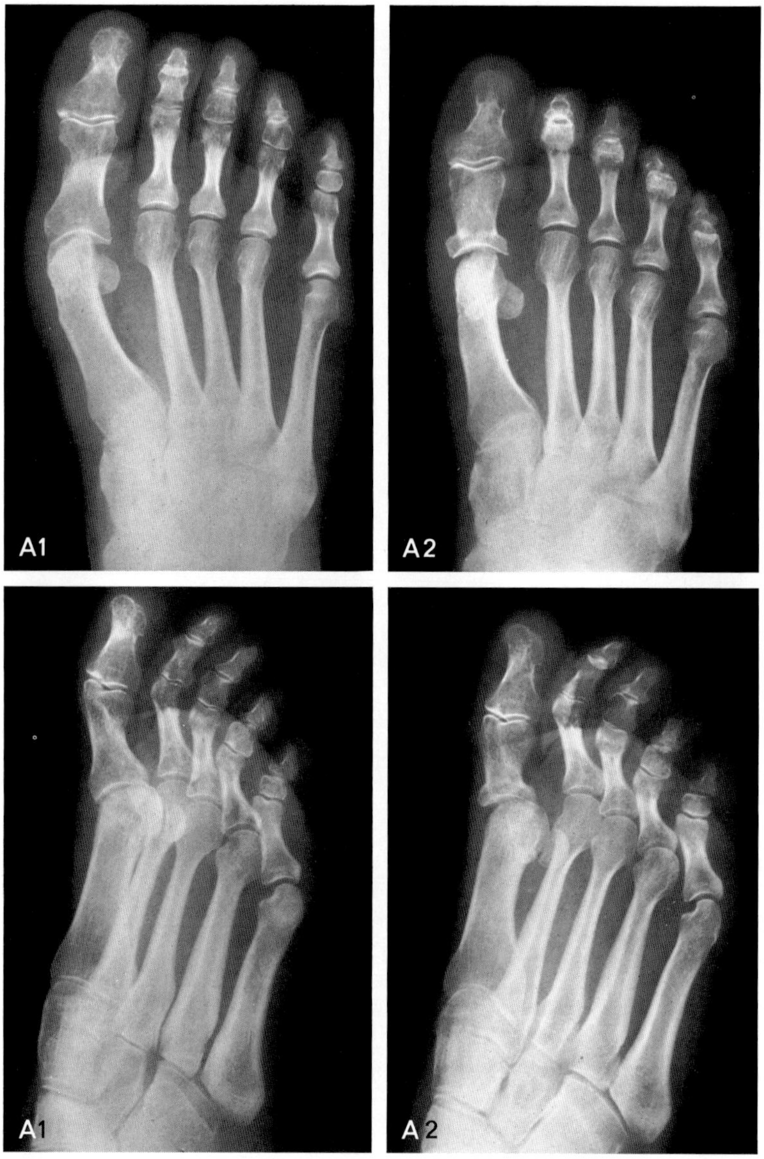

Fig. 25.5 A–K. Failed operative procedures for hallux valgus. **A** *1* Sequelae of Schède operation: arthritis, contracture, pain in first metatarsophalangeal joint; *2* after metatarsophalangeal arthroplasty with hat-shaped graft. ▷

B–K see pp. 367–371

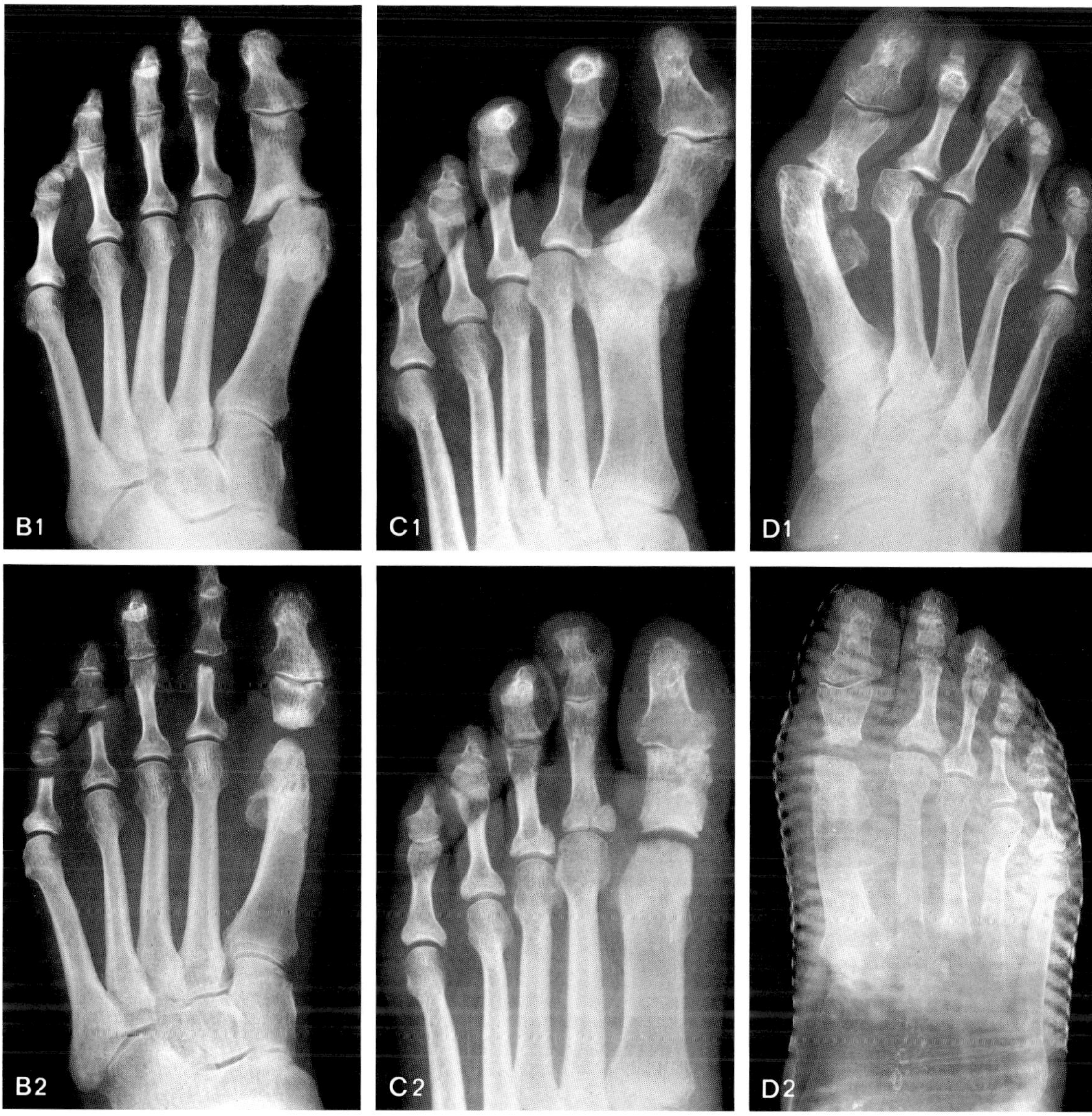

Fig. 25.5 *(continued).* **B** *1* Sequelae of Lelièvre-Keller Brandes operation: painful arthrosis, ankylosis; *2* after metatarsophalangeal arthroplasty with capsular interposition. **C** *1* Sequelae of modified McBride operation: painful hallux varus; *2* after metatarsophalangeal arthroplasty using cork-shaped graft. **D** *1* Sequelae of Keller Brandes operation: recurrent hallux valgus; *2* after metatarsophalangeal arthroplasty with cup interposition prosthesis, correction of lateral digital deviation

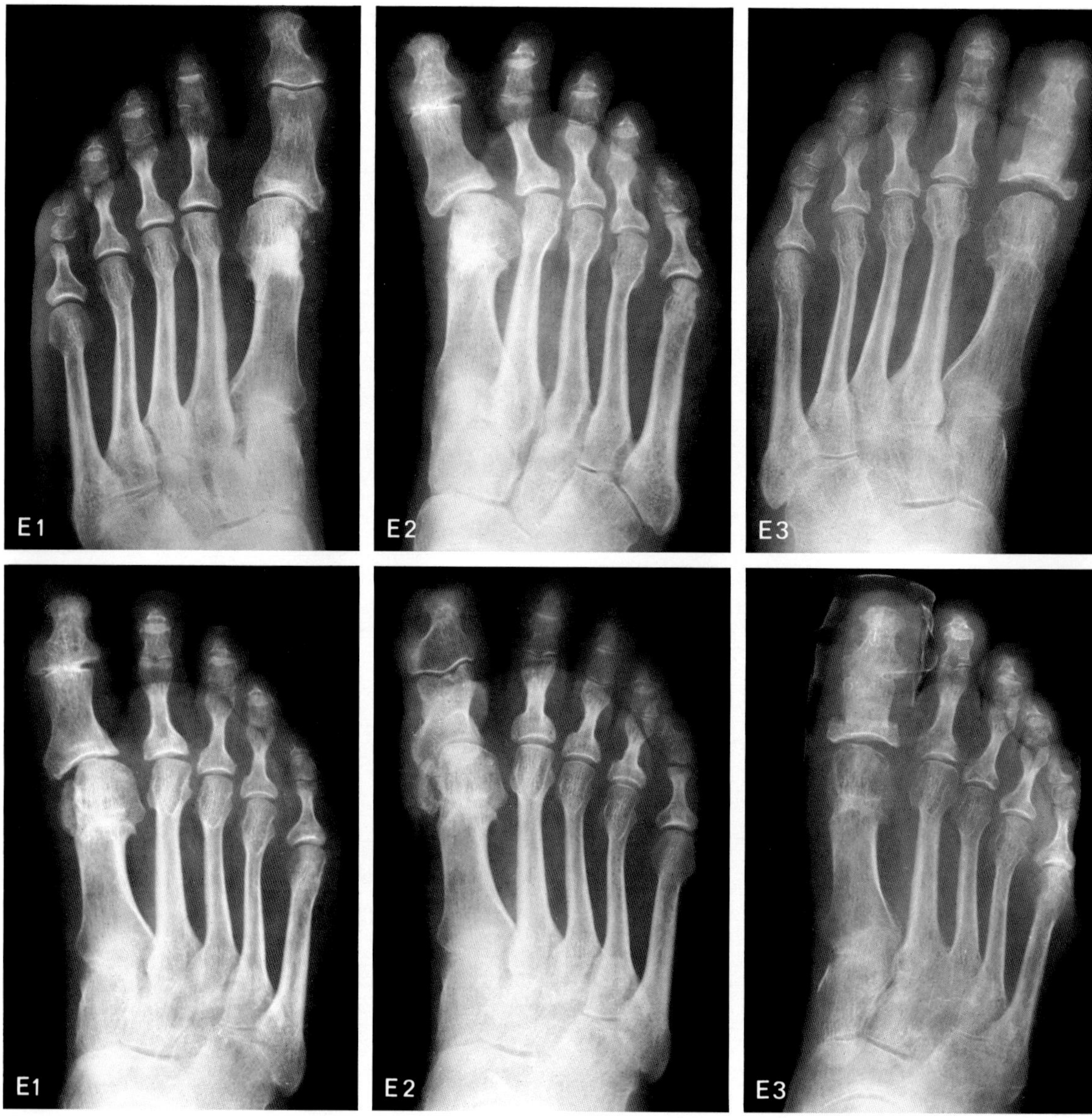

Fig. 25.5 *(continued).* **E** *1, 2* Sequelae of McBride operation: slight hallux varus *(1)* and extensus *(2)*, diminution of articular range of motion, pain on walking, overloading with callus formation under second metatarsal head; *3* after arthrolysis, metatarsophalangeal arthroplasty with hat-shaped graft, basal osteotomy of metatarsal. **F** *1* Sequelae of modified McBride operation: persistence of hallux valgus; *2* after correction of hallux valgus by metatarsophalangeal arthroplasty using cork-shaped graft. **G** First-degree hallux valgus. *1* Preoperative; ▷ *2* sequelae of Keller Brandes operation: painful contracture on account of insufficient resection from base of proximal phalanx, leading to convex forefoot; *3* after correction of hallux valgus by arthroplasty with hat-shaped graft, realignment of central three metatarsal heads by head-shaft enclavement; *4* iatrogenic arthroplasty with hat-shaped graft: interposition of cup prosthesis

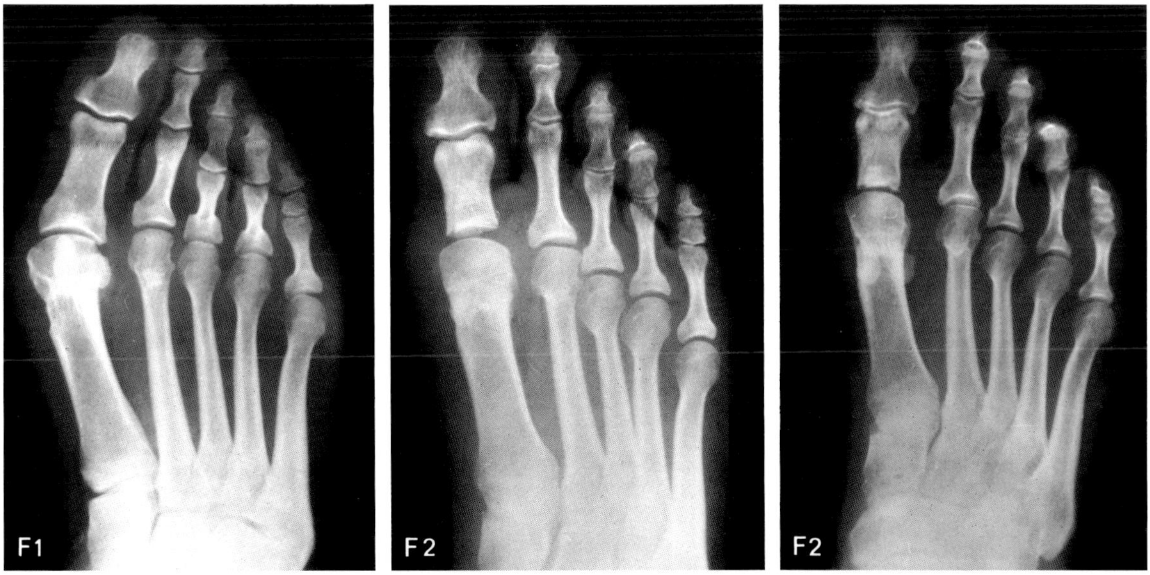

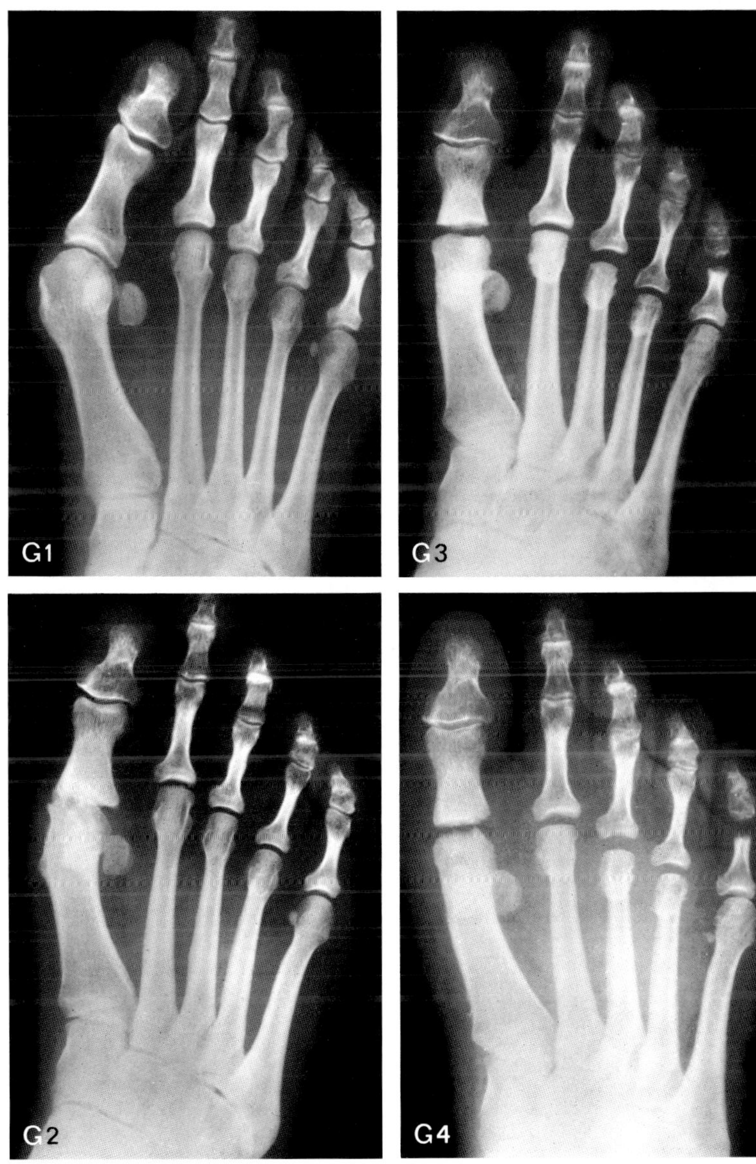

Fig. 25.5 F, G. Legend see p. 368

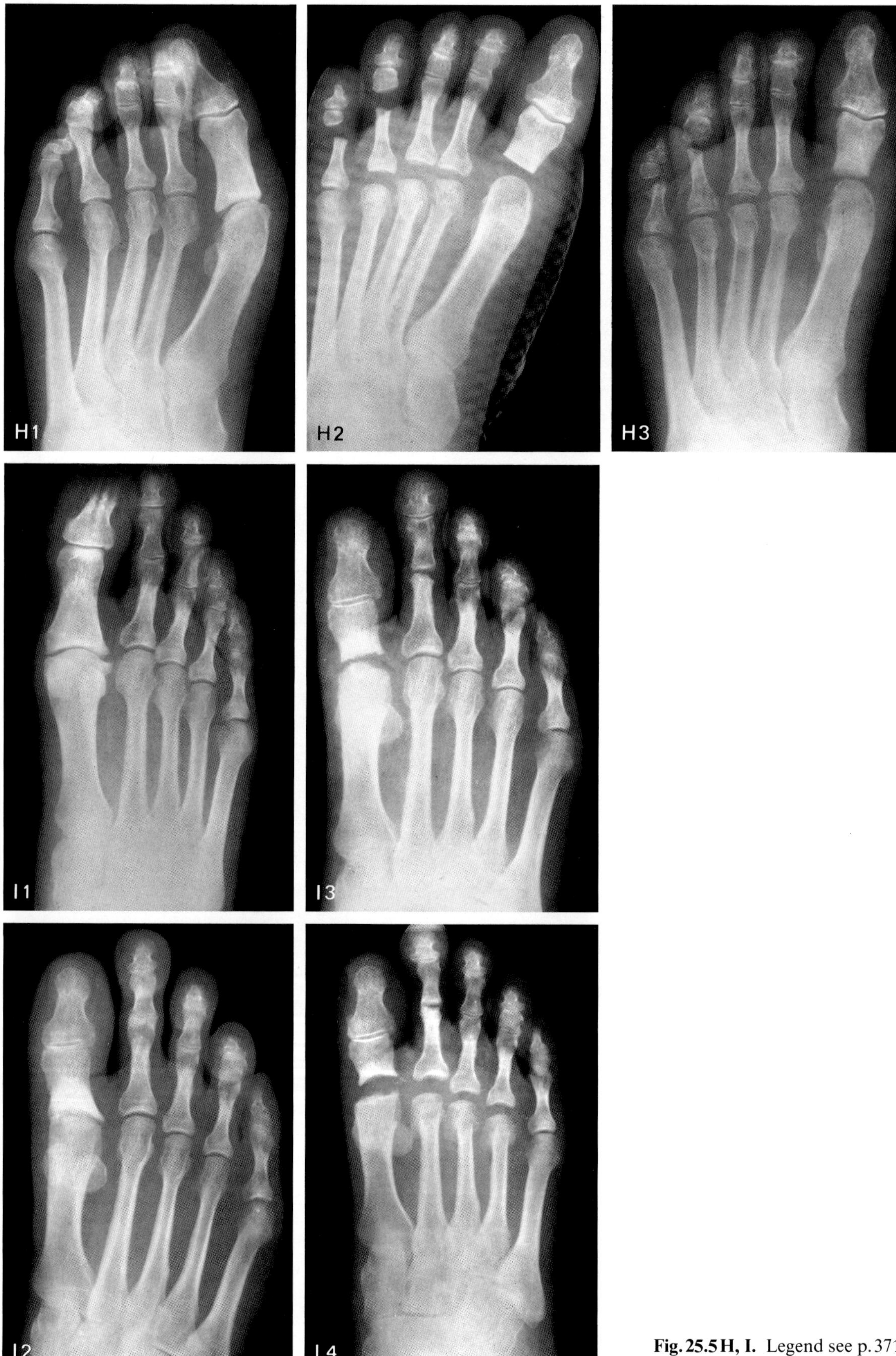

Fig. 25.5 H, I. Legend see p. 371

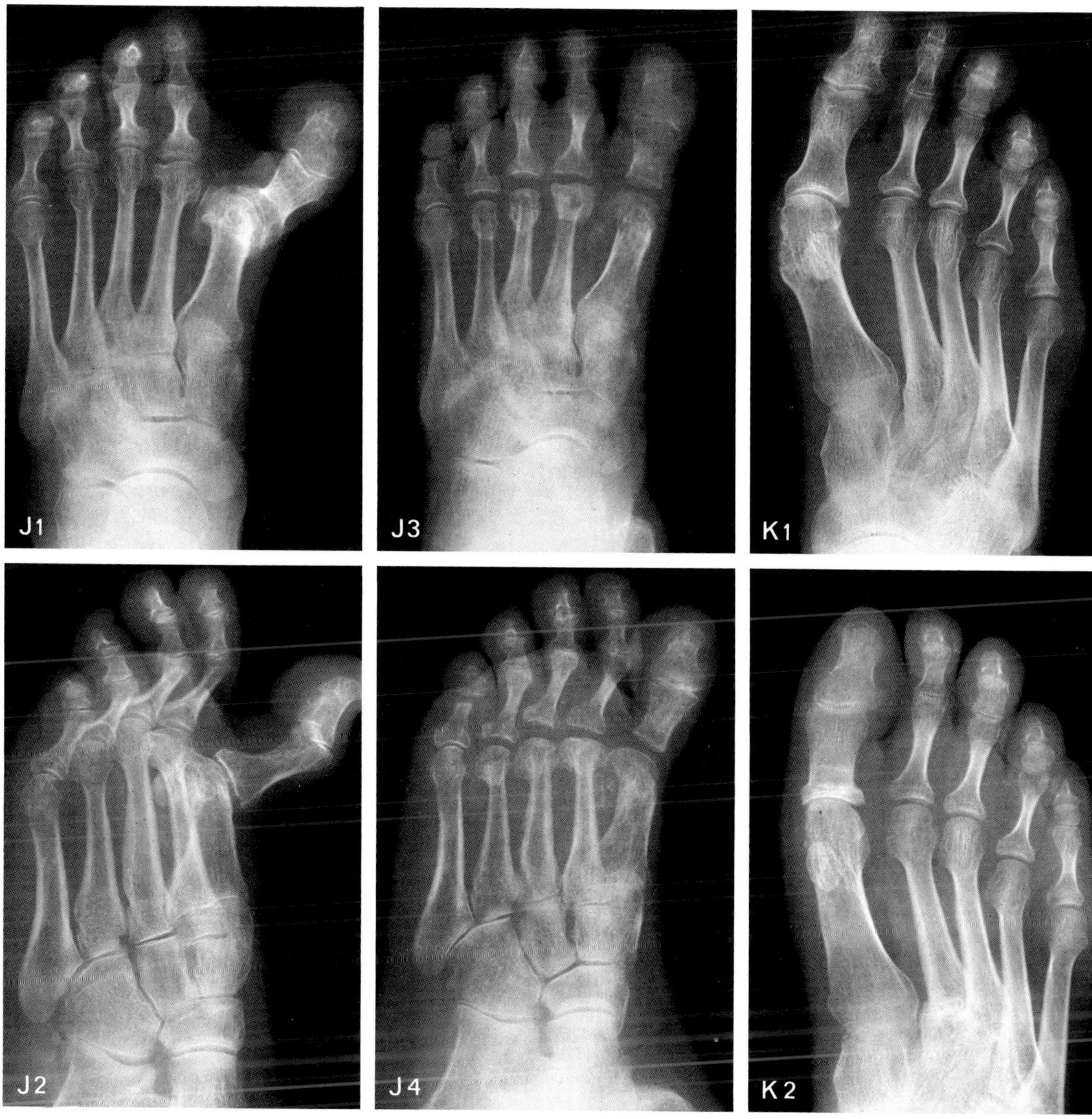

◁ **Fig. 25.5** *(continued)*. **H** *1* Sequelae of Schède operation: hallux valgus, convex forefoot, painful arthrosis; *2* after correction of hallux valgus by arthroplasty with cup prosthesis, realignment of central three metatarsal heads by head shaft enclavement; *3* good correction, adequate range of motion, normal forefoot loading. **I** First-degree hallux rigidus. *1* Preoperative; *2* ankylosing arthrosis after successive arthroplasties with insufficient resection of phalanx; *3* after arthroplasty of metatarsophalangeal joint with cup endoprosthesis: development of central metatarsalgia; *4* after removal of cup prosthesis and realignment of metatarsal heads by head-shaft enclavement: restoration of comfort and good range of movement. **J** *1, 2* Sequelae of Hueter-Mayo operation: arthrosic hallux varus, convex forefoot; *3, 4* after correction by arthroplasty using interposition cup prostheses, realignment of central three metatarsal heads by head-shaft enclavement. **K** *1* Sequelae of McBride operation: painful persistent hallux valgus; *2* after correction by metatarsophalangeal arthroplasty using hat-shaped graft

Elongation of extensor hallucis longus and the extensors of the other toes may be necessary.

25.4.2 *Damaged Cartilaginous Surface of Phalangeal Base*

The choice is between metatarsophalangeal arthroplasty by interpositional cup prosthesis and implantation of a homograft with interpositional cup prosthesis or cutaneous graft (de Wulf 1978) (Fig. 25.6). The forward convexity of the great metatarsal head should be corrected, and as before, attention to the loading of the central three metatarsal heads is important.

25.4.3 *Gross Resection of Metatarsal Head*

As much as a third or even a half of the metatarsal may have been excised (Fig. 25.7). The condition is unstable and hypermobile with severe convex forefoot formation. The second metatarsal head may project some 20 mm beyond the remaining part of the first metatarsal. Severe problems of overloading will occur, with corns and callosities or even ulceration. Claw deformities of the middle three toes develop, and contractures of the metatarsophalangeal and interphalangeal joint capsules and the associated tendons and skin complete a sorry picture.
Surgical management comprises correction of the convex forefoot by means of arthroplasty in order to restore the function of the great metatarsophalangeal joint. Attention must be directed to the proximal phalanx and the first metatarsal itself.
With regard to the proximal phalanx, operative intervention may not be necessary, but if the articular cartilage is intact and there is significant valgus of the toe (this must be corrected), the phalangeal base may be used as an autograft. If the cartilage is damaged, insertion of a phalangeal autograft, after removal of the superficial cartilaginous surface using the technique described by Valenti is appropriate. If the base of the phalanx is severely damaged, interposition of a cup prosthesis may be the only solution.
As regards the first metatarsal, when the length of the remaining bone allows, it may be possible to preserve as much as possible by means of trimming and modelling the head appropriately and then shortening the outer four metatarsals by enclavement. This is only acceptable when it does not result in too much loss of length of the antetarsus. In more extreme cases, when more than a third or even a half of the length of the first metatarsal has been lost, correction of the round forefoot cannot be achieved in this way, and lengthening of the first metatarsal is necessary. While insertion of a prosthesis is a possibility, much preferable is the implantation of an iliac graft modelled so as to reconstitute the bone and adapt its length to suit that of the outer metatarsals, which may have to be shortened somewhat by enclavement (Fig. 25.7 D).

Operative Technique. A graft of some 40–60 mm in length and 15–20 mm in diameter is taken from the region of the anterior superior iliac spine. The end of the graft is modelled so as to resemble the shape of a metatarsal condyle 15–20 mm in diameter and 15–30 mm in length. The proximal end of the graft is fashioned so as to provide a spike 30–40 mm in length, the diameter of which is tailored to the exact dimension of the medullary canal of the stump of the first metatarsal. The spike inserted into the medullary canal provides adequate stability, and after restoration of the length of the first metatarsal, realignment enclavement of the central three metatarsal heads should be performed (Regnauld 1968).
In extreme cases, when even more of the first metatarsal has been lost, perfect realignment of the forefoot is impossible and the only solution is the continuous use of a monoblock insole with a retrocapital bar and a Martorell anterocapital bar.

25.5 Metatarsophalangeal Complications of Lesser Toes

Painful arthrosis may result after unsuccessful treatment of Freiberg-Köhler osteochondritis by head-shaft enclavement. If the joint had been affected by rheumatoid arthritis or ankylosing spondylitis, osteolysis or pseudarthrosis of the enclaved head may develop subsequent to operation, perhaps due to walking too early or to trauma.
Operative correction comprises reshaping of the metatarsal head using an interposition cup prosthesis. Exceptionally, a metatarsal prosthesis may be necessary, careful realignment of load bearing of the metatarsal heads being assured.

25.6 Resection of Metatarsal Heads of Lesser Toes

Symptoms are produced by displacement of the toes in various directions, rigidity at the fibrosed metatarsophalangeal joint regions, irregular osteophyte formation, and the formation of plantar calluses under the stumps of the amputated metatarsal heads (Fig. 25.8 A, C).

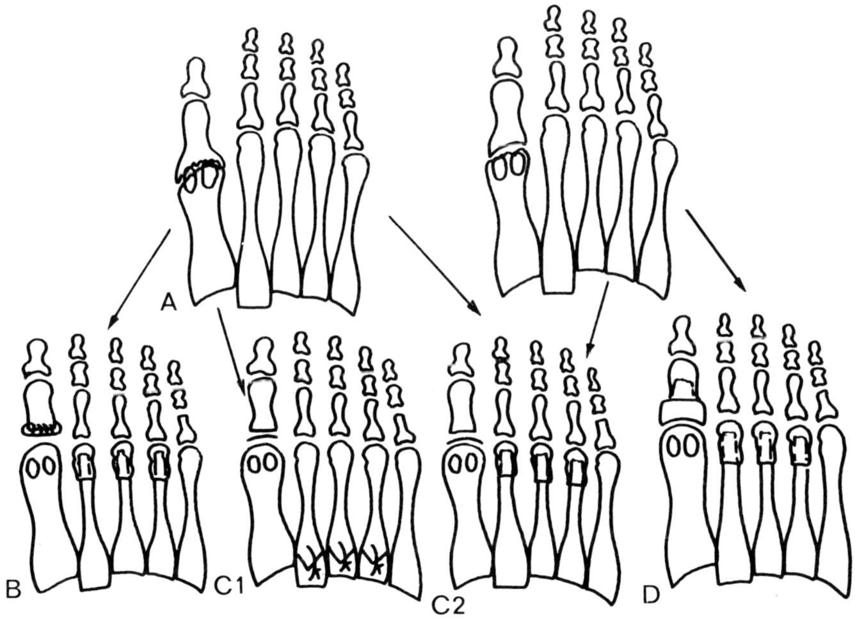

Fig. 25.6 A–D. Treatment of sequelae of Hueter-Mayo operation. **A** Before further treatment. **B** Cutaneous arthroplasty (de Wulf). **C** Cup arthroplasty accompanied by *1* metatarsal osteotomies or *2* enclavement realignment of central three metatarsal heads (Thys). **D** Arthroplasty by graft without cartilage (Valente) and enclavement realignment of central three metatarsal heads

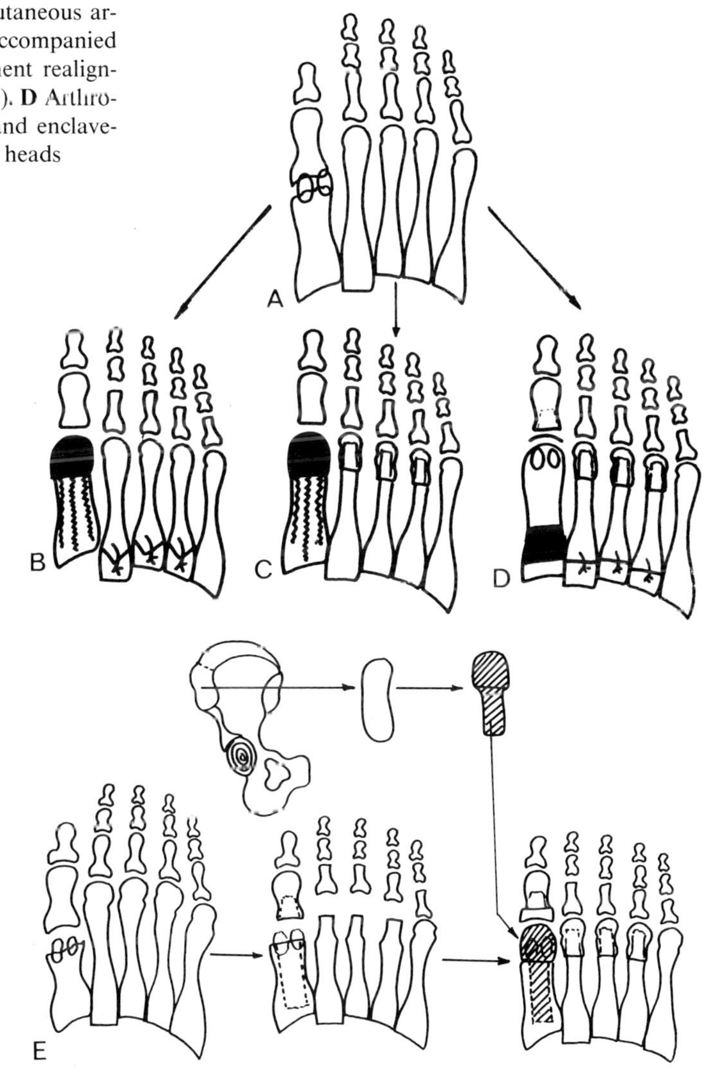

Fig. 25.7 A–D. Treatment of shortened first metatarsal **A** Sequelae of Hueter-Mayo operation. **B** Destruction of base of proximal phalanx, loss of distal third of metatarsal. Treatment: limited resection of base of proximal phalanx, insertion of metatarsal prosthesis (Regnauld) and either *1* metatarsal osteotomies (Thys) or 3 enclavement realignment of central three metatarsal heads (Regnauld). **C** Base of phalanx intact, loss of more than one-third of metatarsal shaft Treatment: arthroplasty using cork-shaped or hat-shaped graft and cup prosthesis, metatarsal prosthesis for great ray, enclavement realignment or metatarsal osteotomies of central three rays. **D** Implantation of an iliac graft. **E** Implantations of an iliac graft

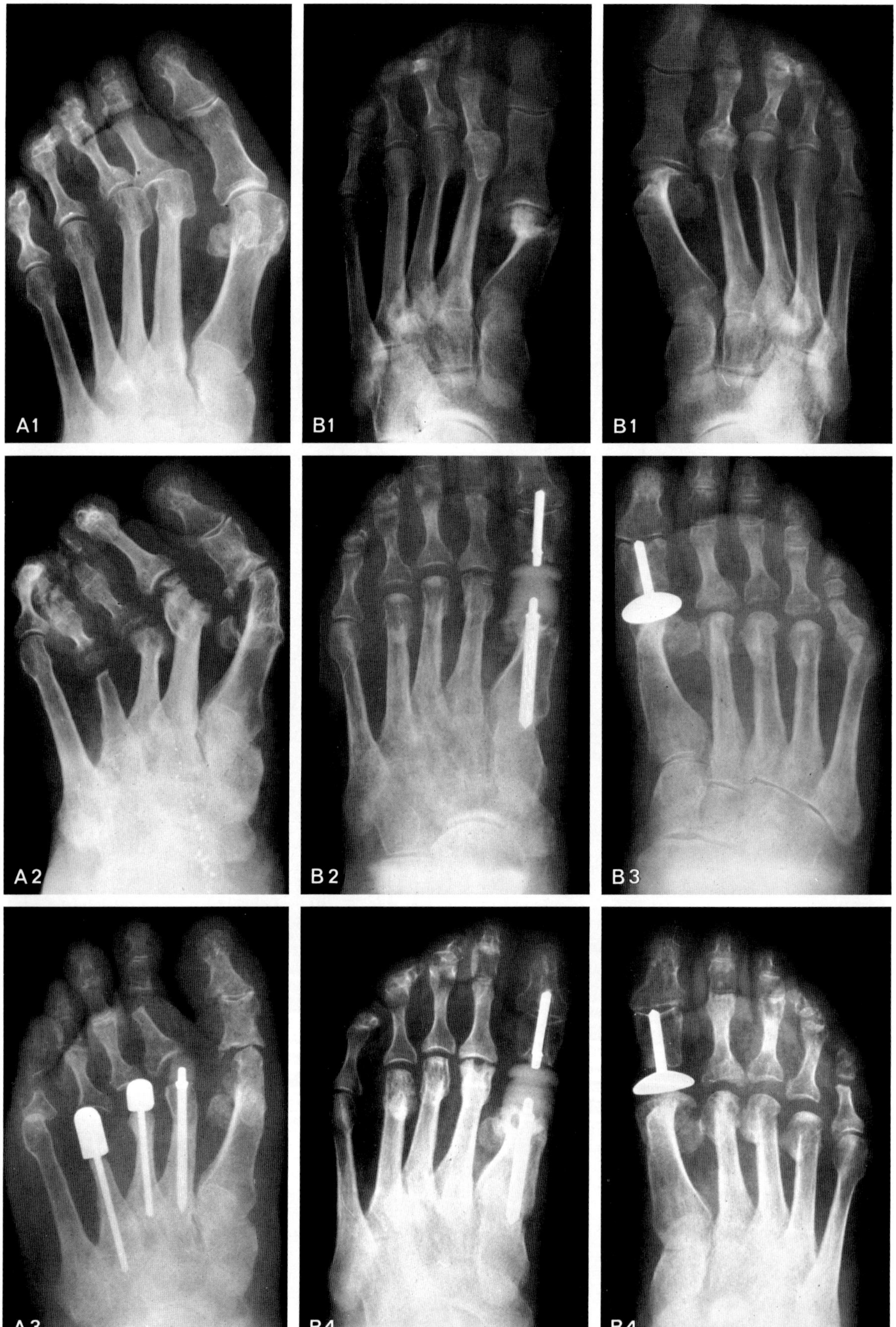
A1
B1
B1
A2
B2
B3
A3
B4
B4

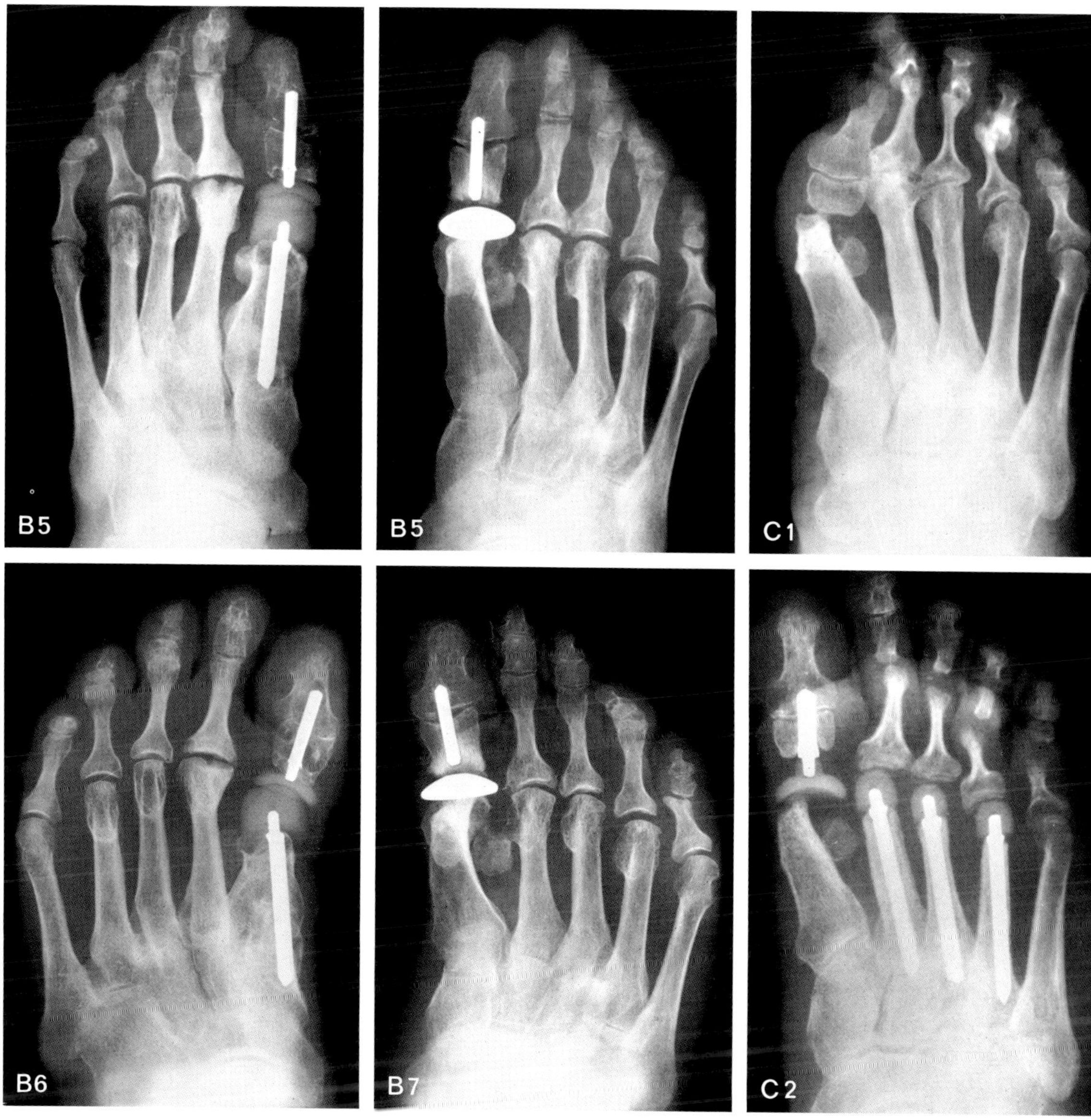

◁ **Fig. 25.8 A–F.** Painful forefoot syndromes following unsuccessful operative procedures. **A** Convex triangular forefoot with second-degree hallux valgus, metatarsalgia with central callus formation, claw toes. *1* Preoperative; *2* after resection of metatarsophalangeal joints: irregular deformities; *3* after reconstitution of metatarsophalangeal joints by correction of hallux valgus, implantation of metatarsal head prostheses. **B** *1* Sequelae of Hueter-Mayo resection of first metatarsal head: convex forefoot; *2, 3* reconstitution by realignment of metatarsal heads by enclavement, implantation of prostheses, tendinous elongation: *2* left foot, 1974; *3* right foot, 1975; *4* appearance 1975; *5* appearance 1977: good realignment of metatarsophalangeal joint, excellent mobility; *6, 7* appearance 1981: despite morphological alterations of metatarsal heads on left side, excellent function, painless loading, and subject was able to walk 4 km each day. **C** *1* Sequelae of Lelièvre realignment with irregular resections; *2* after reconstitution of forefoot by realignment and insertion of articular prostheses which allow uniformity of loading and comfort. **D–F** see pp. 376, 377

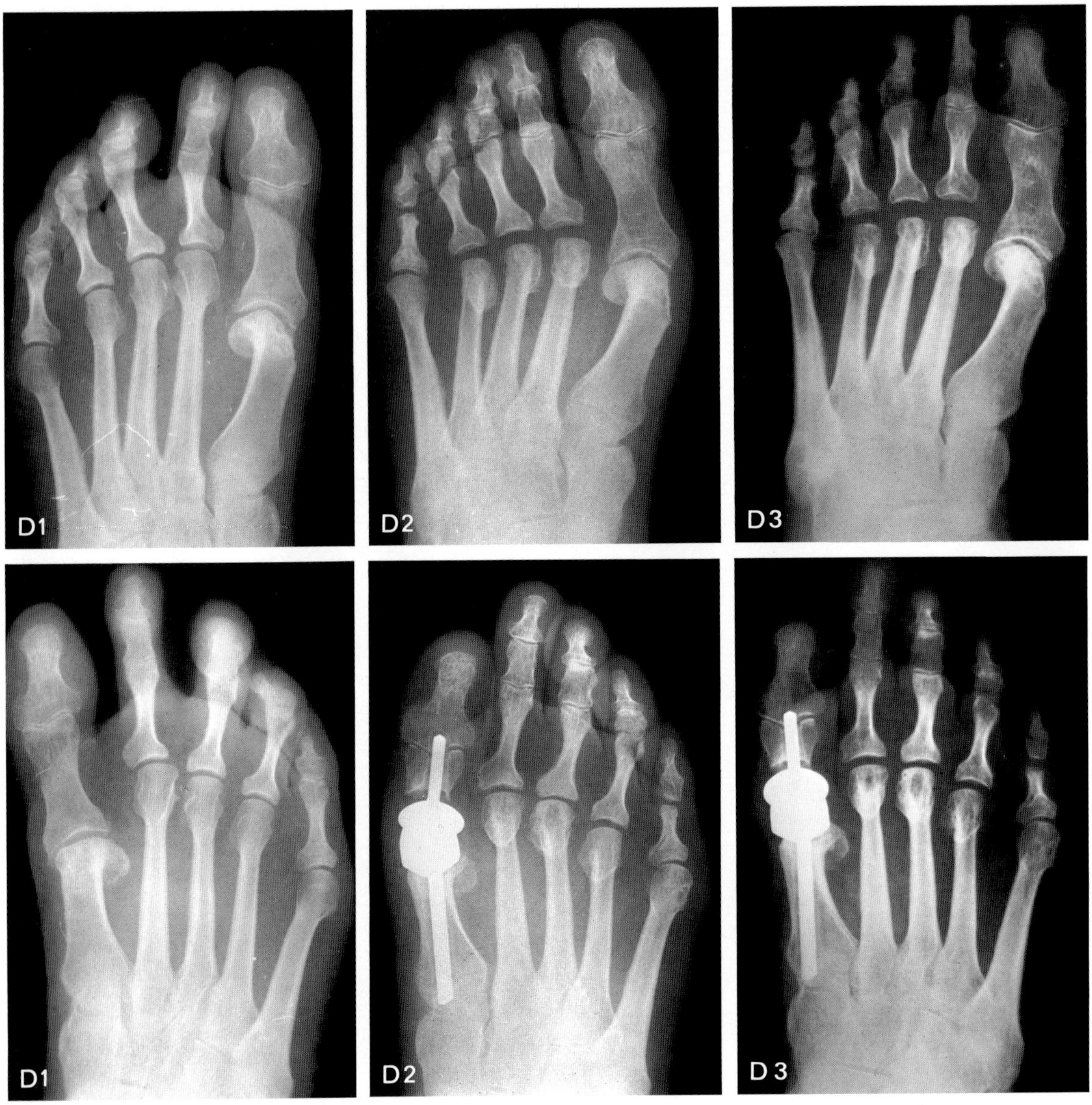

Fig. 25.8 *(continued)*. **D** *1* Sequelae of operative treatment: convex forefoot metatarsalgia under central metatarsal heads, median callosity formation, walking impossible; *2* 1977: realignment of central three metatarsals by head-shaft enclavement, on the right side articular prostheses; *3* postoperative; *4* appearance 1978; *5* appearance 1980: on left side good realignment of metatarsals, but on right side some alteration in shape of middle of third metatarsal head. Despite latter, loading pain-free and gait satisfactory. **E** *1* Sequelae of Hueter-Mayo operation: convex forefoot, central callus formation, painful arthrosis of first metatarsophalangeal joint; *2* after modified Burutaran operation (elongation of first metatarsal, arthroplasty of first metatarsophalangeal joint using cork-shaped graft); *3* good loading-bearing distribution of forefoot and mobility of first metatarsophalangeal joint. **F** *1* Sequelae of Hueter-Mayo procedure: convex forefoot, central callosity formation with metatarsalgia; *2* after metatarsophalangeal arthroplasty using hat-shaped graft, head-shaft enclavement of central three metatarsals ▷

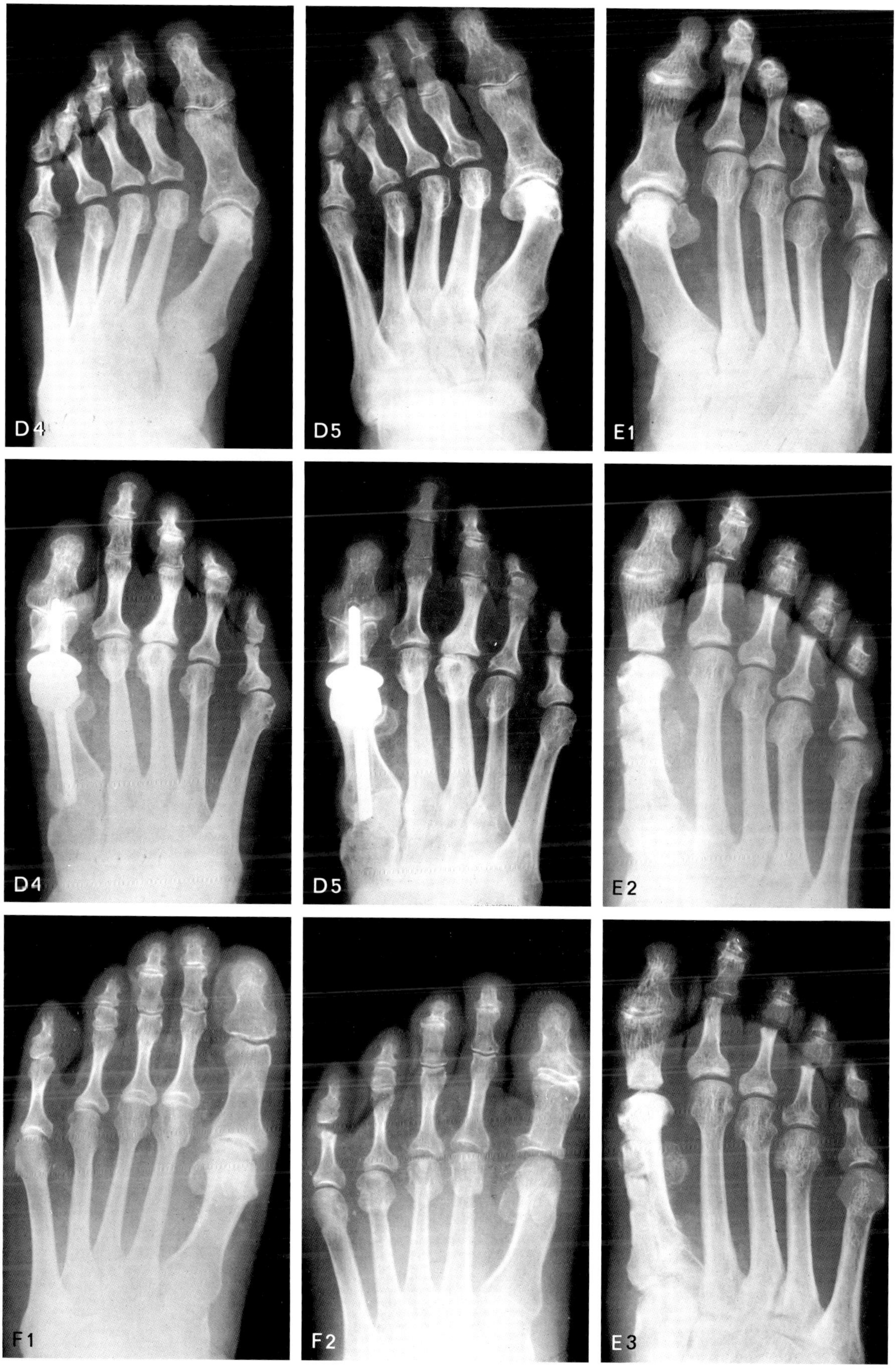
D4
D5
E1
D4
D5
E2
F1
F2
E3

Treatment comprises arthroplasty by careful excision of the osteophyte formations, detachment of the residual joint capsules and elongation of the associated flexor and extensor tendons followed by the insertion of homografts by enclavement onto the metatarsal stumps or by the implantation of cup prostheses so as to reform a joint (Figs. 25.9, 25.10). Subsequently, relative equinus of other metatarsals must be corrected by osteotomy or enclavement. The combination of different excisions in these cases necessitates an individual approach to every foot for obvious reasons. Sometimes surgery must be complemented by permanent use of supporting insoles.

In the case of resection of all three central metatarsal heads, iatrogenic cavus forefoot is likely to develop (see Chap. 9.3).

25.7 Hohmann-Wallet Procedure

The treatment of the distressing sequelae of the Hohmann-Wallet procedure is summarised in Fig. 25.11.

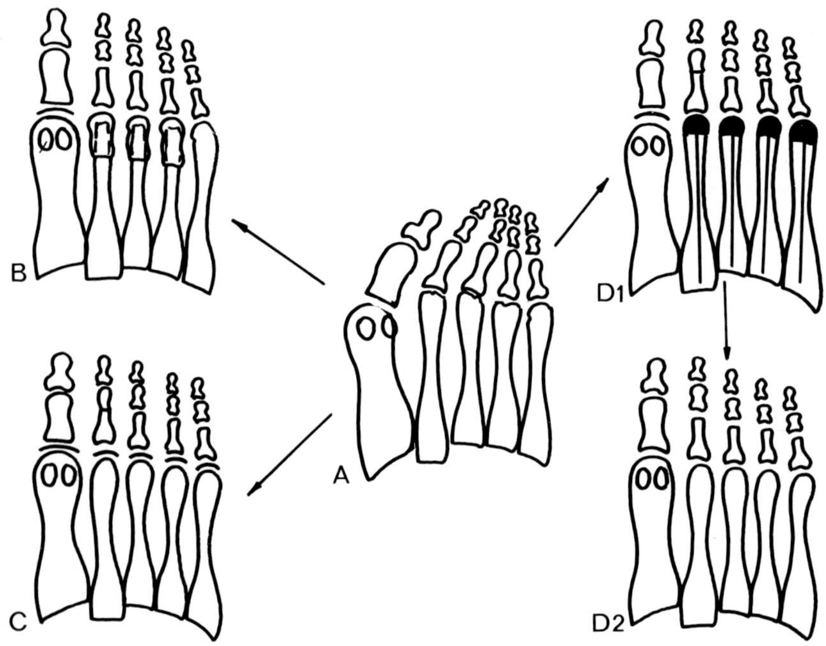

Fig. 25.9. A Sequel of Lelièvre realignment procedure. **B** Enclavement homografts of central three metatarsal heads and insertion of cup prosthesis in first ray (Regnauld). **C** Cup arthroplasty of all five rays. **D** *1* Metatarsal prostheses of second to fifth rays and cup arthroplasty of first ray; *2* removal of prostheses after 1 year

Fig. 25.11 A–D. Sequel of Hohmann-Wallet procedure. **A** Before further treatment. **B** After metatarsal homografts. **C** After realignment of metatarsals (Lelièvre) and cup arthroplasties. **D** After insertion of metatarsal head prostheses (and basal osteotomies if necessary) ▷

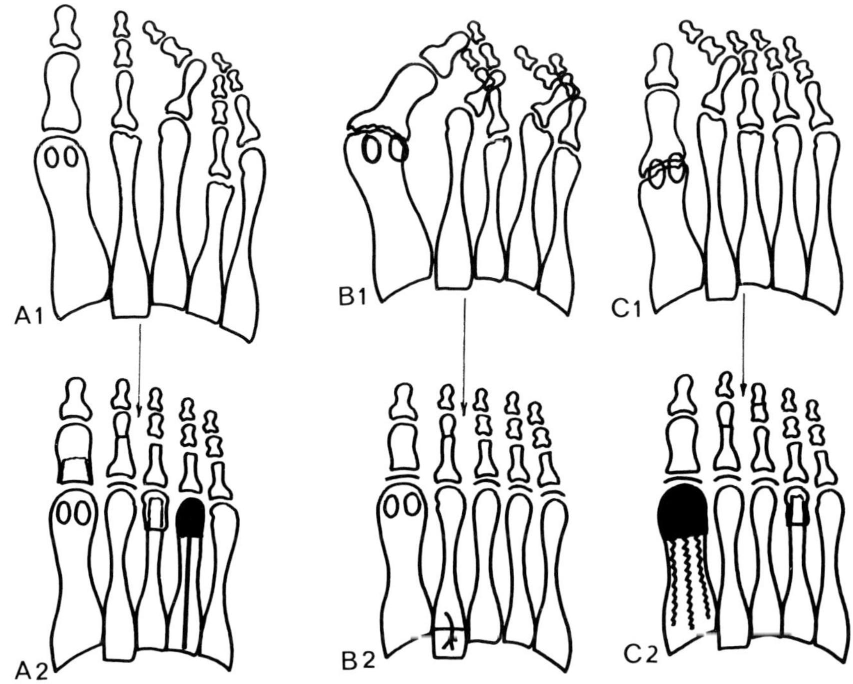

Fig. 25.10 A–C. Examples of sequelae of poorly executed attempts at realignment. **A** *1* Before re-operation; *2* after autograft arthroplasty in great ray, remodelling and cup arthroplasty of second metatarsophalangeal joint, realignment enclavement of third metatarsophalangeal joint, insertion of metatarsal prosthesis in fourth ray. **B** *1* Before re-operation; *2* after cup arthroplasty of great metatarsophalangeal joint, realignment of second metatarsal (Lelièvre), remodelling (Clayton), cup arthroplasty of lesser metatarsophalangeal joints and metatarsal basal osteotomy if necessary. **C** Sequelae of Hueter-Mayo operation: *1* Before re-operation; *2* after insertion of metatarsal prosthesis in first ray, cup arthroplasty in first to third rays, selective realignment of second and third metatarsals, realignment enclavement in fourth ray, arthroplasty or arthrodesis of interphalangeal joints as indicated

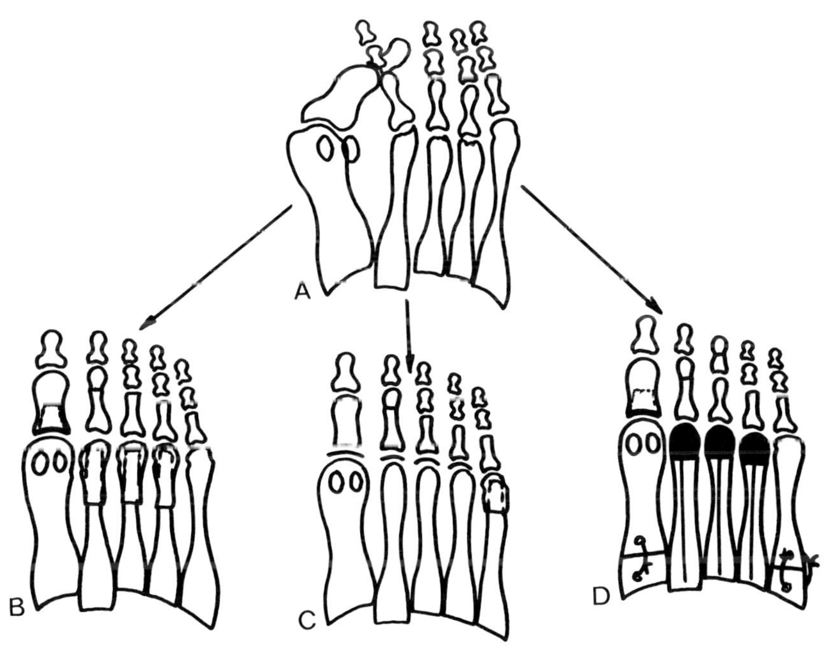

IV Congenital Abnormalities

Congenital abnormalities of the foot may be divided into displacements, malformations, and the presence of supernumerary bones.
Congenital displacements (Chap. 26) are normal postures of components of the foot present at birth and probably associated with abnormalities of pressure in utero. Laurence (1966) attributes most cases to prolonged immobilisation of the foetus in an abnormal position on account of the environment. He classifies the displacements as follows:

Simple unidirectional: pes talus, pes valgus, pes varus and pes adductus
Complex multidirectional: pes equinovarus and congenital vertical talus (convex flat foot)

Congenital malformations (Chap. 27) are anomalies of structural development directly dependent upon genetic factors which are ill understood. They may be classified as follows:

Aplasia: ectrodactyly, ectrometatarsia and ectropodia
Hypoplasia: micropodia and brachypodia
Hyperplasia: macropodica, macrometatarsia and macrodactyly
Polyplasia: polymetatarsia and polydactyly
Symplasia: syndactyly and synostosis
Congenital deviations: clinodactyly (permanent deviation in one direction) and camptodactyly (permanent flexion of digits)

Os intermetatarseum (Chap. 28) is a supernumerary bone which occurs with sufficient frequency to warrant brief discussion.

26 Congenital Displacements

26.1 Pes Talus

In pes talus (sometimes called pes calcaneus), there is persistent hyperdorsiflexion of the foot usually neutral with respect to the leg (simple talus) but sometimes associated with some valgus of the subtalar joint (talovalgus).

26.1.1 Etiology

Pes talus is probably associated with oligohydramnios or a narrow pelvis. The foot is compressed against the anterior border of the leg until birth, when it presents in this posture. The condition may be unilateral or bilateral (Fig. 26.1).

26.1.2 Clinical Features

Spontaneous plantarflexion is absent in the affected infant. On attempted plantarlexion the foot displays obvious tendinous contracture anteriorly with bowstringing under the dorsal skin and sometimes dislocation of the peronei in front of the lateral malleolus. The plantar aspect of the foot may face forwards; if there is an associated valgus component, however, it faces outwards. It appears flat or convex and is abnormally elongated on account of the prominence of the heel (varus component is very uncommon with the talus). The anterior border of the foot sometimes leaves an imprint on the tibia, provoking a tibial recurvatum. When viewed from its plantar aspect, the foot tapers from a broad metatarsus anteriorly to a narrow heel but the general axis is directly in line with that of the tibia.

Stretching of triceps surae leads to flaccidity on palpation, and excitation of the muscle provokes only a small contractile response.

Tenting of overlying skin is due to the contraction of tendons internally (tibialis anterior and tibialis posterior), centrally (extensor hallucis longus and extensor digitorum longus) and laterally (the peronei, sometimes with dislocation).

Radiography shows the morphological integrity of the skeletal components of the foot with the general dorsiflexed posture, particularly of the talus, with which the metatarsals are in alignment. The calcaneum appears to be displaced forwards with lowering of its body.

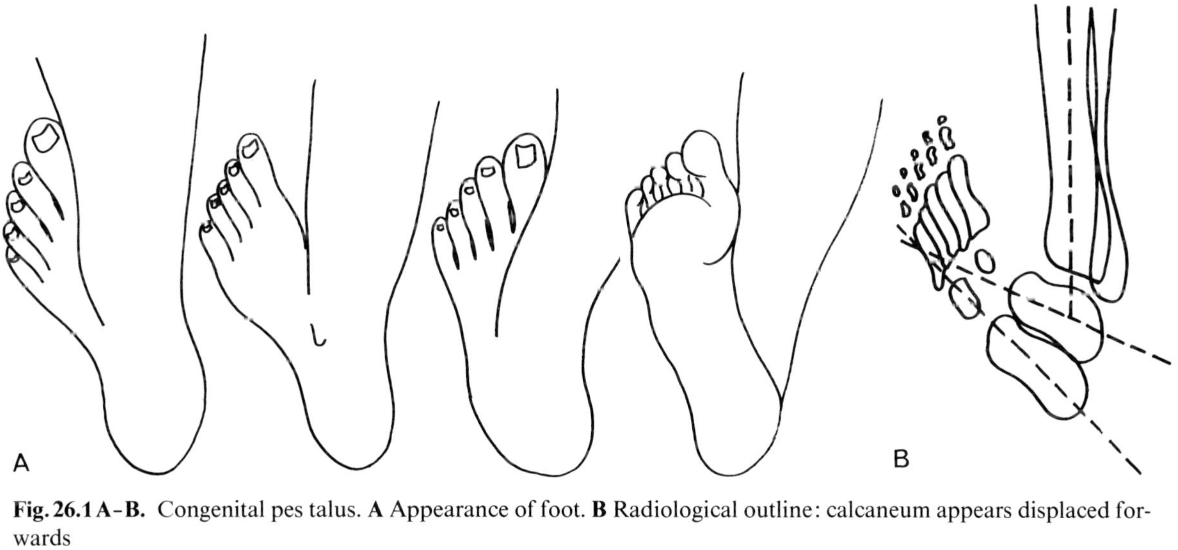

Fig. 26.1 A–B. Congenital pes talus. **A** Appearance of foot. **B** Radiological outline: calcaneum appears displaced forwards

26.1.3 Treatment

Pes talus is a benign condition which can be corrected very easily provided appropriate measures are undertaken within the first few days. In the absence of treatment, cutaneous, tendinous and capsular contractions can become irreversible and render the condition resistant to correction.

Conservative. Conservative management comprising manipulation is usually successful (Fig. 26.2). This should begin as soon as possible after birth and be progressive, gentle and purely corrective; the whole foot should be maintained by the manipulator's index finger supporting the plantar aspect of the heel to the toes so as to avoid a false correction at the midtarsal region and a consequent posterior cavus. Progressively, over perhaps 15–20 days, restoration of a normal range of movement is achieved. Treatment should be completed by the application of a plaster of Paris boot or a simple splint as described by Saint Germain. These devices should be worn after each manipulation, thereby maintaining the correction obtained, at least 90° or 100° plantarflexion with respect to the axis of the leg.
Bensahel recommends that manipulation should be succeeded by active exercises with active re-education of muscles which have been stretched or relaxed thereby reassuring proper balance of the ankle. Electrophysiotherapy may help. Bensahel (1977) described an orthosis exerting elastic traction to the foot into plantarflexion which allows early kinesitherapy and spontaneous rapid mobilisation. Restoration of an adequate range of movement and power assures future normal gait.

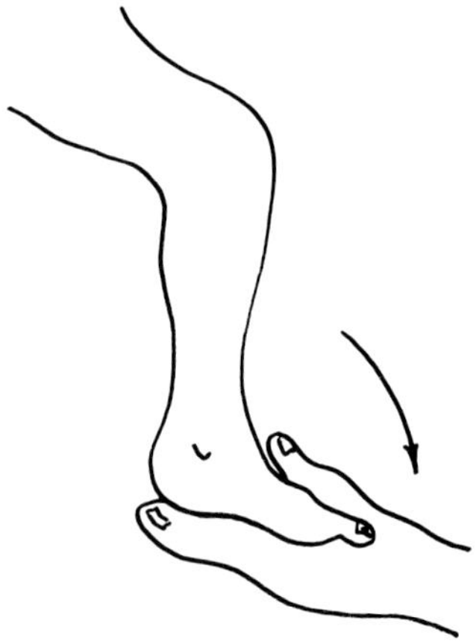

Fig. 26.2. Congenital pes talus: treatment by manipulation

Operative. It is rare that operative treatment is needed, as the conservative measures detailed above are usually successful. In the resistant case, the following measures are necessary: Elongation of contracted tendons of the antero-external compartment (tibialis anterior and the toe extensors), reduction of dislocation of the peronei and repositioning them in their retromalleolar gutter (the Lannelongue operation), shortening of tendo Achillis when re-education of triceps surae proves inefficacious and hemitransplantation of the tendon of peroneus brevis and extensor hallucis longus to tendo Achillis if there is a deficiency of triceps power. In the adult or adolescent it is rare to find pes talus, but the condition may occur, however, in the presence of a posterior cavus foot with extreme elongation or paralysis of tendo Achillis. In such instances, operation comprises (a) arthrolysis of the ankle joint associated if necessary with subtalar cuneiform wedge resection with the base positioned posteriorly, thereby correcting the talus position of the calcaneus and (b) midtarsal wedge resection with the base plantarwards if there is an associated pes planus or with a dorsal base if there is a midtarsal cavus. To this bony adjustment, the tendons must be corrected by, as appropriate, either shortening of tendo Achillis or reinforcement of tendo Achillis by transplantation to it of peroneus brevis, flexor hallucis longus or tibialis posterior.

26.2 Pes Valgus

26.2.1 Description

Pes valgus can exist in isolation, and is most frequently the consequence of external rotation of the lower limb, possibly associated with a habitual prone position during sleep. There is general abduction of the longitudinal axis of the foot relative to the normal axis of horizontal propulsion, valgus of the heel and midtarsus and sometimes associated genu valgum.

26.2.2 Treatment

This postural abnormality should be corrected early, because it may lead to pes planovalgus or genu valgum of a more marked degree. Treatment is essentially conservative, comprising manipulations, corrective splints, the wearing of a supple shoe with a high shank and perhaps the use of corrective stimulating insoles for the first 6 months of life.

26.3 Pes Varus

26.3.1 Description

Pes varus is relatively common. It often occurs unperceived, as the convexity of the external border of the foot and the slight adduction of the forefoot only become apparent on walking. When walking commences, however, the disturbance due to intoeing attracts the parents' attention. A high-shank shoe usually corrects the posture and provokes normal gait.

There is general varus of the foot with adduction of the midtarsus, forefoot and toes, exaggerated internal concavity and external convexity of the foot generally and a normal transverse position of the tarsus (but sometimes a vertically disposed calcaneum). Usually there is decreased tone of the peroneal muscles.

Radiography confirms the slight adduction of the midtarsus. The metatarsus is in line with the midtarsus and there is no metatarsus varus.

26.3.2 Treatment

Conservative management should be initiated as early as possible because the condition can become associated with a varus calcaneum. Manipulation, re-education of the peronei and the use of a Saint Germain splint re-establishes normal posture in most instances. At the age of walking, the wearing of a shoe with an internal extended border associated with a pronating anterior wedge, beginning as soon as walking commences, achieves correction by the age of 1 year.

In the occasional case when, despite these measures, the varus persists, surgical management is necessary. It takes the form of calcaneal osteotomy (Dwyer 1959) involving removal of a wedge with the base externally, thereby re-establishing the lateral equilibrium of the tarsus.

26.4 Pes Adductus

26.4.1 Description

The adduction posture stems from the tarsometatarsal joint line (Fig. 26.3). There is a marked vertically aligned groove on the inner border of the foot and a comparable convexity at the cuboidometatarsal region.

In most instances the hindfoot is normal and the tarsus is aligned with the leg. However two variants exist:

1. *Pes planovalgus*. This form (Fig. 26.48) was described by Dengler (1936). In addition to the associated valgus posture of the calcaneum, there is digital divergence, most marked in the first commissure due to particular adduction of the first ray; there is only light varus or normal alignment of the other toes (e.g. Fig. 16.17).
2. *Pes cavovarus*. The calcaneum is in varus and there is cavus of the metatarsus, i.e. inversion of the tarsus and of the metatarsus varus. This relates to an incompletely corrected equinovarus club foot. The condition usually affects the great metatarsal predominantly, progressively diminishing across the foot to the fifth metatarsal. It is often associated with limitation of dorsiflexion of the ankle joint, in which case it represents compensation by the forefoot.

The appearance is striking because the foot is short. It seems compressed at the Lisfranc joint line

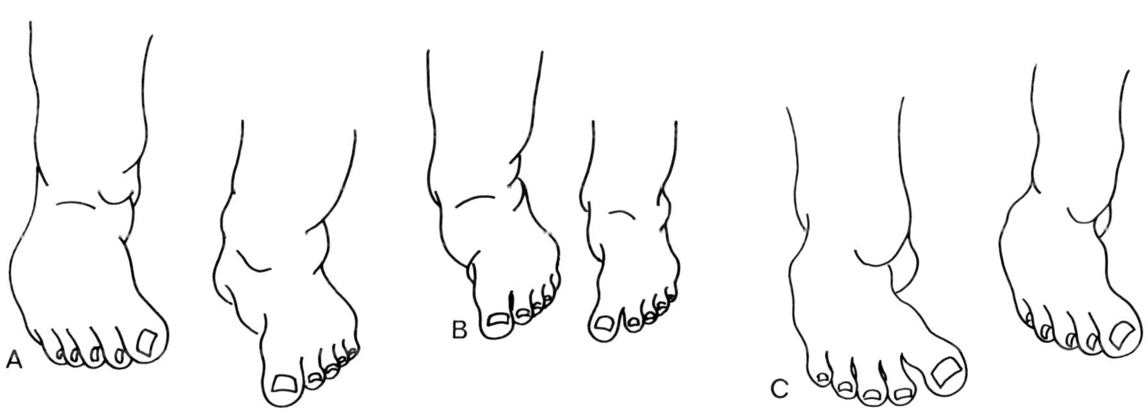

Fig. 26.3. A Isolated pes adductus with normal tarsus. **B** Pes adductus with planovalgus deformity. **C** Pes adductus following congenital equinovarus club foot

with widening of the forefoot, which is usually in valgus and adducted. The hypertrophy of the tarsometatarsal region leads to the inversion of the forefoot in cavovarus and adduction. The pes adductus may be simple or, as mentioned above, may present with flattening of the longitudinal arch or in the varus form, the sequel of a club foot.

Fairly frequently there is valgus of the tarsus and lowering of the midtarsus. Dengler (1936) emphasises this feature, which is seen during walking and is much commoner in males. In other instances, there is cavovarus affecting the tarsometatarsal region and inversion of the forefoot, entailing adduction, pronation and equinus of varying degrees affecting the first metatarsal. This is the inadequately corrected equinovarus club foot.

Whatever the original cause, the pes adductus or the metatarsus varus affect the configuration of the tarsometatarsal joint and the internal displacement of the antetarsus generally. The orientation of the transverse axis of the tarsometatarsal joint is more oblique than normal in relation to the long axis of the foot. The conformation of the articular planes of the tarsometatarsal joint is such that the cartilaginous surfaces look forwards, increasingly lower and outwards from the first to the fifth rays, and there is paradoxical displacement of the antetarsus into adduction; this stems from angulation of the base of each metatarsal and from rotation of the metatarsals on their longitudinal axes, these deformities increasing progressively from the first to the fifth metatarsals.

Previously regarded as a rare malformation, pes adductus has been described by numerous authors: Cramer, Helburg, Jochimspahl, Hirsch, Frohlich, Blumenphal and Broca. The classical form, i.e. pure pes adductus, was described by Laurence and Bensahel.

26.4.2 Clinical Features

The child is usually brought for consultation because its parents are worried by its clumsy gait, frequent falls, tangling of the feet together, difficulty in shoes and tendency to turn the feet inwardly.

Characteristic features are the convexity of the external borders with hypertrophy of the cuboid, which may appear subluxed outwardly, a dorsal curve marked by projection in staircase fashion of the bases of the metatarsals, and the folding of the internal border at the tarsometatarsal joint, marked by a vertical groove. The presence of associated planovalgus or cavovarus (perhaps with adduction and equinus of varying degrees) distinguishes the two variants detailed above. In the incompletely corrected equinovarus club foot, there may be hypertonia and contracture of the abductor of the great toe.

The forefoot adduction is variably obvious and accompanied by a straight appearance of the first metatarsal, which is both adducted and in slight supination. The central metatarsals are curved slightly downwards and inwards, while the fifth metatarsal is straight, adducted and lies, unusually, below the adjacent fourth metatarsal. After the age of 6 years, a characteristic staircase appearance may present at the bases of the metatarsals due to internal angulation at the diaphyso-epiphyseal junctions.

On palpation, there is no hypertrophy of the leg muscles, but contracture of the abductor of the great toe. Often, the great toe is hypermobile and prehensile, the child being able to grasp objects. The absence of contracture of triceps surae is apparent except in cases of relapsed or incompletely treated equinovarus club foot or the association of pes planus. The calcaneum is in the correct position and posture, and there is no tarsal varus. The ankle joint is normal, and the posterior intertarsal joints are only involved in the case of varus club foot. There is contracture of the plantar aponeurosis. The long and short peroneal muscles are usually weak.

Radiography shows the degree of metatarsus varus, the disturbance of posture between the metatarsals and toes, the curvature in equinus and varus of the middle metatarsals, the adduction and sometimes equinus of the great metatarsal (if this is a cavovarus foot), and the diminution of angle of declination of the great metatarsal (if there is pes planus) (Fig. 26.4).

The straight alignment of the fifth metatarsal is apparent, together with the general inward and downward angulation of the metatarsus, contrasting with the straight alignment of the anterior and posterior tarsus. Films show the exact site at which the angulation arises; this is usually at the tarsometatarsal joint, exceptionally at the midtarsus or the naviculocuneiform joint line (Bensahel 1977) or even at the basal apophyses of the metatarsals. The appearance is striking due to inversion of the metatarsals, which instead of being side by side in a straight line are superimposed in a semilunar alignment when viewed from the side, from the front or back, or from above or below. There is also lateral epiphyseal hypertrophy at the bases of the metatarsals, causing progressively increasing deviation into adduction from the fifth to the first ray.

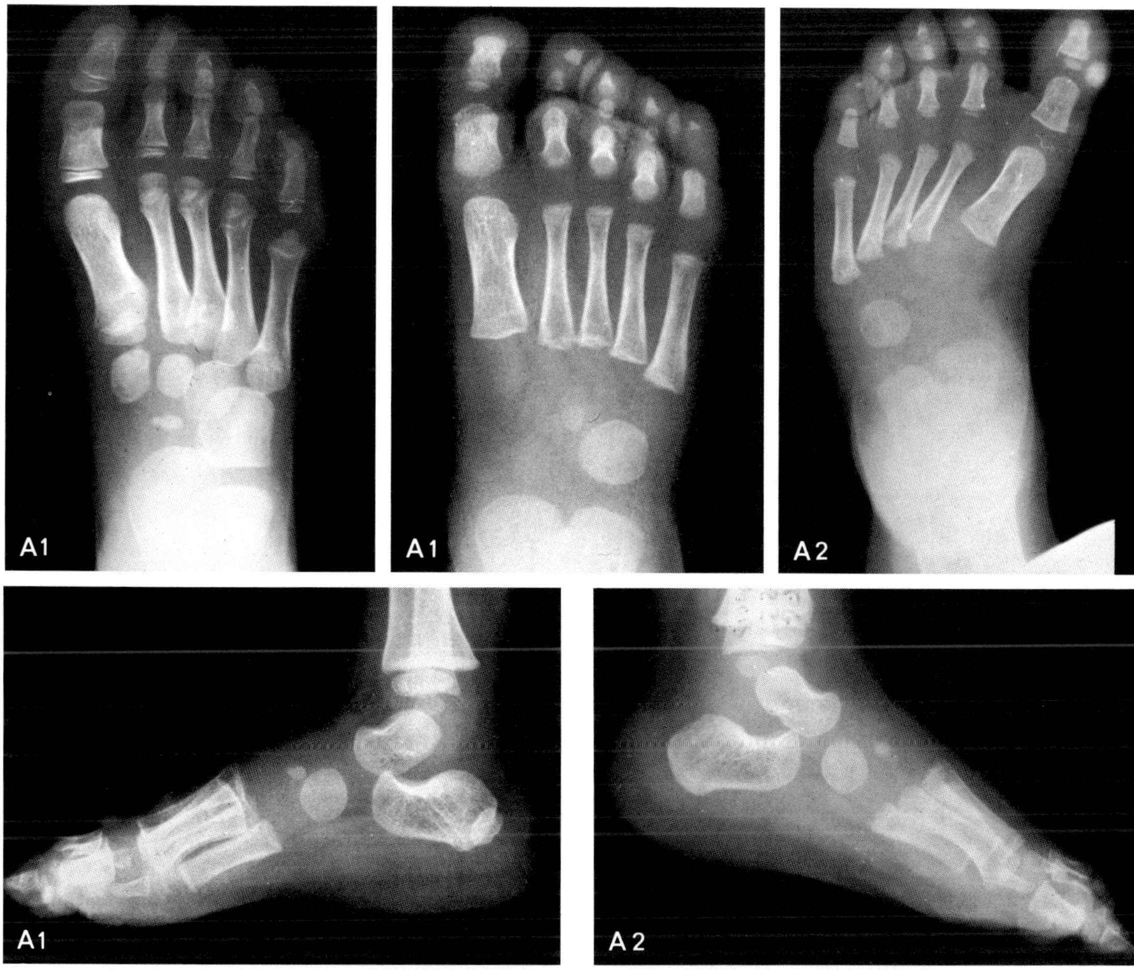

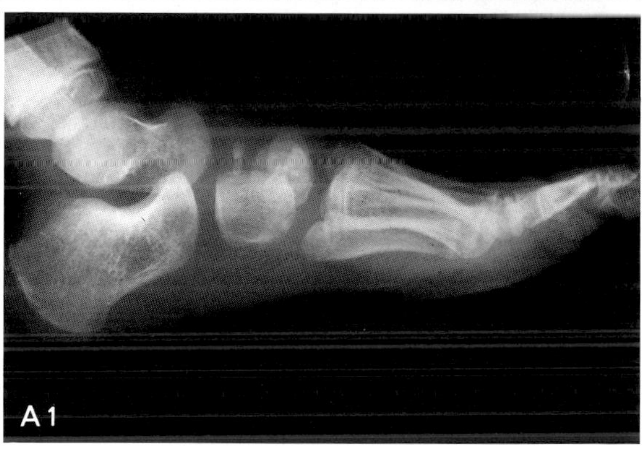

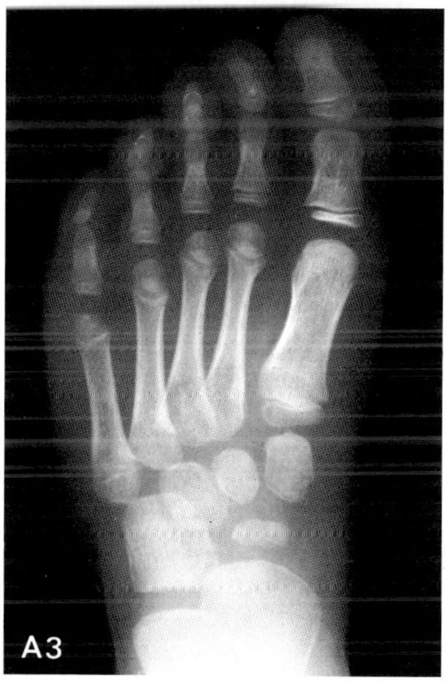

Fig. 26.4 A–H. Pes adductus in children and adolescents. **A** *1* Normal feet; *2* left pes adductus: note tarsal integrity; *3* good correction at 6 years. **B–H** see pp. 388–392

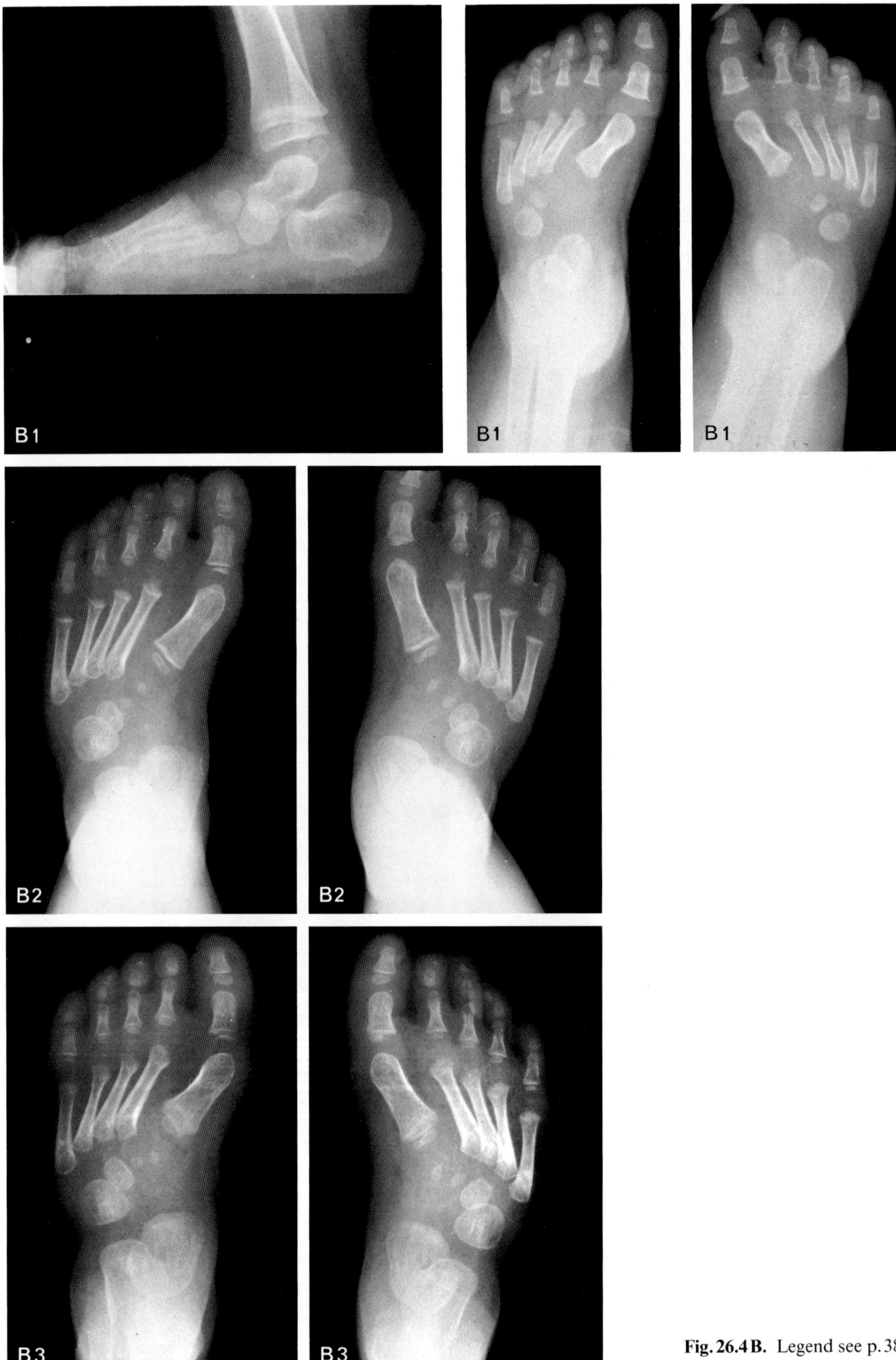

Fig. 26.4 B. Legend see p. 389

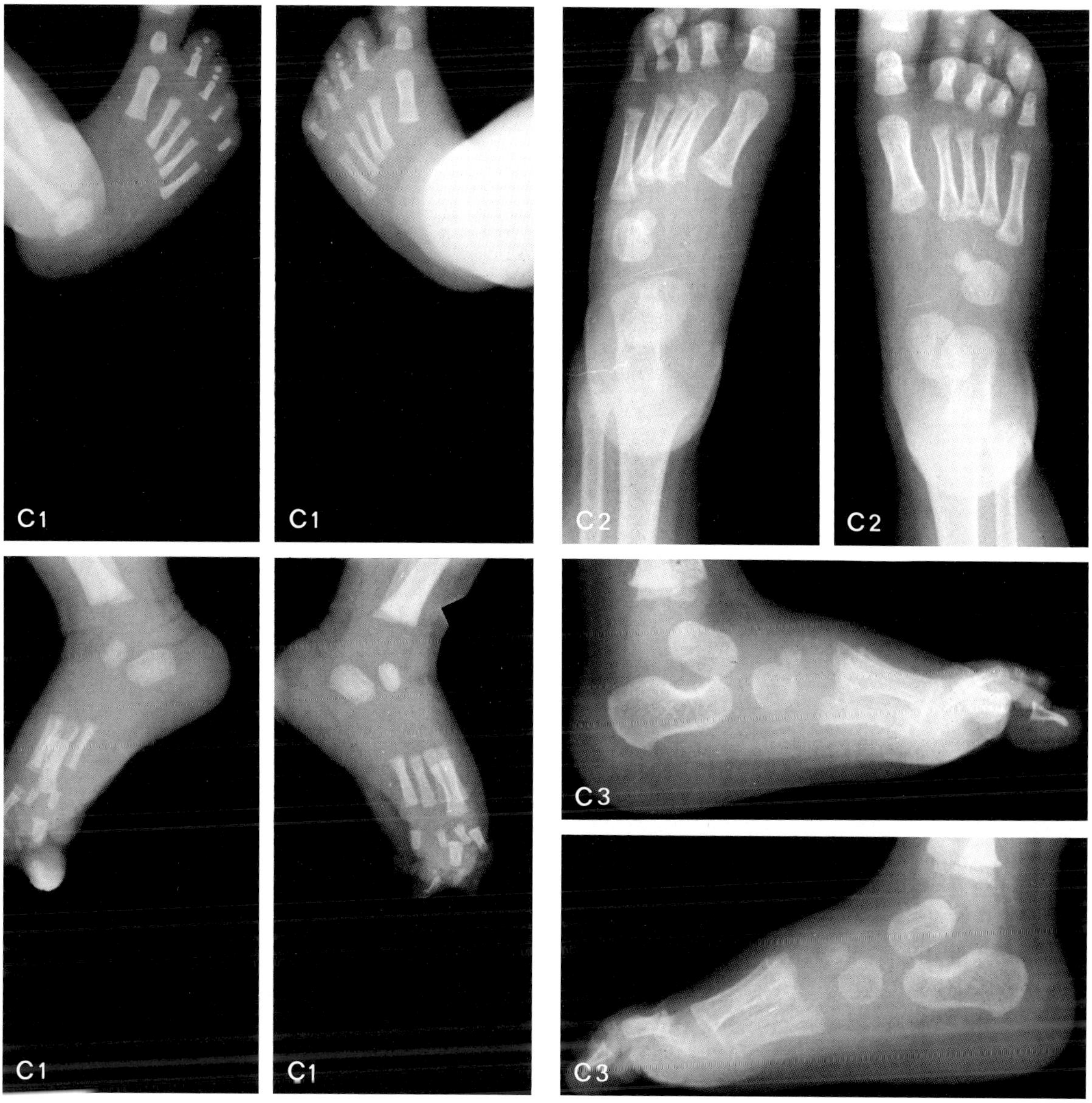

◁ **Fig. 26.4** *(continued).* **B** Pes adductus and pes planovalgus (Dengler): *1* Lateral view; *2, 3* weight-bearing and non-weight-bearing dorsoplantar views. **C** Bilateral mild pes adductus: *1* Age 5 days; *2* good correction at age 2 years; *3* persistence of slight equinus of antetarsus during dorsiflexion of foot on leg

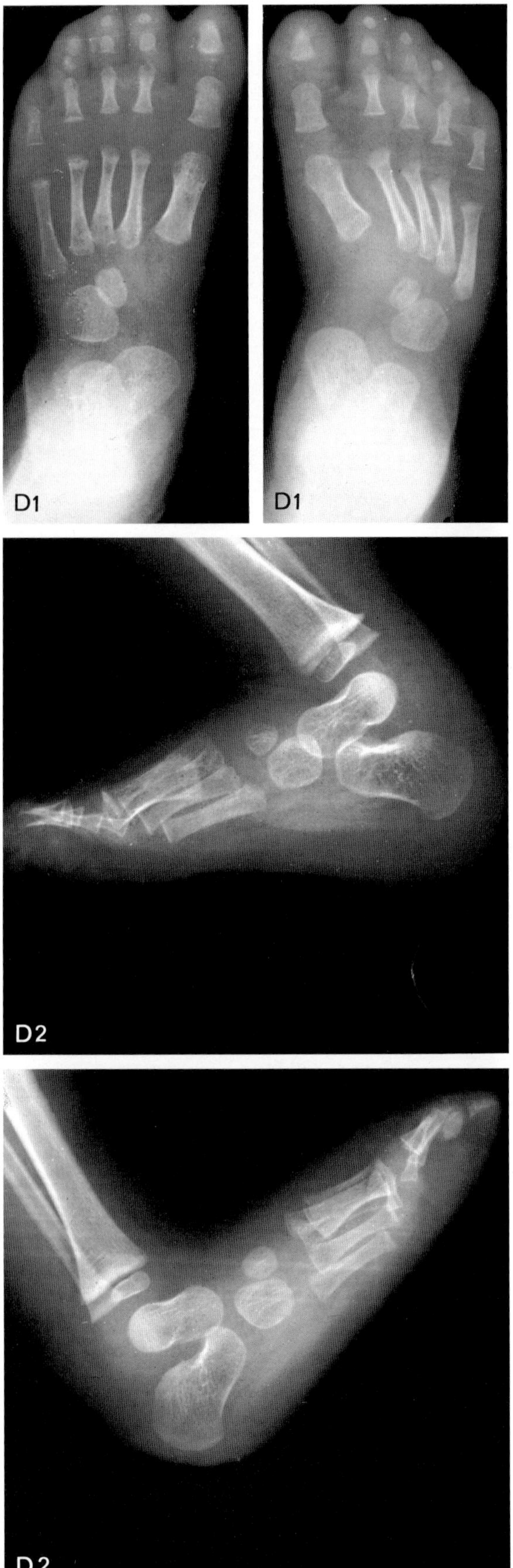

Fig. 26.4 *(continued).* **D** *1* Pes adductus in right foot; ▷ *2* normal appearance of tarsus in both dorsiflexion and plantarflexion. **E** Bilateral pes adductus: marked adduction and supination of forefoot, tarsal integrity, limitation of dorsiflexion of antetarsus

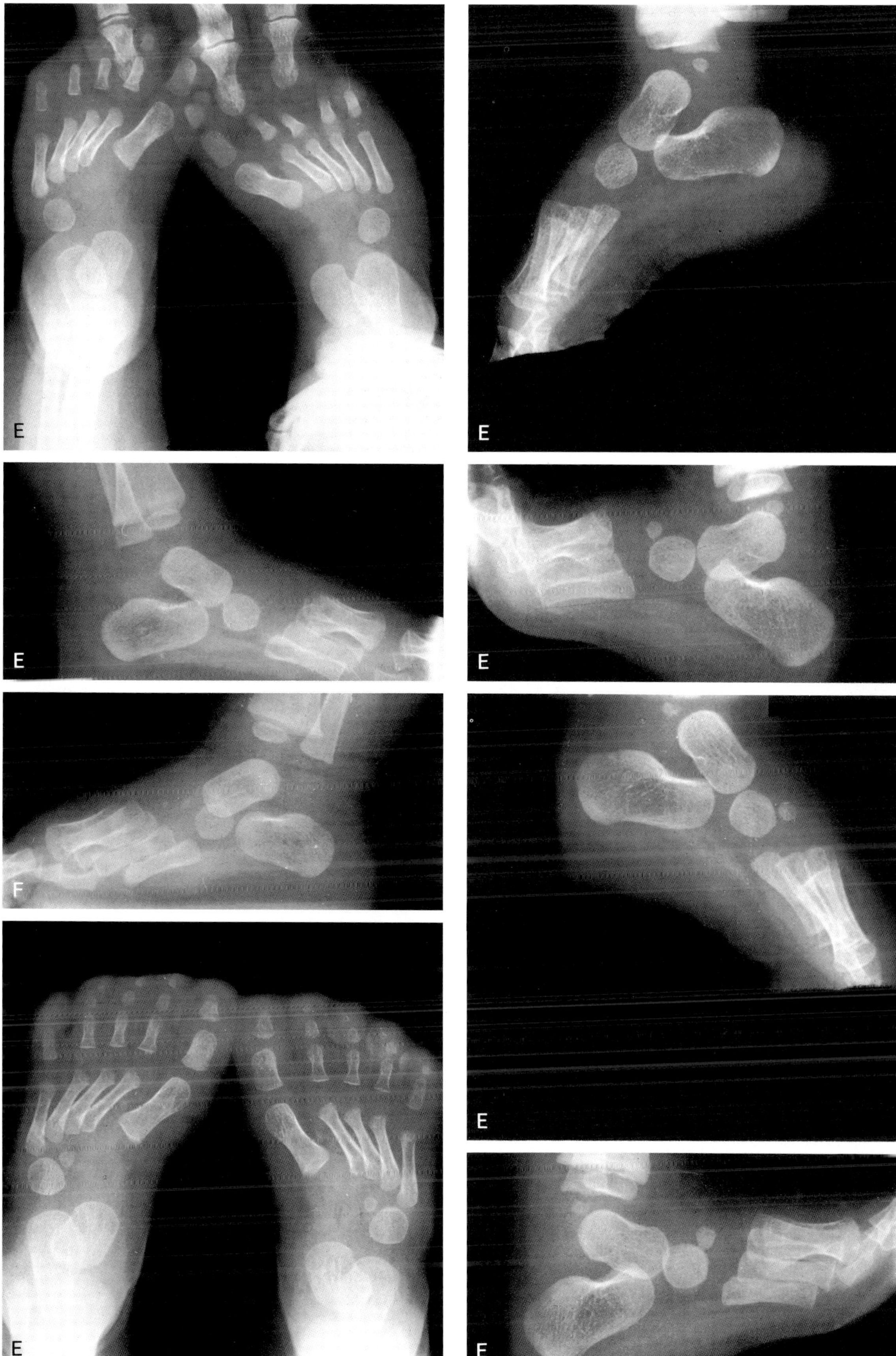
E
E
E
E
F
E
E
E

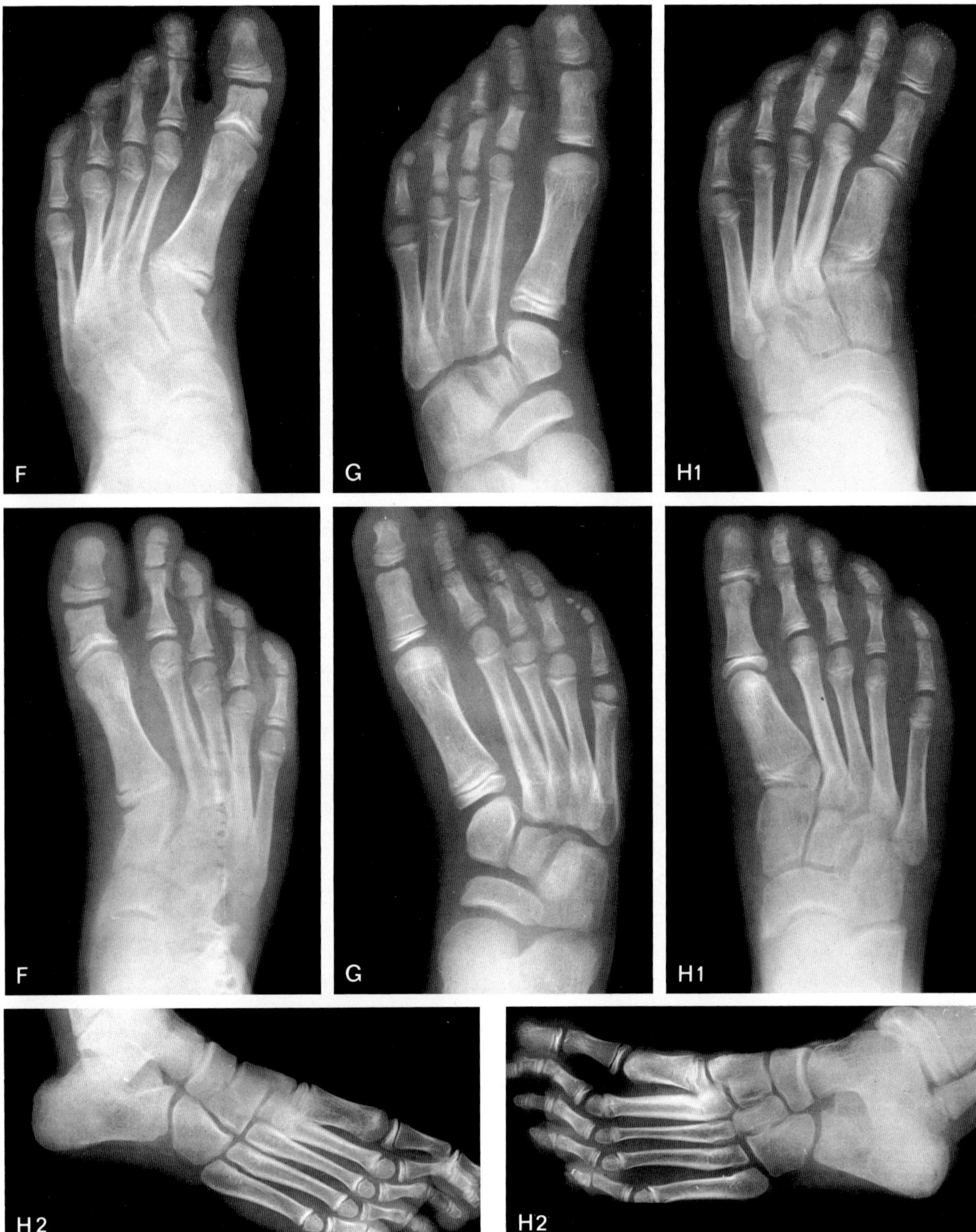

Fig. 26.4 *(continued).* **F, G** Untreated pes adductus: adduction, supination, angulation at necks of metatarsals leading to inversion. **H** Pes adductus associated with congenital brachymetatarsia of first metatarsal: *1* Dorsoplantar views; *2* lateral views

26.4.3 *Treatment*

Conservative. Whether the adductus is pure or associated with planovalgus or cavovarus, the treatment is from the outset conservative, comprising manipulation and splinting which must be pursued for several months until re-establishment of completely normal tarsometatarsal alignment is achieved. Conservative management is easier when the child has commenced walking (Laurence 1966; Bensahel 1977).

Operative. In resistant cases – up to the age of 6 years, after which time deformation of the bases of the metatarsals is likely – the Heymann operation (1958) allows a perfect stable reduction. Capsulotomy of the five tarsometatarsal joints is performed through a transverse incision over the Lisfranc joint line, preserving the external aspects and thereby allowing correction by hinging at these points (Fig. 26.5). The liberation allows slight overcorrection into abduction, following which the correction is maintained by plaster casts for 3–5 months. If there is any instability of the joints at the time of operation, internal fixation with a pin may be necessary. Should radiographs show marked deformation of the metatarsal bases with adduction angulation, precisely calculated proximal wedge osteotomies with the bases orientated dorsally and externally re-establish alignment more effectively. In adulthood, either osteotomy-arthrodesis of the tarsometatarsal joint line or multiple corrective metatarsal osteotomy using the Lelièvre procedure (1952) is usually appropriate. Occasionally, midtarsal naviculocuneiform or cuboidal osteotomies with elongation of the tibialis

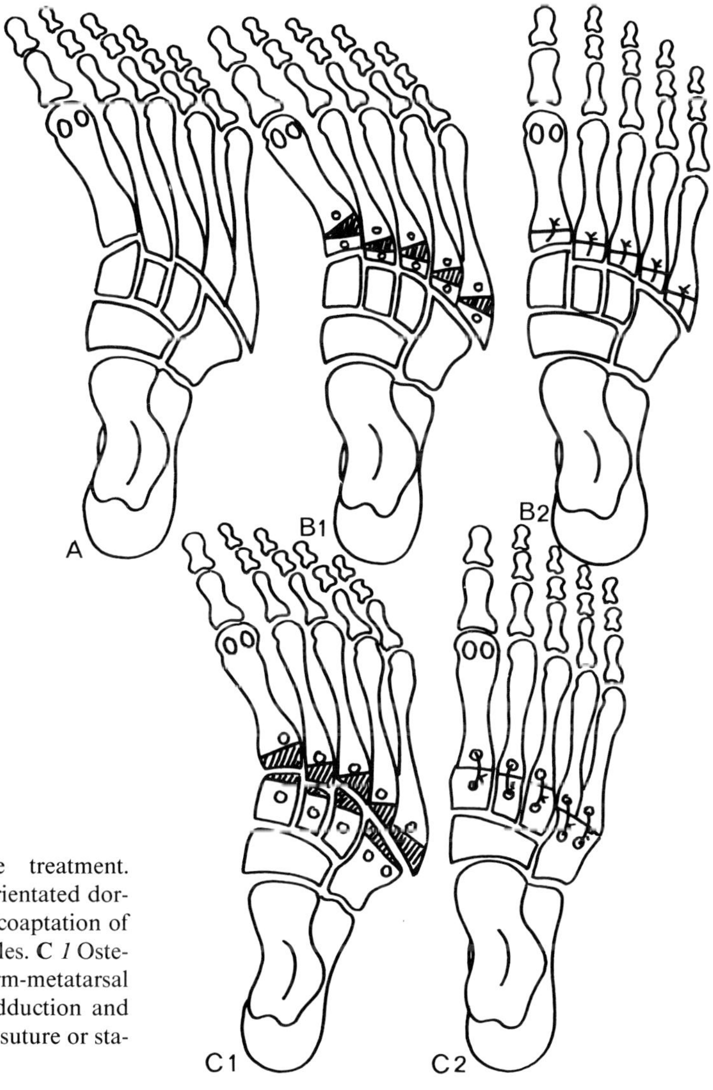

Fig. 26.5 A–C. Pes adductus. **A** Before treatment. **B** *1* Wedge basal osteotomies with bases orientated dorsolaterally; *2* correction of adduction and coaptation of osteotomies by intra-osseous suture or staples. **C** *1* Osteotomy through Lisfranc joint line: cuneiform-metatarsal and cuboidometatarsal; *2* correction of adduction and coaptation of osteotomies by intra-osseous suture or staples

muscles, the flexors and triceps surae are necessary.

26.5 Pes Equinovarus

The equinovarus club foot is by far the commonest significant type of *complex* malposition, the other type being the rare congenital vertical talus (Sect. 26.6). Broca (1914) defined club foot as a condition in which faulty posture involves both the leg and the foot, and the foot has lost its normal pattern of loading. Pes equinovarus is determined in utero by osteoarticular displacement and tissue contractures of an asymmetrical and serious nature which are irreversible and lead to the abnormal loading.

26.5.1 Etiology and Description

The pathogenesis may be associated with any of the following:

1. Faulty posture due to muscle shortening, fibrous contracture and alteration of the joint surfaces
2. Disturbance of tonicity and balance of the muscles of the foot
3. Arrest of development with persistence of the foetal attitude of the foot
4. Failure of normal outward rotation of the foot (Sudder; de Wulf; Jeanneney)
5. Congenital osteoarticular aplasia and capsulotendinous atresia leading to an inversion posture

Bensahel (1977) records an incidence of one infant in 800. It is the second most frequent congenital abnormality (18%), the most frequent being congenital dislocation of the hip (73%). Male children are predominantly affected (Scaglietti), the ratio being 2:1. Slightly over half the cases are bilateral. Equinovarus club foot accounts for 80%–85% of all cases of club foot.

The condition may begin without any malposition of the various bones of the foot, perhaps commencing development in utero from malformation associated with some sort of osteogenic atrophy. This may start at about 5 months of gestation, the deformity being associated with faulty position or narrowness of the intra-uterine environment. (Laurence 1966; Bensahel 1977). Spina bifida has been invoked, but obvious associations of club foot with this condition are unusual. Moreover, the club foot of spina bifida is peculiar in that it comprises a cavovarus foot in which the cavus predominates and the equinus is located in the metatarsus.

Böhm (1929) observed that in club foot associated with delay in development of the bony centres of ossification of the tarsus (notably the navicular, the medial cuneiform and the calcaneal tubercle), these features lead to a particularly severe presentation, with a strong tendency to relapse. Müller observed a similar delay affecting the medical cuneiform and remarked that compensatory hyperplasia associated with atrophy of the navicular constituted opposition to reduction of the foot and was a factor predisposing to relapse after treatment.

Lombard (1946) regarded the cause as muscular disbalance. This would lead to capsuloligamentous abnormalities and secondarily to the bony deformities.

It must be admitted that at our present state of understanding we do not know the prime cause. The concept of faulty position imposed by compression in utero is logical, but only one in 800 infants is affected. If malposition of the bones of the tarsus delays development of bony nuclei, it is not known what mechanism produces this effect; not all club feet present such phenomena. It is possible that there is a hereditary factor, for in 31% of club feet there is such a tendency; Mastromarino (1936) established that 11% of children with club foot are born of parents who have the same deformity, in 20% of cases there is a familial history, and 21% of cases seem to relate to other congenital disease or to dystocia. The remaining 48% of cases display no relevant family history.

If the cause is imbalance between muscle groups, the origin is again unclear in most instances. The possibility of a causative factor in the central nervous system acting through neuromuscular imbalance is supported by the tendeny to relapse during adolescence or even adulthood. On the other hand, club feet which are well corrected initially tend to remain stable, and *all* club feet which are insufficiently corrected tend to relapse. The majority of authorities conclude that it is a genetic factor which is involved in the etiology of equinovarus club foot.

Whatever the site or cause of the underlying condition, equinovarus club foot may be described with relevance to muscular, capsuloligamentous and bony involvement.

26.5.1.1 Muscular Involvement

There is hypertonia of the posterior muscles innervated by the fourth lumbar and first sacral roots, the anterior tibial muscles (fourth lumbar root), triceps surae, flexor digitorum longus (first sacral root) and the internal muscles of the foot (second sacral root). This is associated with hypotonia of the extensors and the peronei (fifth lumbar root), which according to Bensahel may be pseudoparalysis caused by stretching over a long period of time.

26.5.1.2 *Capsuloligamentous Contracture and Hypertrophy*

Posteriorly, there is contracture of the posterior capsule of the ankle joint and of the talocalcaneal joints, and of the posterior talofibular ligament. *Anteriorly*, Faraboeuf (1893–1895) emphasised contracture of the annular anterior ligament of the tarsus. *Medially*, there is contracture of the posterior and middle fasciculi of the deltoid ligament. On the *plantar aspect*, there is contracture of the plantar aponeurosis and the calcaneocuboid ligaments.

26.5.1.3 *Bony Abnormalities*

The *talus* is plantarflexed. It remains aligned with the longitudinal axis of the foot, but only the posterior part of the ankle articular surface remains in the mortice. The anterior extracapsular part of this surface is hypertrophied, while postero-internally the intra-articular segment is atrophied. The talar head protrudes on the dorsolateral aspect of the instep of the foot. Its angle of declination is more than 40%.

The calcaneum is dorsiflexed and adducted, lying under the head of the talus. In its supinated position, its external surface presents on the sole of the foot.

The *navicular* is atrophied and dislocated into an adducted position on the supero internal or internal aspect of the head of the talus or even on to the neck of the talus, approximating towards the medial malleolus.

The *cuboid* is hypertrophied, supinated and adducted. It comes to lie underneath instead of beside it.

The *cuneiforms* are completely supinated, lying one above the other. There is often atrophy of the intermediate and lateral cuneiforms with hypertrophy of the medial cuneiform.

The *metatarsus* in general is adducted and supinated, leading to very abnormal load bearing.

The *ankle joint* is empty in its posterior part, being occupied only by the posterior atrophied area of the talar surface. Its transverse axis is disturbed by posterior displacement of the lateral malleolus, which produces external torsion of the mortice. Dorsiflexion of the talus is impossible, partly because of the antero-external hypertrophy of the articular surface; it cannot enter the mortice, and develops what Adams (1866) described as a transverse bar at the dorsal portion of the talar mass, just in front of the tibial shaft.

Additionally, a cavity (Nelaton 1890) develops at the external portion of the talar mass in front of the lateral malleolus. Capsuloligamentous contractures also contribute to the loss of movement (the posterior tibiotalocalcaneal ligaments, the posterior talofibular ligament, the annular anterior ligament of the tarsus and the interosseous ligament). These are accentuated by contracture of triceps surae. This malposition of the talus in the ankle mortice is a prime factor in the equinus component of the deformity.

The *subtalar joint* is supinated, in equinus and in adduction as a result of relative malposition of the talus and the calcaneum – the two bones diverge in a fashion converse to that seen in a planovalgus deformity – and contracture of tendo Achillis (Mömburg) which is associated with true aplasia of the external half of the tendon and which therefore exerts a supinating effect on the calcaneum. There is contracture of the posterior and medial ligaments of the tibiotalocalcaneal complex, the Y-shaped ligament and the plantar aponeurosis.

The *naviculocuneiform joint* is completely dislocated. Its main transverse axis becomes vertical, while the *talonavicular joint* is distorted by dorsal dislocation and internal displacement. The joint line is filled with fibrous tissue which is also well developed on the dorsal aspect of the space between the talus and the navicular. This fibrous mass restricts movement and opposes reduction, a fact emphasised by Judet et al. (1976) and Viladot (1972). As a result of the equinus posture of the calcaneum and supination of the cuboid, the *calcaneocuboid joint* is fixed in plantarflexion; all dorsiflexion and abduction is impossible. Thus the deformity at the naviculocuneiform joint (adduction and supination) is due not only to distortion of the four articular surfaces which it comprises, but also to dorsomedial capsular thickening between the talus and the navicular, contracture and hypertrophy of the Y-shaped ligament and contracture of the annular anterior ligament of the tarsus and the plantar calcaneocuboid ligament. There is also muscle contracture affecting tibialis anterior, tibialis posterior and flexor hallucis longus. Contracture of the plantar aponeurosis, the short flexor muscles and the subcutaneous tissue on the inner side of the foot in general completes the rigid displacement.

The *tarsometatarsal joint line* presents with its main transverse axis vertically aligned, and there is hypertrophic development of the external portion of each of the metatarsal bases. This posture further aggravates the supination and adduction of the forefoot from the bony deformities and muscular contractions already described (extensor digitorum longus, abductor hallucis, the short plantar muscles and flexor hallucis longus) and the capsuloligamentous contracture and involvement of the skin on the inner and plantar aspects.

26.5.2 Clinical Features

The equinovarus club foot exhibits the triad described by Faraboeuf (1893–1895) (Fig. 26.6):

1. *Varus:* The foot presents significant inward angulation with respect to its longitudinal axis, characterised by convexity of the outer border, whose summit lies at the cuboid, and by concavity of the inner border, in which angulation is marked by a beaked groove or transverse fold at the level of the navicular. The varus is associated with obvious cavus due to plantar angulation of the foot, this being marked by a prolongation of the internal fold on to the plantar aspect.
2. *Equinus:* This stems from the ankle joint and extends into the tarsus, associated with fibrous thickening on the postero-external aspect (Seringe 1976). Thickening extends into the deep aponeurosis of the leg, the external annular ligament, the fibrous sheaths of the peronei and the middle fasciculus of the lateral ligament of the ankle.
3. *Supination and adduction:* These displacements emphasised by Delpech, are associated, with the result that the plantar aspect of the foot looks inwardly. The deformity develops at the level of the subtalar joint through rotation of the calcaneum and compounds the adduction-supination of the forefoot, accentuated by inversion of the bones of the midtarsus and metatarsus.

Further features include bulging of the medial aspect of the heel pad, vertical disposition of the plantar aspect of the forefoot, general shortening of the foot, separation of the great toe from its neighbours and external torsion of the ankle mortice, which may amount to 40°–50° in the horizontal plane, associated with posterior displacement of the fibular malleolus and relative forward displacement antero-internally of the medial malleolus.

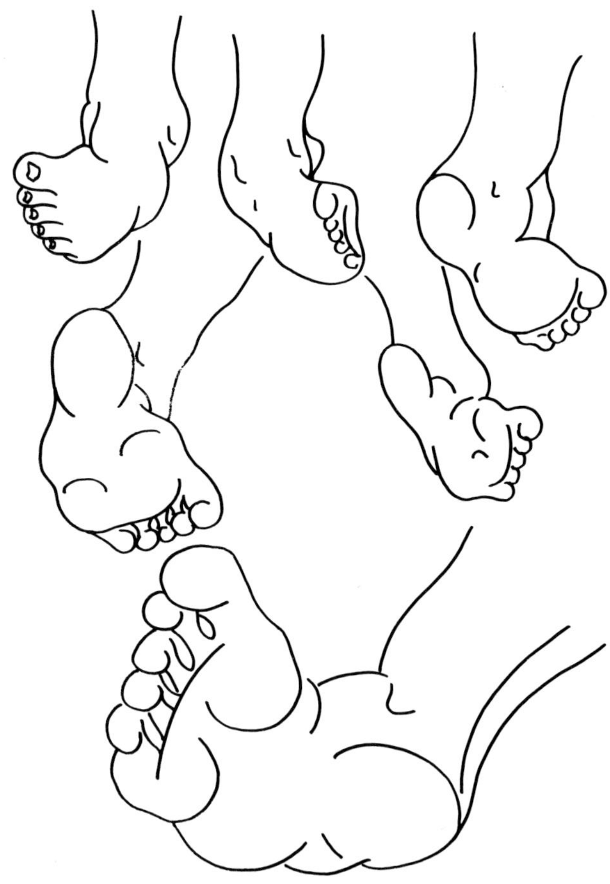

Fig. 26.6. Clinical features of equinovarus club foot

The torsion results in external deviation of the longitudinal axis of the talus, and appreciation of this is essential in measuring the significance of subsequent displacements. The club foot must be assessed with the hand and not with the eye stated Faraboeuf (1893–1895). It is for this reason that palpation must be carried out extremely gently by experienced hands, thus ensuring that the muscles remain relaxed (Maschas 1954); any sudden manoeuvres of reduction will augment the hypertonia and fix the deformities, perhaps giving an impression of irreducibility. With care, the position of all the bones of the foot can be appreciated and an understanding of the alignments of the various joints can be achieved.

An effort should be made to appreciate the following particular components by palpation: the postero-external torsion of the mortice, the exact position of the talus, the degree of irreducibility of talar equinus, the degree of abduction of the longitudinal axis of the calcaneum and the degree of supination (of the calcaneum at the subtalar joint) and of adduction-supination of the forefoot. The development of the heel should be assessed together with the contact or separation between the posterior parts of the talus and the tibia. The medialised or superior position of the navicular with respect to the talus and the medial malleolus must be measured.

The degree of tonicity of different muscle groups can be felt with respect to contracture of the postero-internal tendons (triceps surae, the tibialis muscles, flexor hallucis longus and flexor digitorum longus), in contrast to the hypotonia of the peronei and the extensors.

These careful examinations will distinguish true equinovarus club foot from a benign variety produced by deformation in utero which is easily correctable. Privat [cited by Broca (1914)] described a homely test consisting of placing the infant in front of a bright fire to provoke relaxation; true club feet exhibit their poor position, in contrast to correctable club feet, which reposition spontaneously. This careful coaxing of correction is most important in assessing prognosis and allows classification into three groups:

1. *Easily reduced.* The foot is long and supple, and equinus, adduction and supination components are less than 20°. The condition responds readily to manipulation and splintage (Dal Monte 1976).
2. *Partially reducible* with residual contracture affecting all components. Equinus, adduction and supination each amount to 20°–45° (Dal Monte 1976), and failure to correct by conservative means within 3 months is an indication for surgery.
3. *Irreducible* with peristent significant contracture. In a long foot, all components exceed 45°, but in the short foot even deformity of only 20° may be incorrectable by non-operative methods; surgical management is then necessary (Dal Monte 1976).

26.5.2.1 Radiography

Three views are essential (Fig. 26.7). The *dorsoplantar* view shows the divergence or parallelism of the axes of the talus and the calcaneum, the juxtaposition of centres of ossification and the projection of the talar and calcaneal axes with respect to the metatarsals, above all the first metatarsal. In the normal foot, the divergence of the centres of ossification of the calcaneum and talus forms an angle of 45°, with the talar axis projecting inwardly with respect to the great metatarsal. In the club foot, there is superimposition of the talar and calcaneal centres of ossification or diminution of the normal divergence, the two bones often even lying parallel. There is also internal angulation at the tarsometatarsal joint, so that the talar axis falls outside that of the first metatarsal. The metatarsus is seen to be inverted into adduction and supination.

The *lateral view* displays the degree of equinus associated at the ankle joint (Fig. 26.8). In *maximum dorsiflexion* in the normal foot, the angle between the talus and the tibia is about 90°, that between the talus and the calcaneum 45°. The cavity of the sinus tarsi is clearly visible. In contrast, in the equinovarus club foot, the angle between the tibia and talus is more than 90° while that between the talus and the calcaneum is reduced or reversed due to anterior divergence. Most frequently, the axes of the talus and calcaneum are parallel and the cavity of the sinus tarsi is hidden. The lateral view in *full plantarflexion* demonstrates the degree of mobility of the ankle joint, the absence of posterior talocalcaneal divergence (i.e. the axes are parallel) and the absence of migration of the calcaneum underneath the talus compared with the lateral view in maximum dorsiflexion.

Radiological examination is essential before, during, and regularly after treatment so that the quality of reduction achieved by whatever method of treatment has been chosen can be assessed accurately.

26.5.3 Treatment

All authors are agreed that treatment should begin as soon as the condition is diagnosed at birth (Sayre); Roederer stated that results depend directly on how early treatment is instituted. It is also agreed that when correction has been achieved, it should be checked vigilantly, both clinically and radiographically, until walking begins.

26.5.3.1 Conservative

Treatment is always conservative at the outset, but if complete correction has not been achieved by the age of 3 months the need for surgical management is indicated. Whatever method is used, the correction must be consolidated subsequently by shoes with insoles during the day and by splints at night. Re-educative measures and very occasionally re-operation are necessary during the period of observation. It may be stated here that whatever method of conservative treatment is chosen, the result may be spoiled by three factors (Bensahel 1977; Laurence 1966): the resistance of the foot to manipula-

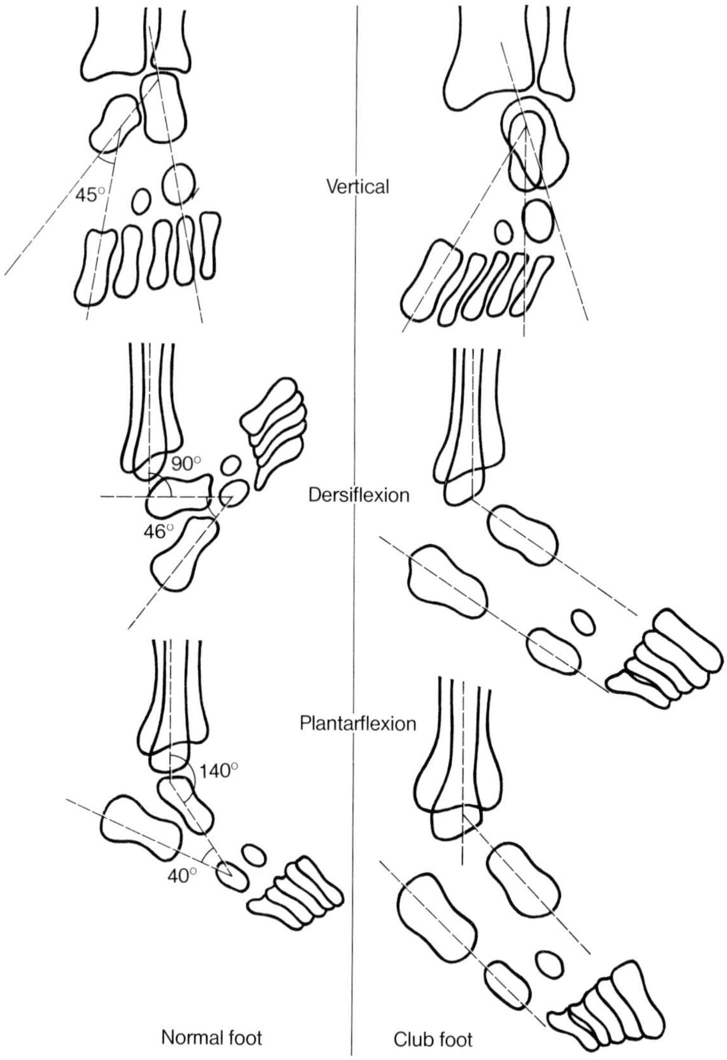

Fig. 26.7. Three essential radiographic views of equinovarus club foot

tive reduction, the absence of any natural spontaneous corrective influence and the tendency to partial or total relapse. It is for this reason that parents must understand the need for long-term treatment and supervision until the termination of growth.

Conservative treatment must begin early, must be gentle, must exclude any forceful manipulation which would damage especially the talus and must be progressive. The foot is coaxed little by little and maintained by splintage according to the components corrected, namely, adduction, supination, varus, and equinus. The passive manipulative measures must be completed by active re-education so as to restore muscle balance and achieve a range of movement similar to the normal. Regular radiological assessment ensures objective proper alignment of the bones.

Laurence (1966) recommended podoscopic examination, which assures good loading distribution and a proper rolling action of the foot with normal heel strike on the heel, and this accompanied by normal shoe wear gives evidence of a functionally satisfactory state.

Broadly, there are three types of conservative management:

1. The method described by Kite (1930), comprising application of a plaster cast which is successively wedged
2. Manipulations followed by corrective plaster casts
3. Manipulations actively and passively associated with the Denis Browne splint (1937 a).

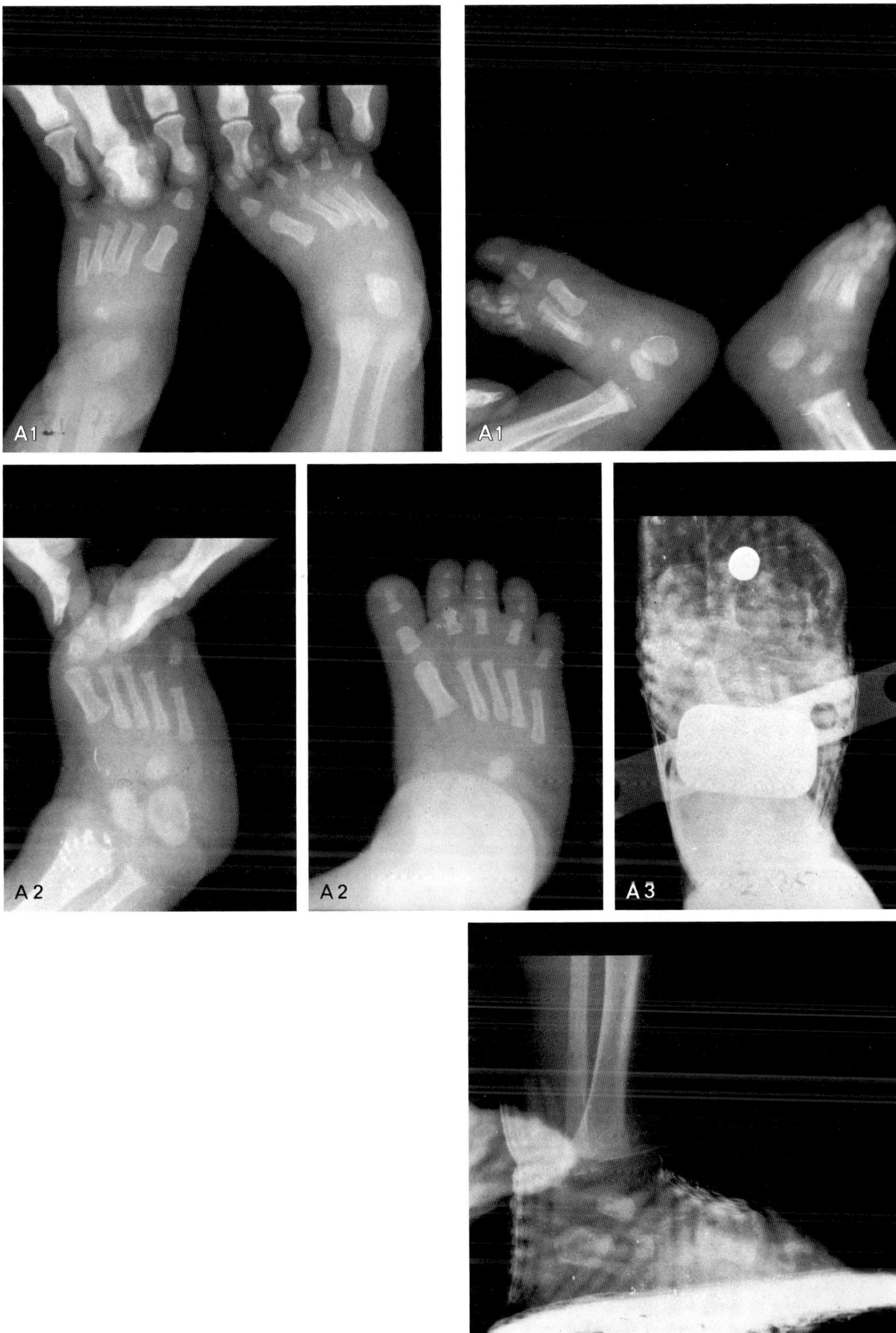

Fig. 26.8 A *1–3*. Legend see p. 401

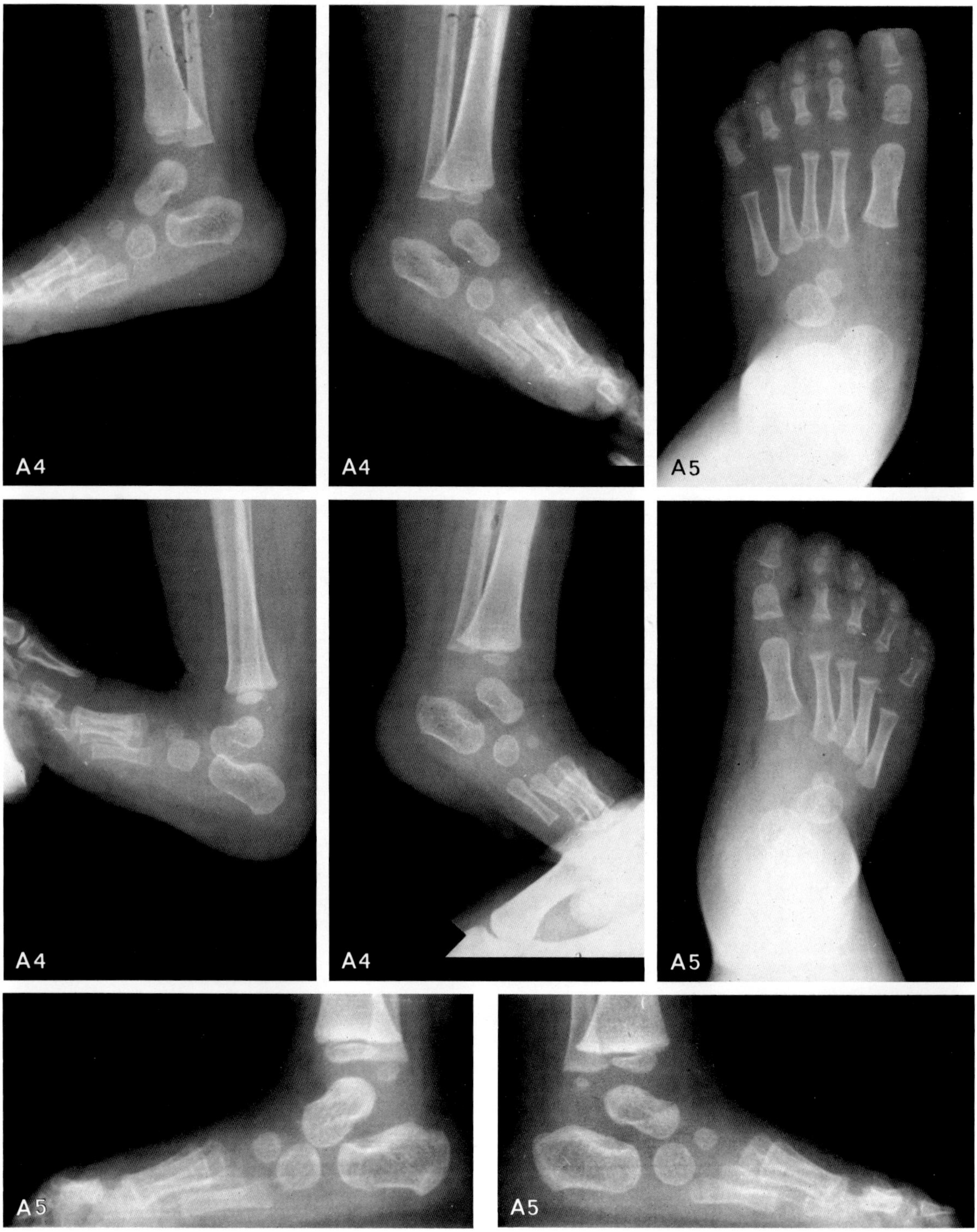

Fig. 26.8 A *4, 5*. Legend see p. 401

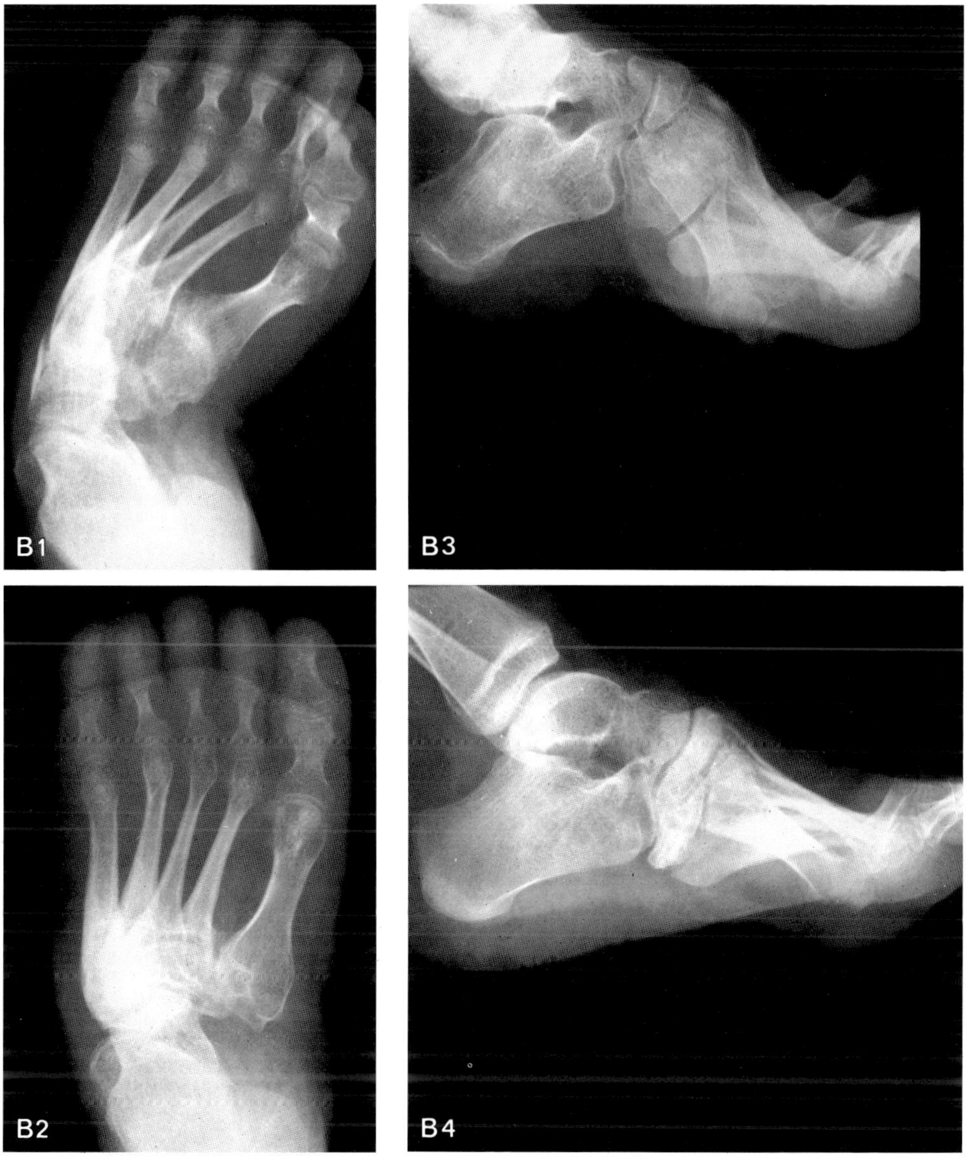

◁ **Fig. 26.8 A–D.** Congenital malformations: pes equinovarus. **A** Pes equinovarus of right foot. *1* Dorsoplantar and lateral views: adduction, supination, superimposition of talus and calcaneum, parallel alignment of axes of talus and calcaneum; *2, 3* 2 months later, before and after treatment by manipulations and Denis Browne splint; *4* 9 months after treatment; *5* 17 months after treatment. **B** Pes equinocavovarus in a 13-year-old child as a sequel of pes equinovarus. *1, 3* Preoperative; *2, 4* after osteotomy of midtarsal region. **C**, **D** see pp 402, 403

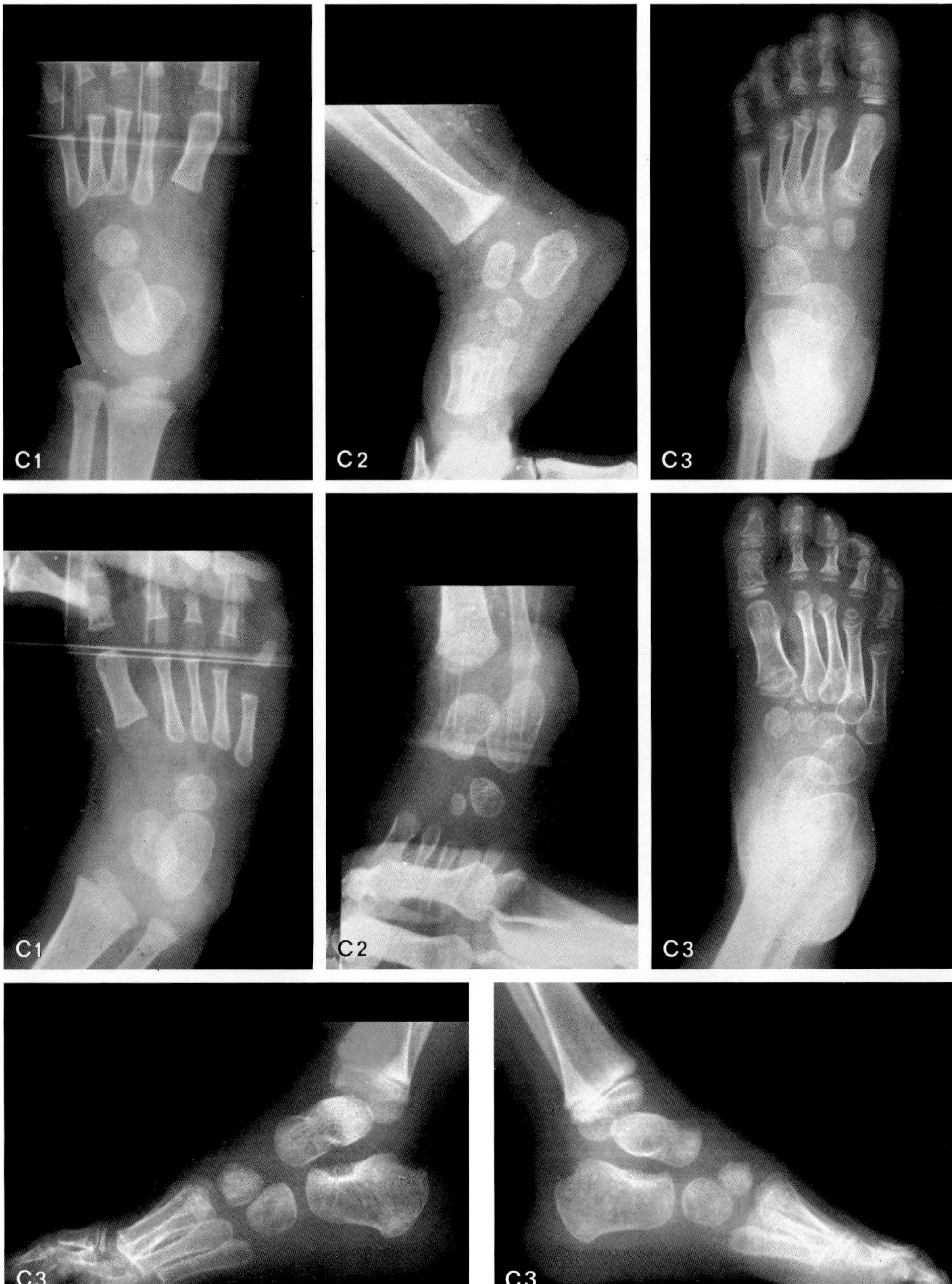

Fig. 26.8 *(continued)*. **C** Mild right pes equinovarus. *1* Pretreatment views; *2* after treatment by manipulations and Denis Browne splint; *3* 3 years 8 months after treatment.

D Normal left foot, right talipes equinovarus. *1–3* Preoperative views; *4* after correction by medial release ▷

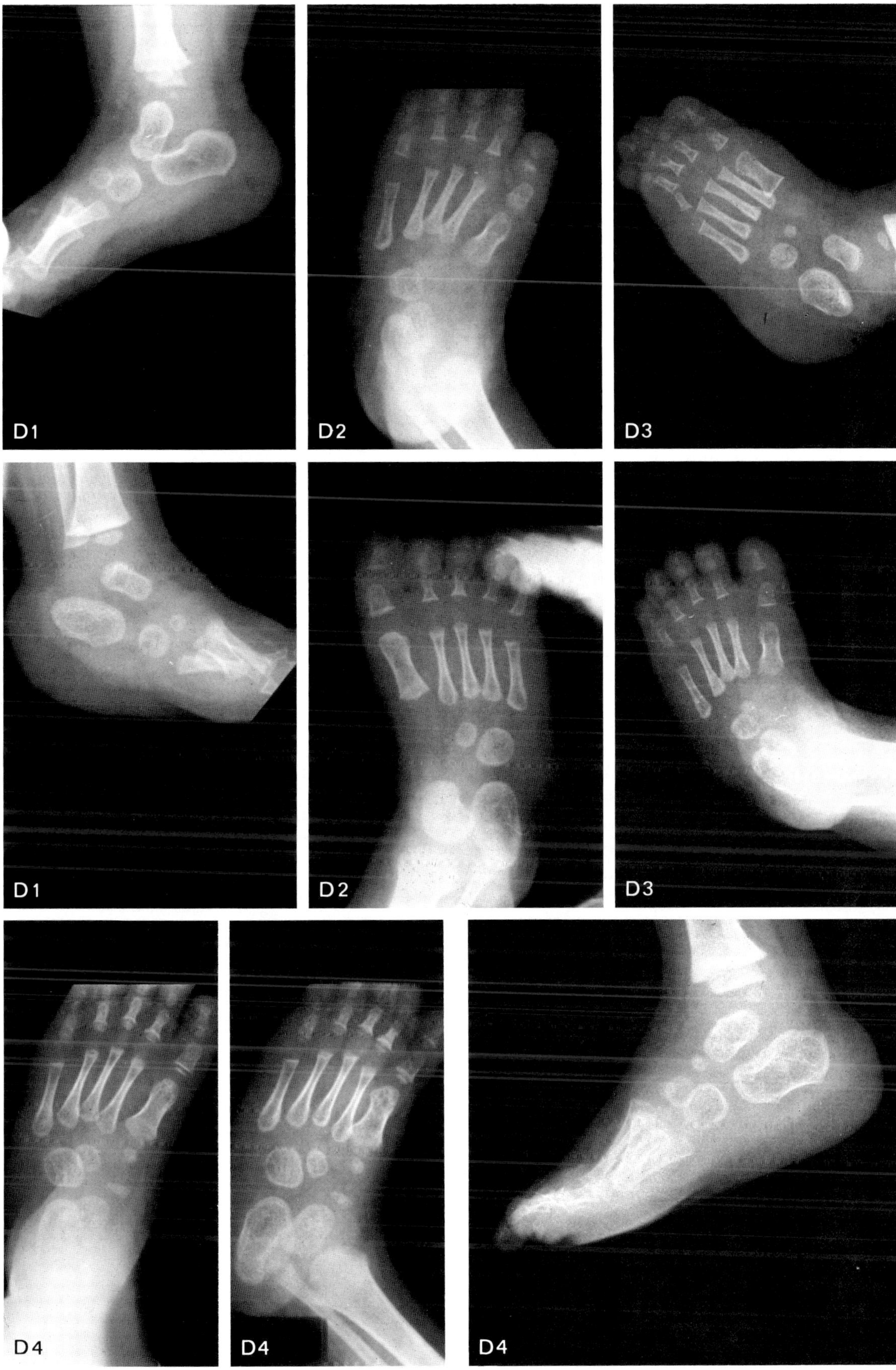
D1
D2
D3
D1
D2
D3
D4
D4
D4

It seems that the majority of modern authors, especially Laurence (1966) and Bensahel (1977) consider the third method as being most efficacious. Whichever is chosen, the inversion (varus, adduction and supination) must be corrected before the equinus component. The technique of manipulation is crucial, success resting in maintaining whatever correction is achieved by splintage.

The manipulator devotes attention first to the inversion, treatments being performed once or twice daily. Initially, the foot is kept the whole time in equinus, otherwise the manipulation risks producing a torsional deformity of the tibia and fibula. One hand grasps the forefoot, the other the heel, the tarsus and the instep. The two hands, opposing each other, first exert an abducting action, bringing the forefoot and midtarsus into a proper position, then correction of the supination, leading the midtarsus and antetarsus into a pronated position, acting cautiously so as to avoid flattening of the longitudinal arch. The result is elongation of the musculotendinous elements of the inner side of the foot (tibialis posterior, the short flexor and abductor of the great toe) and correction of the concavity of the internal border of the foot, thereby mobilising the talonavicular joint line. Correction of the varus posture of the calcaneum is achieved by stretching the medial ligament of the ankle by means of exerting pressure on the posterior tarsus while supporting the ankle mortice. Simultaneously, the subtalar joint is persuaded into better alignment by stretching triceps surae while pressing on the posterior tuberosity of the calcaneum. The calcaneum is twisted about a vertical axis so as to lead the anterior process into its proper external position, while the body of the calcaneum swings around the longitudinal axis, leading the bone into a pronated posture.

The second aim, correcting the equinus, must relate to the calcaneum, which is to be brought into its normal dorsiflexed posture. This entails stretching of tendo Achillis, which can be achieved by exerting gentle pressure from the thumb and index finger over its insertion while supporting the leg (Broca 1914). Marique recommended the use of skeletal traction through a transcalcaneal pin. If the calcaneum cannot be brought down, a high tenotomy of tendo Achillis (Petit 1947) or even release of the ankle and subtalar joints (Hauser 1966) may be necessary. Correction by the manipulative measures described is succeeded by splintage, by means of either a plaster cast or the Denis Browne device.

26.5.3.1.1 The Kite Method

Manipulation is performed early but is succeeded by further correction in a plastèr cast, achieved by wedging. Treatment lasts from 6–8 months; the plaster must be changed every 20 days during the early months and then more frequently, twice per month, until complete correction is achieved. As always, active re-education and massage must follow.

The first manipulation aims at correcting the adduction and replacing the head of the talus inwardly without any attempt to correct equinus. A plaster cast is applied and kept on for 8 days. Wedging of the plaster is then performed; a segment is removed transversely at the summit of the convexity of the outer border of the foot, the posterior border of the segment being level with the talar head. The size of the segment varies according to the rigidity of the foot and requires experience in assessment. The apices of the wedge are situated superiorly on the dorsum of the foot and inferiorly on the plantar aspect. The foot is gently stressed into abduction so as to close the wedge and maintained thus until the 16th day, when a new plaster is applied. At about the 24th day a further wedge resection is conducted in this plaster so as to gain further longitudinal correction of the foot.

Once this has been achieved, the stage of correction of supination begins. An appropriate manipulation is performed and a new plaster cast applied which maintains the abduction stress with as much correction as possible. After 8 days, and then again at 15 days if necessary, triangular resections of the plaster are made on the external aspect at the hindfoot so as to correct the varus of the tarsus. When the adduction and the supination have been corrected, the plaster is removed and manipulations are directed at the equinus component. After manipulation a new plaster is left on for 8 days, following which an anterior transverse wedge at the level of the ankle joint is removed and gradual correction of the equinus is commenced. By degrees, complete correction is achieved, following which plaster immobilisation is conducted for some 3 months. After removal of this cast, manipulations, massage and active re-education are pursued assiduously. Sometimes the equinus cannot be corrected properly, in which case high tenotomy of tendo Achillis will be necessary, usually allowing complete gentle reduction of the last component of deformity in two or three stages.

I have achieved excellent results with the Kite (1930) method of treatment, but it is undoubtedly difficult. There is also the danger of over-forceful correction which can lead to damage to the ankle articular surface of the talus; if this surface flattens, the result will undoubtedly be a restricted range of movement of the ankle and failure to achieve good function of the foot generally. Flattening of the anterior margin of the tibia and of the talar articular surface is a tragedy. Treatment can advantageously be followed by the use of the Denis Browne splint, which encourages better muscular re-education.

26.5.3.1.2 Manipulations and Plaster Casts

This method is in some ways similar to the Kite method, but does not employ the technique of wedge resection. First adduction, then supination and finally equinus are corrected by successive manipulations, following each of which a corrective plaster cast is applied. Usually these manipulations are performed every 8–10 days. After full correction, plaster immobilisation with changes each month should be continued for 3 months. Each period of immobilisation is followed by a session of massage, active re-education and proprioception. The main indication now appears to be failure of the Denis Browne splint to correct the equinus component of the deformity.

26.5.3.1.3 The Denis Browne Splint

This method has become increasingly attractive. The use of the Denis Browne splint follows passive and active manipulations. Ideally, it is easier if the infant is kept in hospital during the first 6 weeks of treatment. Denis Browne (1935, 1936) stated that forced correction and plaster immobilisation should never be employed. The principle is one of preservation of active muscular contraction, thereby avoiding osteoporosis and muscle atrophy, which he ascribed to plaster immobilisation. Treatment begins within a few days of birth, with correction successively of the supination of the forefoot, the adduction of the midtarsus and the equinus of the ankle joint. The sessions of manipulation are followed by application of the Denis Browne foot plates, applied with the transverse bar bent progressively so as to encourage abduction and pronation of the feet.
Laurence (1966), and Bensahel (1977, Biename, and Bourden described very accurately their method of fixaton of the foot to the plates by three metatarsal bands to the heel and the midtarsal region; the adduction and the metatarsus varus were controlled by the metatarsal component, the varus and the internal angulation of the midtarsal region by the midtarsal band and the supination of the hindfoot by the talar band. These bands maintain the foot accurately and permit autopassive mobilisation, encouraging active correction of the deformities. Regular manipulations are performed in addition to the use of the Denis Browne splint, at first daily and then at progressively greater intervals according to the rate of correction until once per week is all that is necessary. The splints are used until the child walks, under the close supervision of the parents, the kinesitherapist and the surgeon. The correction of the equinus is the last source of concern.
The two disadvantages of the Denis Browne method are the tendency for metatarsus varus to develop and persistent contracture of triceps surae. Accordingly, it is necessary to be aware of the occasional need to use a corrective plaster cast with respect to the equinus after appropriate manipulation or perhaps high tenotomy of tendo Achillis. Even posterior capsulotomy of the ankle or subtalar joint may be necessary. After such measures, plaster immobilisation or a Saint Germain splint stabilises the correction until walking is commenced.

26.5.3.2 Operative

The indications for operative treatment relate to failure of conservative management. Some club feet, as observed above, are resistant, and in these cases it is essential to avoid the damage, particularly to the talar surface (Dimeglio and Pons 1976), and the subsequent aplasia of the front of the ankle joint which will inevitably result from the nutcracker effect of manipulations. Further, as emphasised by Judet et al. (1976), normal structural development of the foot will not occur until proper alignment has been achieved, and in resistant cases surgical release is the only way of restoring the initial alignment.
Padovani (1978) stated that if conservative methods have not achieved correction by the age of 3 months, surgical intervention is essential. The foot must be properly aligned and there must be a good range of movement of the ankle joint, especially dorsiflexion. Radiography must show proper divergence between the axes of the talus and the calcaneum in both lateral and anteroposterior views.
Two prerequisites are that any form of elongation of tendo Achillis should be avoided until correction of adduction and supination has been

achieved (Scholder 1971b) and that any operative measure must be preceded by accurate identification of the zones of main contracture. These may be posterior, medial or related to specific tendons or muscles or the plantar aponeurosis. Seringe (1976) stressed the importance of a postero-external node of fibrous tissue fixing the calcaneum at the external annular ligament, the peroneal tendon sheaths and the calcaneofibular joint.

Clinical identification of all the possible bony abnormalities and confirmation by radiological examination must be conclusive. Exact identification of the main sources of deformity dictates the site of surgical attack.

The surgical procedure must be adapted to the nature of the specific residual deformities. Pure inversion persisting in a club foot after orthopaedic treatment for 3 months necessitates (preferably before the age of 5 years, sometimes at 5–12 years and in exceptional cases in adolescence) the classical complete soft tissue release procedures as described by Ombredanne, Nove Josserand, Codivilla, Leveuf and Bertrand, and more recently by Dal Monte, Judet, Laurence, Padovani, Seringe and Viladot, to name but a few. As well as those in pure inversion, there exist club feet in which, despite well-conducted manipulative treatment, there persist variable displacements such as supination of the subtalar joint, adduction and cavus of the midtarsal region, supination with varus of the forefoot, metatarsus varus, or pure equinus, absence or limitation of dorsiflexion of the foot, and adduction and internal rotation of the hindfoot or forefoot.

26.5.3.2.1 Technique

Surgical correction of these residual displacements involves a medial release appropriately adapted to the type of correction required. The essentials of soft tissue release depend upon the age of the child.

Medial Release in the Infant

Many authors, notably Dal Monte (1976), advise as follows in the infant of up to 3 months.

1. A posterior longitudinal incision is made parallel to tendo Achillis. Through this approach are performed the following procedures:
   - Bayonet elongation of tendo Achillis, taking care to preserve the outer part of the insertion of the tendon into the calcaneum.
   - Median longitudinal incision of the deep fascia, allowing inward retraction of the posterior tibial neurovascular bundle and the tibialis posterior and flexor tendons. This in turn permits cautious posterior arthrotomy of the ankle and subtalar joints using fine, curved, blunt-nosed scissors, thereby restoring the two joint spaces exactly. Always beware mistaking the diaphyso-epiphyseal line for a joint interspace.
   - Repair of tendo Achillis (with the foot at right angles to the axis of the leg), either with interrupted sutures of the two tendinous tongues, or with two catgut sutures above and below, permitting sliding of the two tongues of the tenotomy as described by Dal Monte (1976).
   - Suture of the sheath of tendo Achillis and the subcutaneous tissue.
   - Closure of the skin with oblique sutures directed from below outwardly (Dal Monte 1976); this allows relaxation of the medially contracted skin and of its lateral tension.
2. A medial incision is made from the diaphysis of the first metatarsal to the medial malleolus (Dal Monte 1975). This exposure allows:
   - Elongation by Z-plasty successively, from above downwards and from superficial to deep, of the tendons of tibialis posterior, flexor digitorum longus and flexor hallucis longus
   - Release of the posterior insertion of abductor hallucis and of the short flexor tendon of the great toe
   - Posterior division of the medial two-thirds posteriorly of the plantar aponeurosis

     After careful identification of the joint lines, one proceeds to:
   - Capsuloligamentous dorsal, plantar and medial arthrotomy of the Chopart joint line using fine curved scissors, division of the plantar expansion of the insertion of tibialis posterior and, if necessary, division of the Y-shaped ligament
   - Arthrotomy of the subtalar joint anteriorly, protecting the middle fasciculus of the deltoid ligament of the ankle
   - Arthrotomy of the naviculocuneiform joint line if this proves necessary

As a result of these releases, the navicular can be restored to its proper position. Dal Monte (1976) insists on certain points of technique: never force and never strip unnecessarily; suture the tendon under tension; commence arthrotomy with a knife and complete it with prudent, gentle and limited use of fine, curved, blunt-nosed scissors. The suture of sliding tendon elongation

(Dal Monte) of flexor hallucis longus, flexor digitorum longus and tibialis posterior is effected with the tendons under tension, the foot being realigned at right angles to the axis of the leg.
3. After suture of the subcutaneous and cutaneous layers, Dal Monte insists on the strict criteria of reduction. The correction is adequate when, at the end of the operation, finger pressure applied to the outer border of the forefoot without force leads to a good general realignment of the foot.
4. A plaster splint holding the knee in semiflexion is maintained for 5 days. A complete plaster holding the knee in semiflexion is then applied and changed every 20 days for 2 months. Corrective manipulations and massage are performed at each change.
5. After 3 months, the use of Saint Germain splints allow manipulations twice a week until walking commences.
6. When the infant begins to walk, the use of the Saint Germain splints is continued at night and shoes with insoles bearing an external pronating band consolidate the correction during the day. However, the foot must be surveyed regularly up to the age of 15 years.

Medial Release in the Child

In the child aged 5–12 years, the medial release described by Codivilla (1904) is appropriate.

The most important aspect is the mobilisation of the calcaneum. A complementary procedure relates to the midtarsus and antetarsus and is completed by occasional elongation and release of the tendons.

With respect to the ligaments there are certain "untouchables" essential for the stability of the foot, including the middle fasciculus of the medial ligament of the ankle; the interosseous ligament of the sinus tarsi, which guarantees balance and proprioceptive adaptation of the foot to inequalities of the ground; and the Y-shaped ligament of Chopart, which maintains the plantar arch. Section of any one of these leads to irreversible iatrogenic overcorrection.

The posterior tendons must be elongated to their new length with the foot at right angles to the leg. Padovani (1978) insists on this requirement and emphasises the dangers of excessive elongation of triceps surae, which leads to a posterior cavus foot. The tendons must be sutured under light tension posterior to the medial malleolus, not at the level of their angulations inferiorly.

This operation again requires several incisions giving direct access to the regions of concern:

- A longitudinal medial incision commences at the inferior third of the leg at the summit of the medial retromalleolar gutter and descends, curving under the medial malleolus and then running longitudinally along the medial border of the foot as far as the head of the first metatarsal. It may have to be associated with a rotation flap when there is severe contracture leading to a medial and plantar fold (Bensahel 1977).
- An anteriolateral malleolar incision skirts the posterior and inferior margins of the lateral malleolus and runs inferiorly to the dorso-external aspect of the midtarsus.
- A third incision is made on the outer aspect of the calcaneocuboid joint if it is thought necessary to transpose tibialis anterior laterally. In practice, I recommend splitting of the tendon and transposition only of the outer part, so as to avoid the risk of creating a valgus deformity of the midtarsal region.

All three incisions are not always necessary. Accurate clinical and radiological assessment of the sites requiring release is essential.

Posterior Release. This includes the following components: (a) Elongation of tendo Achillis may be performed in the usual Z-fashion, preserving the lateral part of the insertion of the tendon onto the calcaneum, or in V-fashion at the musculotendinous junction, as described by Vulpius (1920). Green also described a technique of tendinous elongation (Green 1942; Banks and Green 1952). (b) Elongation of tibialis posterior, flexor hallucis longus and flexor digitorum longus is performed in the retromalleolar area. In some instances it may be more appropriate to perform these elongations distally to the medial malleolus. (c) The deep aponeuroses of the leg and of associated tendinous sheaths are released. (d) Capsuloligamentous release must be performed under direct vision and comprises division of the posterior capsule of the ankle and medial or posterior capsulotomy of the subtalar joint, which may have to be extended through the external approach in order to release the whole of the posterior aspect. Division of the posterior tibiocalcaneal ligament and the posterior talofibular ligament has to be performed through the lateral incision. Padovani (1978) has stressed the importance of progressive attempts at reduction during operation. It must first be ascertained that the calcaneum is reduced into a normal externally rotated position underneath the talus and with respect to the axis of the leg, ensuring that the talar head becomes palpable at the internal border of the foot, this being the main criterion of completed reduction.

Medial Release. Elongation of tibialis posterior will have been performed during a posterior release and must be accompanied by section or disinsertion of abductor hallucis. Tibialis anterior must be released, perhaps associated with its hemitransplantation or even complete lateral transposition. The plantar aponeurosis must be released on its medial aspect. The capsuloligamentous release may include the posterior fasciculus of the medial ligament of the ankle, the medial capsule of the posterior part of the subtalar joint, the tibionavicular ligament and the dorsal and medial aspects of the talonavicular ligament, but the plantar calcaneonavicular ligament must always be preserved. Medial release must be completed by excision of the fibrous mass of tissue overlying the navicular in front of the head of the talus (Judet et al. 1976; Viladot 1972) and by reposition of the navicular in front of the talar head after its release from the medial malleolus and after mobilisation of the talonavicular joint, the naviculocuneiform joints and, if necessary, the medial aspect of the tarsometatarsal joint.

External Release. The somewhat surprising need for attention to the outer side of the foot has been emphasised by Seringe (1976). It is necessary sometimes to release fibrosis causing adherence of the tendon sheaths of the peronei to the calcaneofibular ligament and mobilise the postero-external aspect of the subtalar joint. This may be completed by division of the anterior annular ligament and of the calcaneofibular component of the lateral ligament, which blocks reduction. It is rarely necessary to section ligaments of the inferior tibiofibular joint to allow reposition of the talus in the mortice. These procedures may enable final reposition of the calcaneum in perfect equilibrium (i.e. external rotation and light valgus). In ensuring stability of reposition of the navicular, it can be valuable to place a large transosseous suture of absorbable material across the talonavicular joint in a vertical tunnel parallel to the medial aspect of the navicular.

In cases exhibiting cavus deformity and abnormally low and inverted malposition of the cuboid, section of the inferior calcaneocuboid ligament may be necessary so as to open the external aspect of the calcaneocuboid joint as well as that of the naviculocuneiform joint. Exceptionally, resection osteotomy of some of the substance of the cuboid may be necessary to shorten the outer aspect of the foot; the same can be achieved by shortening the neck of the talus with or alternatively by calcaneal osteotomy with a wedge resection based laterally (Dwyer 1959). Calcaneocuboid arthrodesis should be considered in the older child or adolescent.

Having achieved repositioning of the calcaneum, the talonavicular joint, and the calcaneocuboid joint, with proper vertical longitudinal and lateral alignment, repairs of the elongated tendons are performed under light tension with the foot held at 90° to the leg.

Relapses occurring between 3 and 18 months of age usually comprise overall inversion of the foot and will respond to medial release followed by plaster immobilisation for several months and subsequent re-educative measures. Later cases, up to the age of 5 years, may involve one or two components of deformity and may require release of the calcaneum, the subtalar joint or the midtarsal region. Very occasionally, release of the tarsometatarsal joint is necessary for metatarsus varus. Between 6 and 12 years of age, complete release may have to be accompanied by Dwyer calcaneal osteotomy (1959) or calcaneocuboid arthrodesis.

Most cases of persistent varus arise in the midtarsal region in feet which are still supple. Simple hemitransplantation of tibialis anterior associated with elongation of the internal tongue suffices, completed if necessary by elongation of tibialis posterior. Persistence of a varus metatarsus can stem from the subtalar joint of the midtarsal region. Tendinous elongations posteriorly, transplantation more externally of tibialis anterior, Dwyer calcaneal osteotomy with excision of an externally based wedge and cuboidectomy or arthrodesis of the calcaneocuboid joint suffice to correct the deformity, provided surgical treatment is followed by re-education, a plaster cast for 2 or 3 months and corrective insoles. Sometimes the varus component arises in the tarsometatarsal joint. Here, the Heymann operation (1958), comprising extensive release of the dorsal and interosseous components of the Lisfranc joint, is usually adequate, but on occasion must be completed by osteotomy of the bases of the metatarsals and tenotomy of the abductor of the great toe. Elongations of tendo Achillis, tibialis posterior, flexor hallucis longus and flexor digitorum longus are also required, together with the transposition more externally of tibialis anterior.

If despite good alignment there is some instability of any joint complex, it may be preferable to fix these under direct vision with temporary Kirschner wires.

A final plaster cast must be applied to maintain correction only, without exerting any corrective pressure, which would always be prejudicial to the formation of a good scar; in addition, the danger that plaster pressure will produce superficial necrosis and subsequent stiffness should not be underestimated. The plaster is a container and not a corrector.

Staples should be used only in very exceptional circumstances; it is better to insert temporary Kirschner wires across the calcaneum into the tibia, through the talus into the navicular, or across the calcaneum, cuboid and metatarsus.

Hemitransplantation of tibialis anterior into a more lateral site on the fifth metatarsal, cuboid or lateral cuneiform is preferable to external transplantation of the whole tendon.

There may be problems with cutaneous closure at the end of the procedure, usually in the form of deficiency of compliant skin on the medial aspect; this can necessitate a rotation flap. Other procedures have been advised: for example, the compensation procedure proposed by Glicenstein and Bensahel (1978) provides in one stage a good-quality scar without tension. When skin deficiency appears likely, a rotation flap incision extending on to the dorsum of the foot, or a transposition on the outer aspect of the foot, allows redistribution of skin tension.

Plaster immobilisation for from 30 to 90 days with radiographic postoperative checking should be succeeded by active re-education, kinesitherapy, massage and proprioceptive exercises. Additionally, a plastic or Saint Germain splint should be used at night for several months, and during the day shoes normal but for a high anklet containing an orthopaedic insole with a pronating external wedge should be the rule. The slightest deterioration must be sought until the conclusion of growth; active exercises and sport should be encouraged.

26.5.4 *Treatment of Relapsed Pes Equinovarus*

Relapses are common when initial correction has not been complete or subsequent follow-up inadequate (Figs. 26.9, 26.10). Surgical treatment is usually necessary unless the displacement is minor, in which case re-educative measures or short periods in a plaster cast or in shoes with corrective insoles may prove adequate.

Persistant metatarsus varus and supination of the forefoot will lead to insufficiency or faulty loading antero-externally. The use of corrective insoles with a physiological shoe incorporating a pronating subcuboid wedge or a pronating external band over a period of years suffices in many instances to coax the forefoot to normal loading, i.e. the presence of a normally elevated cuboid and a normal angle of declination of the great metatarsal, as emphasised by Hendrix (1962). The frequency with which this correction can be achieved by conservative measures indicates great caution in choosing surgical treatment. This applies especially to residual or relapsing metatarsus varus associated with supination.

The persistence of metatarsus varus in a foot which has become rigid is a much stronger indication for surgery, comprising a lateral procedure such as the Heymann operation (1958), shortening of the outer border of the foot or arthrodesis of the tarsometatarsal joint, removing a wedge based externally and dorsally. Accompanying this, a medial operation consists of eleongation of flexor hallucis longus (which I prefer to its transposition onto the neck of the great metatarsal); this preserves the possibility of plantarflexion of the great toe and avoids the development of hallux erectus. Only occasionally will osteotomy of the great metatarsal be necessary to increase its angle of declination, and in general this is poorly indicated. While it may re-establish good loading of the forefoot, it encourages a generally varus posture and accentuates the supination of the midtarsus by preventing elevation of the external part of the longitudinal arch. It may be necessary to recognise that the renal cause of this metatarsus varus relates to limitation of dorsiflexion of the ankle joint.

The persistance of pure equinus of the tarsus at the ankle joint demands elongation of tendo Achillis, which must be carefully calculated to avoid creating a posterior cavus foot. Sometimes it is not adequate and must be completed by posterior capsulotomies extended medially from the ankle (preserving the middle part of the medial ligament of the ankle and the subtalar joint) and by release of the fibrous tissue posterolaterally, section of the posterior talofibular ligament (especially if there is true talar equinus) and elongation of tibialis posterior, flexor hallucis longus and flexor digitorum longus. If the articular surface of the talus does not enter the mortice, arthrolysis of the ankle joint and the inferior tibiofibular joint, while somewhat drastic, allows complete dorsiflexion.

The choice of treatment for pes equinocavovarus in adolescence is dictated by the degree of rigidity. In a supple foot, it may be correctable by Dwyer calcaneal osteotomy associated with elongation of tendo Achillis and tibialis posterior and lateral transplantation of tibialis anterior, in intermediate

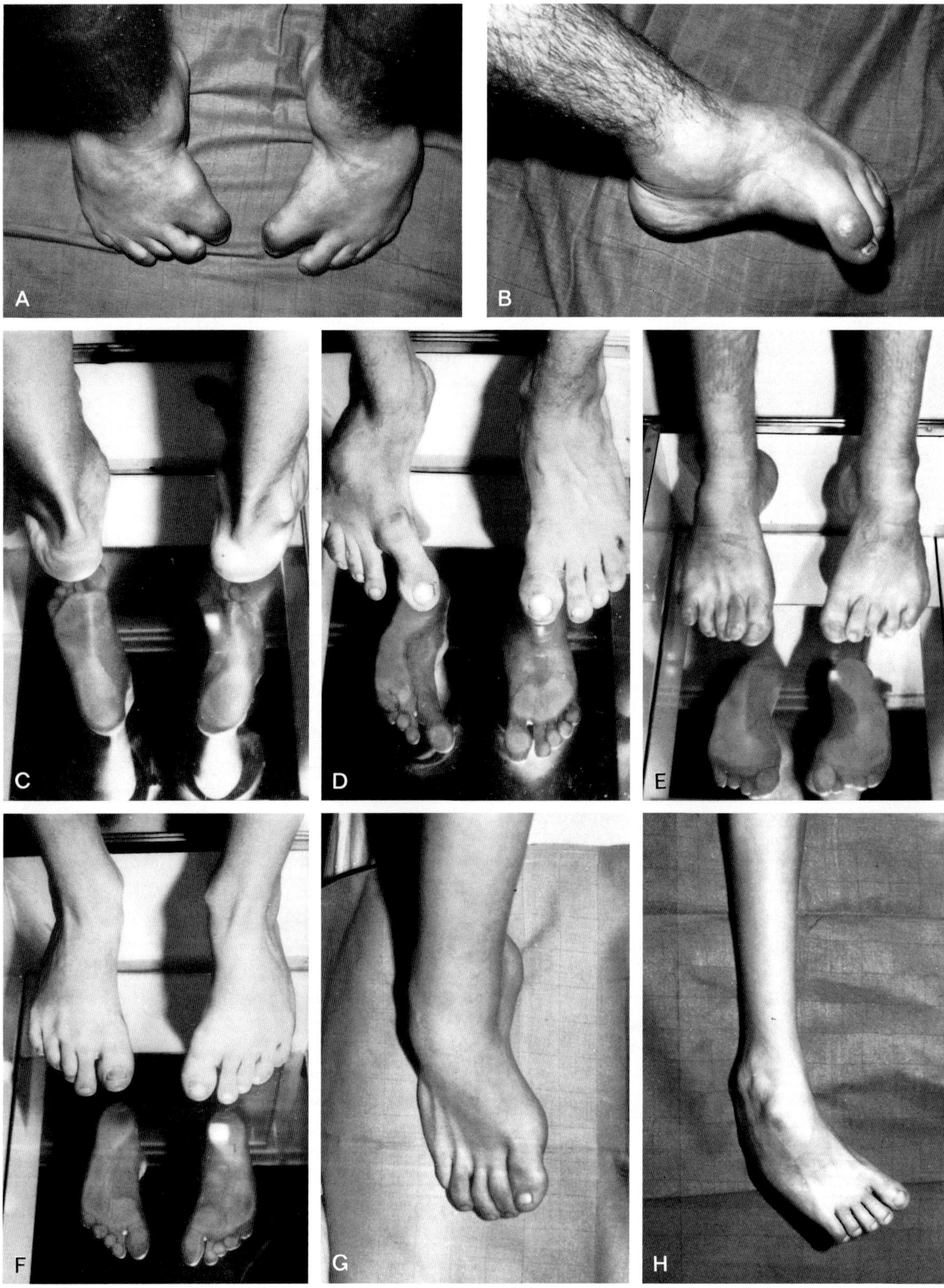

Fig. 26.9 A–J. Sequels of club foot. **A, B** Club foot in the adult. **C, D** Pes cavus with metatarsus varus and hallux varus with flexion. **E, F** Pes adductus. **G, H** Pes cavovarus in adolescence. **I, J** Pes cavovarus in adulthood. **I, J** see p. 411

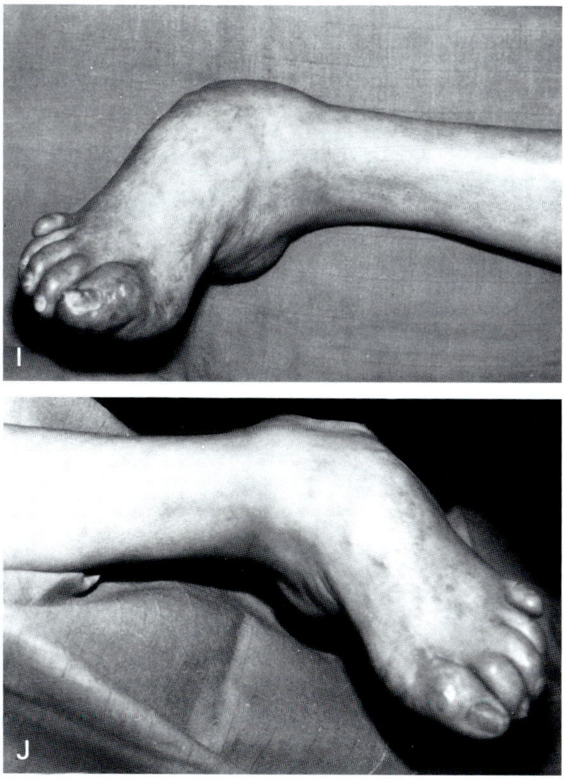

Fig. 26.9 I, J. Legend see p. 410

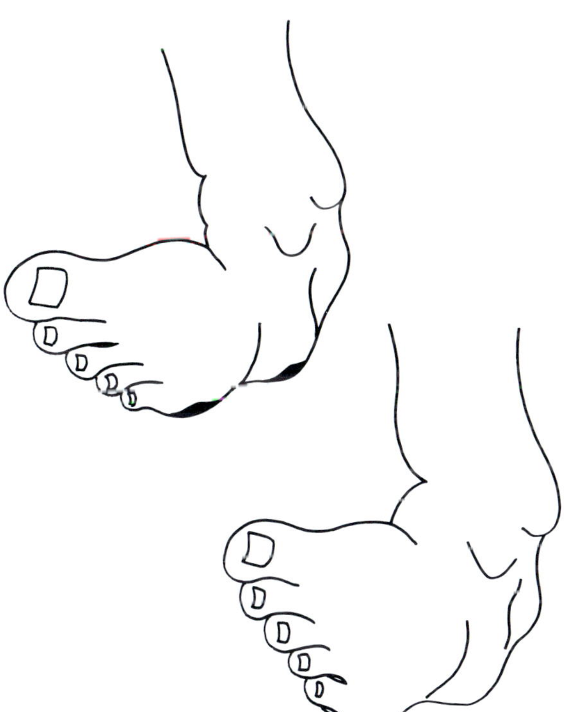

Fig. 26.10. Relapsed equinovarus club foot

cases by double arthrodesis of the subtalar and midtarsal joints (provided the ankle is normal), or in extreme cases by resection of part of the tarsus depending on the site of maximum deformity.

In the adult, irreducible equinus leads to serious disturbance of loading on account of subcuboidal and external submetatarsal callus formation. The calluses are hyperkeratotic and permanently inflamed, and despite the use of special shoes, ulceration with infection is common (Fig. 26.11). Talectomy should be avoided, as it considerably diminishes the height of the tarsus and the heel and does not allow shoes supporting the side of the heel to be worn. Greatly preferable is midtarsal tarsectomy, located according to the site of maximum deformity; even though this can significantly shorten the foot generally, it allows good static loading. Calcaneal osteotomy or arthrodesis of the midtarsal and subtalar joints with wedge resections judiciously orientated in order to correct supination, varus and cavus may be chosen.

I strongly recommend careful assessment of the ankle joint in relapsed equinovarus club feet in adolescence or adulthood. The morphology of the talar surface should be assessed clinically and radiologically. Most frequently, it is found that the antero-external portion of the articular surface of the talus is hypertrophied, especially in adults, following the law of Delpech, i.e. when there is no pressure on bone, it hypertrophies. Re-introduction of the talar articular surface into the mortice is impeded, and the site of the hypertrophy explains both the equinus posture and the varus component. Surgical treatment is indicated and comprises exploration through an anterolateral incision to identify the exact morphological abnormality preventing full integration of the talar articular surface into the mortice. The excess bone can be resected progressively together with associated osteophytes of the neck of the talus, and only after it is ensured that full dorsiflexion at the ankle joint is possible is surgical attention directed to other components.

In the adult, it is usually possible to correct all components, this sometimes involving working down the foot even into the toes, but the procedure may take as long as 2 h. At the end of the operation, general realignment of the foot and restoration of amplitude of ankle movement should have been achieved.

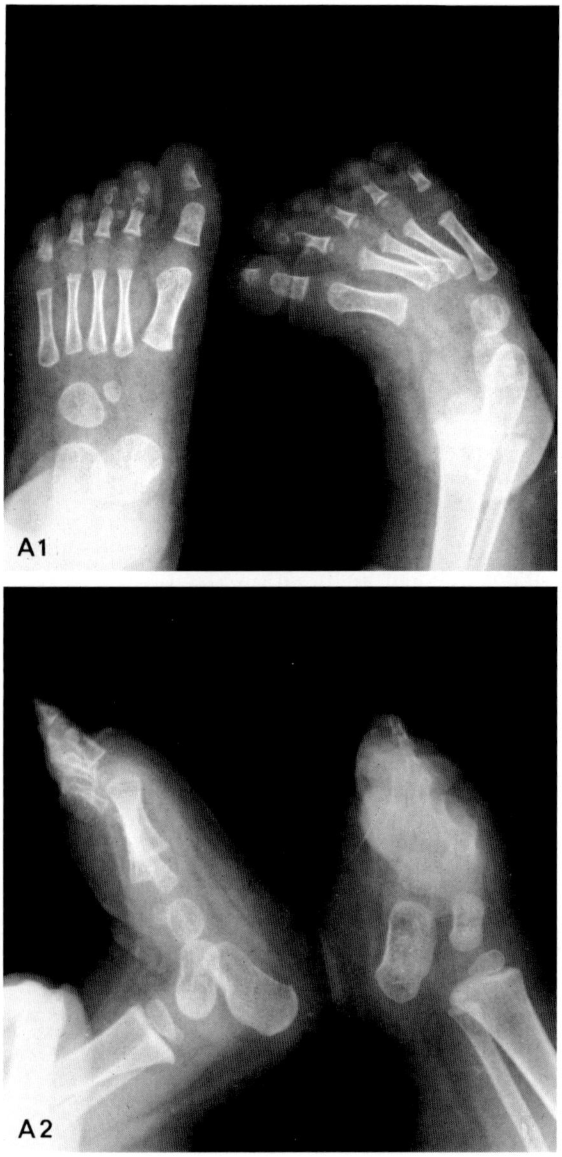

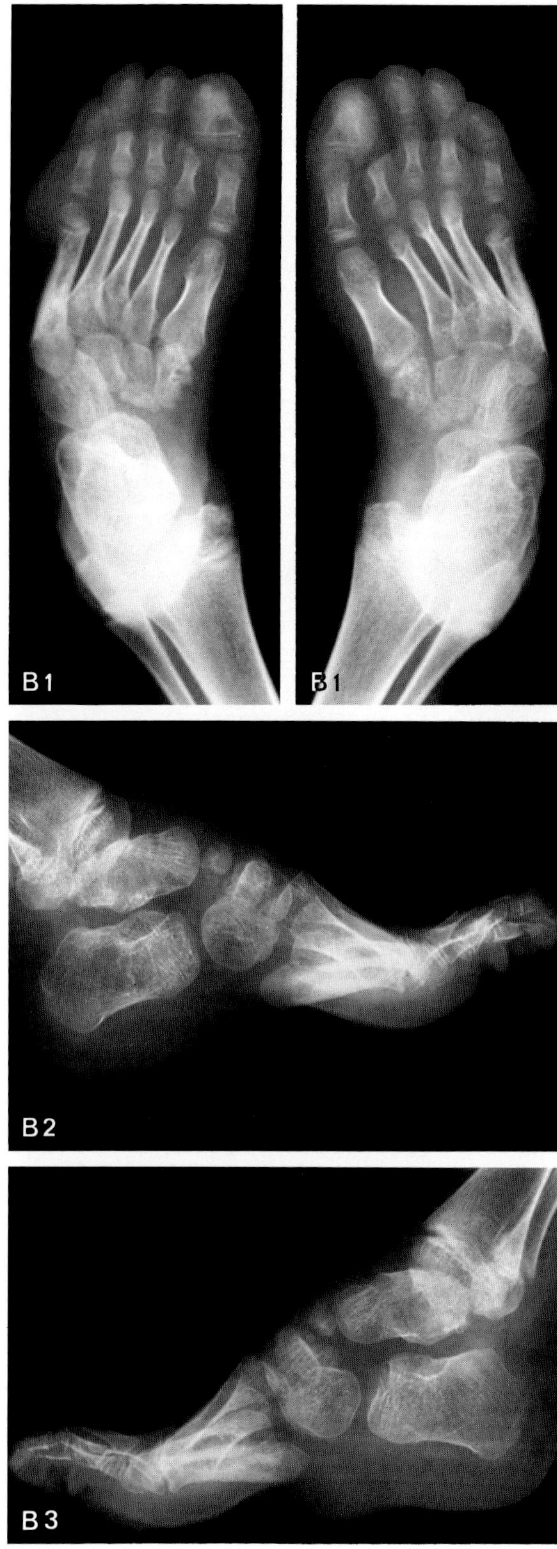

Fig. 26.11 A–E. Congenital malformations: results of congenital talipes equinovarus. **A** *1, 2* Right talipes equinovarus, normal left foot. **B** *1–3* Results of bilateral talipes equinovarus with complete absence of reduction of tarsus, midtarsus, and antetarsus. Right foot *(2)*: flattening of articular surface of talus. Left foot *(3)*: persistent equinovarus due to failure of talus to re-enter ankle mortice. Bilateral loss of dorsiflexion at ankle. **C** Talipes equinovarus. *1–4* Reproduction of varus and antetarsal supination due to equinus and absence of dorsiflexion of foot on axis of leg provoked by significant damage to talar articular surface in ankle mortice. **D** Pes equinocavus as a result of displacement following talipes equinovarus. Walking was impossible. *1* Preoperative; *2* treatment by midtarsal osteotomy, arthrolysis of ankle joint and elongation of tendons, reducing the equinus and allowing loading in suitable orthopaedically prescribed shoes *(3)*. **D–E** see pp. 413, 414

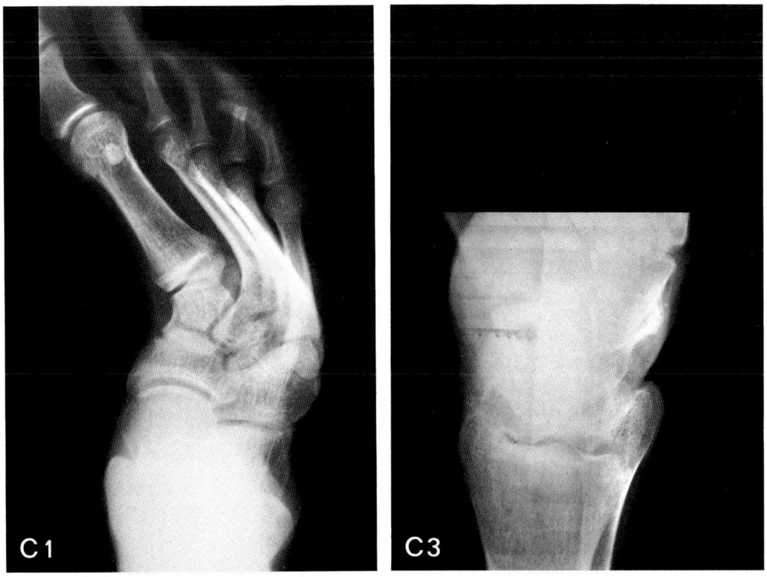

Fig. 26.11 C, D. Legend see p. 412

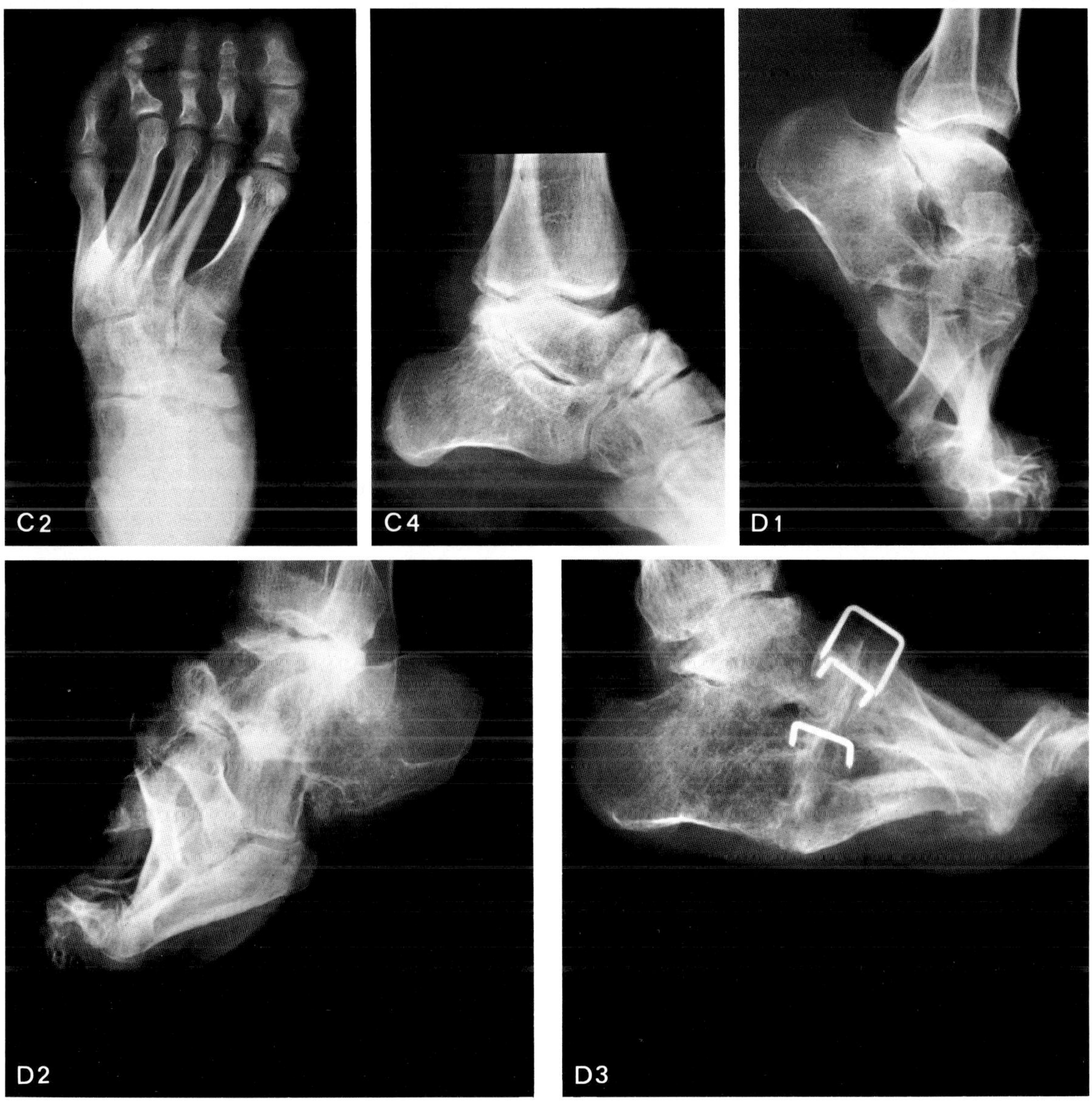

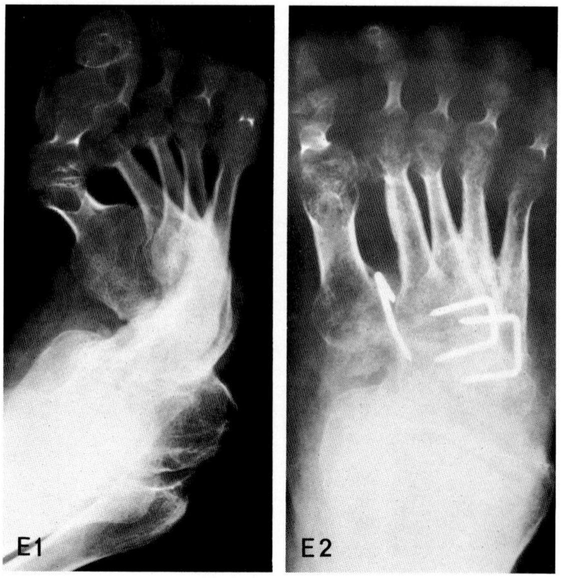

Fig. 26.11. *(continued).* **E** Pes equinocavovarus of extreme degree resulting from hypertrophy of anterolateral aspect of talar articular surface. *1* Preoperative; *2* after arthrolysis of ankle, trimming of talar articular surface, midtarsal osteotomy realigning foot

26.6 Congenital Vertical Talus (Convex Planovalgus Foot)

26.6.1 Description

In common with the preceding congenital equinovarus club foot, congenital convex planovalgus foot is multidirectional and includes primitive or secondary aplasia of the navicular bone (Figs. 26.12, 26.13). The position of the navicular and the talus is inverted; in the convex planovalgus foot, the navicular comes to lie above and outside the head of the talus. The talus is plantarflexed and adducted. In the equinovarus club foot, the navicular is lower and more inwardly situated than the head of the talus, and the talus itself is orientated outwardly and is dorsiflexed. In congenital vertical talus it seems that the vertical alignment of the talus is the primitive, generative factor of the convex planovalgus foot (Böhm 1930).

This rare malposition was described for the first time by Henke (1859), and then by Lamy (1910), who named it "valgus congenital convex foot",

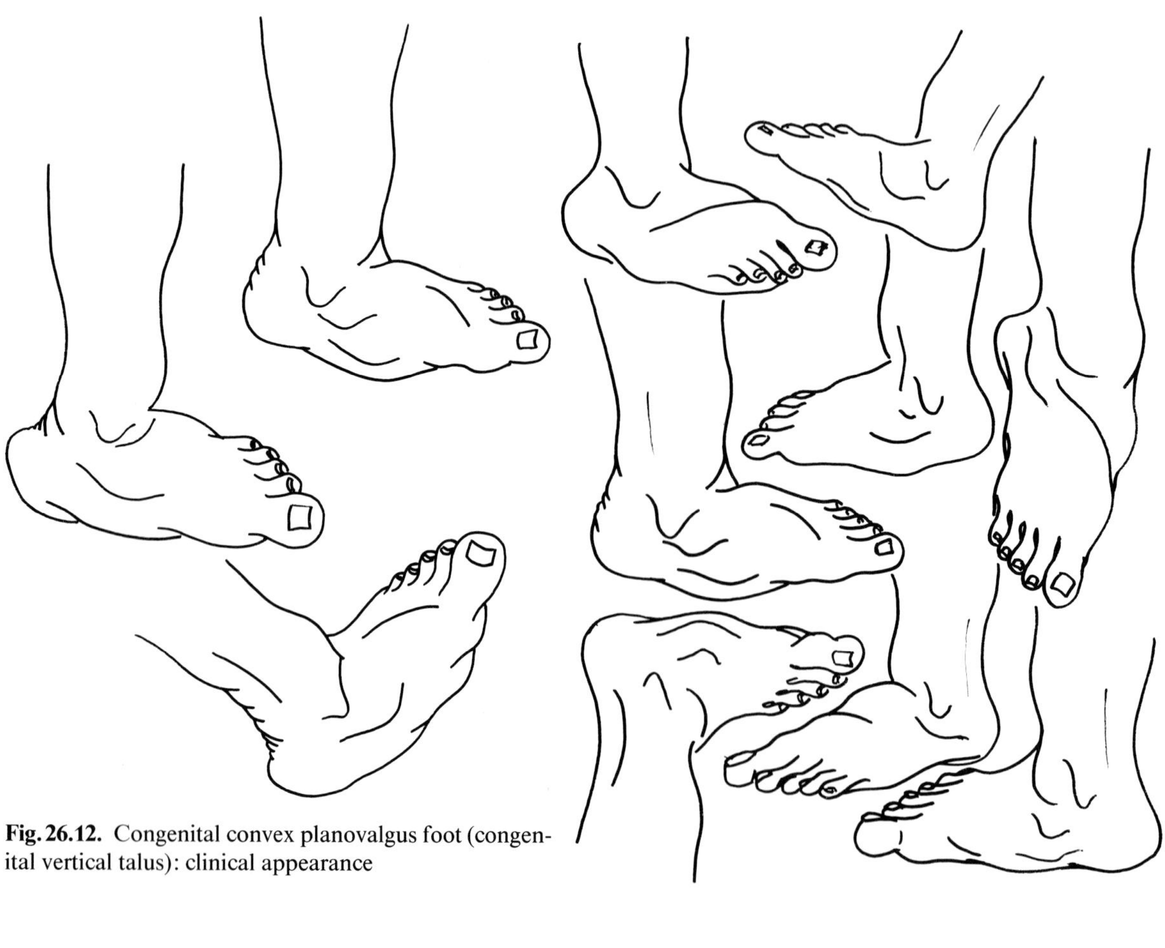

Fig. 26.12. Congenital convex planovalgus foot (congenital vertical talus): clinical appearance

Bossi (1904), Josserand (1914), Leveuf (1946), who called it "convex congenital valgus foot", and Rocher and Rigaud (1956), who called it "ice pick foot".

The malposition is very different from the acquired planovalgus foot on account of the convex aspect of the sole of the foot, analogous, according to Leveuf (1946), to the rocker of a rocking horse; also, the general pronation of the forefoot contrasts with the supination of the forefoot in the acquired planovalgus foot.

The deformity is characterised by irreducibility, which is apparent at the outset. Frequently there are other congenital abnormalities (Rigault 1972) involving the hand, the hip, the spine or the other foot, or features of arthrogryposis. Occasionally, there is spina bifida occulta.

26.6.2 Etiology

Two observations may be cogent: Dega (1971) emphasised the arrest of horizontalisation of the talus normally occurring after the 3rd month of intra-uterine life, while Leveuf (1946) drew attention to the predominant hypertonia of triceps surae (first sacral root) and the extensors and peronei (fifth lumbar root).

Dega's observation relates to the fact that during the first 2 months of intra-uterine life, the talus is vertical, aligned with the axis of the tibia. It then becomes progressively more horizontal and achieves its normal position in the ankle mortice (Paparella-Treccia 1977). In persistent vertical talus, the alignment is maintained by elevation of the calcaneum laterally and dorsal subluxation of the navicular onto the dorsal aspect of the neck of the talus while the cuboid subluxes upwards outwardly and posteriorly. The two midtarsal dislocations of the navicular and the cuboid lead in the long term to valgus pronation of the tarsus and pronation-abduction of the forefoot.

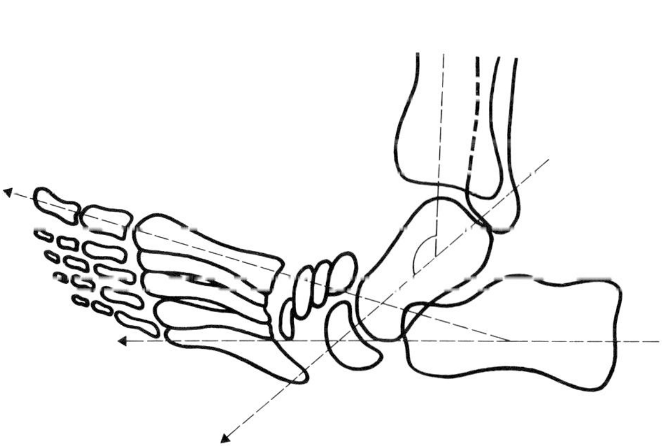

Fig. 26.13. Congenital convex planovalgus foot (congenital vertical talus): outline of skeletal elements

The muscle imbalance theory of Leveuf (1946) apportions blame to hypertonia of triceps surae, the extensors and the peronei, which leads to eversion of the tarsus and dorsiflexion, pronation and abduction of the forefoot. The foot "breaks" in the midtarsus at the talonavicular joint. The muscle hypertonia relates to the fifth lumbar and first sacral segments, but it is not known whether there is a lesion of the cord or whether the abnormality is at a higher level.

Whatever the basic cause, the vertical alignment of the talus and accompanying displacements of other bones and the hypertonia seem to be related and must be treated together.

26.6.3 Clinical Features

From birth, the foot has a flat appearance and is in valgus and the sole is convex. Eversion is marked. The foot is generally displaced outwards with respect to the axis of the leg and rests principally on its inner border at the midtarsus and metatarsus. The tarsus rests on the ground only at the extremity of the heel. "Ice pick" (Rocher and Rigaud 1956) and "rocker bottom" (Leveuf 1946) are both apt terms (Fig. 26.12).

Posteriorly the tarsal equinovalgus is indicated by elevation of the heel and by a dorsolateral submalleolar depression. This depression is reduced in the somewhat older infant by projection of the peroneal tendons, while in the baby the tendinous elevations are perceived only by palpation and are masked by the thicker adipose tissue. There is rupture of the midtarsal hinge of the talonavicular joint line, evidenced by internal and plantar convexity and by the double dorsal and external angulations.

Along the inner aspect of the foot there are three bony projections: the medial malleolus, the head of the talus, situated directly and underneath it, and the anterior process of the calcaneum, which is prominent in the midtarsal region. These three projections constitute overall convexity of the inner aspect of the sole of the foot, so forming the rocker. The summit of the triple convexity is at the talonavicular joint line.

On the outer aspect there is a double dorsolateral concavity which is vertical with respect to the midtarsus and longitudinal with respect to the tarsus. Its summit is located at a depression on the dorsum of the foot under the lateral malleolus and it is elevated somewhat in the older infant by bowstringing of the peroneal and extensor tendons.

There is double eversion of the forefoot as a result of pronation and abduction which is accentuated by dorsiflexion of the metatarsus. The angulated dorsum of the foot therefore seems shorter while the plantar aspect appears elongated. In the untreated case, an adduction component of the metatarsus supervenes towards the 5th year of life, due to reflex attempts to stabilise the valgus and convexity of the midtarsus.

Palpation clarifies the osteoarticular features. There is equinovalgus of the calcaneum, the posterior process of which is clearly elevated with respect to the general line of the sole of the foot, in contrast to the anterior process, which comes to lie much more under the heel than normal due to the plantarflexion; a triple convexity in the tarsometatarsal region centred over the talonavicular joint; vertical alignment of the talus with its prominent head medially; dorsal dislocation of the navicular onto the dorsal aspect of the neck of the talus (although this may be difficult to palpate on account of thickness or tension in the tissues); upward posterior subluxation of the cuboid; and eversion of the forefoot, as evidenced both by the abduction, pronation and dorsiflexion of the metatarsals with respect to the midtarsus and by their reduced angle of declination, this becoming progressively more noticeable from the first to the fifth rays. The loss of joint motion is most marked at the ankle joint and talonavicular joint. Plantarflexion is much reduced compared with dorsiflexion of the foot.

Evidence of muscle imbalance is given by the contracted hypertonic triceps surae and the hypertonia of the peroneal tendons, which bowstring under the skin; peroneus brevis fixes the elevation and eversion of the external border of the cuboid and the base of the fifth metatarsal (therefore the whole foot), and peroneus longus fixes the great metatarsal in adduction. Hypertonia of the extensor muscles exaggerates dorsiflexion and abduction, which fixes the forefoot in eversion and accentuates metatarsal pronation, while stretching of tibialis anterior and the posterior tendons accentuates their hypotonicity.

Commencement of walking is usually delayed some 8 months beyond normal. Usually there is no evidence of discomfort, but it is obvious from the general valgus of the foot that a disability exists, and this is reflected in abnormal wear of the shoes in the somewhat older child.

Podoscopy does not add anything to clinical diagnosis, only confirming a plantar print reflecting the head of the talus.

Radiography (Figs. 26.14, 26.15): The essential features are the vertical alignment of the long axis of the talus, the eversion of the forefoot, the subluxation or dislocation of the talonavicular joint onto the neck of the talus, the horizontal divergence of the axes of the talus and calcaneum, and the equinus posture of the calcaneum with diminution of areas of contact at the subtalar joint.

In the dorsoplantar view, there is overall external displacement of the foot with respect to the mortice of the ankle; the tarsometatarsal angulation with its summit at the talonavicular joint is clear with distal metatarsal abduction, and there is divergence of the talocalcaneal horizontal axis, showing abduction of the calcaneum, and adduction with hypertrophy of length of the neck of the talus. An empty space appears between the talus and the cuneiform joints, due to the navicular dislocation, and the metatarsus is abducted.

In the lateral view, the vertical divergence of the talocalcaneal joint is shown by the fact that the vertical axis of the talus is orientated downwards and forwards and forms an angle of approximately 120°–180° with respect to the tibia; it is exceptional for it to be directly in line with the tibia. There is an obtuse angle between the axis of the talus and the first metatarsal. The calcaneum is either horizontal or in equinus with its anterior process depressed, and its longitudinal axis projects below that of the metatarsus. The reduced area of contact between the subtalar joint surfaces may be obvious (Bensahel 1977), while dislocation of the talonavicular joint may be difficult to appreciate in the infant because the navicular ossification centre is not yet apparent. The midtarsus is seen to be lower, this relating to the superimposition of the head of the talus onto the cuboid; the metatarsus is in general horizontal, perhaps associated with inversion, and its axis of alignment forms an obtuse angle with the equinus of the tarsus at the sinus tarsi region.

The foregoing describes the pathognomonic features of congenital vertical talus. However, Rigault (1972) emphasised correctly that the degree of divergence between the talus and the calcaneum is very variable. There are many degrees of this malformation. In some there is a good range of dorsiflexion of the talus when it is stressed, while in others the equinus of the talus persists. In yet others, there is a false abducted valgus equinus foot. Rigauld described three types with respect to severity of the overall malformation:

Type 1: Absence of talocalcaneal divergence with significant equinus of the calcaneum. It is the least common.
Type 2: Marked talocalcaneal divergence without equinus of the calcaneum. This is intermediate in incidence.
Type 3: Marked talocalcaneal divergence and equinus of the calcaneum. This is the most frequent type.

The diagnosis must be made at birth, for whatever the indications for conservative or surgical management, all authors agree on the necessity for the very early institution of treatment.

26.6.4 *Treatment*

26.6.4.1 *Conservative*

Lelièvre and Bensahel state that early treatment by manipulative correction will lead to fairly good rehabilitation of the foot. Manipulations should be performed in the hospital environment, at first daily and later at progressively longer intervals. The first aim should be to correct abduction and dorsiflexion of the metatarsus, bringing it into normal alignment with the talus with some degree of pronation (Lelièvre 1952). After this, the tarsal equinus should be corrected, and finally the angulation of the midtarsus. It is often necessary during conservative management to perform elongation of triceps surae. Fixed splinting after each manipulation maintains the corrections. Use of shoes with insoles during the day and splints at night should continue for a long period after the child begins walking.

26.6.4.2 *Operative*

26.6.4.2.1 Child Under 5 Years

Failure of conservative management, with persistent displacements of the talus, the calcaneum and the medial cuneiform, demands medial release and realignment of the foot as indicated by Judet et al. (1966). The procedure comprises three phases: (a) correction of the subtalar dislocation and reseating of the dislocated talar head on the sustentaculum tali, thereby correcting the valgus posture of the calcaneum; (b) reposition of the navicular on the end of the talar head after excision of the mass of fibrous tissue on the pretalar aspect; and (c) correction of the calcaneal equinus after elongation of the peroneal tendons, the extensors and tendo Achillis. The fixation should be maintained by a Kirschner wire and plaster immobilisation for some 6–8 weeks. A talocalcaneal screw can be used for this purpose [the so-called horseman operation of Judet (1972)].

26.6.4.2.2 Child Over 5 Years

Dega (1971) has described an osseous procedure comprising exposure of the talonavicular joint through a midline incision, reinsertion of tibialis anterior onto the dorsal aspect of the navicular and medial cuneiform, reinsertion of tibialis posterior onto the plantar border of the navicular or onto the medial cuneiform, resection of the head of the talus and then, through a lateral longitudinal incision, Z-elongation of tendo Achillis and the peronei. Cuneiform osteotomy of the body of the calcaneum, with a wedge based plantarwards located under the sinus tarsi, completes the procedure. The correction of the talocalcaneal divergence is thus facilitated. The calcaneum is maintained by a thin Küntscher nail which is introduced from the plantar aspect of the calcaneum, traverses the bone and gains purchase on the posterior cortex of the tibia. The plantar arch is reconstituted, and the correction is consolidated by protection in a plaster cast for some 8 weeks. This procedure allows sinking of the posterior process of the calcaneum and reduction of the dorsal dislocation of the cuboid and of the medial cuneiform, and re-establishes a longitudinal plantar arch and a balanced foot (Figs. 26.16, 26.17).

Operative Technique. I favour the original concept of Dega (1971), Judet (1972), Rigault (1972) and Leveuf 1941). The operation proceeds in five stages.
Stage 1: A longitudinal medial incision beginning 3 cm above and behind the medial malleolus curves and follows the medial border of the foot as far as the tarsometatarsal joint line. Tibialis posterior is identified and detached from the navicular. The subtalar joint is opened medially, and on incising the talonavicular joint, the upward and outward displacement of the navicular is clearly identified. The medial cuneiform is adjacent to the "empty space" seen on radiographs which is really occupied by a mass of fibrous tissue in the gap between the talus and the medial cuneiform. The fibrous mass should be dissected very carefully from the surfaces of the displaced navicular and cuneiform, preserving capsular tissue between the front of the talus and the back of the cuneiform.

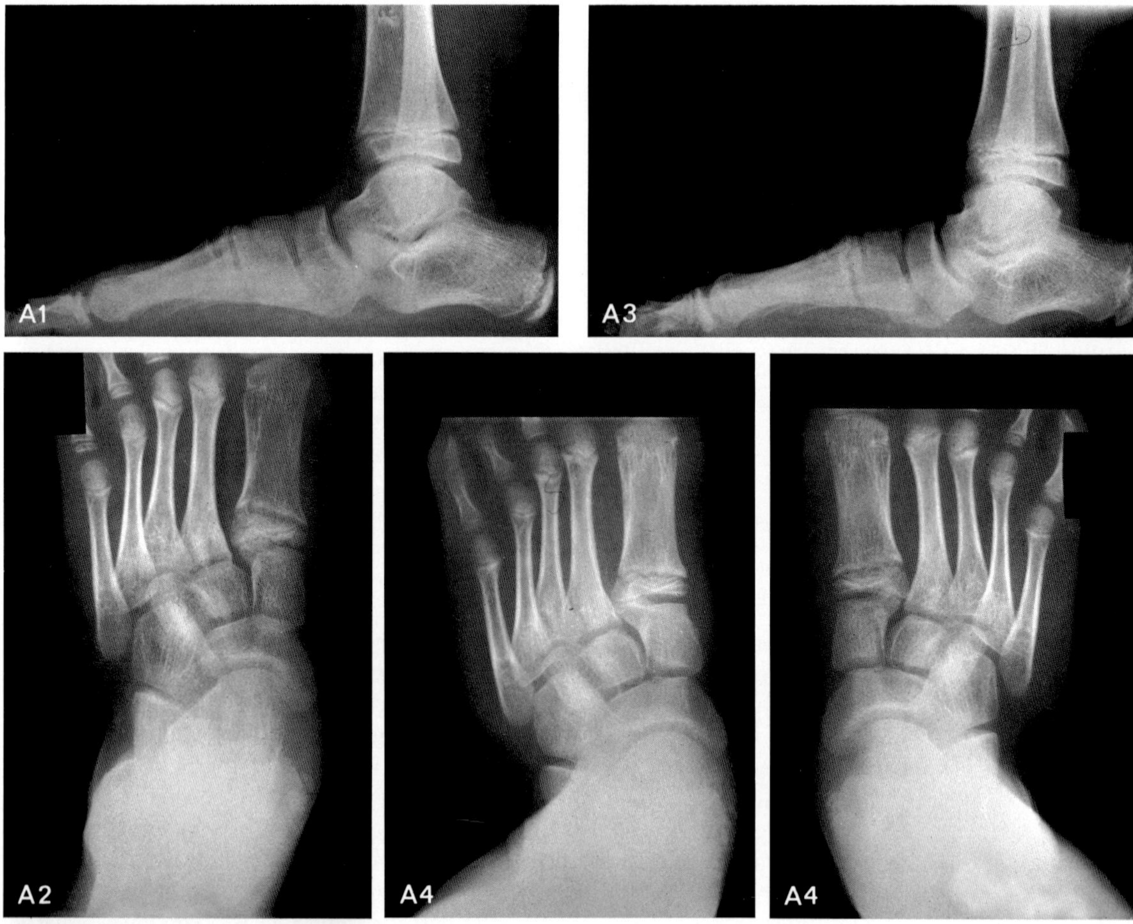

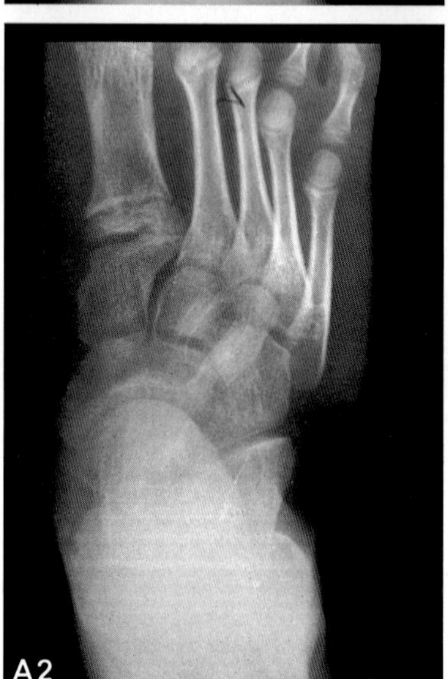

Fig. 26.14 A–C. Congenital pes planovalgus. **A** *1* Right foot, weight-bearing ▷ lateral view: lowering of midtarsal region, superimposition of navicular and cuboid; *2* left foot, weight-bearing lateral view: shortness of neck of talus, equinus of talus; *3* right foot, dorsoplantar view: midtarsal angulation, adduction of neck of talus; *4* left foot, dorsoplantar view: abduction of cuneiform-cuboidal mass. **B** *1* Left foot, weight-bearing lateral view: shortness of neck of talus, lowering of midtarsus; *2* right foot, weight-bearing lateral view: superimposition of navicular and cuboid, horizontal alignment of calcaneum, early convexity of the plantar longitudinal surface; *3* both feet, weight-bearing dorsoplantar view: abduction of cuneiform-cuboidal mass compensated by supination and light adduction of metatarsus. **C** Right foot. *1* Weight-bearing lateral view: lowering of naviculocuboidal mass, equinus of neck of talus; *2* non-weight-bearing lateral view: dislocation of navicular onto dorsal surface of neck of talus, equinus of calcaneum; *3* weight-bearing lateral view: lowering and plantar convexity of midtarsal mass, dorsal subluxation of navicular onto neck of talus, which is in equinus and aplastic; *4* lateral and dorsoplantar views of midtarsus: atrophy of navicular, aplasia of head of talus and navicular; *5, 6* weight-bearing and non-weight-bearing lateral views: midtarsal angulation, aplasia of navicular, abducted axes of cuneiforms

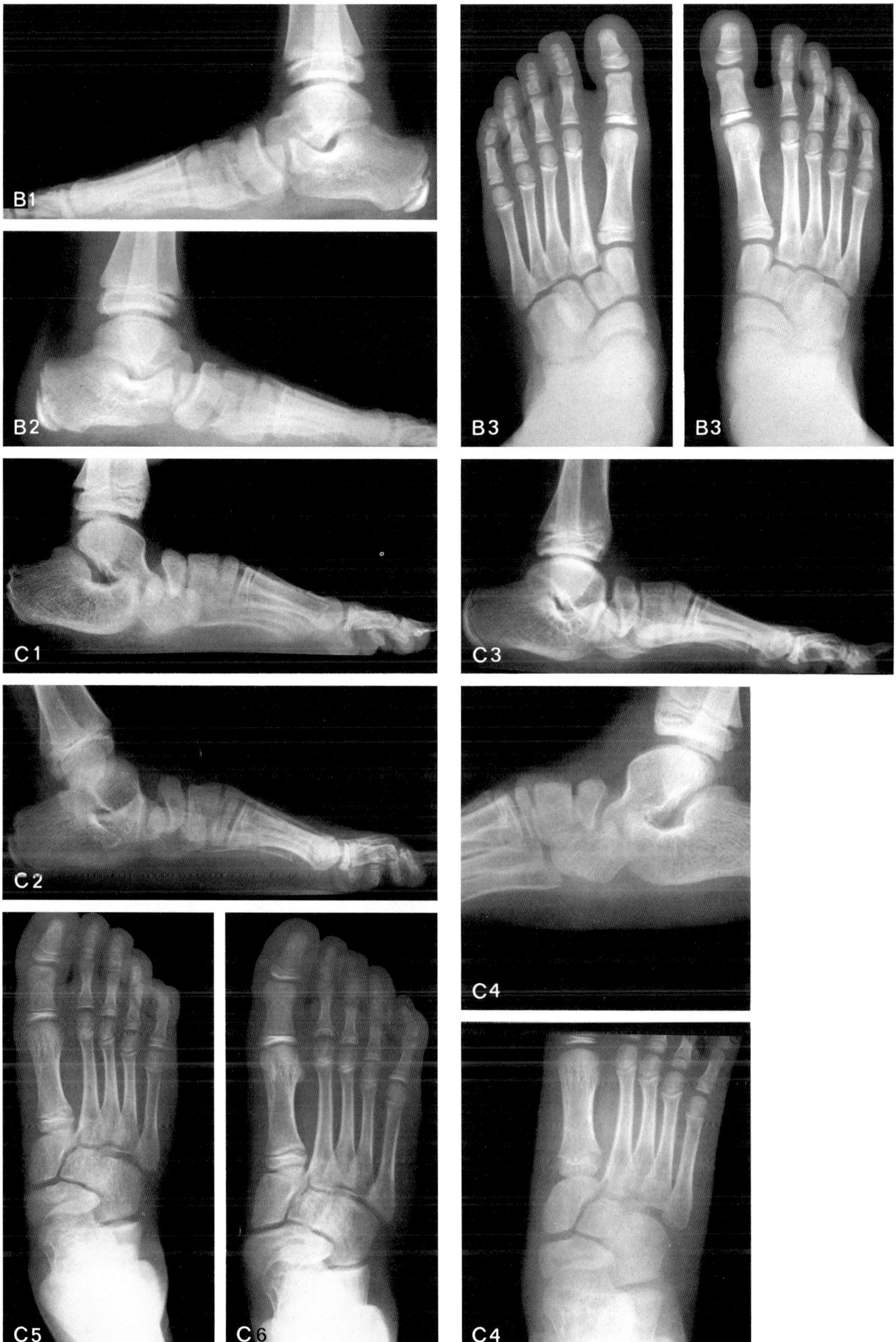
B1
B2
B3
B3
C1
C3
C2
C4
C5
C6
C4

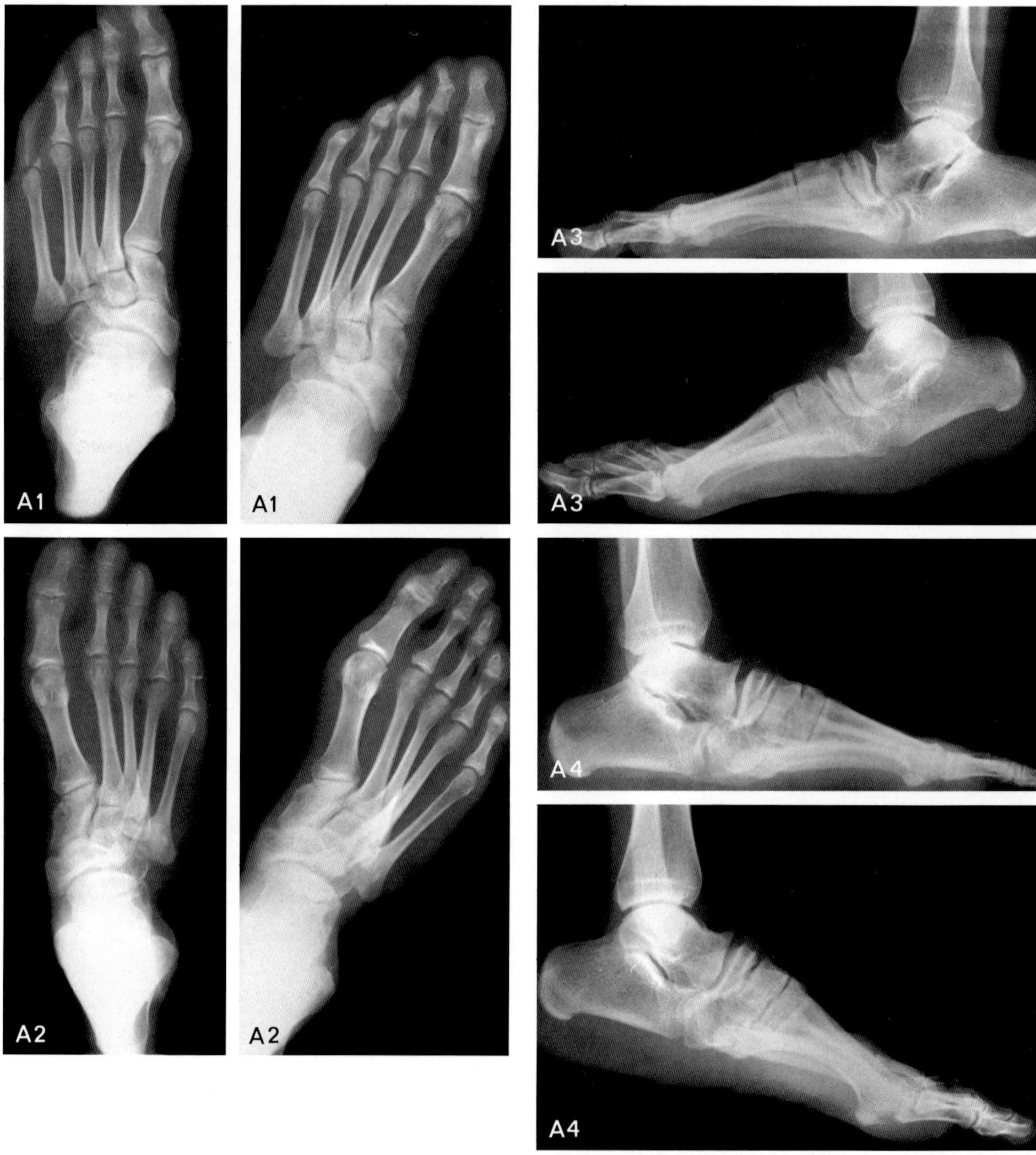

Fig. 26.15. A Adolescent congenital pes planovalgus. *1* Left foot, weight-bearing and non-weight-bearing dorsoplantar views: weight-bearing view shows medial displacement of midtarsus, subluxation and medial hypertrophy of navicular; *2* right foot, weight-bearing and non-weight-bearing dorsal views: findings as in left foot; *3* left foot, weight-bearing and non-weight-bearing lateral views: collapse of midtarsal mass leading to convex plantar aspect of foot, equinus of calcaneum, navicular dystrophy; *4* right foot, weight-bearing and non-weight-bearing lateral views: findings as in left foot. **B** see p. 421 ▷

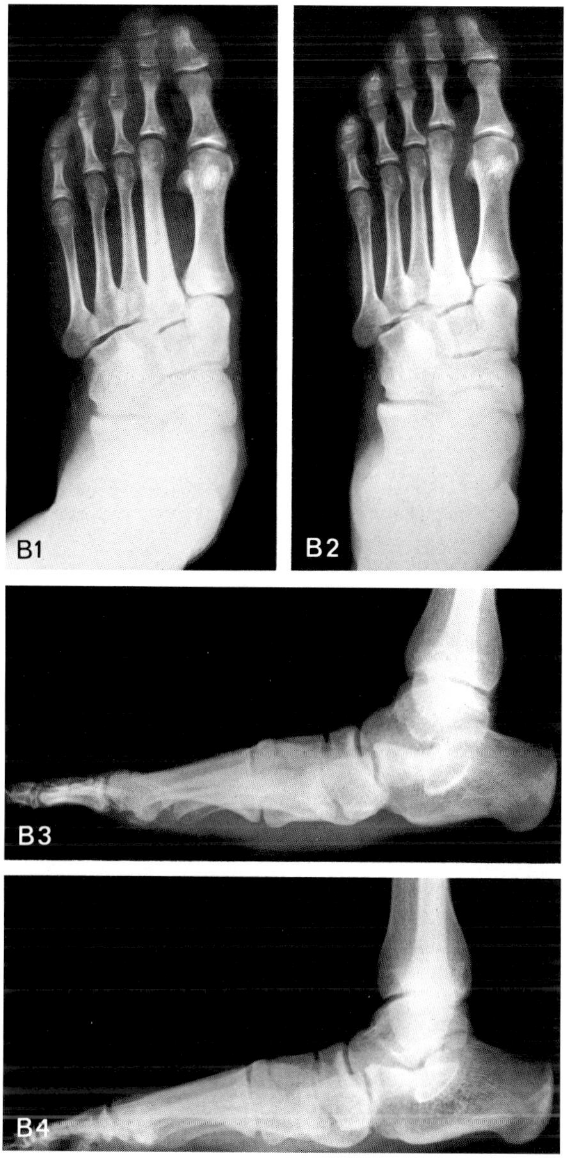

Fig. 26.15 *(continued)*. **B** Congenital pes planovalgus, left foot. *1, 2* Weight-bearing and non-weight-bearing dorsoplantar views: medial displacement of midtarsal mass; *3* non-weight-bearing lateral view: plantarflexion and shortness of talus, horizontal alignment of calcaneum; *4* weight-bearing lateral view: complete flattening of midtarsal mass, superimposition of navicular and cuboid

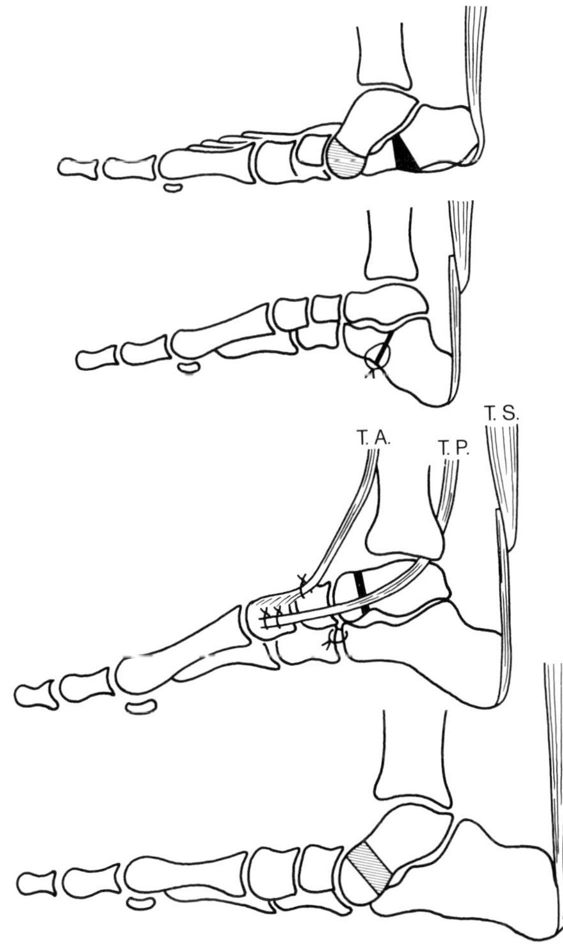

Fig. 26.16 A, B. Treatment of congenital vertical talus. **A** Resection of head of talus, plantar osteotomy of calcaneum, elongation of tendo Achillis (Dega). **B** Elongation of tendo Achillis, transfer of tibialis anterior *(T. A.)* to navicular, transfer of tibialis posterior *(T. P.)* to neck of talus, semilunar resection of plantar calcaneonavicular ligament (Pisani) and of talonavicular component. *T. S.*, triceps surae

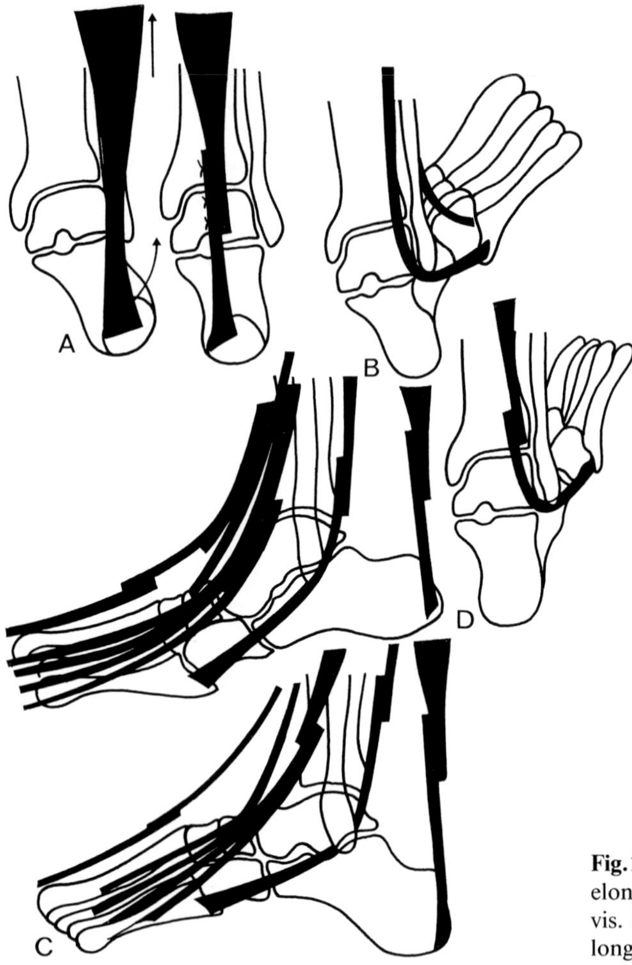

Fig. 26.17 A–D. Treatment of congenital vertical talus by elongation of tendons. **A** Triceps surae. **B** Peroneus brevis. **C** Extensor hallucis longus and extensor digitorum longus. **D** Peroneus brevis

Stage 2: An external longitudinal incision is made in the middle axis of the retromalleolar gutter, extending from the inferior third of the leg and descending obliquely below and parallel with the peroneal tendons, and elongation of triceps surae or tendo Achillies and of both peroneal tendons is performed. Peroneus tertius should be included if necessary. The origin of extensor digitorum brevis on the outer aspect of the calcaneum is elevated, as are the whole of the lateral ligament of the ankle joint and of the subtalar joint anteriorly, while the posterior talofibular ligament and the posterior capsule of the ankle joint are divided. During this extensive arthrotomy, great care is taken not to open the subtalar joint posteriorly, as this area provides the pivot on which correction of the talocalcaneal horizontal divergence will be effected (Judet et al. 1966). By means of this mobilisation the talocalcaneal displacement can be corrected, bringing the head of the talus into its proper position on the sustentaculum tali. The reposition is unstable. If necessary, the tendons of extensor hallucis longus and extensor digitorum longus may be elongated through a more anterior incision.

Stage 3: The repositioned talus and calcaneum must be stabilised while the dorsal dislocation of the navicular is corrected and the navicular is held between the head of the talus and the medial cuneiform. The situation can be rendered more stable by means of appropriate orientation of the articular surface by transverse osseous resection through the neck of the talus. Sometimes, rigidity of the talonavicular joint line indicates impossibility of realignment, and in these instances resection of the head of the talus is necessary (Dega 1971).

Stage 4: The operation concludes with stabilisation of the navicular in its proper place by insertion of the tibialis posterior tendon into its medial tubercle, reconstitution of the capsules of the talonavicular and naviculocuneiform joints and semilunar resection of the plantar calcaneonavicular ligament and the Y-shaped ligament followed by suture according to Rodgvelle (1976) [cited by Pisani (1979f)]. The navicular is further stabilised by a suture passed in a loop across the neck of the talus, the tuberosity of the calcaneum and the periosteum of the cuneiform. The distal insertion (into the medial cuneiform) of tibialis anterior is brought onto the dorsal face of the navicular and held by a transosseous stitch. Arthrorisis of the subtalar joint has been advocated for persisting instability of the calcaneal correction, but in general it is not effective and may be impossible on account of the aplasia of the sinus tarsi, which precludes insertion of a graft or even a prosthesis. The calcaneum can be kept under the talus by means of a talocalcaneal screw [the horseman operation of Judet (1972)].

Stage 5: With the foot held at 90° to the leg, suturing to correct the lengths of the various tendons is carried out.

During closure, the lateral ligamentous layers are left unsutured, while in the medial aspect the repair is firm. Haemostasis is most careful. When the stability of the reshaped foot has been assured, with particular attention to the formation of the longitudinal arch, the skin is closed over suction drainage.

A plaster cast is applied to maintain the foot in a neutral position, supporting the cavus in the midtarsal region, for 1 month. Thereafter, re-education is undertaken and walking is allowed only with an orthopaedic insole comprising an internal dome, the prescription of which exceeds by 2–3 mm the height of the correction obtained.

It remains to emphasise the importance (stressed by Judet, Rigault and Leveuf) of the great care and attention to detail which is necessary for operative success.

26.6.4.2.3 Adult

In patients over the age of 18 years, one would still attempt the soft tissue release described above, but osteoarticular deformation of the midtarsus may make this impossible. In these circumstances, and in later adulthood, correction must be achieved by wedge tarsectomy across the midtarsus and subtalar regions or by the triple arthrodesis described by Viladot and by Torner.

These operations assure good correction of the malformation and a balanced foot, despite suppression of the articular function of the hindfoot.

27 Congenital Malformations

Congenital malformations are dependent upon ill-understood genetic factors. Their presentations are polymorphic, and treatment is often difficult or impossible. No attempt will be made here to identify underlying causes, but some indication of appropriate conservative or operative measures will be given for each of the various types encountered.

27.1 Aplasia

Aplasia may be *transverse*, characterised by deficiency of a segment of the foot, posing problems regarding footwear and therefore relieved to some extent by special shoes and insoles (Fig. 27.1 e, f, h, k). Alternatively, the condition may be *longitudinal*, affecting one or several rays, restricted to the toes or extending proximally into the tarsus (Fig. 27.2). Of the longitudinal defects, hemimelia or lobster claw foot seems the most frequent, and is characterised by a defect which divides the foot into two claw-like elements extending into the midtarsus. The medial claw is constituted by the first ray, perhaps in association with the second and third rays, while the fifth ray, perhaps in association with the fourth ray, forms the outer component. The hemimelia may be accompanied by a planus deformity with horizontalisation of the tarsus and midtarsus, especially involving the calcaneum, and complicated occasionally by tarsal synostosis or a syndesmosis involving bones of the tarsus and midtarsus. Alternatively, there may be an unbalanced cavus deformity, in which case the foot is slender, spider-like, lax, unstable and painful. The hemimelic foot, whether planus or cavus, is painful on account of the distortion imposed on joints, especially the ankle and subtalar joints, and the existence of calluses under the sharp points of loading in the metatarsal region.
Treatment: Insoles adapted to relieve the points of overloading and support the other parts of the foot must be carefully made for the individual. Surgery is indicated only for correction of gross divergence of the hemimelic claws which makes it impossible to wear shoes. Operation will involve osteotomy or arthrodesis, correcting deformities and restoring a straight forefoot more amenable to future use of insoles and adapted shoes.

27.2 Hypoplasia

Hypoplasia may be micromelic (involving diminution in volume of the metatarsals or phalanges) or brachymelic (involving shortening of the long axes of the bones). Both occur in the same patient (Fig. 27.1 a–d). The condition is met most frequently in the fourth ray and with decreasing frequency in the second, first and third rays. The metatarsal alone, the toe or the whole ray can be involved (Figs. 27.3, 27.4). Hypoplasia leads to a syndrome of loading insufficiency and associated overloading of the neighbouring metatarsals (Fig. 27.5 g–i). *Treatment* is palliative, involving chiropody and use of appropriate insoles protecting the zones of overloading. Surgery is indicated only occasionally to realign the metatarsal heads, usually by shortening the normal metatarsals (by head-shaft enclavement), but occasionally, if appropriate, by elongation of a hypoplastic metatarsal (see Chap. 12).

27.3 Hyperplasia

Hyperplasia may involve the whole foot, which is then hypertrophied in height, width and length; when it involes one foot, there is obviously difficulty with footwear because of the different sizes needed (Fig. 27.5 m). In some instances, one or several bones of the antetarsus may be involved, especially the second and third metatarsals. More commonly, macrometatarsia is accompanied by macrodactyly of the corresponding toes (Fig. 27.5 a–f).
The difficulties with shoes are accompanied by a painful syndrome of overloading in this convex macromelic forefoot. Finally, macrodactyly can involve one or several toes both in length and circumference. The first, second and third rays are affected in decreasing order of (Fig. 27.6).

Treatment: Surgery is often valuable and comprises shortening of one or more metatarsals by means of basal osteotomy according to Mau (1940) and Thys (1974b) or realignment head-shaft enclavement (Regnauld 1968). A broad toe can be treated by longitudinal splitting of the integument and bones, reduction of volume of all components, and resuturing.

27.4 Polyplasia

Duhamel (1973) has made a valuable study of polyplasias. Polymetatarsia and polydactyly can exist together or in isolation, and may be unilateral or bilateral (Figs. 27.7, 27.8). Supernumerary rays are often complicated by polysyndactylies and hyperphalangias (Fig. 27.5 n). The abnormal width of the foot results in difficulties with footwear. Depending on the number of supernumerary rays, the condition may be termed hexadactyly (Fig. 27.5 j), heptodactyly or octodactyly.
Treatment is surgical and comprises excision of the supernumerary rays.

27.5 Symplasia

Symplasia may involve the skin or other tissues down to bone (Fig. 27.5 a–f, k, l).

27.5.1 Cutaneous Syndactyly

This is a mild malformation which often leads to no serious inconvenience, amounting only to a webbing of the affected toes. It can be partial (uniting only the proximal segments of two neighbouring toes) or complete (uniting all the phalanges). Occasionally the syndactyly is extensive, involving all five toes, and in this case the term "palm foot" is appropriate.

27.5.2 Osteocutaneous Syndactyly

This term covers synostosis of phalanges of varying degrees associated with hyperphalangia which may be bifid or duplicated.

27.5.3 Synostosis

The bones at all levels of the feet can be involved. At the toes, there may simply be syndactyly of varying degrees, in the metatarsals there may be duplication of bones with partial or total fusion of two metatarsals, in which case there is often hypoplasia of one or both, while in the tarsus, the classification offered by Meary and Roger (1969) is appropriate (Figs. 27.9–27.11): talonavicular, calcaneonavicular, talocalcaneal, calcaneocuboid, calcaneotalonavicular, cuneiform-cuboidal or cuneiform-metatarsal. There is also the extreme example of syndesmosis affecting all the bones of the tarsus and midtarsus. The result is foot pain on account of unnatural strain placed on neighbouring normal joints, contractures, and features of overloading with callus formation.

27.6 Clinodactyly

Clinodactyly is relatively common, affecting, in order of frequency the first, fifth, third, fourth and, only exceptionally, the second toe.
In the great toe, there is a transverse lateral deformity (see Chap. 18). Congenital hallux varus (see Chap. 18), which appears at the age of 2–3 years, must be differentiated in adulthood from acquired post-traumatic or iatrogenic hallux varus.
In the third toe (Fig. 27.13), the clinodactyly is secondary to congenital swan-neck deformity of the second toe (transverse malalignment of the distal phalanx or, more rarely, the intermediate phalanx).
In the fourth toe (Fig. 27.13), the deformity is usually secondary to clawing or medial clinodactyly of the neighbouring third toe. It amounts to a transverse malalignment of the toe, usually from the proximal interphalangeal joint, sometimes from the distal joint.
Treatment is described in Chap. 17.

27.7 Camptodactyly

Camptodactyly is equivalent to the classical swan-neck deformity of the second toe described in Chap. 17.

27.8 Hallux Varus

Congenital hallux varus, presenting at the age of 2–3 years, must be distinguished from the acquired forms (see Chap. 18).

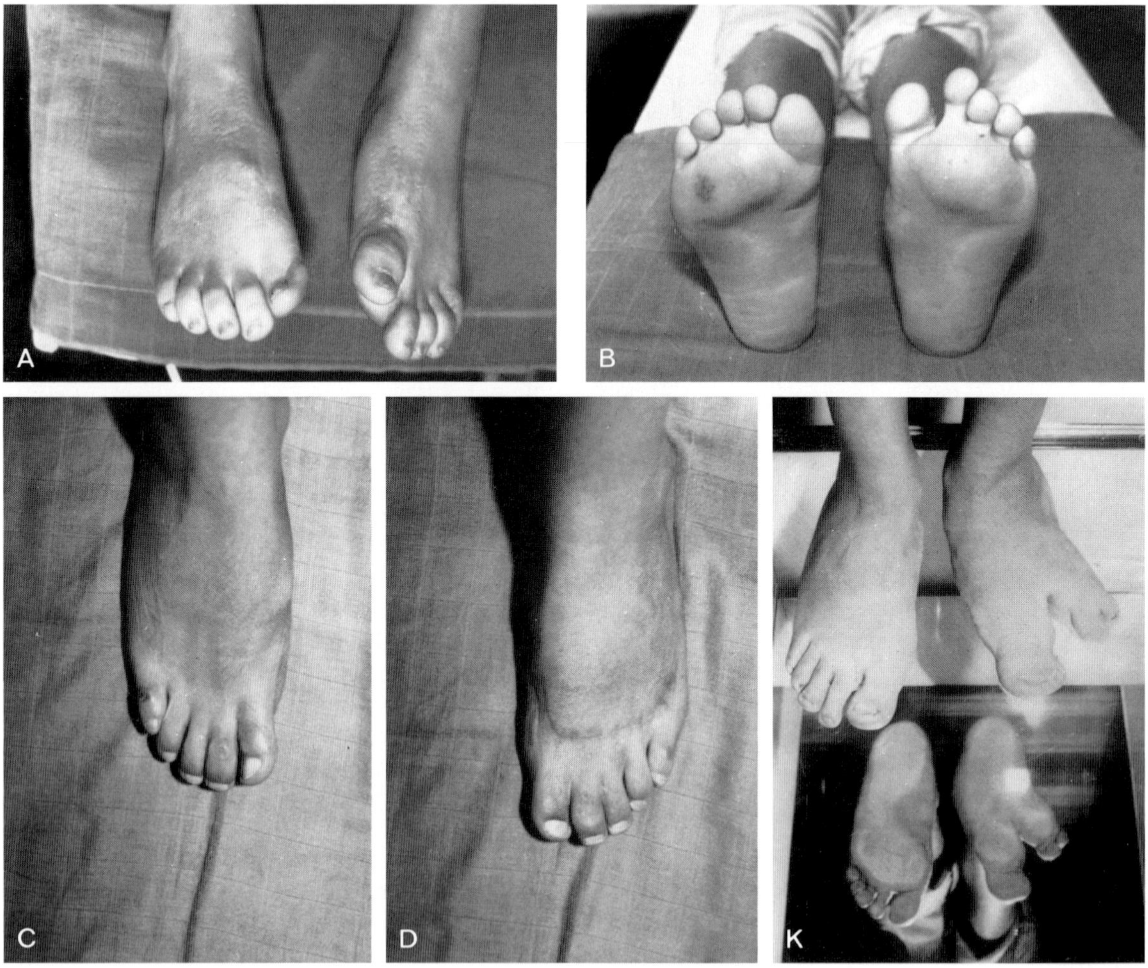

Fig. 27.1 A–J. Congenital malformations. **A–D** Aplasia of first metatarsal, congenital convex forefoot. **D** Following operative treatment. **E, F, H, K** Hemimelia. **G, I, J** Polymetatarsia of great ray with hallux varus. ▷ **J** Appearance after operative treatment of left foot in **I**. **E–J** see p. 427

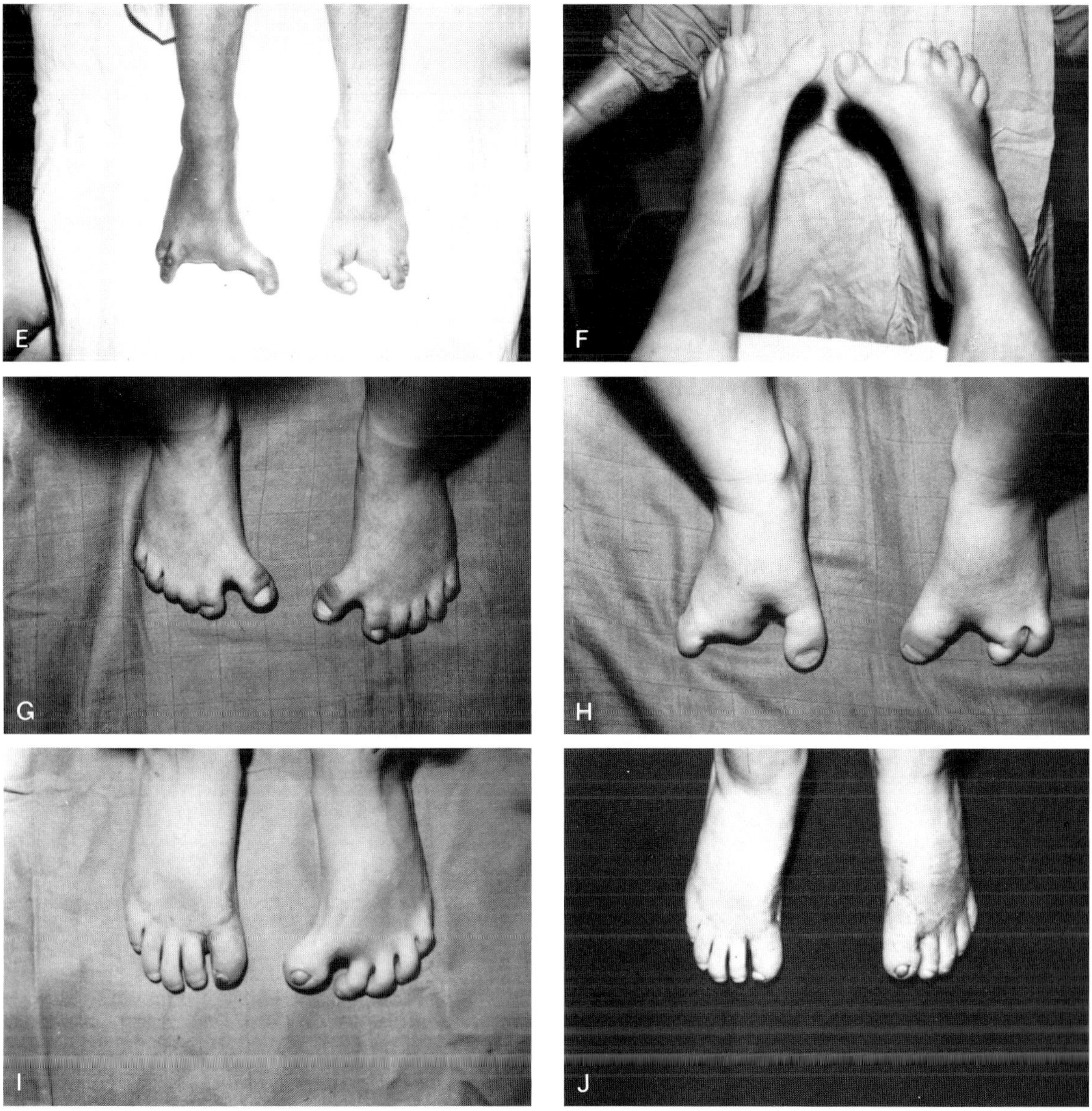

Fig. 27.1 E–J. Legend see p. 426

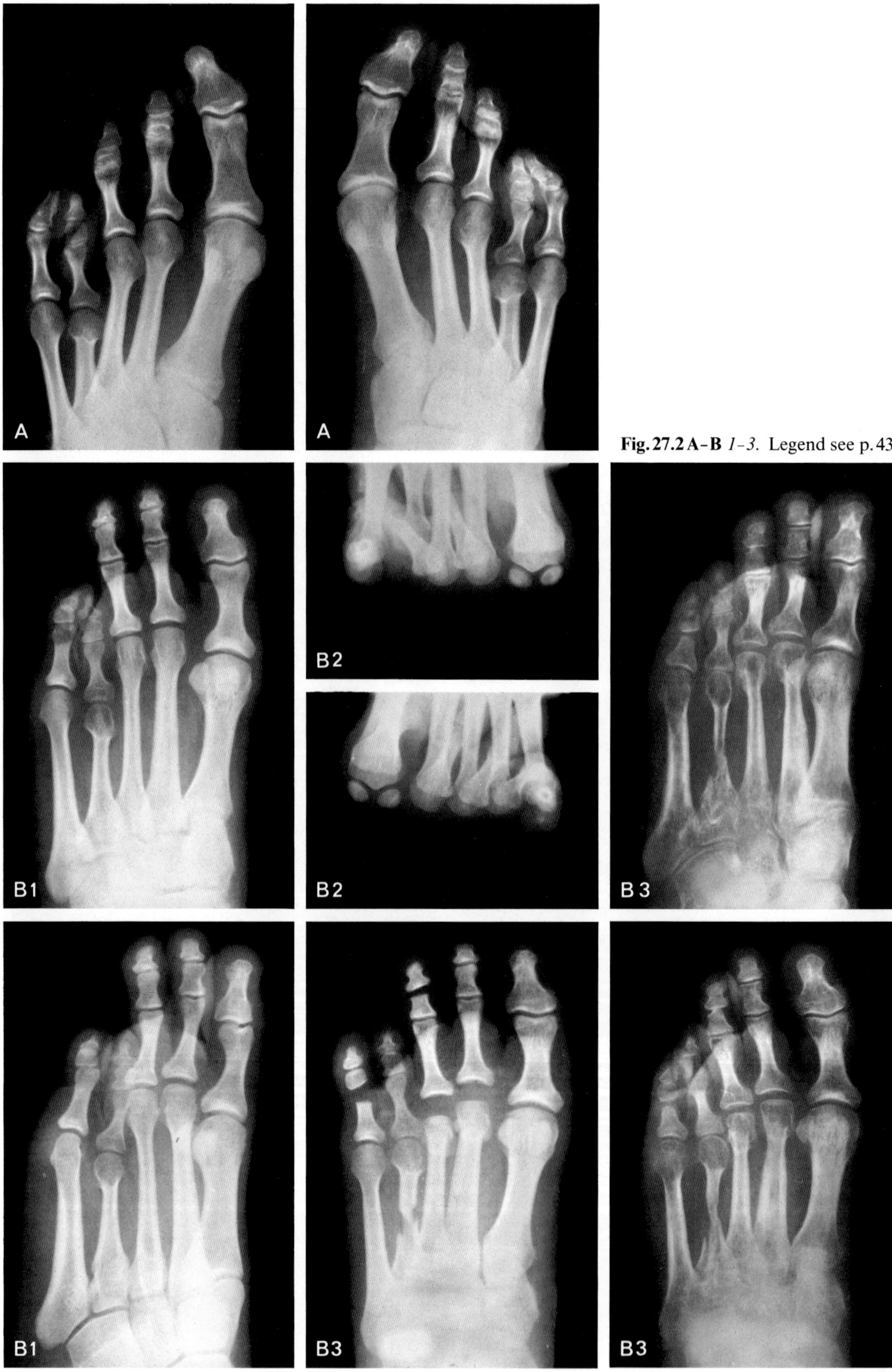

Fig. 27.2 A–B *1–3*. Legend see p. 430

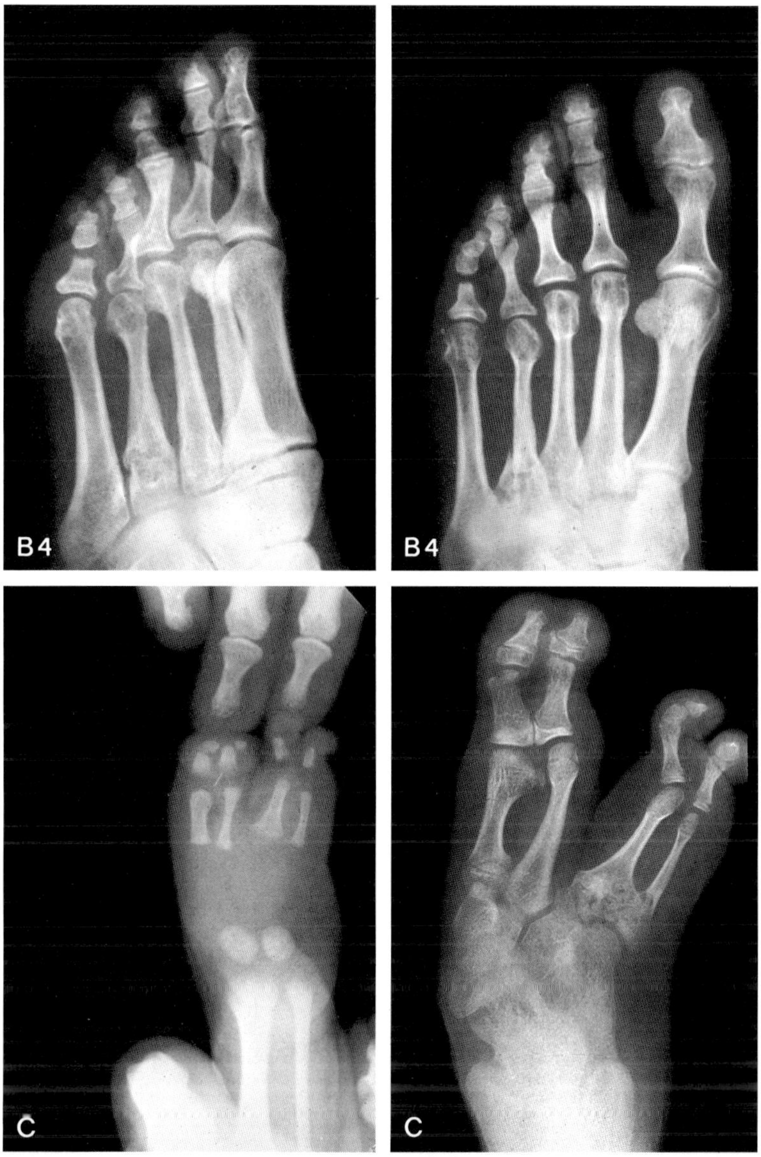

Fig. 27.2 B *4*, C. Legend see p. 430

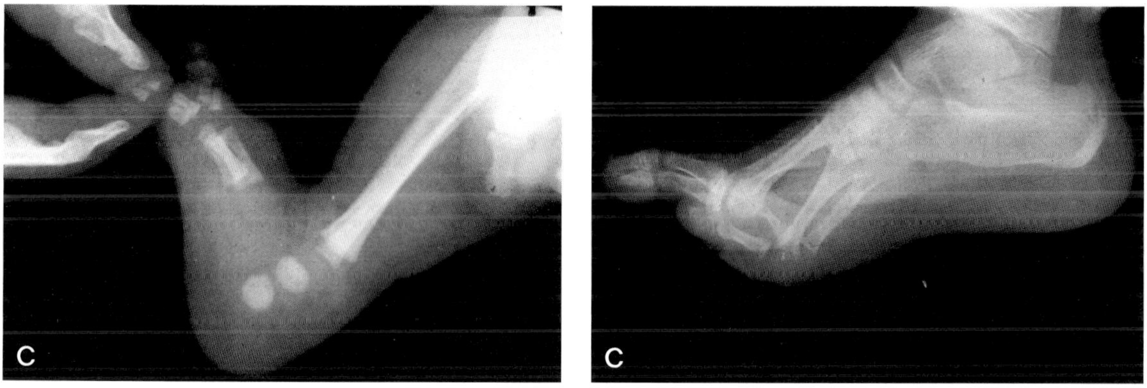

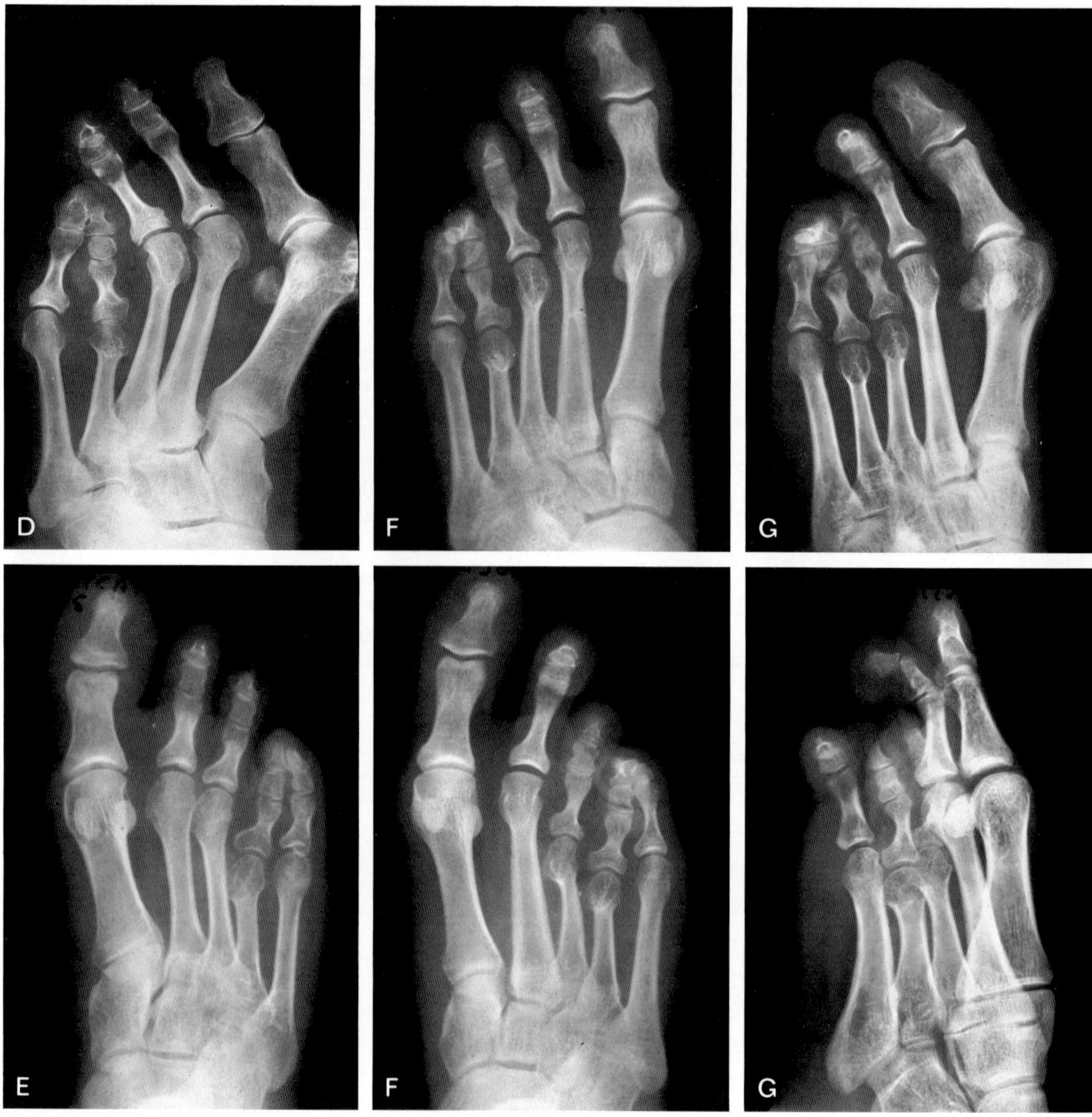

Fig. 27.2 A–G. Congenital malformations: brachymetatarsia and longitudinal hemimelia. **A** Bilateral fourth brachymetatarsia. **B** Shortness of fourth ray caused by brachymetatarsia: normal toe, underloading of fourth metatarsal head. *1, 2* Preoperative; *3* after realignment head-shaft enclavement of second and third metatarsals, elongation of fourth metatarsal by longitudinal osteotomy; *4* consolidation of second, third and fourth metatarsals. **C** Longitudinal hemimelia: aplasia of third ray, syndactyly of first and second toes and of fourth and fifth toes, synostosis of calcaneum and cuboid, equinus of fourth and fifth metatarsals, clawing of fourth and fifth toes. **D, E** Fourth brachymetatarsia. **F** Fourth brachymetatarsia in left foot, third and fourth brachymetatarsia in right foot. **G** Third and fourth brachymetatarsia. **A–C** see pp. 428, 429

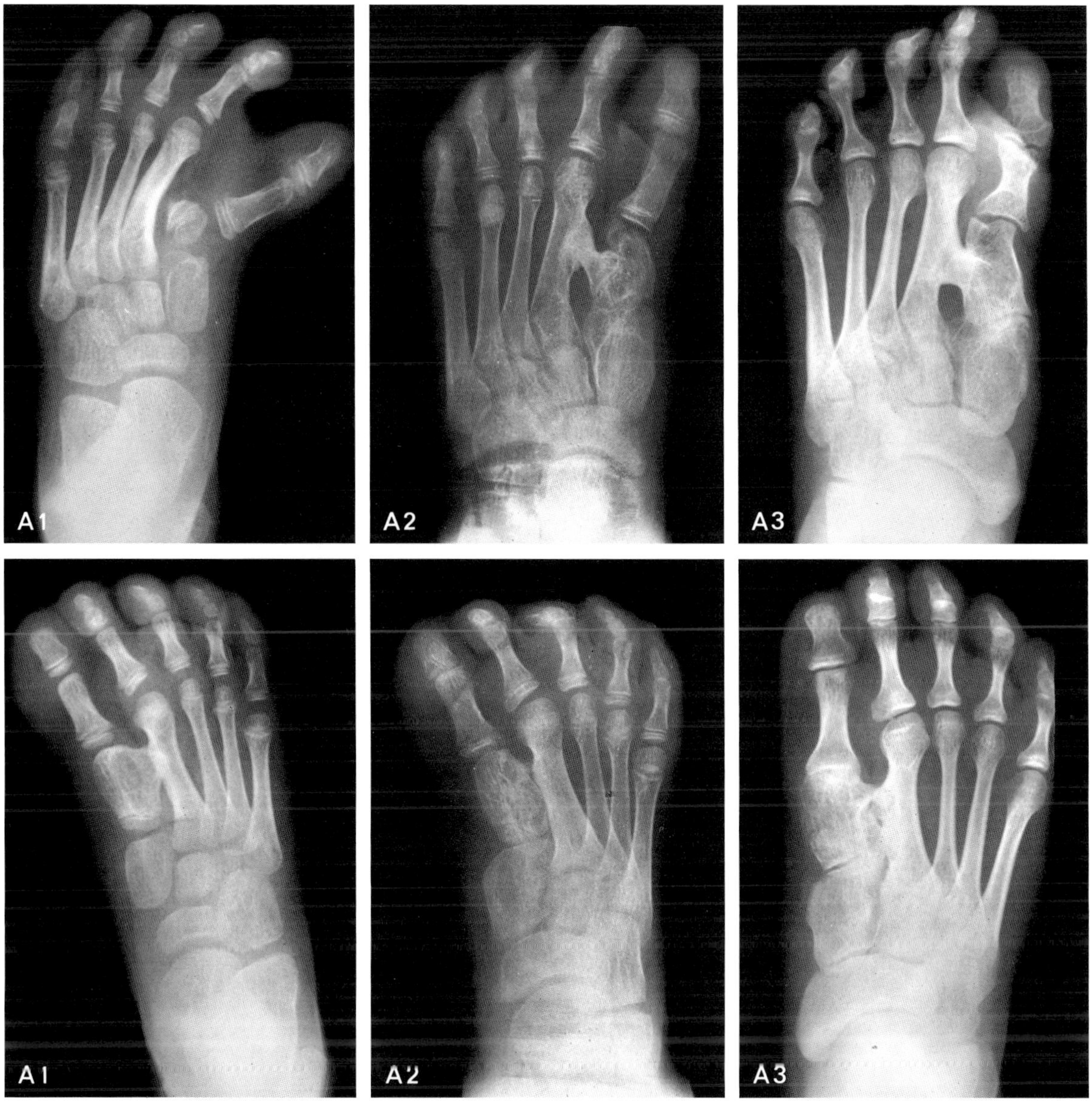

Fig. 27.3 A–G. Congenital malformations: forefoot dysostoses. **A** *1* Left foot 1970: partial aplasia of first metatarsal, varus of great toe, varus of first metatarsal, metatarsus varus, medial metatarsal incurvation; *2* right foot 1974: first brachymetatarsia with hypertrophy synostosis of first and second metatarsals; *3* 1974: increased hypertrophy of first metatarsal; *4, 5* development of foot over 10 years: by 1980, convex forefoot with overloading of central metatarsal heads. **A** *4*–**G** see pp. 432–435

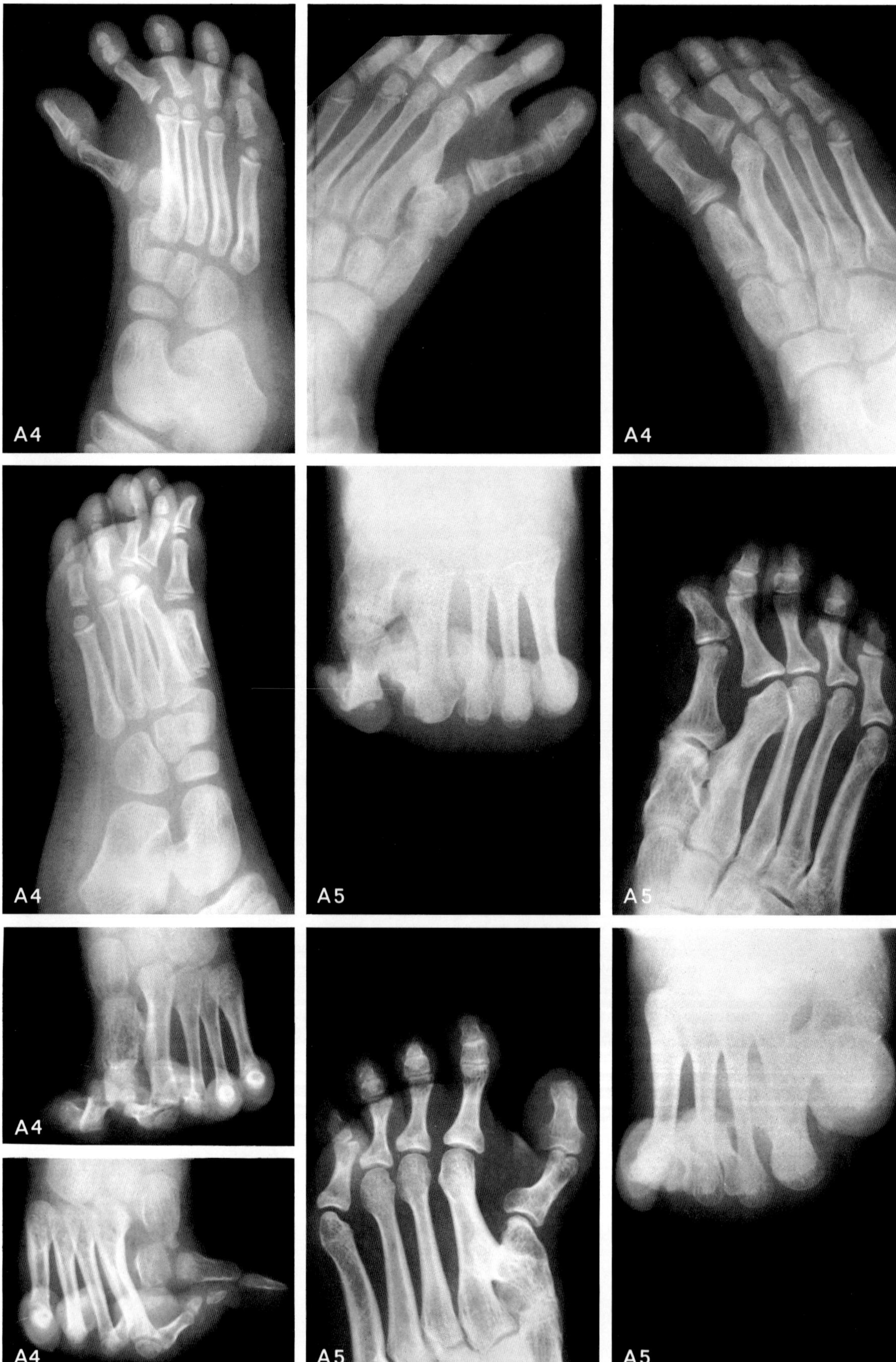
A4
A4
A4
A5
A5
A4
A4
A5
A5

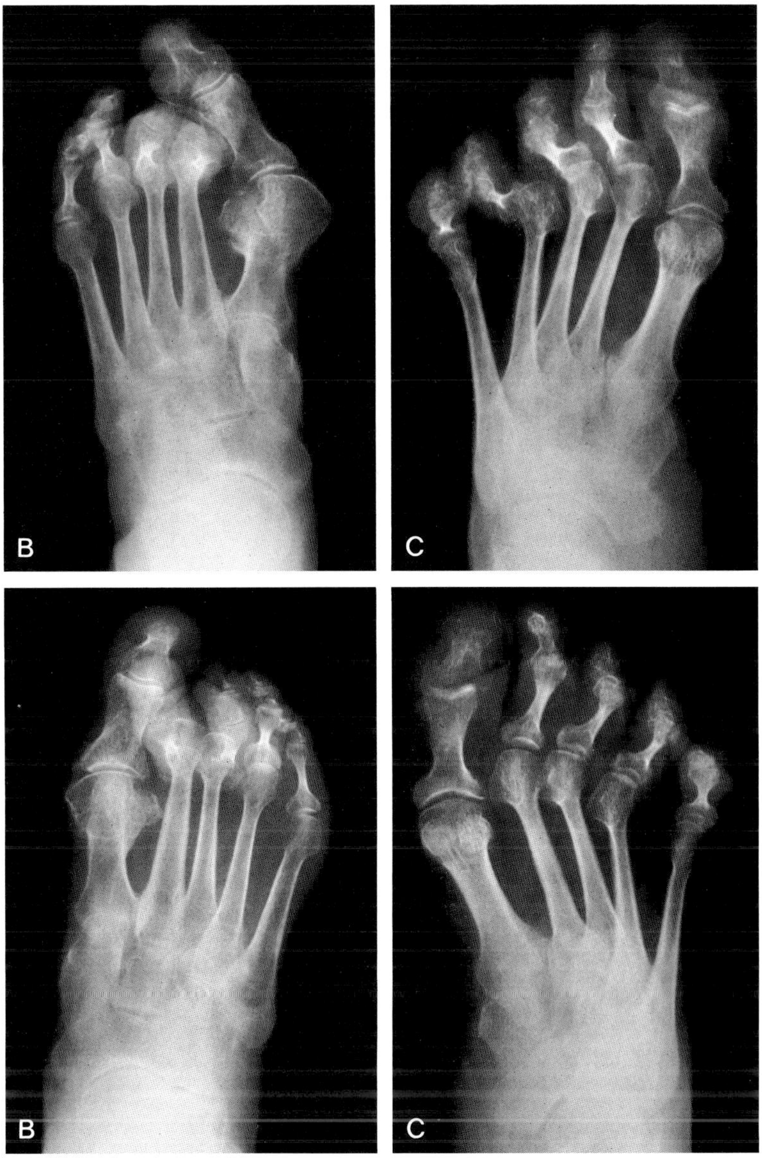

Fig. 27.3 *(continued)*. **B, C** First brachymetatarsia leading to convex forefoot syndrome

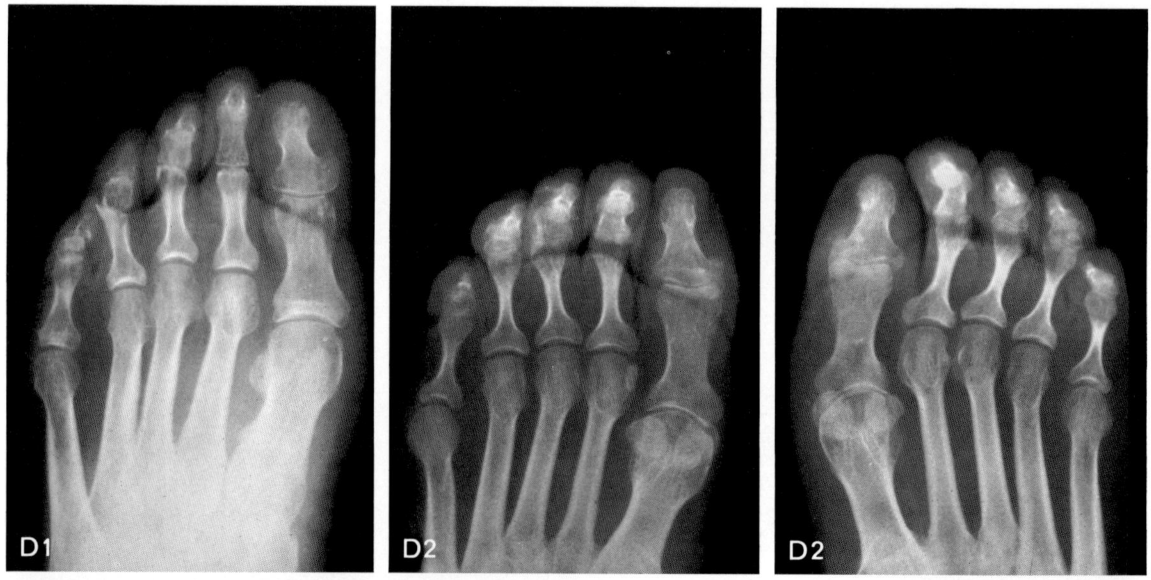

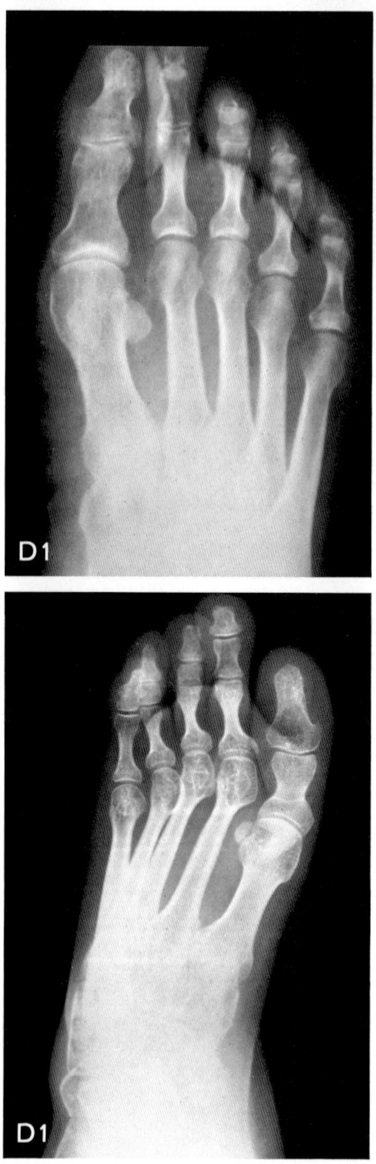

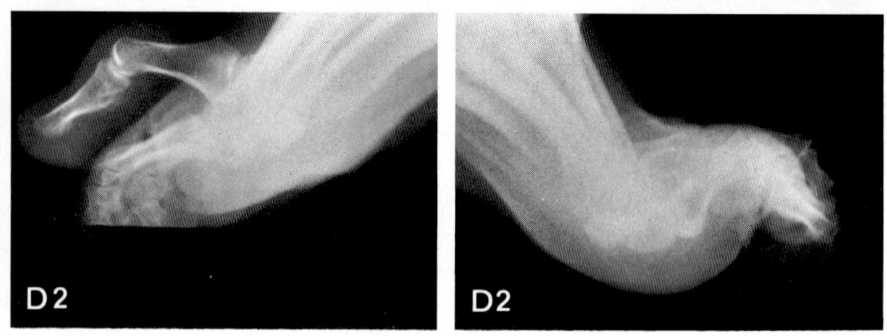

Fig. 27.3 *(continued)*. **D** *1* Congenital convex forefoot syndrome with shortness of first metatarsal; *2* short first metatarsal leading to convex forefoot. **E** Congenital hemimelia of lobster-claw variety: syndactyly of first and second rays and of fourth and fifth rays, absence of third toe. **F** Aplasia of second and third toes. **G** Bilateral dysostoses. Left foot: lobster-claw deformity with syndactyly of third, fourth and fifth toes, absence of second toe. Right foot: lobster-claw deformity with hallux varus, metatarsophalangeal synostosis of second ray, absence of second and third phalanges of second toe, absence of third toe ▷

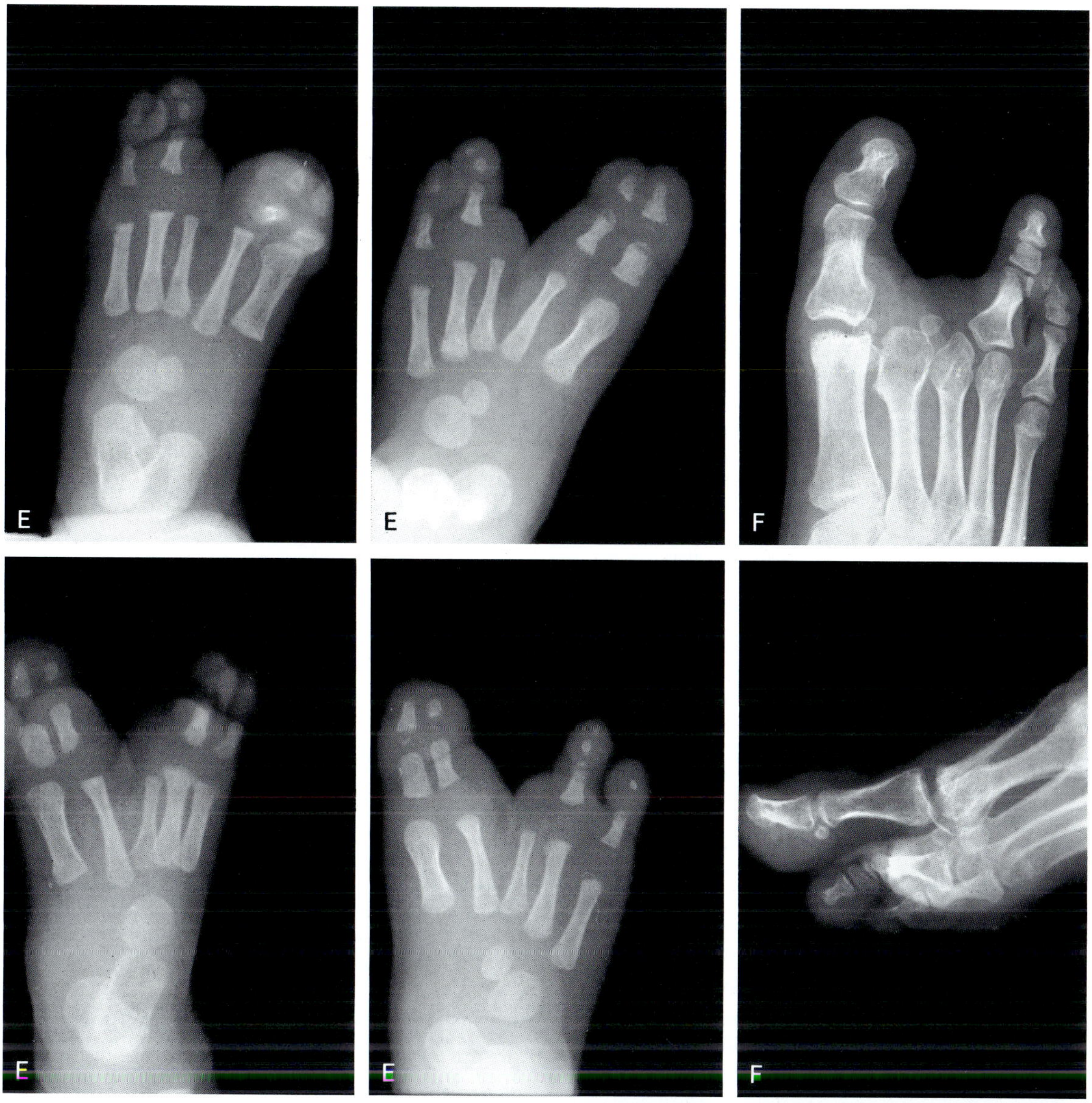

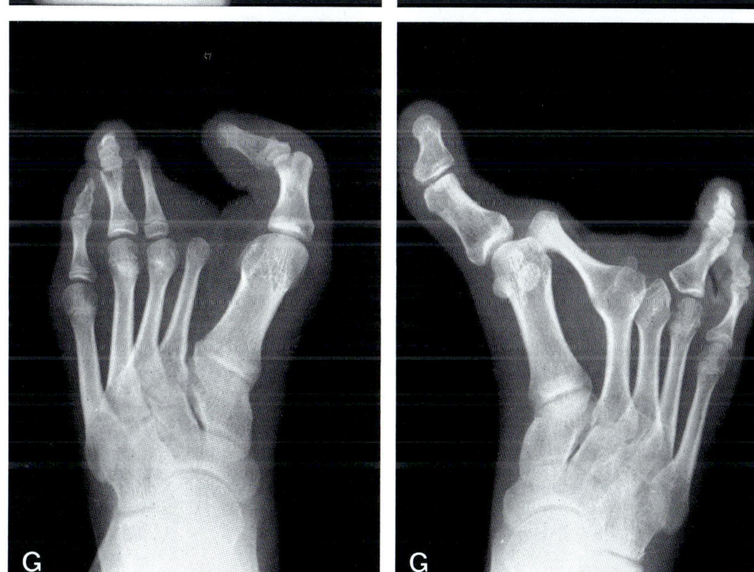

Fig. 27.3 E–G. Legend see p. 434

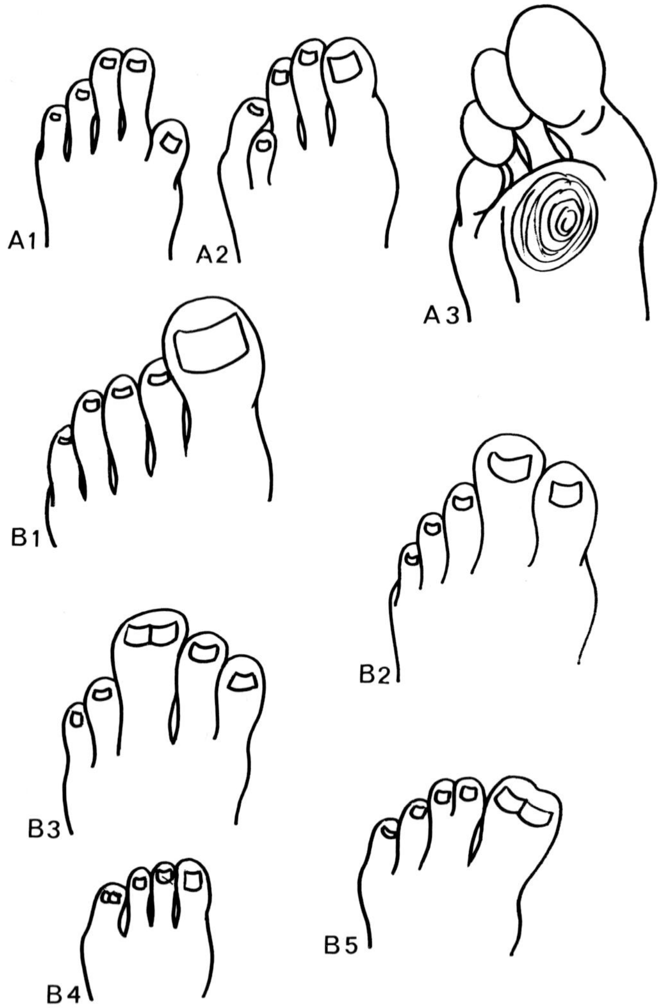

Fig. 27.4. A Hypoplasia: *1* First ray; *2* fourth ray; *3* fourth ray with central callosity formation. **B** Hyperplasia: *1* First ray; *2* second ray; *3, 4, 5* with syndactyly and/or bifid nail

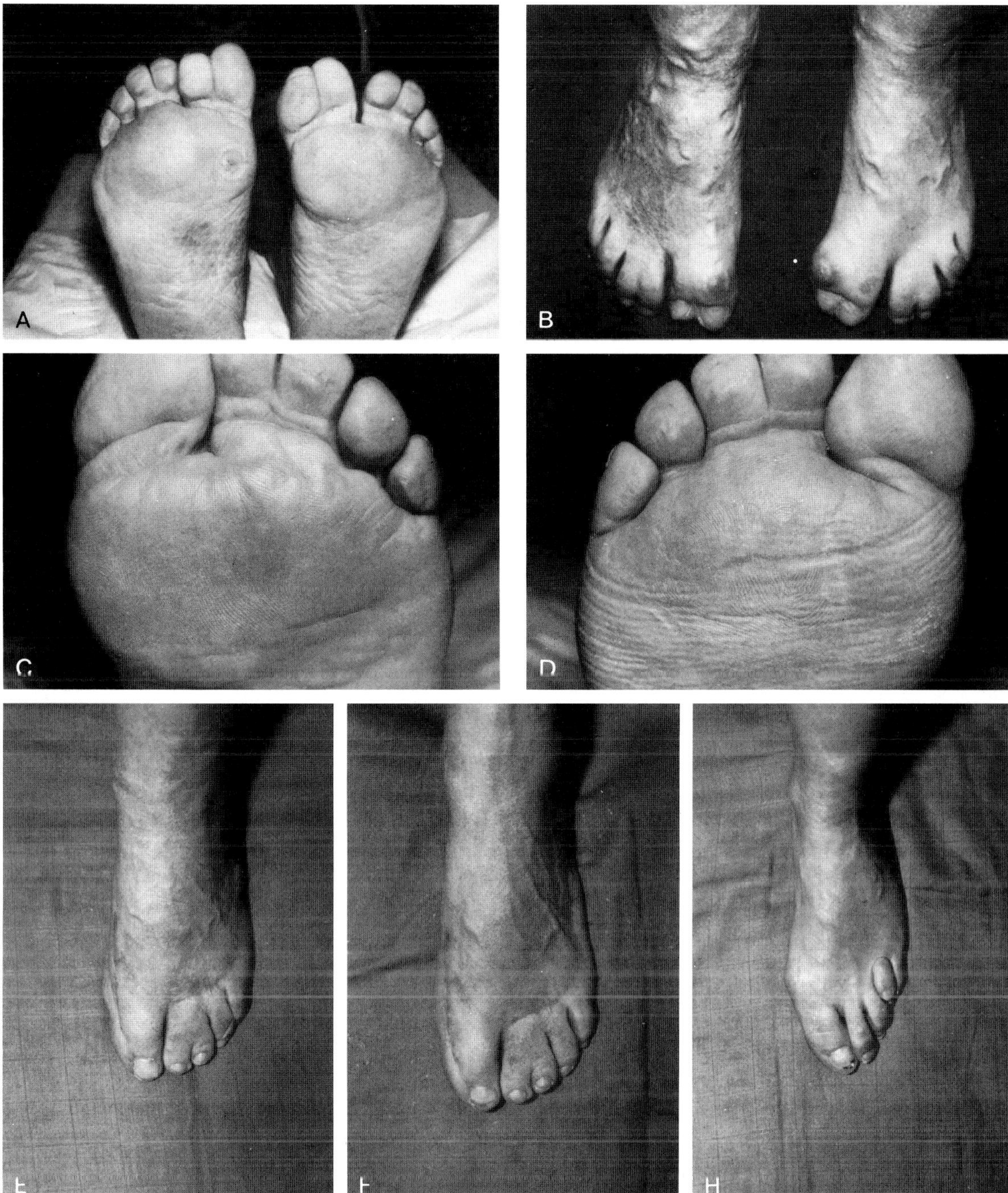

Fig. 27.5 A–N. Congenital malformations. **A–F** Polyplasia involving metatarsals and toes: hyperplasia of second and third metatarsals and syndactyly of first to fourth toes: **A, B** Preoperative appearance: **C–F** postoperative appearance. **G, H** Aplasia of fourth ray: dorsal aspect. **I** Aplasia of fourth ray: plantar aspect, showing callus formation. **J** Hexadactyly. **K** Pes adductus. **L** Polydactyly-syndactyly with hallux varus. **M** Macropodia of third ray. **N** Supernumerary fifth toe. **G–N** see p. 438

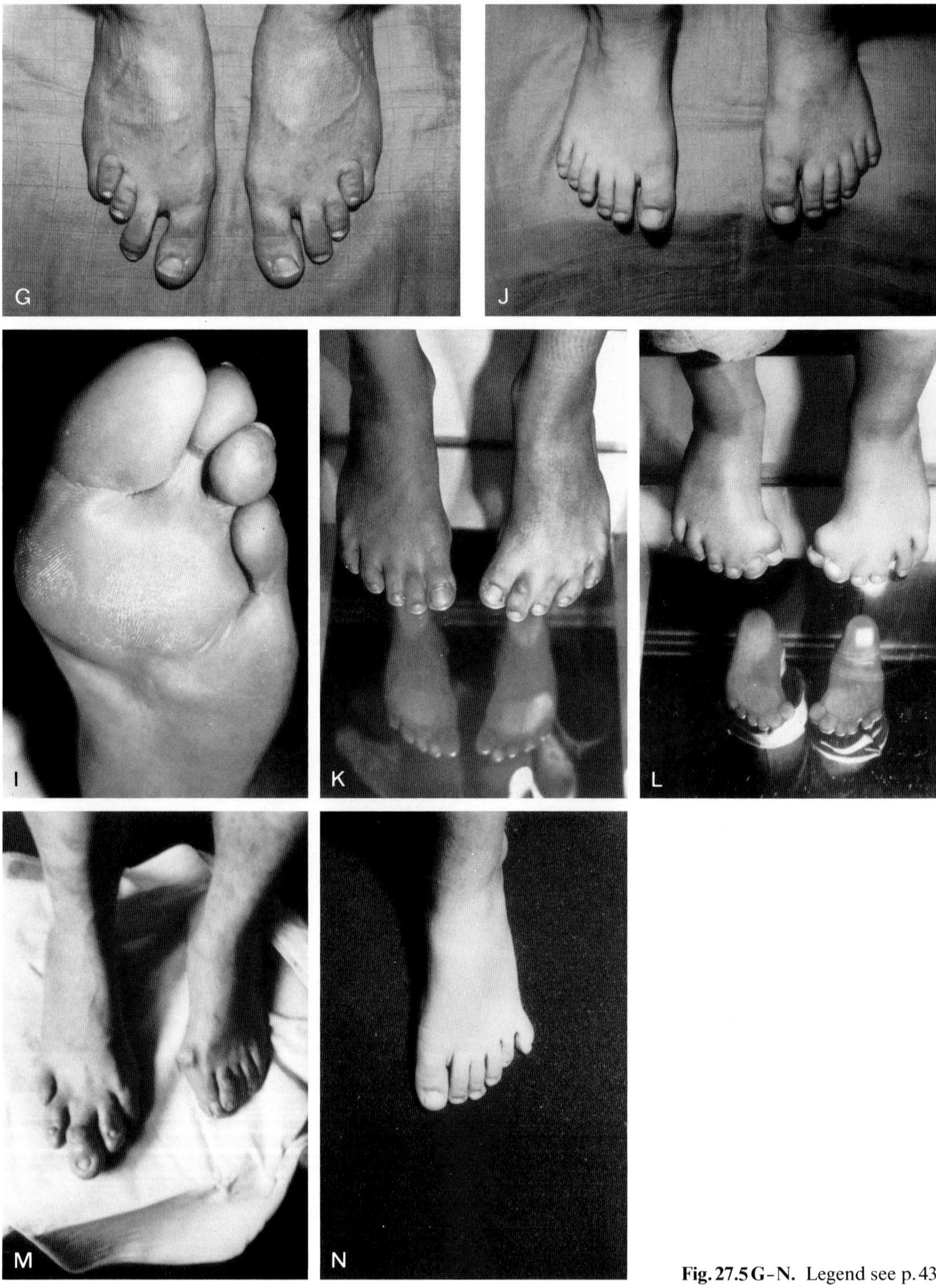

Fig. 27.5 G–N. Legend see p. 437

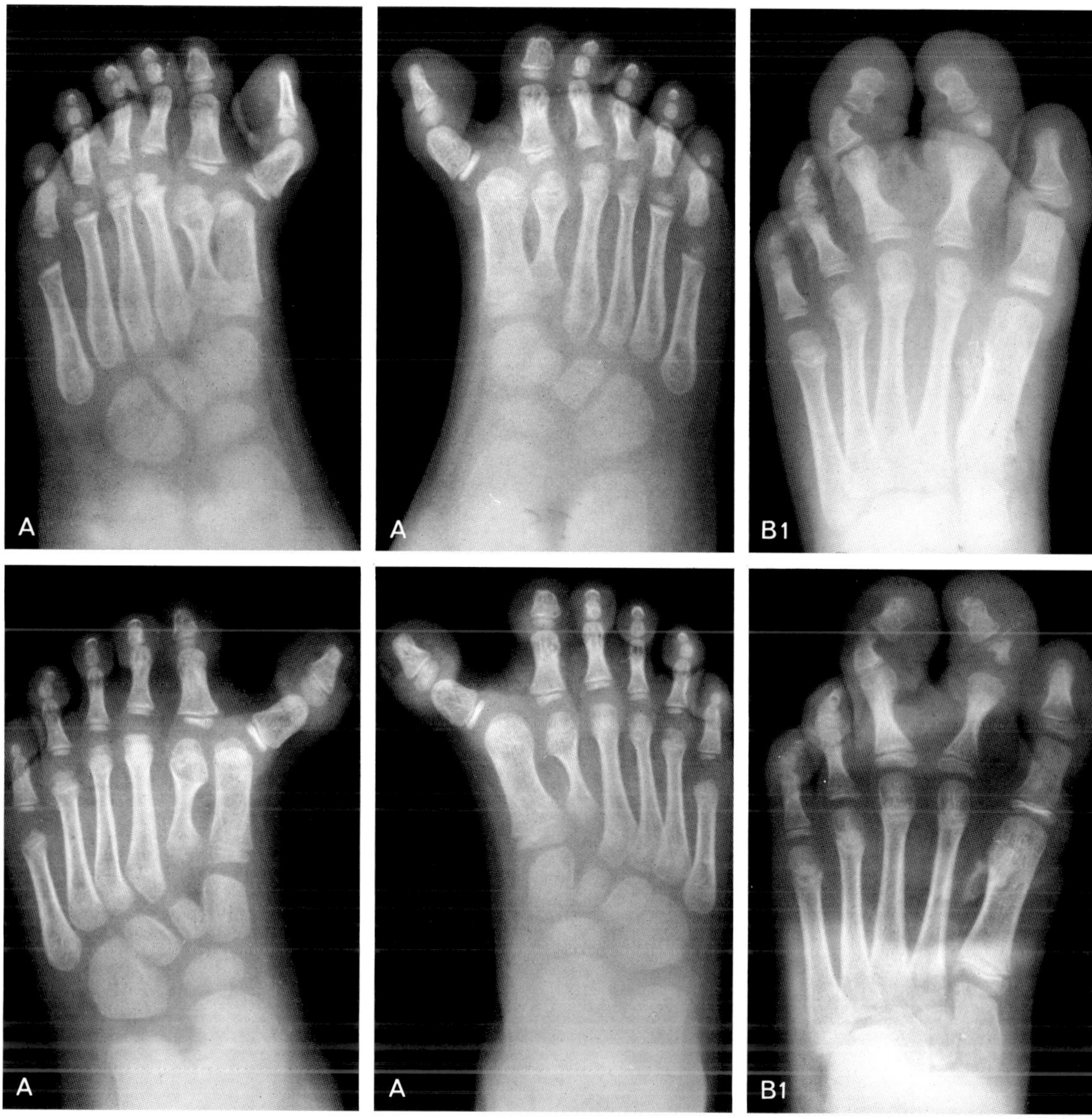

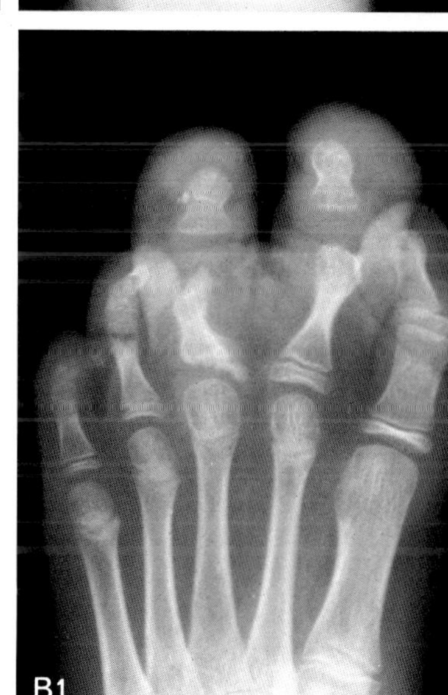

Fig. 27.6 A–G. Congenital malformations: dysostoses. **A** Bilateral hallux varus and supernumerary second ray. **B** *1* Macrodactyly and brachyphalangia of second and third toes, convex forefoot due to frontal protrusion and hypertrophy of condyles of second and third metatarsal heads; *2* correction of convex forefoot syndrome by head-shaft enclavement of second and third metatarsals. **C** Supernumerary metatarsophalangeal joints and hallux varus. *1* Preoperatively; *2* postoperatively. **B***2*–**G** see pp. 440–443

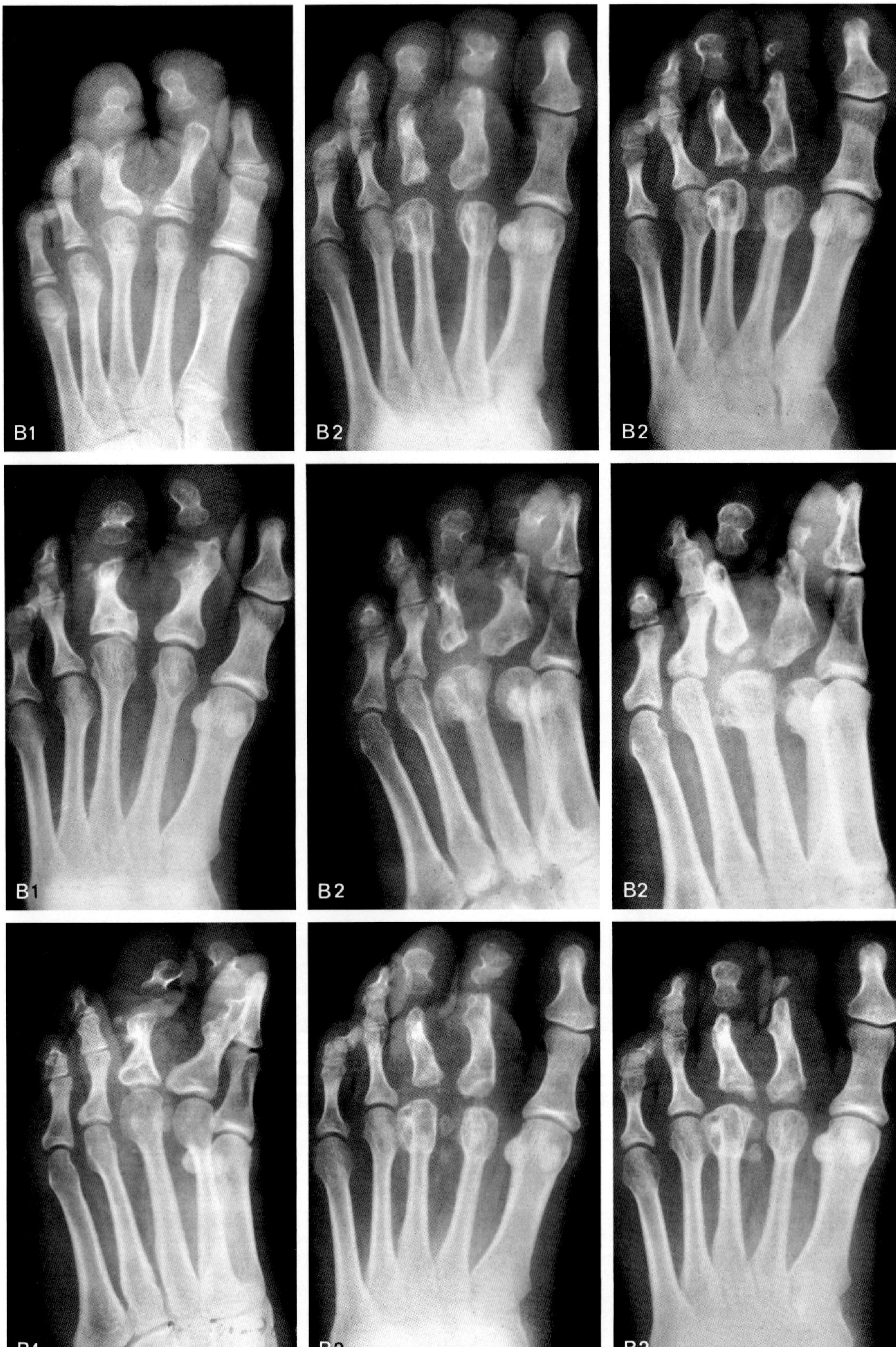
B1
B2
B2
B1
B2
B2
B1
B2
B2

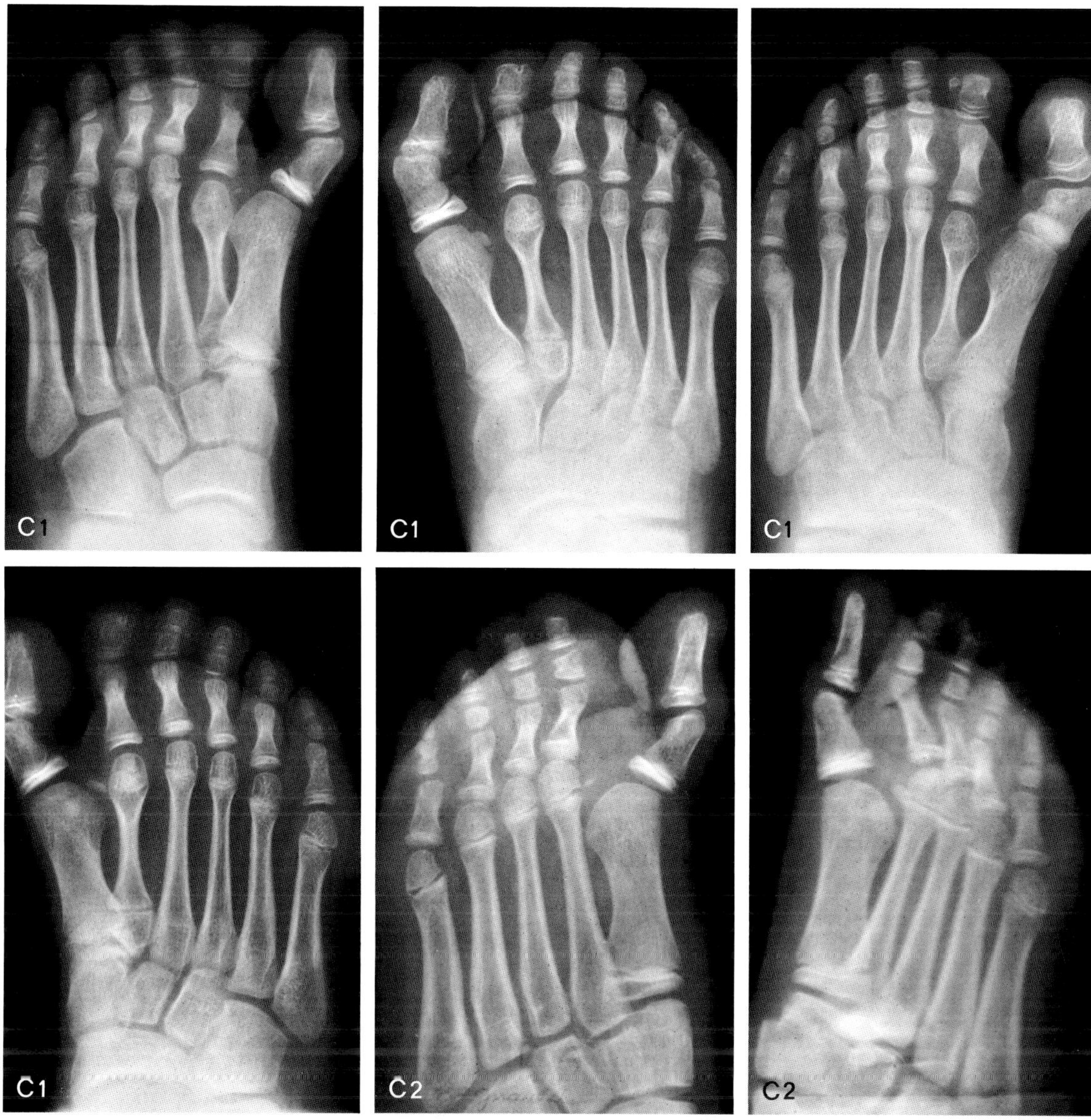

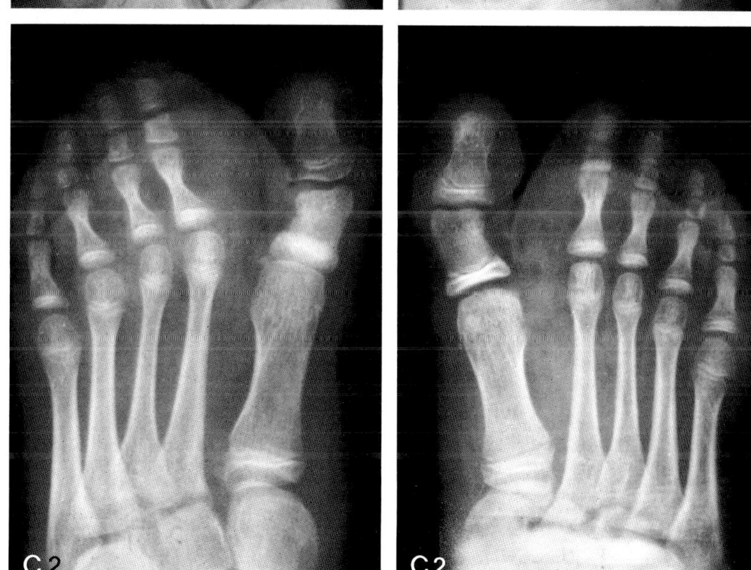

Fig. 27.6 B–C. Legend see p. 439

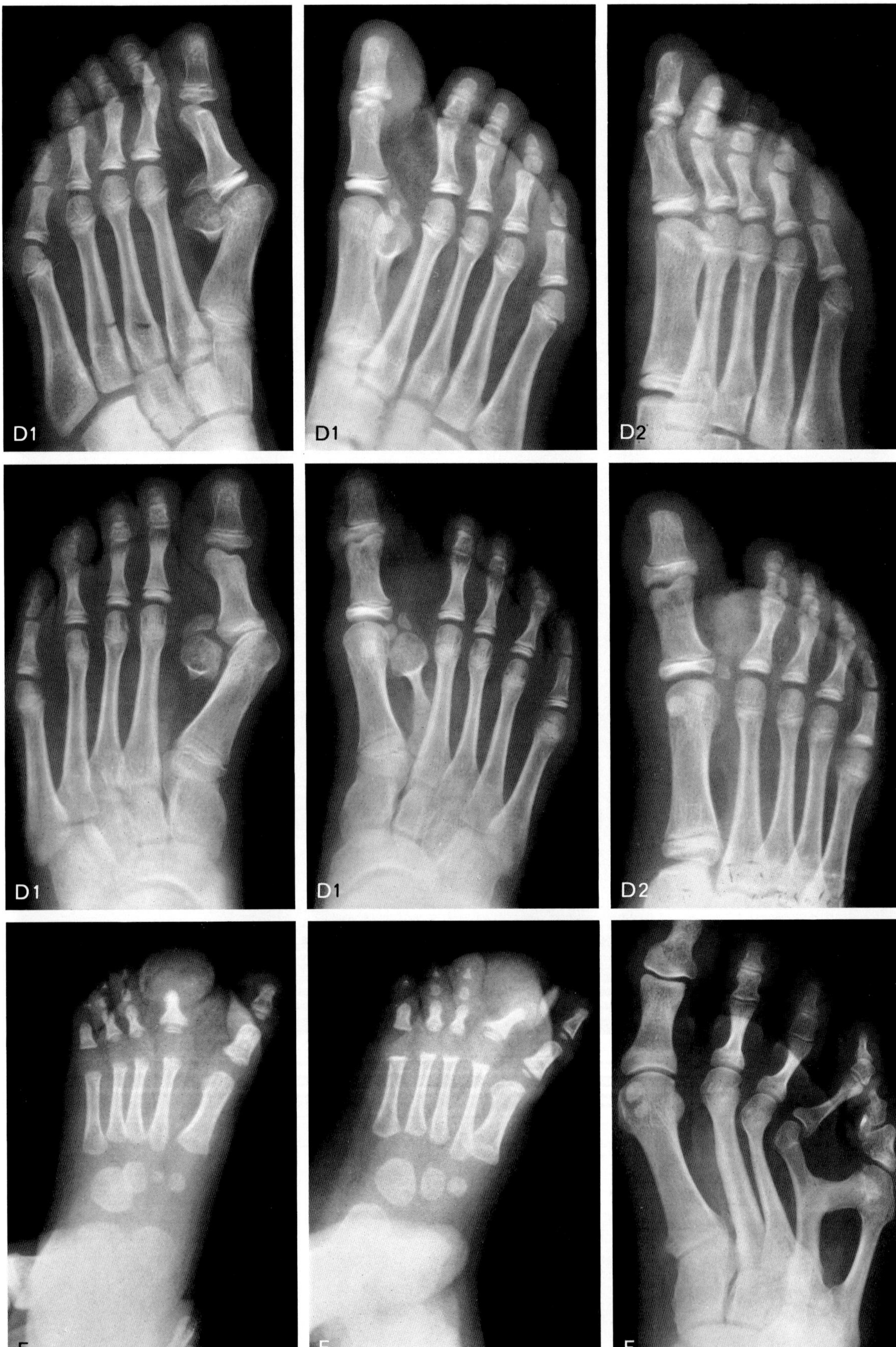
D1
D1
D2
D1
D1
D2
E
E
F

◁ **Fig. 27.6** *(continued)*. **D** *1* Development of supernumerary second ray; *2* postoperatively. **E** Macrodactyly of second toe with soft tissue distal hypertrophy and brachyphalangia of proximal phalanx, absence of second and third phalanges. **F** Intermetatarsal synsostosis of fourth and fifth rays, brachyphalangia of fifth toe. **G** Macrodactyly and brachyphalangia of fourth toe

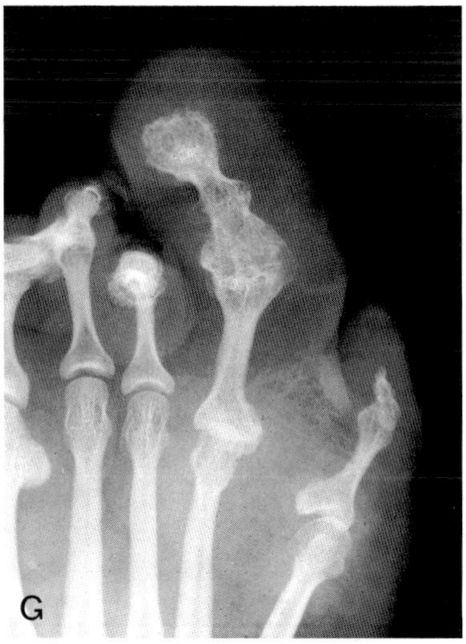

▽ **Fig. 27.7 A–H.** Congenital malformations: dysostoses of first ray. **A** Bifidity and basal syndactyly of great toe, supernumerary metatarsal segment in first interspace. **B** *1* Left foot: duplication of first metatarsal, metatarsus varus; *2* right foot: partial duplication of first metatarsal. **C–H** see pp. 444–447

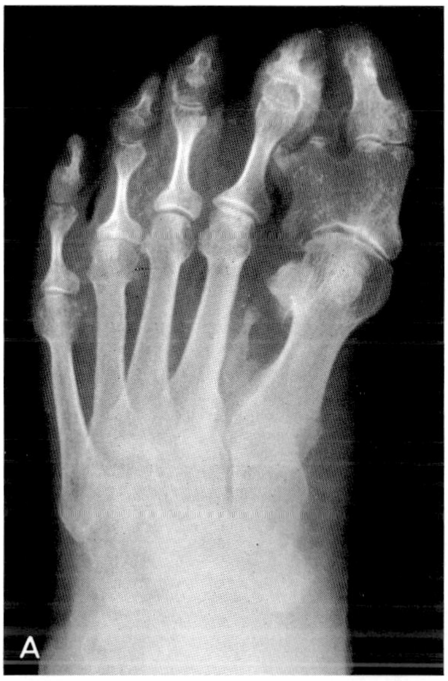

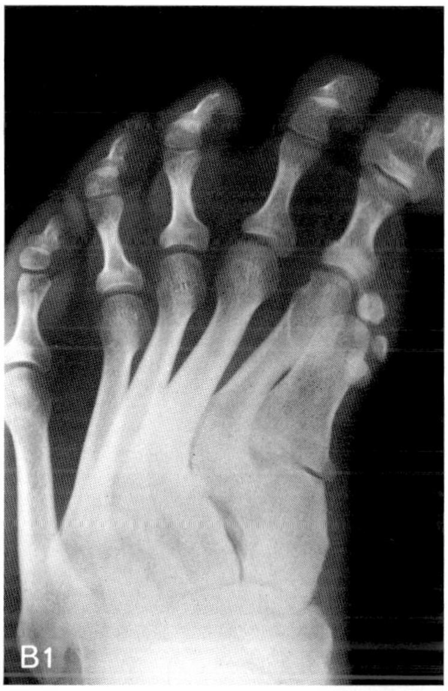

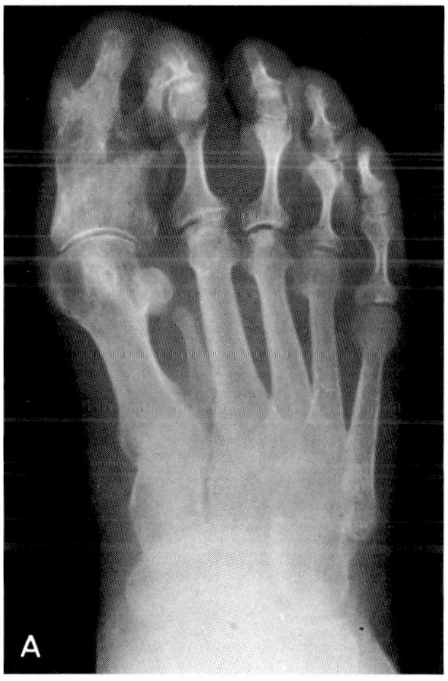

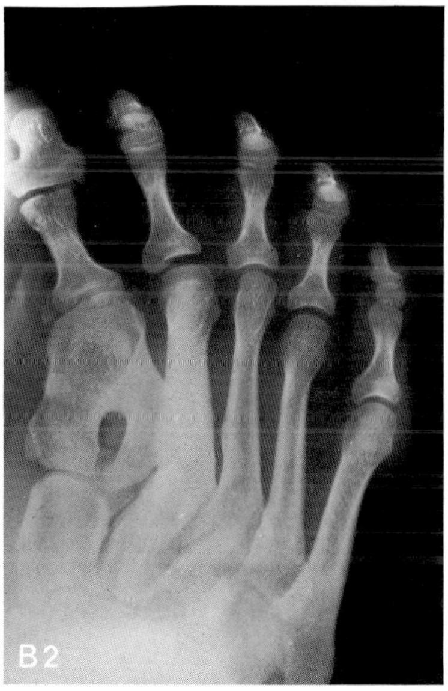

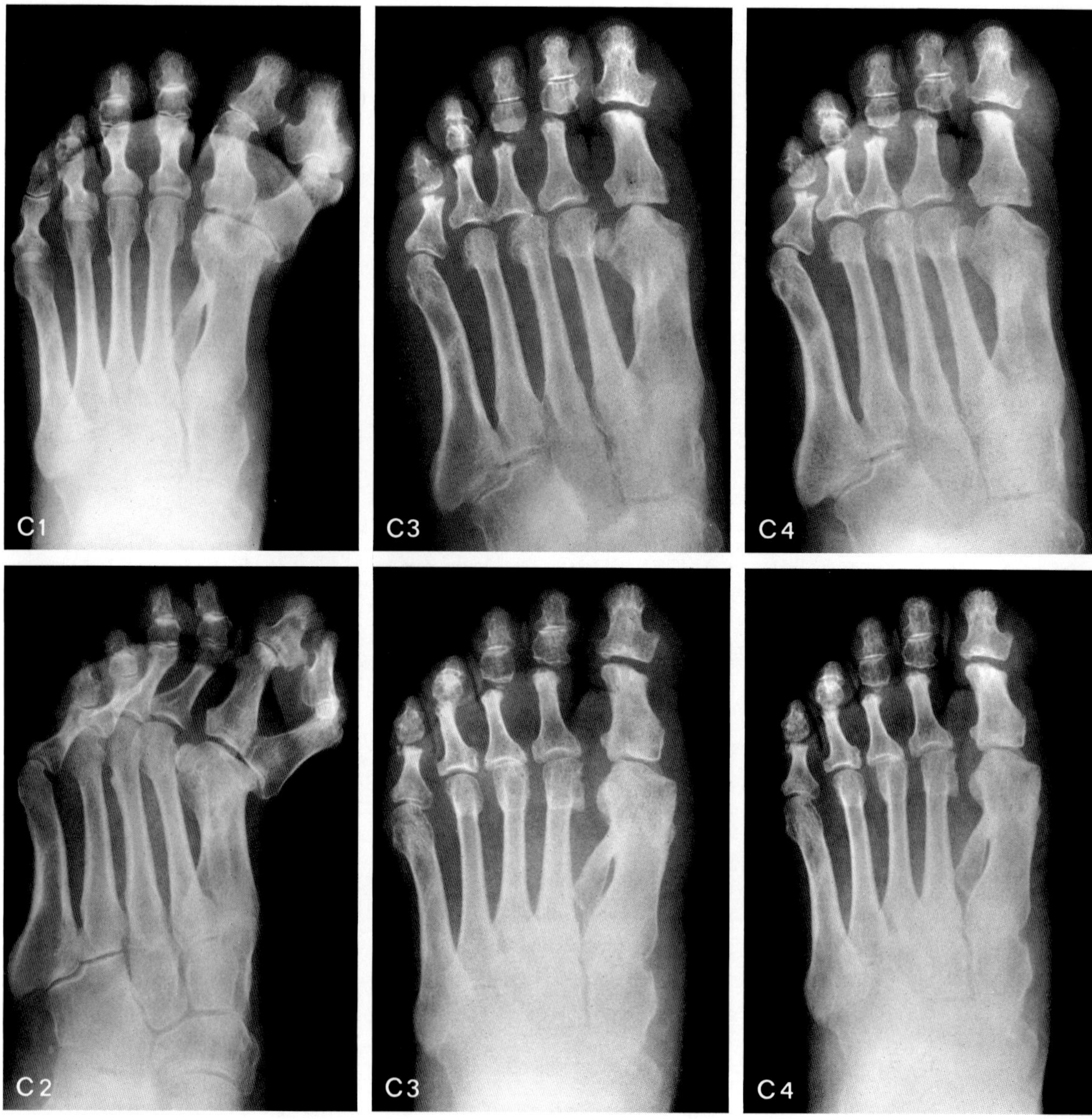

Fig. 27.7 *(continued)*. **C** Left foot. *1* Bifid great toe, partial duplication of first metatarsal, convex forefoot; *2* clawing of bifid great toe; *3* after resection and trimming of bifid great toe, interphalangeal arthroplasty of all five toes, realignment of second, third and fourth metatarsal heads by head-shaft enclavement to correct convex forefoot; *4* three months after operation

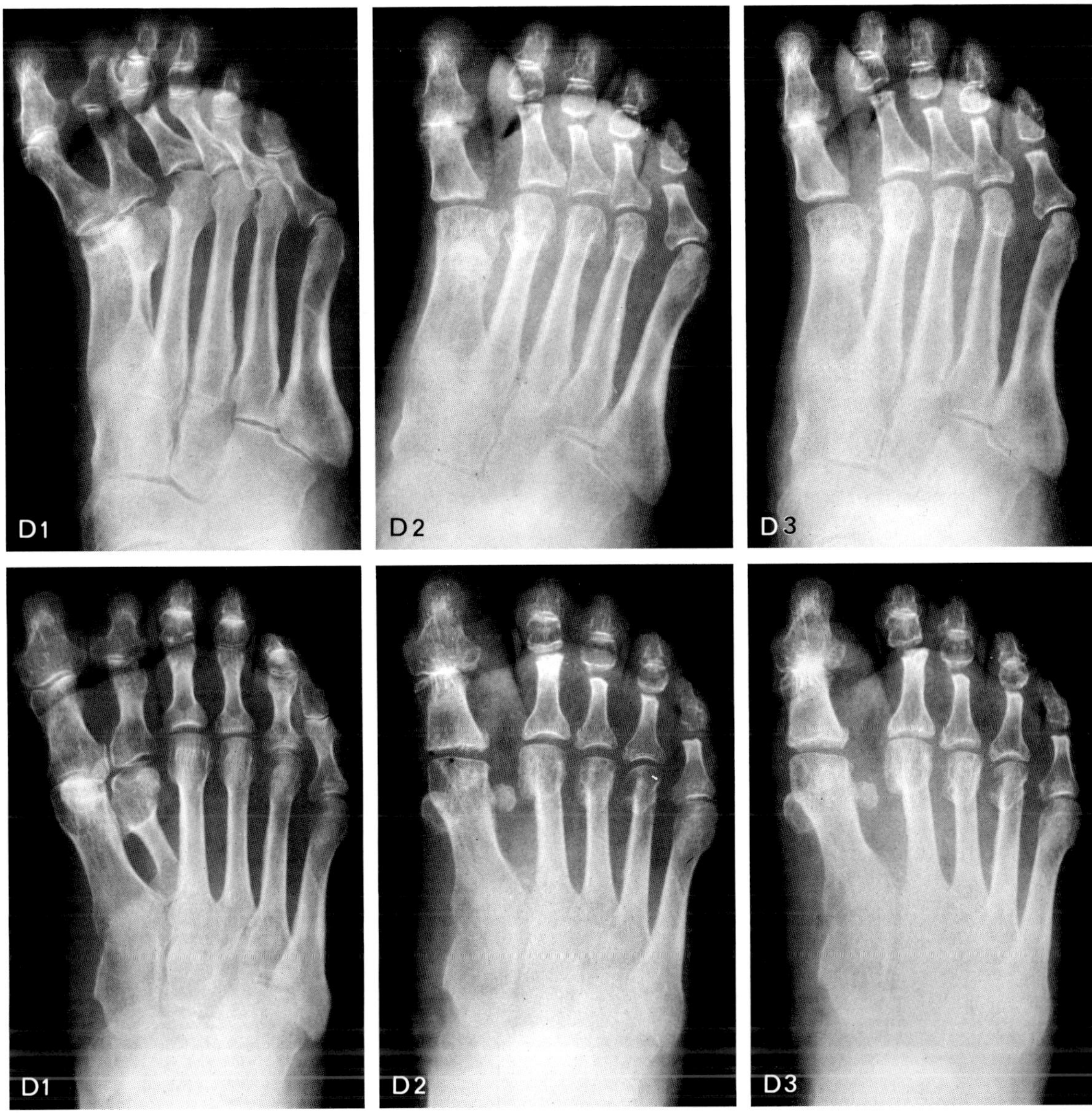

Fig. 27.7 *(continued).* **D** Right foot (same patient as **C**). *1* Syndactyly of great toe, bifid phalanges, complete duplication of great toe, convex forefoot due to frontal protrusion of central metatarsal heads; *2* after resection and trimming of supernumerary second ray and of great toe, arthrodesis of interphalangeal joint of great toe, arthroplasty of second to fifth toes, realignment enclavement of second, third and fourth metatarsal heads to correct convex forefoot; *3* three months after operation

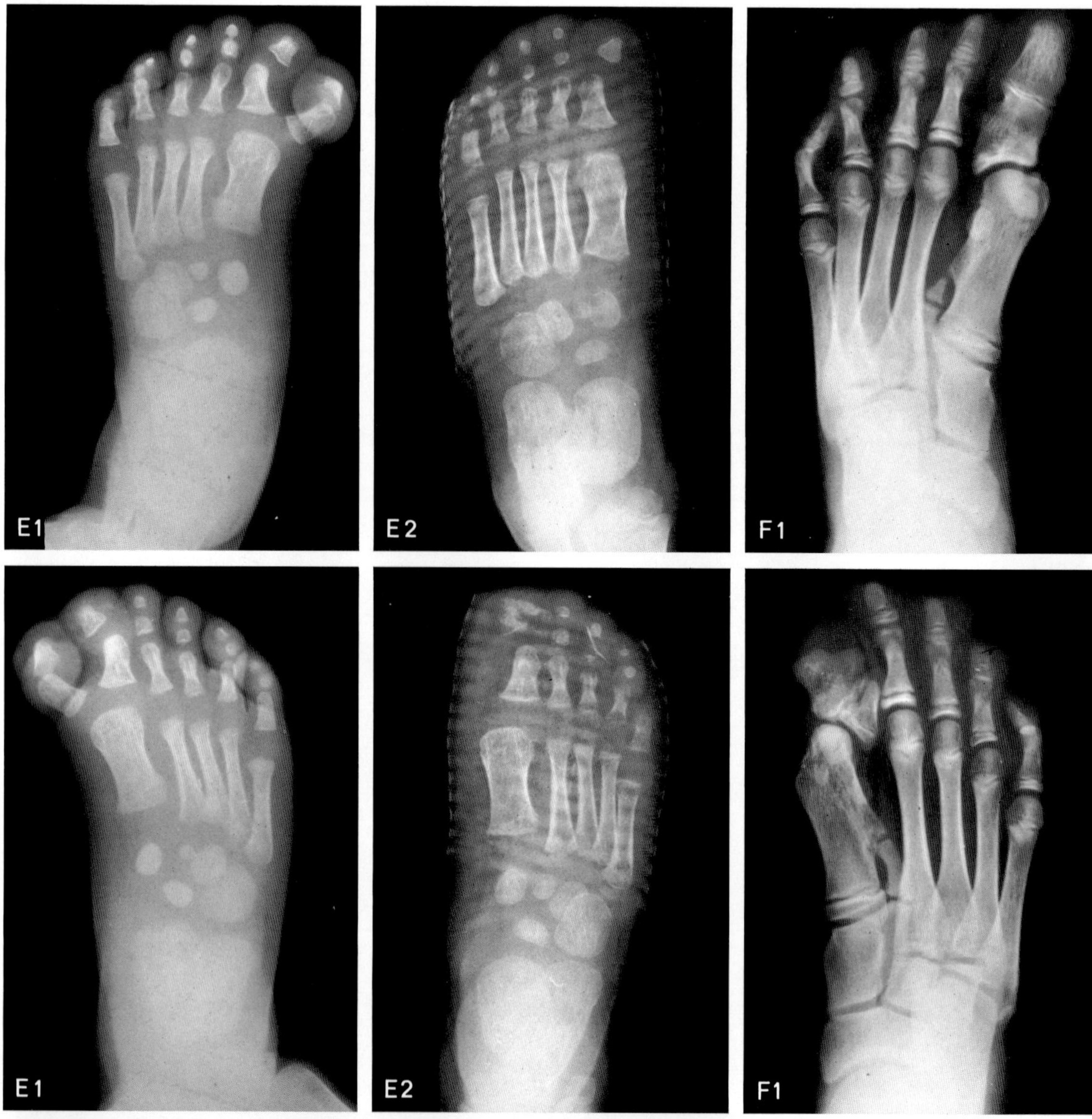

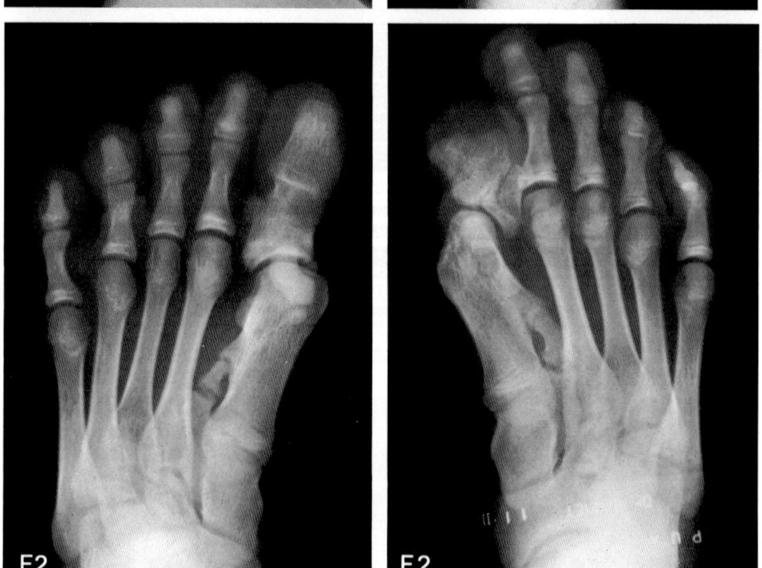

Fig. 27.7 *(continued)*. **E** Brachymetatarsia of supernumerary great toe. *1* Preoperative; *2* after remodelling by excision of supernumerary toe. **F** *1* Brachyphalangia of great toe and partial duplication of first metatarsal; *2* same patient 2 years later

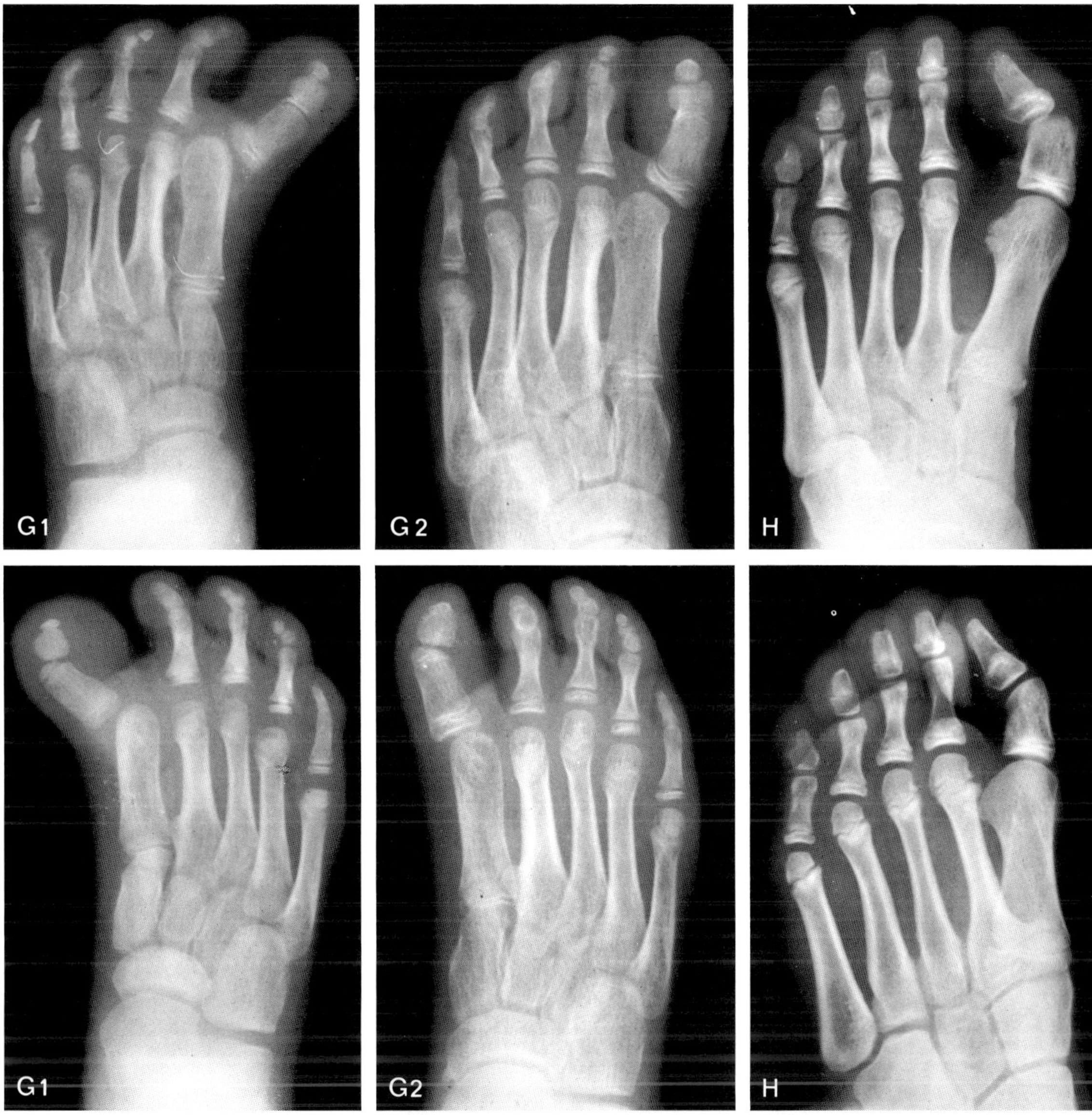

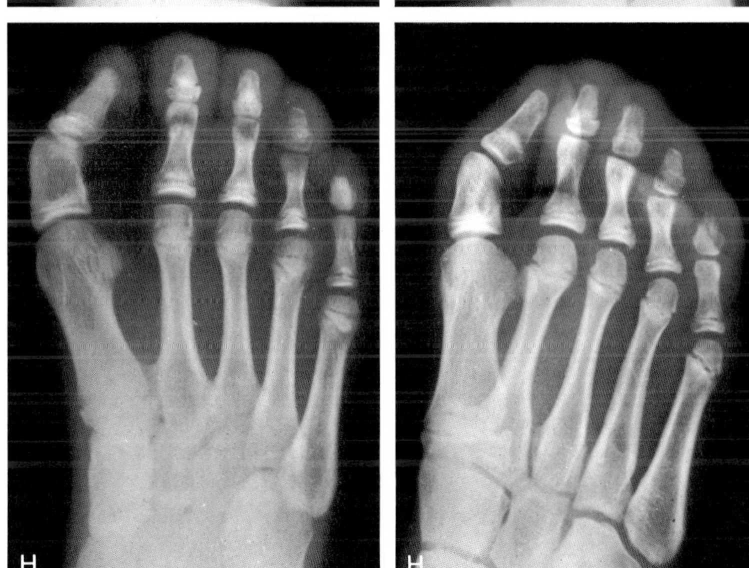

Fig. 27.7 *(continued)*. **G** *1* Hypertrophy of great toe with congenital hallux varus; *2* same patient 2 years later. **H** Congenital transverse lateral deformity of great toe

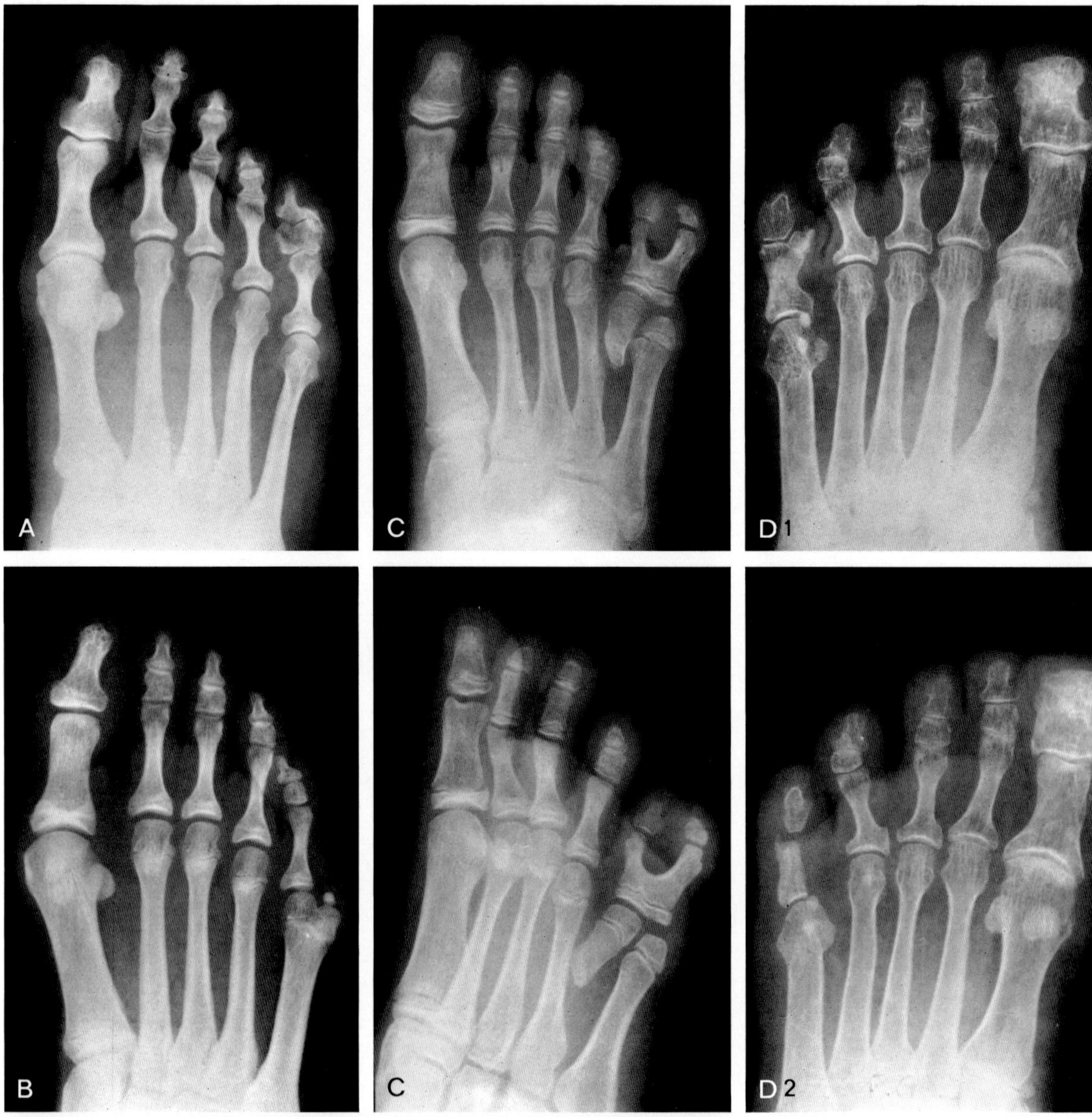

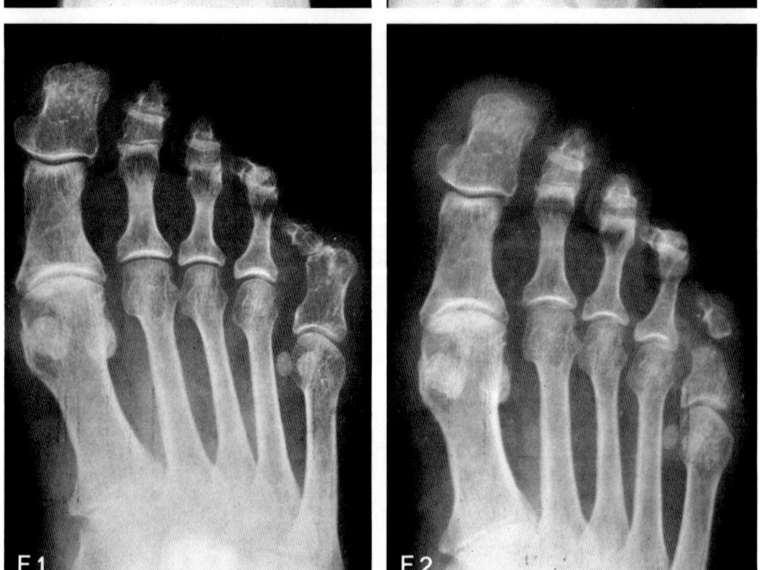

Fig. 27.8 A–M. Congenital malformations: metatarsal and phalangeal dysostoses. **A** Brachyphalangia of middle phalanx of fifth toe. **B** Bifid condyle of fifth metatarsal. **C** Supernumerary metatarsal of fourth ray, bifid fifth toe with basal syndactyly. **D, E** Brachydactyly and brachyphalangia of first and fifth toes. *1* Preoperative appearance; *2* postoperative appearance. **F** Partial duplication of proximal phalanx of fifth toe. **G** Supernumerary syndactyly of fifth toe. **H** Supernumerary fifth ray with duplication of metatarsal. **F–M** see pp. 449–451 ▷

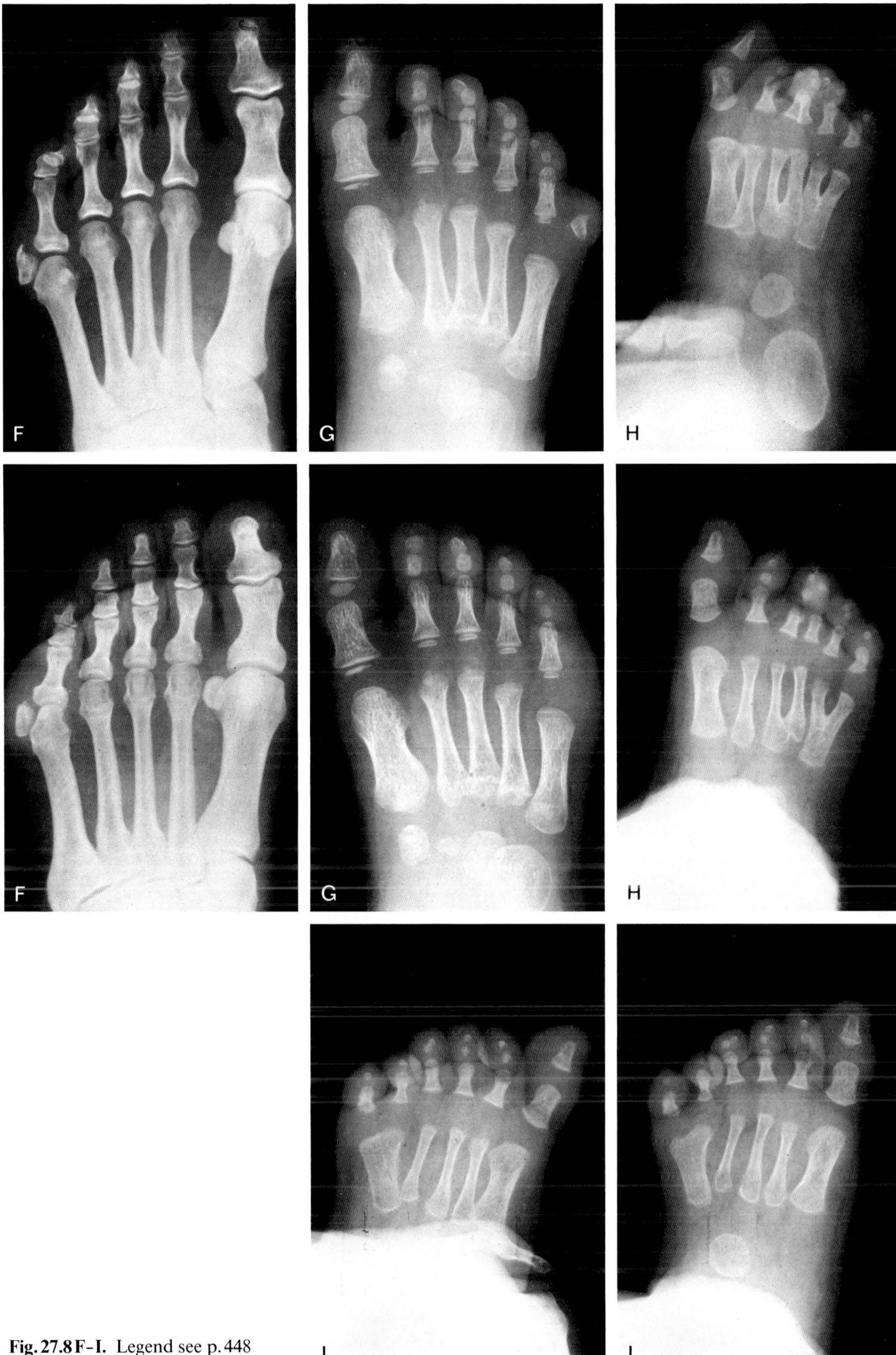

Fig. 27.8 F–I. Legend see p. 448

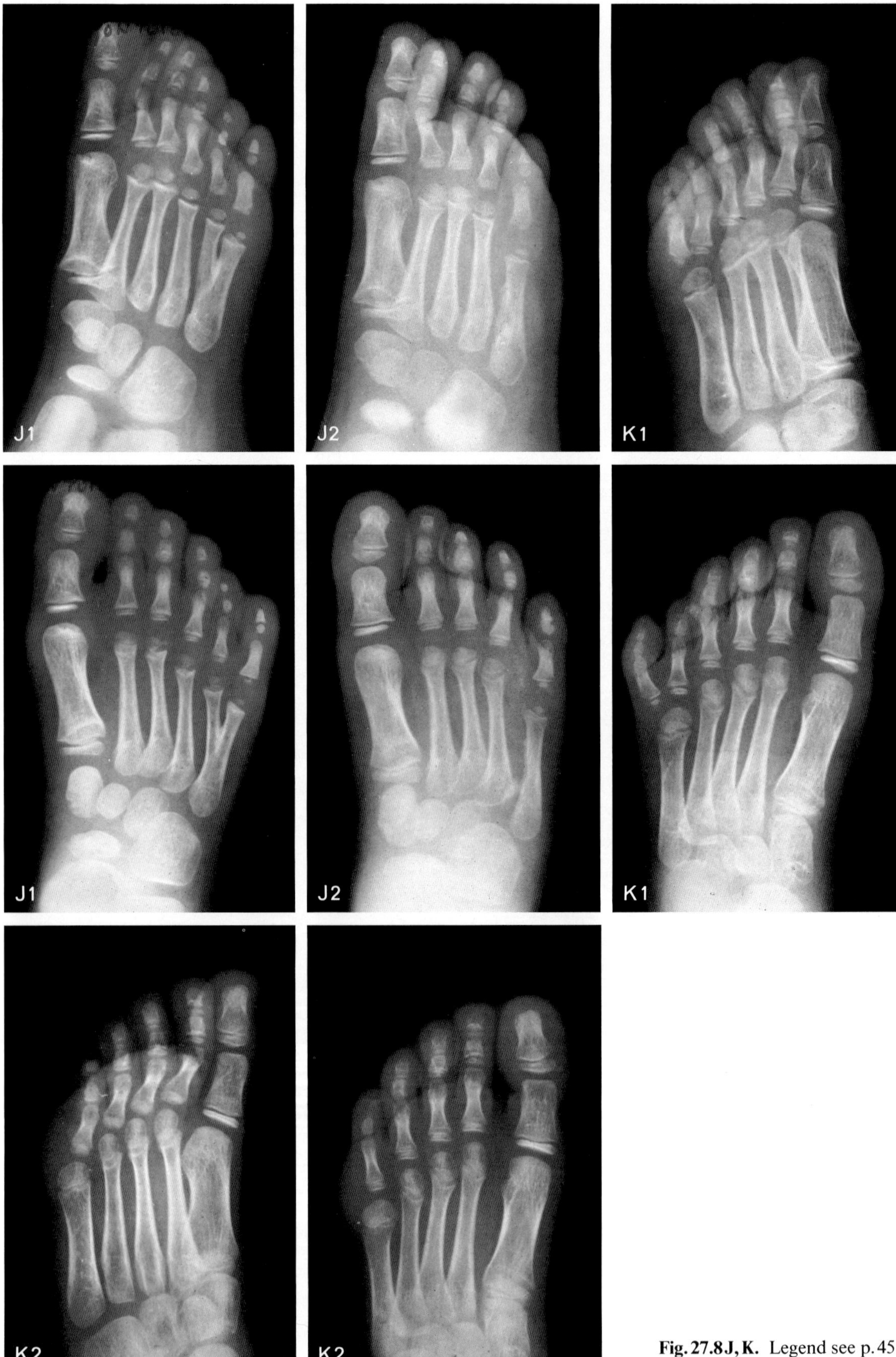

Fig. 27.8 J, K. Legend see p. 451

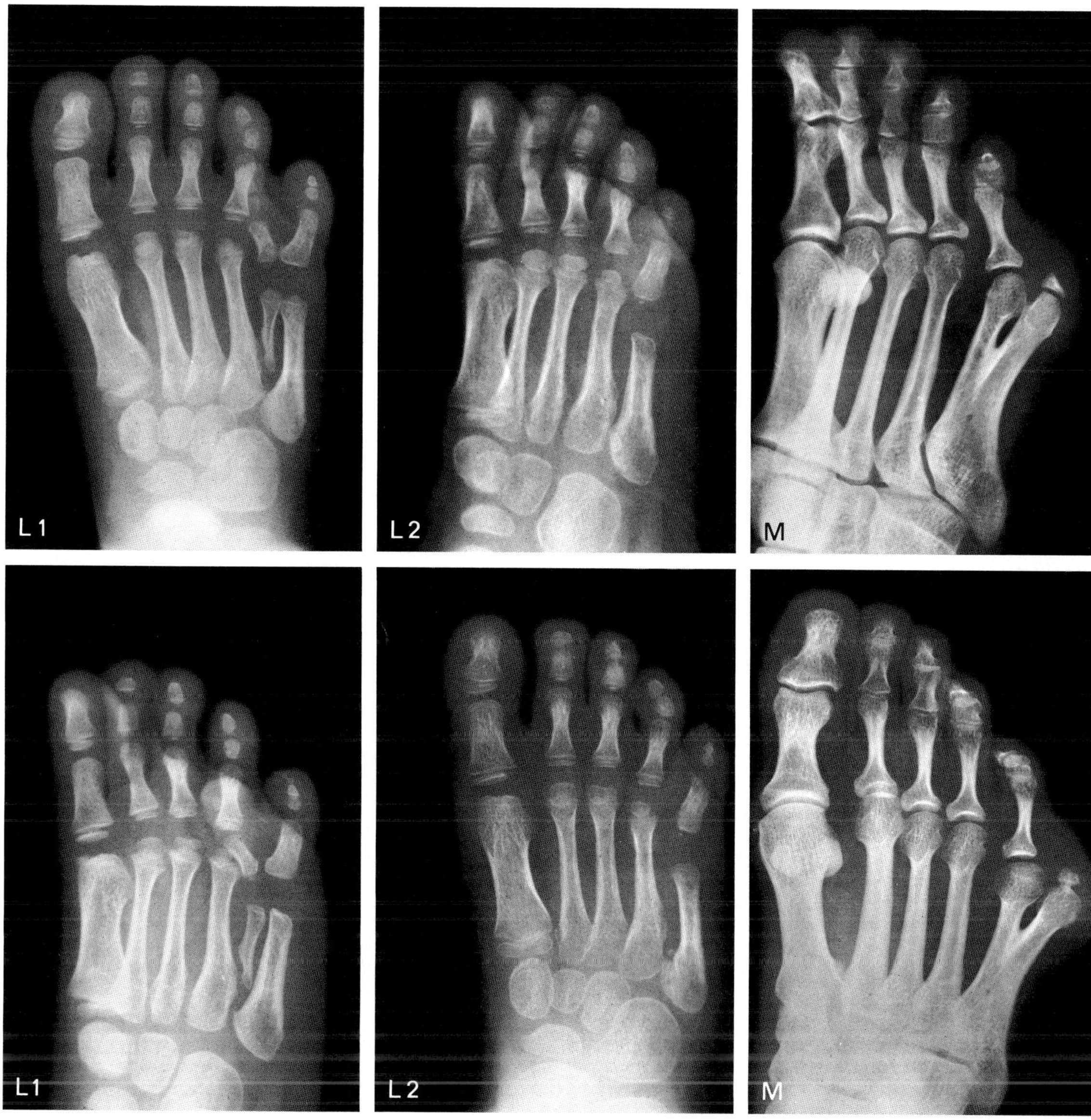

◁ **Fig. 27.8** *(continued)*. **I** Syndactyly and brachymetatarsia of fifth ray. J Duplication of fifth metatarsal and supernumerary toe. *1* Preoperative appearance; *2* postoperative appearance. **K, L** Supernumerary fifth toe. *1* Preoperative appearance; *2* postoperative appearance. **M** Duplication of fifth metatarsal

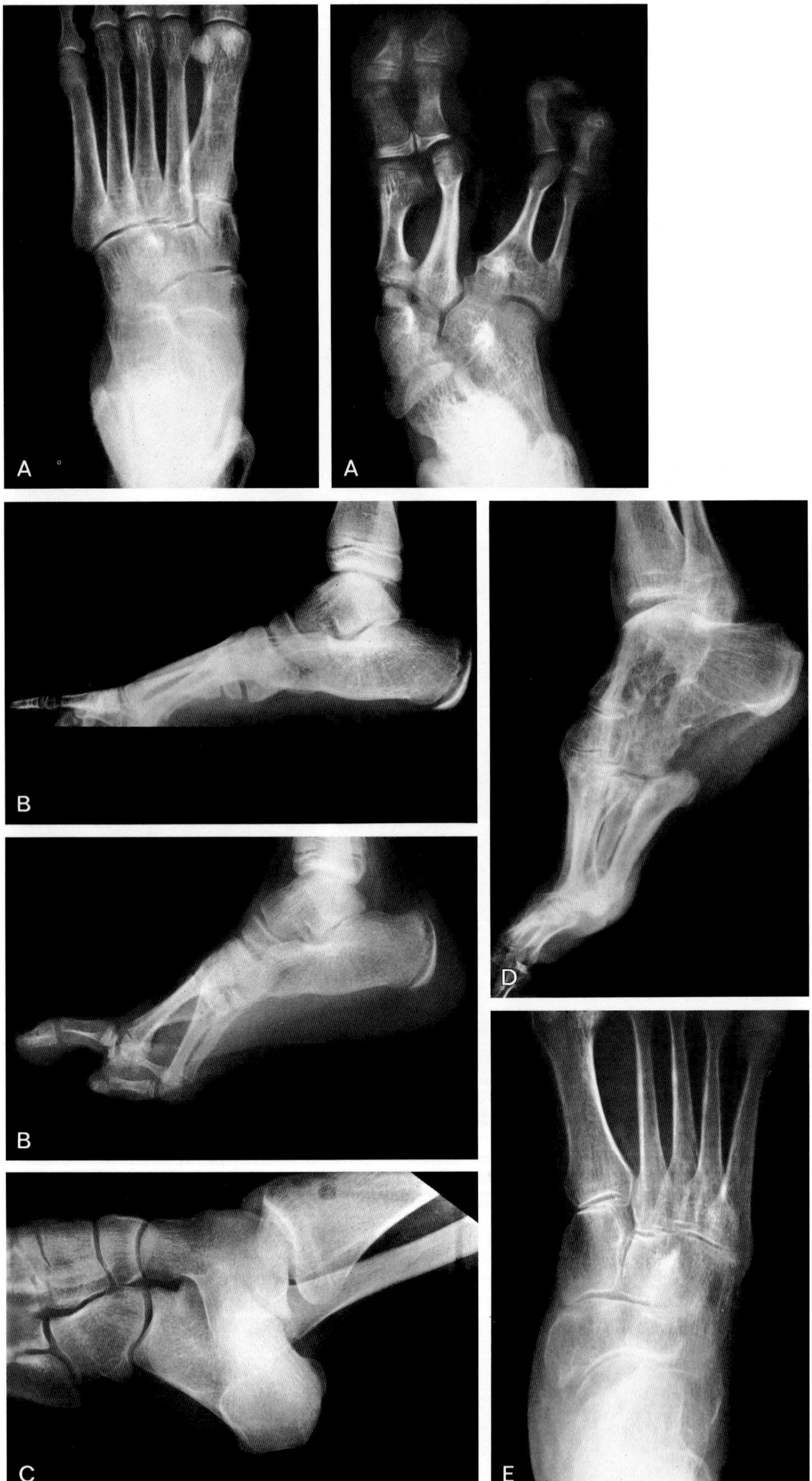
A
A
B
B
C
D
E

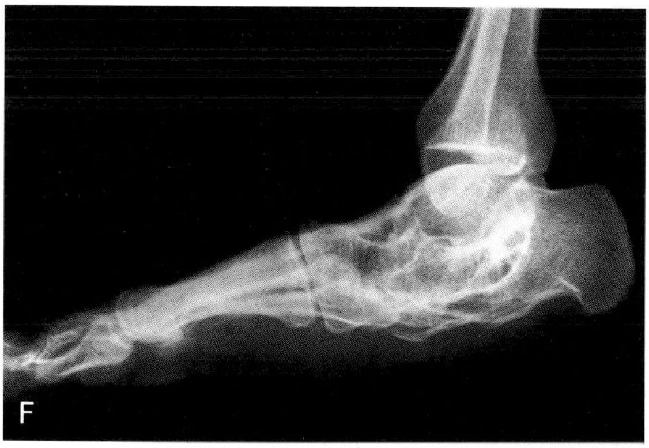

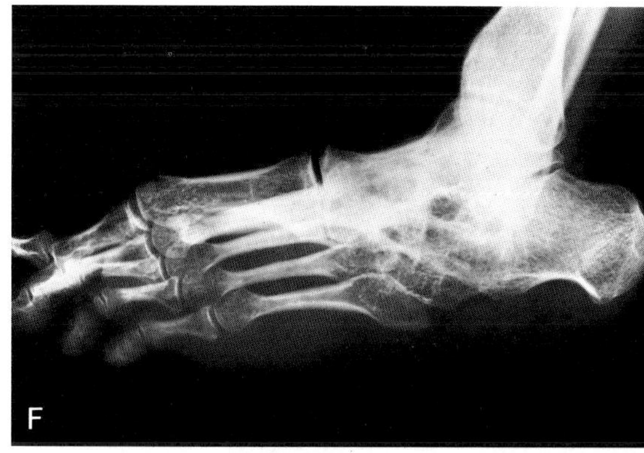

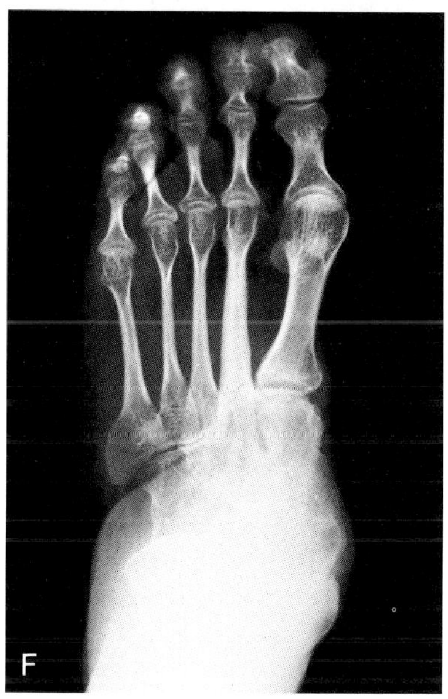

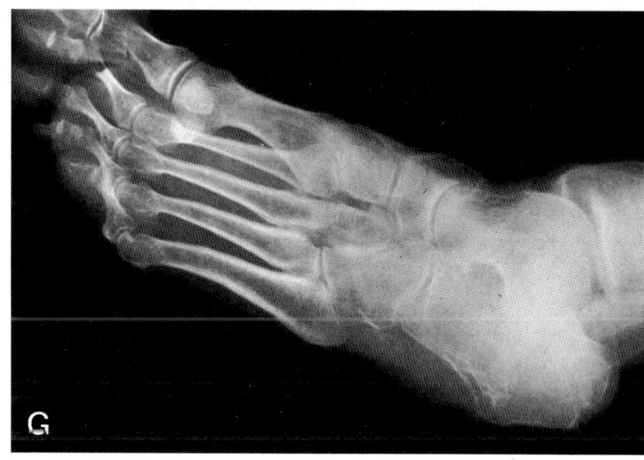

Fig. 27.9 A–G Congenital synostoses. **A** Calcaneocuboid synostosis. **B** Calcaneocuboid synostosis with lobster-claw deformity. **C** Talocalcaneal synostosis. **D** Talocalcaneonaviculocuboid synostosis. **E** Cuneiform-cuboidal synostosis. **F** Tarsomidtarsal synostosis of tuberculous origin. **G** Lateral cuneiform-metatarsal synostosis

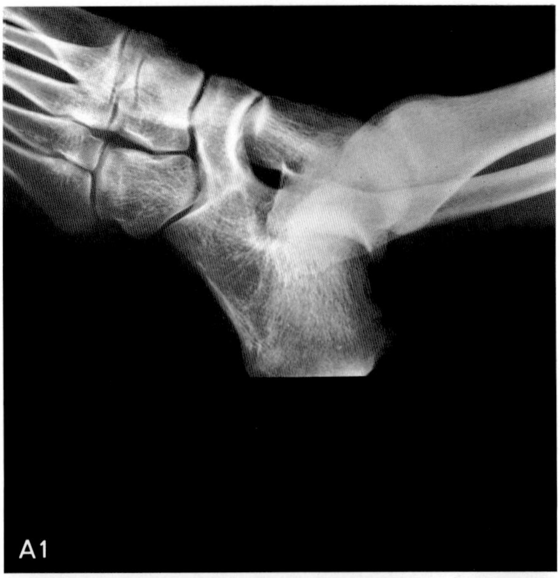

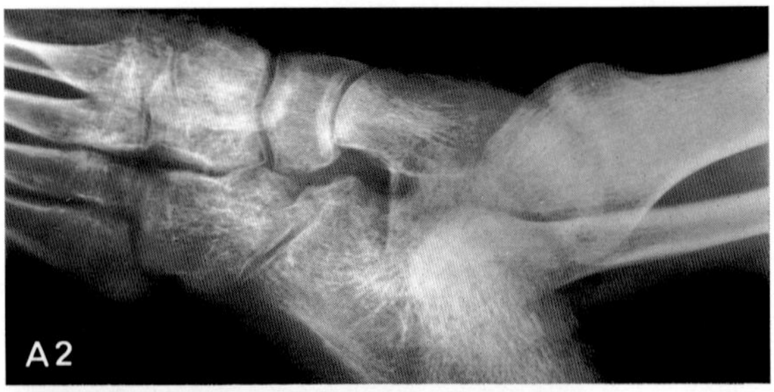

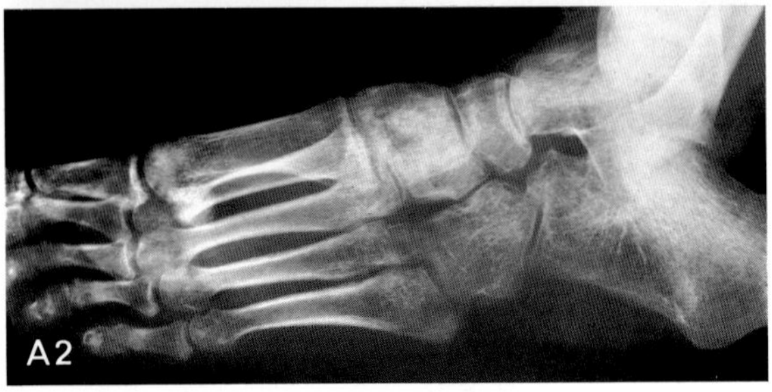

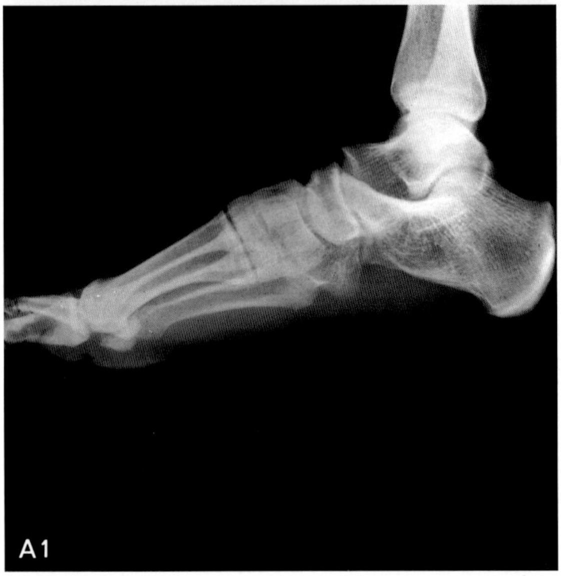

Fig. 27.10 A–C. Calcaneonavicular synostoses. **A** *1* Pre-operative; *2* after resection of synostosis. **B** Bilateral synostoses. **C** Painful pes planovalgus due to fracture of synostosis. **B, C** see p. 455

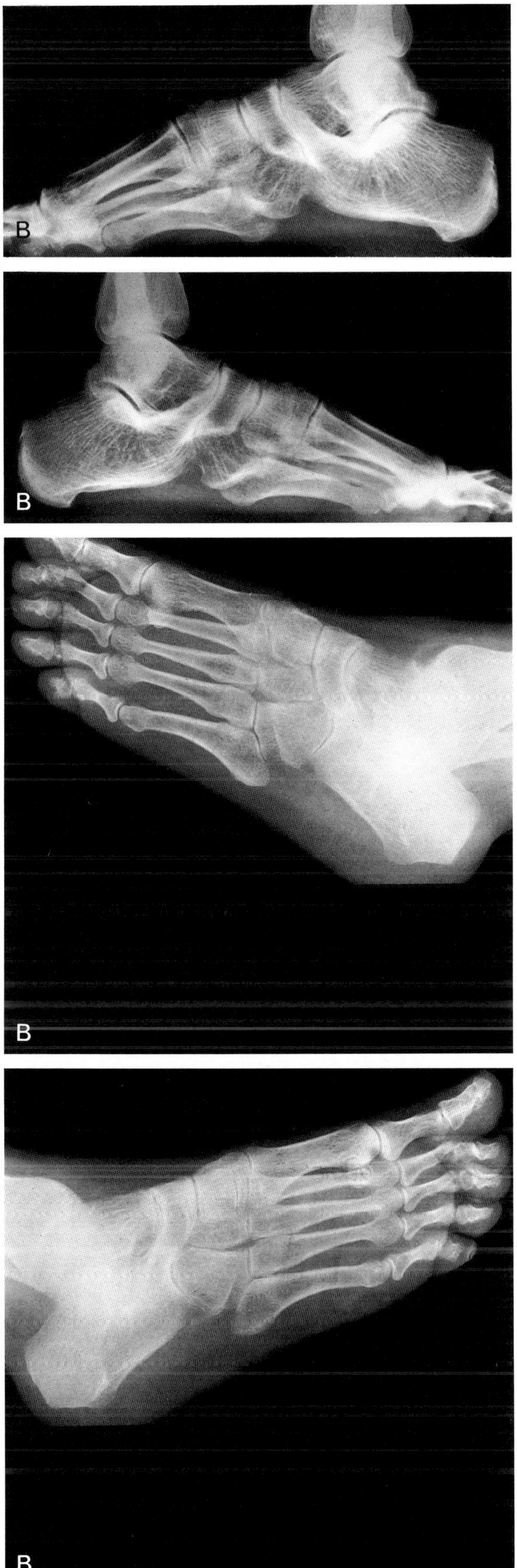

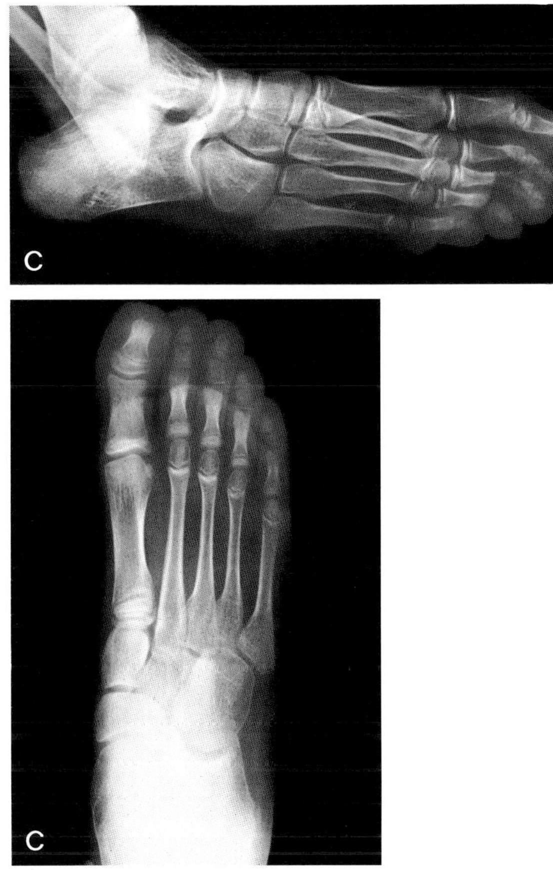

Fig. 27.10 B, C. Legend see p. 454

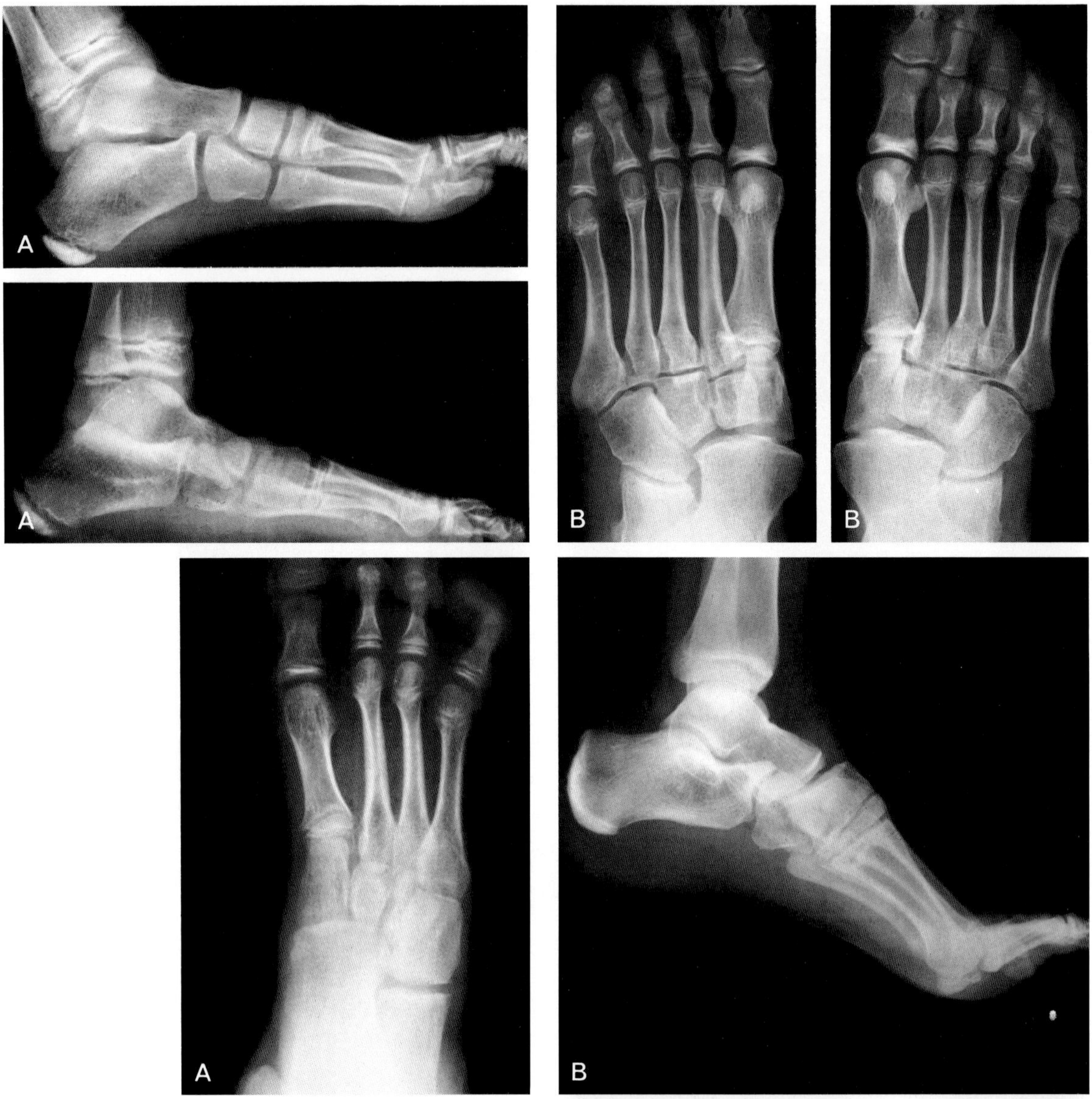

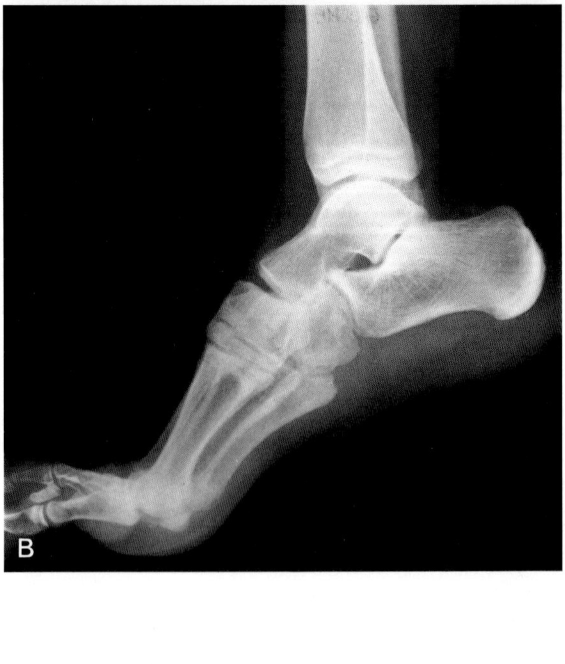

Fig. 27.11 A–D. Talonavicular synostosis. **A–C** Three examples of talonavicular syndesmosis. **D** Talonavicular syndesmosis with pes planovalgus. *1, 2* Dorsoplantar views before and after shortening resection osteotomy and correction of pes planus; *3, 4* lateral views before and after operation. **C, D** see p. 457

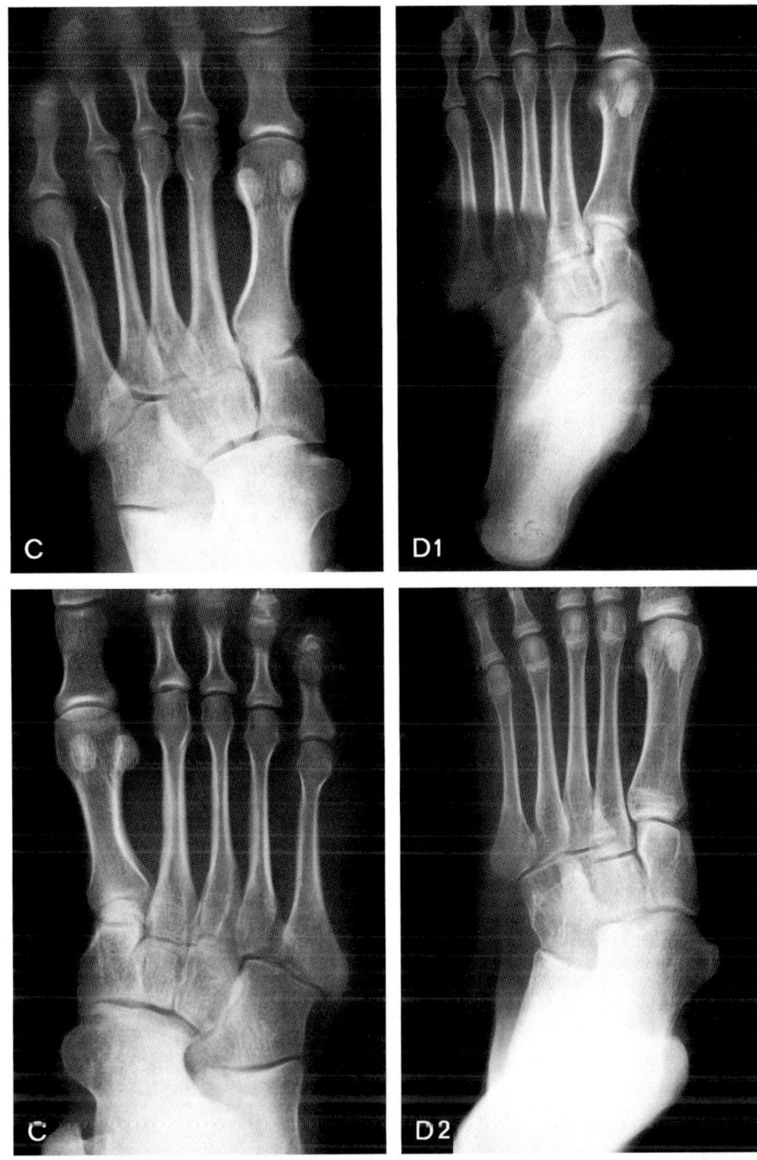

Fig. 27.11 C, D. Legend see p. 456

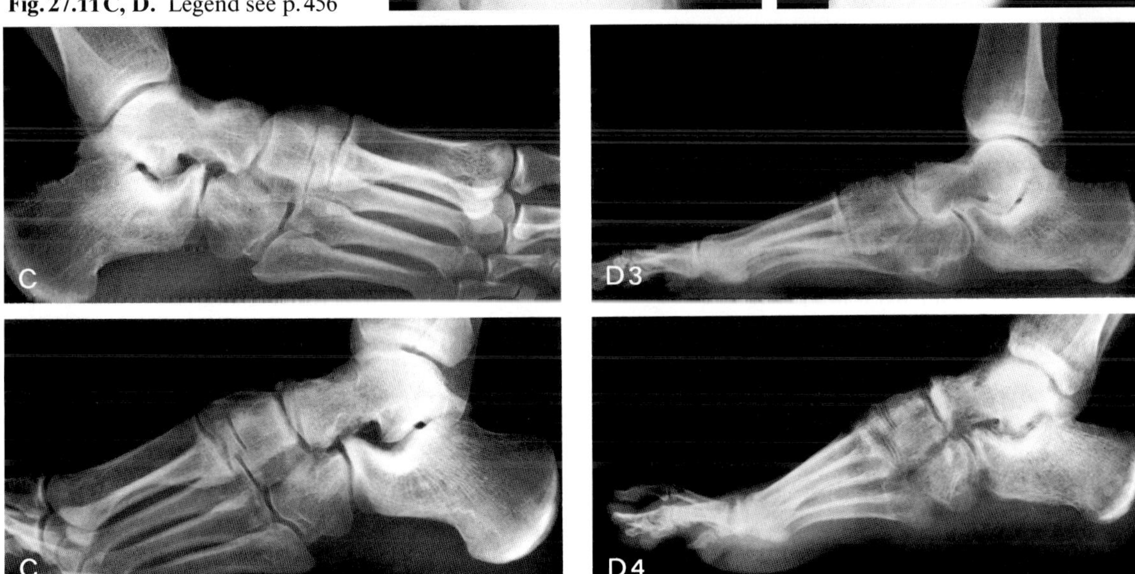

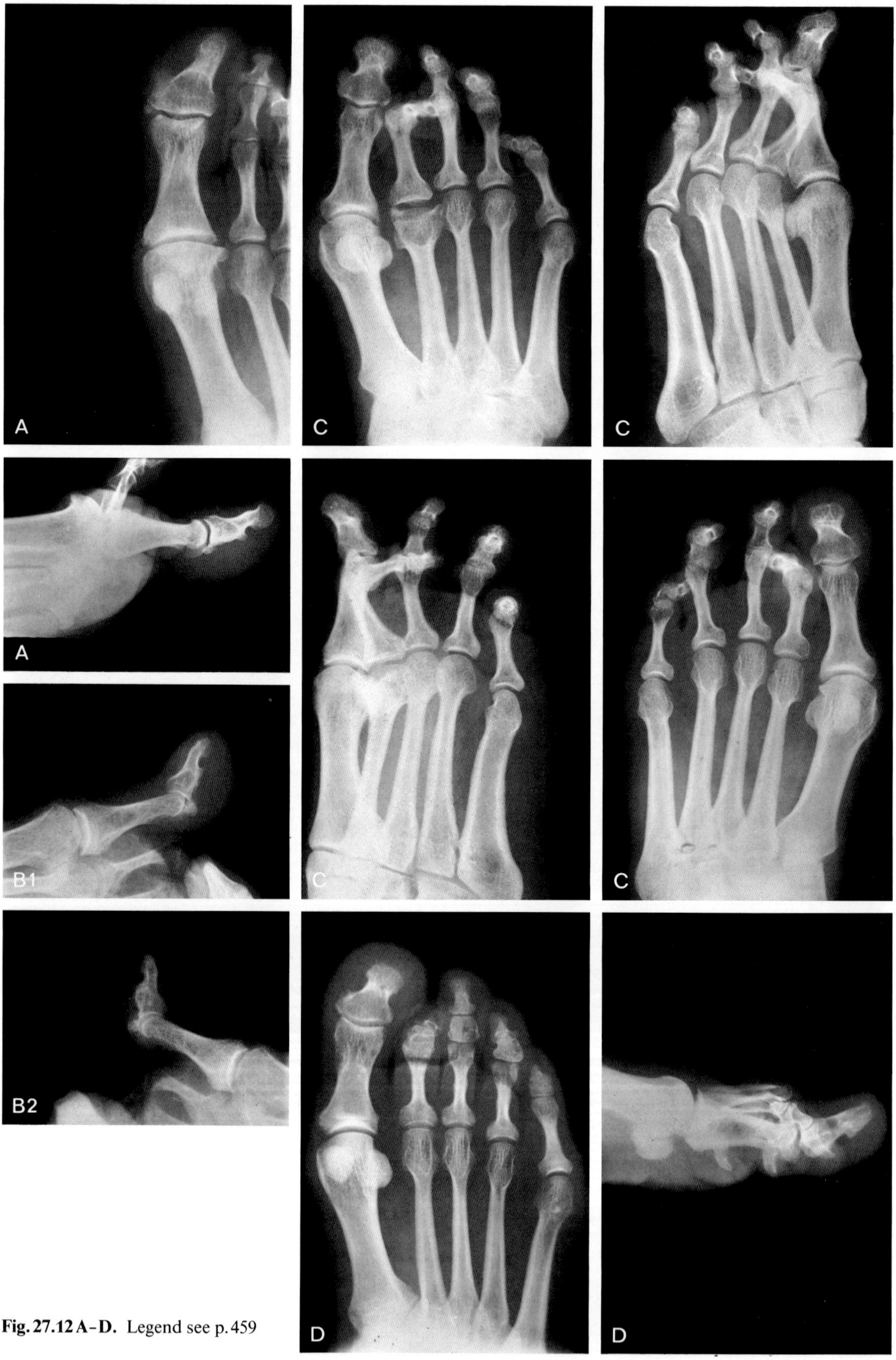

Fig. 27.12 A–D. Legend see p. 459

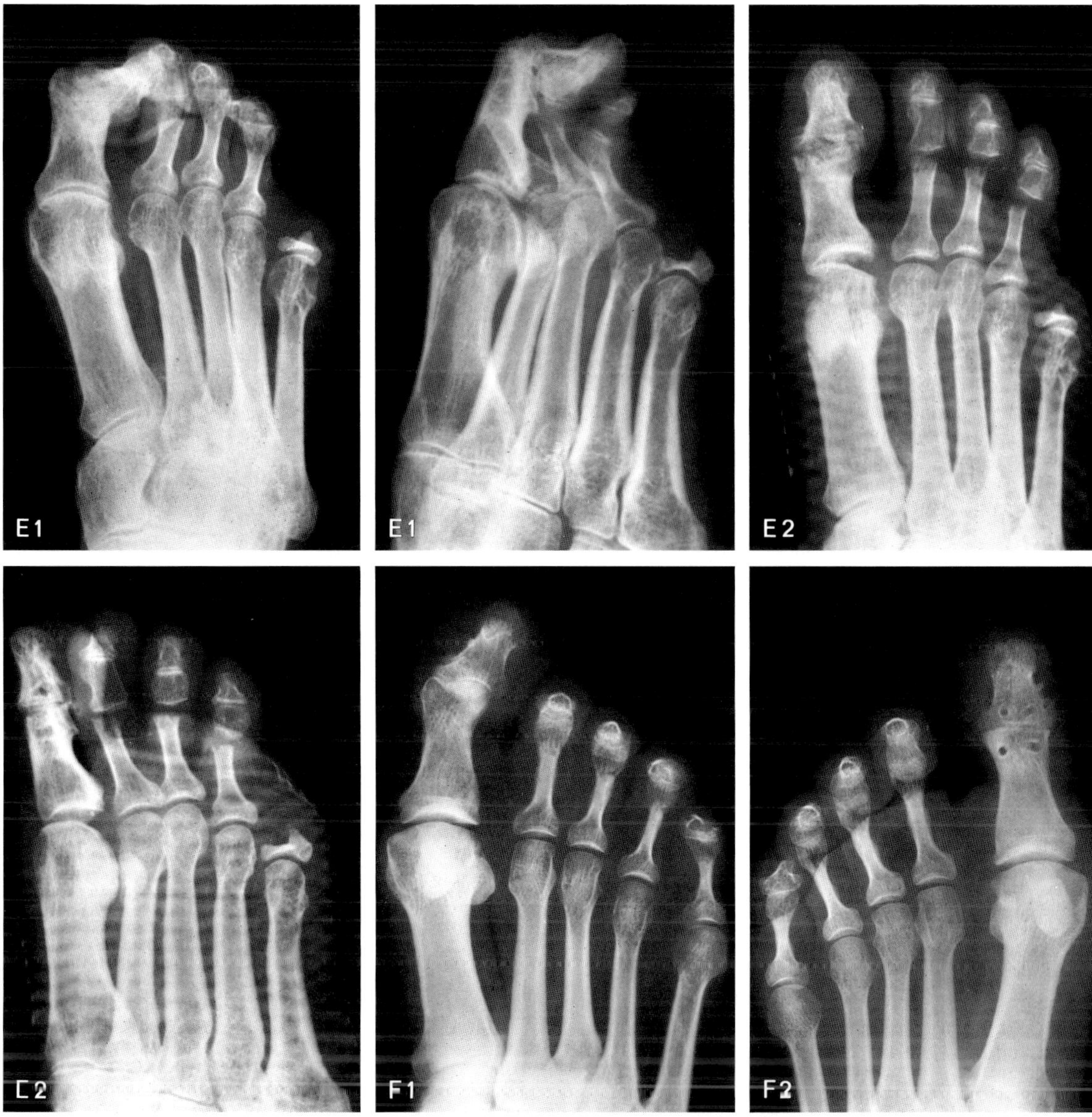

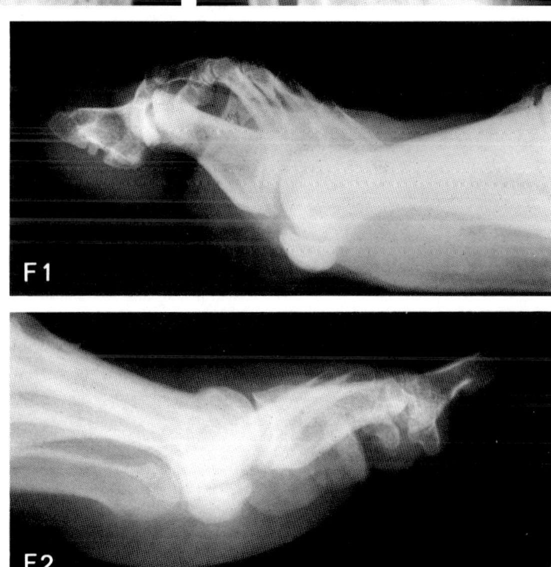

◁ **Fig. 27.12 A–I.** Congenital displacements of the toes. **A** Basal anomaly of distal phalanx of great toe. **B** *1* Hallux erectus involving distal phalanx; *2* phalangeal sesamoid with first-degree hallux rigidus. **C** Camptodactyly of second toe, swan-neck deformity. **D** Transverse deformity of great toe with erectus, camptodactyly (swan-neck deformity) of second toe. **E** Transverse deformity of great toe with flexus and digital clawing associated with aphalangia of fifth ray. *1* Preoperative; *2* after arthrodesis of interphalangeal joint of great toe, arthroplasties of second, third and fourth toes. **F** Transverse deformity of great toe with flexus of distal phalanx, claw toes. *1* Preoperative; *2* after interphalangeal arthrodesis of great toe. **G–I** see p. 460

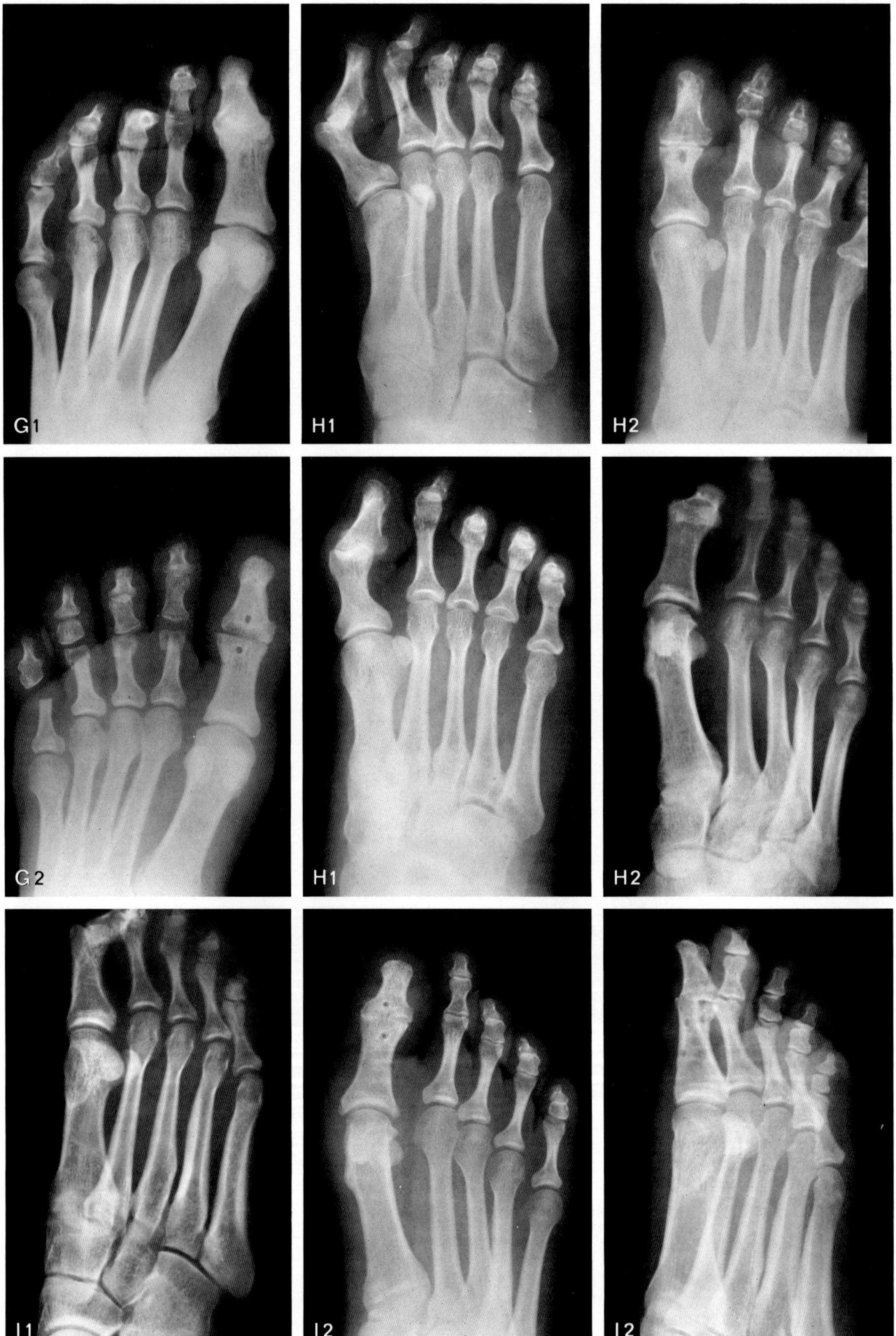
G1
H1
H2
G2
H1
H2
I1
I2
I2

◁ **Fig. 27.12** *(continued).* **G** Transverse deformity of great toe, claw toes. *1* Preoperative; *2* after arthrodesis of interphalangeal joint of great toe, arthroplasty by head-shaft enclavement of second, third and fourth toes, arthroplasty of fifth toe. **H** Transverse deformity with clawing of great toe, clawing of lesser toes. *1* Preoperative; *2* after arthrodesis of interphalangeal joint of great toe. **I** Distal clawing of great toe. *1* Preoperative; *2* after arthrodesis of interphalangeal joint

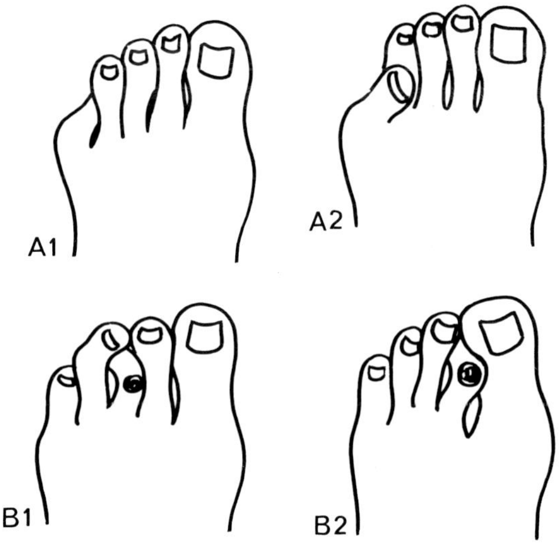

Fig. 27.13. **A** Clinodactyly: quintus varus: *1* Infraductus; *2* supraductus. **B** *1* Clinodactyly of fourth toe associated with swan-neck deformity of third toe; *2* Swan-neck deformity of second toe ▷

28 Os Intermetatarseum

The os intermetatarseum is, according to Faber (1934), a supernumerary ossicle or an osteophyte developing in the commissure between the first and second metatarsals and articulating with both metatarsals and with the medial cuneiform bone. It is a rudimentary vestigial structure, not an accessory apophysis of the cuneiform. Its reported frequency of occurrence varies between anatomists: thus Pfitzner (1892; quoted by Faber) states an incidence of 12%, while Faber records only 1.2%. I estimate the frequency as being 2%–3%.

There is a small articular surface between the os intermetatarseum and the three bones of the commissure. It results in some broadening of the space between the first and second metatarsals [Young 1910 (cited by Mouchet and Mouthier 1926); Wheeler 1933].

The patient occasionally consults for sharp pain localised to the dorsal aspect of the foot at the site of the os intermetatarseum, describing the pain as a tearing, burning or cracking sensation during standing, aggravated by walking and by certain types of shoes. Sometimes there is a neuralgic component, which may be due to irritation of local nerves.

Radiography proves the presence of the os intermetatarseum.

Treatment is specifically surgical, comprising removal, and is usually curative.

V Trophic Disorders

29 Plantalgias of Vascular Origin

29.1 Venous Insufficiency

Chronic venous insufficiency occurs in obesity and during the menopause and is associated with varicose veins, varicose ulcers and inflammatory phlebitis. It becomes associated with perimalleolar oedema and is aggravated especially in the heavy individual, by prolonged standing on the thickly engorged soles of the feet.

Pain in the plantar tissues is diffuse and of a tension type; the patient complains of general heaviness of the lower limb, affecting both leg and foot, as well as of burning of the forefoot, experienced as much on the dorsum as on the plantar aspect. Intercurrent cramps, episodes of paraesthesiae during day and night, sensations of bony grating and the restless legs syndrome (Ekbom) are other accompanying features. The latter is capricious in onset, often bilateral and intense; it is never confined to the foot, but also involves the leg, and is manifested by motor twitching, sudden irregular movements which seem to compel the patient to move the limb about.

Treatment is essentially conservative:

a) General measures are directed towards proper diet and weight reduction; diuretics and medicaments for augmenting venous tone may be helpful.
b) Local measures include the treatment of varicose ulcers and varicose veins, the application of supporting bandages and appropriate physiotherapy.
c) It may be appropriate to employ a physiological supporting insole comprising an internal dome and a retrocapital bar made of thick, soft, supporting material. Occasionally, a stabilising insole comprising an internal dome, a supinating wedge under the inner heel and a pronating wedge under the outer aspect of the metatarsus may be tolerated and effective.

29.2 Arterial Insufficiency

29.2.1 *Raynaud's Disease*

Raynaud's disease comprises attacks of paroxysmal pain occuring in two phases. Firstly, there is acute ischaemia with pain of a paraesthetic type and numbness of the toes, which are pale and cold. This is succeeded by the onset of intense pain of a pricking, tingling or lancing type, especially aggravated by cold. In the long term, a permanent trophic disorder results and gangrene can occur.

The etiology is neurological, and the condition is seen with hemiplegia, paraplegia, vascular disorders, arterial hypertension, atheroma, Buerger's disease and arteriovenous aneurysm. Another etiological factor is collagen disease, including scleroderma, polyarteritis nodosa, lupus erythematosus and various blood disorders, due to microtrauma from the shoe in individuals doing constantly heavy work.

Treatment relates to the etiology:

a) General treatment comprises measures avoiding cold, administration of vasodilation, transcutaneous corticosteroid therapy and massage.
b) Insoles comprising thick layers of cork or felt should be inserted into comfortable shoes to encourage warmth.
c) Surgical management is directed towards improvement of the blood supply and may involve sympathectomy.

29.2.2 *Arteritis*

There are numerous causes of arteritis. Symptoms may be directed towards the antetarsus, or may be diffuse, involving the whole foot and lower limb. The sensations experienced are like freezing, cramps or fatigue, with plantalgias associated with acute vasomotor crises.

Treatment is of the arteritis itself when possible.

29.2.3 *Erythema Pernio*

In erythema pernio (chilblains) the pain is localised to the site of the lesions on the sole of the foot. The lesions comprise small erythrocyanotic plaques 1-5 mm in diameter, rounded and well circumscribed which are precipitated by cold damp weather or overtight rubber shoes. They appear in front of or below one or more metatarsal heads or under the intercapital spaces. Usually pink-violaceous in appearance, they may be brownish-violet or white in the centre. Often they are misdiagnosed as corns or verrucas, especially as they may be of long duration, but the evidence of poor footwear and their occurrence during winter, together with the characteristic pricking, itching, pinching or burning pain exaggerated by damp cold but relieved by warmth and massage, should clarify the diagnosis. Obviously the lesions are more painful on standing and walking.

The cause of these lesions is not understood, but they are seen much more in older people in whom the peripheral circulation is impaired.

Treatment includes Oligosol (Labcatal, Montrouge), vasodilators, vitamin D, flavinoids, and dry warmth together with advice on proper shoes, woollen socks, massage in the mornings with alcohol and talc, and anti-inflammatory creams. Anticoagulants are occasionally advised. With proper treatment, cure within 8 days can be expected.

30 Neurodystrophic Metatarsalgia

Neurodystrophic metatarsalgia is related to the algodystrophic reflex syndrome. It is also known as Sudeck's atrophy, and has been given numerous other names, including angioneurodystrophic decalcification, Sudeck-Leriche syndrome, neurotrophic rheumatism or arthropathy, painful foot with oedema and decalcification, sympathetic dystrophic reflex, painful idiopathic decalcification of the foot (Ravault et al. 1959; Ravault and Bouvier 1966), Destot (1911), bony atrophy, post-traumatic algic osteoporosis (Leriche and Fontaine 1930) and algodystrophic sympathetic syndrome (de Seze and Ryckewaert 1954). The painful condition may affect the extremities of the upper or lower limb. Authors agree that it is due to disturbance of the neurovegetative innervative reflexes, usually of the peripheral nociceptive type but sometimes central in origin.

The condition is found in adults of all ages, especially those who have active, arduous jobs or other activities exposing the foot to respective microtrauma; 70% of cases occur in such subjects (Ruffié et al. 1964; Ravault and Bouvier 1966). Men and women are affected equally. The problem is more often unilateral than bilateral.

30.1 Etiology

The commonest precipitating cause is trauma of the lower limb, involved in some 50%-75% of cases. This may be a sprain, contusion, fracture, minimal trauma followed by prolonged immobilisation, microtrauma provoked by prolonged standing or walking, or a sequel to operation on the foot. Prolonged immobilisation, especially following trauma, appears to be an important factor.

Sometimes there are postural disorders of the foot; Mostini (1962) stated that a cavus foot of some description was present in 80% of cases.

Other etiological factors include local infection, vascular disorders, arteritis, venous thrombosis, frostbite, burns and neurological diseases, including parkinsonism and sciatica. Psychological disorders may be seen: neurovegetative dystonia, anxiety, emotional disturbance or asthenia. Lejeune et al. (1966) stated that such conditions mitigate towards an unfavourable prognosis.

In a significant proportion of patients no specific etiology can be found and the condition must be called idiopathic (Ravault et al. 1959, 1966). Indeed, Gougeon (1965) and Gougeon and Seignon (1978) stated that 15%-20% of cases were idiopathic, while Lejeune et al. (1966) placed the incidence even higher, at 50%.

Despite the multiplicity of precipitating causes, neurodystrophic metatarsalgia is a rare condition. Bony atrophy does not explain the entire pathogenesis of the syndrome.

According to Leriche and Fontaine (1930) and Terrasse et al. (1959), the majority of authors recognise the reflex sympathetic etiology as most convincing. The disturbance of arteriocapillary circulation relates to vasomotor arteriolar control. Capillary stasis brought about by contraction of the precapillary sphincters causes local anoxia.

30.2 Clinical Features

There are four main groups of clinical features:

1. Painful loss of function (stage I in both Ravault and Steinbrocker classifications)
2. Progressive vasomotor disturbance, described by Chambers and Zweifach, occurring in three phases: vasodilatation, vasoconstriction and vasomotor atony
3. Trophic disturbances (Ravault stage II, Steinbrocker stages II and III)
4. Generalised osteoporotic changes in the extremities of the limb

The condition is slow to develop and apparently benign. There is always a symptom-free interval between the accident and the onset of pain (Denis 1961-1974). Medical treatment comprising sympatheticolytic ganglion-blocking and general physiotherapy measures is effective. The development of the radiographic signs is extremely slow and later recalcification often incomplete.

The clinical development of the syndrome can be divided into three periods: the onset, the established condition and a phase of recovery.

30.2.1 Onset

The onset can be sudden and characterised by pain localised to the foot, the forefoot or even only one toe. More frequently, it is gradual, with an interval of quiescence between the event precipitating the syndrome and the development of the symptoms (Denis 1961-1974).

The pain is associated with loss of function and develops progressively. It is often moderate, but sometimes hyperalgic, with sympathetic characteristics of acute crushing, burning or compression sensations. It is aggravated by loading and shoe pressure, but relieved by rest. It may extend over the whole of the forefoot or be restricted to one ray or toe. Occasionally, the tarsus or midtarsal region is involved. The pains are of varied plantar or dorsal distribution and sometimes radiate into the leg. The diffuse character marks this period of onset.

There is local swelling due to oedema, and the foot appears white, red or cyanotic, usually with local tenderness, predominantly on the dorsal aspect. Genuine inflammation can occur, and the ranges of joint movements throughout the foot can be impaired.

The vasomotor disorder is apparent from the condition of the integument, which is warm - or sometimes hypothermic - with a red appearance, associated with increased sweating. Sometimes there are circulatory features, with augmentation of the oscillometric index.

The blood chemistry is normal, but there may be a moderate rise in the erythrocyte sedimentation rate.

Radiographic examination should include comparison with the opposite foot. The radiographic appearance is usually normal with respect to the skeletal structures, and Gougeon (1965) and Denis (1961-1974) have stressed the latency in the development of radiographic signs, although oedema of the foot and the soft tissues can be detected. Early decalcification may be apparent, however, with the development of a punctate or "tigering" appearance due to the onset of osteoporosis. Occasionally a glassy appearance occurs with geodic forms. This decalcification, if seen, always respects the integrity of the joint margins. According to Denis, the radiographic signs will become apparent not before 6 weeks after the onset of clinical symptoms. The tigering appearance described by Vacuolar involves the heads of the metatarsals and the bases of the phalanges.

30.2.2 Established Condition

The established condition may last for some months, perhaps as much as a year. There is loss of function, and pain is less severe but more constant in character and remains present during standing. Pain is aggravated by activity, and is accompanied most importantly by increasing articular stiffness diffusely throughout the foot, with a tendency to contracture of capsulotendinous structures. The intensity of subjective symptoms is in contrast with the physical signs. The features of vasoconstriction progressively replace those of vasodilatation seen in the earlier phase of development. Oedema is diminished, but atrophy of muscle previously masked by the oedema is now more apparent. Sometimes there is wasting of the leg muscles. Contracture of the aponeurosis and joint capsules is sometimes associated with adhesions of tendons to their synovial sheaths, particularly affecting the metatarsophalangeal and interphalangeal joints, which become stiff and cold with a tendency to clawing. All attempts at mobilisation of the foot produce violent discomfort, and this becomes the overriding feature of the established phase. The skin is cold, atrophied and tightly stretched, while the nails are flattened, brittle, hard, striated and sometimes thickened; they lose their pink coloration, becoming pale or violaceous. The amount of hair on the foot may increase or diminish.

The oscillometric index diminishes in parallel to the temperature of the skin.

In most instances, routine blood parameters, including the erythrocyte sedimentation rate, remain normal.

Two relatively new paraclinical examination methods show promise in aiding diagnosis. These are scintigraphy and telethermography, which can be used to assess the condition and follow the progress of treatment.

30.2.2.1 Radiography

The usual classical radiographic signs may be remarkably slight, but the relative absence of signs does not exclude the diagnosis. The essential feature is the appearance of osteoporosis, which, though it begins with the onset of the condition, may not be radiographically detectable until a long time afterwards. According to Ecoiffier and Geerts

(1956), the calcium content of the bone must be reduced by some 30% before radiographic signs are apparent. Ruffié et al. (1964) drew attention to a predilection for involvement of the calcaneum, the anterior tarsal bones, the metatarsals, the bases of the proximal phalanges and the sesamoids.

The osteoporosis may be patchy, being characterised by clearly defined microgeodic zones of rounded configuration contrasting with the homogeneity of the neighbouring osteoporotic areas, giving the bony architecture a spotted, punched out or tigered appearance. More rarely, there are true geodic formations which amalgamate extensive initial microgeodes. Above all, the metatarsal heads and the styloid of the fifth metatarsal are involved in this way.

Alternatively, there may be homogeneous osteoporosis leading to a glassy flocculent appearance, a general bony transparency. The osteoporosis as seen on X-ray always respects the joint spaces. Occasionally it extends into the leg, even as high as the knee or the hip, indicating a generalised reaction.

Lejeune et al. (1966) summarised the radiographic signs of osteoporosis into four groups:

(a) simple increase of radiographic lucency,
(b) the appearance of so-called stains,
(c) the appearance of glassy bones, and
(d) a coned appearance of the bony trabeculae, which appear enlarged and sometimes very mature. These different pictures can appear successively.

The diagnosis of the established state rests on the classical triad of features described by Leriche and Fontaine (1930): painful loss of function, typical vasomotor and trophic disturbances associated with extensive osteoporosis, but conservation of the joint spaces on radiographs.

30.2.3 Phase of Recovery

The final development will depend upon the effect of treatment. Serre et al. (1977) observed that the algodystrophic reflex could extend to the knee or even as far as the spine, in which osteoporosis could produce frank fish-tailing of the outline of the vertebral bodies.

With effective treatment, there is permanent recovery of articular mobility and disappearance of oedema and vasomotor disturbance. However, a decalcified foot stays a decalcified foot, and some degree of discomfort during loading and walking can persist for as much as a year or even 2 years. Again, mild oedema, perhaps localised, wasting of the calf muscles and contracture due to synovial sheath irritation can be most troublesome. Bureau states that any sort of arthroplastic intervention for the claw toes should be avoided while any degree of trophic change remains. This includes contracture of the plantar ligaments and plantar aponeurosis, which can be associated with a painful cavus foot, while occasionally there may be development of a planovalgus foot due to overrelaxation of involved ligaments.

In parallel with these features, the osteoporosis is extremely slow to regress, and reossification can take several years. How long this recovery takes depends on the severity of the symptoms and signs at the onset.

While the degree of calcification may become normal or nearly normal, there always remains a rather coarser trabecular pattern of the bone with development of some osteophytes.

As will be stated later, treatment needs to cover a very long period, and there are cases in which some degree of symptoms or signs may persist for 2–10 years. The most frequent residua of the condition are articular contracture and a tendency to limp, according to Lelièvre.

30.3 Atypical Forms

In addition to the usual presentation of this condition, examples of atypical varieties are as follows:

a) A painful decalcified foot in which the osteoporosis is evident radiologically but without other signs
b) A painful hyperalgic forefoot followed by inflammation
c) An oedematous decalcified foot as described by Ruffié (1964) with diffuse oedema and pain during walking, the osteoporosis being various in distribution
d) An algodystrophy of such extensive and diffuse distribution that it affects the whole lower limb
e) An idiopathic form described by Ravault et al. (1959) and Ravault and Bouvier (1966) which supervenes without apparent cause
f) A permanent non-resolving form described by Coste and Piguet (1956) in which contracture predominates without any sign of improvement

30.4 Differential Diagnosis

Diagnosis has been seen to depend in general upon the history of (a) a traumatic episode leading to osteoporosis which does not involving joint spaces, and (b) the absence of systemic signs of inflammation, reflected in blood chemistry. The tendency is to recovery following the evolutive cycle described. The following conditions should be excluded:

a) Osteoporosis due to inflammatory arthritis (staphylococcal or gonococcal infection, in which the joint spaces are narrowed or the joint surfaces eroded)
b) Osteoporosis due to tuberculous arthritis, in which there is a blurring of the articular space, the diagnosis being finally determined by biopsy
c) Neurological conditions, including tabes dorsalis and hemiplegia, in which the homogeneity of the decalcifying process predominates in the extremities, sometimes with osteolysis and periarticular osteophytosis
d) Diabetes, in which the condition is bilateral, the joint spaces are eroded, and there is evidence of vascular calcification
e) Gout, with its preceding history, the biochemical abnormalities, the more frequent pseudogeodic appearance, and the near-diagnostic therapeutic test of colchicine administration

30.5 Treatment

It must be stated at the outset that the following treatments should be avoided (Gougeon 1965): immobilisation in plaster casts, any form of surgical intervention, exploration or biopsy and excessively vigorous early physiotherapy.
Correct treatment comprises three aspects:

1. Efforts to avoid contracture and muscle atrophy by means of local injection of corticosteroids, infiltration with local anaesthetic in the tarsal canal, massage and gentle, progressive, prudent physiotherapy [emphasised by Ravault et al. (1959), and Ravault and Bouvier (1966)]. Active re-education hydrotherapy and thermal cures are valuable.
2. Control of the vasomotor disturbance. Kinesitherapy, beta blockers (except in patients receiving anticoagulants), electrophysiotherapy (ionisation, lumbar radiotherapy, ultrasound), calcitonin (50–160 units daily or two or three times a week during the developmental and static stages only), sympathetic block, intra-arterial cocaine, vasodilators, hormone therapy, calcium, vitamin D and ganglion and neurone blockers.
3. Treatment must be continued for long periods of time.

Treatment may be augmented by physiological supportive insoles which comfort the foot and avoid painful residua.

31 Perforating Plantar Ulcer

The term "perforating ulcer" was first proposed by Vesignié d'Abbéville. The first description was made by Nelaton in 1852: "a torpid ulceration, painless, without tendency to spontaneous cure, of neurotrophic origin with a protruding epidermal border which is cornified and whitish in colour" (Figs. 31.1, 31.2).

The perforating plantar ulcer supervenes in a foot afflicted by a permanent disorder of superficial and deep sensitivity. It occurs in areas of load bearing and consequent ischaemia, therefore affecting mostly the forefoot and the heel (the latter less commonly). The so-called pseudo-perforating ulcer is of mechanical origin and is a complication of infection of a callosity or corn or plantar keratoma. Otherwise, the perforating ulcer constitutes a very well-defined entity. The local disturbances resulting from plantar tissue involvement comprise ulceration, loss of sensation, indolent healing, oedema, cyanosis and abnormal sweating of the skin. The trophic disorders of the deep soft tissues and underlying bones comprise synoviocapsular or ligamentous necrosis, osteoporosis, osteolysis, osteophyte formation, sometimes osteosclerosis or osteonecrosis, arthropathy and perhaps even gross loss of tissue from vascular complications. There may be local ischaemia with paradoxical hyperthermia.

These local signs may be accompanied by general disorders, of which vascular insufficiency is the principle sign. Neurological features are usual, and will be described under the specific disease entities involved. The general condition of the patient may be severely affected.

In general, following the contributions of Bauman and Gerling (1963) concerning leprosy, and those of Lelièvre (1952) and Huriez (1971), the majority of authors agree that the main cause of the condition is overloading of the tissues. The perforating ulcer is characterised histologically by complete destruction of the dermis, thickening of the surrounding dermis with hypertrophic papillae, extensive local vascular and nervous lesions surrounding the lesion, endarteritis of a proliferative or obliterative nature, interstitial neuritis and degenerative disease.

31.1 Etiology

Perforating plantar ulcers are found as complications in the following conditions (order of frequency): diabetes, Bureau-Barrière disease (1955), tabes dorsalis, Thévenard's acropathy (1942), syringomyelia, spina bifida, leprosy, various forms of arteritis, sciatic paralysis and, rarely, ainhum. Huriez and Duprez established that 40% of perforating ulcers were of diabetic origin, 12% were due to alcoholic neuritis (Bureau-Barrière disease), 5% occurred in tabes dorsalis and 43% related to other etiologies.

31.2 Clinical Features

The features of the specific diseases will be dealt with in subsequent sections of this chapter but certain generalisations can be made.

The condition presents between the ages of 30 and 50 years in the zones of weight bearing of the foot, exceptionally of the plantar arch. Sensory disturbance, usually analgesia, affects the site of the lesion and the surrounding skin. Often the ulcer begins with a callosity, keratoma or corn under one, two or three metatarsal condyles, the posterior tuberosity of the calcaneum or the base of the fifth metatarsal or on the plantar aspect of the great toe. A zone of hyperkeratosis becomes rapidly inflamed, with the development of a painless abscess or subjacent bursitis. A corn, however, may become very painful, hypothermic, and phlyctenoid around the peripheral zone. The peripheral area of the main lesion becomes oedematous, and within a relatively short period of time, perhaps a few days, the general swelling ruptures, allowing release of pus or seropurulent fluid, following which any pain resolves. This is the classical plantar whitlow of the collar stud variety. There are instances where the suppurative process evolves without any discomfort. Without treatment, the sinus matures and extends centrifugally, the typical whitish hypertrophy of the borders develops and a constant seropurulent discharge, sometimes yellowish, sometimes

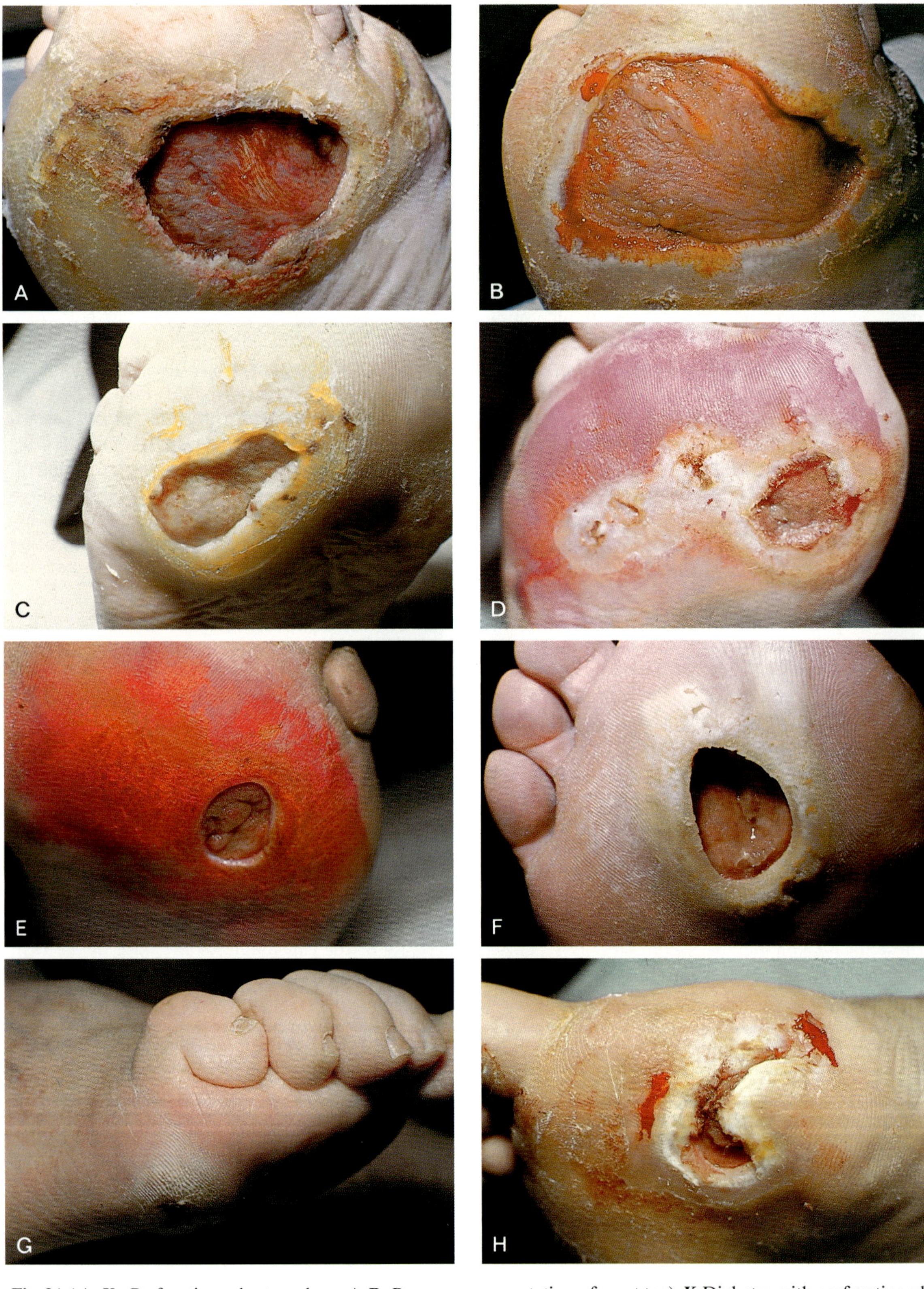

Fig. 31.1 A–K. Perforating plantar ulcer. **A, B** Bureau-Barrière disease. **C, D** Bureau-Barrière disease and alcoholic polyneuritis. **E, F** Diabetes. **G** Ulcerated callus. **H** Distal callus on great toe. **I** Thévenard's disease (with amputation of great toe). **K** Diabetes with perforating ulcer following bruising of great toe (amputated). **J** Thevenard's disease. **I–K** see p. 472 ▷

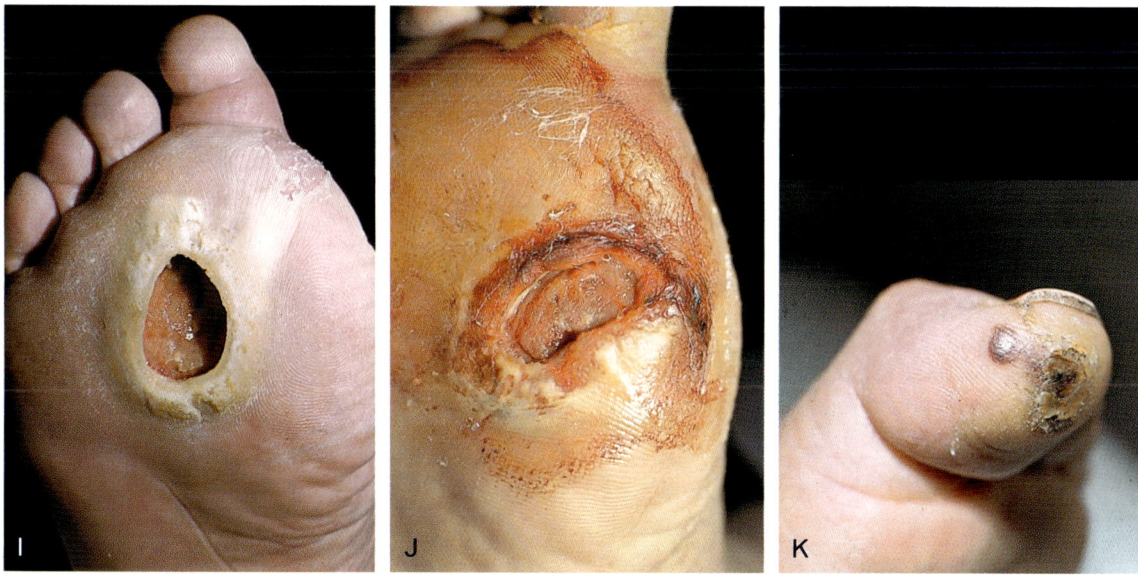

Fig. 31.1 I–K. Legend see p. 472

yellowish-green, sometimes serosanguinous, ensues. The lesion deepens progressively, the impression of depth being accentuated by the hypertrophy of the borders, and the typical perforating ulcer entity is established. The skin, tendinous sheaths, capsules of joints and synovium and finally underlying bone surface become involved.

Typically, the established perforating ulcer is round with a central reddish crater, sometimes violaceous, carpetted by little bulges of tissue containing purulent material, covered with whitish filaments and easily bleeding when disturbed, together with small radial fissures and old granulations. In the centre of the crater, which tends to bulge, there is an opening of variable size, but generally punctiform and narrow, out of which flows the sometimes offensive discharge. Probing confirms direct contact with the bone, with para- or intra-articular involvement. Occasionally the central opening of collar stud formation is not present. The steep sides of the whitish hypertrophied cornified borders slope towards the cornified periphery of the initial callosity. The borders are clearly delineated and lined by the readily bleeding granular surface. The indolence with respect to healing is very characteristic, and the likely outcome is progressive extension of the lesion leading to arthritic irreversible changes.

In addition to the perforating ulcer, a generalised oedema develops throughout the forefoot, with swelling of the retromalleolar gutters and the dorsum of the foot and an appearance of succulent tumifaction. There is sometimes local heat or, in contrast, general coldness of the foot. The surrounding skin lesions include erythema, eczema and frank desquamation. Loss of sensation of the sole of the foot, sometimes extending to the ankle region like a shoe, may be accompanied by a particularly hard consistency of oedema in the ankle region with a violaceous, greyish or deep-grey colour of the skin. The sweating disorder is usually hyperhidrosis. There is clawing of the toes and the nails are also involved, with onychauxis, onychorrhexis, onychogryphosis, and onychomycosis.

The indolence of healing is associated with an element of indifference on the part of the patient due to the loss of normal sensation. The most common complaint by patients relates to the inconvenience of frequent changes of surgical dressings.

Later complications associated with infection include lymphangitis, phlebitis and frank gangrene, The swollen appearance of the foot becomes increasingly marked, as does the discoloration and general thickening of the skin. The podgy hammer toes are particularly typical.

31.3 Diagnosis

The indolent perforating ulcer is usually recognisable. What remains is to ascertain the underlying cause, which is usually general in nature.

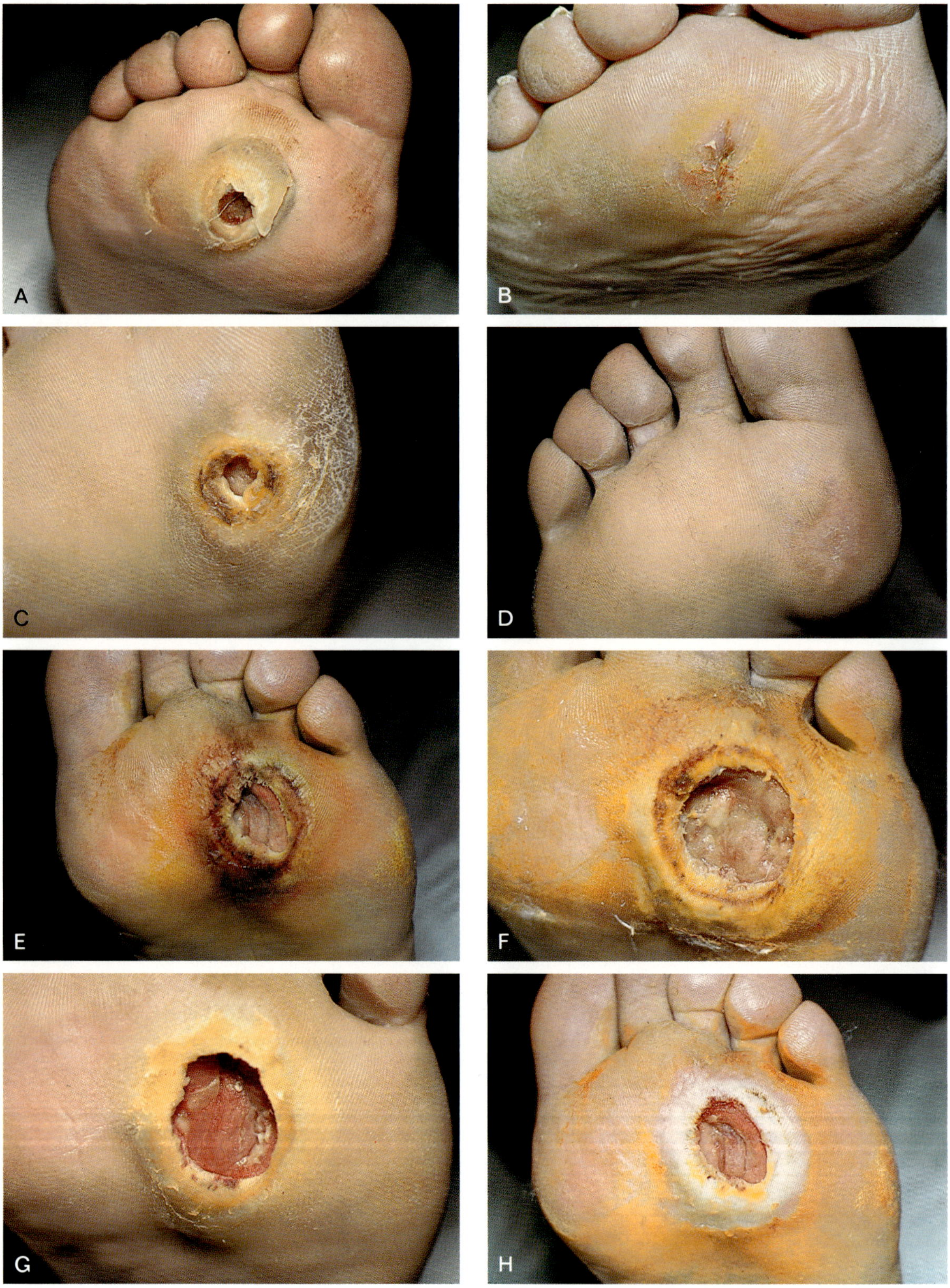

Fig. 31.2 A–M. Perforating plantar ulcer. **A, B** Diabetic ulcer, before and after early treatment. **C, D** Diabetic ulcer, before treatment and after complete cure. **E–J** Diabetic ulcer associated with equinus of third metatarsal. **E–H** Development during local treatment over 6 months. ▷ **I, J** Cure after osteotomy of third metatarsal. **K–M** Tabes dorsalis. **I–M** see p. 475

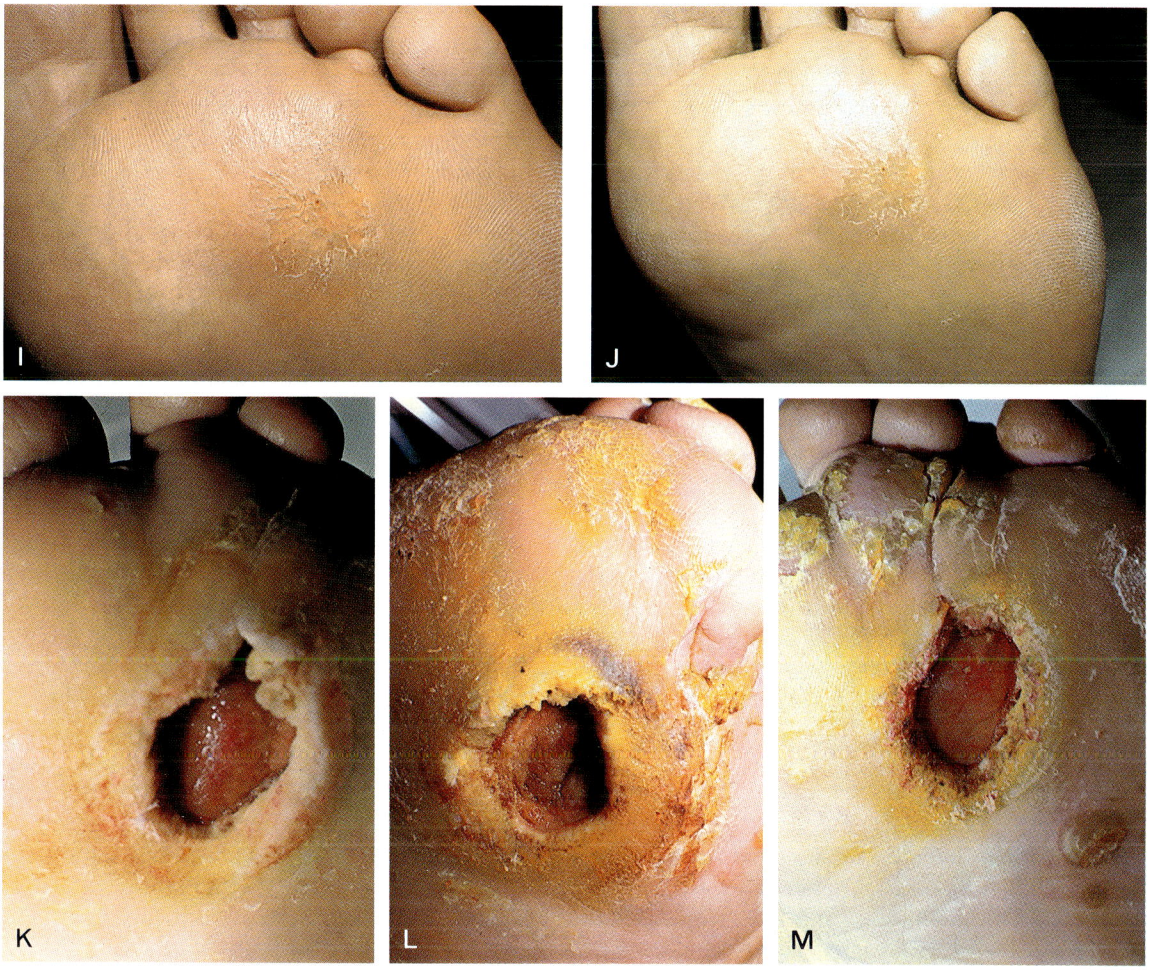

Fig. 31.21–M. Legend see p. 474

31.3.1 Past Medical History

Diabetes, syphilis, alcoholism, poor hygienic conditions, visits to countries in which leprosy is endemic some 2–3 years previously, known or occult spina bifida, family history of Thévenard's disease, syringomyelia and sciatic palsy are all relevant.

31.3.2 Morphological Abnormalities of Foot

The following conditions may be found: irreducible pes cavus, elective equinus of the metatarsus, bony swellings under the base of the proximal phalanx of the great toe or on the plantar aspect of the interphalangeal joint of the great toe, perhaps related to abnormalities of the sesamoids, which themselves may protrude abnormally. Posterior paralytic pes cavus may be obvious, while restriction of movement of the ankle joint, perhaps held in equinus, may be due to arthrosis, past trauma or a poorly orientated arthrodesis.

31.3.3 Vascular Supply

Oscillometry and arteriography may be necessary. The vascular supply must be assessed most carefully before undertaking local or general therapy.

31.3.4 Laboratory Tests

Laboratory tests relate to the specific diseases likely to underlie the perforating ulcer. Blood sugar, liver function, prothrombin index, total cholesterol and albumen-globulin ratio tests, the Wassermann reaction and a search for Hansen bacillae in the mucous glands of the skin are all investigations to be considered.

31.3.5 Neurological Examination

Neurological examination is of paramount importance. Discovery of the absence of motor involvement in diabetes, muscle atrophy due to involvement of the external popliteal nerve in leprosy or the typical paralyses of syringomyelia leads to early diagnosis. Ataxia may be present in tabes dorsalis, and is bilateral in amyotrophy but asymmetrical in syringomyelia. Of more immediate significance is the loss of deep sensation sometimes seen in Thévenard's disease and in diabetes. Tabes dorsalis is accompanied by diminution of pain on deep tendinous or bony pressure. The distribution of pain is not radicular in leprosy, but is so in syringomyelia. Superficial sensitivity may be increased in tabes dorsalis, while there is dissociation of temperature and tactile sensation in syringomyelia. Total anaesthesia or just loss of sensation of heat and cold occurs in Thévenard's disease. Leprosy is characterised by loss of sensation of heat and touch, but this begins distally with a tendency to progression proximally along the limb.

31.3.6 Joint Involvement

Destructive or hypertrophic osteoarthropathy is usually painless and may be associated with hypermobility of the joint with subluxation or dislocation, especially in tabes dorsalis. There is usually no arthropathic involvement in leprosy. Rapid development with significant hypertrophy of the joint and spontaneous dislocation is characteristic of syringomyelia. Destructive and atrophic osteoarthropathy is seen in Bureau-Barrière disease. Diabetes mellitus tends to lead to lytic osteoarthropathy of a particularly destructive pseudo-inflammatory type. Characteristic of Thévenard's disease are lytic osteoarthropathy with destruction of the epiphyseal region, dislocation and geodic vacuolar or splitting erosions of slow evolution presenting over several years.

The *radiographic features* of the arthropathies may be diagnostic:

a) Tabes dorsalis. Brailsford (1929) [cited by Kerbrat (1974)] described three stages: joint effusion, destruction of the joint, reconstruction. The signs of destruction and repair are disordered, occur simultaneously and involve the knee more frequently than the foot.
b) Diabetes mellitus. Perforating ulcer formation usually precedes arthropathy, in which there is destruction of the joints with no tendency to repair. The arthropathy affects predominantly the midtarsal region, then the forefoot, and finally the tarsus. The osteolytic lesions are geodic in form, and fractures may occur together with patchy osteoporosis and occasionally evidence of spontaneous amputation.
c) Bureau-Barrière disease. This condition (Bureau and Barrière 1955) is characterised by perforating ulcer preceding any arthropathy. It is the metatarsophalangeal and interphalangeal joints which are destroyed, with marked osteolysis and atrophy.
d) Thévenard's disease. In this condition (Thévenard 1942) the arthropathy is early and mutilating, accompanied by osteolytic lacunar or vacuolar lesions affecting the phalanges and the metatarsophalangeal joints. The osteolysis predominates without evidence of repair and without periostosis (Kerbrat 1974). It is destructive and extensive.
e) Leprosy. The osseous involvement comprises clear round lacunae in the spongy bone and epiphyseal lesions in the loading zones. The latter are erosive, geodic, atrophic, osteolytic and osteoporotic, ending in progressive amputation.
f) Lateral popliteal nerve palsy. The perforating ulcers are associated with osseous lesions located towards the fifth metatarsal head and then involving the fifth metatarsal diaphysis.
g) Spina bifida. The bony lesions are essentially osteolytic.
h) Syringomyelia. Osteolytic epiphyseal lesions with clear contours and associated with peripheral osteophytosis are characteristic. General osteoporosis and areas of osteosclerosis are always present.

The overlap of the various radiological findings is considerable and the importance of history-taking and laboratory examination cannot be underestimated.

31.3.7 Differential Diagnosis

The differential diagnosis between a pseudo-perforating ulcer and a true perforating ulcer is made on the basis of the history of the development of the lesion from secondary infection, irradiation (perhaps as much as 20 years previously) leading to an excruciating neuralgic type of pain, electrical injury or the excessive use of carbon dioxide snow or silver nitrate for cutaneous lesions.

31.3.8 Trophic Disorders

The evidence of trophic disorders may be characteristic: in tabes dorsalis, Thévenard's disease and leprosy, sudden painless episodes of oedematous swelling may occur, perhaps with bruising; the condition subsides after several days. In Thévenard's disease and leprosy, cyanosis of the extremities is common. Increased sweating is characteristic of Thévenard's disease and syringomyelia. Loss of sweating is seen in leprosy, accompanied by atrophy of the skin, loss of pigmentation, evidence of nodular hypertrophy of the nerves and various forms of mutilation. Local hyperthermia may be seen in diabetes, while bullas, erythema, vesicle formation and scleroderma are sometimes present in syringomyelia.

In the toes, perforating lesions involving the phalanges are seen in arteritis, leprosy and Bureau-Barrière disease.

A perforating ulcer under the navicular is usually a complication of the midtarsal arthropathy of tabes dorsalis or diabetes mellitus associated with flat foot or the cubic foot described by Charcot (1868) involving crumbling of the midtarsal region.

It should be mentioned that ulceration can occur as a sequel to radionecrosis at any site following treatment of a verruca or other cutaneous tumour.

31.3.9 Postural Disorders of Foot

In the majority of cases there is a disturbance of the longitudinal or transverse orientation of the foot, leading to selective overloading. Thus, an unperceived equinus of the metatarsus may precipitate a perforating ulcer of the forefoot in an otherwise normal foot. A number of specific variations are worthy of record:

- Elective equinus of the first metatarsal accompanying a first-degree pes cavus, perhaps in reaction to pes cavovarus, can lead to ulceration under the first metatarsal head.
- A perforating ulcer may develop in the median callosity in the convex or triangular forefoot.
- Alternatively, fixed equinus or isolated protrusion of one of the metatarsal heads may lead to an isolated lesion.
- In the varus foot with inversion or a supinated forefoot ulceration can occur under the fifth metatarsal head. In the cavus forefoot, ulceration can occur under the first and fifth metatarsal heads, while in the varus foot, cavovarus foot or varus club foot of congenital origin, the fifth metatarsal head may be involved.

Perforating lesions of the hindfoot are the least frequent, but may be seen in pes planus, where the calcaneum has a horizontal disposition, and posterior paralytic pes cavus, in which it is vertically orientated; either of these conditions can lead to diminution of the zone of loading of the calcaneum and increased local pressure in the region of the postero-inferior tuberosity. In these cases the calcaneum does not rest on the ground by means of its normal posterior and plantar border, due to paralysis of triceps surae and the extensors and hypertonia of the short plantar muscles.

31.4 Treatment

Whenever possible, any general disease present should be treated.

31.4.1 Local Treatment

The limb should be immobilised and elevated to reduce oedema and all loading should be avoided. Rigorous hygiene and local application of anti-infective dressings are essential. Antiseptic dressings should initially be cicatrising, alternating with cleaning of the wound of exudate. Prudent excision should be repeated at monthly intervals, the cutaneous cornified margins of the ulcer being reduced. After control of infection, dressings of physiological saline with cicatrising tulle gras should be alternated with drying dressings. The length of time for which the different dressings are applied should be adjusted to the progress of healing. Local massage to stimulate the scarred area and hypothermic treatment complete the local therapy.

31.4.2 General Medical Treatment

General medical treatment comprises administration of antibiotics against infection, vasodilators and eutrophics, all complementing the appropriate medical treatment of the general underlying condition.

31.4.3 Surgical Management

Any surgical treatment should be most circumspect. Especially in conditions like diabetes mellitus, the possibility of worsening the lesion should be appreciated. All surgery should be conducted under general antibiotic cover, and major surgery

is indicated only in the presence of displacements of the foot which manifestly aggravate or precipitate the lesion mechanically.
Surgery is usually limited to cleaning and curettage or resection of an arthropathic joint, excision of sequestra or realignment of metatarsals if the general state and the condition of local tissues allow osteotomy of the bases. After correction of any osteoarticular deformity, attention can be directed to the lesion itself by means of a simple split skin graft or some local flap procedure. Again, caution should always be adopted because of the likelihood of slow healing, even after correction of skeletal disorders. Bony corrections may be prejudiced by the presence of osteoporosis. Complementary cancellous bone grafting may be necessary.

Broader surgical procedures may be indicated in certain cases:

- Revision arthrodesis to correct fixed equinus resulting from ill-aligned arthrodesis of the ankle
- Midtarsal osteotomy or wedge metatarsal osteotomy to correct longitudinal fixed cavus
- Low sympathectomy (Lazorthes) to improve circulation

31.4.4 Orthopaedic Insoles

Carefully adapted and fitted to proper shoes, orthopaedic insoles aim to support the whole foot in a uniform fashion. They must be padded or excavated to protect zones of overloading and be made of firm but compressible materials so as to cushion the atrophied tissues.

31.4.5 Rehabilitation

Rehabilitation often entails the patient changing to a sitting job. Also important are strict attention to hygiene; persistent education in the choice of good shoes, as well as insoles; dietary measures; when indicated, a careful antidiabetic regime with the avoidance of alcohol and other toxic drugs; and careful attention to weight control.

31.5 Specific Neurological Diseases

31.5.1 Bureau-Barrière Disease

Bureau-Barrière disease (Bureau and Barrière 1955) is caused by hyperplasia and congestion of the sympathetic ganglia of the lumbar region, with cellular alterations characterised by excess pigment (pyknosis and chromatosis), leading to alteration of the terminal elements of the cutaneous supply, notably of the foot. Damage occurs from microtrauma. Associated disorders include metabolic disturbances, often due to chronic alcoholism, which encourages the spread of the neurological lesion. There is no evidence of medullary syringomyelic lesions, ascending neuritis of the Guillain type, hyperactivity of the sympathetic nervous system, the extensive progressive syndrome described by Barré, disturbances of the vasa nervorum affecting the vascular supply (Van Bogaert) or angioneural hyperplasia of the superficial layer of the dermis.

31.5.1.1 Clinical Features

Bureau-Barrière disease is non-familial, non-hereditary and affects predominantly males of 40 years or older. The subject is frequently a chronic alcoholic exhibiting vulture-like facies, an air of flamboyancy, tremor, tenderness of muscles, injection of the conjunctivae, painful hepatomegaly and disturbance of liver function. His state of hygiene is often poor and he has a history of deficient diet. Often he works in cold or humid conditions, and the use of poor footwear contributes to the development of relevant foot abnormalities.
Cardinal features relevant to diagnosis include the absence of any medullary involvement, the lack of relationship of disease distribution to any particular dermatome, the absence of evidence of any spinal dysraphism (Brenner) and the exclusive involvement of the lower limbs. The disease is characterised by the association of trophic and sensory disorders.
The *trophic* disorders relate to ulcers on the foot following benign trauma such as a sprain or frostbite. Repeated excoriation of the skin may be followed by the appearance of blisters or phlyctenular haemorrhages, or by the ulceration of a plantar callus already present for a long time. (Fig. 31.1 a–d). These cutaneous lesions are recurrent with poor tendency to healing. They develop within a few days, weeks or months and form a perforating plantar ulcer, which is the usual presenting symptom. Like the classical perforating ulcer described by Nélaton (see beginning of chapter), this ulcer is insensitive, and situated under one or several metatarsal condyles, on the plantar aspect of the interphalangeal joint of the great toe, on the external border of the foot or related to the posterior tuberosity of the calcaneum at the heel.

The *sensory* disturbances comprise a diminution of the sensations of touch, pain and temperature, with a tendency to spread progressively as far as the upper third of the leg. Sometimes there are paradoxical pains of a spontaneous causalgic type. Occasionally, there is dissociation of temperature and pain rather like that seen in syringomyelia. These sensory disorders are not radicular in distribution, but are bilateral and roughly symmetrical in all ways. There is usually no reflex disturbance, but sometimes diminution or disappearance of the ankle jerk is found. The plantar cutaneous response is normal. Muscle wasting or tenderness of the muscle masses may be a feature. Bowel and bladder function normally. There is no vascular disturbance, and oscillometric findings are initially normal.

In contrast with other disorders, the skin is shiny and pale-pink at the outset and then becomes coloured with a brown pigment, later associated with hyperkeratosis. Pigmentation and keratosis coexist and contrast in colour. The nails lose their brilliant lustre and become thickened and irregular. Their surface becomes striated or sometimes thin and they take on a dirty-white or greyish coloration. There may be hyperhidrosis of the toes or of the entire foot relating to the sympathetic imbalance. Viewed grossly, the foot becomes deformed, swollen, shortened and widened. This process is progressive and is accompanied by progressive development of osteoarticular lesions. Deformations which may develop are: convex forefoot with a perforating median ulcer under the middle metatarsal heads; elective equinus with keratotic lesions due to overloading leading later to perforating ulcers; cavus forefoot with perforating ulcers under the first and fifth metatarsal heads; irregular displacements of the metatarsophalangeal joints with curling of the toes.

The evolution of the condition is progressive and apparently irreversible, with relapses and remissions alternating over many years.

Radiographic appearance varies according to the degree of evolution of the condition (Fig. 31.3). There may be generalised osteoporosis of the foot; irregularities in the contours of the bones; progressive sinking of the forefoot due to rarefaction and to resorption of the epiphyseal region, affecting predominently the metatarsals and the phalanges; metatarsophalangeal arthritis; destructive distal epiphyseal osteolytic lesions without any tendency to repair; occasional gross amputations of toes; and dislocations of the metatarsophalangeal joints. The osteonecrotic features appear to be irreversible.

Findings of laboratory investigations include abnormal liver function and a negative Wassermann reaction.

31.5.1.2 Treatment

No treatment is likely to alter the irreversible nature of the disease, which progressively destroys particularly the skeleton of the forefoot.

Efforts at local amelioration include cleaning and disinfection of the lesions and removal of bony fragments as they separate. Attention should be paid to diet, liver failure should be treated, and the patient should have prolonged periods of rest. Lumbar sympathectomy and sympathetic block seem to bring no benefits.

31.5.2 Tabes Dorsalis

Tabes dorsalis is due to degeneration of the posterior columns of the spinal cord and of the sensory nerve trunks with wasting. There is general neuritis, atrophy of motor and sensory fibres, sympathetic lesions and demyelination. A long history of syphilis may be elicited, but usually diagnosis depends on serology.

Perforating ulcers associated with tabes dorsalis are accompanied by features including visceral disorders, occular abnormality, joint involvement and the ataxia described so admirably by Déjerine in 1906, which is made more obvious by abruptness of movement during walking. The foot is lifted abnormally high and more suddenly than usual; it falls equally suddenly, striking the ground with the heel. In more advanced cases the legs are flung abruptly upwards and outwards like those of a puppet. The normal reflex action of walking is lost, and the subject has to consciously control his gait. There is a tendency for the victim to walk with his head inclined forwards, looking down at the ground, as if there were a need to see the results of his efforts. This ataxia signals the onset of a perforating ulcer (Duchenne de Boulogne 1858).

The perforating ulcer is often an early sign of tabes dorsalis. It usually develops in the pre-ataxic period, and when it is associated with loss of ankle and knee reflexes, loss of deep sensation, hypotonia, Argy'l Robertson pupils and a positive Romberg sing, the diagnosis is usually clear. Visceral disorders include gastritis and urinary problems with impotence, while sympathetic involvement is manifested by hyperhidrosis, augmentation of the oscillometric index with increased amplitude of the pe-

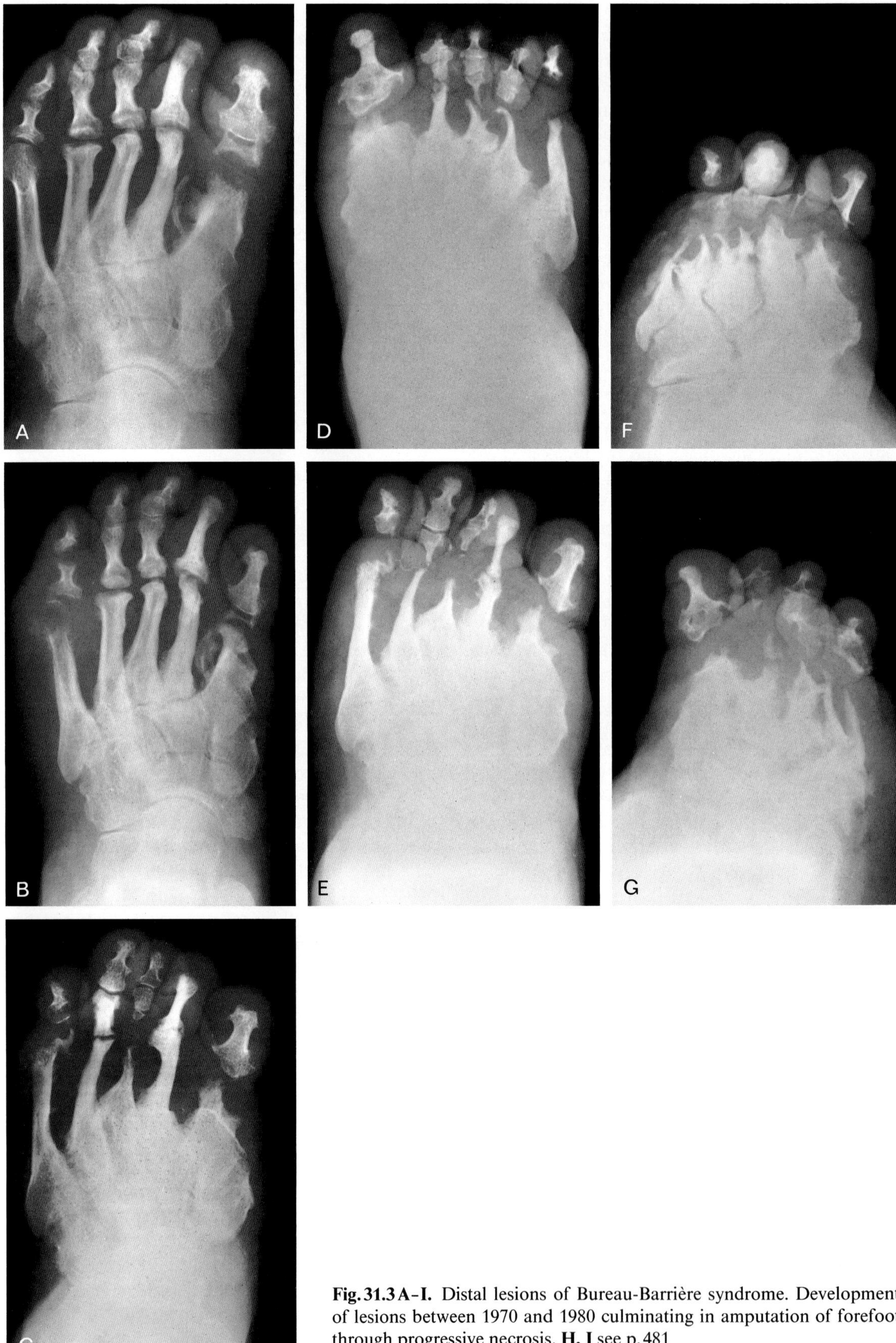

Fig. 31.3 A–I. Distal lesions of Bureau-Barrière syndrome. Development ▷ of lesions between 1970 and 1980 culminating in amputation of forefoot through progressive necrosis. **H, I** see p. 481

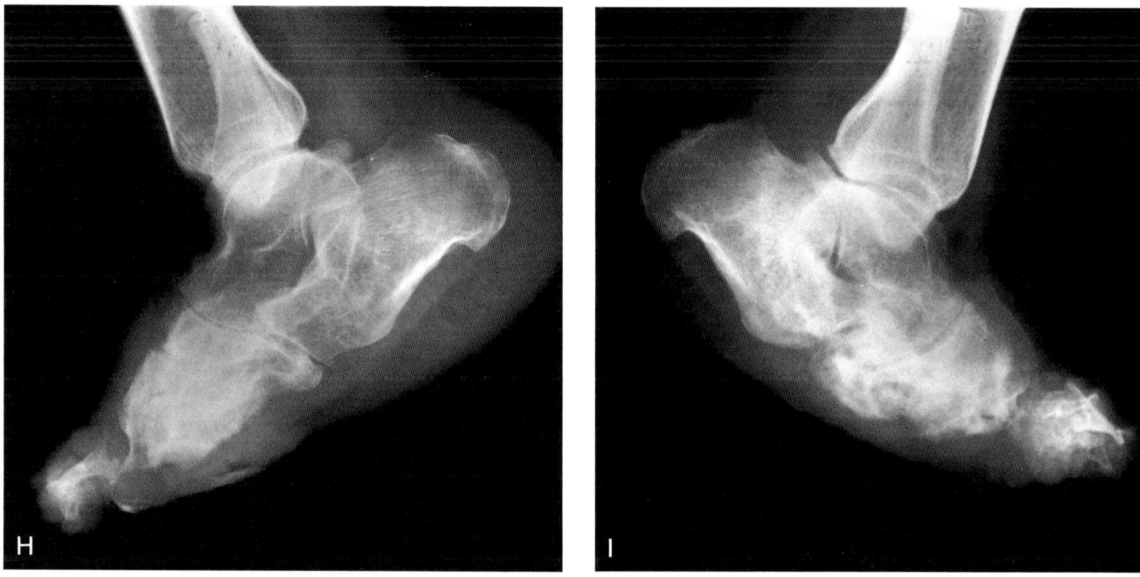

Fig. 31.3 H, I. Legend see p. 480

ripheral pulses, and trophic crises with oedema which comes on suddenly and painlessly, is associated with bruising and resorbs after several days or weeks (Bascourret). Humoral findings include a positive or negative Wassermann reaction, and raised levels of albumen and lymphocytes in the cerebrospinal fluid. The Vernes test and the Kahn and Meinicke reactions are positive.

The perforating ulcer most frequently affects the undersurface of the first metatarsal head, but may relate to others. The midtarsal region at the talonavicular, the navicular bone or the cuneiform may also be involved. The ulcer is usually of sudden onset, painless except in the pseudo-inflammatory variety, and is hypertrophic with associated articular swelling. There is local oedema extending to the ankle and the leg, with hyperhidrosis. The joint primarily affected is hypermobile in all directions, with a crackling sensation on palpation indicating destruction of the joint. There is no apparent functional disability, despite synovial and capsular thickening. Nail involvement includes friability and onycholysis. There are few or no vascular changes.

Radiographic features include central diffuse geodic osteoporosis and contrasting peripheral hyperostosis. There is rarefaction and necrosis of the distal epiphyses and arthropathic dislocation or subluxation. The arthropathy is characterised by the three features described by Brailsford (1929) [cited by Kerbrat (1974)]: hydrarthrosis, destruction and construction. The destructive signs include erosion of the bone and the patchy osteoporosis described above, with thinning of the joint space and progressive destruction of cartilage. The osteonecrosis has been likened to barley sugar in morphology. There is epiphyseal amputation. The constructive signs are contemporaneous with the destructive features and include osteosclerosis, especially in the epiphyses, and marginal exuberant osteophytosis with fragmentation or fracture leading to intra-articular sequestra. Finally, osteochondromatosis occurs in islands of varying size.

The joint involvement confers upon the tabetic foot a particular shape. Most frequently this is the "midtarsal foot" described by Alajouanine; the "cubic foot" of Charcot, in which there is particular destruction of the talonavicular joint line, leading to a flattened, thickened, shortened foot with abduction of the metatarsus; the equinovarus club foot configuration described by Joffroy, with arthropathic destruction of the inner part of the midtarsus; or the "Chinese foot" of Damasquino, in which osteonecrosis of the cuneiforms predominates.

31.5.3 Thévenard's Disease

Mutilating ulceration of the extremities constitutes a clinical entity clearly defined by Thévenard in 1942. The disease is familial, hereditary and associated with lesions of the posterior root ganglia. It has no infectious, biochemical, tubercular, syphilitic or alcoholic connections. The disease affects very young men (only exceptionally appearing before puberty or after the age of 30 years) and is characterised by trophic cutaneous and bony lesions associated with superficial sensory impairment which progresses centripetally and is not responsive to any known treatment.

Historically, this condition has been confused with syringomyelia. It has been variously described as: isolated affectation of the bones of the foot (Nélaton); symmetrical gangrene and familial acropathy of the feet (Bruns); perforating familial plantar ulcer (Schultze); neuropathic familial bony atrophy (Smith); perforating ulcer of the foot with bony atrophy of familial character (Tolantius and Reimann); and mutilating symmetrical arthropathy of the lower limbs (Van Bogaert). Thévenard (1942) defined the condition as ulcerative mutilating familial acropathy.

31.5.3.1 Clinical Features

The disease presents with trophic sensory disturbances which are detected after the development of a typical perforating ulcer. There may be myalgia of the lower limbs with numbness or cramps in the calves, twitching, digital contractures, or vasoconstrictive or vasodilatory episodes affecting the toes with the development perhaps of ecchymoses, or haematomata under the nails. The association of the trophic sensory disturbance with other reflex motor abnormalities is characteristic. The disease is localised to the lower limbs and involves both the skin and the bones.

Cutaneous lesions are the first manifestation of the disease. Small phlyctenae appear after walking, cutting the toenails or wearing shoes, most often without apparent cause. They are painless and may be ascribed to cold. Thévenard noted the exceptional occurrence of transitory episodes of swelling or pruritis. After several hours, the phlyctenae rupture and ulcerate.

The superficial ulceration is flat to begin with, but then deepens and spreads to produce a classical perforating ulcer with irregular sharply delineated borders and a rounded deep painless crater of violaceous appearance in the floor, associated with infection (Fig. 31.1 i). Hyperhidrosis is very common. Hyperkeratoses or haematomata under the nails, various disturbances of the nail form, such as onycholysis and onychogryphosis, and even an ochrous pigmentation of the lower third of the leg may be seen. The cutaneous lesions are followed by bony involvement, deformities, and sometimes gangrene with spontaneous amputation of the digits.

The onset of the bony lesions is variable: sometimes they occur simultaneously with the cutaneous lesions (Price), sometimes a long time after the ulceration (Fig. 31.4). In general they are distal in distribution, bilateral and, in the forefoot, initially affect the metatarsal and proximal phalanges especially in the first and second rays. They spread centripetally, eventually involving the midtarsus and then the tarsus. The development is sometimes insidious, but in other cases there may be acute inflammatory episodes like suppurative arthritis, associated with various osteolyses. Claw deformity, contracture of associated tendons and dislocation of the metatarsophalangeal joints develop concurrently, and the mutilating aspect of the condition is seen in spontaneous amputations. Serious infective episodes further complicate the development, while destructive osteolytic bone lesions in the midtarsus and tarsus may lead to the appearance of the cubic foot of Charcot or the elephant foot of Gobell and Runge, in which gross oedema extending into the leg is particularly significant. Thévenard described extensive ulceration involving the calcaneum and even the distal extremity of the tibia. Circulatory failure occurs gradually over a period of years, as evidenced by loss of peripheral pulses.

The objective sensory disturbances include paraesthesia, pain or numbness, but the most frequent feature is the loss of superficial sensation. A stocking distribution may extend to any level up to the knee. Dissociation of the sensations of pain and temperature (pseudo-syringomyelia) was observed by Gobell and Runge.

Motor disorders may become associated with the trophosensory features described above; they are of no great significance and are limited to loss of reflexes. There are no urogenital complications.

Radiographic examination of the foot shows lytic lesions in the epiphyses, beginning as generalised osteoporosis without sclerosis or periostosis (Kerbrat 1974). Small rounded vacuolar images a few millimetres in diameter appear in the heads of the metatarsals and the bases of the corresponding phalanges, slowly increasing in number to import a moth-eaten, tigered and then lacunar appearance. They eventually become confluent, leading to complete destruction of one or several metatarsal heads, which crumble like barley sugar and disappear. The osteolytic process is extensive, involving many joints, although only exceptionally the bones of the tarsus.

In the diaphyses, there is narrowing and sometimes the development of ensheathing periostitis, leading to bizarre deformations, especially when spontaneous fractures occur.
In the very advanced stages, the metatarsus and tarsus are involved and the foot collapses and widens. Thévenard emphasised the apparent melting of the bones in the tarsus.
Radiographic follow-up of the cases shows distinct periods of deterioration perhaps separated by lengthy (up to 10 years) intervals of quiescence.

31.5.3.2 Treatment

Only symptomatic treatment is of any benefit. Attention to hygiene, careful choice of shoes, and wearing of appropriate insoles to relieve pressure, especially under the perforating ulcers, are useful palliative measures. Surgical management is rarely indicated.
There is no known useful treatment for the establishing underlying disease itself.

31.5.4 Syringomyelia

Lumbosacral syringomyelia is an extremely rare disease which was so named by Ollivier (1837) and extensively investigated by Enderlé (1933). It is characterised by destructive cavity formation in the intramedullary region developing into a fibroglioma or an appendimoglioma involving the posterior grey matter and progressively invading the anterior horns and lateral tracts of the spinal cord. The etiopathology has been much discussed. Leyden regarded the disease as a congenital, hereditary abnormality of development, Minor suggested that it was traumatic in origin with the development of haematomyelia, and Guillain suggested an ascending neuritis. Infection has been invoked by Levaditi, Lepine and Schoen, while central necrosis of an intramedullary neoplasm was described by Bielschowsky, Guillain, Schmitt and Bertrand.
The condition predominantly affects men between the ages of 20 and 40 years. It involves the lower limbs, is symmetrical, and develops slowly. There is sensory disturbance associated with trophic signs and variable reflex motor disorders. No evidence of compression of the cord is seen. The first obvious sign may well be a perforating plantar ulcer. The involvement of the lower limbs has been variously named plantar familial perforating abscess (Nélaton 1852), symmetrical familial gangrene with arthropathy (Bruns), lumbar familial syringomyelia (Guillain and Thévenard 1929), familial trophic necrosis of the lower limbs (Gobell and Runge), familial myelodysplastic syndrome (Enderle) and trophic myelodysplasia of the foot (Kienbock). More than 40 references are available in the medical literature. In particular, Van Bogaert (1940) gave a particularly telling description of the trophic cutaneous osteoarticular pathology, emphasising the irreversibility of the bony destruction and the classical sign of dissociation of the sensations of pain and temperature.

31.5.4.1 Clinical Features

With respect to the foot, it is the cutaneous, muscular or osteoarticular trophic disorders which lead to consultation. In the beginning, there may be one or several simple keratotic plantar lesions situated under one or several metatarsal heads of otherwise normal appearance and without ulceration. Frequently the foot is abnormally shaped, flattened or in cavus – leading to misdiagnosis of overloading from morphological causes. A more unusual manifestation is hyperaemia with alternation of areas of redness or pallor leading to cyanotic discoloration of the toes, the forefoot or the whole foot as far as the ankle. Disorders of hair growth on the dorsal aspect of the foot or ankle, dystrophic changes in the nail, with longitudinal grooving, onychauxis and onychorrhexis, and sweating disorders, with hyperhidrosis or anhidrosis associated with a shiny or even sclerodermatous appearance of the skin, may all occur. Ulceration, when it occurs may be accompanied by sensory disorders and later by pseudo-inflammatory arthropathy. The more typical cutaneous lesions comprise painless areas of gangrene of the extremities, erythematous lesions, and vesicles and bullae on the plantar aspect of the toes or on the dorsum of the foot, as well as the scleroderma-like lesions.
The osteoarticular lesions sometimes present as the first sign or contemporaneously with the skin lesions. They comprise painless spontaneous fractures which are reluctant to heal because of associated severe osteoporosis. The osteoarthropathies supervene in a generally swollen foot. They may be indolent or, occasionally, rapidly developing but are in general irreversible. Osteoarticular destruction with dislocation increases the general swelling of the foot. They bony changes are symmetrical and are seen predominantly at the instep and in the interphalangeal joints. They are painful only in the early phase of the disease. The pain is experienced in the toes, on the plantar aspect of the foot or in

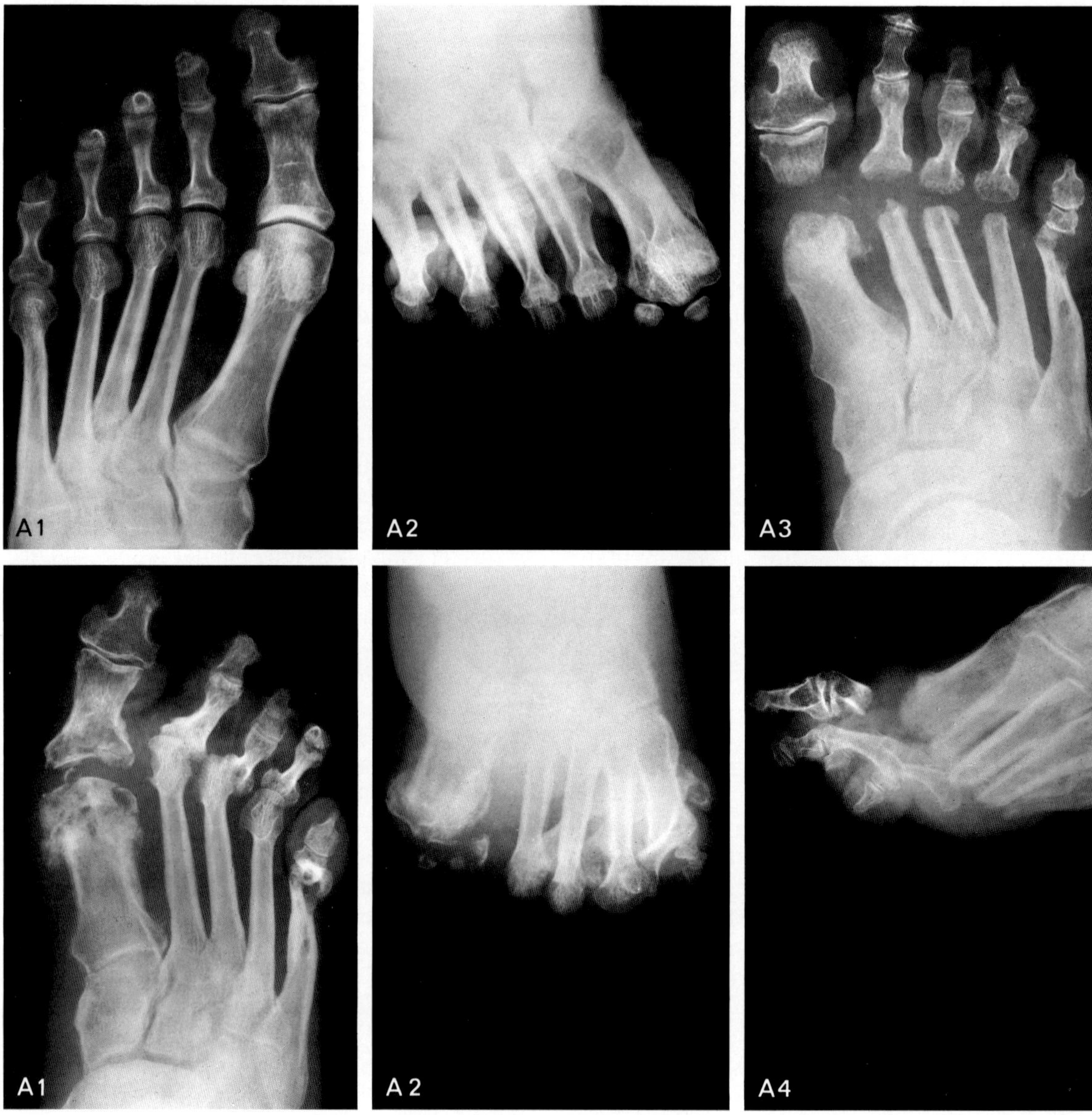

Fig. 31.4 A–E. Perforating plantar ulcer. **A** Diabetic perforating ulcer, osteonecrotic arthropathy of first metatarsophalangeal joint and of second, third and fourth metatarsal heads, convex forefoot. *1, 2* Preoperative; *3, 4* dorsoplantar and lateral views after Lelièvre realignment. **B** Diabetic arthropathy with perforating ulcer. **C** Ulceration and osteolysis of toes following Volkmann ▷ syndrome. **D** Thévenard's disease: osteonecrosis of fifth metatarsal head, mutilating ulceration of toes, plantar perforating ulcer. **E** Thévenard's disease: mutilating ulceration of toes, perforating plantar ulcer. **B–E** see p. 485

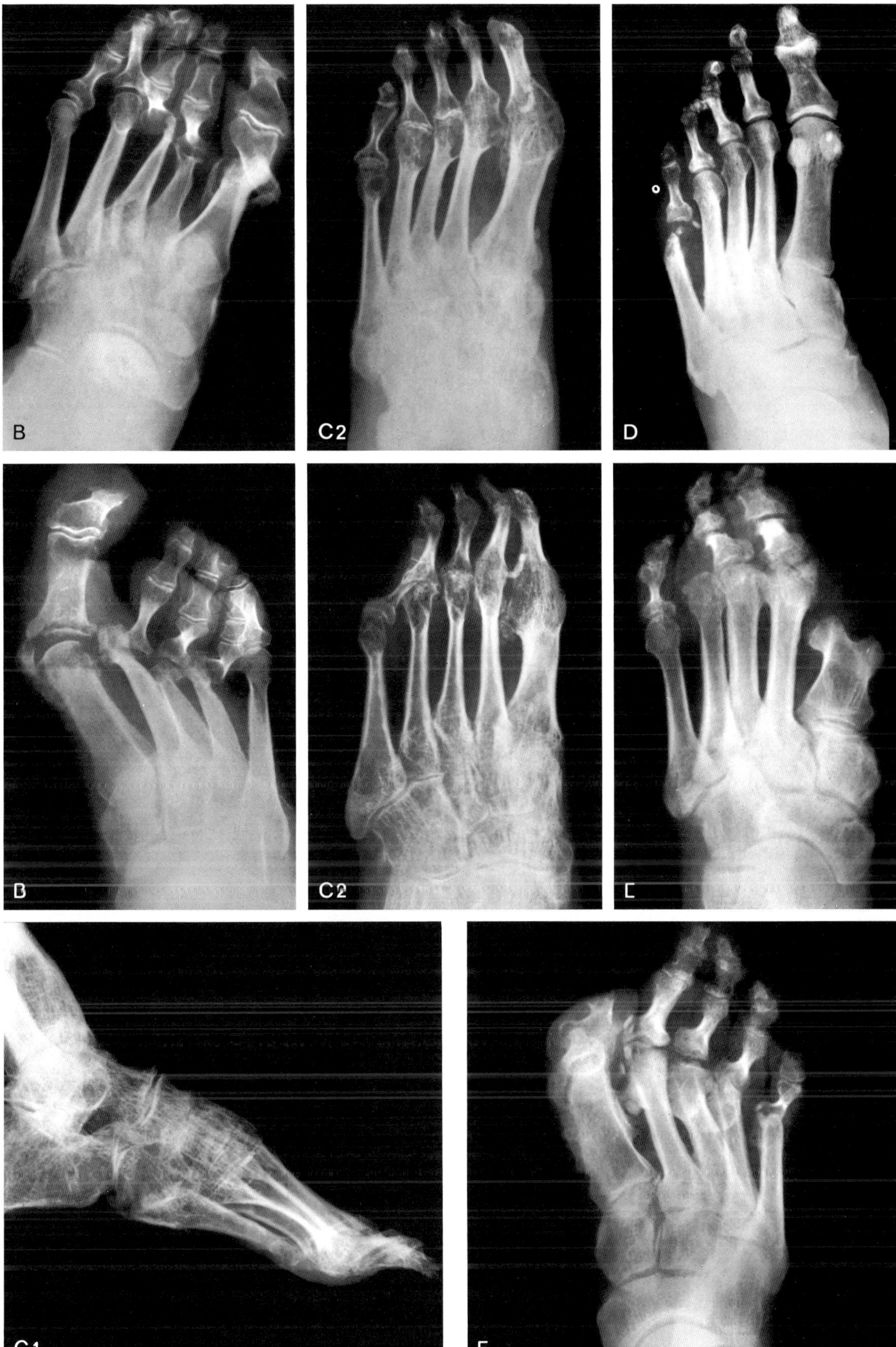
B
C2
D
B
C2
C1
E

the tarsus, particularly during walking; it may be lancinating, dull or diffuse. Increased sensitivity to heat may be localised to the great toe and the medial border of the foot (Van Bogaert).

While the dissociation of the sensations of pain and temperature is the cardinal neurological sign, there are instances (Van Bogaert 1940; Guillain et al. 1926) in which these features are absent, while exaggerated tendon reflexes at the ankle, perhaps with clonus, and a positive extensor response may be present. Bilateral muscular atrophy, weakness or a spasmodic paraplegia with extensor plantar responses, genito-urinary disturbances and even involvement of the upper limbs may lead to diagnosis. Cranial nerve involvement is unusual, but can comprise visual disturbance, dysphagia, dysphonia, vertigo, and aural manifestations.

In the established case, the patient may present with a perforating ulcer, pseudo-inflammatory arthropathy and erythematobullous eruptions. In these instances, investigations must include a search for neurological sensory and motor signs, a full vascular examination, including oscillometry and arteriography, laboratory tests for hyperglycaemia, serology for syphilis and a bacteriological study.

Radiographic examination will confirm any overall deformity of the foot and will show epiphyseal osteolysis with clear contours leading rapidly to complete destruction; osteophytic peripheral lesions with osteoporosis, osteolysis, or sometimes osteosclerosis subchondrally with cartilage fragments in the joints; spontaneous fractures which may be unperceived by the patient because of their painlessness and which unite with difficulty because of the associated osteoporosis; pseudo-tabetic or pseudo-inflammatory arthritis in some cases; and, characteristically, atrophy of the distal parts of the metatarsals and the proximal phalanges, with melting away of the distal third of the metatarsal shafts and thinning in a flame-like fashion of the proximal phalanges without expansion of the medullary area of the bone and without hypertrophic periosteal reaction (Van Bogaert). Tarsal ankylosis involving the midtarsal region or cuneiform-metatarsal joint line, with complete disappearance of the joints, even extending to the metatarsophalangeal and interphalangeal areas, was emphasised by Van Bogaert.

The inconstancy of the classical signs may make syringomyelia difficult to diagnose. This is especially the case if the trophoneuropathic aspect of the disease presents first.

31.5.4.2 Treatment

No specific treatment can be advised for the central lesion. Only local palliative measures for the perforating ulcers are of value and comprise, as in other diseases, careful attention to hygiene, dressings for the ulcers, and the use of suitable insoles sparing the damaged areas.

32 Diabetes Mellitus

Trophic signs and symptoms characterising the diabetic foot can be the presenting features of the generalised disease, but usually there is an overlap with a known condition, often with unstable ketosis. The presentation can be extremely polymorphic, and while in earlier times involvement of the foot was considered rare, the majority of modern authors recognise its real frequency and gravity, the latter shown by the associated osteo-angioneuropathic disorders. Mirouze (1968) estimated that one diabetic in ten suffers from foot problems.

32.1 Etiology

Robillard et al. (1968) describe thickening of the vasa nervorum, a degenerative process present early in diabetes which is responsible for neuropathy. Together with the generalised metabolic aspects of the condition, this is responsible for the progressive, irreversible anatomical and functional damage in all organs involving the parenchymal tissues which are suffering from the metabolic disturbance due to loss of balance between peripheral need for insulin and the insulin-secreting capability of the pancreas (Butturini 1968). The osteopathic dystrophic foot with its tendency to infection is just one manifestation, comprising the following aspects.

Endocrine Metabolic Disorder. Butturini (1968) and Mirouze (1968) have described the changes in calcium phosphate metabolism on bony matrix, the parenchymatous alterations due to protein metabolism, diminution of utilisation of glucose by the neurons and Schwann cells, reduced synthesis of cholesterol and fatty acids by the marrow and or cholesterol by the sciatic nerve, and inhibition of acetylcholine, all occurring when hyperglycaemia is above 2 g/100 ml. Recordier and Serratrice (1965) suggest that there may be a preexisting genetic or acquired fragility of nerves due to enzymatic abnormality; they point out that the neuropathies which appear during poorly controlled diabetes after stress, coma or some other precipitating event lead to anatomically evident primary neuronal degeneration. The association of certain exogenous neurological syndromes with alcoholism or malnutrition is analogous (Recordier and Serratrice 1968).

Vascular Involvement. Thickening of the vasa nervorum (Wolkman and Wilder) leads to a neuropathy, developing at the typical age for arteriosclerosis, and frequently to acropathy. The main arteries, especially the posterior tibial and dorsalis pedis vessels, become obliterated to varying degrees by calcification of Leriche. Bony rarefaction is caused by the arteriosclerosis (Butturini). There is diabetic micro-angiopathy of the peripheral vessels. Arteriosclerosis of the vasa nervorum and segmental demyelinisation of nerve fibres lead together to the dystrophic neurological disorder. The demyelinisation extends to the posterior columns of the spinal cord, with consequent sensory degeneration, as well as involving the motor root ganglia and, to a lesser degree, the anterior root ganglia of the peripheral nerves.

The dystrophic osteoneuropathic lesions are dominated by a tendency to infection associated with the tissue fragility, oedema, poor circulation and neuropathy. The risk is enhanced by the abnormality of glucose metabolism, especially when the diabetes is poorly controlled. The early control of infection is essential, because infection disturbs the control of the diabetes, thereby establishing an increasingly acute form of the disease entity.

32.2 Clinical Features

The site of the foot lesions is variable, but in 77% of cases they are in the midtarsus. A further 22% of cases involve forefoot, 3% the tarsus (Kerbrat 1974). The lesions may be uni- or bilateral and affect men and women equally. As stated above, the foot lesions can be the presenting manifestation of the disease, but more frequently they occur after a long, poorly controlled course.

Frequently the foot is shortened, wide, lowered generally, damp and cold (except during acute infectious episodes). Sometimes it is inflamed, with an appearance of pseudogout, during an acute phase. Cavus deformity may be confined to the first ray with a normal forefoot, in which case a perforating ulcer develops under the first metatarsal head. When the cavus is more general, a convex forefoot is seen, determining the site of ulceration under the central paddle of the middle three metatarsals. Occasionally the foot is flat, with crumbling of the convexity of the external border and a dorsal arch like a necklace around the tarsometatarsal joint. This is a sign of midtarsal osteopathy. The general rigidity of this type of foot makes walking difficult.

From the beginning, sudorific disturbance may comprise excessive sweating or dryness of the skin of the plantar aspect, with crevices developing between squames and frequent episodes of superficial infection occurring. The tissues may be succulent, greyish and moist, ideal for certain infections, notably athlete's foot. Loss or abnormal growth of hair may occur on the dorsal aspect of the interphalangeal joints, especially on the great toe, together with dystrophic nail lesions with dryness, onychauxis and onychorrhexis, perhaps with frank infection. Usually the arterial pulses are preserved.

The cutaneous ulcers are of either vascular origin due to infarction or trophic origin due to the neurological deficiency, and lead to the perforating plantar ulcer with classical steep borders, purulent floor and granulations and underlying one metatarsal head or the heel. The cutaneous ulcers are necrotic, deep lesions of a gangrenous type, almost always infected (Fig. 31.1 e, f, j, k; Fig. 31.2 a–j).

Ischaemic gangrene usually develops in a toe at the nail bed, perhaps from a fungus infection, initially presenting as a small, congested, violaceous area which is not painful. It extends progressively over the body of the foot and then into the leg. The gangrene is usually wet and is associated with general congestion of the foot with local warmth. Blisters or vesicles filled with contaminated exudate rupture and lead to an infected eschar. Bacteria are nearly always aerobic, the most frequent being *Staphylococcus aureus, Proteus* spp., *Pseudomonas* spp. and *Escherichia coli,* but anaerobic involvement with *Clostridium welchii* does occasionally occur. Fungus infections with *Candida albicans* may also be seen.

The neurological deficit is constant. It is associated with superficial and deep sensory loss, subjective paraesthesiae, a sensation of engorgement and intermittent sudden and intense pains or permanent discomfort of a causalgic type associated with intense vasodilatation (Dreyfus). Sensory disturbances affect pain as well as temperature, and the widespread peripheral neuropathy is reflected also in loss of the senses of position and vibration and loss of tendon reflexes. A stocking distribution may extend up as far as the knee.

In the early stages, the peripheral circulation remains good, but then cutaneous infarctions occur, leading to lesions like chilblains or to more extensive pink or violaceous patches. These lesions are sometimes painful to a greater or lesser degree, sometimes completely painless. A pustule develops which swells and ulcerates, and a perforating ulcer is likely to form. The ulceration can affect any of the weight-bearing zones of the foot and can be associated with ischaemia at the levels of the main arterial supply or the microcirculation. Distal lesions tend to migrate proximally with the ever-increasing risk of frank gangrene.

Osteopathic lesions may be of a vascular type, with sequestration and fracture, of a neurological type, with destrucitve lesions of the tarsus or midtarsus, or may be due to infection and associated with ischaemia and altered sensation. It becomes increasingly difficult, both clinically and radiologically, to determine whether vascular, neurological or infectious causes predominate.

Radiography (Figs. 31.4 A, B, 32.1). There is a general osteopathic, destructive, lytic tendency without signs of healing. Occasionally, signs of bony reconstruction may resemble Paget's disease (Mirouze 1968) or fibrous osteitis with exostosis formation.

In the joints, fragmentation of the surface varies in degree and involves the first and fifth metatarsophalangeal joints, which may appear hypertrophic with exostosis formation or have a gouty appearance with images of clearness in the condyles or lytic thinning of the metatarsals like barley sugar. Atrophy of the bone with lacunae, osteoporosis, thinning of the cortex, elongation and atrophy of the spongy trabeculae and widening of the medullary canal can occur (Mirouze 1968). The lytic lesions erode the cortex and produce the "outline image" described by Azerad et al. (1963). Dislocation and telescoping of the diseased parts can give a sensation of crepitus like a bag of nuts. The osteoporosis can be diffuse, affecting all areas of the foot, but at the outset may arise in discrete areas and spread progressively.

Destructive lesions usually begin in the navicular and the head of the talus, spreading to the cuboid, the bases of the metatarsals and the phalanges with severe involvement of the metatarsophalangeal joints.

The bony involvements and osteoarticular disease were described by Recordier and Serratrice (1968) as the diabetic neurogenic foot, characterised by involvement of the soft tissue comprising blistering, perforating ulcer, necrosis and then gangrene. The osteopathic lesions can be acute, associated with fever, and rapidly succeed the cutaneous ischaemic, neurological and infective signs. It is the evolution over several months or years with repeated remissions that leads to the shortened thickened "cubic" foot described by Charcot (1868).

Laboratory Examinations. Bacteriological examination of exudate usually yields a positive culture while blood investigations reveal secondary anaemia. Hyperglycaemia and glycosuria are essential to the diagnosis. Occasionally, examination of the cerebrospinal fluid reveals an augmentation in the protein level.
The metabolic disturbance characterised by diabetes mellitus and the polymorphism of the multiple lesions of the foot distinguish the diabetic foot from other neurological disorders described in earlier chapters.

32.3 Treatment

In general it is important to recognise that because of the fragile state fo the tissues and the possibility of general complications of septicaemia, urinary infection and ketosis, surgical management is to be viewed with great caution. Antibiotic treatment is often less than effective on account of the oedematous spongy tissues with their poor blood supply; the dangers of enhancing the vicious circle involving local complications and the general metabolic state cannot be overestimated.
The diabetic condition must be controlled by appropriate diet and insulin therapy.
Locally, rigorous immobilisation, elevation, avoidance of loading, massage and articular re-education must accompany the management of any perforating ulcer present. With regard to the latter, the peripheral margin of white, thickened skin should be excised as far as the limit of frank granulation tissue so as to avoid bleeding. Antiseptic dressings should then be applied, followed by cicatrising agents with physiological saline and tulle gras. In more severe lesions, a short period of dressing with trypsin may be valuable.

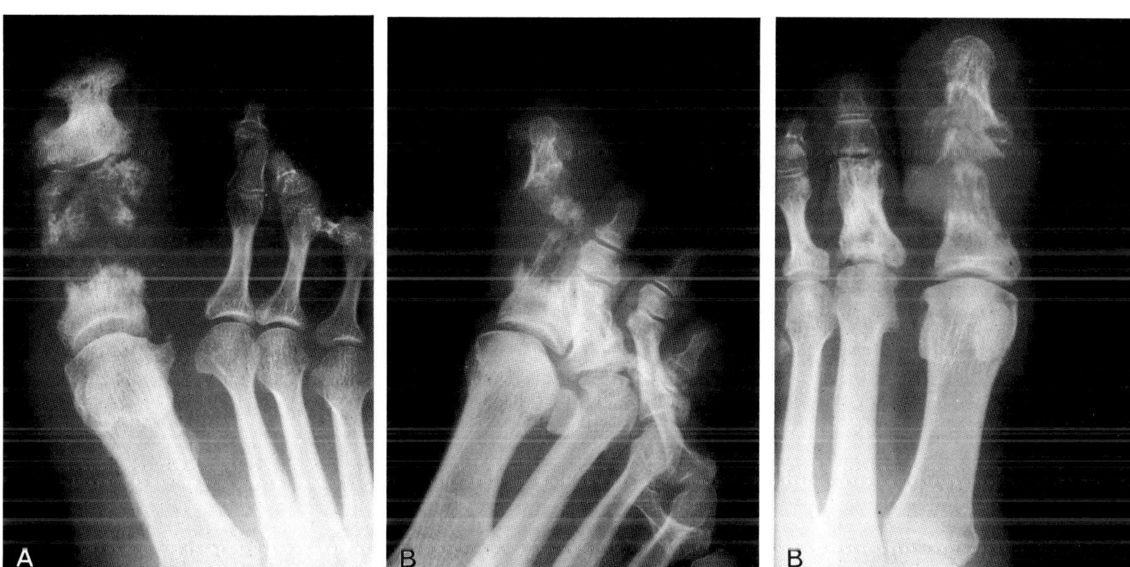

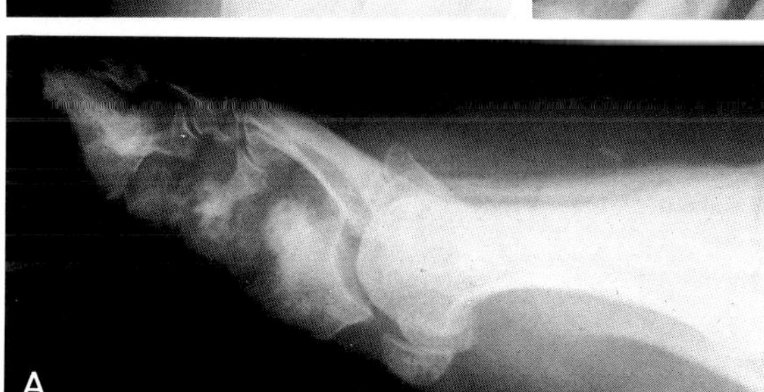

Fig. 32.1 A–E. Diabetic perforating plantar ulcer. **A** Osteonecrosis of proximal phalanx and perforating plantar ulcer of great toe. **B** Osteonecrosis and perforating plantar ulcer of great toe. **C–E** see p. 490, 491

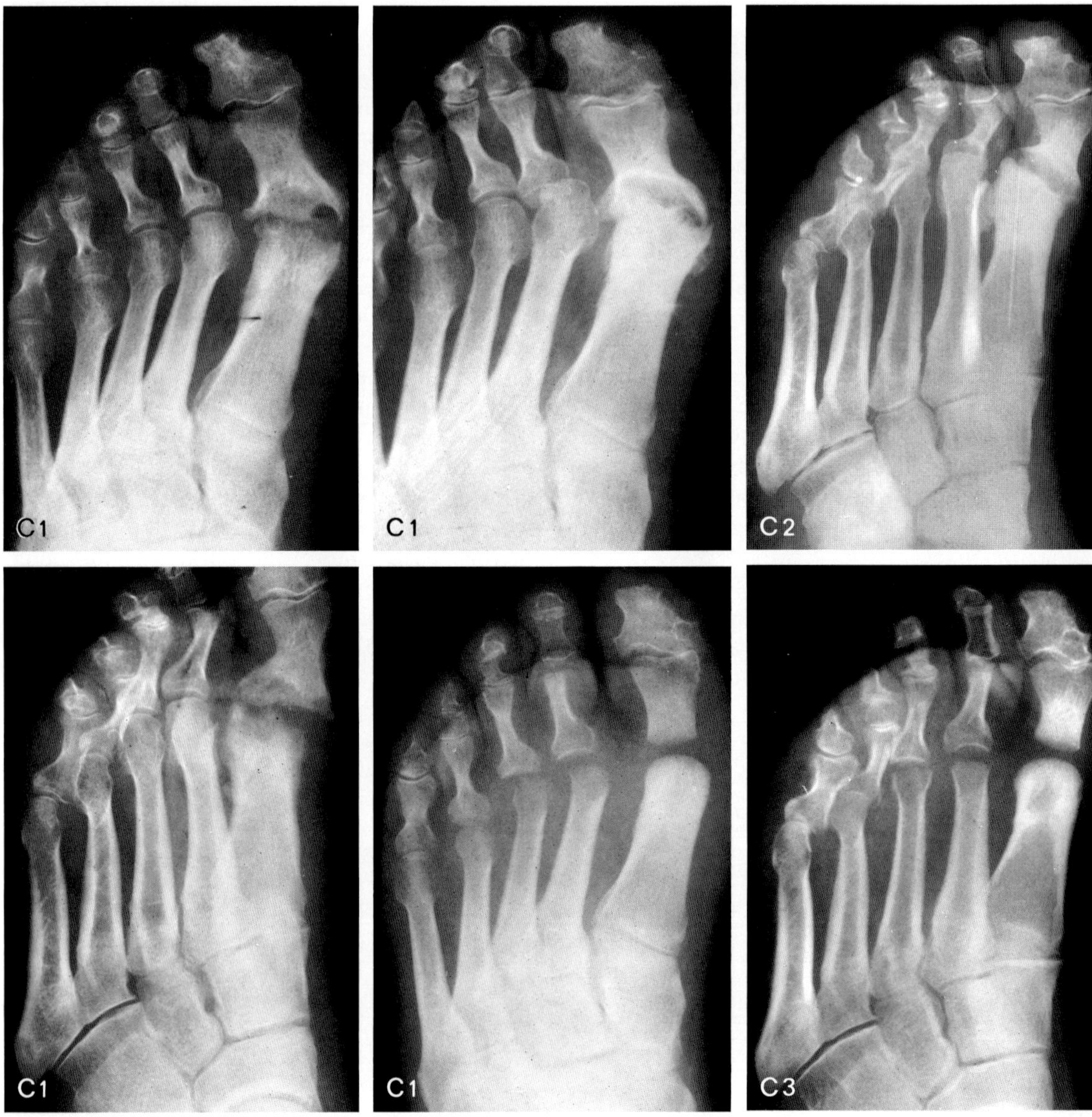

Fig. 32.1 *(continued)*. **C** *1* Perforating plantar ulcer under first metatarsal head, arthropathy of first metatarsophalangeal joint; *2* convex forefoot, arthropathy of first metatarsophalangeal joint; *3* after Lelièvre realignment. **D** Geodic osteonecrosis of base of fifth metatarsal. *1, 3* Preoperative; *2, 4* after resection. **E** Diabetic arthropathy of naviculocuneiform joint ▷

Systemic administration of antibiotics or intra-arterial infusion of Transcycline (rolitetracycline) may be indicated. Vasodilators, perhaps introduced by the lumbar procedure of Leriche, may be of benefit, as may intra-arterial xylocaine, cortisone and antibiotic administered as described by Stotter. Anticoagulation by continuous intravenous infusion of heparin may be indicated.

Limited excision or amputation of toe, sequestrectomy, excision of a joint and the transmetatarsectomy described by MacKittrick are exceptional requirements. Cutaneous autografts to cover ulcerated areas are sometimes useful in the absence of infection.

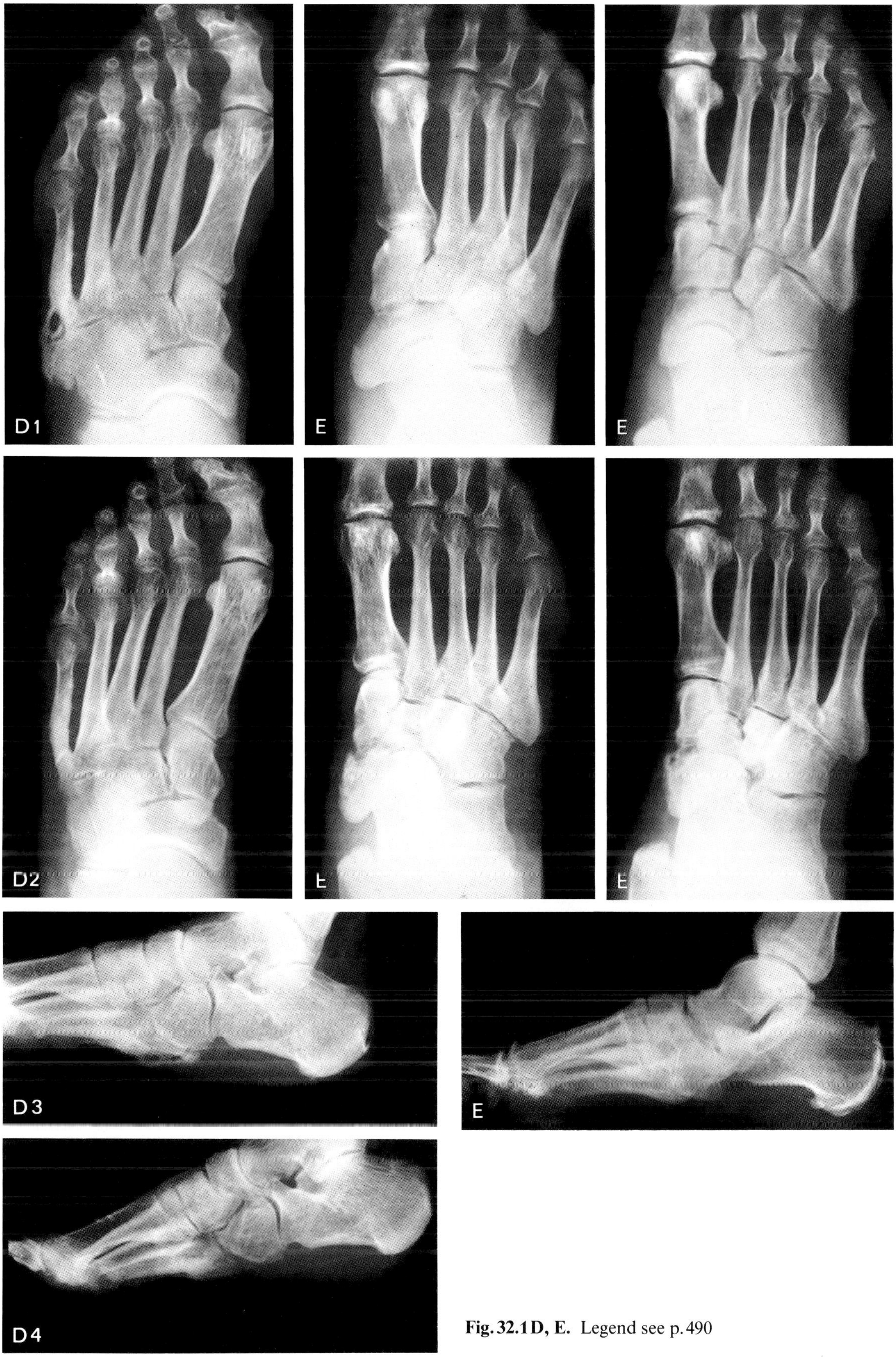

Fig. 32.1 D, E. Legend see p. 490

VI Entrapment Syndromes

33 Tarsal Tunnel Syndrome

Tarsal tunnel syndrome is a painful motor and neurotrophic disorder caused by compression of the posterior tibial neurovascular bundle. It was first described by Pollock and Davis in 1932 as a disorder of compression of the posterior tibial nerve consecutive to trauma. Other authors include Fahlung (1946), Roaf (1946), Ward (1948), Keck (1962), Lam (1962), Sidney (1963), Mumenthaler et al. (1964), Ficat (1966) and Serre et al. (1965).
The tibiotalar calcaneal canal of Richet (1957) is narrow and predisposes to intrinsic and extrinsic compression of the elements it contains. The divisions of the nerves and vessels are variable, and the intimate relationship with perivascular sympathetic fibres, the frequency of bony and joint lesions in the region, the synovial tissue and the intimate relationship of the contents all led Ficat (1966) to describe this as a "trigger zone".

33.1 Etiology

While the syndrome can appear spontaneously, in the majority of instances there is a predisposing event. The most frequent is trauma, such as a bimalleolar fracture, fracture of the distal third of the tibia, the calcaneum or the talus, or sprains of the lateral or medial ligaments of the ankle. I have seen the syndrome develop five times after fracture and twice after sprains of the medical ligament. It may follow operations on the tarsal region, such as subtalar arthrodesis and transcalcaneal osteotomy, or arise from contracture of scars. Other causes include synovitis of varying origin. Synovial cyst of the posterior tibial tendon lipoma formation in the medial gutter as described by Richet. The condition may also be provoked by trophic disorders, as in the neurotrophic foot of Bureau-Barrière (1955), diabetes mellitus, alcoholic polyneuritis or elephantiasis. Ficat (1966) cites one example of the last-named.

33.2 Clinical Features

Ficat (1966) and Kohn Tebner and Carnevale (1971) describe a triad of clinical signs comprising neurological, vascular and local features; however, it is unusual for all three to be present simultaneously. Trophic complications can also occur.

33.2.1 Neurological Disorders

The neurological disorders are essentially sensory in type, comprising spontaneous nocturnal and diurnal pain which is mechanical in character and is aggravated by walking, by local palpation or pressure, especially percussion, and plantarflexion of the foot and of the toes, especially in forced pronation. The pain may stay localised to the retromalleolar gutter or to the medial aspect of the instep of the foot, but may diffuse throughout the tarsus, radiating in many directions. Sometimes hypalgesia or anaesthesia may predominate, while on other occasions there is hyperaesthesia of variable intensity and distribution, perhaps surrounding an area of hypalgesia. There may be numbness in the area covered by the sock, terminating quite suddenly just above the malleoli, or localised to a cuff round the two retromalleolar gutters, and the patient may describe the foot as feeling dead or complain of local burning, often worse at night. Pain may radiate into the calf. Distal radiation of pain may follow the territory of any of the nerves including those going into the sole of the foot, the forefoot, the toes and the plantar calcaneal area, and may be aggravated by local compression. The presence of objective sensory disturbance makes the diagnosis easier. Motor disorders are variable and inconstant. They may comprise diminution of the power of the toes, involving both dorsiflexion and plantarflexion, and the patient may complain that he cannot control movements easily, especially in the great toe. Diminution of amplitude of movements may be the only feature. The condition in which the great toe overlaps or underlies the second toe during forced plantarflexion was attributed by Ficat

(1966) to a neuropraxis of the medial plantar nerve supplying the abductor of the great toe. The patient may have difficulty in abducting the toes during dorsiflexion, and there may be motor weakness of the short plantarflexor muscles.

33.2.2 *Vascular Impairment*

Vascular impairment is manifested by the formation of oedema of varying degree and distribution which may present different features when accompanied by trophic disorder. Sometimes the oedema is localised to a segment of the ankle or the foot, such as the tarsal region generally or the retromalleolar gutters, more medially than laterally, but it may extend into the leg; indeed, in some cases the whole foot and leg are involved. The oedema in the retromalleolar gutter is painful on pressure and may develop a woody painful texture accompanied by trophic disorders such as sweating and varicosities. In chronic forms, the pain may resemble that caused by the polyneuritis in disabling arteriosclerosis.

33.2.3 *Trophic Disorders*

Trophic disorders comprise excessive or reduced sweating of the sole of the foot, cyanotic discoloration of the skin of the dorsum of the foot and the toes and of the medial aspect of the ankle and local warmth or coldness of part or all of the foot, while in most instances the posterior tibial pulses are normal.

Radiographic examination may reveal some postural problem, residua of trauma or localised osteoporosis of varying degrees, perhaps involving the whole foot.

Although it is unusual for all the above clinical features to present, the existence of one or more of them should draw attention to the possibility of the tarsal tunnel syndrome. The diagnosis will be clarified by the paraclinical investigations detailed in Sect. 33.3. Differential diagnosis is from algodystrophy, sciatica, interdigital neuroma, peripheral neuropathy, diabetes mellitus, mutilating ulceration of the extremities, leprosy, gout, rheumatoid arthritis and other inflammatory conditions.

33.2.4 *Clinical Forms*

There are numerous clinical forms:

a) The topographical forms are localised to the territory of the nerve affected by compression or involve more than one of the three territories of the branches of the posterior tibial nerve.
b) Ficat has distinguished three neurological forms – pure sensory, pure motor and combined – without pain, an irritative form with burning pain worse during the day or during the night, and mixed forms.
c) Vascular or trophic disabilities may dominate the picture. These are usually post-traumatic, but may also be associated with perforating ulceration, diabetic neuropathy, elephantiasis or leprous neuritis (Bourrel et al. 1976).
d) Spontaneous forms are due to diminution of volume of the tarsal tunnel and consequent strangulation of the posterior tibial nerve (Keck 1962), varicose dilatation of the contained veins or fibrous thickening of the roof of the canal (Lam 1962). Joubert asserts that augmentation of volume of any one element of the canal or prolonged stretching of the structures in the enclosed space can be responsible.
e) Post-traumatic forms are most numerous, as mentioned earlier (Sect. 33.1). Fibrosis in haematoma or oedema or the projection of callus into the region following bony injury can be the causative factor.
f) Humoral forms may be due to a synovial cyst of the tibialis posterior sheath or to inflammatory synovitis. I have seen two cases where lipoma was responsible.

33.3 Paraclinical Examination

Arteriography frequently displays no abnormalities, but there is sometimes a funnel-shaped stenosis due to stricture of the arterial lumen, arterial spasm or arteriovenous aneurysm. There may be a simple communication in the retromalleolar region (the system of Lazorthes).

Phlebography shows regular stenosis of the posterior tibial veins and arrest in the pre-canal area.

Neurography localises the obstruction to the level of compression of the posterior tibial nerve.

Electromyography may be valuable in diffuse presentations. De Sèze et al. (1970) described in detail how this investigation should be carried out. The chronaxy for muscles in the territories of the medial and lateral plantar nerves must be measured on both sides, along with the excitability of triceps surae, the short extensors and tibialis anterior on the affected side and motor nerve latency on the affected side in comparison with the opposite side. Neurogenic atrophy in the muscles innervated by the plantar nerves contrasts with normal curves obtained in electromyograms of muscles innervated by the lateral popliteal nerve. A positive augmentation of latency of the motor nerves (7–12 ms) arising from the medial and lateral plantar nerves is of major diagnostic importance, but normal curves do not exclude the diagnosis of tarsal tunnel syndrome.

33.4 Treatment

33.4.1 Conservative

Rest, use of a supportive insole in the presence of static pes planus or pes cavus, weight reduction if indicated, administration of anti-inflammatory agents (indomethacin and phenylbutazone) and local infiltration of corticosteroids into the tarsal canal are all valuable measures. Kinesitherapy with massage aims to reduce oedema and actively re-educate the muscles of the foot, especially of the toes, ankle joint and subtalar joints, and may relieve symptoms permanently. Failure of conservative measures indicates the need for operation.

33.4.2 Operative

Operative treatment comprises two essential procedures: neurolysis of the posterior nerve and its branches and complete section of the fibrous layers compressing the tarsal tunnel structures. Vascular involvement is an indication for periarterial sympathectomy. Angiography may have given evidence of venous congestion or arteriovenous aneurysms demanding appropriate exploration, and if there is tenosynovitis, synovectomy should be performed.

Operative Technique. Operation is performed in a bloodless field under general anaesthesia. An incision is made behind and below the medial malleolus, following the axis of the retromalleolar gutter overlying the trajectory of the tarsal tunnel. Cellular tissue in the subcutaneous region is incised, and from above downwards the flexor aponeurosis is displayed together with the flexor retinaculum and the muscle mass of the abductor of the great toe. The plantar cutaneous nerve is protected.
The aponeurosis of the leg and then the anterior annular ligament are sectioned from above downwards, and with the aid of a retractor directed below and inwards the muscle mass of the abductor of the great toe is reclined so as to display clearly the flexor retinaculum. After incision, the contents of the canal are displayed. Above, in the retromalleolar osteofibrotic tissue, are located, from distally forwards, the tendons of flexor digitorum longus and flexor hallucis longus, between which are located (a) more deeply, the posterior tibial nerve, usually dividing into its two terminal branches; and (b) covering the nerve medially, the posterior tibial artery and veins. Below the malleolar region in the osteofibrous tissue, from behind forwards, from below upwards and from superficial to deep, are located the external plantar pedicle, comprising the external plantar veins, artery and nerve, flanked behind by the nerve to the abductor of the fifth toe; the internal plantar pedicle, comprising the internal plantar veins, artery and nerve (from below upwards); and finally the tendon of flexor hallucis longus.
Whatever the nature of the lesion to be decompressed, whether using a dissector or a grooved director, it is necessary to liberate and to individualize each of the elements of the canal, to open each of the compartments and to identify any compressive bands.
A number of different lesions may be identified:

- Thickening of the internal annular ligament.
- Generalised thickening of the connective tissue of the canal involving all elements in a sort of cellulitic mass.
- Multiple venous dilatations, many of which can be resected to advantage.
- Apparent compression of the posterior tibial artery between multiple branches of nerves.
- Zones of inflammation or thickening of the connective tissue at the level of the division of the posterior tibial nerve.
- Occasionally, a fusiform swelling which can be identified as a neuroma.
- Slight oedema of the posterior tibial nerve, which is also more yellow in colour than normal and hypertrophied. Following neurolysis in such cases, neuralgia disappears.

Cyst or lipoma formation.
Occasionally, no abnormality can be found and yet operative decompression is successful.
After careful haemostasis, the annular internal ligament is closed without tension. Suction drainage should be employed. After closure of the skin, a light compressive dressing is applied. Ice treatment in the operated region and administration of anti-inflammatory agents should be followed on the day after operation by mobilisation of the ankle. Walking is allowed on the 10th day.

34 Sinus Tarsi Syndrome

The sinus tarsi syndrome was identified and named by O'Connor (1956) [cited by Brown (1960)]; later writers include Hauser (1962), Debrunner (1960, 1963), Blasnick (1963), Komprda (1966) and Navarre (1966).

34.1 Anatomy and Etiology

The sinus tarsi is a funnel-shaped transversely disposed region lying between the subtalar joints, the talocalcaneal junction posteriorly and the talocalcaneonavicular joint anteriorly (Fig. 34.1). The axis is oblique, being directed medially and posteriorly. Medially the sinus tarsi is narrow, while laterally it develops a flared base in front of the lateral malleolus. The roof is concave, formed by the neck of the talus, and likewise the calcaneal floor is excavated. The sinus is traversed by the fasciculi of the interosseous talocalcaneal ligament, which varies in configuration (Fig. 34.1); it is generally tightened by supination and relaxed by pronation (Lanz and Wachsmuth 1938; Lapidus 1963), and is filled with cellular fatty tissue containing small vessels and autonomic nerve fibres. It appears to constitute a zone of reflex proprioception for the foot generally, and contributes to the balance of the tarsus. It has been named the "eye of the foot" by Valenti (1980a).

In 50% of cases, according to Komprda (1966), the sinus tarsi syndrome supervenes without any earlier predisposing cause. In other cases there is a previous event, notably trauma, in which a sprain of the ankle or subtalar joint or a fracture of the malleoli, calcaneum or neck of the talus may be responsible.

A fairly frequent cause is valgus posture of the calcaneum associated with pes planus or pes cavus, and in this context, spasmodic flat foot, if it occurs, can very frequently be relieved by infiltration of the sinus with local anaesthetic. Sometimes there is a varus calcaneal posture associated with a cavus foot in inversion (Hauser 1962), this being provoked by forced unaccustomed walking. Rheumatoid arthritis and osteoarthritis of the talonavicular joint or ankle joint are exceptional causes. Of note is the fact that arthrosis of the subtalar joint has never been proved to cause the syndrome. Iatrogenic causes are again rare: Komprda (1966) has suggested that the syndrome can result after metatarsal osteotomy for hallux valgus, and I have seen the condition following treatment of pes planovalgus deformity by osteotomy of the talar neck. Valenti (1980a) recorded incidence of the syndrome after Grice (1952) arthrolysis performed without curettage of the sinus, in this case associated with contracture of the peronei and the extensor digitorum brevis. Neurological etiology was invoked by Hauser (1962), who described an interdigital neuroma accompanied by the syndrome. Algodystrophic syndrome of the forefoot following a simple sprain of the ankle may be manifested by sinus tarsi syndrome (Valenti 1980a).

The general conclusion is that the syndrome is produced by tearing, rupture of herniation of the posterior capsule of the subtalar joint, by partial or complete tearing of the interosseous ligaments in which hyaline degenerative lesions of the collagenous tissue or associated vessels can be identified. O'Connor (1956) [cited by Brown (1960)] emphasised partial or total rupture of the interosseous ligament, while Hauser (1962) maintained that in all cases there was rupture or inflammation of the subtalar joint capsule, sometimes with arthritis of the joint. Debrunner (1960) identified multiple lesions involving the interosseous ligament, the capsule of the associated joints, the lateral tibiotarsal ligaments and sometimes osteophytes of the subtalar joint. Blasnick (1963) described chronic synovial inflammation, while Komprda (1966) demonstrated the degenerative hyaline lesions of the collagenous tissue. Brown (1960) could identify no specific lesion in this syndrome.

I have often observed partial rupture of the interosseous ligaments, sometimes with lytic atrophy. In other cases there has been tearing of the posterior subtalar joint capsule. On one occasion a capsular hernia was manifest in the sinus itself.

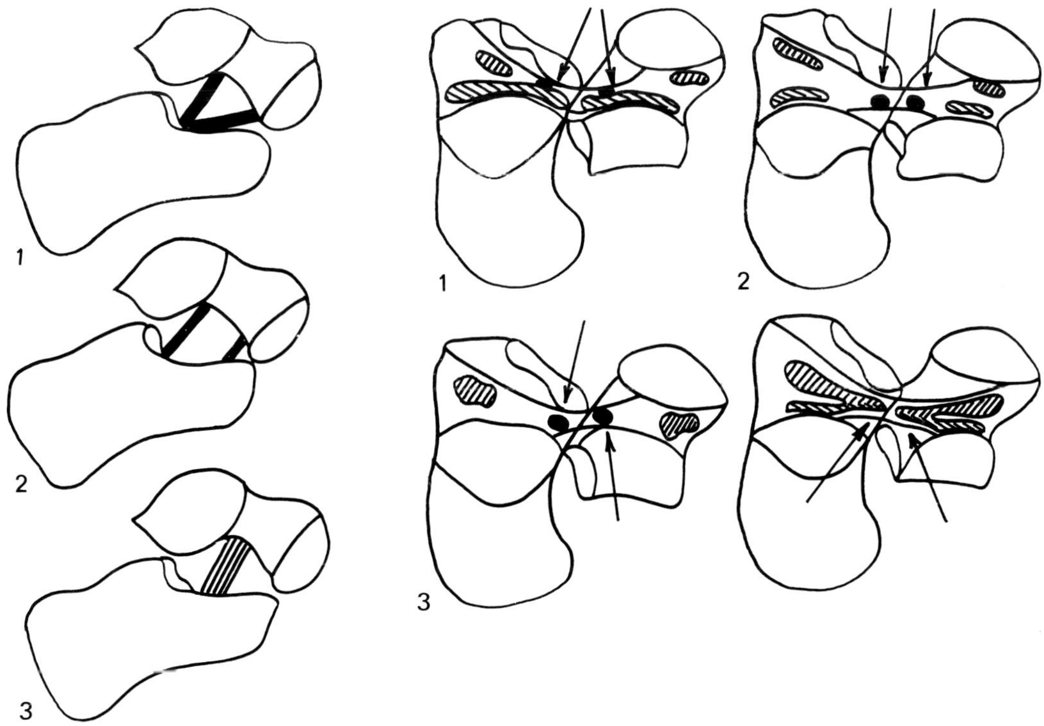

Fig. 34.1. Structure of the interosseous talocalcaneal ligament showing three variations in configuration of its main fasciculi (Valenti)

34.2 Clinical Features

The sinus tarsi syndrome affects adults only, predominantly those between the ages of 40 and 60 years, never being seen in subjects under 20 years of age. It is seen four times more frequently in women than in men, and affects with particular frequency active individuals who walk or stand a great deal or practise sport regularly.

The syndrome is characterised by localised pain towards the outer aspect of the sinus tarsi; this is a pathognomonic sign. The pain can appear insidiously, without apparent cause, and is frequently associated with clinical imbalance of the calcaneum in pes planus, pes planovalgus or pes cavovarus. A history of some predisposing accident may be given. The use of supporting insoles may previously have given relief from the pain, and this can be significant in the presence of a valgus or varus calcaneum. The pain irradiates from the external orifice of the sinus to the medial malleolus, to the plantar aspect of the calcaneum or, more rarely, to the heel, leg, or outer aspect of the instep. The pain is most frequently of a stretching, burning or twisting variety. There is a neuralgic character, with occasional episodes of paraesthesia which preclude activity. Sometimes the presentation is more imprecise, with a sensation of instability of the foot. Less frequently, there is metatarsalgia. The pain or disability is always aggravated by activity and can occur exclusively at night or first thing in the morning.

There is local tenderness over the outer aspect of the sinus tarsi, sometimes spreading to the plantar aspect of the body of the calcaneum under and behind the medial malleolus. I have noted that the sinus tarsi syndrome can be associated with plantar calcaneal talalgia or occur in the presence of a subcalcaneal spur. Komprda (1966) emphasised the presence of perimalleolar oedema.

Examination of the foot shows a free range of movement of the subtalar and talocalcaneonavicular joints except in those cases in which marked spasm is a feature. Quite commonly there is pes planus, less usually balanced pes cavus or pes cavorarus.

Radiographic examination usually shows no abnormality, unless there has been a previous trauma such as a fracture, but occasionally ankle or talonavicular arthrosis is revealed. No author has described any association of arthrosis of the subtalar joint or instability of the ankle due to ligament rupture with the condition.

The differential diagnosis includes peroneal tenosynovitis, the plantar talalgia syndrome, the tarsal canal syndrome and, in some cases of very severe pain, sciatica.

34.3 Treatment

34.3.1 Conservative

Conservative measures should always be advised initially. Rest, supportive bandaging and the use of the appropriate insole for a planovalgus, cavovalgus or cavovarus deformity may allay symptoms quite quickly. Administration of anti-inflammatory agents such as phenylbutazone and indomethacin and weekly local injection of corticosteroids and xylocaine into the sinus tarsi are beneficial. Massage and proprioceptive re-educative exercises as advised by Freeman et al. (1965) are especially effective in traumatic cases. In two-thirds of cases, this type of management will bring amelioration of symptoms.

34.3.2 Operative

In cases in which severe symptoms persist despite conservative treatment, Brown (1960) and Komprda (1966) have advised complete excision of the elements of the sinus tarsi. I myself find such major intervention illogical; it deprives the interosseous ligament of its proprioceptive function.

Operative Technique. I advise the following procedure: A curvilinear lateral incision is made under general anaesthesia with a bloodless field, and through this incision is performed conservative curettage of the fatty neurovascular tissue of the sinus, preserving the integrity of the interosseous ligament itself. When there is an obvious partial rupture, this area may be excised. Any torn or inflamed part of the capsule of the subtalar joint should also be excised, and after careful haemostasis, the cutaneous layer only is closed. A compressive dressing is replaced after a few days by an elastic support which allows early weight bearing and walking.

35 Morton Neuralgia

Morton neuralgia comprises a painful paroxysmal syndrome emanating from the intercapital metatarsal region and was described in 1876 by Thomas G. Morton (not to be confused with Duddley Morton, who described the convex forefoot; see Chap. 10).

The intolerable pain is localised to the affected interspace and radiates into the foot generally, associated with cold sweating. It is due to compression of a nerve, sometimes by the development of a true neurofibroma, by ligaments or by the metatarsal condyles; a cyst, serous bursa or bony protuberance can be responsible. Betts (1940) offered a further description of the syndrome, while Nissen (1948) attributed it to ischaemia of the nerve due to plantar digital arteritis.

35.1 Anatomy and Etiology

The majority of Morton neuralgias supervene in feet affected by postural abnormalities, particularly in the precavus or cavus foot with convex forefoot or varus or valgus of the heel. Sometimes isolated depression of a particular metatarsal head causes extrinsic compression of the nerve. In the majority of histological examinations are found some degree of endarteritis of the vascular bundle and some specific nerve lesion, such as a neuroma. Occasionally there is simple generalised thickening of the nerve as if due to compression irritation.

The results of histological examinations described by Leroux and Gordeeff (1970) suggest a compressive cause, and the following types of lesion have been described:

1. A true plexiform neuroma, varying in size from the size of a pea to the size of a small nut, associated with fibrous scarring and hypertrophy.
2. Multiple plexiform neuromata with interstitial fibrosis, dense and rich in collagen, surrounding the hyperplastic nerve filaments and the vascular filaments, which exhibit some degree of arteriosclerosis or endarteritis or discrete fibrotic lesions.
3. Occasional lesions comprising dense sclerosis associated with a fatty mattress including vascular formations and small nerve elements.
4. Neuromatous hyplasia with diffuse and extensive fibrosis.
5. The association of dense fibrosis with distortion of nerve elements, which appear to be stretched, sensitive Pacchionian corpuscles, and the whole embedded in cellular adipose tissue lobulated with multiple fibrous bands having a rich vascular supply but showing some evidence of degeneration.
6. A conglomeration of sclerosed tissue surrounding hyperplastic nervous elements and multiple tactile corpuscles or vessels with lesions of parietal fibrosis, the whole area forming an interstitial fibro-elastic mass.

Some authors, notably Lelièvre, Gauthier and Dutertre, Dubois and Wolkas, have found this syndrome quite frequently, but I regard it as a relatively rare occurrence. Many metatarsalgias which at first sight seem to possess clinical features of Morton neuralgia are in fact metatarsalgias of disordered loading confused with Morton neuralgia because of their site in the forefoot.

35.2 Clinical Features

The painful neuralgic syndrome affects, in order of frequency, the third, second, first and fourth intercapital spaces. The pain is severe and sudden in onset with no apparent cause. It may begin while walking with a stumble or while wearing shoes which are too tight. It is intolerably intense and ir radiates into the body of the foot or, more frequently, distally into the toes corresponding to the space concerned. Sometimes it spreads to the heel and calf, depending on how far forward the lesion is sited in the space affected. The pain is sometimes described as like a violent electric shock, analogous to that experienced when striking the ulnar nerve at the elbow, but can be of a burning type with a sensation of stretching of the intermetatarsal space. It lasts characteristically for a few seconds.

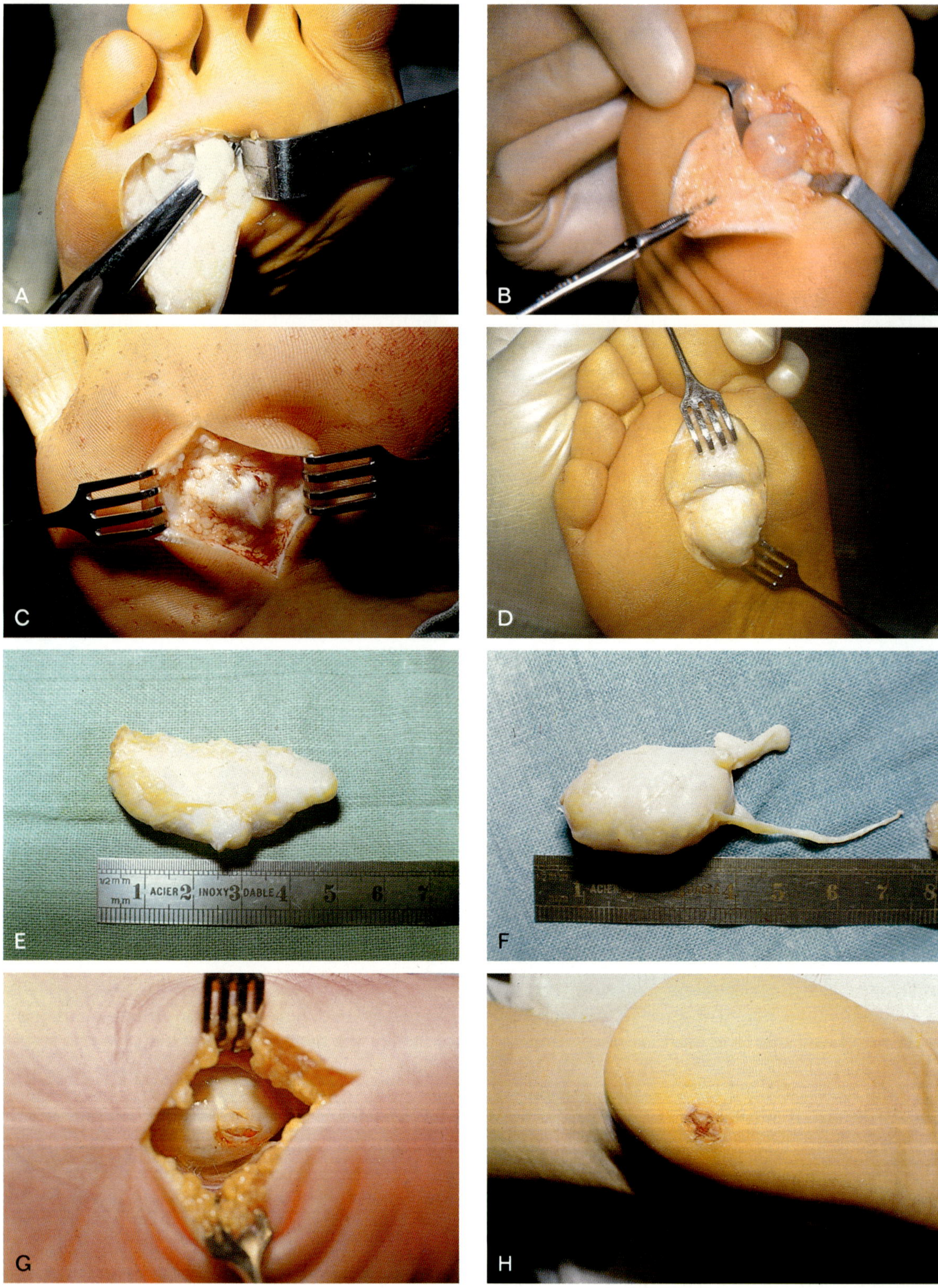

Fig. 35.1 A–K. Tumours of forefoot. **A–F** Plantar neuromata. **G** Plantar neuroma, size of a pigeon's egg. **D** Intercapital cyst. **H** Melanoma. **I** Callus formation over extensor hallucis longus. **J, K** Synovial cyst of first intermetatarsal space. **H–K** see p. 503 ▷

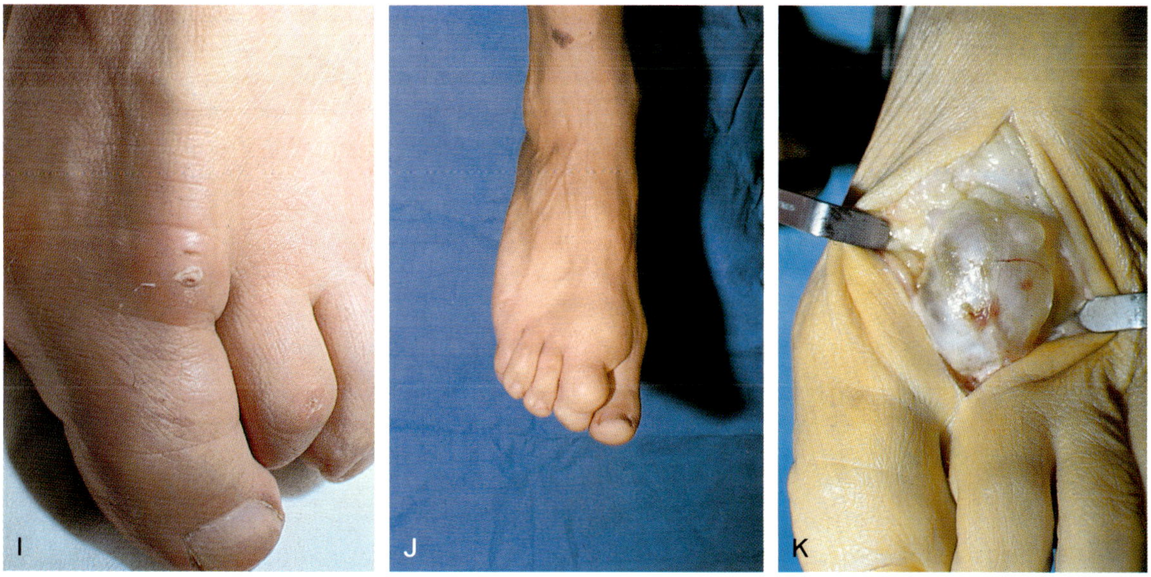

Fig. 35.1 I–K. Legend see p. 502

A diffuse ache lingers for some minutes in the forefoot and the subject is apprehensive about putting weight on the foot or even putting on his shoe.

Palpation defines precisely the site of any neuroma present, by detecting a corresponding small swelling. Compression of the forefoot collaterally produces the pain, which disappears very suddenly when compression is relieved. According to Mulder (1951), the latter feature is a pathognomonic sign; Lelièvre (1952) interprets it as always indicating the presence of a hygroma or serous bursa, rather than compression of a true neuroma. It permits exclusion of symptoms due to isolated depression of a metatarsal head. Further, if the pain is due to capsular inflammation or a bursitis secondary to metatarsal head overloading, it does not possess the sudden intense onset characteristic of true Morton neuralgia; the two should be distinguished clearly. However, Morton neuralgia and metatarsalgia can coexist, especially in the presence of a convex forefoot or a cavovalgus foot. Condylar metatarsalgia is more diffuse, whereas Morton neuralgia is localised and has characteristic radiation.

Podoscopy in Morton neuralgia may show longitudinal displacement: a balanced cavus, cavo valgus or cavo varus foot. *Podometry* will exclude isolated metatarsal head overloading and may confirm generalised overloading of the central metatarsal heads. Obviously, the presence of isolated or central metatarsal head overloading indicates a different form of treatment. Should a neuroma coexist with one of these conditions, excision can be performed at the same time as operative correction of the mechanical aspect.

35.3 Treatment

35.3.1 Conservative

Medical treatment consists of administration of anti-inflammatory agents and infiltration of the space concerned with local anaesthetic. Insoles should comprise a subcapital or perhaps retrocapital bar or be of the physiological monoblock type. Use of such insoles may balance and support the foot, therefore allowing the source of irritation to settle.

35.3.2 Operative

Failure of conservative measures demands excision of any neuroma present. Nissen (1948) and Lelièvre (1952) advised exploration via the plantar approach but I have avoided this method during the last 15 years because of its tendency to produce keratotic painful scars. The plantar approach should be used only if a neuroma exists in the intermetatarsal space behind the condyles. Occasionally such lesions can be large, as big as a pigeon's egg (Fig. 35.1).

Operative Technique. The dorsal approach is preferred. Excellent exposure can be achieved through a 3-cm longitudinal incision over the intercapital space concerned if the assistant flexes the metatarsophalangeal joints while pressing upwards on the tissue of the ball of the foot. The neurovascular bundle can then be seen clearly, having been displaced dorsally in the space being explored. Resection, whether of a fusiform swelling of the nerve or of a rounded oval pea- or nut-sized local neuroma, can be accomplished. After careful haemostasis the skin is sutured. Walking is possible after 2 days, with progression to full weight bearing by the 10th day.

VII Rheumatic Diseases

36 Rheumatoid Arthritis

Of the rheumatic inflammatory conditions affecting the foot (rheumatoid arthritis, ankylosing spondylitis, psoriatic arthritis and gout), rheumatoid arthritis is the commonest. While the origin remains uncertain, viral and immunological etiologies have been proposed, it is known to affect all peoples commonly living in damp or temperate climates. Women aged 30–40 years are affected most commonly (75% of cases). The inflammatory condition involves the connective tissue, generally leading to extremely incapacitating arthropathies. Most authors agree that the foot is affected in 80%–96% of cases.

With respect to the joints, a proliferative synovitis develops, forms a pannus which progressively destroys the cartilaginous tissues, invades the bone and periarticular tissues and softens the associated capsule and tendons.

36.1 Clinical Features

At the onset, diagnosis may be uncertain because of the polymorphic distribution of clinical and biological signs. Radiographic signs may develop early, initially in the metacarpophalangeal joints and then in the joints of the foot. In the hand, the joints of the thumb and index finger are usually the first to become involved. In the foot, it is the second and third metatarsophalangeal joints followed by the fifth, and this distribution is regarded as pathognomonic by Forestier and Robert (1940) and Coste et al. (1968). Subsequently, a symmetrical polyarthritis develops progressively, with swelling of the periarticular tissues and progressive articular contracture; the symptoms present mostly in the morning, settling at first during the course of the day. Occasional features include (a) more classical acute polyarthritis of the thumb, index finger and metatarsophalangeal joints, (b) acute mono-arthritis of a larger joint such as the wrist or the ankle, and (c) acute mono-arthritis of a metacarpophalangeal or metatarsophalangeal joint. The arthritis may be of sudden onset with fusiform swelling, local redness and a sensation of tension or burning. Mobility is conserved but painful.

In the foot, the condition is manifested by dorsal swelling over the joints affected; by scattered pain exacerbated by loading or pressure, including the sesamoid-metatarsal articulation (Denis 1974c); and by tenosynovitis of tibialis posterior, the long flexors, the peronei or the extensors. These symptoms may occur concurrently. There may be pain under the hindfoot. Braun (1975b) has drawn attention to the development of Achilles bursitis, a rare early sign (1.6% of cases), or plantar fasciitis (15%). Francon (1959) described involvement of the great metatarsophalangeal joint like pseudo-gout.

Systemic signs comprise general weight loss, asthenia and a subacute febrile condition.

Over a few months or even years, the more classical picture of rheumatoid polyarthritis becomes established and diagnosis is easy (Debeyre and Denis 1966). Postural disorders present due to deformity, while the foot generally has a pink, violaceous or whitish appearance and is moist or succulent, with persistent swelling around joints and atrophy of the overlying skin, which while supple loses its elasticity. The foot may develop a balanced planovalgus posture with some rigidity, which becomes irreversibly fixed. Pronation of the calcaneum is accompanied by breakdown of the midtarsal region, which becomes internally displaced with its summit at the navicular or more frequently the medial cuneiform. A general abduction of the metatarsus confers on the forefoot a classical triangular configuration, with digital displacements giving it a windswept appearance. Occasionally the foot assumes a false cavovalgus posture; podoscopic examination seems to show collapse of the vault of the medial longitudinal arch and internal displacement of the metatarsus, but in reality the combination of metatarsal abduction and convex forefoot which brings the patient to consultation on account of its painful rigidity is simulating this image. Pain comprises a localised metatarsalgia or more often a diffuse anterior tarsalgia, affecting more the internal and plantar aspects of the foot. I have not seen cavovarus deformities in rheumatoid arthritis, but they have been described by Allieu et al. (1975–1977) in six cases and I have seen them in ankylosing spondylitis. It is clear that in such a polymorphic condition with wide distribution, any deformity can occur.

Although the disease predominates in one area of the foot, it will be found that most joints are involved. Thus, the ankle exhibits periarticular swelling inflating the retromalleolar gutters and causing pain related to the posterior joint line as well as the subtalar joint. The oedema sometimes causes the tissues to bulge over the heel cup of the shoe, and there is restriction of amplitude of movement of the ankle joint. The midtarsal joints are easily palpable on account of atrophy of the capsular and subcutaneous tissues and exhibit impaired mobility. Evidence of tenosynovitis of tibialis posterior may be obvious, and in relationship to the calcaneum, pain under the heel is due to plantar bursitis, fasciitis or involvement of the Achilles tendon.

Rheumatoid involvement of the forefoot leads to various deformities determined by articular, capsulotendinous and cutaneous involvement:

1. Primary involvement of the first ray, with hallux valgus of second or third degree and secondary displacement of the neighbouring toes, which become clawed and develop calluses over the bony prominences, likely to become inflamed or infected.
2. A classical windswept deformity of the five toes accompanied with a light varus of the great metatarsal but no valgus of the fifth metatarsal. This is usually associated with a cavovalgus foot with displacement of the extensor tendons leading to lateral metatarsophalangeal subluxation.
3. A triangular forefoot with medial clinodactylies of the toes associated with significant varus of the first metatarsal and valgus of the great toe. Valgus deformity of the fifth metatarsal causes development of a tailor's bunion on the outer surface of the fifth metatarsal condyle with varus deformity of the little toe, which usually underrides the fourth toe. A partridge eye develops at the site of pressure on the fourth toe and very painful para-ungual external keratoma forms on the fifth toe. The clawing of the second, third and fourth toes leads to a windswept lateral deviation which rapidly becomes irreducible due to lateral subluxation or dislocation of the metatarsophalangeal joints fixed by tendinous contractures involving the long and short extensors, principally the latter. The distal phalanges of the toes can present clinodactylies or camptodactylies of varying types associated with painful callus formation and inflammation. Cutaneous plantar atrophy is marked under all of the metatarsal condyles, which nevertheless remain well aligned in the horizontal plane.
4. The very typical form described in item 3 above is of a flat triangular configuration; much less commonly a convex triangular form can coexist with a cavovalgus foot. It is always associated with marked atrophy, and the projections of the condyles into the tissues of the foot are marked by longitudinal furrows separating the painful individual calluses. There is displacement of varying degrees of the first and fifth rays, lowering and marked protrusion of the central three metatarsal heads and subluxation progressing rapidly to total fixed dislocation of the central three metatarsophalangeal joints with associated clawing of the toes. This becomes fixed by contracture of the integument and the long and short extensor tendons; the toes look much shorter because they are submerged in the swollen subcutaneous dorsal fat of the metatarsophalangeal region. This type of rheumatoid forefoot presents the greatest difficulties in correction due to the contractures.

Whatever the type of deformation of the forefoot, some degree of articular mobility remains, although it is restricted. Thus at the great metatarsophalangeal joint, plantarflexion is mainly limited. In the second, third and fourth metatarsophalangeal joints there is a permanent dorsiflexion which cannot be corrected because of the dislocation and dorsal contractures. In the fitth metatarsophalangeal joint, dorsiflexion is very limited, perhaps absent, but the toe preserves some degree of active plantarflexion; here, the restriction of dorsiflexion is due to destructive lesions of the fifth metatarsal head. The toe is usually in infraductus with respect to the fourth toe, but can be in supraductus. The interphalangeal joints are generally fixed in plantarflexion.

Together with the deformities described and the involvement of joints and tendons of the hindfoot, a general state of fatigue and weakness with sensitivity to cold and chronic weight loss or, occasionally, obesity are associated with this debilitating illness.

36.2 Radiography

In the forefoot (Figs. 36.1–36.3), early radiographic signs are seen at the metatarsophalangeal joints. In the central three joints, a band-like transparency across the epiphyseal region with central cortical linear configuration indicates central osteoporosis of the metatarsal heads. It is associated with slight narrowing of the joint interspace, and premonitory signs of epiphyseal destruction are thinning of the cortex, subchondral marginal lytic lesions and slight interruption of the joint contour (Kerbrat 1974). At the fifth metatarsal head particularly, early involvement is a radiographic sign of great diagnostic value. This was emphasised by Forestier and Robert (1940), who described localised geodic areas of decalcification and epiphyseal notching of the fifth metatarsal head. Coste et al. (1968) proposed a classification of this Forestier sign comprising five stages:

Stage 1: Epiphyseal localised decalcification of the outer margins of the metatarsal.
Stage 2: Geodic outlines, perhaps isolated and only the size of a pinhead, in the spongy or subcortical bone. These may be multiple and grouped under the other margin of the inferior part of the condyle.
Stage 3: Confluent geodic areas lending a nibbled appearance to the contours of the metatarsal head.
Stage 4: Lytic lesions affecting the epiphysis on the inferior aspect, spreading collaterally and then involving the whole circumference, which changes in shape to resemble a truncated cone.
Stage 5: An appearance of amputation of the head, which is reduced to a configuration like a pencil point.

These radiographic signs are associated with fusiform periarticular soft tissue shadows indicative of synovial hypertrophy, and contrast with the thinning of the cortical linear margin and increased translucency of the metatarsal heads. The absence of osteophytes, except in later cases where osteoarthrosis supervenes, is notable (Galmiche 1972).

At a later stage, in addition to the local joint destruction radiographic examination reveals the grosser deformities of the foot which reflect the clinical descriptions given above. Stages 4 and 5, comprising lysis and apparent amputation of the metatarsal heads together with the windswept deformity of the toes, may be gross. The interphalangeal joints may show a hatchet deformity with various dislocations or sometimes fusions. The heads of the phalanges are sometimes impacted into the corresponding bases, as described by Coste et al. (1968).

In the hindfoot, general narrowing of joint spaces and, in contrast with the forefoot, some osteophytosis anteriorly and posteriorly at the ankle may be seen. This has been described as a pheasant-head appearance of the posterior part of the talus. Dorsal osteophytosis may be seen at the navicular cuneiform joint region. In the calcaneum, a destructive rheumatoid erosion may be seen (Braun et al. 1970), comprising posterosuperior calcification and geodic erosions which give a striking frilled appearance to the bone edge without any evidence of reconstruction. Inferiorly, notching in the region of the plantar tuberosity relates to serous plantar bursitis (Lenoir) or a large erosion of circular outline without surrounding bone reconstruction as described by Braun (1975a, b, 1978).

Besides the inflammatory changes, subacute lesions are evident in the form of macrogeodes or juxta-articular pseudotumours of two types (Kerbrat 1974): they may appear as active macrogeodes with irregular contours, polycyclic and condensed, or as static macrogeodes with central calcifications (Jayson), homogeneously bright and displaying bony trabeculae with regular contours and bony condensations. These features are met above all in the metatarsophalangeal joint regions and communicate with neighbouring joints.

In contrast to radiography, which is important in diagnosis and in following the evolution of the condition, isotope technetium scanning is useful in the surveillance of treatment.

36.3 Laboratory Investigations

The general blood count exhibits anaemia of the normochromic or hypochromic type, but the white cell count is non-specific. Elevations in erythrocyte sedimentation rate, fibrinogen level, reactive protein C, alpha gammaglobulins and IgA, IgC and IgM immunophoresis are indicative of the inflammatory process but not specific to rheumatoid arthritis. In three-quarters of cases there is a positive test for rheumatoid factor in the Rose Waaler reaction (1/64) and the latex fixation test (1/160). The latter are often negative at the beginning of the disease but when positive indicate its severity. The rosette rheumatoid test is positive when six lymphocytes per 1000 give a rosette image. Indirect immunofluorescence tests give positive results in 30% of cases due to the presence of nuclear antibodies. A search for Hargrave's cells is positive in less than 5% of cases.

Examination of aspirated joint fluids show a significant diminution in the complement level and an increase in white cells suspended in liquid poor in mucin content.

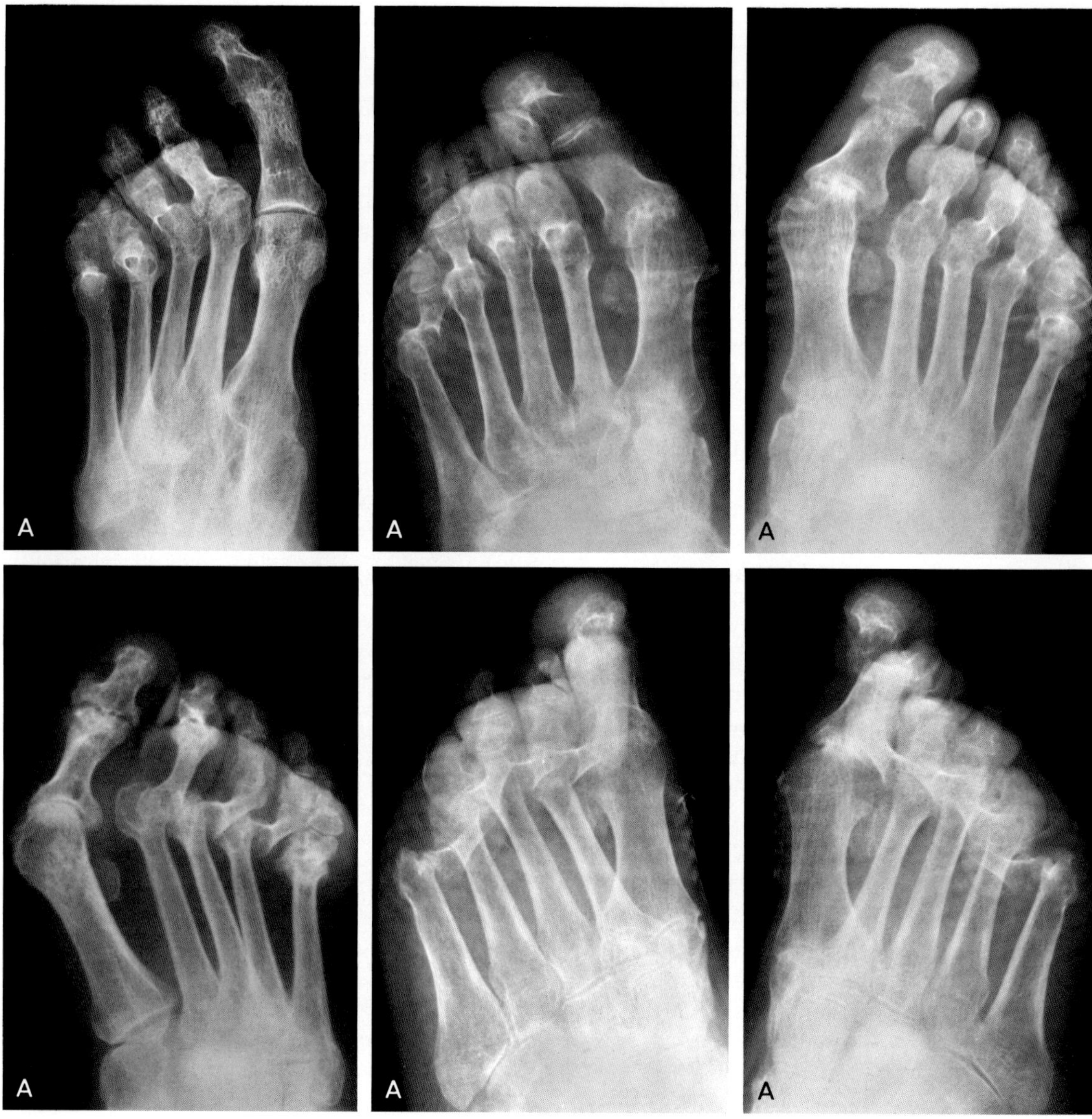

Fig. 36.1 A–C. Rheumatoid arthritis in forefoot. **A** Progressive development of arthropathy leading to ankylosis of ▷ metatarsophalangeal joint. **B, C** see pp. 511–513

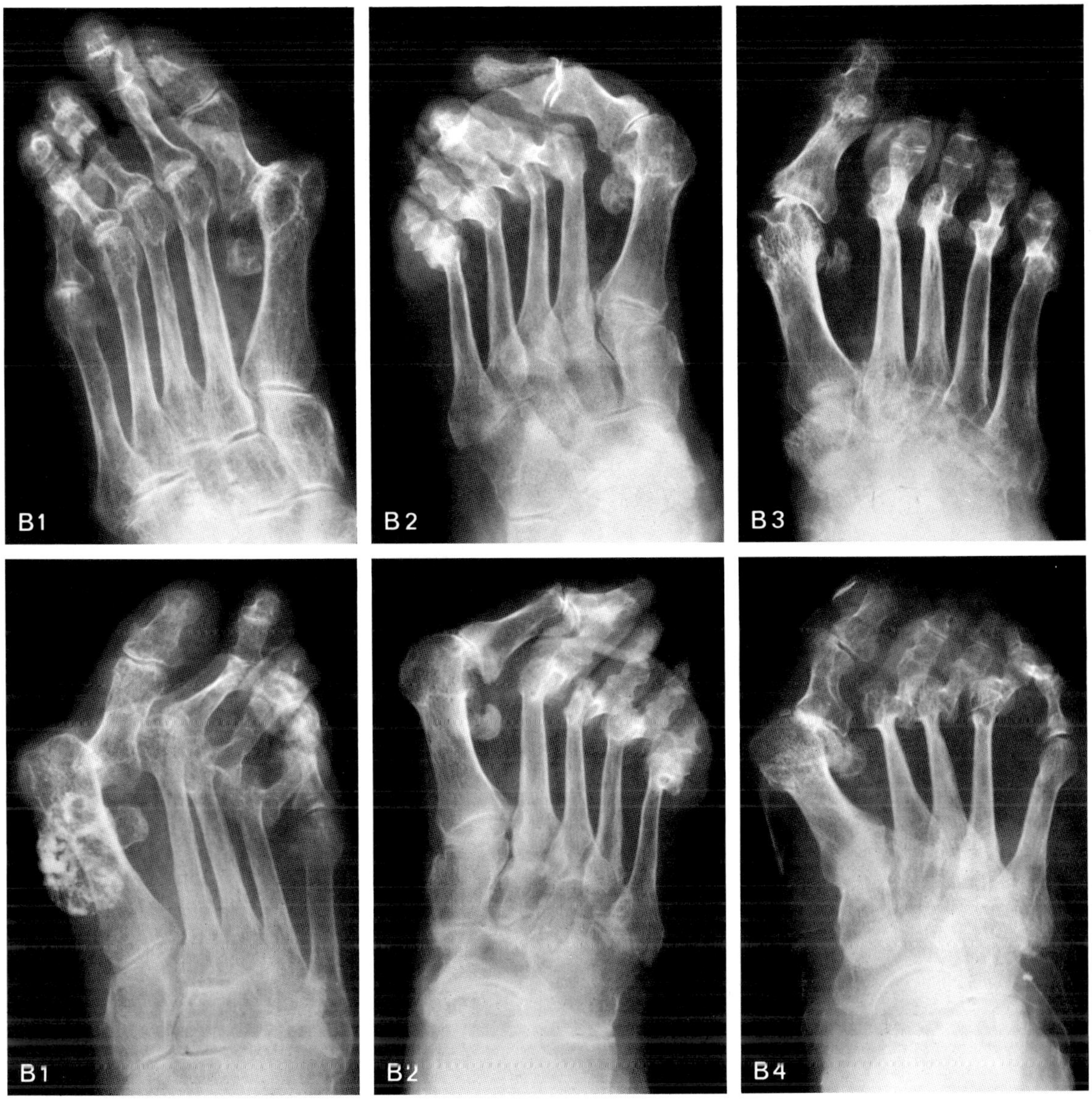

Fig. 36.1 *(continued)*. **B** Examples of windswept deformity, dorsolateral dislocation

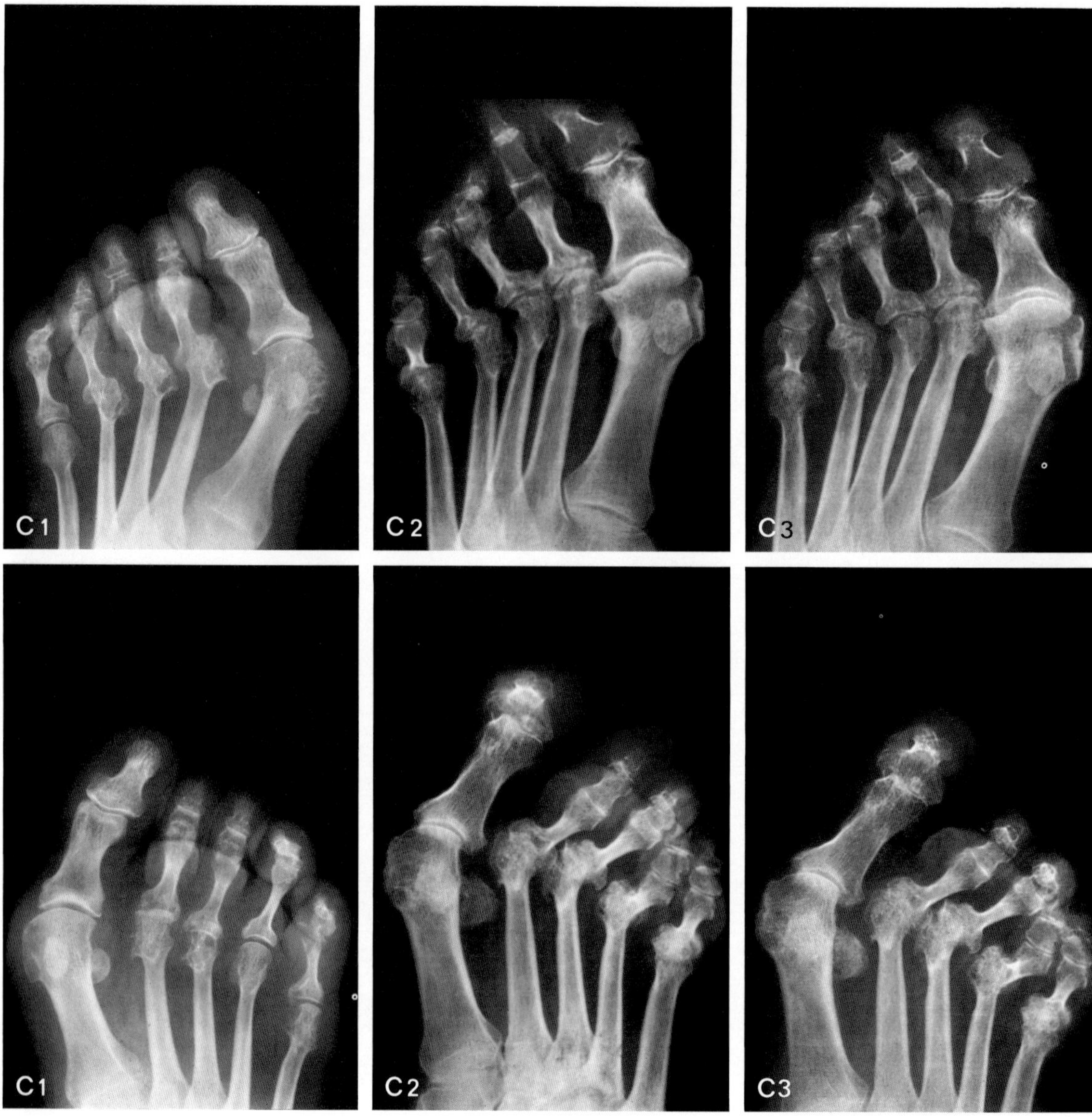

Fig. 36.1 *(continued).* **C** *1–6* Examples of dislocations with involvement of epiphyses of varying degree ▷

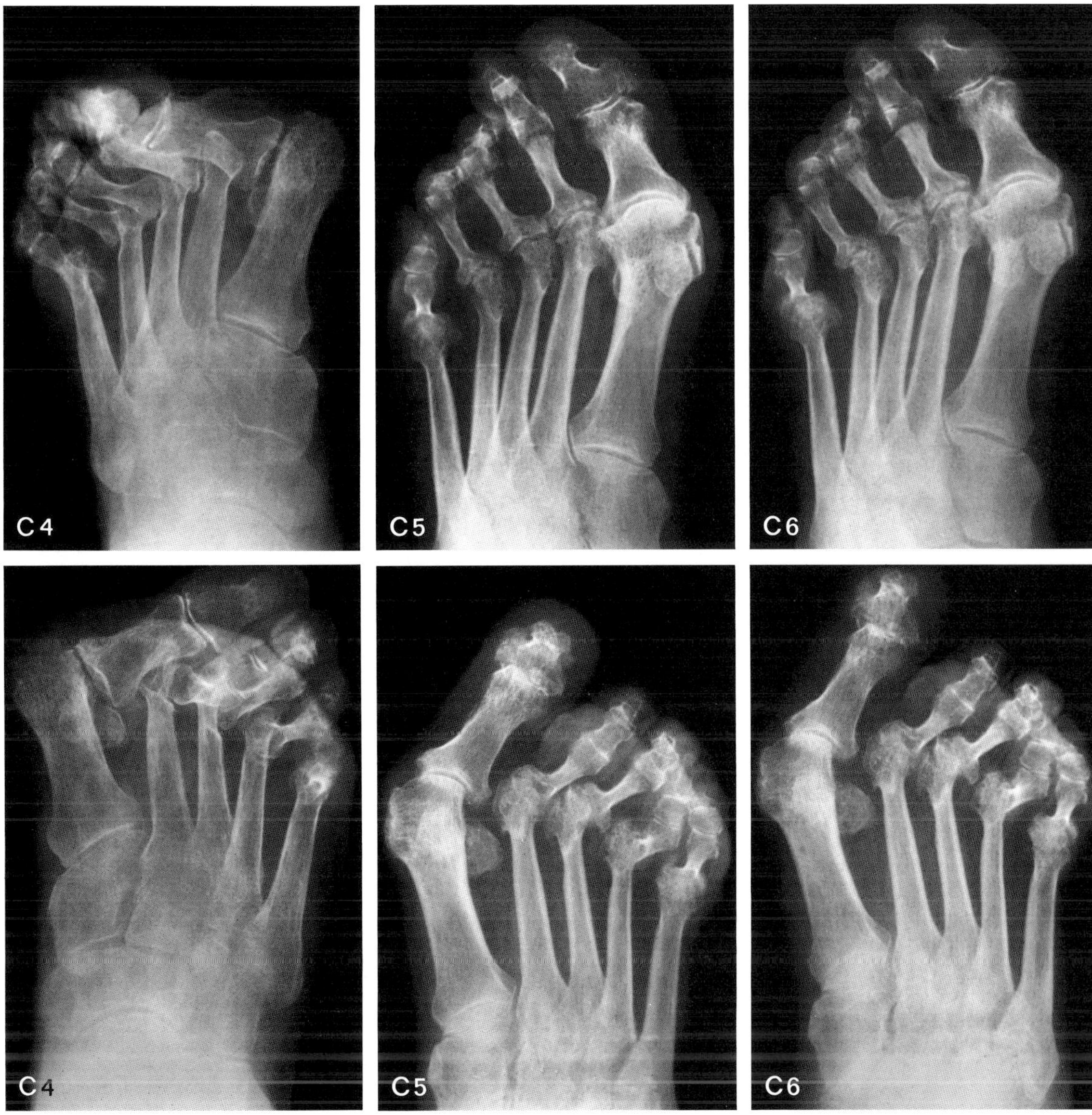

Fig. 36.1 C *4–6.* Legend see p. 512

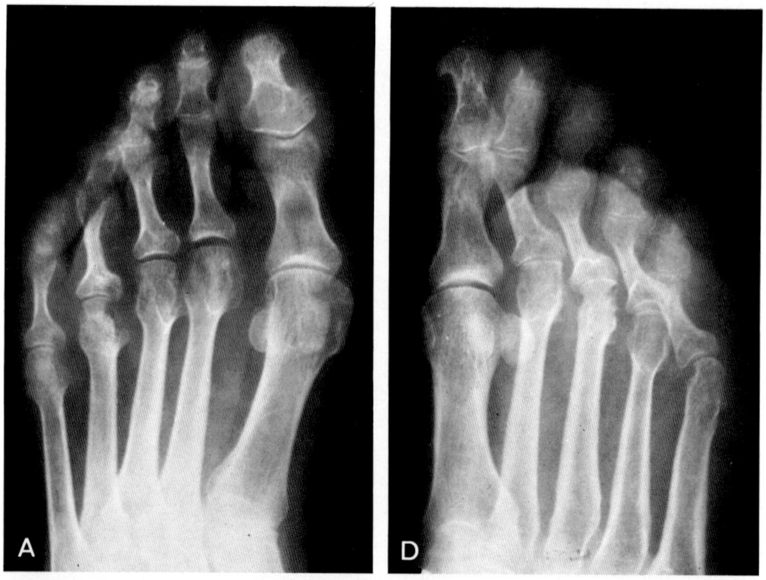

Fig. 36.2 A–E. Legend see p. 515

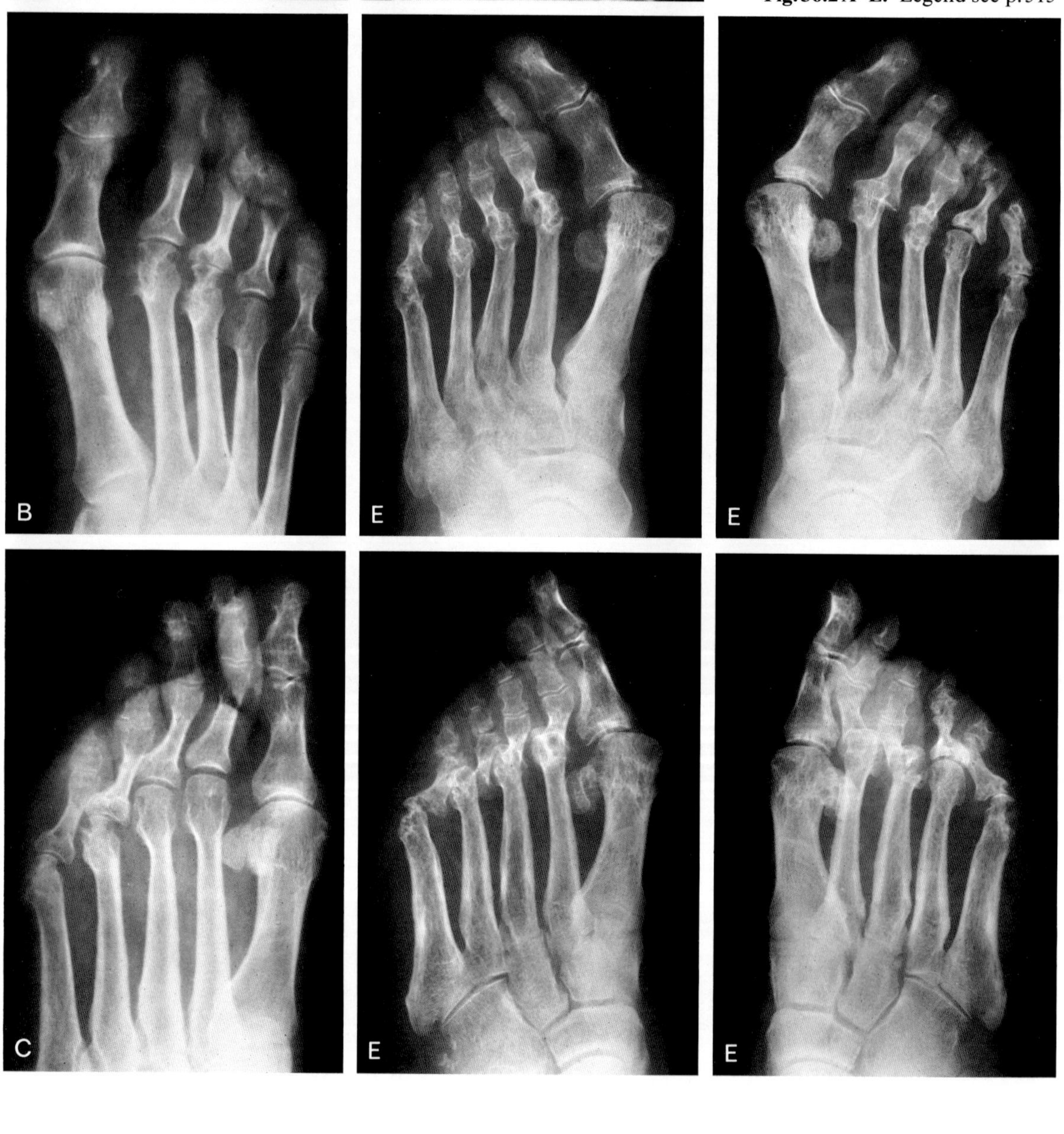

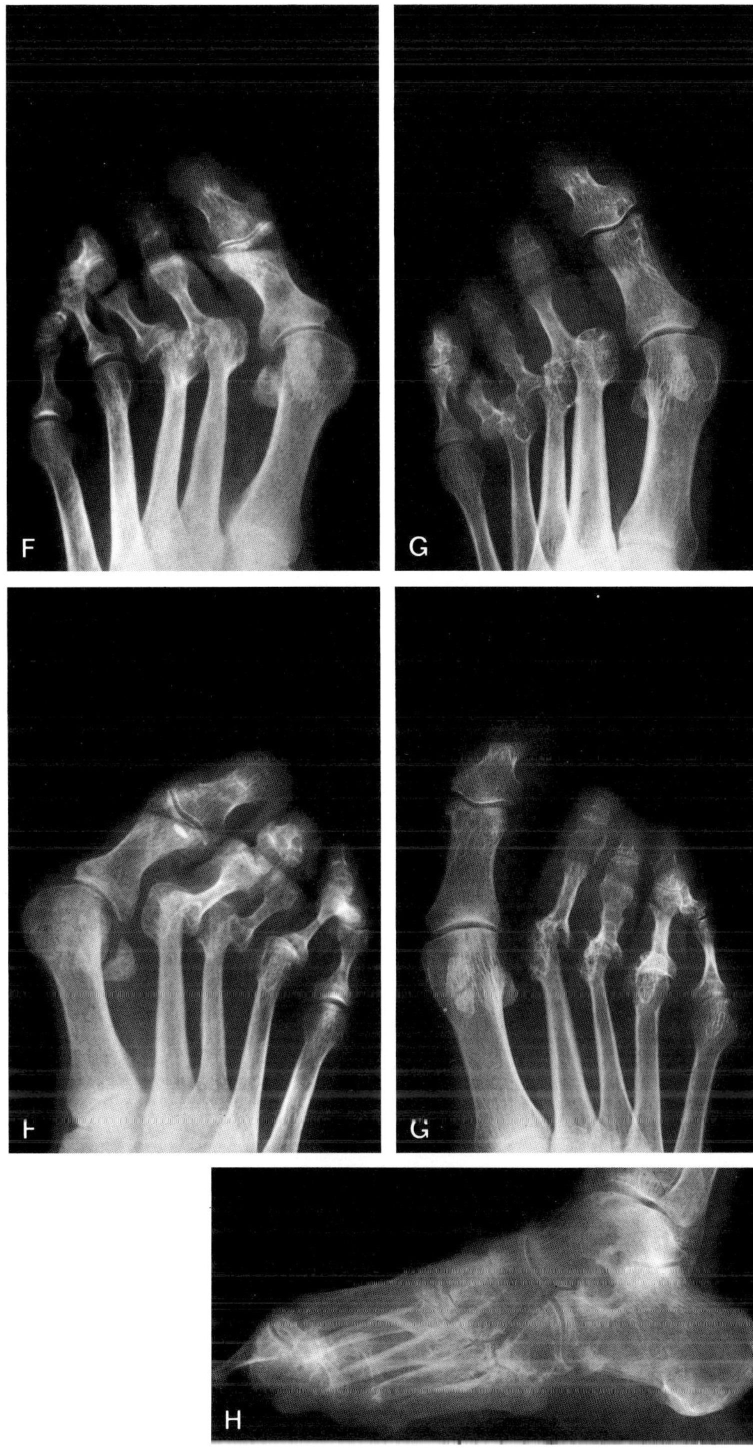

◁ **Fig. 36.2 A–K.** Rheumatoid arthritis in forefoot. **A** Geodic lesions in third, fourth and fifth metatarsal heads. **B** Lesions in second, third and fifth metatarsal heads. **C** Involvement of third, fourth and fifth metatarsal heads. **D** Lesions in second, third and fifth metatarsal heads. **E** Osteolysis involving all five metatarsal heads, dorsolateral dislocation of bases of phalanges, commencement of metatarsophalangeal arthropathy. **F** Lateral windswept deformity of toes. **G** Metatarsophalangeal arthropathy, dorsolateral dislocations, destruction of second, third and fourth metatarsal joints. **H** Microgeodic lesions at Lisfranc region, metatarsophalangeal arthropathy. **I–K** see p. 516

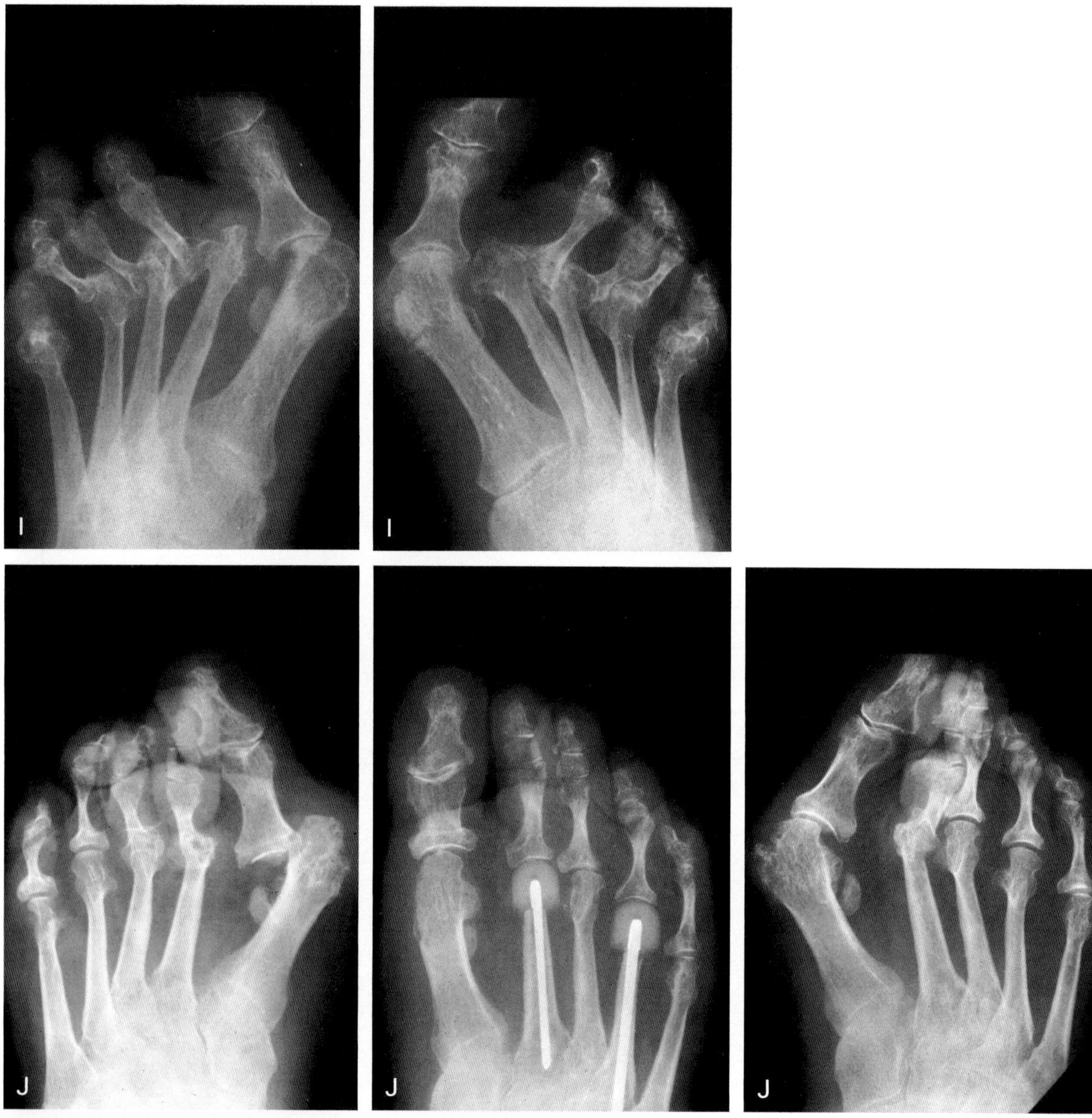

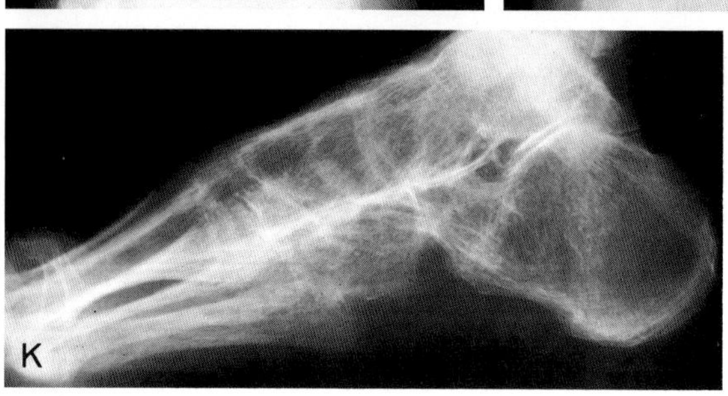

Fig. 36.2 *(continued)*. **I** Classic rheumatoid forefoot. **J** Example of surgical reconstruction of simple triangular forefoot in rheumatoid arthritis by correction of hallux valgus with hat-shaped graft and realignment by implantation of prostheses in second and fourth metatarsals. **K** Generalised rheumatoid arthritis tending to fusion of tarsal and midtarsal joints

Fig. 36.3 A–C. Surgical treatment of a case of rheumatoid arthritis. Convex triangular forefoot with frontal protrusion of central metatarsal heads, arthritic process involving all midtarsal and metatarsophalangeal joints with severe destruction of metatarsal heads and lateral dislocations of toes. **A** Before surgery. **B** Right foot, lateral view 1 year after metatarsal realignment (Lelièvre), cup interposition arthroplasty of first metatarsophalangeal joint (note also involvement of joints of mid-foot). Left foot, 2 years after same procedures. **C** see p. 518

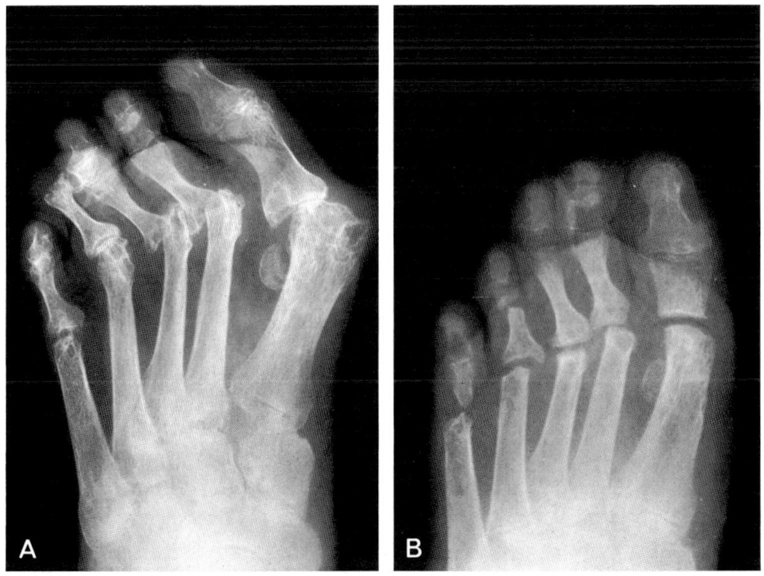
A
B

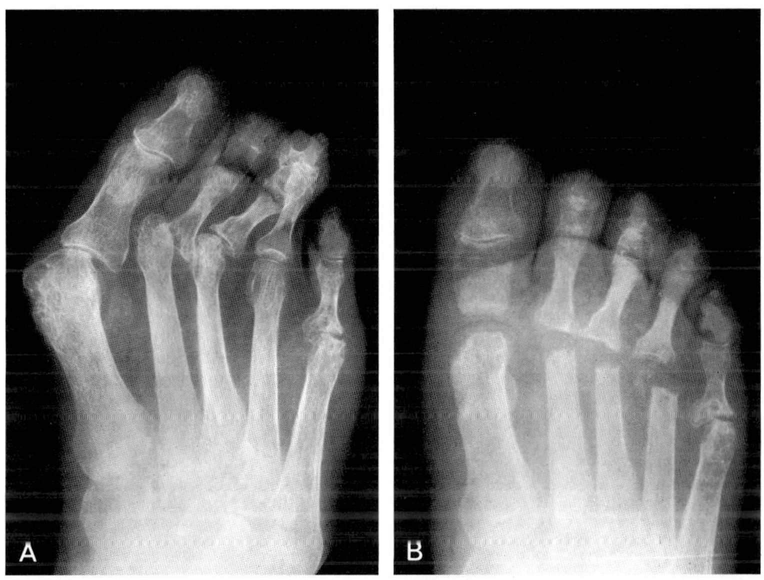
A
B

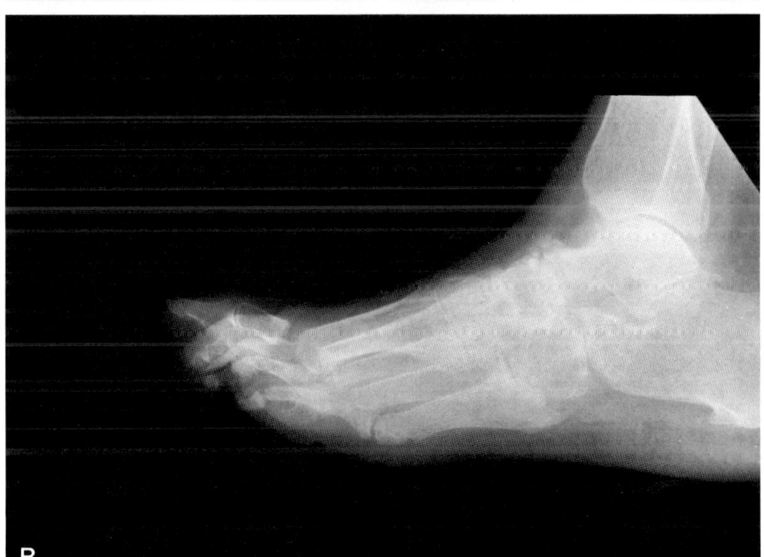
B

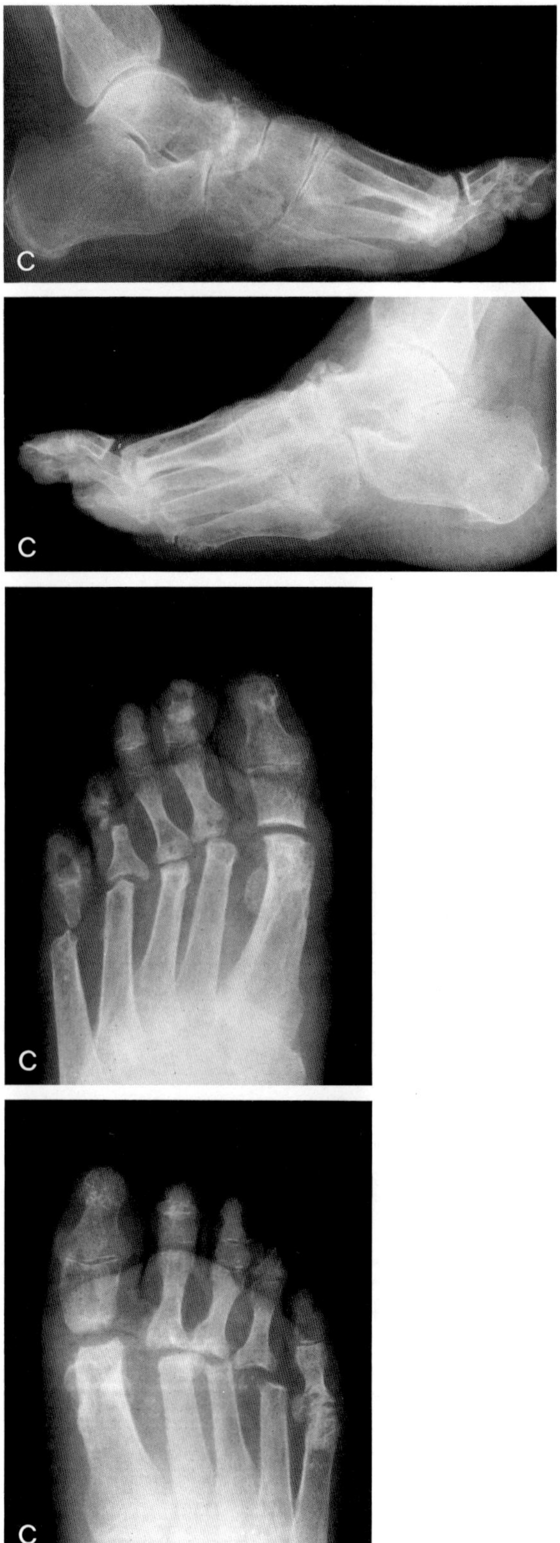

Fig. 36.3 *(continued).* **C** Right foot, 2 years after operation: lateral view shows involvement of intertarsal and metatarsophalangeal joints. Left foot, 3 years after operation: the cup prostheses were left in place because they were well tolerated

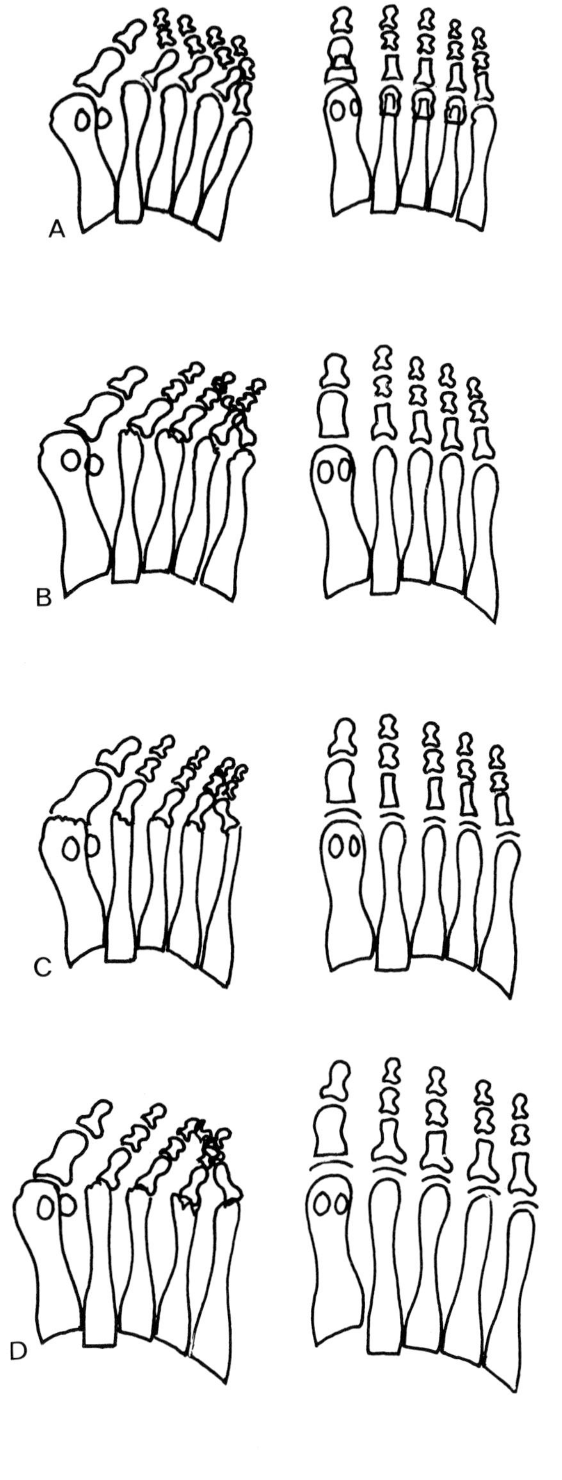

Fig. 36.4 A–D. Surgical treatment of rheumatoid arthritis. **A** Metatarsal head-shaft enclavements (Regnauld). **B** Metatarsal realignment (Lelièvre). **C** Clayton operation with cup arthroplasties (Regnauld). **D** Lelièvre realignment with cup arthroplasties (Regnauld)

36.4 Treatment

36.4.1 General Measures

Rest during acute episodes is essential, while prevention of infection and trauma, and measures against pain form a general background to care. Contractures should be avoided as far as possible by gentle physiotherapy conducted during non-acute periods, and care should be taken to avoid production of deformities by inappropriate insoles or other splintage.

36.4.2 Medical

Analgesics, especially salicylates if tolerated, should be tried first. Subsequently, gold therapy and administration of antimalarial agents, non-steroidal anti-inflammatory drugs, immunosuppressive agents and penicillamine are advised. Chemical synovectomy with osmic acid and treatment with radioactive agents such as yttrium, gold, erbium or rhenium are specialist forms of therapy.
I recommend medical care comprising injections of corticosteroids and anti-inflammatory agents, but these should be administered by a rheumatologist.
The patient with rheumatoid disease of the foot is frequently referred for management of postural deformities which have resulted from the destructive articular processes, but such specific treatment needs to be carried out against a stable background of medical care.

36.4.3 Orthotic

Careful selection of shoes is essential. These should be adapted to the abnormal shape of the foot and possess a supple upper which is both large and high. They should be fitted with supportive insoles padded by India rubber or soft latex carefully moulded and excavated to relieve pressure under the prominent metatarsophalangeal joints. General chiropodical measures, including attention to corns and bursitis, are only palliative but nevertheless valuable.

36.4.4 Operative

Arthrodesis of destroyed joints is applicable more in the hindfoot, where fusion of the subtalar joint, the midtarsal joint and the Lisfranc joint line may be indicated. However, caution is advised, because the osteoporosis and slowness of bony fusion can make arthrodesis uncertain.
Stabilising procedures of a more functional nature in the forefoot are very valuable (Fig. 36.4). During the phase of onset, when the metatarsal heads are intact or little involved, even in the presence of displacements of the metatarsophalangeal joints, realignment head-shaft enclavement associated with correction of clinodactylies of the first and fifth rays and elongation of the tendons can lead to stabilisation of the foot and much better load-bearing capacity. In the majority of cases, however, the metatarsophalangeal arthopathies do not allow enclavement procedures and one of the following solutions may be necessary:

1. Metatarsal realignment as described by Lelièvre (1952), by which uniform zone of loading of the metatarsal heads can be re-established.
2. Lelièvre realignment or the Clayton operation (1960a, b) with the interposition of cup prostheses (Regnauld and Grassin 1975) (Fig. 36.5). The realignment is complemented by the cup prostheses and mobility of the metatarsophalangeal joints is re-established. Resection of the bases of the proximal phalanges can be added to the cup prosthesis method (Fig. 36.6). Attention must be directed to the length of the tendons, and arthrodeses of the interphalangeal joints may also be necessary.
3. Temporary implantation of metatarsal prostheses into the second, third, fourth and fifth metatarsals after realignment (Regnauld and Grassin 1975). This operation allows realignment of the five metatarsal heads and a good stable range of toe movement so that an almost normal rolling action during walking can be achieved. There is no excessive shortening of the foot (Figs. 36.7, 36.8), and normal shoes can be used. The metatarsal prostheses must be removed after 1–2 years and their excision allows an articular cavity due to which the metatarsophalangeal joint mobility is preserved, allowing continuation of a useful range of dorsiflexion and plantarflexion.

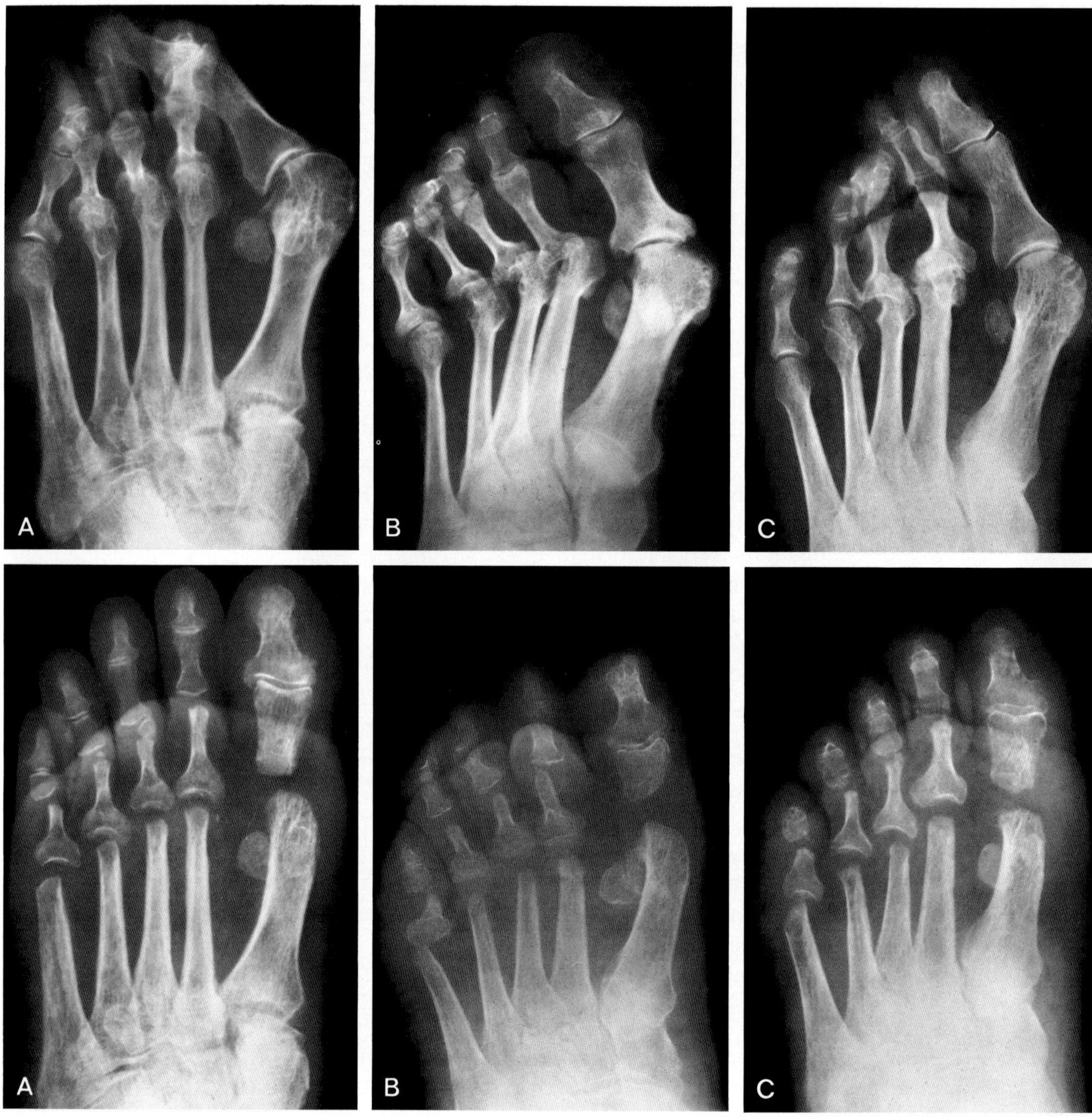

Fig. 36.5 A–H. Surgical treatment of rheumatic conditions of forefoot. **A–E** Preoperative and postoperative appearances in five patients with rheumatoid arthritis treated by Lelièvre realignment of forefoot. **D–H** see ▷ pp. 521–523

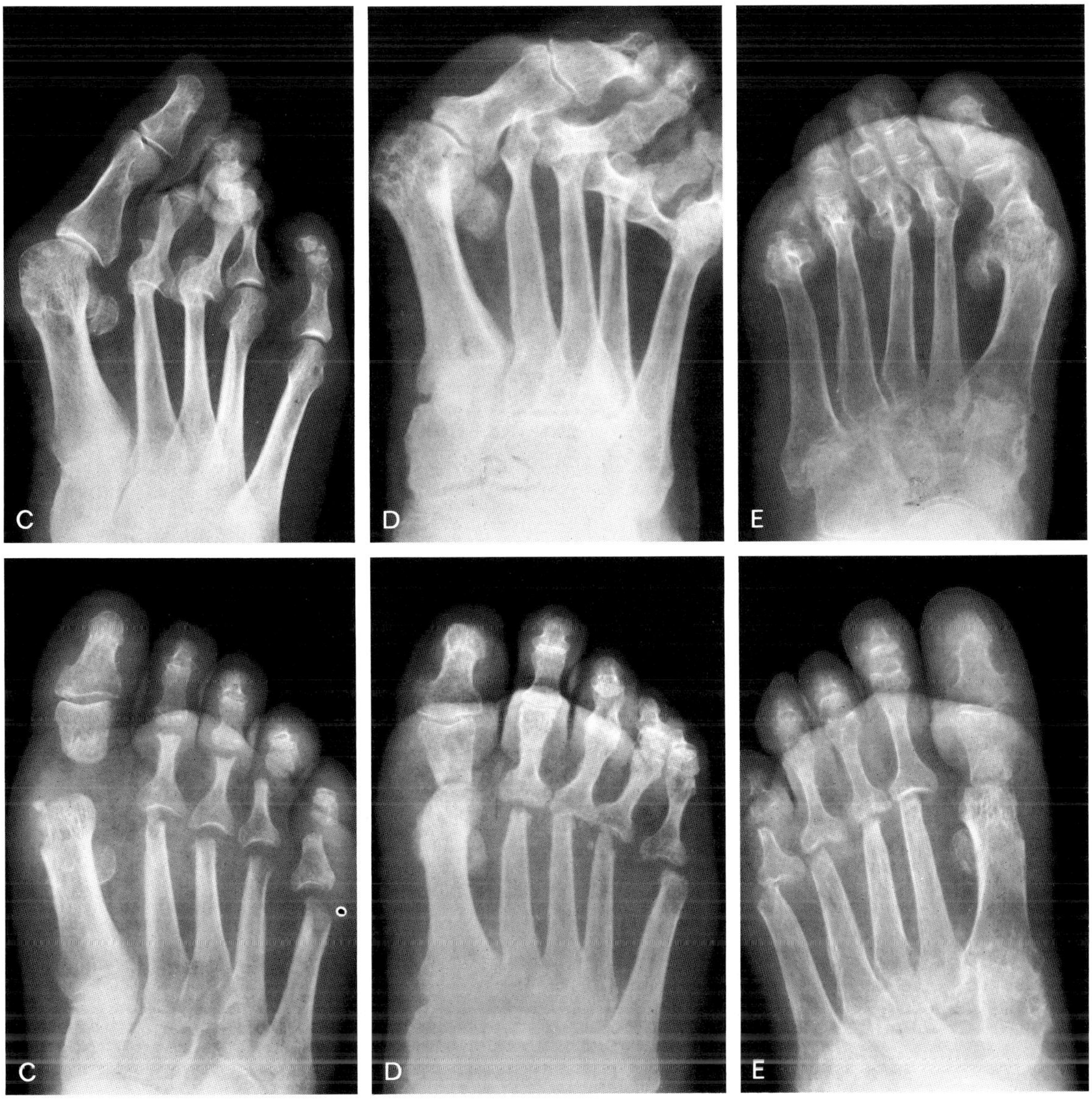

Fig. 36.5 C–E. Legend see p. 520

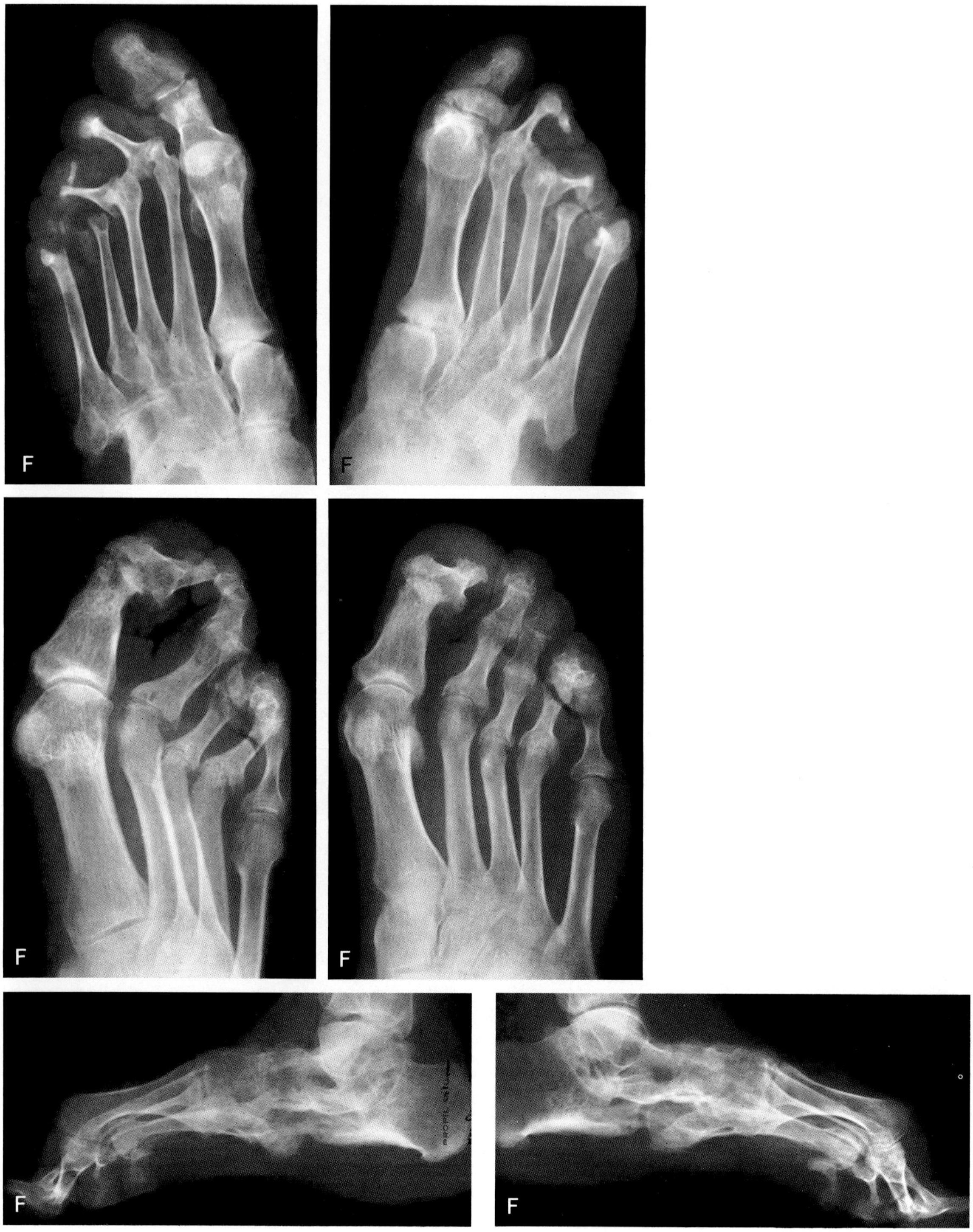

Fig. 36.5 *(continued)*. **F** Ankylosing spondylitis: internal and external lateral views. **G** Rheumatoid arthritis with dislocation of foot. *1* Before surgery; *2* left foot after Lelièvre metatarsal realignment; *3* right foot after metatarsal realignment with implantation of metatarsal prostheses. **H** Metatarsophalangeal arthropathy due to gout. ▷ *1* Before surgery; *2* left foot after head-shaft enclavement in 1970; *3* right foot after implantation of metatarsal prostheses in 1971

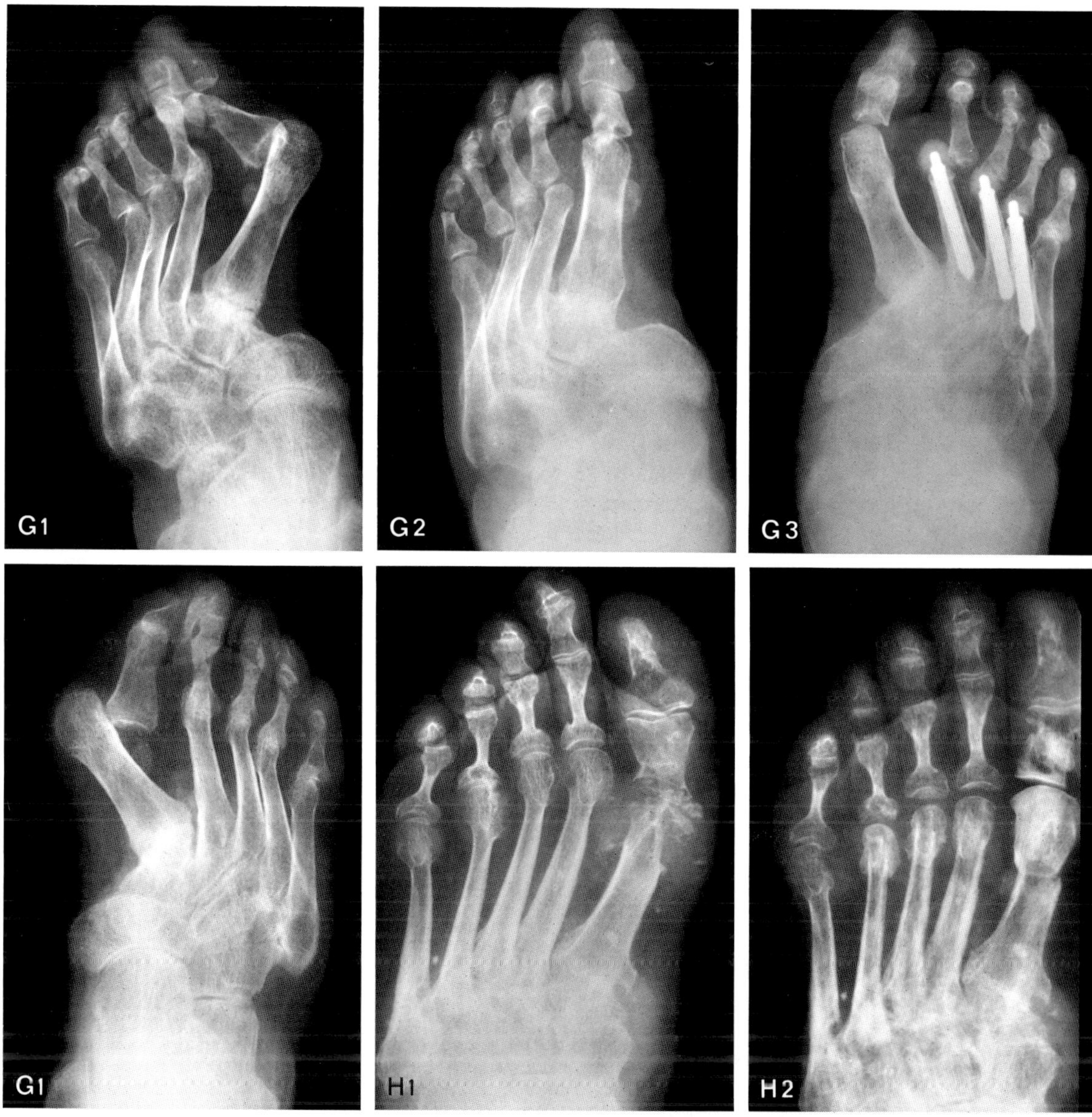

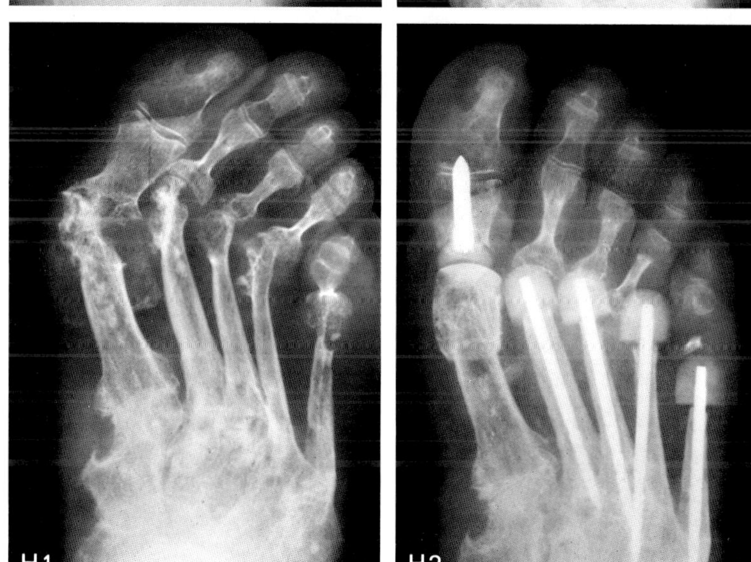

Fig. 36.5 G–H. Legend see p. 522

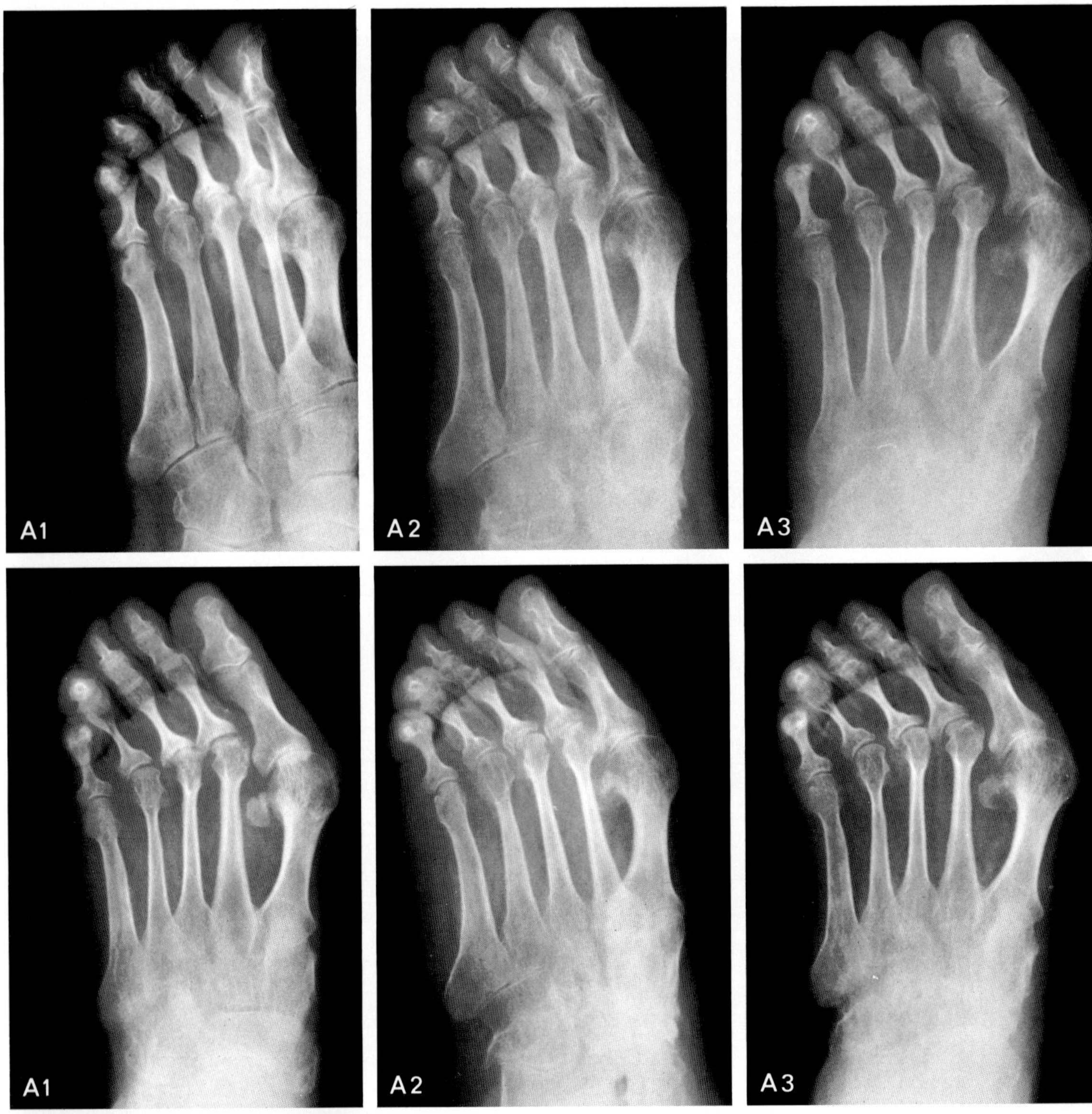

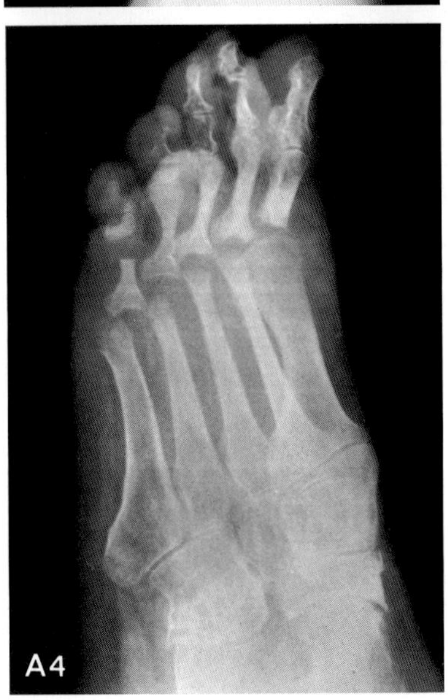

Fig. 36.6 A, B. Development and surgical treatment of chronic rheumatoid ▷ arthritis in a 40-year-old patient. **A** Left foot. *1* February 1978: metatarsophalangeal arthritis, hallux valgus, lateral windswept deformity, osteonecrosis; *2* December 1978: further development; *3* November 1980: further development; *4* after correction of hallux valgus with graft, Lelièvre realignment of second to fifth metatarsals, interposition of cup prostheses, elongation of long and short extensor tendons, arthroplasty of fifth toe; *5* appearance a year after operation. **B** Right foot: metatarsophalangeal arthritis, hallux valgus, lateral windswept deformity, osteonecrosis (especially marked in second metatarsophalangeal joint). *1* Before surgery; *2* after correction of hallux valgus by arthroplasty with graft, head-shaft enclavement of second, third and fourth metatarsals, elongation of long and short extensor tendons; *3* a year after operation: good general alignment of metatarsophalangeal joints, ankylosis of second metatarsophalangeal joint necessitating interposition of a cup prosthesis

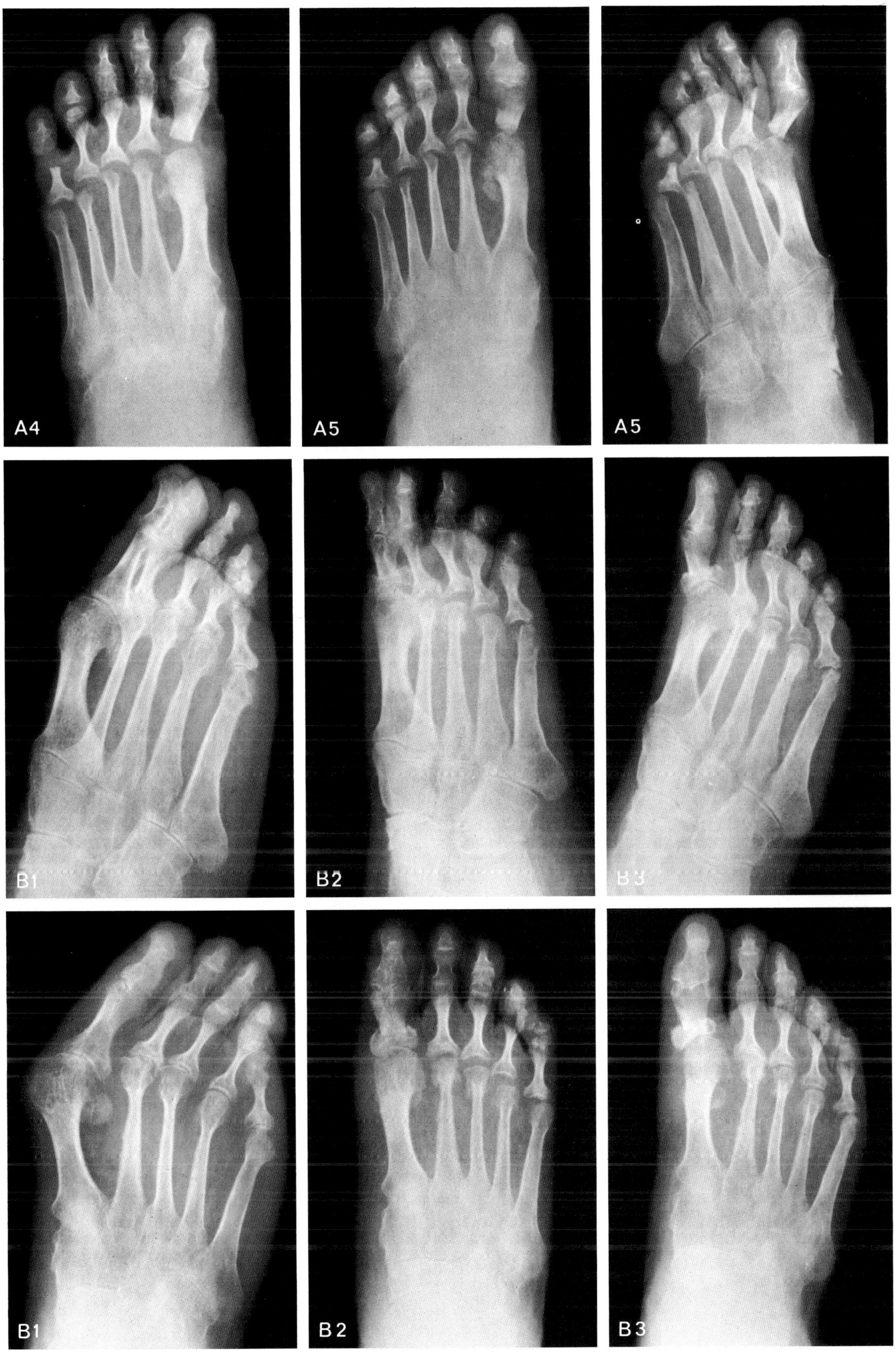
A4
A5
A5
B1
B2
B3
B1
B2
B3

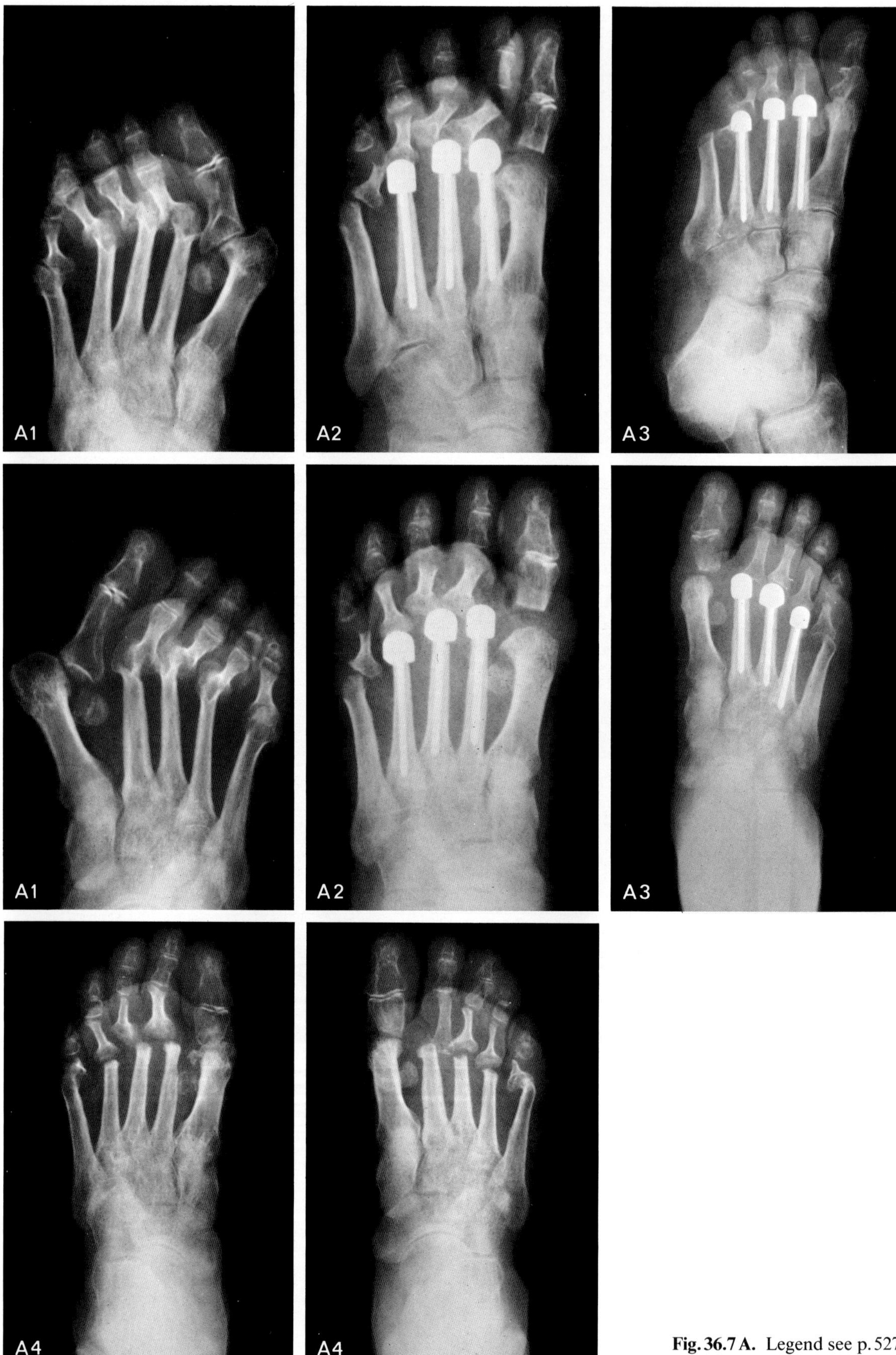

Fig. 36.7 A. Legend see p. 527

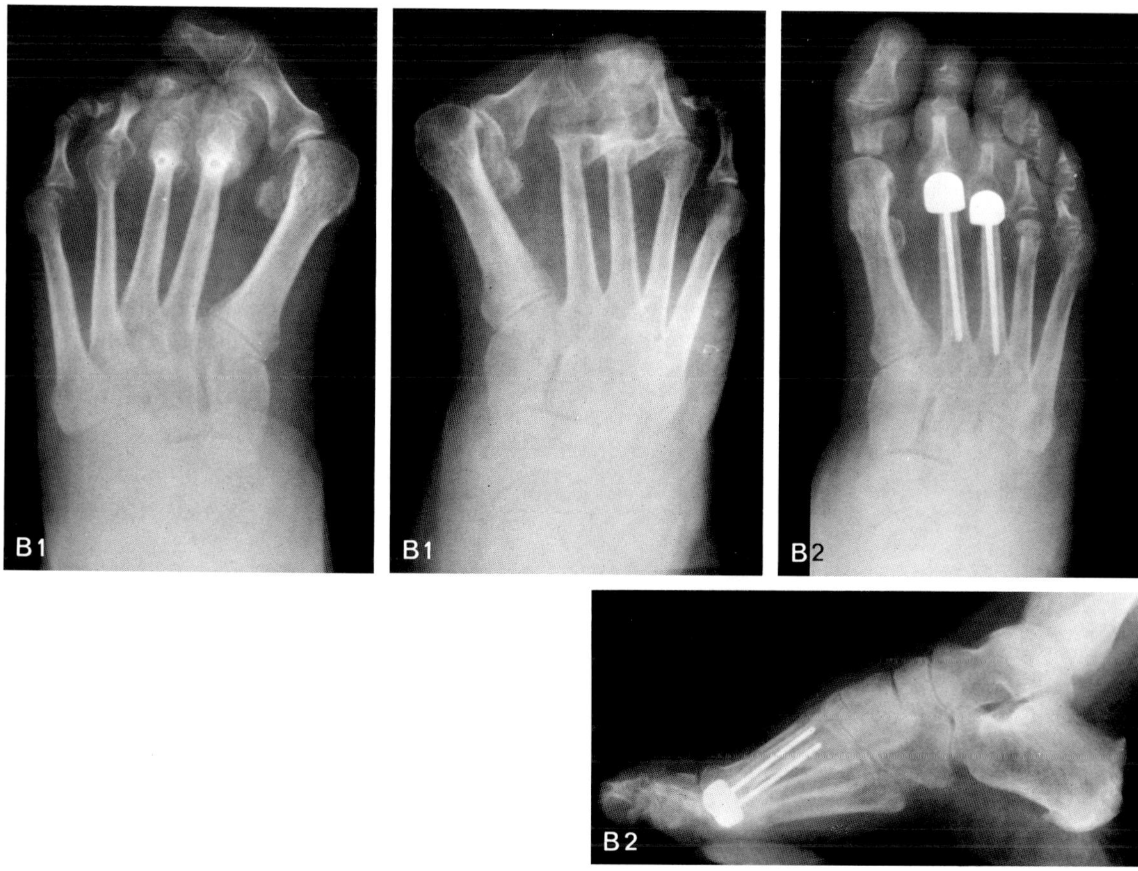

◁ **Fig. 36.7 A, B.** Surgical treatment of rheumatoid arthritis in simple triangular forefoot (Locke syndrome). **A** Metatarsophalangeal dislocation, lateral windswept deformity, metatarsophalangeal arthropathy. *1* Before surgery; *2* left foot after Lelièvre realignment of metatarsus, correction of hallux valgus and interposition of a cup prosthesis, implantation of metatarsal prostheses in second, third and fourth metatarsals; *3* right foot after same procedures; *4* both feet after removal of prostheses 2 years later. **B** Irregular dislocation, third-degree hallux valgus, clawing and varus deformity of toes. *1* Before surgery; *2* right foot 6 months after correction of hallux valgus by metatarsophalangeal arthroplasty using cup prosthesis, metatarsal prostheses for second and third heads, neck-shaft enclavement of fourth metatarsal, arthroplasty of second, third and fourth proximal interphalangeal joints, elongation of long and short extensor tendons, detachment of insertions of long and short flexor tendons of toes

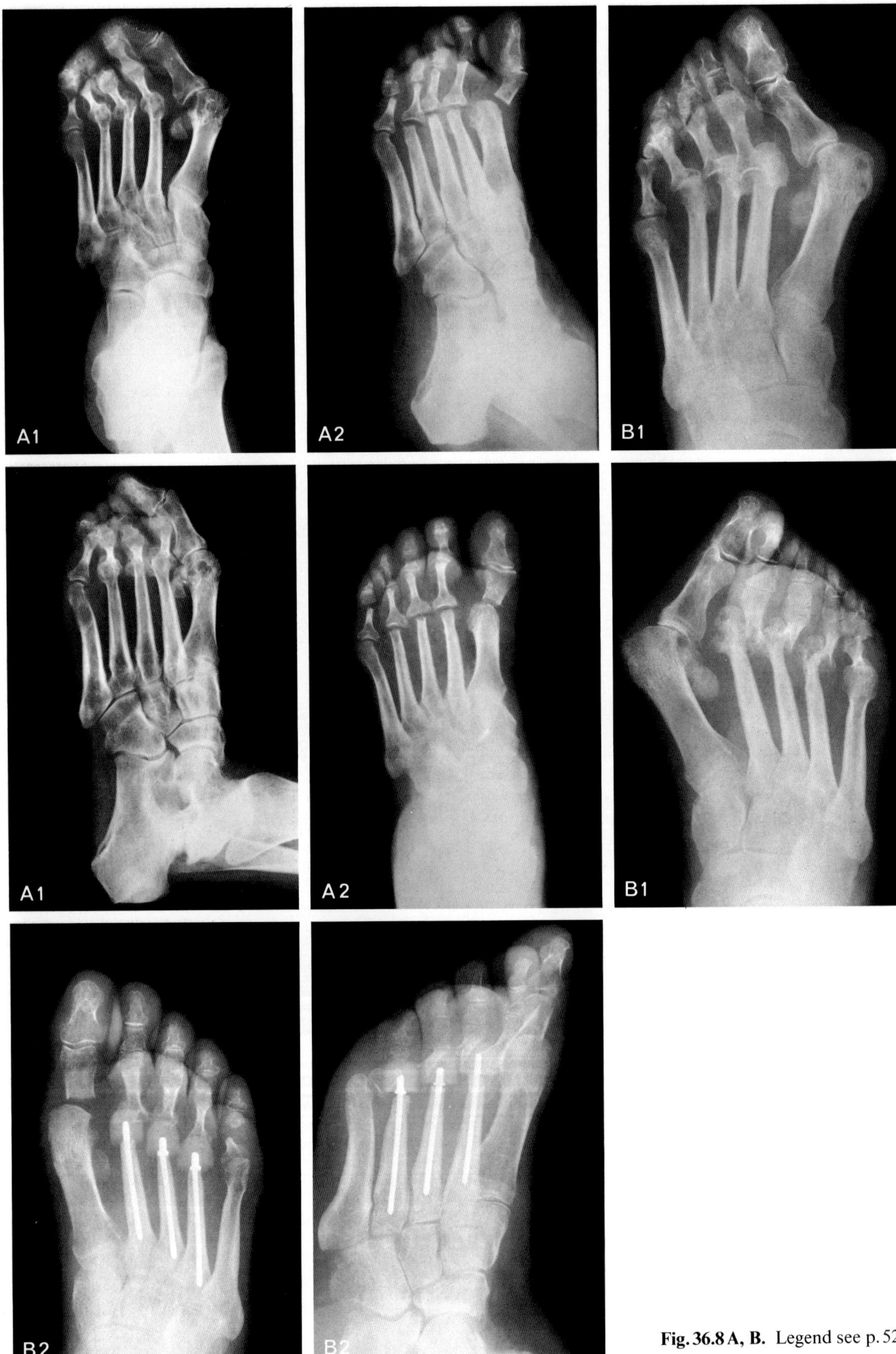

Fig. 36.8 A, B. Legend see p. 529

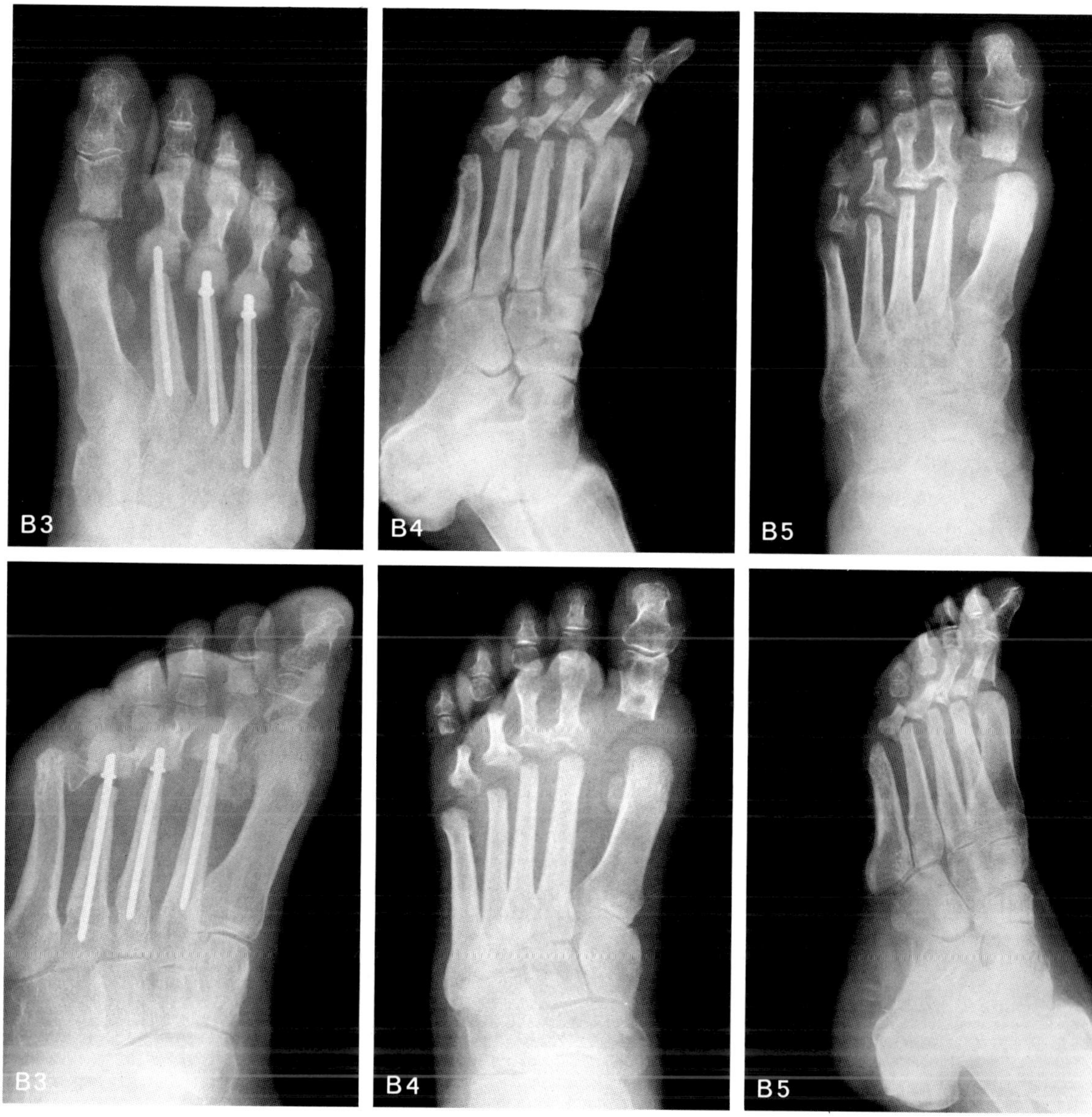

◁ **Fig. 36.8 A, B.** Surgical treatment of rheumatoid arthritis. **A** Left foot: flat forefoot with ankylosis of the metatarsophalangeal joints, lateral windswept deformity, claw toes. *1* Before surgery; *2* after Lelièvre realignment of first to fourth metatarsals, interposition of cup prostheses, arthroplasty of proximal interphalangeal joints of second to fifth toes, elongation of long and short extensor tendons. **B** Left foot: hallux valgus, metatarsophalangeal dislocation with dorsolateral dislocation, involvement of condyle. Right foot: metatarsophalangeal joint arthropathies. *1* Both feet before surgery; *2* right foot 8 days after arthroplasty of first metatarsophalangeal joint using cup prosthesis, insertion of metatarsal prostheses in second, third and fourth metatarsals; *3* right foot 3 years after operation; *4* left foot 8 days after realignment and modelling (Lelièvre) of metatarsal heads, elongation of long and short extensor tendons, arthroplasty of all metatarsophalangeal joints using cup prostheses; *5* left foot 2 years after operation

37 Ankylosing Spondylitis

Ankylosing spondylitis, otherwise known as rhizomelic spondylosis or rheumatoid spondylitis, is a disease of unknown origin, although recent work has determined a genetic factor: the leucocyte group W27 is found in many patients. According to Bontoux (1967) it can occur simultaneously with or after an attack of psoriasis, Reiter's syndrome (1916) or Crohn's disease. It was first described by Connos in the seventeenth century and was more precisely defined by Strumple, von Bechterew and Marie.

The condition is characterised by a chronic, extensive, inflammatory rheumatic condition leading to ankylosis of symmetrical distribution. It occurs in young men from 18 to 40 years of age, mostly around the 25th year. The principle sites involved are the sacro-iliac joints, the spine and, in 6%-20% of cases, the foot, where the calcaneum, the midtarsus and exceptionally the forefoot are affected.

Serre et al. (1970) stressed the predilection towards the outer four metatarsals.

37.1 Clinical Features

The disease begins most frequently in the lumbosacral region, where the onset of pain is localised to the intervertebral lumbar joints and the sacro-iliac joints. The pain irradiates from the small of the back into the buttocks and thighs. It is at first episodic, occurring with maximum intensity during the night, causing insomnia and succeeded by stiffness on getting up which settles with activity. Pains may also arise from arthritis in the knee or foot; all areas may become involved, or the arthritis may remain localised to one site. Iritis can be an accompanying feature.

In 40% of cases the presenting symptom may be pain in the foot, and Simon, Claustre and Serre have emphasised the frequency of bilateral, symmetrical talalgia localised posteriorly or posteromedially. Pain in the foot in a young man indicates further investigation.

More rarely, there can be pain in the back and the intercostal joints, mono-arthritis of a hip, knee or ankle or, at the other extreme, panarthritis of an algodystrophic type. Occasionally, the toes and metatarsophalangeal joints are the primary site, but in the majority of cases, these anterior lesions occur in more advanced stages.

In the *established condition* the earlier features are more permanently present and peripheral pain relates especially to the hips, the shoulders, the knees and the feet. Braun (1975b) emphasised bony hypertrophy around the calcaneum and midtarsus together with destructive lesions in the forefoot. Tendinoperiostitis around the calcaneum and midtarsus is characterised by intermittent chronic and increasingly severe episodes of pain exacerbated by pressure or movement. Progressive stiffness leads to total ankylosis.

Biochemical examination exhibits a paucity of signs, except for the elevated erythrocyte sedimentation rate. Synovial biopsy shows discrete hyperplasia of the basal layers of the synovium, cellular infiltration, islands of ossification in the synovial and capsular tissues, sclerosis and endarteritis obliterans.

Radiography: In the spine, ossification of the intervertebral joints results in syndesmoses, beginning in the dorsolumbar region and spreading progressively to involve the whole column, which straightens, flexes and angulates (Bontoux). Bony ankylosis of the posterior articular joints occurs. The spinal involvement is typical and indicates the need for radiographic examination of other joints of the thorax, especially the costovertebral, sternoclavicular and acromioclavicular joints.

Lesions of different types occur around the calcaneum in ankylosing spondylitis, psoriatic rheumatism and non-specific urethritis. In ankylosing spondylitis the lesions are limited to exostoses of varying contours, perhaps diffuse on the plantar aspect of the bone. There is little associated destruction and the hypertrophy is not marked. Above, some demineralisation and patchy condensation of bone can be seen (Braun). The calcaneum may appear spongy or barbed due to the microgeodic erosions. The zones of demineralisation may be limited to serous bursae or may be sited along the posterior border of the bone.

Ankle and midtarsal arthritis is indicated by narrowing of the joint spaces, osteoporosis alternating with osteophytosis, the latter being particularly marked at the ankle and dorsal aspects of the midtarsal joints. The dorsum of the foot appears distorted by the protrusions of the osteophytes and has even been likened to a hedgehog. The appearance is not, however, pathognomonic of ankylosing spondylitis. Occasionally, there is evidence of decalcification associated with an inflamed foot.

In the forefoot, the arthritic process is more destructive than in the hindfoot, involving, according to Simon, Claustre and Serre, the outer four metatarsophalangeal joints (Fig. 37.1 A–D).

The interphalangeal joint of the great toe can be involved, but its metatarsophalangeal joint usually remains unaffected. The lesions are similar to those seen in rheumatoid arthritis in the epiphyseal regions, where osteoporosis, subchondral lysis, and narrowing of the joint space occur successively, followed by the appearance of erosions with notching and cupping leading to subluxation, dislocation and various deformities. The forefoot is sometimes in varus, sometimes in plantarflexion, or, more rarely, has a windswept appearance.

37.2 Treatment

37.2.1 General

General treatment is essentially a rheumatological problem, comprising administration of anti-inflammatory agents (especially pyrazoles and indomethacin) and local corticosteroids, occasional chemical or radioactive synovectomy, radiotherapy, and analgesics.

Physiotherapy consists of respiratory exercises and careful mobilisation to prevent deformity following the stiffening of the joints; the latter is performed especially during periods of remission, perhaps with the use of a lumbosacral support.

37.2.2 Insoles

Orthopaedic insoles are designed to stabilise, support and protect the foot. In no instance must they be corrective. Pain from metatarsalgia and calluses can be avoided by appropriate support or excavation for prominent metatarsal heads. The insoles should be very well padded, supple and thick.

37.2.3 Operative

Operative intervention is indicated only in cases of serious disability and is undertaken after stabilisation of the disease process. Arthroplasty of the hip and knee will contribute to comfort in the foot. Arthrodesis of the ankle joint may be indicated.

Interposition cup arthroplasty of the metatarsophalangeal joints, perhaps after Lelièvre (1952) realignment procedures, offers a solution when the metatarsal heads are destroyed, and may also be useful after continued iatrogenic symptoms following the resection of metatarsal heads and phalangeal bases advised by Clayton (1960a, b).

The Lelièvre and Clayton operations performed alone are likely to lead to fresh ankylosis and more metatarsophalangeal displacement. The interposition cup arthroplasty preserves mobility. In extreme cases, the implantation of intramedullary metatarsal head prostheses is the last resort, but success depends on the state of the metatarsal shafts, which may be severely atrophied.

I am of the view that surgical treatment is more efficacious if undertaken during a stable controlled period of the general condition but before extensive ankylosis has occurred. At such a time, synovectomy and capsulotomy, with or without the interposition cup prostheses, have some chance of success.

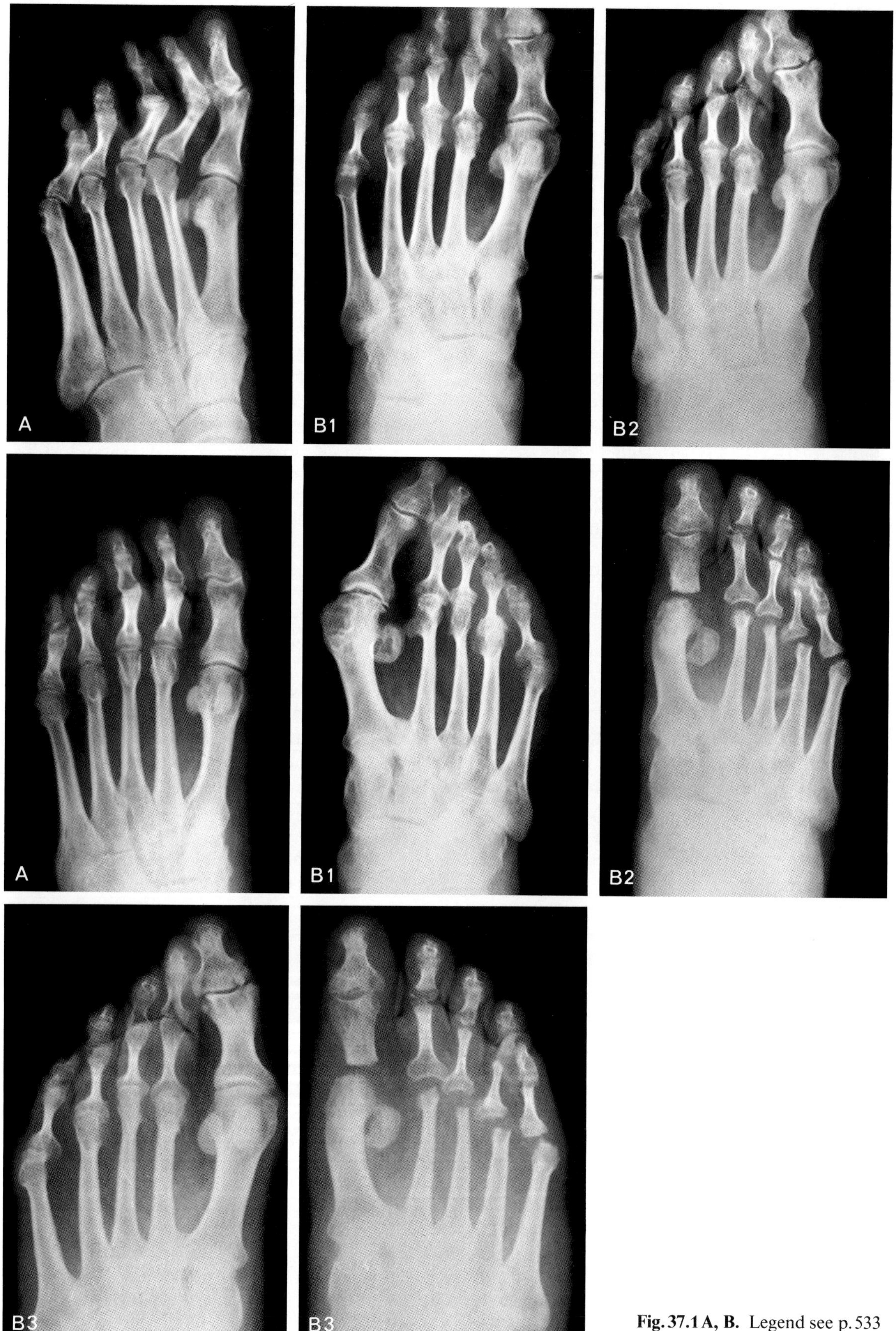

Fig. 37.1 A, B. Legend see p. 533

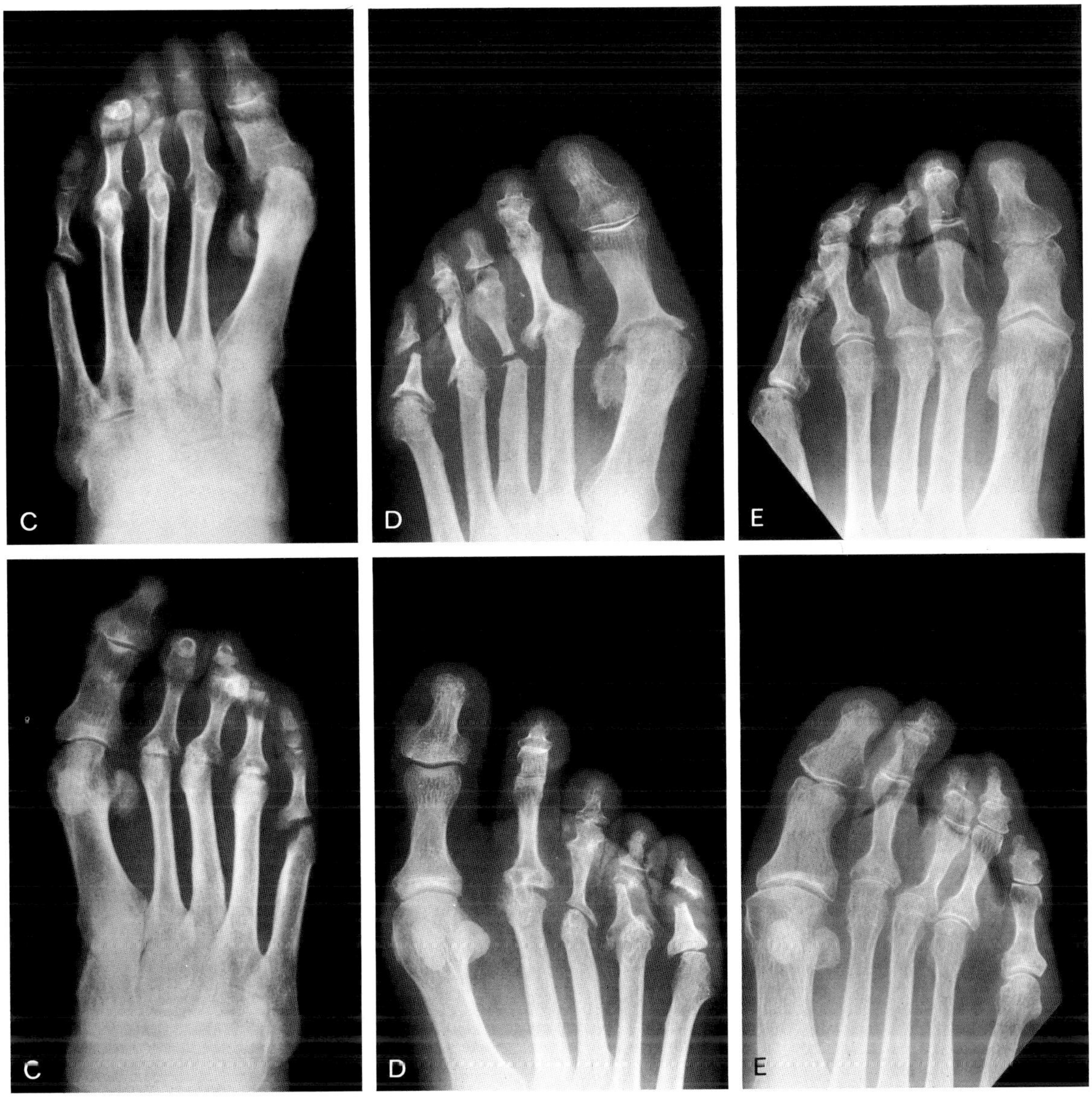

◁ **Fig. 37.1. A** Ankylosing spondylitis: early notching of condyle most marked in fifth ray. **B** Ankylosing spondylitis with ankylosis of metatarsophalangeal joints. *1* Before surgery, *2* 2 weeks after realignment, interposition of cup prosthesis in first metatarsophalangeal joint (right foot); *3* 2 months after operation. **C** Rheumatoid arthritis with telescoping of metatarsophalangeal joints. **D** Psoriatic arthritis with arthropathy of metatarsophalangeal joints. **E** Rheumatoid arthritis of 3 years' duration with developing lesions

38 Psoriatic Arthritis

Psoriatic arthritis was first described in 1880 by Besnier and Bourdillon; other descriptions were made by Sherman (1952), Loyau (1958), Avila (1960), Wright (1961), Fehr (1967) and Dryll (1973). Bret drew attention for the first time to involvement of the toes.

Psoriatic arthritis is rare, amounting to only 5% of the total incidence of polyarthritis (Coste 1946). Both sexes are affected, but the condition is somewhat more common in men at about the age of 30 years. The characteristic lesions of the nails occur most frequently some 10 years after the skin manifestations. Occasionally, articular involvement precedes or is simultaneous with the cutaneous lesions. Psoriatic arthritis supervenes in 3%–5% of cases of psoriasis (Bontoux). It is not contagious or hereditary, but Lang regarded it as being due to a parasite.

Joint involvement is most marked in the hands, feet, sacro-iliac joints and cervical spine. The condition is asymmetrical, with some features of osteoarthritis; the radiographic signs of osteolytic lesions of the joints (Fournié 1975) are frequently late. There is an absence of abnormal results in biochemical tests, in contrast to rheumatoid arthritis and ankylosing spondylitis. Irregular exacerbations are characteristic, and the condition ranges from relatively benign to very disabling.

38.1 Clinical Features

38.1.1 Cutaneous Manifestations

The skin lesions prove the psoriatic origin of the condition. The mucous membranes are not involved. The distribution of the lesions is as follows:

1. The central parts of the extensor surfaces of the limbs, especially the elbows and knees (Chatelain 1896), display desquamating, powdery lesions of varying thickness, stratified and accompanied by flaking. They are white in colour – matt, yellowish or shiny – and rest on a dermis which is usually dry and either brilliantly smooth or creased, but is sometimes slightly moist, and is reddish-brown, contrasting with the surrounding healthy skin and giving a characteristic haemorrhagic appearance.
2. On the scalp, there is characteristically scurf or accumulation of squames on an irregular surface covered by hair which is dryer than normal. There may be a single plaque, extending over the whole scalp and projecting beyond it, delimited on the forehead and the back of the neck by a curved red line.
3. The eyelids may become affected by stiff, dry lesions, leading to ectropion.
4. On the hands and feet, the palmar or plantar surfaces can be involved but the dorsal aspects are spared, the squamous eruptions stopping at the borders of the dorsal skin. The thickening and rigidity of the epidermis impedes movement. Bazex et al. (1966) described the lesions as plantar postular trychophytoid psoriasis in the region of the interdigital commissures, in the form of either carbuncles or simple keratoderma.

38.1.2 Nail Lesions

Bret was the first to describe the nail lesions. There may be onyxis (Bazex et al (1966), or the changes may comprise opaque pigmentation or dry ecchymoses of thickened rugose areas situated in the substance of the nail, giving a punctate, furrowed or transversely striped appearance. The nails are fragile. These lesions can appear in isolation or simultaneously with the cutaneous manifestations. Meynadier and Guilhou (1977) described the histological features of the nail, which include hyperkeratosis of the subungual region which is the source of onycholysis and haemorrhages into the nail bed, and the alterations of the nail surface. When the lesions are proximal, there are transverse striae or little pin-head sized depressions ("pitting") like those on a thimble. When they are distal, there are patches of leuconychia and the nail becomes opaque. When the lesion is total, the nail disappears and is replaced by a hyperkeratotic crust.

Like the cutaneous lesions, the nail involvement progresses chronically with exacerbations, episodes being separated by remissions of several weeks, months or even years.

38.1.3 Osteoarticular Involvement

At the *onset,* osteoarticular lesions involve predominantly the hands, feet, sacro-iliac joints and cervical spine, but any area can be affected. The hip joint is usually spared, but even there an occasional isolated arthritis can occur.

Painful stiffness with associated brachalgia of variable intensity spreads downwards from the cervical spine to involve the lumbar spine and produce sciatica. The sacro-iliac joints are commonly bilaterally involved, and this sacro-iliitis is a feature of great diagnostic importance if it is associated with interphalangeal arthritis of the toes and fingers (Fournié 1977).

In the foot, lesions are very common; and in 85% of cases they involve the forefoot, in 72% the calcaneum, in 24% the tarsus and in 16% the heel (Fournié 1977). The condition is variable in onset, often insidious, and progressive. Most commonly only a few joints are involved, although some cases are more widespread, like rheumatoid arthritis. The pain produced is inflammatory in character, sharp and interspersed with subacute episodes. There is redness of the overlying periarticular tissue but no local elevation of temperature. The lesions are most commonly localised to the distal interphalangeal joints and are asymmetrical in 50% of cases. In the hindfoot there may be inflammatory talalgia of the subcalcaneal spur.

The condition develops slowly over several years or decades into established psoriatic arthritis, and was described by Coste (1946) as "mummifying polyarthritis".

In the *established state,* the foot presents trophic and arthritic features. The skin is withered, wrinkled, thin, adherent to the underlying tissues and without elasticity. The subcutaneous layer is extremely atrophied. Painful swelling of the affected joints is accompanied by stiffness or even ankylosis. The hands are less frequently involved than the foot. Deformity at the metatarsophalangeal joints is uncommon, but the interphalangeal joints become stiff and the toes develop dorsal and distal calluses which are particularly painful because of the subcutaneous atrophy. Clawing may develop, involving both interphalangeal joints, and occasionally the digits have a windswept appearance, usually outwardly. Transverse displacement with infraductus or supraductus may be seen, as may inverted clawing. The latter bayonet deformity comprises dorsiflexion of the proximal phalanx, plantarflexion of the middle phalanx and marked dorsiflexion of the distal phalanx. The digital deformities are rarely uniform, so that the five toes vary in shape.

In the metatarsophalangeal joint there is fixed dorsiflexion, perhaps with lateral deviation, held by fibrous contracture of the capsules and tendons. The integument generally becomes rigid and ankylosed.

In the hindfoot, the heel may be deformed by irregular thickening of the posterior tuberosity of the calcaneum. The subtalar and ankle joints are arthritic with loss of range of movement; the subtalar joint may develop a fixed valgus posture, giving the impression of a contracted rigid flat foot.

The patient is characteristically kyphotic and stiff and complains of lumbago and sciatica, but the hip joint is spared for a long time.

Radiography: The interphalangeal joints exhibit destruction, leading to an appearance of cupping or mushrooming of the bases of the distal phalanges and the heads of the proximal phalanges. A "pencil point" or "barley sugar" appearance is seen, with frequent resorption of the tufts of the distal phalanges. Ankylosis of the interphalangeal joints is characteristic (Avila et al. 1960). The appearance of the great toe, with osteophytosis of the interphalangeal joint and resorption of the tuft of the distal phalanx, is also characteristic (Figs. 37.1 F, 38.1 A).

In the metatarsophalangeal joints there is a polymorphic, asymmetrical picture comprising osteolysis of the metatarsal heads with ulceration and fusion leading to the same barley sugar appearance. There is radiographic evidence of accompanying modelling and attempts at reconstruction, together with excavation, flattening and widening of the phalangeal bases and thinning of their lateral apophyses. Epiphyseal periostitis of a spiculate or band-like nature may be seen. Intra articular ankylosis of the fifth metatarsophalangeal joint is particularly significant, but bilateral fusion of the great metatarsophalangeal joints can also occur (Recordier et al. 1975). Hallux valgus may be seen.

In the sesamoids there is frequent hypertrophy of an irregular notched appearance but otherwise without any specific character.

The calcaneum exhibits periostitis which may be very marked, irregular, and confined to the plantar aspect of the body of the bone (Fournié 1977). Sometimes the great tuberosity is irregularly thickened, leading to plaque-like armour-plating under

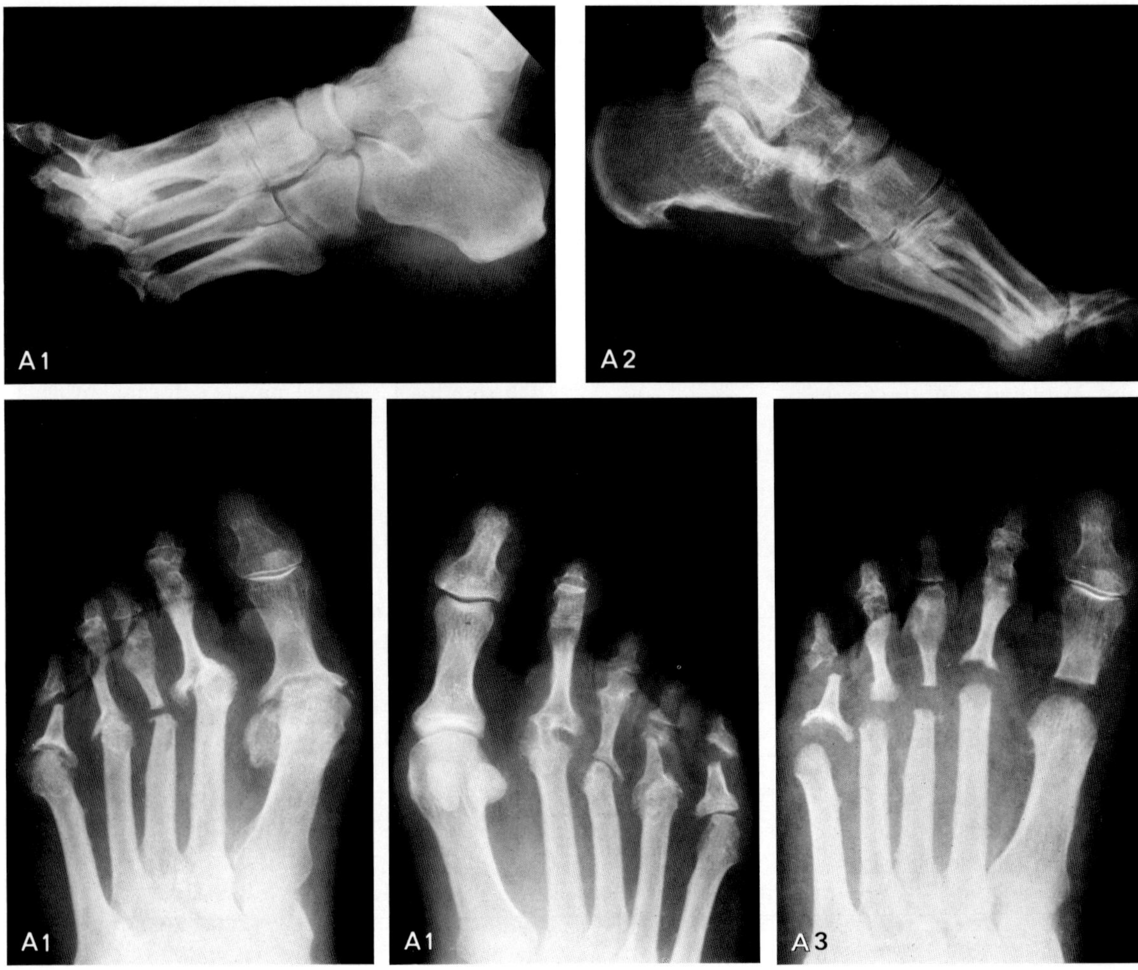

Fig. 38.1 A, B. Surgical treatment of psoriatic arthritis. **A** *1* Metatarsophalangeal arthropathy, metatarsophalangeal and interphalangeal osteolysis, telescoping of second metatarsophalangeal joint; *2* right foot, lateral view: arthritic process in naviculocuneiform joint; *3* left foot, dorsoplantar view: Lelièvre realignment of all metatarsals; *4* left foot, lateral view: interposition cup prostheses of first to fourth metatarsophalangeal joints; *5* left foot: appearance 6 months after operation. Right foot: onset ▷ of arthropathies; *6* left foot: appearance 2 years after operation. Right foot: development of arthropathies. **B** Right foot: early psoriatic arthropathy, osteonecrosis of condyles, dorsolateral subluxation of second to fifth metatarsophalangeal joints. *1* Before surgery; *2* 2 years after Lelièvre realignment. **A** *4–6*, **B** see p. 537

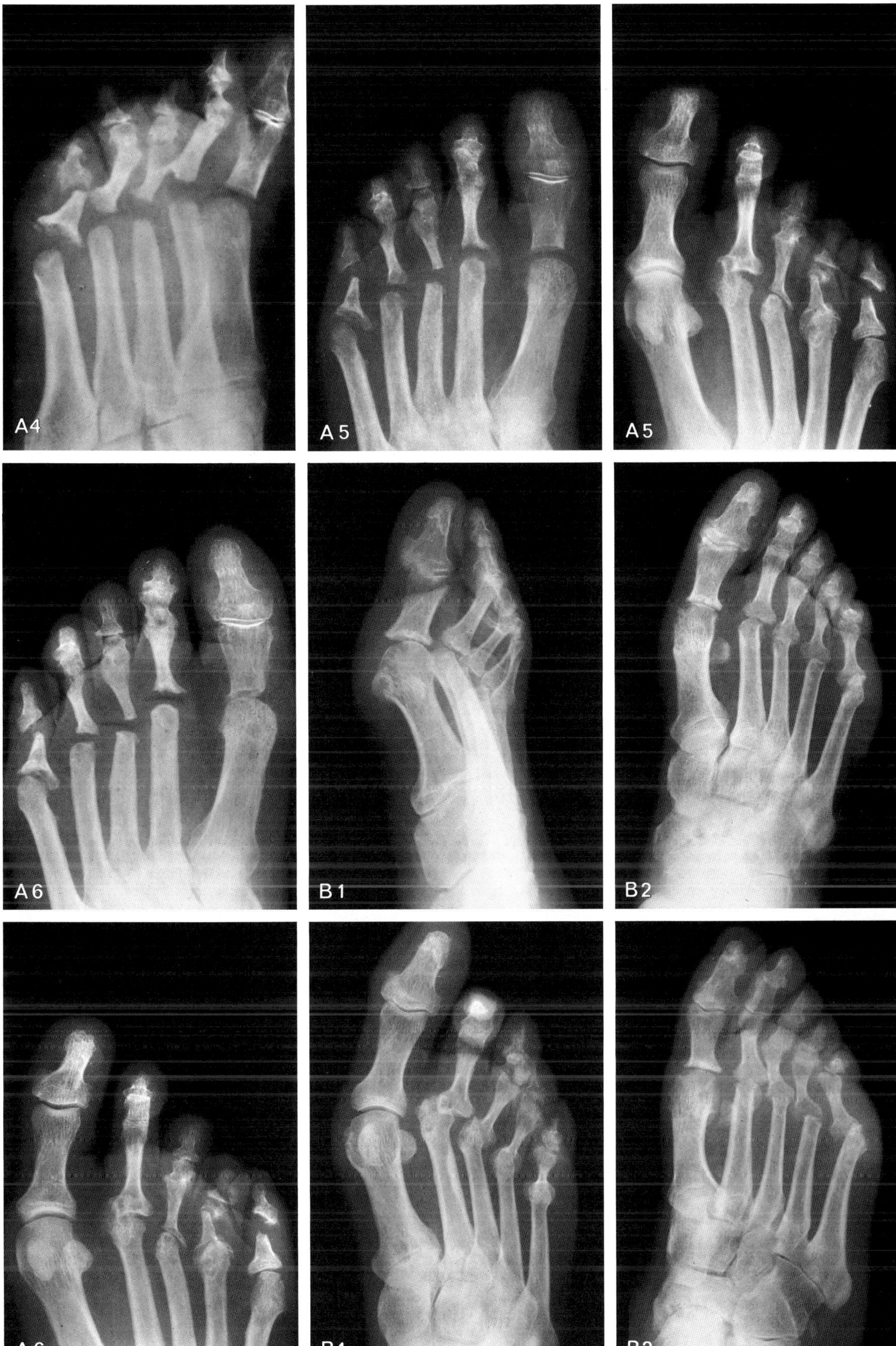
A4
A5
A5
A6
B1
B2
A6
B1
B2

the postero-inferior aspect prolonged to two extremities by spurs under the retrocalcaneal area (Braun 1975b). The bone may have a multiple spiny appearance.

The intertarsal joints may show alternating signs of fusion or osteolysis, giving the subtalar joint, for example, a "hairy" appearance. Involvement of the talonavicular joints may be uni- or bilateral, and geodic erosions of the cuboid may be seen. The ankle can be similarly afflicted.

In the hands, fusion and osteolysis with the characteristic resorption of phalangeal tufts are the main features. They are analogous to those of the foot but less frequent.

The sacro-iliac joints exhibit symmetrical sacroiliitis, especially significant when related to the signs of interphalangeal arthritis (Fournié 1975).

In the cervical spine, marginal osteophytosis affecting the bodies (in contrast to ankylosing spondylitis) and images of ossification of the paravertebral tissue with a flowing contour, but without contact with vertebral body or a disc, are features which Bywaters and Dixon (1965) regarded as particularly indicative of psoriatic arthritis.

Biochemical Investigations: Fournié (1975) noted the frequency of the antigen HLA-B27 and remarked that the presence or absence of rheumatoid factor was not of diagnostic importance. The erythrocyte sedimentation rate is elevated fairly constantly. There is no elevation of the blood immunocytes, unlike in rheumatoid arthritis (Delbarre).

Synovial biopsy reveals sclerosis and thickening of the walls of the small vessels, but there are no specific findings in the synovial fluid (Fournié 1975).

In conclusion, the diagnosis of psoriatic arthritis depends upon the coexistence of the arthritic process with cutaneous psoriasis; the association of pelvic and spinal arthritis with involvement of the limbs, above all the distal interphalangeal joints; the radiographic criteria described above (Avila et al. 1960) and the asymmetry of these seronegative lesions.

38.2 Treatment

38.2.1 Medical

Medical care comprises administration of analgesics (especially salicylates), indomethacin, antimalarials, phenylbutazone and, in severe cases only, corticosteroids.

38.2.2 Insoles

Orthopaedic insoles are especially important; they are fitted to large, comfortable, supple shoes and designed to support the foot. They should be made of thick, spongy, supple material. They are usually of the physiological monoblock type, but occasionally incorporate a retrocapital or subcapital bar according to the site of pain on loading.

38.2.3 Operative

Surgical indications are exceptional on account of the tendency for ankylosis to occur after any form of operation in these feet. Disorders of loading of the metatarsophalangeal joints can be treated by Lelièvre realignment or by Clayton resection of the metatarsophalangeal joints with interposition cup prostheses, or metatarsal head prostheses if there is longitudinal cavus (Fig. 38.1C–F). At the interphalangeal joints, arthrodesis to re-establish axial digital alignment may be indicated, while in the intertarsal joints, arthrodesis is the only means of relieving pain or progressive deformity.

39 Gout

Gout is a disease of multiple presentation. Joint involvement is common, and signs in the foot often constitute the first manifestation. The cardiovascular system, the alimentary tract, the liver and the kidneys are also affected by the overload of urates and uric acid due to both excessive production and deficient elimination (Sorensen 1969).

Historically, the disease is interesting. Almost exclusively males are afflicted, including such famous names as Seneca, Michaelangelo, Pitt, Calvin, Luther, Baron, Franklin, Darwin, Newton, Lamartine, Chateaubriand, the Medicis and the Bourbons. Hippocrates stated that it was never found in women or in children before puberty. In the sixth century, Alexander of Talles proved the efficacy of colchicine in the management of the acute crisis, but it was Sydenham (1693) who gave the first accurate clinical description. Scheele (1776) discovered uric acid. Wollaston (1797) showed that the tophus was constituted by sodium urate, while Garrod (1848) detected the accompanying hyperuricaemia. Horbaczewski (1889) and subsequent modern authors progressively elaborated our knowledge of purine metabolism. More recently, McCarthy and Hollander (1961) demonstrated that acute gout is provoked by the precipitation of microcrystals of uric acids in the joints and that it is the phagocytosis secondary to this which causes the painful inflammation.

Of great importance is our present knowledge that early efficacious treatment of the acute episode and subsequent control leads to cure and avoids the appearance of the disabling chronic gouty foot (Gutman et al. 1971). Thus, a disease known for thousands of years and causing great disability in the foot can now be controlled by medical therapy although the basic metabolic disorder will persist in these patients (Mostini 1979).

Typically, gout affects the man of about 40 years of age. It occurs in all races, more commonly in sedentary people, big eaters and those prone to lithiasis, arthrosis, eczema and obesity. There is a familial trend on the paternal side. Consideration of gout can be divided into the acute attack and the chronic sequelae of ill- or non-treated acute episodes.

39.1 Acute Gout

39.1.1 Clinical Features

The description made by Sydenham (1693) remains accurate. The victim goes to bed in good health but is awakened at about two o'clock in the morning by intense pain, usually in the big toe, less commonly in the heel, the ankle or the ball of the foot. The pain is comparable in intensity to that of a dislocation and the affected spot feels as if it has been dowsed with cold water. The pain then assumes a violent stretching character as if the ligaments were being torn, yielding to a feeling of burning and then a sensation of pressure. Sometimes, the pain is so acute that the patient cannot bear the weight of the bedclothes resting on it, or even the vibrations of a person walking about the room. The night passes in torment.

This acute painful arthritis of the great toe supervenes almost always on latent asymptomatic gout, of which it is the first clinical presentation. The left great toe is more often affected than the right. Local inflammatory signs comprise warmth, swelling of the integument, with shiny violaceous skin, and vasodilatation of the peripheral veins of the foot. An apparent abscess can develop (no attempt should be made to incise it) with variable fever oscillating between 38° and 40° C, shivering and general distress. The conjunctivae may be injected, and gastro-intestinal and cardiovascular symptoms prevail. The regression of the attack leads to a general relaxation, and the patient is able to sleep again. The local signs persist for a while after the acute attack. The swelling of the tissues does not pit like typical oedema.

The acute episode can affect other parts of the foot in a similar way: the midtarsal region, the instep, the heel, the malleoli, the Achilles tendon or, most rarely, the extensor tendons. Whatever the site, the patient's good general health contrasts with the severity of the local symptoms.

The crisis lasts for some 2–10 days and then settles progressively over a further period of several days to 2 weeks. After the 2nd day, the wine-red discoloration of the great toe changes to bright red, then violet. The shiny skin looks varnished like that of an onion with folds and grooves and later desquamation. The latter is accompanied by itching which occasionally becomes intense and leads to further injury from scratching.

During the acute episode, the erythrocyte sedimentation rate may be elevated and the hyperuricaemia may exceed 70 g/100 ml. Joint aspiration fluid contains microcrystals of urate.

Radiography after the crisis often shows no abnormality, but occasionally reveals small vacuolar erosions in the head of the first metatarsal indicative of previous undiagnosed episodes.

The asymptomatic period after settling of the crisis is extremely variable, and successive attacks may be delayed for months or years. Coste (1946) stresses the diagnostic importance of the gross severity of the attack and the completely symptom-free intermissions. Subsequent attacks can involve other joints in irregular distribution, including the knee and the elbow, and can be precipitated by trauma of any nature, even emotional, as well as by an overtight shoe, excessive physical activity and overeating, especially with spirits or other alcoholic beverages. The possibility of an attack following a completely unrelated surgical procedure should not be forgotten. The differential diagnosis is from other acute arthritic conditions with an elevated erythrocyte sedimentation rate, especially a particularly acute onset of rheumatoid arthritis or ankylosing spondylitis. The latter typically afflicts a subject under 30 years old and the pain and inflammation are less acute than in gout.

39.1.2 Treatment

Early and prolonged medical management is vital in order to avoid the late tophaceous arthropathic complications of chronic gout.

Pain can be controlled early by the administration of 4 mg colchicine on the first day and then 3 mg and 2 mg on successive days. Anti-inflammatory drugs are efficacious (phenylbutazone or indomethacin). Subsequently, the hyperuricaemia must be controlled by the administration of uricosuric agents, e.g. probenecid, and inhibitors of uric acid synthesis, e.g. allopurinol and thiopurinol. A dietary regime excluding nucleoproteins, purines and alcohol must be instituted.

In a particularly severe attack, ACTH may be administered with the colchicine.

39.2 Chronic Gout

In most cases, the relationship between chronic tophaceous gout and previous acute episodes is obvious. However, the relationship is extremely variable in time, and there are cases in which the chronic condition apparently develops insidiously. The interval between the first crisis and the onset of the chronic phase can be 5, 10 or even 25 years.

Chronic tophaceous gout in the foot amounts to a destructive polyarthropathy with osteolysis and without reconstructive processes, and leads to displacement of joints, which are filled by urate granulomata. Cartilaginous arthropathy characterised by osteolytic lesions, extends to the subchondral bone.

39.2.1 Clinical Features

The following parts of the foot are affected in descending order of frequency: the metatarsophalangeal, interphalangeal and metatarsosesamoidal joints of the first ray; the corresponding joints of the other rays; the midtarsal joint; the tarsometatarsal joint line; the talonavicular joint; the calcaneocuboid joint; the ankle and the calcaneum. The parts affected are swollen, irregular and bossilated, and the tophi show up white under the skin surrounded by pink, red or cyanotic areas which become greyish in the cutaneous depressions between the stretched areas (see Fig. 17.4G–I). Pain is provoked by shoe pressure and aggravated by loading, as well as being produced by the hypermobility, which may reach neuropathic proportions, and associated deformities. Stiffness or ankylosis can develop from the excessive swelling.

The appearance of the forefoot varies: The metatarsophalangeal joints may preserve their alignment or develop a dorsal subluxation and lateral or medial deviation. Hallux valgus is less common than hallux rigidus. At the interphalangeal joints, clawing and variable degrees of permanent swelling are seen. The longitudinal arch of the foot is normal or occasionally in cavus, flattening only when osteolytic arthropathies predominate at the midtarsal region.

Radiographic examination reflects the variable clinical features. Notably, there is an absence of osteoporosis. Alteration of joint cartilage leads to narrowing of the joint space, and vacuolar rounded areas of erosion are visible in the subchondral areas of the bones, being at first only a few millimetres in diameter. Notches in the diaphyso-epiphyseal areas can be small and multiple in a "honeycomb" pattern or larger (10–30 mm), isolated and spear-shaped. These geodic epiphyseal lesions coalesce, leading to more widespread areas of osteolysis which remain clearly defined and have sclerotic borders. They can measure some centimetres in diameter and are associated with marginal osteophytes. The association of the first and fifth metatarsophalangeal joints and the interphalangeal joint of the great toe is characteristic (see Fig. 36.5 H). Displacement of the metatarsophalangeal joint is delayed for a long time, commensurate with the clinical development of calluses and local pressure pain.

In the midtarsal region, the joint spaces are narrowed and marginal osteophytes may be present. Osteolysis of the joint surfaces may also be present. If large, the osteophytes may be obvious on the dorsum of the foot (hedgehog foot).

The calcaneum exhibits a discrete type of subcalcaneal spur, a retrocalcaneal exostosis or a diffuse appearance like "armour plating" over the posterior aspect (Kerbrat 1974).

39.2.2 *Treatment*

General measures include control of the acute attacks or disordered purine metabolism together with dietary restrictions, as described in Sec. 39.1.2. Protection from overloading of areas with callosities, usually under the metatarsal heads, can be achieved by the use of orthopaedic insoles in made-to-measure shoes of soft leather with large uppers and firm shanks.

Surgical management comprises occasional removal of tophi when their volume or site is producing severe pressure symptoms, the resection of a retrocalcaneal exostosis when it impedes shoewear and reconstructive operations when metatarsophalangeal arthropathy has led to severe disability. Lelièvre and Clayton realignment procedures of the metatarsals with interposition cup prostheses are most valuable. Amputation of toes should always be avoided.

VIII Treatment

40 Insoles

Orthotic measures - insoles and special shoes - are essential adjuncts to all other methods of treatment of foot disorders. In order for the measures to be effective, certain requisites must be observed:

1. The diagnosis of the condition to be treated must be established and understood.
2. The insole should be prepared under the supervision of the orthopaedist.
3. The insole should be constructed according to a prescription which describes the various features required for the foot concerned. This includes details of any shoe adaptations necessary after preparation of the insole itself. Parts of the shoe (e.g. the heel cup) against which the corrected or stimulated foot may bear require appropriate reinforcement.
4. The condition of the insole must be checked by the orthotist regularly every 4-6 months and new prescriptions prepared by the orthopaedist as frequently as necessary. The need for a change of insole depends upon the condition for which it is prescribed.

Insoles can be classified according to the mechanism of action they exert on the foot or according to the condition they are designed to treat. Both classifications will be offered, together with appropriate examples, in the following account. Insoles are generally made out of leather, but for delicate painful feet, softer material like foam rubber, rubber incorporating particulate leather, or felt can be used. Thermoplastic materials are available.

40.1 Mode of Action

Insoles are designed to *correct* a deformity, to *support*, to *relieve load* locally or to *compensate* for a fixed deformity either originating in the foot itself or resulting from some abnormality above (e.g. leg length inequality, vertebral abnormality). The elements of which the insole is constructed may be described according to the direction of action and the stimulating, stabilising, supporting, blocking or other function they may exercise.

40.1.1 Corrective Elements

The corrective elements of an insole exert their action in a foot deformity by producing a change in position of the foot so that consequent neuromuscular control produces a corrective influence. They may be said to exercise a *stimulating* dynamic action. Subsequently, the correction achieved can be protected by a less stimulating, or *stabilising* dynamic insole.
Mechanical effects exerted on different areas of the foot can be conveniently subdivided into posterior, midtarsal, anterior or generally longitudinal. The direction of corrective displacement completes the functional description of the device.

Posterior Supinating Stimulating Wedge. This is a triangular wedge situated under the postero-internal part of the calcaneum (Fig. 40.1 B). It rolls the part but does not push it, and must reach to the midline axis of the foot. It is utilised in the valgus heel of early infancy exercising a proprioceptive corrective influence, and is replaced at about 6 months to 1 year of age by a posterior supinating stabilising wedge. It can be tried in older subjects, but may not be tolerated.

Posterior Supinating Stabilising Wedge. This wedge, which is similar to its stimulating predecessor, is used in maintaining correction or as a means of pain relief in valgus deformity in the adult (Fig. 40.1 B).

Posterior Pronating Stimulating Wedge. The converse of the supinating wedges, this may be used as a proprioceptive corrective agent for the varus heel, as a trial of treatment in older persons, or to secure proprioceptive relaxation of the talocalcaneal complex, which is required in the majority of cases of varus deformity of the tarsus (Fig. 40.1 A).

Posterior Pronating Stabilising Wedge. This wedge is also used in the varus heel, either complementary to its stimulating pronating counterpart or for balancing the hindfoot. It initiates and encourages midtarsal and metatarsal pronation (Fig. 40.1 A).

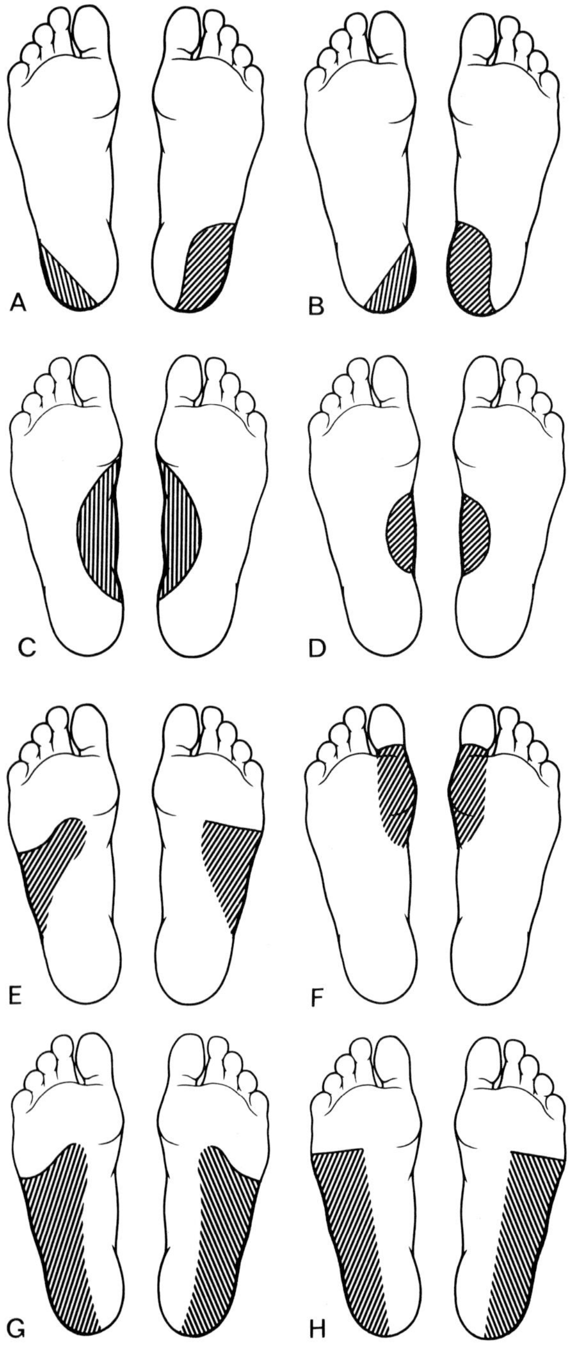

Fig. 40.1 A–H. Corrective elements of orthopaedic insoles. **A** Posterior pronating stimulating wedge, base posterolateral *(left)*, posterior pronating stabilising wedge, base lateral *(right)*. **B** Posterior supinating stimulating wedge, base posteromedial *(left)*, posterior supinating stabilising wedge, base medial *(right)*. **C** Internal dome. **D** Internal dome localised to navicular. **E** Retrocapital anterior pronating stabilising wedge, base lateral *(left)*, subcapital anterior pronating stabilising wedge, base lateral *(right)*. **F** Anterior supinating stimulating wedge, base medial. **G** Retrocapital external pronating bar, base lateral. **H** Subcapital external pronating bar, base lateral

Internal Metatarsal Dome. This may be localised and narrow, exerting exclusively a stimulating action under the navicular in the correction of valgus displacements of the foot, or may alternatively constitute a broad, longitudinal, transversely hemispherical dome extending to the midline axis of the foot with a stabilising action on the plantar arch affecting the whole of the internal border of the foot (Fig. 40.1 C). It is used in the presence of medial displacement in the valgus foot.

Subcuboidal Support. This comprises a triangular wedge based externally under the cuboid and is utilised in the general varus deformities of the foot, in supinated forefoot, and in genu varum. Depending on its height, it can stimulate or stabilise in early supple deformities.

Anterior Supinating Stimulating Wedge. A triangular wedge based medially, situated under the sesamoid of the first metatarsophalangeal joint, this is appropriate for the correction of planovalgus occurring in early infancy by a stimulating action. After the age of 6 months to 1 year, it is changed for a pronating stabilising device (Fig. 40.1 F).

Anterior Pronating Stabilising Wedge. This triangular wedge is based externally, situated under the fifth metatarsal. Its anterior margin may be retrocapital or subcapital according to whether it is necessary to stimulate or stabilise correction of supinated forefoot, metatarsus adductus or generalised eversion of the foot (Fig. 40.1 E, E').

Retrocapital Central Button. This is a small symmetrical rounded projection situated behind the heads of the second, third and fourth metatarsals. It can stimulate and restore vertical and lateral amplitude of movement of the first and fifth metatarsals in the correction of early convex forefoot deformity.

External Pronating Bar. This bar extends along the outer border of the foot from the heel to the retrocapital area (Fig. 40.1 G) or subcapital (Fig. 40.1 H) area of the fifth metatarsal. It is triangular in section with the base situated externally and constitutes a longitudinal corrective element. It is utilised in stimulating or stabilising correction of an overall varus of the foot sometimes associated with other elements of correction.

40.1.2 Supportive Elements

Supportive elements may be designed to support the foot vertically, transversely or longitudinally. Longitudinal support means prevention of longitudinal movement (i.e. horizontal) of the foot in the shoe. Vertical support relates to the midtarsus and the tarsus, while transverse control relates essentially to the position of the heel and the ball of the foot.
These elements are designed to prevent excessive movement of painful joints in cases not severe enough for, or untreatable by, surgical intervention.

Physiological Internal Metatarsal Dome. The term "physiological" is used here to indicate that the height of an element corresponds to that of the part of the foot it is designed to support. This is in contradistinction to the stimulating element, which exceeds this dimension and cannot be tolerated by the unsupple foot. In painful pes planus in the adult, the internal longitudinal arch can be supported, while in other cases, it can resist possible overpronation from stimulating or stabilising elements applied to the outer side of the foot (Fig. 40.2 A).

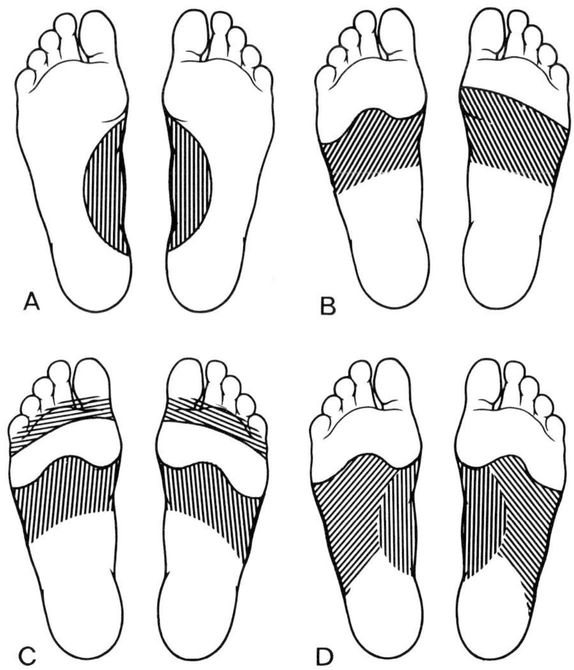

Fig. 40.2 A–D. Supporting elements. **A** Internal midtarsal physiological dome, base medial. **B** *Left:* retrocapital bar; *right:* subcapital bar. **C** Antecapital bar (with retro capital bar). **D** Monoblock physiological insole

Retrocapital or Subcapital Bar. This comprises a flat longitudinal and transverse element the anterior border of which may be retrocapital (forming a rounded edge just behind the plantar aspect of the metatarsal condyles and sesamoids) or may form a subcapital support which elevates specific metatarsal heads (Fig. 40.2 B). The latter is always associated with zones of appropriate cavitation under calluses, keratomata or other forms of plantar cutaneous swellings. It blocks longitudinal movement of the foot in the shoe.

Antecapital Bar (Martorell Martorell 1963). This transverse curvilinear bar affords a blunt ridge situated under the proximal phalanges of the toes in front of the metatarsal condyles (Fig. 40.2 C).
It is always associated with a retrocapital bar (see immediately above), and helps to restrict longitudinal movement of the metatarsal heads. It may be incorporated into the monoblock insole.

Physiological Monoblock Insole. This term applies to an insole carefully moulded to conform with the undersurface of the foot, supporting all areas (Fig. 40.2 D). Accordingly, it will include a midtarsal dome, a retrocapital bar and supports under the cuboid and antero-external aspects of the subcalcaneal region. It distributes loading to all areas, exercises a most valuable control over pain from local overloading, and damps loading of both the tarsus and the metatarsal heads. Its antalgic effect may be striking.

Calcaneal Semicircular Support. This is a horseshoe-shaped element which supports the heel on both sides, relieving local loading under the calcaneum. It is generally useful in cases of painful heel and in those in which stabilisation of the heel is required.

40.1.3 Relaxing and Load-Relieving Elements

Relaxing and load-relieving elements act by changing the posture of a foot so as to alter the loading of an otherwise painful area. Their effect may be beneficial at a distance, e.g. the extension of a supple pes cavus may have the additional effect of relieving an accompanying lumbago. Their mechanism of action contrasts with that of the supportive insole, which is designed to relieve load under specific localised areas of the foot.

Physiological Monoblock Insole. This is similar to that described in Sect. 40.1.2 above (Fig. 40.3 A).

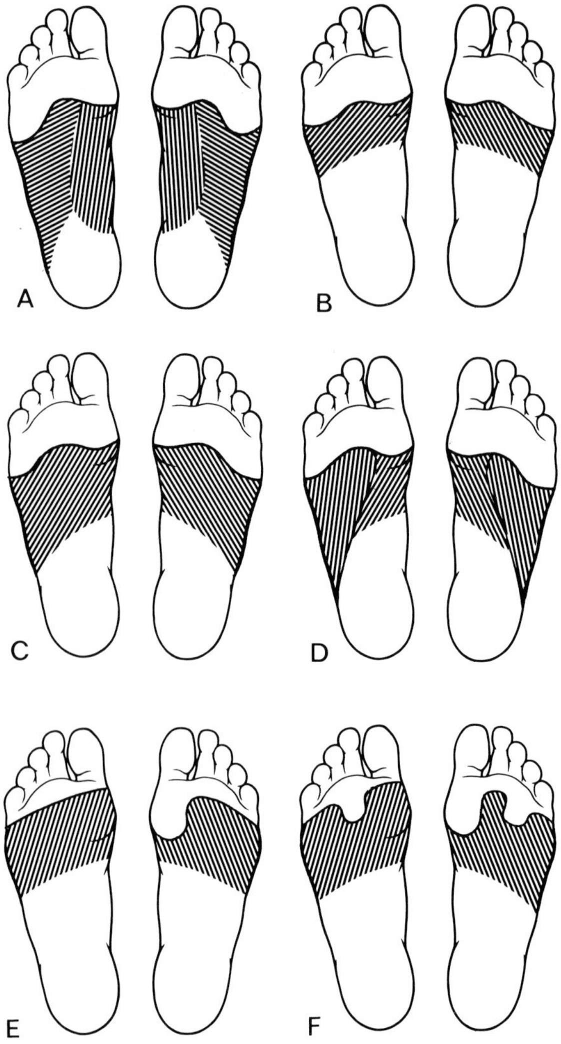

Fig. 40.3 A–F. Relaxing and unloading insoles. **A** Monoblock physiological insole (relaxing and unloading). **B** Retrocapital bar (relaxing and unloading). **C** Compensatory retrocapital bar. **D** Retrocapital pronating bar. **E** Subcapital bar. **F** Subcapital bar with protective excavations

Retrocapital Bar. When designed for unloading or relaxation, this comprises a short bar of which the thickness is calculated to elevate the neck of the fifth metatarsal (Fig. 40.3 B). It also acts as a means of relaxation of longitudinal cavus, thereby relieving pressure under the metatarsal heads.

Compensatory Retrocapital Bar. This is similar to the retrocapital bar for unloading but of greater longitudinal dimension, so as to support the whole of the fifth metatarsal (Fig. 40.3 C). It is valuable in support of longitudinal cavus associated with forefoot pain due to plantar equinus.

Retrocapital Pronating Bar. Here, a pronating wedge is incorporated into the retrocapital bar (Fig. 40.3 d), combining the action of relaxation and load relief with a pronating effect on the metatarsus. This bar is used in metatarsal supination associated with cavovalgus and cavovarus and in localised overloading of the fourth and fifth metatarsal heads in the precavus or cavus foot.

Subcapital Bar. This is useful as a means of relaxation of the hypertonia of the posterior muscles in an early cavus foot, and associated with localised excavations it can relieve local pressure from painful lesions like neuromata, papillomata or miliary corns (Figs. 40.3 E, F).

40.1.4 Compensating Elements

Compensating elements are designed to compensate *intrinsic* displacements of the foot (e.g. associated with trauma, paralysis or operation in the foot or with arthrodesis of the ankle joint) or *extrinsic* displacements (e.g. from leg length discrepancy, dorsolumbar scoliosis, pelvic tilt or unilateral hip dysplasia). Again, there is overlap with the preceding categories.

Physiological Monoblock Insole. When used for leg length compensation, the monoblock can be thickened under the whole of the foot (Fig. 40.4 A).

Retrocapital and Subcapital Bars. See Sects. 40.1.2, 40.1.3 (Fig. 40.4 B, B').

Heel Raise. It should be noted that a heel raise extends under the whole of the heel; it creates anteversion of the pelvis and thus an increase in lumbar lordosis. It must never be utilised in the presence of any painful disorder of the lumbar spine or talalgia accompanied by hyperlordosis, which it will aggravate. The physiological monoblock insole elevating the whole foot is preferable and also relaxes equinus at the ankle joint.

The elements described above are usually combined in a carefully prescribed insole. In certain specific cases, only one element is required, but more commonly several are indicated.

40.2 Therapeutic Indications

With respect to the therapeutic indications, the insole may be classified as corrective, supportive

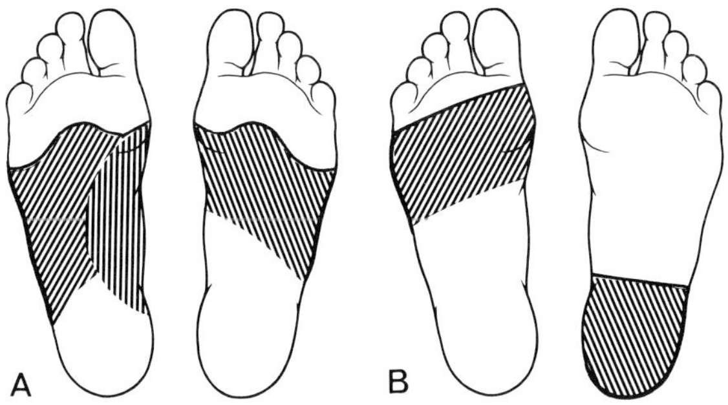

Fig. 40.4 A–D. Compensating insoles. **A** *Left:* monoblock physiological insole; *right:* retrocapital bar. **B** *Left:* subcapital bar; *right:* heel raise

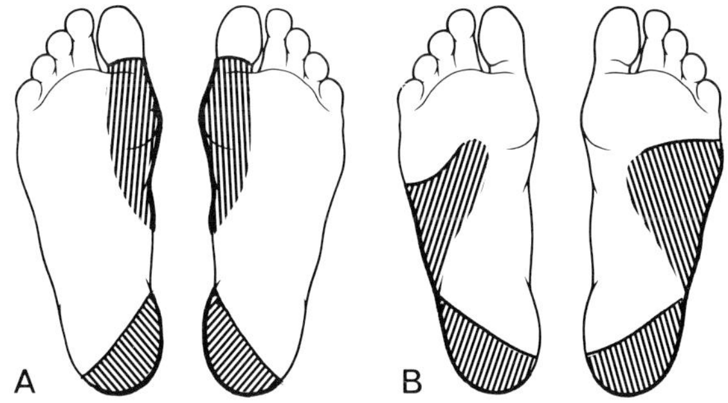

Fig. 40.5 A, B. Stimulating insoles. **A** For planovalgus foot in early childhood. **B** For cavovarus foot

(with antalgic or corrective compensation), relaxing or special.

40.2.1 Corrective Insoles

Corrective insoles can be divided into four types: stimulating, prestabilising, stabilising and consolidating.

40.2.1.1 Stimulating Insoles

Described by Lavigne and Noviel (1975), stimulating insoles are used in the following conditions.

Pes Planovalgus of Early Childhood (Age 3–6 Years). Tarsal pronation is linked to metatarsal pronation. Lavigne and Noviel (1975) emphasise the presence of a spurious supination of the metatarsus in the pes planovalgus of infancy. The appropriate insole is composed of a posterior calcaneal supinating stimulating element with a medial metatarsal internally stimulating wedge (Fig. 40.5 A).
It exercises a reflex proprioceptive action, encouraging dynamic supination of the foot and in contrast provokes re education of the pronating muscles of the forefoot. The action of this insole must be supervised, for its efficacy may be poor or, at the other extreme, it may attain the maximum desired effect within a few months, leading perhaps to overcorrection. Once correction is achieved, the stimulating insole must be replaced by a stabilising insole.

Pes Cavovarus. In this instance, a posterior pronating calcaneal stimulating element is associated with an anterior pronating lateral metatarsal wedge.

40.2.1.2 Prestabilising Insoles

Each of the five types of prestabilising insole has its own precise indications:

a) Planovalgus foot:
   - posterior supinating stabilising wedge
   - anterior pronating stabilising wedge (Fig. 40.6 A)
b) Cavovalgus foot:
   - posterior supinating stabilising wedge
   - pronating retrocapital bar (Fig. 40.6 B)
c) Cavovarus foot:
   - pronating external longitudinal bar associated and incorporated at the level of the metatarsus with a retrocapital pronating bar (Fig. 40.6 C)
d) Varus foot:
   - pronating external longitudinal bar (Fig. 40.6 D)
e) Supinated metatarsus:
   - subcuboidal pronating support (Fig. 40.6 E) or submetatarsal pronating wedge

Prestabilising insoles are useful in the management of supple deformities in children and adolescents and for the same displacement in the young adult, always provided the foot remains flexible. They are not tolerated in the rigid fixed deformity of later adulthood, when supportive insoles are necessary.

40.2.1.3 Corrective Stabilising Insoles

Corrective stabilising insoles exercise their beneficial effect either by gently *stretching* contracted structures or alternatively by *relaxing* them.

Corrective Stretching Insoles. These are used in pes planovalgus in adolescents and adults:

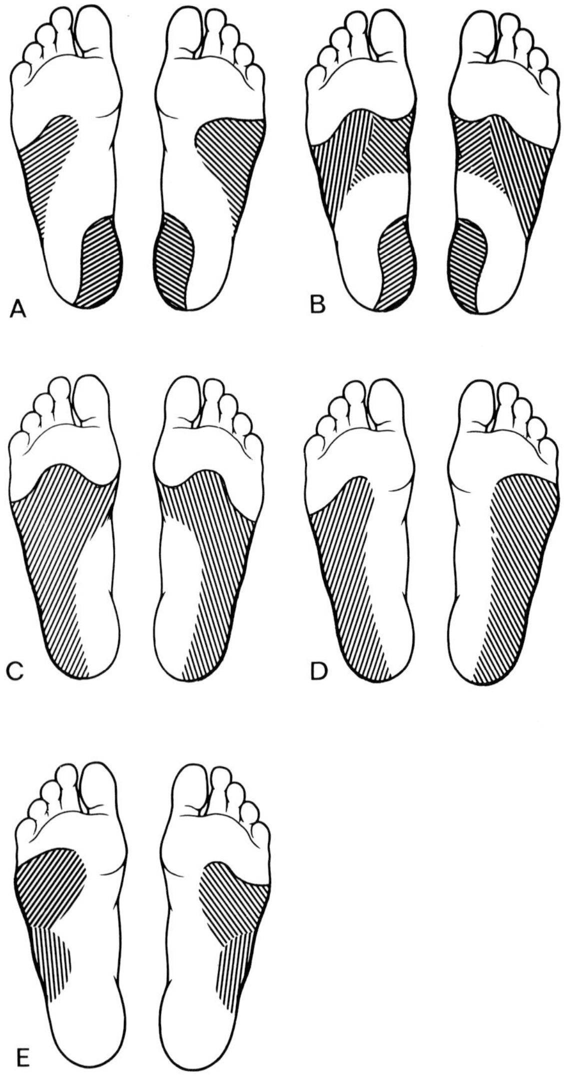

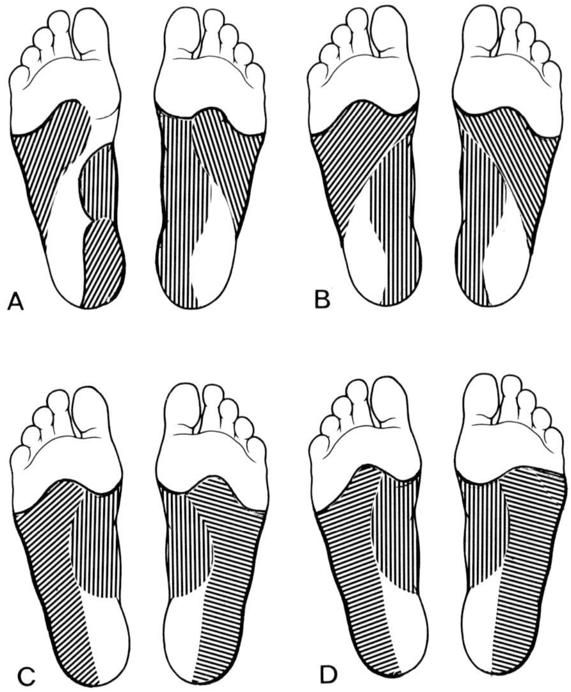

Fig. 40.7 A–D. Stabilising corrective insoles. **A** For planovalgus foot in adolescent or young adult. **B** For cavovalgus foot in adolescent or young adult. **C** For cavovarus foot in adolescent or young adult. **D** For varus foot in adolescent or young adult.

◁ **Fig. 40.6 A–E.** Prestabilising corrective insoles. **A** For planovalgus foot. **B** For cavovalgus foot. **C** For cavovarus foot. **D** For varus foot. **E** For supinated metatarsus

- Posterior supinating stabilising wedge
- Anterior pronating stabilising wedge
- Midtarsal elements comprising perhaps an internal subnavicular button or a medial midtarsal support of which the height is slightly greater than the apparent longitudinal arch of the foot in this area and which completes the action of the anterior and posterior elements above (Fig. 40.7 A)

Corrective Relaxing Insoles. These are of three types:

1. Pes cavovalgus in adolescents and young adults:
   - Posterior supinating stabilising wedge
   - Retrocapital pronating bar
   - Internal midtarsal corrective dome of a height equal to or slightly greater than that of the measured plantar longitudinal medial arch (Fig. 40.7 B)
2. Pes cavovarus in adolescents and young adults:
   - Retrocapital pronating bar
   - Pronating external longitudinal bar

   Sometimes these elements may be accompanied by an internal midtarsal supporting dome of which the height is slightly less than that of the measured medial longitudinal plantar arch, exercising a relaxing longitudinal action and laterally blocking possible overcorrection (Fig. 40.7 C).
3. Varus foot:
   - Pronating external longitudinal band
   - Internal midtarsal dome which allows longitudinal relaxation and prevents possible overcorrection

40.2.1.4 *Insole Consolidating Correction of Pes Planovalgus*

After correction of planovalgus deformity in the child or adolescent, a stabilising insole identical to the prestabilising insole (Fig. 40.6 A) is employed exclusively in order to maintain the correction achieved, for at least a year. The insole is used when correction is indicated by lateral stabilisation of the midtarsal internal displacement and when there is light valgus displacement of the heel due to residual calcaneal pronation. It comprises a posterior supinating stabilising wedge and an anterior pronating stabilising wedge (Fig. 40.8).

40.2.2 Compensating Supportive Antalgic Insoles

Compensating supportive antalgic insoles are so called because they compensate for some painful intrinsic abnormality in the foot by supporting the part. The deformity involved is usually longitudinal.

40.2.2.1 *Pes Planovalgus in Adults*

When pes planovalgus is irreducible and painful, an insole may be prescribed on a trial basis, or permanently if the general state or age of the patient precludes operative treatment. It comprises an internal midtarsal supporting dome, a posterior supinating stabilising wedge and anterior pronating stabilising wedge (Fig. 40.9 A).

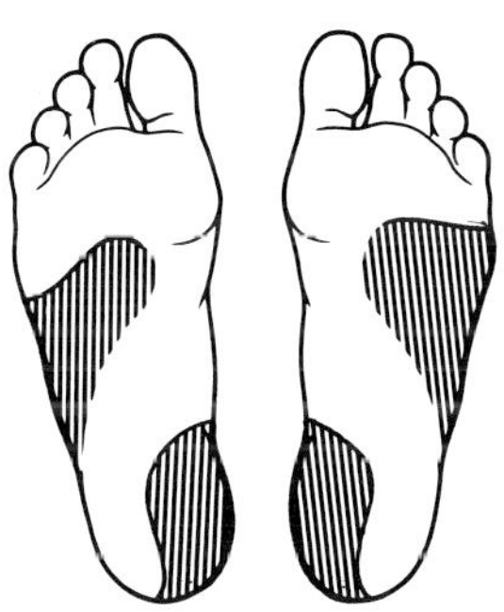

Fig. 40.8. Consolidating insole for planovalgus foot after correction

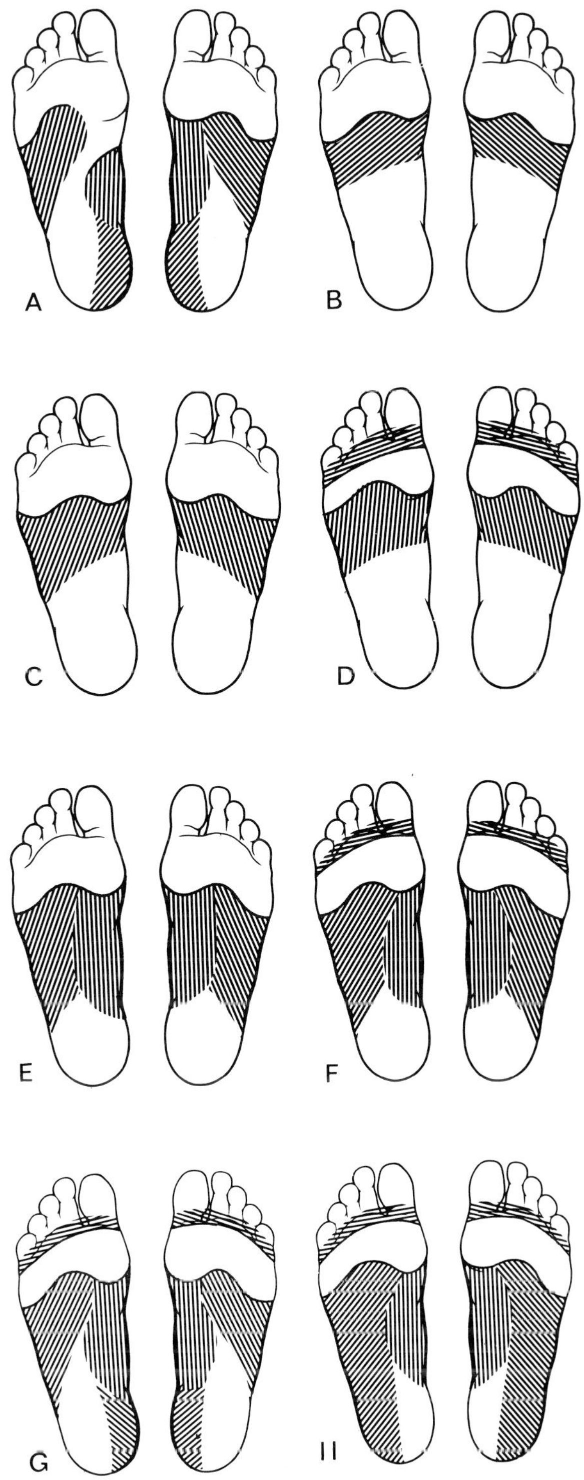

Fig. 40.9 A–H. Compensating supportive antalgic insoles. **A** For planovalgus foot in adult. **B** For early anterior longitudinal cavus (unloading anterior bar). **C** For early anterior longitudinal cavus (supporting anterior bar). **D** Similar to **C** but with antecapital bar. **E** For irreducible anterior longitudinal cavus. **F** Similar to **E** with antecapital bar. **G** Similar to **F** but for valgus deformity. **H** Similar to **F** but for varus deformity

40.2.2.2 Pes Cavus

Supple, Balanced, Anterior Pes Cavus. When there are symptoms of metatarsal overloading in the early stages, the insole comprises a retrocapital compensating load-relieving bar (Fig. 40.9 B, C).
If the metatarsalgia of overloading is more severe, with burning and pricking sensations, the insole should be made up of a retrocapital bar and an antecapital bar (Martorell Martorell 1960) (Fig. 40.9 D).

Irreducible Anterior Pes Cavus in Fixed Valgus or Varus. When one of these conditions is associated with metatarsalgia accompanied by callosity, inflammatory bursitis or keratoma formation under the central metatarsal heads, the insole is designed to restrict longitudinal movement of the foot in the shoe in addition to performing its supportive antalgic role. It then comprises a physiological supporting insole with a retrocapital bar and an antecapital bar (Martorell Martorell 1960) (Fig. 40.9 E, F).

Pes Cavus with Valgus or Varus Posture. The insole should incorporate corrective elements for the additional valgus or varus components (Fig. 40.9 G, H).

40.2.2.3 Additional Elements for Various Forefoot Displacements

In *simple convex forefoot* in the otherwise normal foot or with precavus balanced deformity, seen in young women who wear high heels and in some cases of supple pes cavus, the insole comprises either (a) a retrocapital midline button designed to re-educate the mobility of the first and fifth metatarsals (Fig. 40.10 A) or (b) a retrocapital midline bar (with or without a midline button), which combines supportive and compensatory actions, designed to relax the associated longitudinal cavus (Fig. 40.10 B-E).
In the *convex forefoot with a fixed cavus deformity* associated with metatarsalgia and either a single localised callus or multiple keratomata, the insole comprises a physiological monoblock (Fig. 40.10 G), a retrocapital bar with a central button (Fig. 40.10 C) and a Martorell antecapital bar (Fig. 40.10 F).
In a *flat forefoot with multiple calluses* under all metatarsal heads, and severe symptoms, the insole is identical to that just described except for the absence of a retrocapital central button.
In *cavus forefoot* which is supple and associated with callus formation under the first and fifth metatarsal heads, a relaxing or compensating retrocapital bar may be effective, sometimes accompanied by an internal midtarsal supporting dome. In the presence of severe callus or keratomata, a rigid Lisfranc joint and fixed equinus of any degree of the first and fifth metatarsals, it is more appropriate to use a physiological monoblock insole associated with one or more of the following elements as appropriate: a simple retrocapital bar; a retrocapital bar with median elevation; a Martorell antecapital bar; a subcapital median bar; excavations under the first and fifth metatarsal heads; a retrocapital bar localised to the first and fifth metatarsal heads.

40.2.3 ***Supporting Compensating Insoles for Extrinsic Displacements***

Lumbar Hyperlordosis with Anteversion of the Pelvis. Lumbago and sciatica may be corrected by the use of shoes with raised heels (10-20 mm) associated with a subcapital or retrocapital bar (Fig. 40.11 A).

Leg Length Inequality and Lumbago Due to "Flat Back." A posterior subcalcaneal heel raise, unilateral for leg length discrepancy or bilateral for flat back lumbago, is appropriate.

Pelvic Anteversion with Hyperlordosis Involving Leg Length Discrepancy. Pelvic tilting can be asymmetrical, producing leg length discrepancy. In this case, the appropriate insole is a physiological monoblock with a heel element to correct any valgus or varus (Fig. 40.11 B).
Note: The fitting of the insole should allow for the leg length discrepancy.

Internal Rotation of the Lower Limb with Pes Planovalgus or a Valgus Calcaneum. The insole should comprise a posterior supinating stabilising element, an anterior pronating stabilising wedge and an internal dome or a button under the navicular.

External Rotation of the Pelvis or the Lower Limb. Pes varus with genu varum may respond to a subcuboidal support, an external pronating longitudinal bar (Fig. 40.11 D) or, if there is supination of the metatarsus, an anterior pronating stabilising wedge.
In pes cavovarus with genu varum, any one of the following may be appropriate: (a) a physiological monoblock insole with an external pronating bar and a retrocapital bar (Fig. 40.11 G); (b) a pronating external bar with a subcuboid support; (c) a

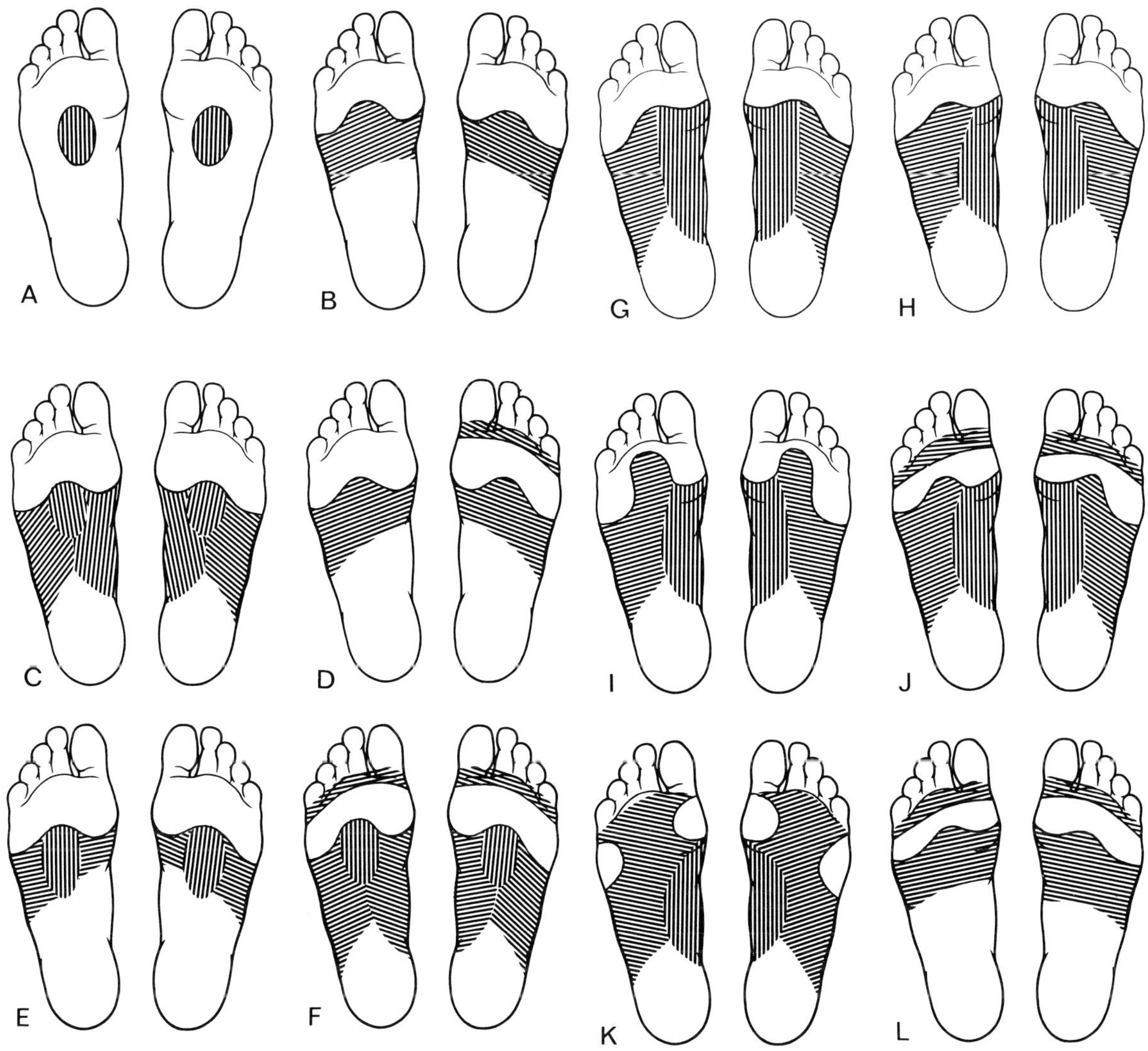

Fig. 40.10 A–I. Insoles for various forefoot displacements. **A–F** Simple convex forefoot: **A** Retrocapital central button; **B** retrocapital midline bar; **C** similar to **G** with central button; **D** retrocapital bar with central support *(left)*, similar to **D** with antecapital bar *(right)*; **E** retrocapital bar with central button; **F** similar to **C** with antecapital bar. **G** Convex forefoot with longitudinal cavus: monoblock physiological insole. **H–L** Forefoot cavus: **H** similar to **G** with simple retrocapital bar. **I** similar to **H** with subcapital central support. **J** similar to **I** with antecapital bar; **K** similar to **G** with subcapital support with excavations for first and fifth metatarsal heads; **L** retrocapital bar supporting especially first and fifth metatarsals and with antecapital bar

pronating external submetatarsal bar (Fig. 40.11 G); (d) if there is accompanying lumbar hyperlordosis with anteversion of the pelvis, a retrocapital bar and a subcapital external pronating element (Fig. 40.11 H).

40.2.4 Load-Reducing Insoles

Load-reducing insoles are designed to relieve pressure under painful areas associated with local pathological alterations in the tarsus, the midtarsus or the metatarsus.

Talalgia. When the pain is in the plantar aspect of the heel, a simple horseshoe calcaneal support suffices. When the talalgia is related to the internal or external aspects of the heel, perhaps associated with serous bursa formation or a traction irritation of the origin of the plantar aponeurosis, the insole must support the whole foot, relaxing the midtarsus and impeding the normal physiological lowering of the plantar arch during walking. In these circumstances it is composed of an internal midtarsal supporting dome or a physiological monoblock stabilising the heel. If there is a valgus component, the insole should incorporate a posterior supinat-

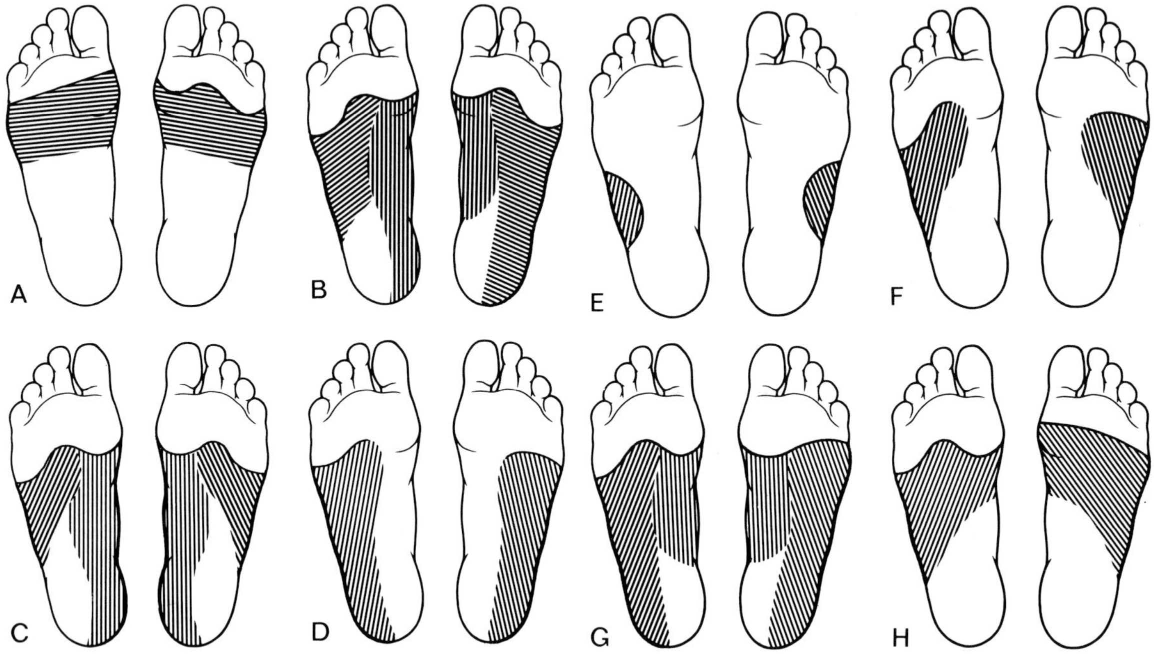

Fig. 40.11. **A** *Left:* subcapital bar for lumbar hyperlordosis; *right:* retrocapital bar for lumbar lordosis. **B** *Left:* monoblock physiological insole with heel element correcting valgus for pelvic anteversion with hyperlordosis; *right:* monoblock physiological insole with heel element correcting varus for pelvis anteversion with hyperlordosis. **C** Insole for internal rotation and pes planovalgus or pes planovarus. **D** Insole with longitudinal pronating wedge for pes varus with genu varum. **E** Insole for subcuboidal support for pes cavovarus with genu varum. **F** Anterior pronating wedge for pes varus with genu varum. **G** Monoblock physiological insole with lateral pronating support for pes cavovarus with genu varum. **H** *Left:* retrocapital bar for accompanying lumbar hyperlordosis with anteversion of pelvis; *right:* subcapital bar for lumbar hyperlordosis

ing stabilising wedge. Conversely, if there is a varus component, the wedge should be posterior and pronating. In both instances, an anterior pronating wedge completes the stabilisation.

Midtarsal Pain Associated with Any Arthritic Condition. The support required is similar to that for talalgia, comprising a monoblock physiological insole with a subcuboidal external button or dome and, if there is a lateral tarsal and midtarsal displacement, elements of stabilisation appropriate to the accompanying eversion or inversion.

Metatarsalgia in Adults. The insoles are extremely varied and relate to the type of displacements present. A simple retrocapital bar with or without an external pronating bar may be appropriate, or an insole designed for a planovalgus cavovarus or cavovalgus foot may be more suitable. In more rigid examples, a physiological monoblock insole with an additional retrocapital or subcapital bar may be indicated.

Subcuboidal Callus Formation Associated with Residual Deformity of Pes Equinovarus or Pressure from Excessive Sporting Activity. Excavations in the subcuboidal region of an insole with a pronating external bar, completed perhaps by a physiological supportive dome in the internal midtarsal region, should be prescribed.

40.2.5 Special Supportive Insoles

The category of special supportive insoles includes those designed to protect the foot afflicted by venous insufficiency, atrophy of the plantar tissues, delicate skin or neurotrophic or dystrophic disorders. They must be adapted to the particular case. They are usually based upon a physiological monoblock insole, which supports the foot generally, and are given excavations under such lesions as calluses and under perforating ulcers from any cause. Further compensation may be achieved by incorporating subcapital, retrocapital or antecapital bars. Examples are given in Fig. 40.10 H–I.
This type of insole needs to be compliant. Appropriate materials include felt covered by layers of varying thickness of soft foam rubber and elasticated leather (a composite material of leather fragments in soft rubber).

41 Instrumentation, Technique, and Surgical Approach

41.1 Instrumentation

Surgery of the foot does not require particularly elaborate instrumentation except for occasional specific procedures. It is convenient to arrange instruments in sets packed in appropriate boxes. The following sets are recommended.
Fig. 41.1–41.5 see pp. 556–558.

41.2 General Technique

The majority of operations should be performed under general anaesthesia with a bloodless field with the tourniquet applied at the inferior third of the thigh or, when the operation allows, at the calf. Caution should be exercised on account of the ischaemic accumulation of toxins and the vascular reactions which may occur on removing the tourniquet. The tissues should always be irrigated with physiological saline, so maintaining as natural an environment as possible.
After closure of the wound, tulle gras should be applied, enclosed in compresses soaked in physiological saline, especially round the toes and forefoot, which maintain the desired correction. Elevation of the leg during the first 6 postoperative days, with ice cooling from the 2nd day onwards, aids the absorption of oedema and relieves pain. Vacuum drainage, especially in cases of extensive dissection, prevents haematoma formation and separation of the tissue planes.

41.3 Surgical Approaches

Careful choice of surgical approach reduces the chances of failure, especially from complications relating to the soft tissues (Fig. 41.6, p. 559). The following descriptions relate in many cases to specific operative procedures, but an understanding of the principles involved will apply usefully to any other procedure.

41.3.1 Great Toe

Shark-Mouth Transverse Incision. This allows easy access for removal of a tumour of the soft tissues of the nail bed or a subungual exostosis, as well as for corrective procedures of the dorsal surface of the terminal phalanx.

Ingrown Toe Nail. O'Donoghue (1940) and Sibley (1945) describe a technique for radical cure of ingrown toe nail necessitating incisions which allows repair of the paronychial tissues and does not hinder growth of a normal nail. The nail body is incised longitudinally 2–4 mm from its margin, and the incision is deepened through the nail bed and soft tissues, extending distally to the end of the nail and proximally to its base. A second incision is then made which curves outside the nail fold, including the granulations of the infected tissue and meeting the first incision at either end. A wedge-shaped piece of nail, its bed and associated skin, including any hypertrophic tissue at the base, are removed by means of a gouge.

Arthrodesis of Interphalangeal Joint. Two transversely orientated incisions are made perpendicular to the long axis of the toe, one a little beyond the level of the interphalangeal joint and the other behind it. A wedge-shaped section of skin and capsulotendinous tissue is excised, allowing coaptation of the excised joint surfaces.

Interphalangeal Arthroplasty. A longitudinal incision extending across the joint permits division of the capsule and exposure of the head of the proximal phalanx, facilitating bony resection.

41.3.2 Lesser Toe

Arthroplasties of Proximal Interphalangeal Joints. These can be performed through longitudinal incisions towards the side of the dorsum, each about 1 cm long and spanning the joint line. Approaches for the second, third and fourth toes should be on

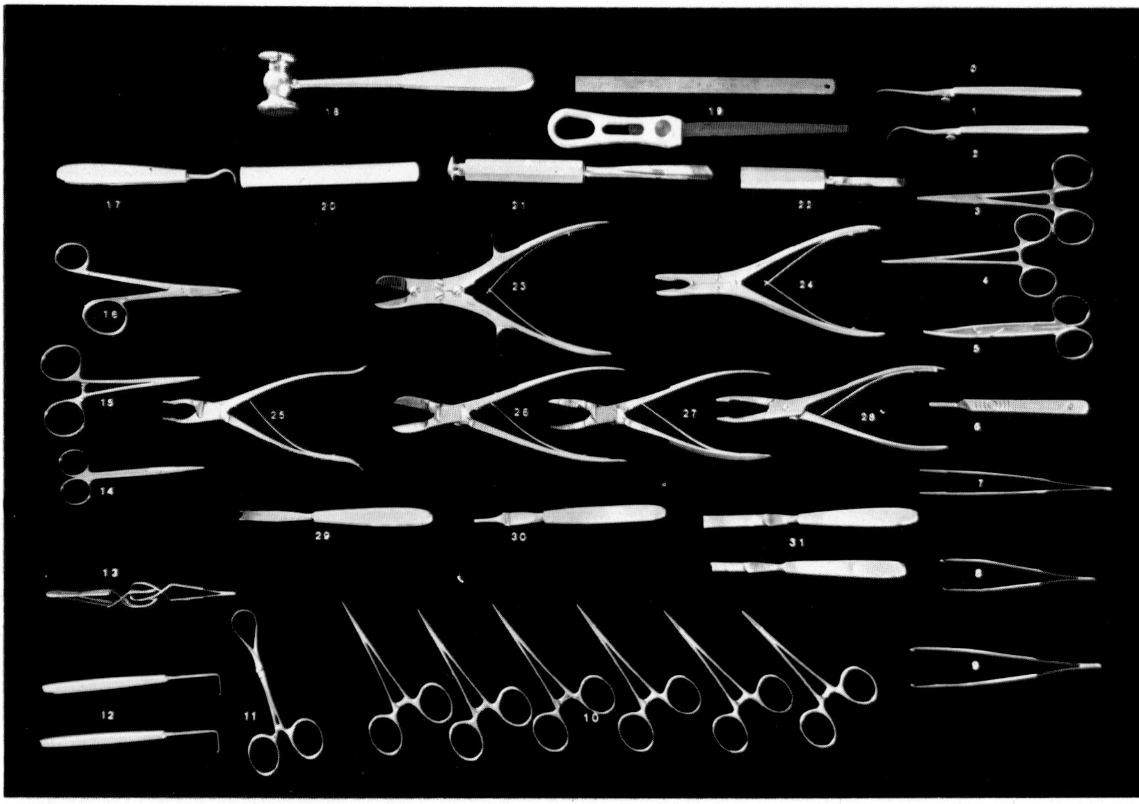

Fig. 41.1. General instrument set

1 1 modified Reverdin suture needle (straight)
2 1 modified Reverdin suture needle (curved)
3 1 pair Willis straight haemostat
4 1 Leriche curved, non-toothed haemostat
5 1 pair Mayo curved scissors (15 cm)
6 2 scalpels (medium and small blade)
7 1 pair de Bakey non-toothed dissecting forceps
8 1 pair Farkas oblique-toothed dissecting forceps (18 cm)
9 1 pair Farkas oblique-toothed dissecting forceps (12 cm)
10 6 Halstead haemostats
11 1 pair Ombredanne forceps
12 2 Chigot retractors
13 2 Finochietto towel clips
14 1 pair fine straight scissors
15 1 pair Halstead straight non-toothed forceps
16 1 pair Thackray scissors/needle-holding forceps
17 1 Regnauld metatarsal hook
18 1 hammer
19 1 metal saw (10 cm)
20 1 Regnauld graft punch
21 1 Lelièvre chisel
22 1 Ombredanne chisel
23 1 pair double-action bone-cutting forceps
24 1 pair double-action rongeurs
25 1 pair Lelièvre phalangeal rongeurs
26 1 pair Liston straight cutting forceps
27 1 pair Lelièvre fine bone-cutting forceps
28 1 pair Dufourmentel fine rongeurs
29 1 Regnauld metatarsal rugine
30 1 straight fine rugine
31 2 Lelièvre rugines (straight and curved)

the outer side, but for the fifth toe it is preferable for the incision to lie medially, thereby avoiding exposure of the scar to shoe pressure. All of these incisions can be prolonged if it is necessary to divide the insertions of the long flexor tendons.

Arthrodesis of Distal Interphalangeal Joint. This requires a transverse dorsal incision for best exposure. Two transverse incisions crossing the dorsal surface and meeting on both sides of the toe allow excision of a crescent-shaped block of skin and capsulotendinous tissue, and after excision of the joint, coaptation of the middle and distal phalanges can be performed.

41.3.3 Forefoot

Procedures on the forefoot are numerous. The structures tend to be slender and fragile, and in

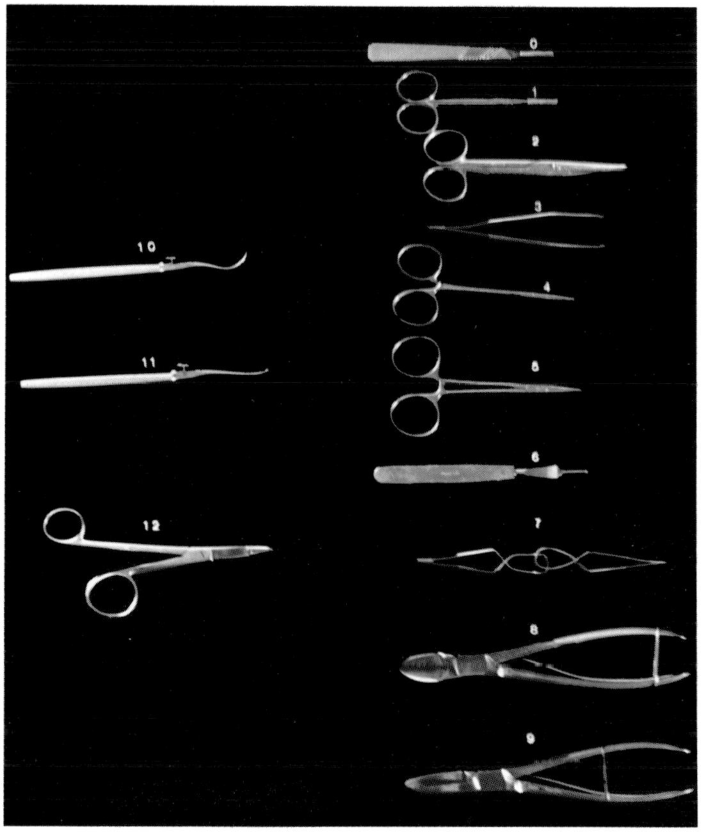

Fig. 41.2. Toe set

0 1 scalpel
1 1 pair fine straight scissors
2 1 pair Mayo curved scissors (15 cm)
3 1 pair Farkas oblique-toothed dissecting forceps
4 1 pair Leriche forceps
5 1 pair Halstead forceps
6 1 straight fine rugine
7 2 Finochietto towel clips
8 1 pair Liston cutting forceps
9 1 pair Dufourmentel rongeurs
10 1 modified Reverdin suture needle (curved)
11 1 modified Reverdin suture needle (straight)
12 1 pair Thackray scissors/needle-holding forceps

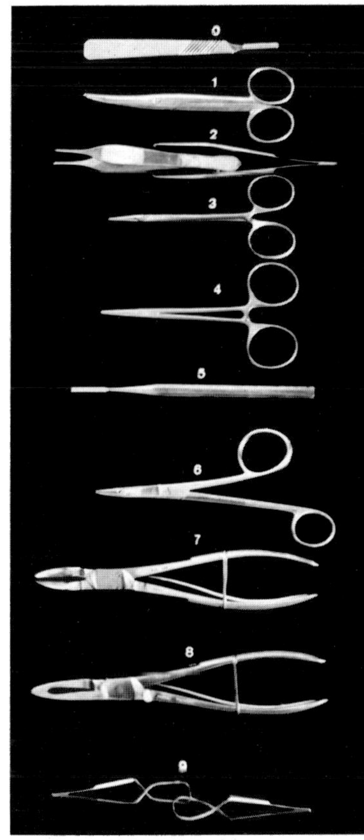

Fig. 41.3. Toenail set

0 1 scalpel
1 1 pair Mayo curved scissors (15 cm)
2 1 pair Farkas oblique-toothed dissecting forceps (12 cm)
3 1 pair Leriche toothed forceps
4 1 pair Halstead straight non-toothed forceps
5 1 Lelièvre fine straight chisel
6 1 pair Thackray scissors/needle-holding forceps
7 1 pair Lelièvre bone-cutting forceps
8 1 pair Dufourmentel fine straight rongeurs
9 2 Finochietto towel clips

particular, the skin on the dorsal aspect at the level of the metatarsophalangeal joints has a somewhat precarious vascular supply; especially here, care is needed for exact positioning of incisions so as to eliminate tension when the approach is too proximal or distal.

Hallux Valgus and Hallux Rigidus. A number of operative incisions have been recommended, but of these the best is a longitudinal one along the medial side of the great toe extending from the head of the proximal phalanx to 2 cm proximal to the head of the metatarsal situated midway between the plantar and dorsal aspects. The incision is deepened to the plane of the capsule, and superficial vessels are ligated. Longitudinal incision of the capsule allows reflection in one layer while preserving the dorsal attachment to the head of the first metatarsal and the periphery of the proximal third of the proximal phalanx. This exposure obvi-

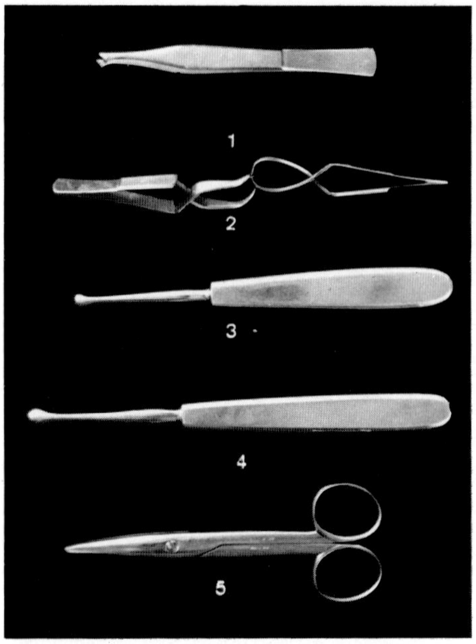

Fig. 41.4. Verruca set
1 1 pair Farkas oblique-toothed dissecting forceps (12 cm)
2 2 Finochietto towel clips
3, 4 2 curettes
5 1 pair Mayo curved scissors (15 cm)

ates excessive retraction and allows realignment of the articular surfaces, correction of subluxed sesamoid bones, elongation of the extensor hallucis longus tendon and repair of the plantar and medial capsule.

Hallux Flexus. The medial longitudinal incision needs to be more extensive than that described above, reaching from the medial aspect on the medial cuneiform bone distally as far as the interphalangeal joint whenever there is an irreducible flexion deformity. This approach gives access to the interphalangeal joint, the metatarsophalangeal joint space and the long flexor tendon (which must be elongated at the base of the first metatarsal), and allows semicircular basal osteotomy of the metatarsal, so that it can be lowered but not shortened. It also allows most other procedures on the first metatarsal bone, including grafting and fracture surgery.

Metatarsal Heads. When depression of the central metatarsal heads is associated with hallux valgus, realignment may be necessary. The transverse plantar incision allows easy access to the joints themselves but does not allow elongation of the ex-

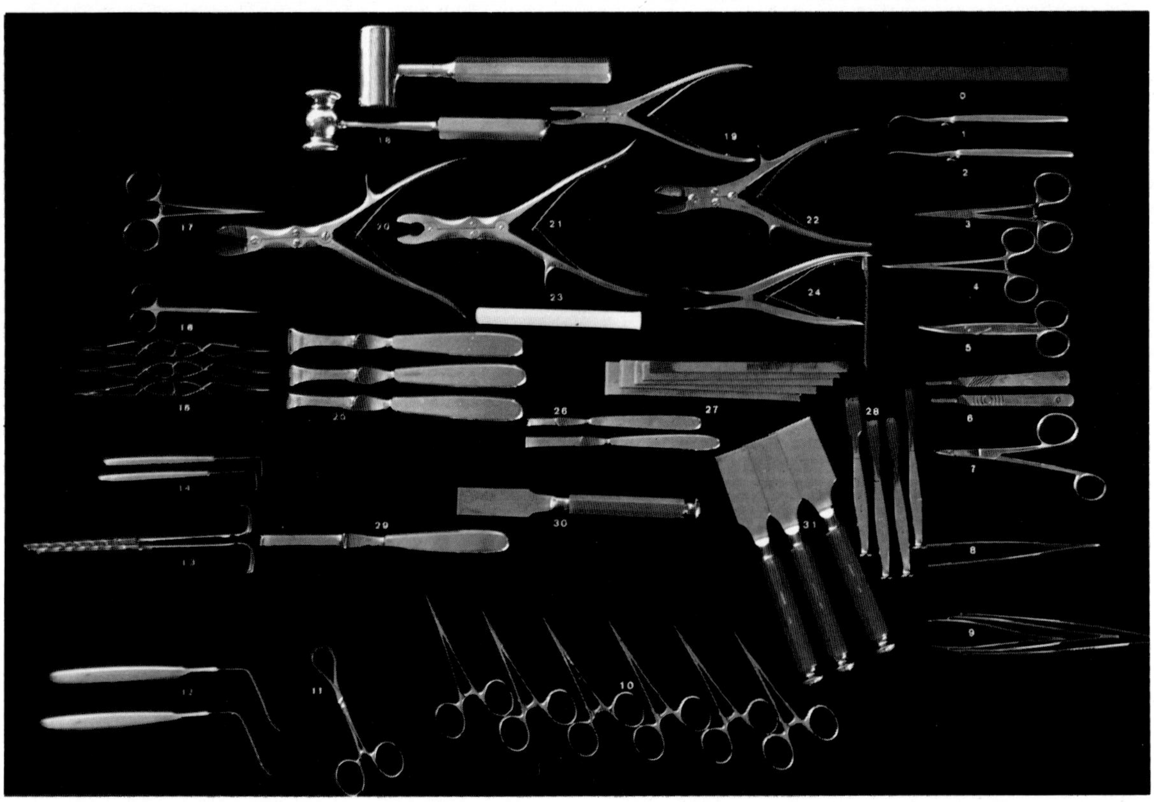

tensor proprius and extensor digitorum brevis tendons. It should be reserved for the simple realignment procedure described by Lelièvre (1952), and care should be taken that it lies in front of the zone of weight bearing of the metatarsal heads behind the digital commissures. Even then, weight-bearing discomfort may occur, and it is for this reason that in general we do not use it. A *transverse dorsal* incision gives excellent exposure of the region. It is made slightly concave posteriorly, exactly over the dorsal prominences of the four outer metatarsal heads, after correction of the position of the toes with respect to the axes of the metatarsals. The longitudinal branches of the dorsal venous arcade can be protected and the extensor tendons and the capsules of the metatarsophalangeal joints can be completely exposed. A *longitudinal* incision on the dorsal aspect of the head of the metatarsal head offers excellent access for resection of the condylar heads or for enclavement. The scar is never exposed to pressure from any part of the shoe even if it becomes keloid, although this seldom happens on account of its orientation in the concavity of the metatarsophalangeal region.

Quintus Varus or Metatarsus Quintus Valgus. Two types of approach may be necessary (see Fig. 19.3). When metatarsus quintus valgus is associated with a bunionette or quintus varus exists, an outer longitudinal incision is made over the external aspect of the fifth toe, crossing the dorsal aspect of the head of the fifth metatarsal, curving inferiorly around the bursa and returning longitudinally along the lateral aspect of the fifth metatarsal. The bursa can be excised together with the underlying exostosis, and correction of the valgus of the fifth metatarsal can be effected by capsulorrhaphy of the fourth and fifth metatarsophalangeal joints. The incision

◁ **Fig. 41.5.** Ankle set
0 1 10-cm rule
1 1 modified Reverdin suture needle (curved)
2 1 modified Reverdin suture needle (straight)
3 1 Willis haemostat
4 1 Leriche haemostat
5 1 pair curved Mayo scissors
6 2 scalpels (medium and small blade)
7 1 pair Thackray scissors/needle-holding forceps
8 1 pair de Bakey dissecting forceps
9 2 pairs Farkas oblique-toothed dissecting forceps (18 and 12 cm)
10 6 Halstead seam haemostats
11 1 pair Ombredanne forceps
12 2 beaked retractors
13 2 claw retractors
14 2 Chigot retractors
15 6 Finochietto towel clips
16 1 pair fine straight scissors
17 1 pair Halstead toothed forceps
18 2 hammers (Ombredanne and MacKeever)
19 1 pair Burky rongeurs
20 1 pair Liston double-action bone-cutting forceps (24 cm)
21 1 pair double action rongeurs (24 cm)
22 1 pair Liston double-action bone-cutting forceps (20 cm)
23 1 Regnauld graft punch
24 1 Lintje retractor
25 3 Lambotte rugines (15, 20 and 25 mm)
26 2 Lelièvre rugines (straight and curved)
27 5 Volkmann chisels
28 4 chisels (blade sizes 6, 8, 10 and 12 mm)
29 1 Merle d'Aubigne curved rugine
30 1 osteotome (25 mm)
31 1 Faraboeuf plain chisel

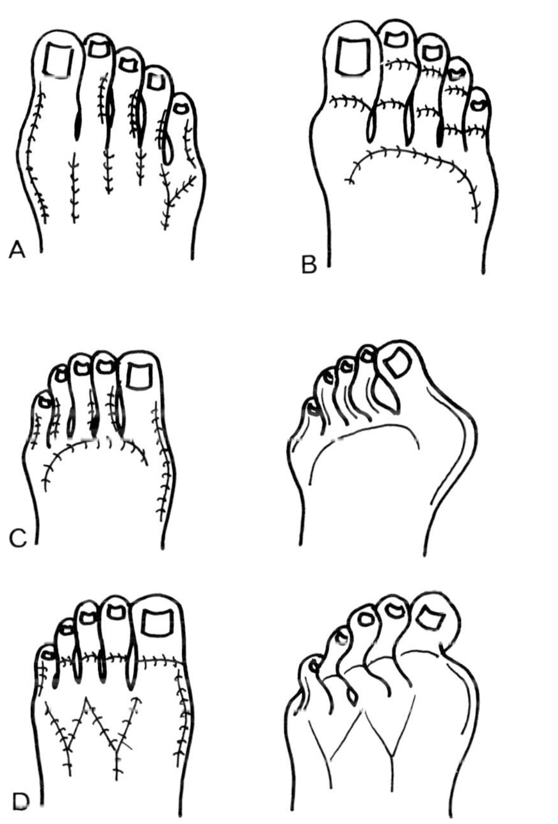

Fig. 41.6 A–D. Examples of incisions in the forefoot. **A** Longitudinal: hallux valgus, hallux rigidus, digital neuroma, claw toes, dorsal tendon elongation. **B** Transverse: interphalangeal and metatarsophalangeal joints. **C** Combined: enclavement, claw toes, first metatarsophalangeal joint. **D** Combined: also showing V-Y incision for relaxation of dorsal skin longitudinally

is situated above the external margin of the forefoot, outside the zone of pressure exerted by the shoe upper, and avoids discomfort from this source. When quintus varus is associated with overlapping of the toe, this external approach is augmented by two cutaneous incisions in an S form between which an area of skin is removed. Coaptation of the borders of the wound aids in the re-establishment of the metatarsophalangeal axis.

Sesamoids. A medial horseshoe incision on the plantar aspect allows access to sesamoids affected by a painful bipartite condition, a fracture or degenerative arthritis. After reflection of the skin and subcutaneous plantar tissue, the sesamoids can be visualised through their thin fibrous covering. Longitudinal incision of the fibrous layer allows resection of part or exceptionally the whole of the sesamoids. The incision is situated outside the weight-bearing zone and does not incur residual discomfort.

Plantar Neuroma. When the nerve irritation is caused by compression from a cyst, lipoma or plantar bursitis, a *plantar* incision is appropriate. A curved cut is made, concave posteriorly and centred midway between the webs of the toes and the metatarsal heads. Elevation of the skin posteriorly allows lateral retraction of the tendon and a longitudinal incision into the space between the metatarsal heads as far as the neurovascular bundles for exposure of the tumour. The development of small keratotic lesions in the scar related to the suture insertions is possible, and accordingly it may be preferable to use the *dorsal* incision, which is situated midway between the metatarsal heads and offers immediate access to the neuroma. If a plantar neuroma responsible for the Morton syndrome (1876) is accompanied by radiation of pain towards the heel, this may be due to the tumour reaching a large size. In this case, a plantar approach situated behind the heads of the metatarsals can be used without fear of involving the pressure zone of the ball of the foot.

41.3.4 Tarsometatarsal Joints

Longitudinal Incision. This can be made on the medial aspect of the medial cuneiform bone and first metatarsal, 6 cm long. It permits excellent access to the base of the metatarsal for osteotomy, which could be necessary for correction of an equinus posture of the bone. At the level of the cuneiform-metatarsal joint, arthrodesis for cavus deformity can be performed. Semicircular transverse trans-cuneiform-cuboidal osteotomy, resecting the whole of the tarsometatarsal joint line, can also be carried out.

Transverse Incision. This is directed obliquely - anterolateral to posteromedial - and permits access to the whole of the Lisfranc joint line. It begins at the dorsal aspect of the base of the second metatarsal and follows the joint line. The small subcutaneous nerves and the vessels of the dorsal arcade can be preserved. After incision of the superficial fascia, retraction of the common extensor tendons and other soft tissues exposes the joint line for resection of the cuneiform-metatarsal and cuboido-metatarsal joints and arthrodesis.

Longitudinal Incision. A longitudinal incision over the dorsal aspect of the base of the fifth metatarsal gives excellent exposure for treatment of a fracture of the styloid process, allowing fixation with a screw.

Proximal Metatarsal Exposure. The base of a metatarsal can be approached through a longitudinal incision 2-3 cm long on the dorsal aspect of the bone concerned. Good exposure of the base is achieved after retraction of the subcutaneous nerves and the extensor tendons, and osteotomy or forage of bone cavities can be performed. Wire fixation is usually necessary after coaptation of the osteotomy surfaces.

41.3.5 Midtarsal Incisions

Midtarsal incisions are used in foot deformities in which the correction relates to the midtarsal region. In a Chopart tarsectomy, a dorsal transverse incision should be used. It begins at the level of the talonavicular joint, descends slightly obliquely, inferiorly, posteriorly and outwards, following the line of the calcaneocuboid joint, terminating over the muscular tissue of extensor digitorum brevis. The superficial fascia is incised and retracted, the extensor retinaculum is partly divided and the extensor communis tendons and neurovascular elements are protected. Excellent exposure of the talonavicular and calcaneocuboid joint is achieved which allows adequate correction of the fixed deformities. When the maximum longitudinal curvature is situated more anteriorly, really metatarsal in origin, a medial tarsal resection should be performed at the expense of the naviculocuneiform joints on the inner side and of the body of the cuboid on the outer side. In this case, the dorsal transverse incision should begin at the inner end of

the dorsal face of the naviculocuneiform joints and descend transversely, obliquely, backwards and outwards to the external face of the midtarsal region, reaching to within 1 cm behind and above the styloid of the fifth metatarsal.
The outer lip of the superficial fascia revealed by this incision includes cutaneous nerves, branches of the musculocutaneous nerve, and these must be isolated on the inner aspect of both extensor hallucis longus and the dorsalis pedis vessels, while on the outer side of the foot, the extensor communis tendons and the branches of the musculocutaneous nerve are more in evidence. The belly of extensor digitorum brevis is retracted laterally, so allowing access for resection of the naviculocuneiform joint and the cuboid as well as fixation of the corrections achieved.

41.3.6 Tarsal Incisions

The many operations described at the tarsus nearly always relate to correction of subluxation or to arthrodesis. The choice of incision depends on the site and on the procedure envisaged:

41.3.6.1 Midtarsal and Subtalar Arthrodesis

The midtarsal and subtalar arthrodesis techniques of Bertrand, Ducroquet-Launay, and Lambrinudi-Boppe (1927), all use the same approach: A curvilinear incision, concave superiorly, starts 1 cm behind and below the tip of the lateral malleolus. It follows the groove formed by the lateral malleolus, crossing the peroneal tendons laterally, and goes below it, descending to within 1 cm of the base of the fifth metatarsal. It then curves backwards so as to become transverse on the dorsal aspect of either the talonavicular joint or the navicular, according to the site of intended bony resection. Retraction of the margins of the incision allows access to the tendons; after opening the sheath, they can be retracted downwards, outwards and posteriorly. In the centre, the peroneal retinaculum is divided in front of its anterior attachment to the malleolus in the axis of the foot so that its inner part can be retracted. The extensor communis tendons and their sheaths are retracted upwards and medially, together with the blood vessels, and the belly of extensor digitorum brevis is stripped from its attachment to the calcaneum, which is retracted downwards and forwards. Good access is offered to the midtarsal and subtalar joint lines, where resections and accurate coaptation are necessary.

41.3.6.2 Pes Planus

Pes planus is a complex deformity involving pronation of the calcaneum accompanied sometimes by an equinus posture and supination of the forefoot with plantar depression of the midtarsus and internal angulation of the tarsometatarsal joint line. The subluxation which results is perpetuated by contraction of triceps surae and aggravated by weakness of tibialis posterior. Several contributing factors need correction through the following recommended incisions:

1. A longitudinal incision situated in the depression between the tibia and the Achilles tendon allows elongation of the tendon while preserving a tongue thereof on the medial side of its calcaneal insertion. This relieves the calcaneum of the tension exerted by triceps surae and allows correction of the heel posture.
2. An external incision concave superiorly, is made over the sinus tarsi on the outer side of the hindfoot, beginning in front of the extensor communis tendon 1 cm below the tibiotarsal interline, crossing the sinus tarsi and terminating 1.5 cm below the tip of the lateral malleolus. Incision of the subcutaneous tissue exposes the sinus tarsi, where arthrodesis will be necessary after mobilisation of the anterior process of the calcaneum as described by Viladot (1975).
3. The third incision, which allows access to the talonavicular region, is longitudinal on the inner aspect of the foot; it begins 1 cm in front of the medial malleolus, descends in the line of the inner aspect of the head of the talus to the navicular and medial cuneiform bones and terminates at the level of the cuneiform-metatarsal joint. This approach allows release of tibialis posterior and mobilisation of the neck and head of the talus and the body of the navicular. It gives good exposure for resection of the anterior process of the talus and the body of the navicular, and transplantation of the tibialis posterior tendon onto the plantar and internal aspects of the medial cuneiform bone is possible.

These three incisions allow simultaneous correction of all the elements constituting the deformities involved in pes planus, essential to the restoration of static and dynamic equilibrium.

41.3.6.3 Calcaneal Varus Deformity

In addition to correction of longitudinal subluxation, Dwyer (1959) described a transverse osteotomy of the calcaneum. This is performed through an approach on the outer aspect of the heel comprising a curved incision, slightly concave from above and anteriorly, which begins 1 cm above the superior border of the calcaneum midway between the posterior border of the external malleolus and the posterosuperior tuberosity, extends obliquely from below forwards, and terminates at the outer border of the foot 3 cm below the orifice of the sinus tarsi. It offers general access to the peroneal tendons, which lie 1 cm posteriorly. The peroneal tendons are retracted superiorly, allowing exposure to the superior and external surfaces of the body of the calcaneum. After periostal incision and stripping along the course of the incision, transcalcaneal osteotomy with removal of a wedge of bone based laterally allows realignment of the calcaneum after coaptation of the joint surfaces.

41.3.7 Ankle Joint

Anterior Approach. This can be employed when the axis of the ankle joint is normal, so allowing easy access. A longitudinal vertically inclined incision along the outer border of the extensor hallucis tendon begins 10 cm above the ankle joint and finishes 5 cm below it. The extensor retinaculum is divided vertically and retracted laterally, together with the extensor communis tendons, while the tendons of extensor hallucis longus and tibialis anterior, together with the anterior tibial vascular bundle, are retracted medially. The capsule of the ankle is incised and stripped from the anterior face of the tibia and from the neck of the talus. Forced plantarflexion of the foot opens the joint anteriorly, exposing the articular surfaces.

Lateral Incision. Merle d'Aubigné (1949a, b, 1951) described an arthrodesis using this approach in cases of gross deformity of the ankle joint. The incision follows the posterior border of the peroneal tendons, commencing 10 cm above the lateral malleolus and curving inferiorly forwards so as to terminate on the anterior part of the calcaneum. The cutaneous layer is retracted and the peroneal tendons displaced outwardly and posteriorly. The fibula is then divided 8 cm above its lower extremity deep to the extensor retinaculum, and the anterior and posterior inferior talofibular ligaments are divided. After section of the posterior talofibular ligament and the posterior part of the calcaneofibular ligament, the lower part of the fibula hinged on the anterior talofibular ligament, which is carefully preserved, can be displaced forwards. This exposes the joint surfaces of the ankle and the internal surface of the fibular malleolus. It is now easy to resect the internal surface of the lateral malleolus and the outer aspects of the articular surface of the talus, followed by accurate corrective resection of the articular surfaces of the tibia and dome of the talus. Following forage, whereby two parallel transverse canals are made across the coapted raw surfaces, fixation can be achieved by two screws, one tibiofibular and the other fibulotalar.

41.3.8 Tendons

Simple longitudinal incisions along the line of the tendons concerned are adequate for procedures such as elongation or shortening. Similarly, the incisions can be related to bony segments into which a tendon may have to be transplanted. An anterior approach in the leg suffices for elongation of extensor communis, tibialis anterior and extensor hallucis longus; the tenodesis uniting the anterior extensor tendons described by Haglund is also performed through this approach. The incision is longitudinal on the anterior surface of the lower tibia, commencing at the anterior border 8 cm above the ankle joint and descending to terminate 2 cm below this line. After incision of the superficial fascia, protecting the anterior tibial neurovascular pedicle, the required structures are exposed.

Elongation or shortening of flexor hallucis is rarely performed as an isolated procedure, being complementary to corrective interventions for clawing of the great toe, hallux rigidus, hallux flexus, and complications following other poorly conducted procedures at the level of the great metatarsophalangeal joint. Three approaches are available:

1. At the metatarsophalangeal region, appropriate to hallux valgus, incision of the flexor sheath between the sesamoids and its insertion exposes flexor hallucis longus for shortening and suture.
2. In the metatarsal region, flexor hallucis longus can be exposed in its plantar segment through a longitudinal incision on the inferoplantar aspect along the line of the first metatarsal. This begins at the sesamoid bones and extends proximally to the tarsometatarsal joint line. Cellular tissue and the plantar aponeurosis are incised and retracted, thus exposing the tendon and the muscle mass of abductor hallucis, which is retracted superiorly while the plantar aponeurosis is retracted inferiorly. Following the plantar border of the abductor tendon, the inner fasciculus of flexor hallucis brevis can be identified. Retraction of

the two heads of this muscle allows exposure of the long flexor which lies between the two fasciculi of the short flexor.

3. Another exposure of value is situated in the inferior third of the inner aspect of the leg. A longitudinal incision situated towards the front of the groove between the Achilles tendon and the posterior border of the tibia, but behind the medial malleolus, allows excellent exposure for elongation of flexor hallucis longus and of tibialis posterior. Thus elongation of tendo Achillis itself is also possible. This approach can be employed for other procedures, for example the tarsal tunnel syndrome, which can be relieved through a longitudinal incision in the mid-part of the groove extended inferiorly to the internal aspect of the ankle between the medial malleolus and the heel. The subcutaneous tissue having been incised above and below, the superficial aponeurosis of the leg, the internal annular ligament and the muscle mass of adductor hallucis are exposed. The plantar cutaneous nerves must be protected. The internal annular ligament is retracted in either direction and the continuity of the canal of Richet (1957) is exposed. Above, at the retromalleolar level, identified from the front backwards are the tendon of tibialis posterior, immediately behind it the tendon of flexor digitorum longus, and the tendon of flexor hallucis longus in its sheath. Descending deeply between these tendons lies the posterior tibial nerve, which is often already divided into two branches, covered internally by the posterior tibial artery and veins. Below the medial malleolus from behind forwards and from below upwards can be identified the lateral plantar neurovascular bundle (vein, artery and lateral plantar nerve) flanked posteriorly by the nerve to abductor digiti minimi. The medial plantar neurovascular bundle (veins, artery and medial plantar nerve) is located anteriorly and superiorly. In the depths of the wound, the tendon of flexor digitorum brevis can be seen.

On the outer aspect of the foot, the peroneal muscles and tendons, the lateral ligament of the ankle, can all be treated through a lateral longitudinal incision. This begins 4 cm above the lateral malleolus descending along its posterior border, crossing the tip and descending in the same line as the tendons obliquely downwards and forwards as far as the base of the fifth metatarsal if the procedure warrants this. In all cases, resection of the cutaneous tissues exposes the lateral malleolus and the tendons. Shortening or tenodesis of the peronei and the Lannelongue operation for restoring stability of the peroneal tendons by elevating a rectangular periosteal layer, can be performed.

41.3.9 Heel

Retrocalcaneal exostoses can be approached through one of two incisions:

1. The approach described by DuVries (1959) and by Maschas (1954) is transversely disposed and follows the horizontal skin creases of the posterior aspect of the heel. It has the advantage of leaving a nearly invisible scar.
2. A vertical longitudinal incision on the outer aspect offers excellent access to the calcaneal tubercles posteriorly with a minimum of periosteal stripping.

In operations for infective sinuses, a transverse posterior incision is suitable. This can be in the form of an ellipse excising the mouth of the sinus, passing through sound tissue and enabling a complete excision of the necrotic focus. Splitting of tendo Achillis allows access to the bony lesion itself, and the tendon can be repaired by simple longitudinal suture, so reconstituting the posterior surface of the heel.

41.3.10 Cutaneous Lesions

On the plantar aspect of the foot, hyperkeratosis can result from scarring after overvigorous electrocoagulation of plantar verucca, radionecrosis, radiosclerosis, radium necrosis, chronic infected callus and perforating ulcer, and from surgical procedures generally. The area can be excised and grafted but the choice of autograft must be made with care. The incision used must be calculated exactly so that the definitive scars which remain will lie between metatarsal heads in front or behind the weight-bearing zones. If this ideal cannot be achieved, the exact coaptation of the lips of the incision and the avoidance of cutaneous infolding necessitate meticulous use of flap rotations and relieving incisions. Infolding inevitably entails the appearance of keloid or keratotic scarring, which ruin the results of this type of plastic work.

Of the many types of incision which can be employed on the sole of the foot, the ones proving most reliable are excision of an isosceles triangle, a rotation flap, Z-plasty, or Hungarian flaps. By using the four-flap technique, a multitude of surgical needs can be satisfied.

42 Corrective Operations for Painful Syndromes of the Forefoot

Throughout this book, while certain immediately relevant operative procedures have been described, frequent reference has been made to techniques applicable to realignment of the forefoot. They are summarised in this chapter for convenience.

It has been emphasised that normal loading of the metatarsal heads depends upon stability of the second, third and fourth metatarsal heads associated with relative mobility of the first and fifth rays. During standing and propulsion, the uniformity of loading must be preserved. Of primary importance is the condition of the hindfoot, where any deformity or abnormality must be corrected before attempts to redistribute load by forefoot procedures; the following account assumes that this prerequisite has been satisfied. Disordered loading of the metatarsal heads of sufficient severity to warrant operative treatment demands redistribution of loading, thereby establishing equality during both static and dynamic functions of the foot.

As regards the distal operations described, a number of comments can be made on the wise choice of procedure. Resection of the central three metatarsal heads for overloading creates an insufficiency of loading and leads to the development of cavus forefoot, which is just as disastrous with respect to the consequent overloading of the remaining first and fifth metatarsal heads. DuVries (1959) practised plantar condylectomy of a depressed metatarsal head, but osteocapsular fibrosis, which follows this procedure, often leads to discomfort and the operation is not advised. Lelièvre (1952), followed by Viladot (1959), also attempted metatarsal realignment by resection of the metatarsal heads involved. This radical procedure has application in the case of metatarsal heads which are severely destroyed by osteolytic processes as seen in rheumatoid arthritis, endocrine disorders, trauma or postoperative failures, but it leads to contracture, fibrosis, osteophytosis and pain and gives no assurance of long-term functional correction; it is definitely contra-indicated in congenital or acquired overloading syndromes in which the metatarsal heads remain anatomically useful. However, anterior overloading syndromes associated with dislocations of the metatarsophalangeal joint and deformities of the toes do require a distal procedure, and for reasons which will be explained below, I am strongly in favour of head-shaft enclavement.

An alternative to local procedures at the distal end of the metatarsals is realignment at or near the metatarsophalangeal joint. Mau (1940), Scherb, Giuntini and Lopez performed a transverse osteotomy, Gagnon (1968) described an oblique osteotomy in the metatarsal diaphysis and Lipstein described a basal V-shaped osteotomy. In cases of frontal protrusion of the prominent metatarsal head, Giannestras (1958) favoured a Z-shaped osteotomy near the base of the affected metatarsal, while Thys (1974b) effected a basal osteotomy of linear or trapezoidal form. I have found the basal V-shaped osteotomy to be the most valuable technique, but the dangers of delayed union at the osteotomy and the importance of absolute perfection in the calculation of the degree of elevation or depression required makes these proximal procedures difficult. A syndrome of insufficiency due to overcorrection is just as disastrous in the long run as the original condition. Certainly, the outcome of basal osteotomies in all five metatarsal heads is very uncertain [Lelièvre (1952) abandoned multiple osteotomies in favour of arthrodesis of the cuneiform metatarsal joints for the cure of anterior cavus foot)] and Thys (1974b) recommended multiple osteotomies confined to the middle three metatarsals, and since 1966 I have performed such procedures in the case of convex forefoot syndrome, especially after the development of podometry by Martorell Martorell (1963) and Steinfort (1975), which has enabled precise calculation of the degree of basal metatarsal resection to be performed. This exact calculation has been confirmed by Thys, Lebrun, Vigneron, van Innis and Detourney (1974). Proximal procedures are excellent for correction of syndromes of overloading associated with disharmony of length, but whenever there is involvement of the metatarsophalangeal joint or destruction of the metatarsal heads themselves, distal procedures are necessary. There will be cases in which both proximal and distal procedures are necessary simultaneously, for instance in irreversible metatarsal obliquities of different degrees associated with capsular and tendinous contractures of the metatarsophalangeal joints and toes. The osteotomies of Thys (1974b) can be associated with metatarsophalangeal arthrotomy to reduce dislocations or deformities at the metatarsophalangeal joints, accompanied by elongations of the flexor and extensor tendons, and arthroplasties or arthrodeses of the interphalangeal joints. Alternatively, and perhaps more attractively, head-shaft enclavement may be more appropriate distally, accompanied by basal osteotomy when it is observed at the end of the distal procedure that elective equinus affects a metatarsal in isolation.

42.1 Metatarsal Realignment

42.1 Indications

The indications for metatarsal realignment (Lelièvre 1952) are irreversible destruction of the head of the metatarsal due to post-traumatic necrosis, osteoarthrosic osteolysis, rheumatoid arthritis, ankylosing spondylitis and gout (Figs. 42.1, 42.2).

42.1.2 Technique

The operation may be performed via the plantar transverse approach described originally by Lelièvre or through the dorsal transverse incision which I favour.

Plantar Transverse Approach. With tourniquet applied, a plantar transverse incision is made midway between the digital commissures and the heads of the metatarsals so as to avoid a scar on the immediate load-bearing area under the metatarsal heads. The incision commences inside the first metatarsal head region and finishes by curving proximally and inwardly in the fourth intercapital space or outwardly to the fifth metatarsal head. A plantar flap is elevated proximally after separating the aponeurotic plantar planes, and on dorsiflexion of the toes the prominences of the outer four metatarsal heads appear in the incision. Short longitudinal incisions are made alongside either aspect of the flexor tendons through the capsules, thereby opening each metatarsophalangeal joint. The capsule is then detached with a fine curved rugine or scalpel, thus displaying the metatarsal head itself. Each metatarsal head is trimmed and rounded, using nibbling forceps, realigning the undersurfaces of the bones in one load-bearing line. The dorsiflexion of the toes is relaxed, the bases of the phalanges become repositioned and the capsule and transverse aponeurotic fibres are sutured. After careful haemostasis, the skin is sutured.

Dorsal Approach. I favour a dorsal incision because it allows correction of contracture of the extensor tendons and avoids the risk of a painful plantar scar; it does not lead to skin necrosis provided the incision is at the correct site. The incision is transverse, overlying the metatarsophalangeal joint lines. Having exposed these, a longitudinal incision is made on either side of each joint and the capsules are detached. The undersurfaces of the metatarsal heads are exposed by plantarflexion and resection can be performed as described above. Contracture of the extensor tendons can be corrected by Z-elongation and any subluxation or dislocation of the phalangeal bases reduced by further capsulotomy. Only the skin requires closure.

42.2 Trapezoidal Osteotomy

42.2.1 Indications

The prime indication for trapezoidal osteotomy (Thys 1974) is disorder of length leading to congenital or perhaps iatrogenic protrusion of metatarsal heads which produces overloading. This is commonly found in convex forefoot when there is selective equinus of the middle metatarsals. In isolation, the procedure is valuable provided there is no fixed displacement of the associated metatarsophalangeal joint involving capsule, tendon or skin (Fig. 42.3).

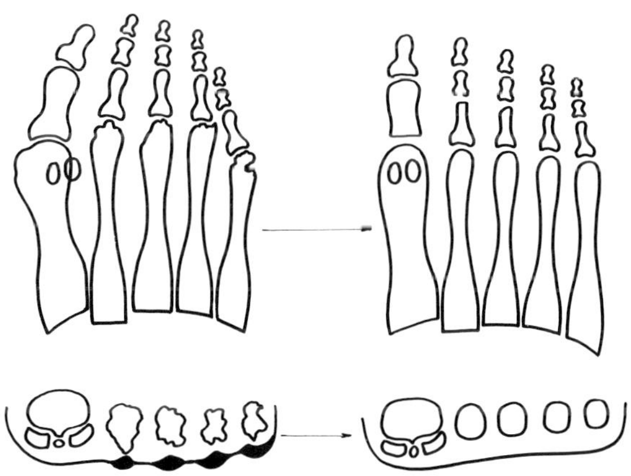

Fig. 42.1. Lelièvre metatarsal realignment

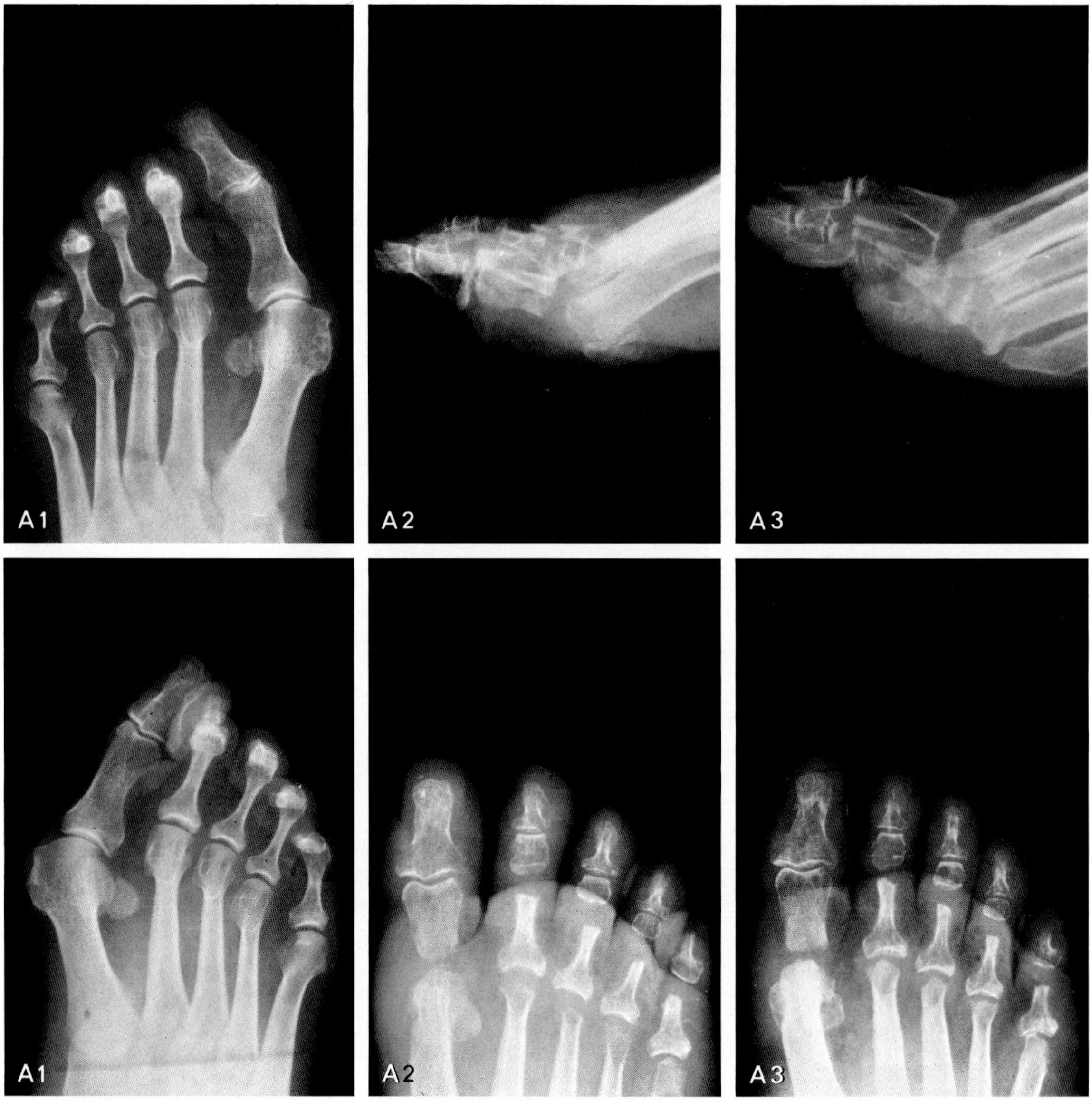

Fig. 42.2 A–D. Lelièvre metatarsal realignment for convex triangular forefoot and simple triangular forefoot with normal plantar arch. **A** Convex triangular forefoot: hallux valgus, frontal protrusion of central metatarsal heads, claw toes, camptodactyly of fifth toe. *1* Before surgery. *2* Six months after metatarsal realignment, correction of hallux valgus by arthroplasty (Lelièvre), arthroplasty of proximal interphalangeal joints of second to fifth toes. *3* A year after operation. *4* Five years after operation: this 55-year-old patient exhibits excellent mobility of metatarsophalangeal joints of all toes despite irregular appearance of metatarsal heads. **B** Convex triangular forefoot: hallux valgus, frontal protrusion of central metatarsal heads, divergence of first and fifth metatarsals, convergence of toes. *1* Before surgery. *2* After metatarsal realignment, correction of hallux valgus, arthroplasty of second to fifth toes. **A** *4*–**D** see pp. 567–569 ▷

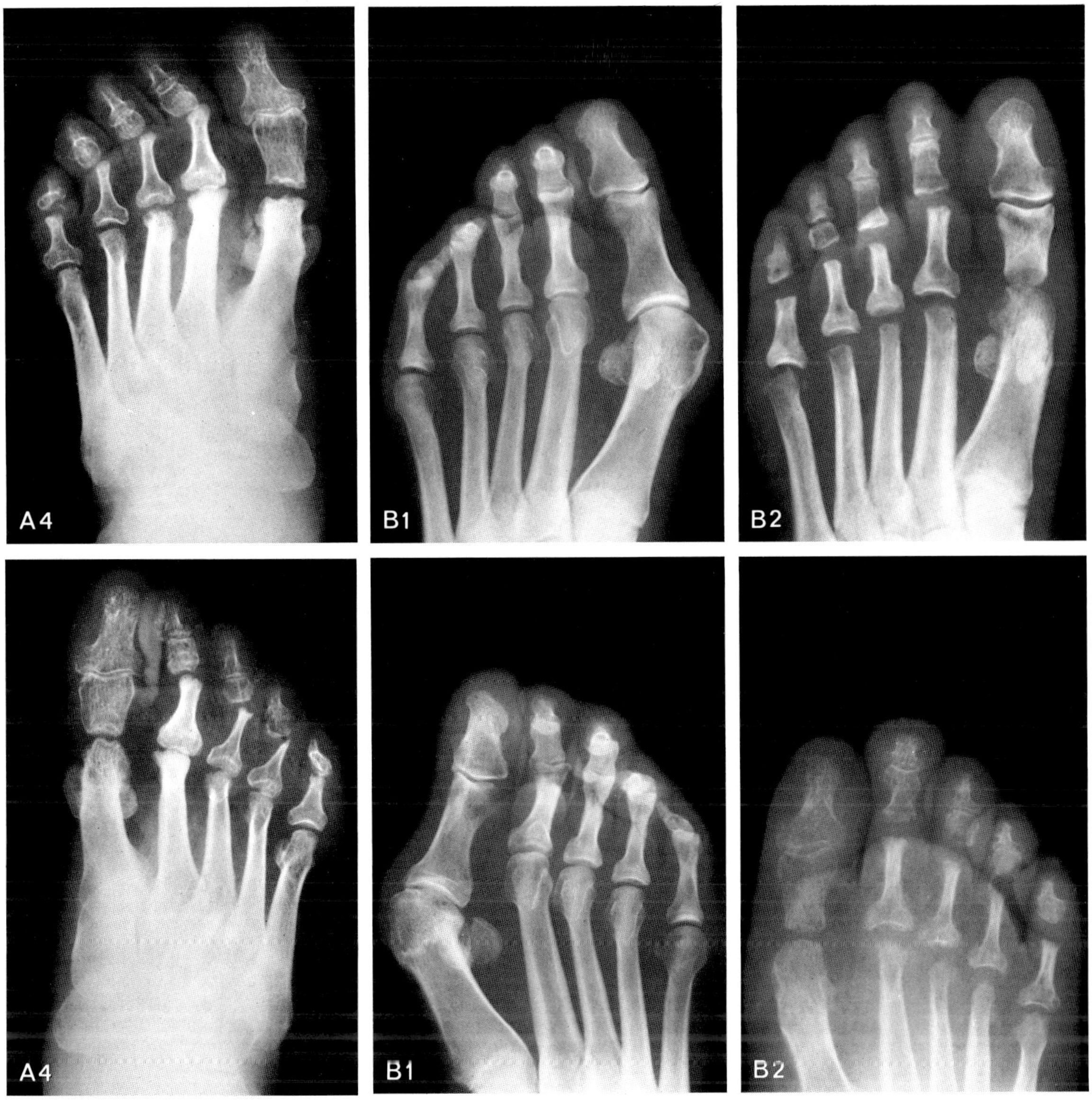

Fig. 42.2 A *4,* **B.** Legend see p. 566

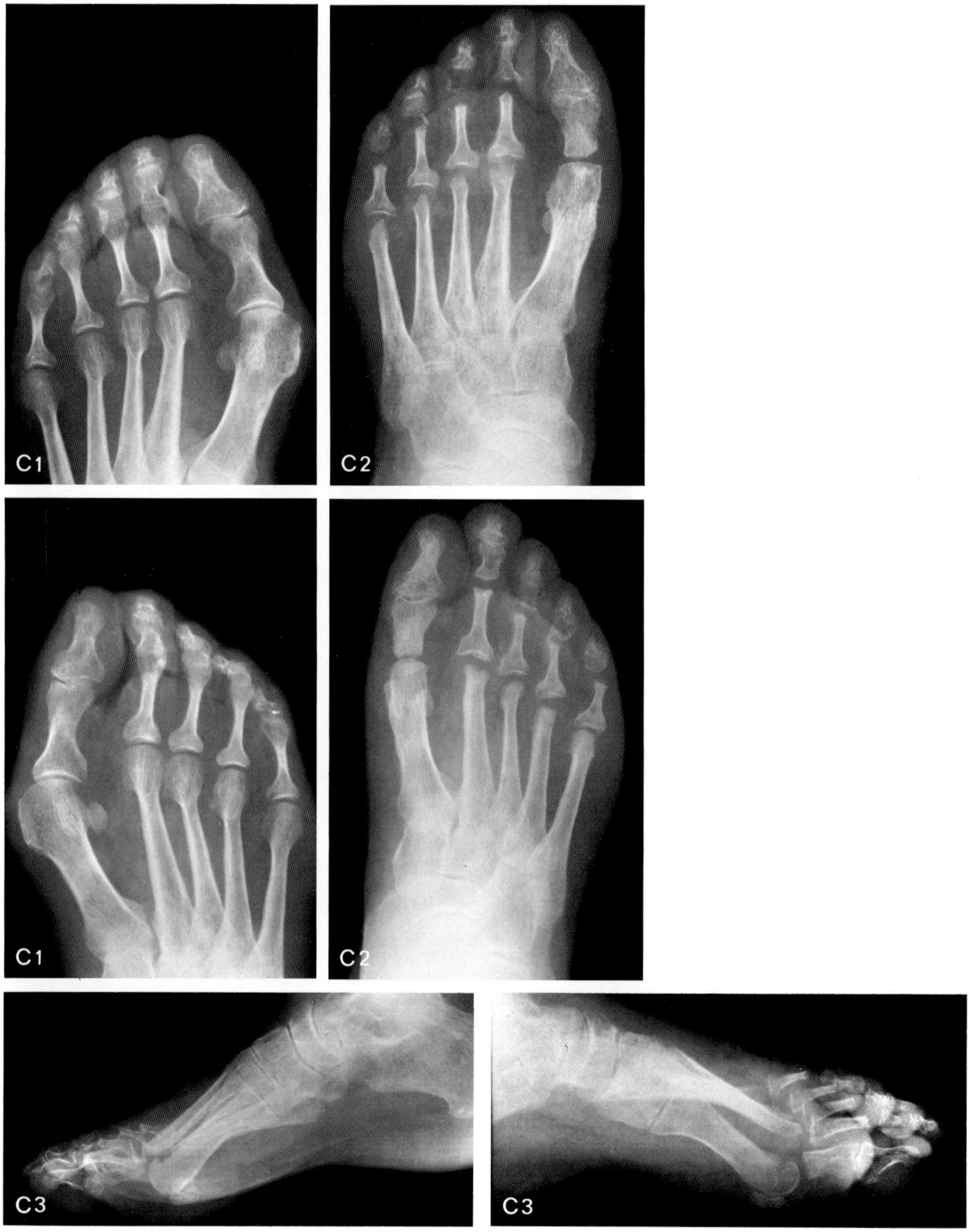

Fig. 42.2 *(continued).* **C** Convex triangular forefoot: hallux valgus with frontal protrusion of central metatarsal heads, distal clawing of toes. *1* Before surgery. *2* After metatarsal realignment, correction of hallux valgus by metatarsophalangeal arthroplasty (Lelièvre), arthroplasties of proximal interphalangeal joints of toes. *3* Oblique view of metatarsophalangeal joints, identifying post-resection metatarsal extremities and pseudarthroses. The result was good, with adequate range of movement and freedom from pain. **D** *1–3* Right foot, simple triangular forefoot: hallux valgus, supraductus in varus of second toe, frontal protrusion of central metatarsal heads: *1* before surgery; *2* a year after realignment, correction of hallux valgus, digital arthroplasties; *3* oblique view: arthroplasties with pseudarthroses. *4–6* Left foot, simple triangular forefoot: *4* before surgery; *5, 6* a year after operation

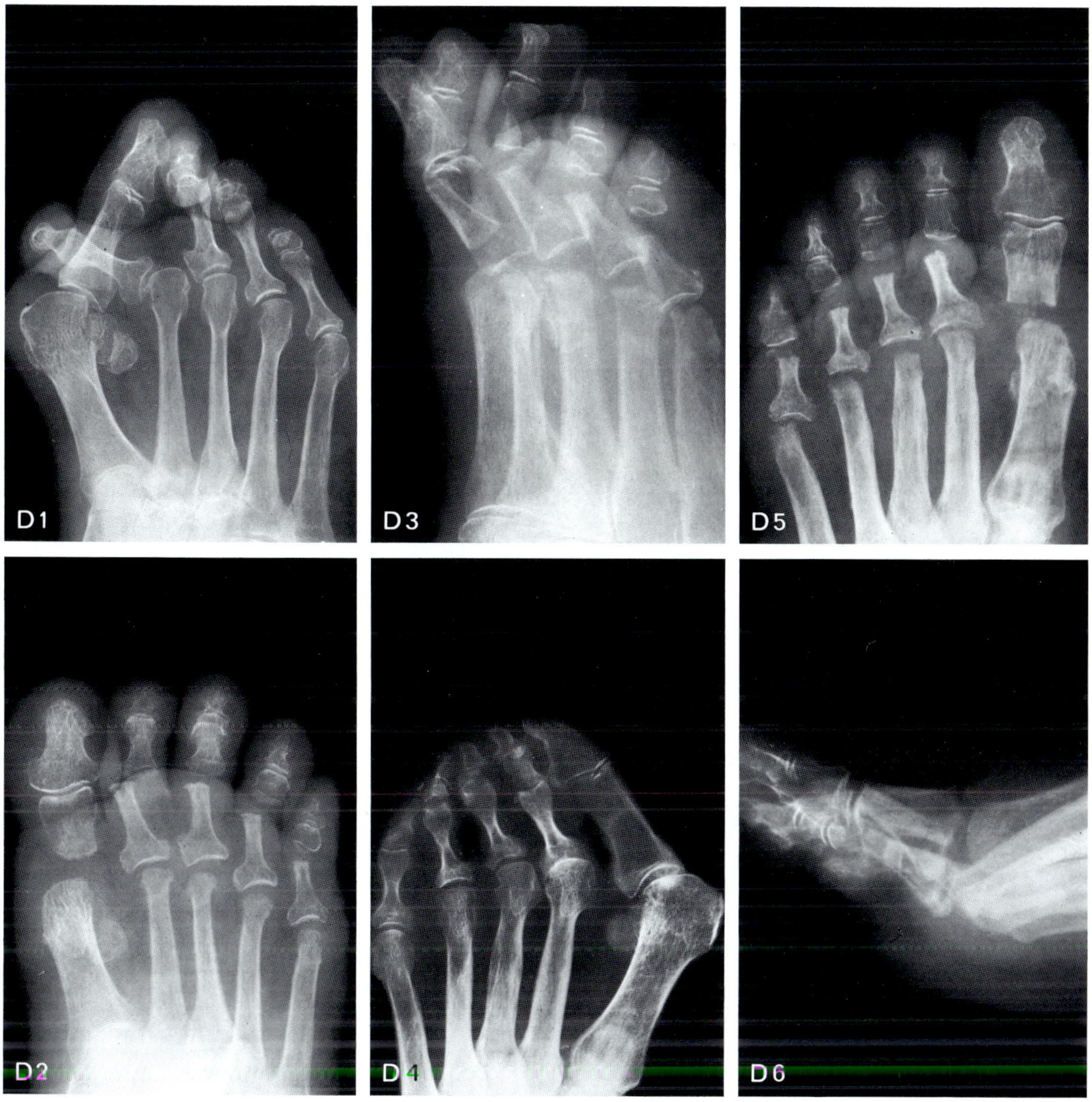

Fig. 42.2 D. Legend see p. 568

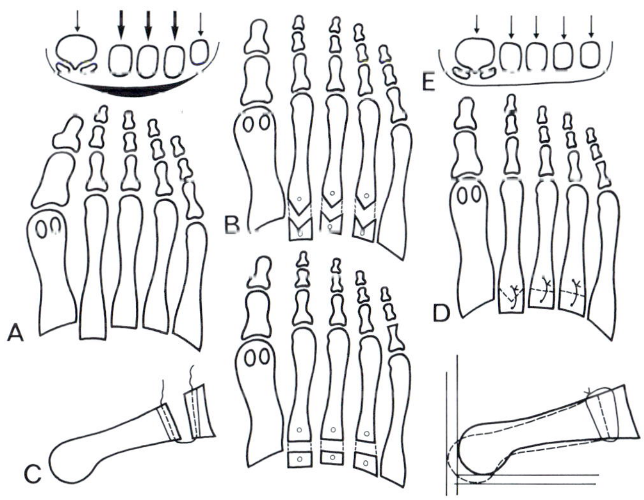

Fig. 42.3 A–E. Metatarsal basal osteotomies. **A** Indications. **B** V-osteotomy technique. **C** Thys technique. **D** Both techniques may be used in the same foot. **E** Desired result

42.2.2 Technique

With tourniquet applied, a dorsal longitudinal incision across the bases of the metatarsals concerned is preferable to a transverse incision, which is more prone to postoperative oedema. Two parallel incisions are necessary when more than three osteotomies have to be performed. The subcutaneous tissue is retracted with vessels, nerves and the muscle mass of extensor digitorum brevis. The periosteum at the site of the osteotomy is slit longitudinally and retracted by periosteal stripping.
The form of the osteotomy must be chosen exactly, depending upon whether correction of length, equinus, or both is necessary.

Correction of Length. For frontal protrusion, a segment of metatarsal shaft base must be resected, and this should be calculated from the dorsoplantar radiograph of the metatarsus. Section of the calculated length is performed using an oscillating saw orientated perpendicular to the long axis of the metatarsal. Coaptation of the bony surfaces should be ensured, and then fixation is achieved by means of a non-absorbable suture threaded through two small holes bored in the sagittal plane through both fragments of the metatarsal. A suture-passer aids passage of the suture material, and on tying, coaptation of the cut surfaces is achieved. The operation is appropriate for the three middle metatarsal heads.

Correction of Equinus. Baropodometry determines exactly the pressure under each metatarsal head and allows precise calculation of the degree of displacement of these. A cuneiform wedge based dorsally can be removed using an oscillating saw following direct calculation of the degree of elevation required from the lateral view radiograph. Coaptation after closure of the wedge can be maintained by a non-absorbable suture passed through tiny drill holes confined to the dorsal cortex only.

Correction of Length and Equinus. Removal of a trapezoidal segment of bone allows correction of both length and angulation. As before, coaptation can be maintained by a non-absorbable suture passed through both surfaces of the bony section. Following fixation of the bone, the periosteum should be repaired and the skin closed. A moulded plaster shoe maintains the correction and should be worn for 10–15 days, during which weight bearing is avoided. From the 16th day an elastic support is allowed and partial weight bearing instituted. Thereafter, active exercises hasten recuperation of function of the metatarsophalangeal joints.

42.3 Head-Shaft Enclavement

This operation (Regnauld 1968) allows perfect reconstruction of the forefoot in many instances. Between 1968 and 1981, I performed 1110 enclavement procedures. The aims are triple: the reposition of metatarsal heads in the same horizontal and frontal planes, the correction of digital displacements with respect to the metatarsals, and the preservation of normal amplitude of joint motion. The procedure consists essentially of section of the metatarsal neck at the base of the head, fashioning of the proximal fragment into a quadrangular tenon, temporary removal of the metatarsal heads and fashioning of a corresponding quadrangular mortice, and reimplantation and proper realignment of the heads. The reposition of the proximal phalanges of the associated toes is facilitated by total capsulotomy.
Head-shaft enclavement can be single or multiple (Figs. 42.4–42.8), the metatarsal heads are completely removed during the procedure and constitute, in effect, autografts. In instances where the

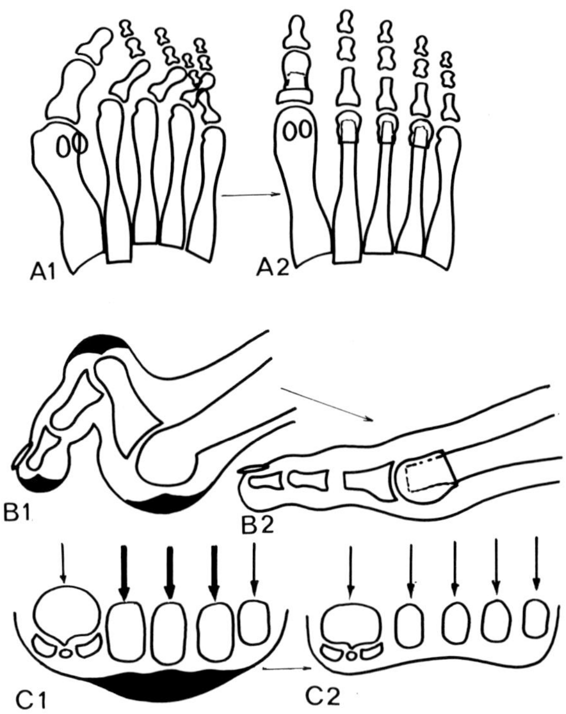

Fig. 42.4. A Central metatarsal head overloading in round forefoot: *1* Before treatment; *2* after metatarsal shaft-head enclavements (Regnauld). **B** Claw toe: *1* Before treatment; *2* after metatarsal enclavement and digital arthroplasty. **C** Central metatarsal head overloading: *1* Before treatment; *2* after redistribution of metatarsal head pressures

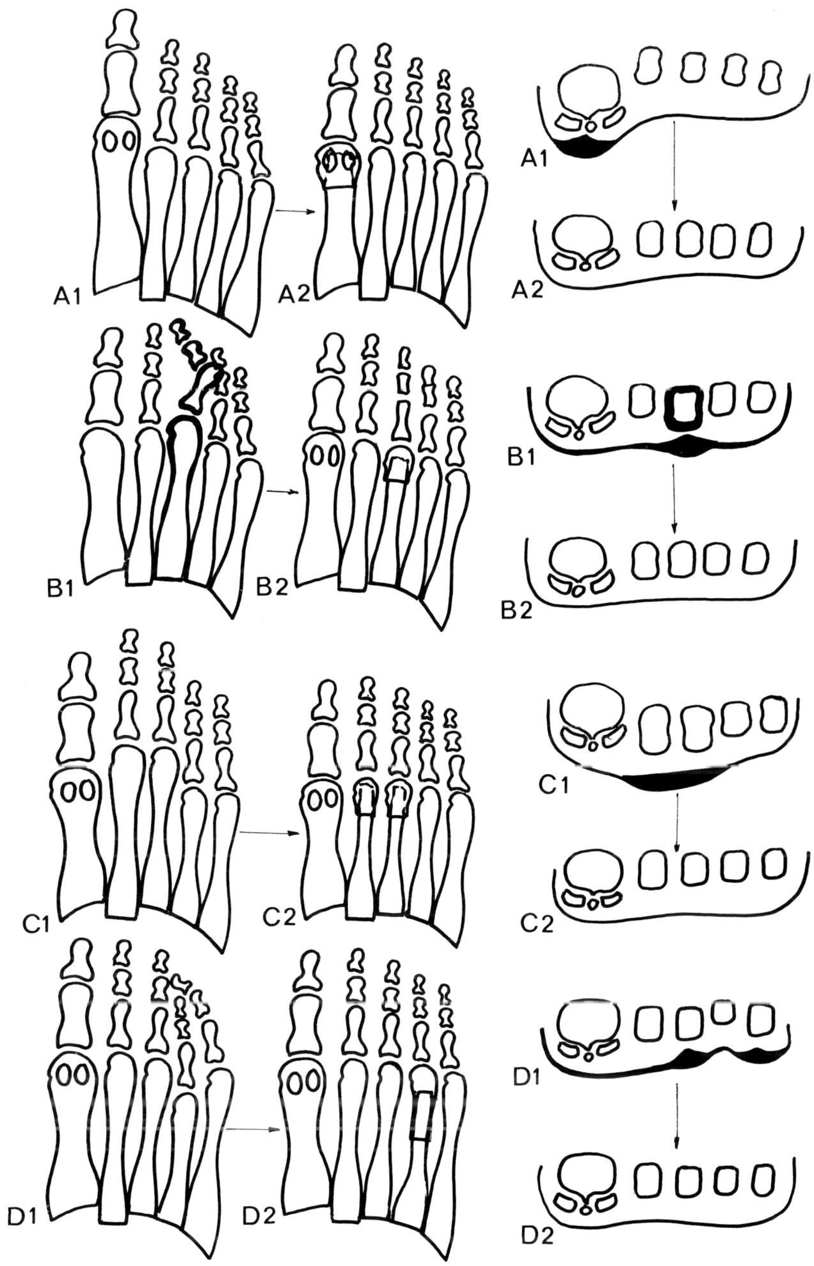

Fig. 42.5. **A** Overloading of first metatarsal head due to excessive length: *1* Before treatment; *2* after realignment head-shaft enclavement. **B** Macrodactyly of third ray: *1* Before treatment; *2* after realignment head-shaft enclavement of metatarsal and reduction of toe. **C** Overloading of second and third metatarsal heads due to excessive length: *1* Before treatment; *2* after realignment head-shaft enclavement (Regnauld). **D** Underloading of fourth metatarsal head: *1* Before treatment; *2* after realignment head-shaft enclavement using a homograft (Regnauld)

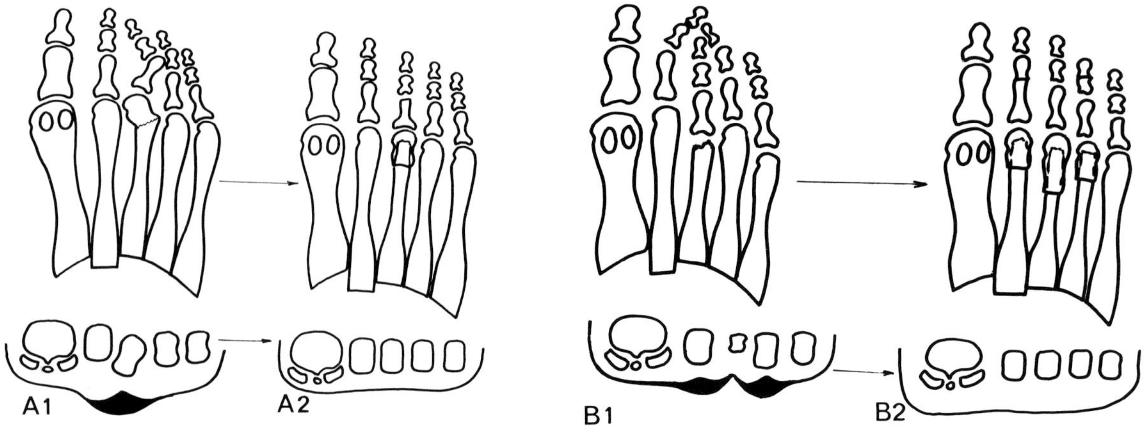

Fig. 42.6. A Overloading of third metatarsal head due to malunion of fractured shaft: *1* Before treatment; *2* after realignment head-shaft enclavement (Regnauld). **B** Underloading of third metatarsal head with secondary overloading of fourth and fifth heads: *1* Before treatment; *2* after realignment head-shaft enclavements, using a homograft for third head in presence of osteonecrosis (Regnauld)

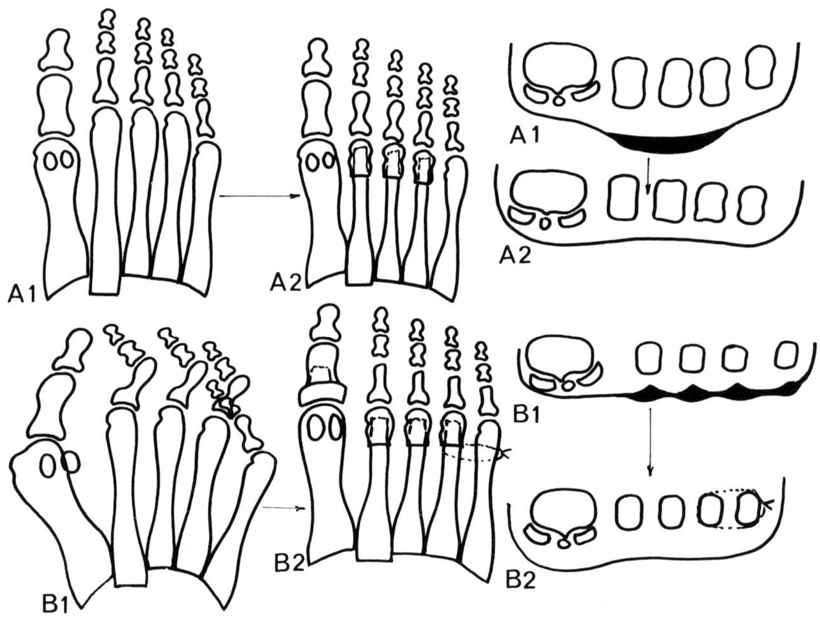

Fig. 42.7. A Round forefoot with overloading of central metatarsals: *1* Before treatment; *2* after metatarsal head-shaft enclavements (Regnauld). **B** Flat triangular forefoot (Locke syndrome) with general overloading of the central three or all five metatarsals, or round triangular forefoot with overloading of the central metatarsals: *1* Before treatment; *2* after correction of hallux valgus and metatarsus quintus valgus and metatarsal head-shaft enclavements

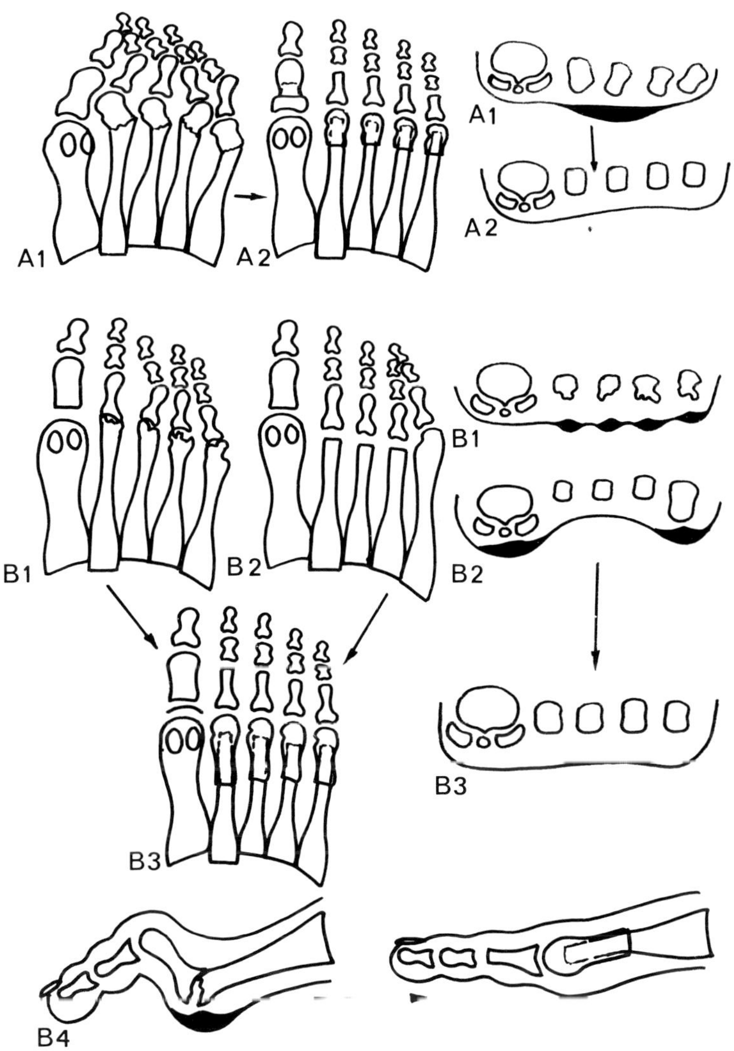

Fig. 42.8. A Malunion of fractured metatarsals, overloading of central metatarsal heads, digital displacements: *1* Before treatment; *2* after realignment enclavement of metatarsal heads, using autografts (Regnauld), to redistribute loading. **B** *1* Localised overloading under irregular ends of metatarsals, due to osteophyte formation, after poor metatarsal alignment in rheumatoid disease of forefoot; *2* iatrogenic forefoot cavus with overloading of first and fifth metatarsal heads after excision of central three metatarsal heads; *3* realignment enclavement of metatarsal heads using homografts, correction of hallux valgus and of lesser toes (Regnauld); *4* lateral view showing correction with homograft

metatarsal heads are too severely damaged for enclavement, homografts taken from cadavers can be used, the damaged heads can be retained and cup arthroplasties performed or prosthetic metatarsal heads can be inserted.

42.3.1 Indications

Single Autografts: Egyptian forefoot with hypertrophy in length of the first metatarsal, isolated frontal protrusion of a metatarsal, macropodia of one or two of the central three metatarsals, congenital aplasia of a central metatarsal (most frequently the fourth), post-traumatic malunited fracture of a metatarsal, post-traumatic metatarsophalangeal arthropathy, arthrosic hypertrophy of Freiberg-Köhler disease, rheumatic conditions with preservation of the gross structure of the metatarsal head, i. e. without osteolytis inflammatory erosion.

Multiple Autografts: Congenital abnormalities [occasionally the forefoot syndrome of Duddley Morton (1935); convex congenital forefoot associated with short first metatarsal, overloading of the middle three metatarsals, or macropodia of the central three metatarsals], convex forefoot, convex triangular forefoot, the triangular forefoot syndrome of Locke, early rheumatoid arthritis, dislocations of the metatarsophalangeal joints, various postoperative iatrogenic failures (see Chap. 25).

Single Homograft: Underloading due to resection of a metatarsal head, third-degree Freiberg-Köhler disease, post-osteitis of a metatarsal head.

Multiple Homografts: Exceptional indications are severe polyarthropathies of the forefoot or multiple deformities associated with poorly orientated Lelièvre realignments or Hohmann-Wallet operations.

42.3.2 Technique

The technique is shown in Fig. 42.9. The skin incision is transverse, lightly concave proximally, over the metatarsal heads required. After haemostasis, pressure under the metatarsal heads and flexion of the toes by the assistant throws the metatarsophalangeal joints into prominence. The capsule is incised longitudinally on one side or the other of the extensor tendons, using a fine scalpel, and detached completely from the metatarsal head, avoiding damage to the interossei. (If the joints are irreducibly dislocated, the extensor tendons can be divided Z-fashion so as to allow elongation after repair at the close of operation.) The capsule is detached similarly from the base of the proximal phalanx.

The neck of the metatarsal is divided carefully and the head removed and wrapped in a swab soaked in physiological saline. The site of section is determined from the dorsoplantar radiograph so as to ensure that the head is properly aligned with its neighbours after enclavement. The procedure applies to any metatarsal head, but usually it is not necessary to remove the fifth one.

The stump of the metatarsal is then shaped so as to form a quadrangular tenon. This can be done with fine rongeurs (e.g. Ombredanne pattern, see Chap. 41), and the size depends on available bone stock. Usually it is 6–8 mm in length.

A mortice of exactly the same dimension as the tenon must now be fashioned in the appropriate metatarsal head. This procedure is started with a drill and finished using a fine rugine. It *must* be directed parallel with the dorsal surface of the metatarsal head. While the assistant steadies the metatarsal shaft with two hooks and holds the toes in plantarflexion, the head is tapped very gently onto the tenon.

It is now possible to check carefully that the metatarsal heads are correctly aligned. The capsule is repaired with interrupted fine absorbable sutured and the skin closed.

After change of dressings on the following day, gentle active flexion and extension is encouraged. Weight bearing is avoided for 7 weeks. No passive manipulation is allowed.

Examples of clinical results are shown in Figs. 42.10–42.12.

42.4 Metatarsophalangeal Interposition Cup Arthroplasty

42.4.1 Indications

Metatarsophalangeal interposition cup arthroplasty (Regnauld and Grassin 1975) is performed when metatarsal heads are too severely damaged, by whatever means, to allow enclavement. It allows continued mobility and functional loading.

42.4.2 Technique

The operation is performed via the same approach as head-shaft enclavement. After exposure, the affected condyle of the metatarsal is trimmed to allow insertion of a high-density polyethylene cup. The cup is fixed either with three or four sutures to the remnants of the proximal capsular attachment or with a transosseous stitch to the phalangeal base. After reposition of the proximal phalanx, perhaps necessitating elongation of the extensor tendons, the capsule is sutured and the skin closed. After exercises are commenced after about a week, and resumption of protected weight bearing ensues at about 20 days. Removal of the cup may be advised after about a year if discomfort is present; otherwise, it can be left, except in the case of the great metatarsophalangeal joint, where it should always be removed. Any residual clawing of the lesser toes must be corrected (Fig. 42.12).

42.5 Prosthetic Replacement of Metatarsal Head

42.5.1 Indications

Insertion of a prosthetic metatarsal head (Regnauld 1974) is the final resort in cases of destruction too severe even for cup interposition arthroplasty. The pathological indications are similar, however (Fig. 42.13).

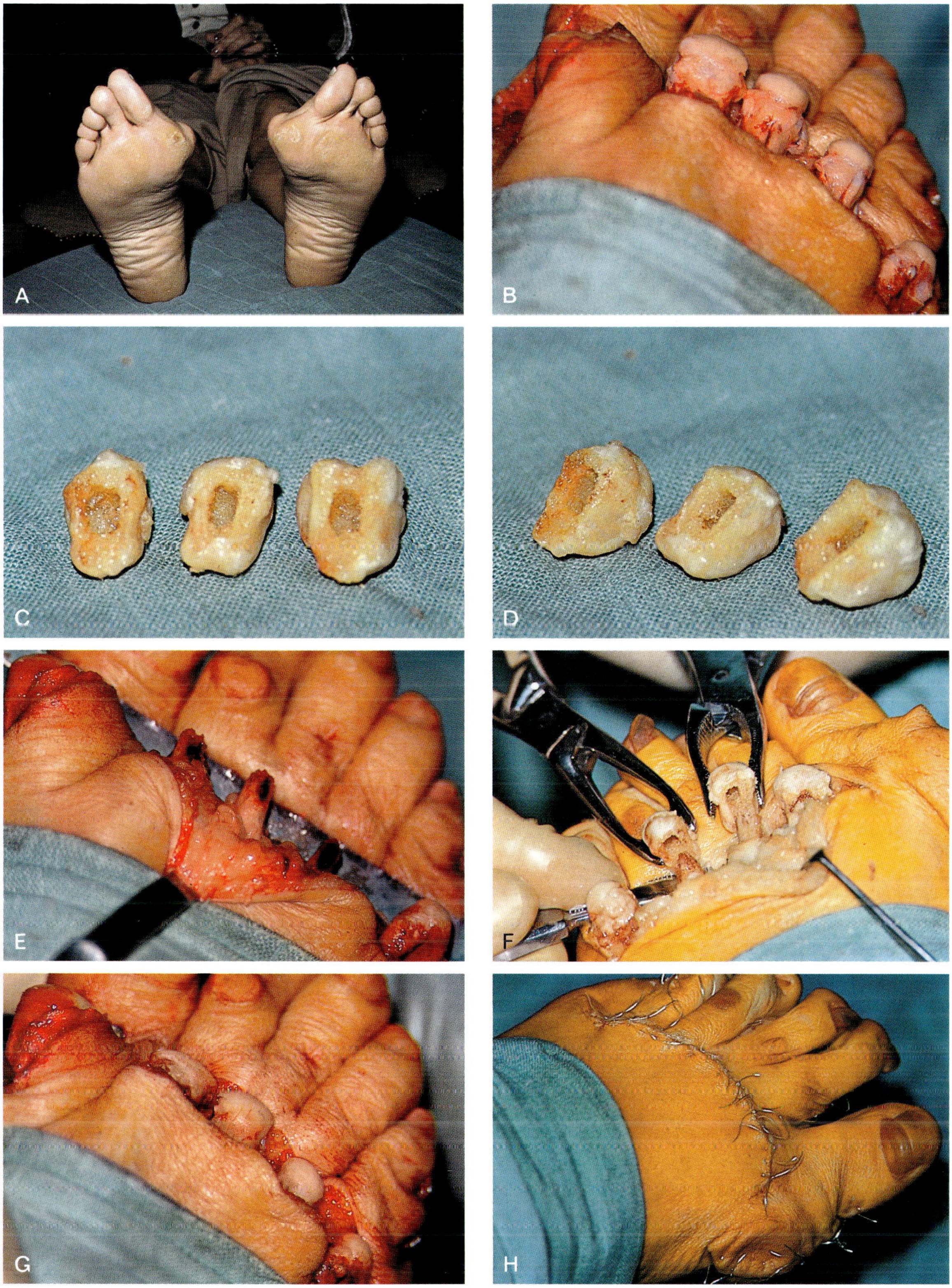

Fig. 42.9 A–H. Head-shaft enclavement. **A** Convex triangular forefoot. **B** Exposure of metatarsal heads and division of neck. **C, D** Fashioning of quadrangular mortice in each condyle. **E** Fashioning of tenon on metatarsal shaft. **F** Implantation of tenon into mortice. **G** Alignment. **H** Skin suture

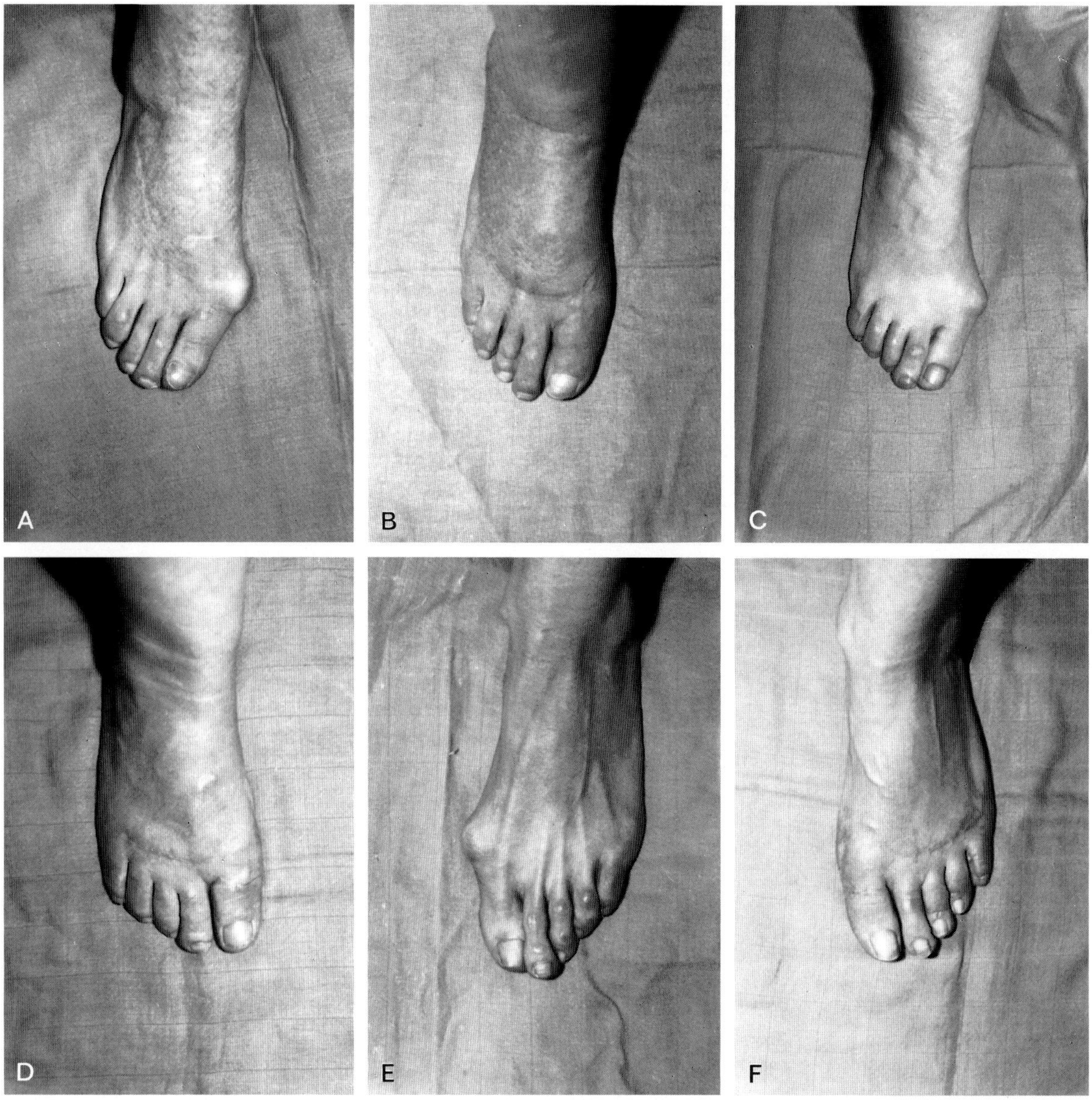

Fig. 42.10 A–L. Correction of convex forefoot, including correction of hallux valgus and claw toes and enclavement of second, third and fourth metatarsal heads. **A** Convex forefoot with second-degree hallux valgus and clawing of fourth and fifth toes; **B** appearance following correction of hallux valgus, arthroplasty of fourth and fifth toes and head-shaft enclavement of second, third and fourth metatarsals. **C** Convex forefoot with second-degree hallux valgus and clawing of outer four toes; **D** appearance following correction of hallux valgus, arthroplasty of proximal interphalangeal joints of the outer four toes and head-shaft enclavement of second, third and fourth metatarsals. **E** Convex forefoot with first-degree hallux valgus and clawing of toes with contracture of extensor tendons; **F** appearance following correction of hallux valgus and claw toes by elongation of extensor tendons, arthrodesis of proximal interphalangeal joints of second toe, arthrodesis of distal interphalangeal joints of third and fourth toes, arthroplasty of proximal interphalangeal joint of fifth toe and head-shaft enclavement of second, third and fourth metatarsals. **G–L** see p. 577

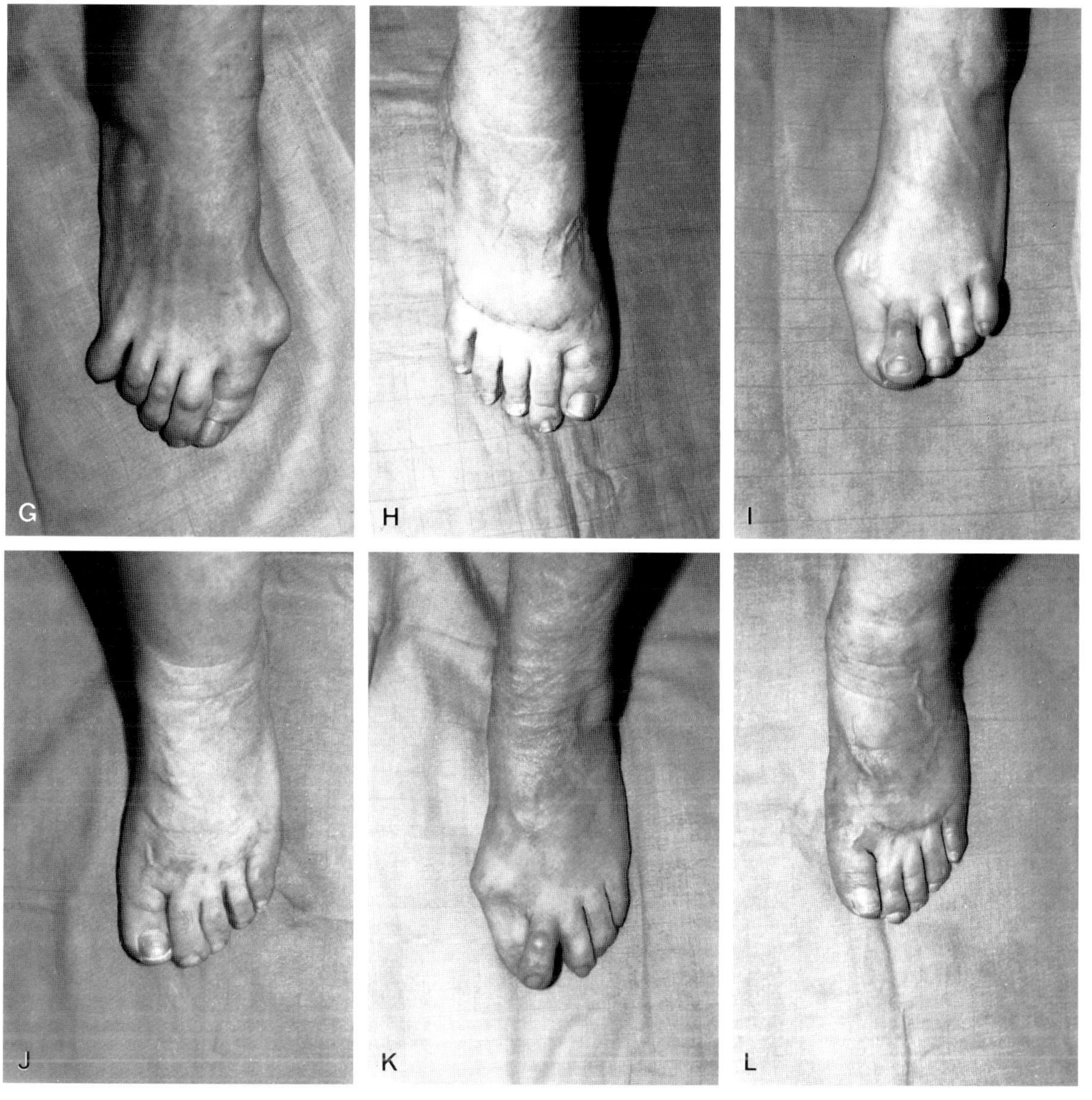

Fig. 42.10 *(continued)*. **G** Convex forefoot with second-degree hallux valgus and clawing of toes; **H** appearance following correction of hallux valgus, arthroplasty of interphalangeal joints and head-shaft enclavement of second, third and fourth metatarsals. **J, K** Convex forefoot with second-degree hallux valgus, superductus of second toe and clawing of fifth toe; **J, L** Appearance of **I** and **K** respectively following correction of hallux valgus, arthrodesis of proximal interphalangeal joint of second toe, arthroplasty of fifth toe and head-shaft enclavement of second, third and fourth metatarsals

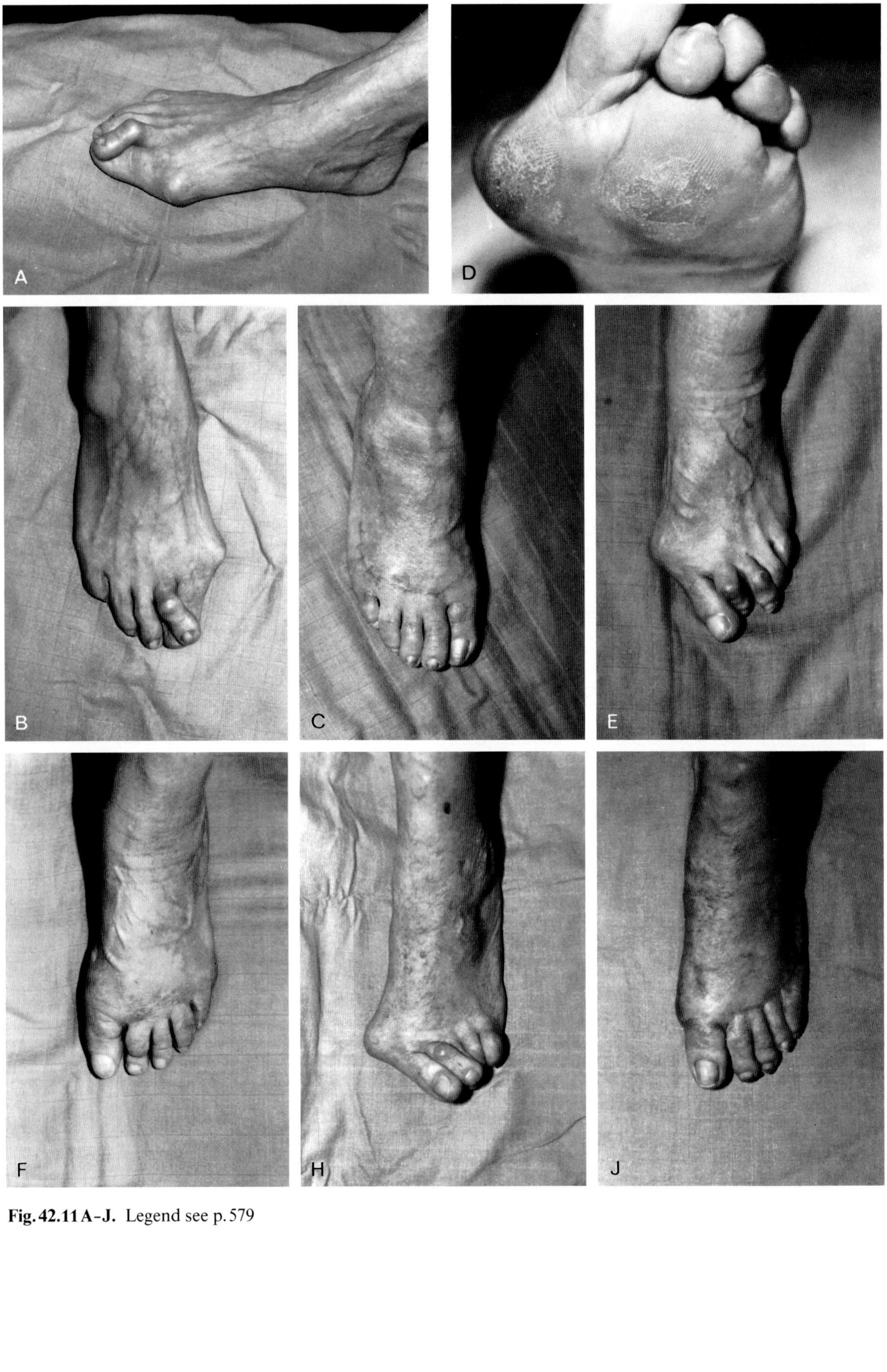

Fig. 42.11 A–J. Legend see p. 579

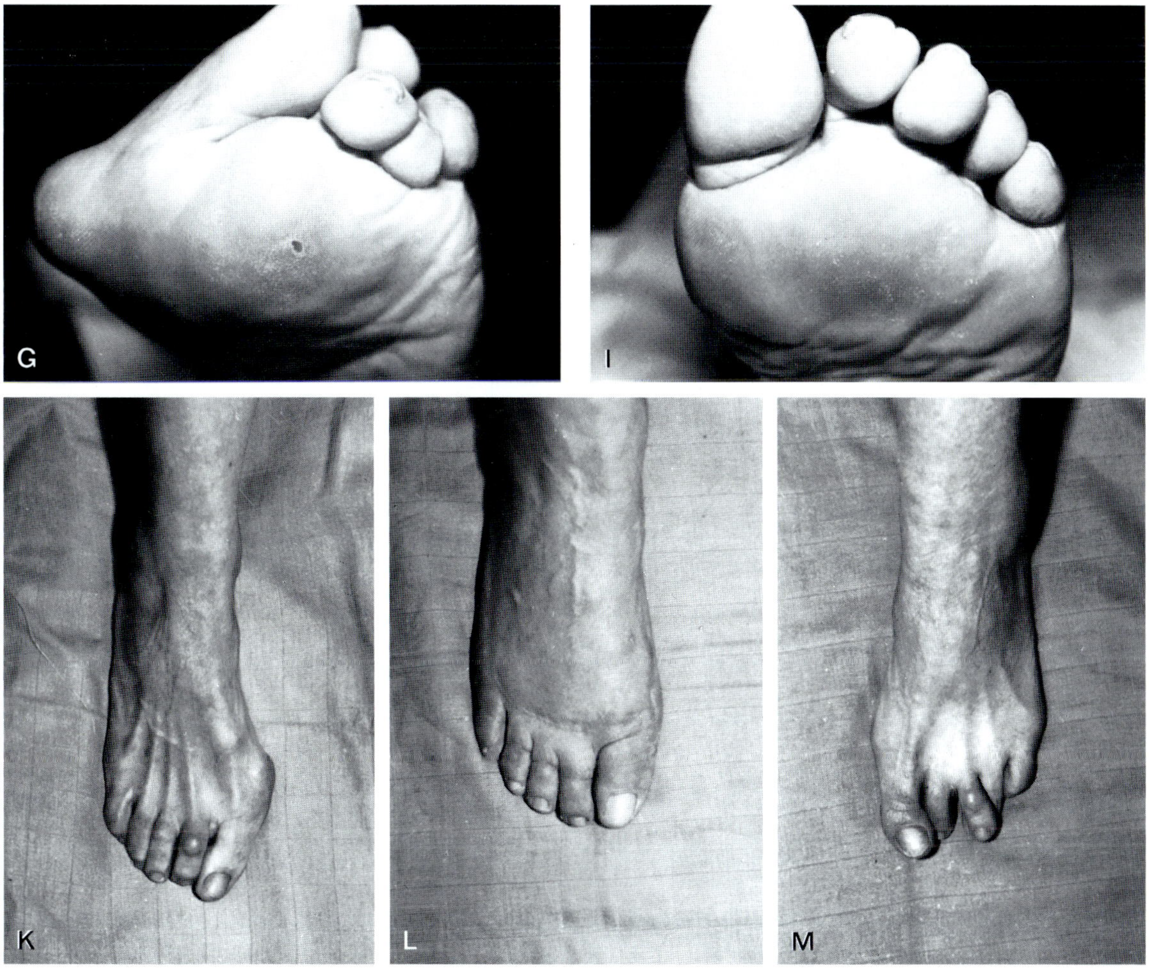

◁ **Fig. 42.11 A–R.** Triangular forefoot syndrome. **A, B** Triangular forefoot with thrid-degree hallux valgus, superductus of second toe in varus and clawing with varus distally of third and fourth toes. **C** Appearance following correction of hallux valgus, arthrodesis of proximal interphalangeal joint of second toe, arthrodesis of distal interphalangeal joint of third and fourth toes, arthroplasty of fifth toe, head-shaft enclavement of second, third and fourth metatarsals and elongation of extensor tendons. **D, E** Triangular forefoot with central callus formation under second and third metatarsal heads, third-degree hallux valgus, digital clawing with valgus of second, third and fourth toes and clawing of fifth toe. **F** Appearance following correction of hallux valgus, arthrodesis of proximal interphalangeal joint of second and third toes, arthroplasty of fourth and fifth toes, head-shaft enclavement of second, third and fourth metatarsals and elongation of long and short extensor tendons (short extensors included because of valgus posture of toes). **G, H** Convex triangular forefoot with plantar callosities and central serous bursa formation, third-degree hallux valgus, valgus superductus of second toe, clawing of third and fourth toes and capsulotendinous dorsal contracture of outer metatarsophalangeal joints. **I, J** Appearance following correction of hallux valgus, arthroplasty of proximal interphalangeal joints of toes, head-shaft enclavement of second, third and fourth metatarsals, elongation of long extensor tendon and of short extensor tendon because of valgus posture of toes. **K** Convex forefoot with second-degree hallux valgus, digital clawing and contracture of long and short extensor tendons. **L** Appearance following correction of hallux valgus, arthrodesis of proximal interphalangeal joints of second, third and fourth toes, arthroplasty of fifth toe, head-shaft enclavement of second, third and fourth metatarsals and elongation of long and short extensor tendons. **M** Convex forefoot with first-degree hallux valgus, infraductus of second toe, valgus superductus of third toe, infraductus of fourth toe and clawing of proximal interphalangeal joint of fifth toe. **N–R** see p. 580

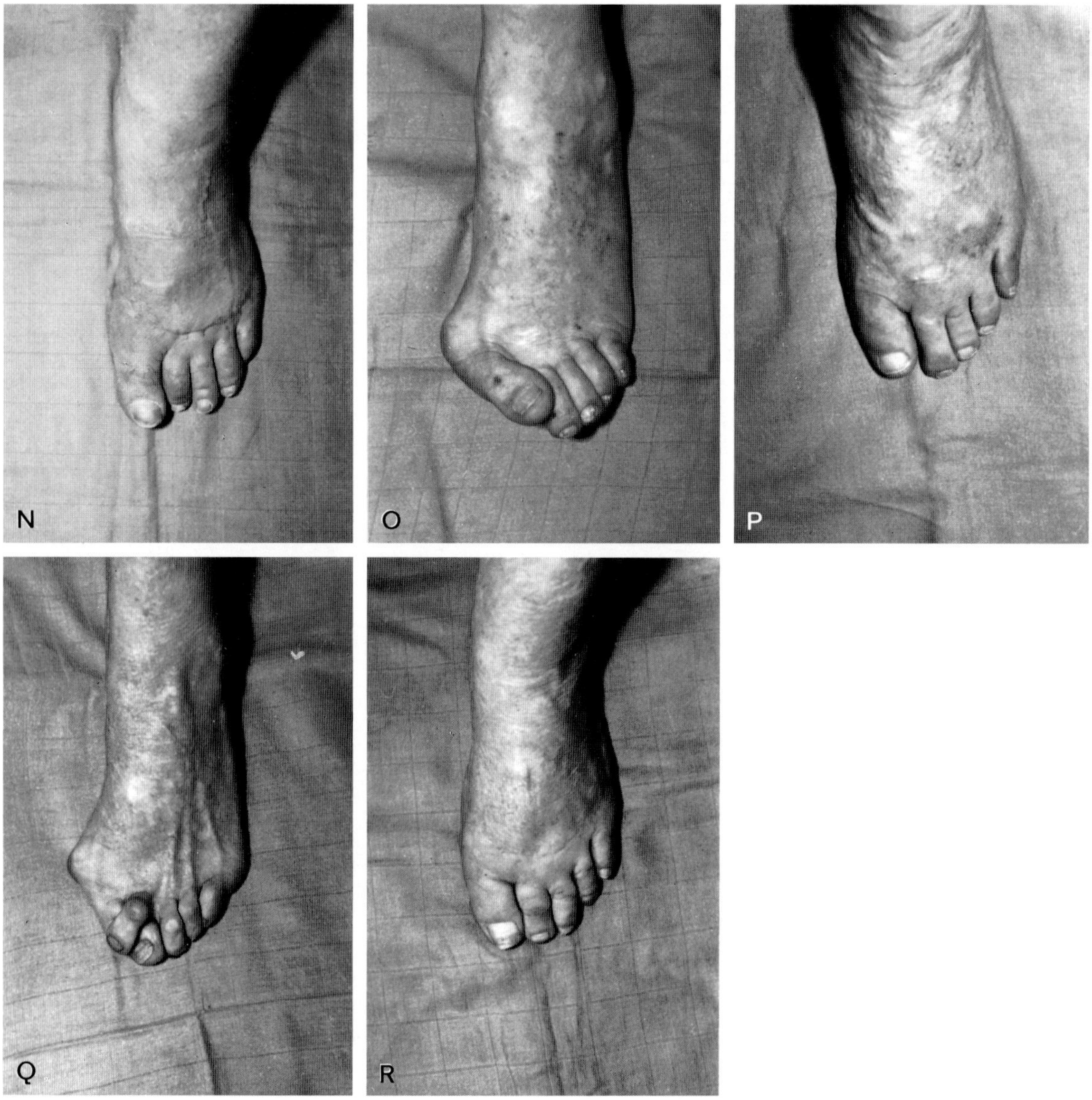

Fig. 42.11 *(continued)*. **N** appearance following correction of hallux valgus, second toe and fourth toe including distal tenotomy of flexor tendon and arthroplasty of proximal interphalangeal joint, arthrodesis of proximal interphalangeal joint of third toe, arthroplasty of proximal phalangeal joint of fifth toe, head-shaft enclavement of second, third and fourth metatarsals and elongation of extensor tendons. **O** Simple triangular forefoot with third-degree hallux valgus, valgus displacement of outer four toes and contracture of extensor hallucis longus; **P** appearance following correction of hallux valgus, arthroplasty of proximal interphalangeal joints of the outer four toes, head-shaft enclavement of second, third and fourth metatarsals and elongation of extensor tendons. **Q** Simple triangular forefoot with third-degree hallux valgus, varus superductus of second toe with clawing of proximal interphalangeal joint, clawing of third, fourth and fifth toes and capsulotendinous contractures involving both extensor and flexor tendons; **R** appearance following correction of hallux valgus, arthrodesis of proximal interphalangeal joints of second, third and fourth toes, arthroplasty of fifth toe, head-shaft enclavement of second, third and fourth metatarsals, flexor tendon tenotomies and elongation of short extensor tendons

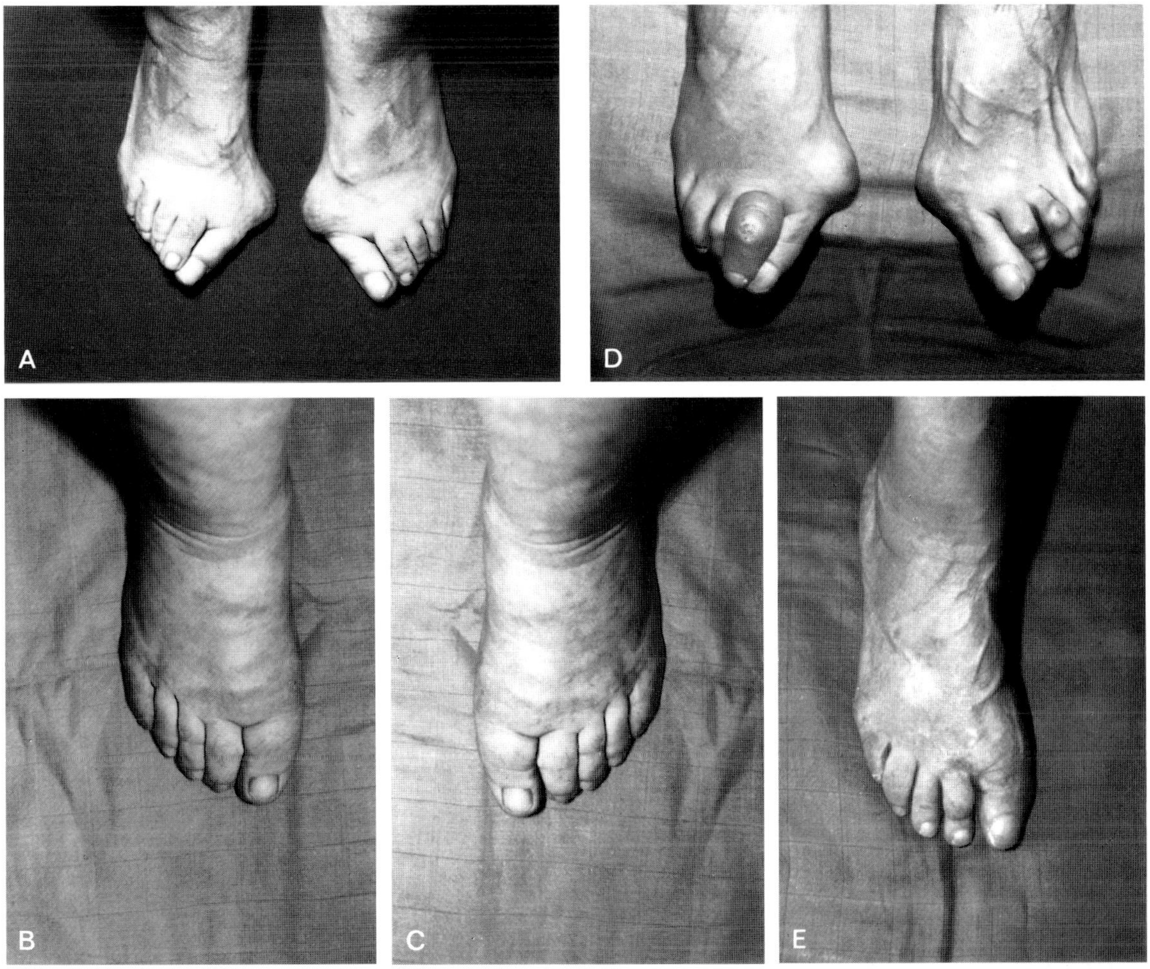

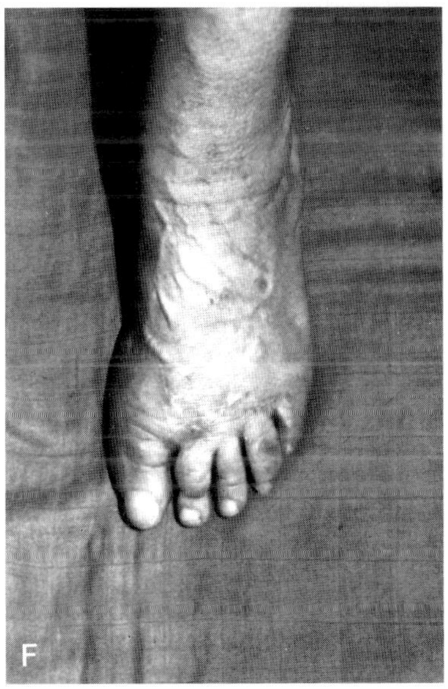

Fig. 42.12 A–L. Treatment of triangular forefoot. **A–F** Simple triangular forefoot: **A** Preoperative; **B, C** postoperative; **D** preoperative; **E, F** postoperative. Operation comprises correction of hallux valgus by arthroplasty with osteocartilaginous graft, arthrodesis of proximal interphalangeal joints of second and third toes, arthroplasty of proximal interphalangeal joints of fourth and fifth toes, head-shaft enclavement of second, third and fourth metatarsals and elongation of long and short extensor tendons. **G–L** see p. 582

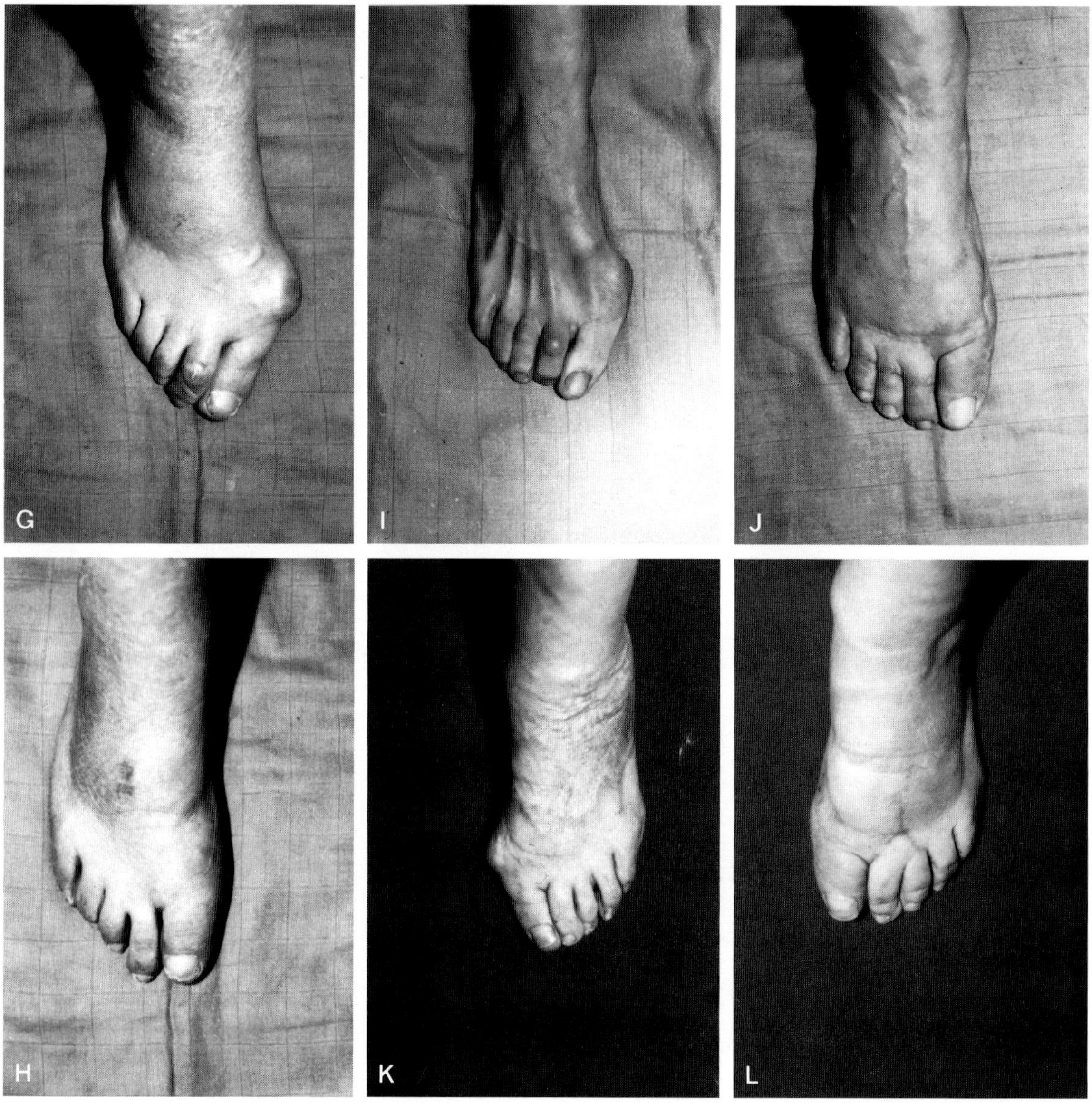

Fig. 42.12 *(continued)*. **G–L** Convex triangular forefoot. **G** Preoperative; **H** after correction of hallux valgus, head-shaft enclavement of second, third and fourth metatarsals and arthroplasty of proximal interphalangeal joints of second and fifth toes; **I** preoperative; **J** after correction of hallux valgus, head-shaft enclavement of second, third and fourth metatarsals, elongation of extensor tendons, arthroplasty of proximal interphalangeal joints of second to fifth toes; **K** preoperative; **L** after correction of hallux valgus, head-shaft enclavement of second, third and fourth metatarsals, arthrodesis of distal interphalangeal joint of second, third and fourth toes and arthroplasty of fifth toe

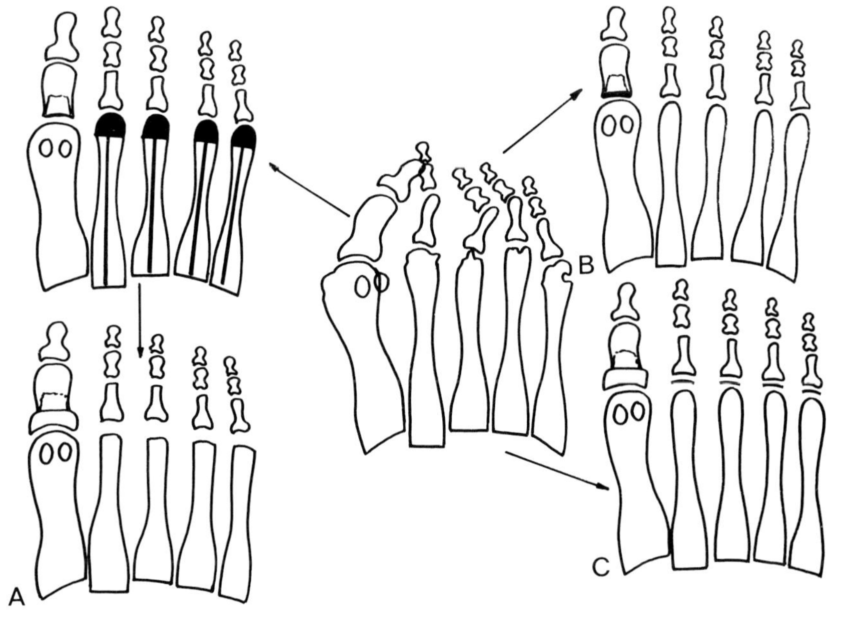

Fig. 42.13 A–C. Techniques of metatarsal realignment. **A** Minimal resection of metatarsal heads and implantation of metatarsal prostheses (Regnauld). **B** Lelièvre method. **C** With cup arthroplasties (Regnauld) and correction of hallux valgus by graft arthroplasty

42.5.2 Technique

Through the same approach as used for head-shaft enclavement, the neck and head of the metatarsal are resected and the metatarsal head prosthesis is inserted into the medullary canal of the proximal residual fragment. The length must be calculated correctly so as to restore frontal and horizontal alignment. The proximal phalanx is repositioned and held by soft tissue sutures, and the skin is closed.

Active exercises commence at about a week, and protected weight bearing can begin at about 20 days. The prosthesis can be removed at 1 year. A space remains but this fills spontaneously, leaving good function.

42.6 Elongation of First Metatarsal for Congenital or Acquired Shortness

42.6.1 Indications

In contradistinction to other authors, who prefer relative shortening of the neighbouring toes (Lelièvre 1952; Thys 1974b), and, sometimes in preference to head-shaft enclavement (Regnauld 1968), Buruturan (1976) advised elongation of the great metatarsal when it displays congenital or acquired shortness. I use the technique only for congenital shortening (Fig. 42.14).

42.6.2 Technique

With tourniquet applied, a longitudinal incision is made over the medial aspect of the great toe, extending from the middle of the proximal phalanx to within 1 cm of the Lisfranc joint line. The incision is deepened in one cut so as to divide the periosteum of the proximal phalanx, the articular capsule of the metatarsophalangeal joint and the periosteum of the first metatarsal. The capsule is detached from the phalangeal base and the metatarsal head. With rongeurs, the medial exostosis of the great metatarsal head is reduced in size and the lateral displacement of the sesamoids released by division of the capsule on their lateral aspect.

The base of the proximal phalanx is divided and the excised proximal fragment preserved in physiological saline. With a curved rugine, the periosteum is stripped around the whole circumference of the metatarsal diaphysis, and after exact calculation, a Z-shaped osteotomy of the bone is performed using a small oscillating saw. The longitudinal component of the osteotomy is horizontal in the axis of the bone, its distal prolongation is transverse and anterior and its proximal part is trans-

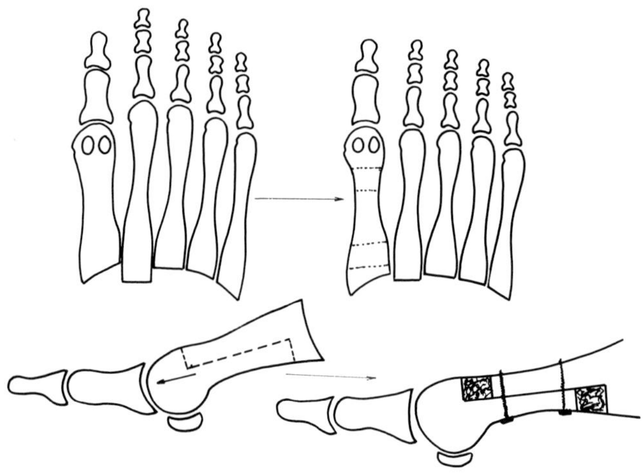

Fig. 42.14. The Burutaran technique of elongation of the first metatarsal

verse and posterior. By means of traction on the distal fragment, the great metatarsal is elongated so that the convexity of the metatarsal head is aligned with respect to the second joint space, the metatarsal head occupying the space vacated by resection of the base of the proximal phalanx. The two segments of the metatarsal are held together by a bone-holding forceps and fixed with two small cortical screws. The two cavities at either end of the osteotomy created by sliding of the fragments are filled by portions of the resected phalangeal base or by corticocancellous grafts taken from the ilium, tibia or fibula. The capsule of the joint is closed carefully as in the technique for hallux valgus. The periosteum of the diaphysis of the metatarsal is repaired, and after meticulous haemostasis the skin is closed.

A plaster cast is applied for 2 months, during which time weight bearing is avoided.

Active exercises commence at the 8th day after operation.

42.7 V-Osteotomy of Metatarsals

42.7.1 Indications

V-osteotomy is indicated in metatarsals where the heads are depressed, protruding or both. It is usually applicable to the central three rays in the simple convex or triangular convex foot. The V-form ensures good stability and healing, which can be delayed when the osteotomy surfaces are flat (Fig. 42.2).

42.7.2 Technique

The approach is through a transverse incision over the dorsal aspect of the metatarsal base concerned, 1 cm distal to the tarsometatarsal joint. A 3-cm incision suffices for one or two metatarsal osteotomies. The extensor tendons, vessels and nerves are retracted carefully, and the periosteum is incised longitudinally and stripped over about 1 cm. Using a fine bone-cutting forceps or a power saw, a V-osteotomy, open anteriorly, is performed at the flare of the metatarsal base. If it is necessary to shorten the bone, a further V-osteotomy is made parallel to the first, the amount of bone to be removed being determined precisely from the dorso-plantar radiograph. With care, the sagittal configuration can be fashioned so as to correct the equinus posture to the desired extent. Approximation of the surfaces is maintained by a transosseous suture passed through the dorsal cortices of the fragments. The periosteum is repaired and the skin closed.

Protected weight bearing is allowed after 2 weeks, and union is followed up radiologically.

43 Afterword

The last page of this book has been turned. Seated at my desk, I let my thoughts wander, and suddenly I relive all that I have experienced, as if at the close of a long and rewarding journey. My eyes take in once more those sentences characterised by restraint and rigor, imbued with a philosophy at once questioning but serene, revealing itself through the choice of thoughts borrowed from distinguished men. Once again, I examine the many illustrations that give emphasis to and clarify the author's ideas, permitting the surgeon to dwell more closely on some detail relating to technique.

What I have just read is not merely a book, it is a summation. Everything that has ever been written on the pathology of the foot has been summarised in these pages, including therapeutic reflections seemingly contradictory or impracticable on the face of it, but lending to the whole a pluralistic character motivated by a desire to seek out the truth.

At the same time, if each of us were to look back and take stock, we could not help but realise that one often "destroys what one reveres and reveres what one destroys". Thus, following the examples of Böhler in the 1930s and Watson-Jones in the 1950s, we condemned osteosynthesis in favor of continuous extension and immobilisation in a cast for the treatment of fractures. Since the 1970s, semi-urgent osteosynthesis has been the golden rule of orthopaedic surgery. Many other examples drawn from visceral surgery would also illustrate this assertion.

Yet all of these examples only confirm Pascal's adage that "today's truth is tomorrow's error". Nonetheless, this saying is only partially true, for each alternative is but another step in the progress of science.

In his book, Dr. Regnauld describes two techniques recommended by him some years ago. These are diaphyso-epiphyseal enclavement of the metatarsals and cuneiform osteotomy of the neck of the talus and the navicular bone with traction of the posterior leg in the treatment of pes planus. Our first impulse is to cry heresy, for it is impossible to hollow out a metatarsal head, which is partially cartilaginous, and enclave it onto the end of the corresponding diaphysis in the expectation that it will form solid callus. It is impossible, as everyone knows, to perform an osteotomy of the neck of the talus without risk of necrosis. And yet, it works! In the words of Teilhard de Chardin, *"Plus je vais et plus je pense que la part du fantastique et de l'impossible est grande dans l'univers"*. Likewise, a magnificent and felicitous propensity towards wonder and discovery pervades this book, which clearly reflects the personal qualities of the author: those of a meticulous and skilled surgeon and tireless worker, with an imaginative mind and a heart sensitive to the sufferings of his fellow man, who embodies the Virgilian dictum *"labor omnia vincit improbus"*.

Henri Courriades

44 Historical Bibliography

1782 Laforest M: L'art de soigner les pieds. Paris

1802 Bourdet J: Dell'arte di curare i piedi. Venezia

1834 Bidault J: Monographie des pieds ou traité de pédicurie descriptive. Naples

1865 Barwell R: On the cure of club foot without cutting tendons. Hardwicke, London

1866 Adams W: Club foot. Churchill, London

1883 Lorenz A: Die Lehre vom erworbenen Plattfuße. Enke, Stuttgart

1888 Blum A: Traité de chirurgie du pied. Asselin et Houzeau, librairie de la faculté de médecine, place de l'Ecole de médecine, Paris

1889 Bessel Hagel F: Die Pathologie und Therapie des Klumpfußes. Petters, Heidelberg

1893 Boegel C: Die Entstehung und Verhütung der Fußabnormitäten auf Grund einer neuen Auffassung des Baues und der Bewegungen des normalen Fußes. Lehmann, München

1895 Walsham, Hughes: Traité des déformités du pied. London

1897 Nasse D: Erkrankungen des Fußes. Enke, Stuttgart

1904 Finochietto E: El pie bot varus equino congenito. Buenos Aires

1933 Wallet A: Atlas de techniques chirurgicales des affections de l'avant-pied. Paris

1934 Hohmann G: Fuß und Bein. Bergmann, München

1935 Morton D: The human foot. Columbia University Press, New York

1936 Debrunner H: Der angeborene Klumpfuß. Enke, Stuttgart

1936 Hauser EDW: Diseases of the foot. Saunders, Philadelphia

1942 Wallet A: Maladies et affections douloureuses du pied. Maloine, Paris

1947 Vidal-Naquet G: Chirurgie du pied. Technique chirurgicale illustrée. A. Legrand, Villeneuve Saint Georges

1947 Marti T: Die Skelettvarietäten des Fußes. Huber, Bern

1948 Massart R: Affections médicales et chirurgicales du pied. Doin, Paris

1950 Hauser EDW: Diseases of the foot, 2nd edn. Saunders, Philadelphia

1951 Hohmann G: Fuß und Bein, 5th edn. Bergmann, München

1952 Lelièvre J: Pathologie du pied. Masson, Paris

1955 Bregegere A: La prothèse podologique étudiée et équilibrée par la base. Ed. Maloine, Paris

1956 Arandés A, Viladot-Perice A: Clínica y tratamiento de las enfermedades del pie. Científico Médica, Barcelona

1957 Debrunner H: Die Therapie des angeborenen Klumpfußes. Enke, Stuttgart

1959 Niederecker K: Der Plattfuß. Enke, Stuttgart

1959 DuVries HL: Surgery of the foot. Mosby, Saint Louis

1959 Lewin P: The foot and ankle. Their injuries, diseases, deformities and disabilities. Kimpton, London

1961 Charlesworth F: Chiropody. Theory and practice, 5th edn. Actinic, London

1961 Wallet A: Podologie. Maladies et affections douloureuses du pied. Ed. Maloine, Paris, 142 pages

1963 Ducroquet JP, Ducroquet P: La marche et les boiteries. Etudes des marches normales et pathologiques. Acta Orthop Belg 31 3: 539

1963 Rabl CR: Orthopädie des Fußes. Thieme, Stuttgart

1966 Dubois JP, Levame JM: Anatomie descriptive du pied humain. Maloine, Paris

1967 Ceccaldi A: Pratique de la rééducation du pied. Masson, Paris

1970 De Doncker E, Kowalski C: Le pied normal et pathologique. Acta Orthop Belg 36: 4-5

1970 Kapandji JA: Physiologie articulaire, Ed. Maloine, Paris

1971 Lelièvre J, Lelièvre JF: Pathologie du pied, 4th edn. Masson, Paris

1972 Dubois JP, Durafourg MP: Physiologie et rééducation fonctionelle du pied. Masson, Paris

1973 Giannestras NJ: Foot Disorders, 2nd edn. Lea & Filbinger, Philadelphia
1974 Regnauld B: Techniques chirurgicales du pied. Masson, Paris
1974 Kerbrat M: Les aspects radiologiques du pied en pathologie générale. Thèse de doctorat en médecine, Université de Brest
1975 Viladot A: Patología del antepie. Toray, Barcelona
1975 Plas F, Viel E: La marche humaine. Masson, Paris
1975 Lavigne A, Noviel D: Traité théorique et pratique de la semelle orthopédique. Scerdes, Boulogne
1976 Cailliet R: Le pied. Rééducation fonctionnelle et réadaptation. Masson, Paris
1977 Paparella Treccia R: Il piede dell'uomo. Verduci, Roma
1977 Valenti V: Le ortesi del piede. Verduci, Roma
1978 Voutey H: Chirurgie orthopédique et rééducation du pied. Masson, Paris
1978 Pierre M: L'ongle. Expansion Scientifique Française, Paris
1978 DuVries HL: Surgery of the foot, 4th edn. Mosby, Saint Louis
1979 De Doncker E, Kowalski C: Cinésiologie et rééducation du pied. Masson, Paris
1980 Montagne J, Chevrot A, Galmiche JM: Atlas de radiologie du pied. Masson, Paris
1981 Montagne J, Chevrot A, Galmiche JM: Atlas of foot radiology. Masson, New York
1983 Galmiche P, Galmiche J: La saga du pied. Erti, Paris

45 References

Abadie P (1971) Déviations latérales du talon. Rev Podol 10: 23-33

Achten MG (1964) Les onychomycoses. Bull Dermatol Syph 71/5: 579-581

Achten G, Wanet-Rouard J, Wiame L, Van Hoff F (1979) Les onychomycoses à moisissures. Dermatologica 159 [Suppl 1]: 128-140

Acton K (1967) Surgical anatomy of the foot. J Bone Joint Surg [Am] 49 (3): 555-567

Adam A (1957) Poliomyélite et paralysies périphériques. Gamm, Bruxelles

Adams AW (1936) Club foot and its treatment. Med Press 193: 348-362

Addante JB (1970) Metatarsal osteotomy as an office procedure to eradicate intractable plantar keratosis. J Am Podiatry Assoc 60 (10): 397-399

Agache P (1973) Particularités de la peau plantaire. Actual Méd Chir Pied 8 (2): 77-83

Agarwal LP, Malik SRK, Mohan M, Khosla PK (1963) Mycotic cornela ulcera. Br J Ophtalmol 47: 109

Agertolm G (1949) Traitement du pied bot par procédé de Denis Browne. Acta Orthop Scand 19 (1): 134-142

Agrifolio E, Rettagliatta F, Pinelli G, Menella G (1964) Considerazioni sul comportamento del circole periferico nell'osteocondrosi posteriore del calcagno. Ann Podol 2: 207-215

Aitken AP, Don Poulsen (1963) Luxation de l'articulation tarso-métatarsienne. J Bone Joint Surg [Am] 45 (2): 246

Alamilla JR (1955) Males de los pies. Paraninfo, Madrid

Alarie R (1968) La part du processus infectieux dans le pied diabétique. Podologie 6: 326

Alban J (1964) Oral Amphotericin B in the management of cutaneous and mucosal candidiasis. Dermatol Trop 3 (4): 217-220

Albanes L (1982) Considerazioni sul trattamento di una non comune deformita del piede: il piede piatto riflesso. Chir del piede, 6, 4: 411-413

Albanese A (1948) Cure delle alterazioni statiche della volta plantare. Relazione al XXXIII Congresso della Soc Ital di Ortopedia e Traumat. Annales SIOT, XXXIII, 40-42

Aleon JF (1972) Luxation de l'articulation du Lisfranc. Thesis, University of Paris

Allan FG (1944) Treatment of flatfoot in children. Med Press Circ 10: 212

Allenbach (1928) Le traitement chirurgical du pied plat. Rapport à la Xe réunion de la soc Française d'Orthopédie, Paris 1928. Revue française d'orthopédie, 15, 6: 650-693

Allieu Y, Claustre J, Simon L (1975-1977) Etude anatomo-clinique et genèse des déformations du pied dans la polyarthrite rhumatoïde. In: Simon L, Claustre J (eds) Le pied inflammatoire, Maloine, Paris, pp 15-27

Almenar Benages L (1966) Cirugia del pie cavo. Facta, Valencia

Almenar Benages L (1970) Patomorfología y patocronía del hallux valgus. Rev Cir Osteo 5: 27

Almenar Benages L, Gomar F (1968) Enfermedad de Freiberg. Rev Cir Osteopat 3: 499

Alonso de Ros J, Vilaret F, Madrigal JJ, Marti Valls J (1972) La operacíon de Steindler ampliada en el tratamiento del pie cavo: revision de 19 casos. Barc Quir 16 (5): 474

Altakoff (1931) Operative und postoperative Behandlung des Plattfußes. Z Orthop Chir 55: 254

Amato P (1971) Patogenía y tratamiento de los dedos en garra. Podologie 6: 286

Amor B (1977) Le pied dans le syndrome de Fiessinger-Leroy-Reiter. In: Simon L, Claustre J (eds) Le pied inflammatoire, vol 1. Maloine, Paris

Amor B (1979) Antigène HLA-B27 et arthrites séro-négatives. Acta Rhum 3: 164-175

Amuso SL, Wissinger HA, Margolis HM, Eisenbeis CH, Stolzer BL (1971) Metatarsal head resection in the treatment of rheumatoid arthritis. Clin Orthop 74: 94

Anapol G (1926) Mechanics in weak and flat feet. Am J Surg 7: 256-258

Anderson B, Roberts SS, Gonzalez C, Chick EV (1959) Mycotic ulcerative keratitis. Arch Ophtalmol 62: 169-179

Anderson LD (1977) Lésions de l'avant-pied. Clin Orthop 122: 18-27

Anderson KJ, Lecoq JF, Lecoq EA (1952) Recurrent anterior subluxation of the ankle joint. J Bone Joint Surg 34-A: 853-860

Anderson KJ, Lecoq JF (1954): Operative treatment of injury to the fibular collateral ligament of the ankle. J Bone Joint Surg 36-A: 825-832

Anderson M, Blair M, Green WT (1956) Growth of the normal foot during childhood and adolescence. Am J Physiol Anthropol 14: 287

Andre JM, Paquin JM (1980) L'appareillage des paralysies du sciatique et de ses branches. Coll Pathol Motrice 4: 258-265

Andre JM, Paquin JM, Albert A, Ory JM (1978) Stimulation électrique fonctionnelle du membre inférieur de l'hémiplégique adulte. Actual Rééd Fonct réadapt. Masson, Paris, 167-171

Andre S (1962) Etude histopathologique des lésions de dégénérescence au niveau de l'articulation sous-astragatienne. Podologie 1: 18-23

Andreasi A, Zanarella G (1977) Il trattamento chirugico delle distorsioni laterali gravi recenti della caviglia e i suoi risultati a distanza. Minerva Ortop 28: 243

Andreasi A, Zanarella G (1977b) L'associazione di lesione grave dei ligamenti esterni della caviglia e frattura del becco della grande apofisi del calcagno nelle "distorsioni laterali della caviglia". Minerva Orthop 28: 571

Angeletti P, Feci A (1967) Hallux valgus. Anatomopathological findings and etiopathogenetic considerations. Arch Putti Chir Organi Mov 22: 392-405

Angles F, Nardi J, Suso S, Lopez Prats F, Cardenal F (1979) Tratamento quirurgico del pie equino valgo espastico. Chir del piede 3 (1): 21-26

Ansel M, Thibaut M (1964) Les principales mycoses cutanées: mycétases et mycétides. Gaz Hopitaux 1: 5-24

Anthony J (1973) L'homme debout. Ses origines préhistoriques. Ann Podologie 8 (2): 3-7

Antoni C, Paul D, Schumann HD (1974) Luxation et fracture-luxation du tarse; résultats du traitement. Zentralbl Chir 99 (51): 1622

Arancia, Rinaldi (1978) Atlas of rearfoot surgery. Futura, New York

Arandes R (1949) A propósito de un caso de enfermedad de Deutschländer bilateral. Rev Esp Reum Enferm Osteoartic 3 (1): 31

Arandes R, Viladot A (1956) Clínica y tratamiento de las enfermedades del pie (pología). Cientifico Médica, Barcelona

Arandes R, Viladot A, Vilanova Montiu X (1958) Biomecánica del calcáneo. Med Clin 21 (1): 25

Arandes R, Viladot A, Vilanova Montiu X (1954) La luxacíon de los dedos del pie. Cir Ginecol Urol 7 (4): 196

Arcq M (1978) Le traitement chirurgical précoce du pied bot varus équin congénital. Chir Piede 2: 197-202

Arlet J, Ruffie R (1961) Etude sur les arthroses tibio-tarsiennes et sur les arthroses astragalo-calcanéennes et astragalo-scaphoïdiennes. Etiologie. Signes cliniques et radiologiques. Rev Rhum Mal Osteoartic 28: 368

Auerbach AM (1970) Review of distal metatarsal osteotomy for hallux valgus in the young. Clin Orthop Relat Res 70: 148

Augé M, Manfra O (1957) Rééducation du pied après arthroplastie du gros orteil. Rev Podol 24: 10-17

Auquier L, Siaud JR (1971) Tendinites nodulaires du tendon d'Achille. Rev Rhum Mal Osteoartic 38: 373

Avila R, Pugh DG, Slocumb CH, Winkelmann RK (1960) Psoriatic arthritis: a roentgenologic study. Radiology 75: 691

Avila de Azevedo M (1964) A propos du syndrome du canal tarsien. Thesis, University of Montpellier

Axhausen G (1909) Die histologischen und klinischen Gesetze der freien Osteoplastik aufgrund von Tierversuchen. Arch Klin Chir 88: 23-145

Axhausen G (1912) Über den histologischen Vorgang bei der Transplantation von Gelenkenden insbesondere über die Transplantationsfähigkeit von Gelenkknorpel und Epiphysenknorpel. Arch Klin Chir 99: 1-50

Axhausen G (1923) Die Köhlersche Erkrankung der Metatarsophalangealgelenke. Med Klin 561

Axhausen H (1923) Der anatomische Krankheitsablauf bei der köhlerschen und der perthesehen Krankheit der Hüftköpfe. Arch Klin Chir 124: 511-542

Axhausen H (1929) Die Aetiologie der Köhlerschen Erkrankung. Beitrag Klin Chir 126: 451-476

Azerad E, Lubetzki J, Stuhl L, Slotine M (1963) Etude radiologique des ostéopathies du diabète sucré. Le pied diabétique. Ann Radiol 6: 421-436

Babin Chevaye J Fractures du calcanéum. Actual Chir Orthop Hop R Poincare 5: 56

Bachmann R (1954) Talushalsosteotomie bei lockeren Knick-Plattfüßen. Z Orthop 85: 449

Baciu C, Brazda A (1971) The surgical treatment of hallux valgus. Z Orthop 109 (5): 888-897

Baciu C, Russu AN, Sgarbura I (1968) Critical considerations on the surgical treatment of hallux valgus. Podologie 6: 165

Bahra H (1966) Report on our hallux valgus operations in the last 5 years. Beitr Orthop Traumatol 13 (10): 650-2

Bailey CC, Root HF (1947) Lesioni neuropatiche del piede in corso di diabete mellito. N Engl J Med 236: 397-401

Baker H, Golding DN, Thompson M (1963) Psoriasis and arthritis. Ann Intern Med 58: 909-925

Baker LD (1954) Princeps surae syndrome in cerebral palsy. Surgery 68: 216

Balasub-Ramaniam P, Silva JF (1971) Tophectomy and bone-grafting for extensive tophi of the feet. J Bone Joint Surg [Am]: 133

Banchero A, Berardi GC, Chiappara P (1975) Possibilità di terapia chirurgica nell'avampiede reumatico. Reumatismo 27: 45-53

Bankaert B (1935) Minor disturbances of the feet. South Med J 2

Banks HH (1977) Le traitement des déformations spastiques du pied et de la cheville. Clin Orthop 122: 110-113

Banks HH, Green WH (1958) The correction of equinus deformity in cerebral palsy. J Bone Joint Surg 40-A: 1359

Banks HH, Panagakosp, Green WH (1968) The correction of severe foot valgus in cerebral palsy. J Bone Joint Surg 50-A: 1479

Baran R (1974) Pathologie ungueale. Encycl Med Chir Paris 10 12885 A 10

Baran R (1978) Les ongles verts ou syndrome chloronychique. Cutis-France 2: 469-474

Baran R (1981) Comment reconnaître et traiter les onyxis et périonyxis mycobactériens. Médicales Fournier Frères, Paris

Baran R, Bureau H, Sayag J (1979) Congenital malalignment of the big toenail. Clin Exp Dermatol 4: 359

Barbera Carre F (1968) El podoestatigrama. Podologie 6: 401

Barbieri A, Federzoni F (1966) Le metatarsalgie da cedimento della volta traversa. Arch Putti Chir Organi Mov 21: 134-150

Barbieri E, García M (1968) Le traitement chirurgical du pied spastique. Podologie 6: 77-92

Barbieri GF (1965) Piede convesso valgo congenito, revisione di indirizzo terapeutico da Miller. Ann Podol 4: 33-43

Barcelo P, Sans Sola (1950) Anatomofisiología y biomecánica del pie. Rev Esp Reum Enferm Osteoartic 6:480

Barcelo P, Vilaseca-Sabter JM (1960) Metatarsalgia. Rev Esp Reum Enferm Osteoartic 3: 528

Barcelo P, Sans Sola L (1950) Metatarsalgia. Rev Esp Reum Enferm Osteoartic 6: 528

Barcelo P, Vilaseca-Sabter JM (1950) El pie doloroso y su relacíon con las variaciones del esqueleto pedico. Las afecciones de los sesamoideos y las ostecondritis pedicas. Rev Esp reum Enferm Osteoartic 6: 496

Barouk LS (1984) Etude comparative de l'utilisation de la chaussure post-opératoire sans appui sur l'avant-pied. Société française de médecine et chirurgie du pied, Nice. Expansion scientifique 1: 24

Barouk LS (1984) Les brièvetés musculaires postérieures du pied de l'infirme moteur cérébral. SOFCOT. Réunion de novembre 83. Rev Chir Orthop 70 [Suppl 2]

Barouk LS, Cadoux J, Benoit Y, Razan-Charensol J, Coste V (1983) La chirurgie du pied de l'I. M. C. à propos de 430 pieds opérés. Symposium international sur la paralysie cérébrale, juin 1983, Toulouse. CRF P Dottin, Ramonville St Agne

Barouk LS, Parcou A, Masse A, Dubois JP, Fouche M (1981) Le chirurgien devant le pied neurologique central. Quest-Médical 34 (17): 1177-1186

Barrett JP, Mooney V (1973) Neuropathy and diabetic pressure lesions. Orthop Clin North Am 4 (1): 43

Barry J, Courriades H (1963) Psychosomatisme et pied plat. Ann Podol 2: 191

Barry J, Courriades H (1968) Contributions à l'étude de certaines ulcérations et hyperkératoses plantaires. Rev Podol 6: 255-264

Barsky AJ (1967) Macrodactily. J Bone Joint Surg 49-A: 1255-1266

Barthalon, Poissonnier (1968) Les pieds qui tournent ou démarches en rotation interne. Gaz Med Fr 75: 1

Bartlett RW (1937) A conservative operation for cure of so-called ingrown toenail. JAMA 108: 1257

Barton NJ (1973) Arthroplasty of the forefoot in rheumatoid arthritis. J Bone Joint Surg [Br] 55: 126

Baruffaldi O, Bignardi A, Boero G (1970) La resezione delle teste metatarsali. Contributo clinico sulla metatarsalgia. Minerva Ortop 21: 298

Basmajian JV, Stecko G (1963) The role of muscles in arch support of the foot. An electromyographic study. J Bone Joint Surg [Am]: 1184

Basora JM (1966) Le pied plat valgus. Podologie 4: 159-160

Bastos Ansart M (1950) Tratado de cirugía ortopédica. Científico Médica, Barcelona

Batchelor JS (1972) Hallux valgus. Acta Orthop Belg 38 (2): 217-8

Bateman JE, Trott AW (1980) (eds) The foot and ankle. Thieme-Stratton, New York

Baudoin P (1966) Contribution à l'étude radiologique de la statique du pied. Thesis, University of Paris

Baumann J (1930) La region de passage de la loge posterieure de la jambe à la plante du pied. Ann Anat Pathol Anat Norm Med Chir 7: 201-209

Baumann JH, Girling JP, Brand P (1963) Plantar pressure and trophic ulceration. J Bone Joint Surg [Br] 45: 4

Bazex A, Dupre A, Christol B (1966) Le psoriasis plantaire. Ann Podol 5: 117-120

Becker F (1974) Contribution à l'étude des entorses graves externes récentes de l'articulation tibio-tarsienne. Thesis, University of Lyon

Bedogni C, Modena M (1964) La resezione delle teste metatarsali nella cure del piede piatto traverso doloroso. Ann Podol 3: 77-88

Bedouelle J (1955) Malformations congénitales du pied. Encycl Med Chir Radiodiagn 15255 B 10

Bell, Grice (1944) Treatment of congenital talipes equinovarus with the modified Denis Browne splint. J Bone Joint Surg [Am] 26: 793-811

Beltramo F (1978) Traitement fonctionnel du pied bot varus équin. Bull Assoc Obstet Pediat Med Périnat 6: 56-57

Benard, Rambert-Perignot, Ecalles (1953) Le pied diabétique. Sem Hop Paris 6. 11. 53

Benassy J (1961) L'ostéogénèse neurogène. Rev Rhum Mal Osteoartic 28: 234-239

Benassy J (1963) L'innervation motrice radiculaire des membres. Rev Rhum Mal Osteartic 31: 110-115

Benassy J (1975) Talalgies et forage du calcanéum. Rhumatologie 27 (3): 127-129

Benassy J (1976) Topographie métamérique motrice du membre inférieur. Cah Reed Read Fonct 11 (3): 81-84

Benezis C (1973) Place de la réadaptation dans le traitement des algodystrophies réflexes du membre inférieur (à propos de 188 observations). Thesis, University of Montpellier

Benichou J (1978) Traitement du pied bot à la naissance. Chir Piede 1 (1-2): 33-38

Bensahel H (1977) Abrégé d'orthopédie pédiatrique. Masson, Paris

Bensahel H (1973) Le pied bot congénital. Acta Med Chir Pied, 8: 1-88

Berardi GC (1965) Traitement chirurgical du valgus calcanéen. Podologie 48: 177-181

Berardi GC, Chiappara P (1964) Considérations sur le pied plat statique. Conc Med Oct: 5757-5760

Berardi GC, Panelli (1960a) Sul trattamento chirurgico del piede cavo. Arch Ist S Corona 12

Berardi GC, Panelli L (1960b) L'osteotomia basale del 1er metatarso nella correzione del piede cavo anteriore. Atti SIOT, 45th Congress, Firenze

Berardi GC, Piccheta F (1966) L'impiego di un nuovo preparato analgesico nell correzione incruenta del piede equino varo supinato congenito. Acta Ortop Ital 12: 175-180

Berardi GC, Chiappara P, Guidi P (1963) L'azione del tricipete surale sul mantenimento della centina plantare. Atti Mem SOTIMI 8 (1): 141-146

Berardi GC, Chiappara P, Lonardo PM (1977) Analisi sperimentale delle possibilità di frattura del calcagno.

Congress, College International de Podologie, Turin, June. Act Med Chir Pied 12: 185–191

Bernard R, Padovani P, Iselin M (1948) Traumatologie, fractures, luxations, entorses, traumatologie générale. Hérel, Paris

Bernau Andreas MD (1977) Long-term results following Lambrinudi arthrodesis. J Bone Joint Surg [Am] 59 (4): 473–479

Berndt AL, Harty N (1959) Transchondral fractures (osteochondritis dissecans) of the talus. J Bone Joint Surg [Am] 41: 988–1018

Bernstein A, Stone JR (1944) March fracture. J Bone Joint Surg 26: 743–750

Berridge FR, Bonnin JG (1944) The radiographic examination of the ankle joint including arthrography. Surg Gynecol Obstet 79: 383–389

Berry TA (1957) Morton's metatarsalgia due to cavernous angioma. J Bone Joint Surg [Br] 39: 124

Berthet G, Charry V (1945) Consultations de podologie. Doin, Paris

Bertola L (1946) Le traitement du pied bot varus équin congital par transplantation tendineuse. Arch Orthop (Bologne) 56 (3)

Bertrand P (1947) La paralysie isolée du jambier antérieur. Rev Orthop Chir 33 (3,4)

Bertrand P (1968) Traitement du pied bot varus équin chez le jeune enfant. Orthopédie traum. Conférences d'enseign. Sociéte Francaise de Chirurgie Orthopédique et Traumatologique. Conc Med Dec: 94–98

Bertrand P (1976) Le névrome plantaire (maladie de Thomas Morton). Phlébologie 29 (3): 245–249

Bertrand PJ (1963) Etude du syndrome d'insuffisance d'appui du 1er rayon du pied. Thesis, University of Paris

Besse D (1979) Pied Plat – Syndrome d'inadaptation à la verticalité. Thesis, University of Bordeaux

Bessel-Hagen (1889) Pathologie und Therapie des Klumpfußes. Heidelberg

Besson J, Wellinger C (1967) L'ostéochondrite disséquante de l'astragale. Rev Rhum Mal Osteoartic 34: 552

Betts LO (1940) Morton's metatarsalgia neuritis of fourth digital nerve. Med J Australia 1: 514–515

Beurey J, Mougeolle JM (1966) Les mycoses du pied en Lorraine. Gaz med Fr 73/18: 3329–3340

Beurey J, Weber M, Percebois G (1969) Etude clinique et mycologique des intertrigos des pieds. Soc Fr Phlébologie 1: 73–79

Beurey J, Weber M, Mougeolle JM (1969) Les mycoses des pieds. Echos de la médecine 11: 40

Bickel WH, Dockerty MB (1947) Plantar neuromas. Morton's toe. Surg Gynecol Obstet 84: 111–116

Bilcsio EA (1951) La métatarsalgie de Morton. Prensa Med Argent 38 (48): 3136–3146

Bingold EC, Collins DH (1950) Hallux rigidus. J Bone Joint Surg (Br) 32: 214–222

Bitar A (1961) Osteotomia dos metatarsianos. Rev Bras Cir 41: 91–92

Bittel M (1965) A propos de 50 interventions pour pieds creux dits essentiels. Thesis, University of Lyon

Bitter T, Jeannet M (1978) HLA-B27 in persistent yet reversible asymetric oligoarthritis (PRAO). Ann Rheum Dis 37: 285

Bittroff R (1926) Zur Frage der entzündlichen Mittelfußerkrankung in Deutschland. Zentralbl Chir 26

Blaimont TP, Burnotte J, Halleux P (1976) Contribution à l'étude de la biomécanique de la cheville. Ann Soc Belg Med Chir Pied, Charleroi, 13–14, CIFOP

Blaimont TP, Baillon JM, Van Elegem P (1976) Possibilités restauratrices du traitement des cals vicieux de la cheville. Ann Soc Bel Med Chir Pied, Charleroi, 173–182, CIFOP

Blasnick J (1963) Syndrome del seno del tarso. Bol Traumatol Soc Arg (also Orthop Traumatol 28: 241–242)

Bloch-Michel M, Cauchoix J, Bourdon R (1960) Les arthropathies du tabès et de la syringomyélie. Rev Prat 10: 2015–2040

Blockey NJ (1955) Peroneal spastic flat foot. J Bone Joint Surg 37-B: 191

Blondin-Walter M (1949) Radiographie de la voute métatarsienne antérieure. J Radiol Electro 30 (9–10): 543–544

Blumenfeld I (1970) Pie diabetico. Actas Trab Com Arg Estud Afecc Pie 35

Blumfeld N, Kaplan, Hicks E (1946) Le traitement conservateur du pied bot varus équin congénital. J Bone Joint Surg 28 (4)

Bocchi L, Zanoli S (1966) Artrodesi nel piede poliomielitico. Podologie 5: 264–265

Böhler L (1922) Die Stellung des Vorfußes beim Plattfuß, Klumpfuß und Hohlfuß. 17e congrès allemand d'orthopédie

Böhler L (1944) Technik der Knochenbruchbehandlung. Maudacher, Wien

Böhler L (1944) Technique du traitement des fractures. Médecine de France

Böhler L (1956) Sudeck's syndrome after closed injury as an unavoidable accident result or a preventable treatment result. Arch Klin Chir 284: 43–53

Böhm M (1929) The embryologic origin of club foot. J Bone Joint Surg 5 (11): 2–227

Böhm M (1929) Pes varus congenital. Z Orthop Chir 51: 409

Böhm M (1930) Pes valgus staticus. Z Orthop 52: 424–452

Böhm M (1930) The development of juvenile pes valgus. J Bone Joint Surg 12 (2): 333–334

Böhm M (1933) Die Disposition zu jugendlichen Deformitäten. Z Orthop Chir 59 (2): 182–209

Boisseau R (1936) Etude du traitement du pied bot varus équin congénital chez le nourrisson, l'enfant et l'adulte. Thesis, University of Paris

Bonhote VH (1953) Bursite rétro-calcanéenne (maladie de Haglund). Thesis, University of Genéva

Bonnel F, Constans JP, Claustre J, Simon L (1983) Anatomie et biomécanique des nerfs plantaires (Intérêt dans le névrome de Morton). Cinésiologie 22: 78–81

Bonney G, MacNab I (1952) Hallux valgus and hallux rigidus. J Bone Joint Surg [Br] 34: 366–385

Bonnin JG (1944) The hypermobile ankle. Proc R Soc Med 37: 282–286

Bontoux D (1967) Spondylarthrite ankylosante. Progrès en rhumatologie, Flammarion, Paris

Bontoux D, Talin d'Eyzak A, Nolen P, Bennaboun (1972) Insuffisance aortique et syndrome de Fiessinger-Leroy-Reiter, J Med Poitiers 3: 183

Boppe (1945) Douleurs et lésions irritatives liées aux variations de forme de la tubérosité postérieure du calcanéum. Rev Orthop 31: 141-148

Boppe, Esteve (1948) Le traitement du pied bot varus équin congénital de la 2e et moyenne enfance. Rev Orthop 402-416

Bordas A (1976) Fracturas del calcaneo. Thesis, University of Barcelona

Borg I (1950) Operation for correction of hammer toe. Acta Chir Scand 100: 619

Borggreve J (1949) Zur operativen Behandlung des kontrakten Spreizfußes. Z Orthop 78: 581-582

Bosch Olives V (1969) Enfermedades de los pies. Monografias Medicas, Barcelona

Bose B (1971) A technique for excision of nail fold for ingrowing toenail. Surg Gynecol Obstet 132: 511

Bose K (1979) A surgical approach for the infected diabetic foot. Int Orthop (SICOT) 3: 177-181

Bosien WR, Stapples S, Russel JM (1955) Residual disability following acute ankle sprains, J Bone Joint Surg 37-A: 1237

Bosse JL (1957) Necrose aseptique post-traumatique de l'astragale. Thesis, University of Lille

Bossi P (1904) Il piede piatto. Biella, Amosso

Boucher M (1949) Le pied décalcifié douloureux. Thesis, University of Lyon

Boudin G, Arfouilloux JC (1970) Paralysie générale et manifestations cérébrales de la syphilis. E. M. C. Neurologie: 17055 A 10

Boudin G, Ricou P, Audebert A (1975) Syphilis médullaire. E. M. C. Neurologie: 17072 A 10

Boulet P, Mirouze J, Pelissier M (1936) Le squelette du pied dans le diabète sucré. Rev Rhum Mal Osteoartic 22: 115-127

Bourdes Y (1936) Clavetage de la tibiotarsienne. Arch Med Gen Trop 4

Bourdillon C (1888) Psoriasis et arthropathies. Thesis, University of Paris

Bourneville DN (1880) Contribution à l'étude de l'idiotie, Arch Neurol Paris 1: 59-91

Bourneville DN (1900) Idiotie et épilepsie symptomatique de la sclérose tubéreuse ou hypertrophique. Arch Neurol 2: 29

Bourrel P, Rey A, Blanc JF, Palinacci JC, Bourges M, Giraudeau P (1976) Syndrome du canal tarsien. A propos de 15 cas purs et de 100 cas associés à la lèpre ou au diabète. Rev Rhum Mal Osteoartic 43 (12): 723-728

Bouvet JM, Hucdebat JM, Benoit J, Ramadier JO (1977) Macrodactylie bilatérale et symétrique des orteils. Rev Chir Orthop 66: 331-334

Braddock GT (1961) A prolonged follow-up peroneal spastic flat foot. J Bone Joint Surg 43-B: 734

Bragadini (1970) Pied diabetico. Actas Trab Com Arg Estud Afecc Pie

Bragard K (1932) Beitrag zur Malakopathie der Mittelfußköpfchen. Arch Orthop Chir 31: 125

Brailsford JF (1959) The radiology of gout. Br J Radiol 32: 472

Branch HE (1937) Pathological dislocation of the second toe. J Bone Joint Surg 19: 978-984

Brandes M (1929) Zur operativen Therapie des Hallux valgus. Zentralbl Chir 56: 2434

Brattstrom H (1953) Tenodesis employing the method of Watson Jones for the treatment of recurrent subluxation of the ankle. Acta Orthop Scand 23: 132-136

Brattstrom H, Brattstrom M (1970) Resection of the metatarsophalangeal joint in rheumatoid arthritis. Acta Orthop Scand 41: 213

Braun S (1971) Le pied en pratique rhumatismale. Eléments du diagnostic. Vie Médic 22: 2701

Braun S (1975 a) Le pied dans les grands rhumatismes inflammatoires chroniques. Rhumatologie 27: 26-32

Braun S (1975 b) Les tarsalgies rhumatismales. Actual Med Chir Pied 12: 22-40

Braun S (1978) L'assise plantaire dite normale. Les assises plantaires anormales et pathologiques. Rev Prat 28 (12): 915-918, 28 (14): 1071-1074

Braun S, Morere R (1973) Réflexions pratiques sur les orthèses plantaires du pied rhumatoïde. Ann Med Phys 26: 3

Braun S, Panahi F (1968) Le pied rhumatismal. Problèmes diagnostiques. Gaz Med Fr 75 (1): 77-94

Braun S, Chatignoux G, Panahi F (1970) Pathologie rhumatismale du calcanéum. Conc Med 92 (6): 1225

Braun S, Ledos S, Moure P (1972) Orthèses plantaires de marche et d'appui. Bull Soc Fr Med Chir Pied Nov: 9

Braun S, Basquin L, Mery L (1980) Considérations sur l'assise du pied normal. Etude statique. Rev Rhumatol 47: 127-133

Braverman IM (1970) Skin. Signs of systemic disease. Saunders, Philadelphia

Bregegere A (1955) La prothèse podologique étudiée et équilibrée par la base. Maloine, Paris

Brenner EA (1970) Consideraciones sobre el pie diabético. Actas Trab Com Arg Estud Afecc Pied 59

Brenner EA (1965) The muscular factor as causal agent of hallux valgus and its recurrence. Rev Ortop Traumatol Latinoam 10: 23-38

Brenner EA (1973) Algunos problemas de la cirugía del antepie. Podologia 8 (2): 192

Brian Thomas F (1974) Levelling the tread-elevation of the dropped metatarsal head by metatarsal osteotomy. J Bone Joint Surg [Br] 56: 314-319

Broca A (1914) Chirurgie infantile. Gsteinhel, Paris

Brokman EP (1937) Modern method of treatment of club foot. Br Med J 2: 572

Brooks DM (1955) The principles of tendon transplantation in the prevention of deformities of the foot. J Bone Joint Surg [Br] 37: 542

Broudeur P, Poinso Y, Mouren P (1968) La métatarsalgie de Thomas Morton. Névrome plantaire. Marseille Méd 105 (3): 223-227

Brousse JP, Braun S, Amor B, Coste F (1966) Etude comparative de quelques types de talalgie et de calcanéite. Sem Hop Paris 42: 795

Brown FB (1943) Sudeck's acute bone atrophy: report of a case. J Med Assoc Georgia 32: 242–244

Brown JE (1960) The sinus tarsi syndrome. Clin Orthop 18: 231–233

Browne D (1934) Talips equino varus. Lancet 2: 969

Browne D (1935) Talips equino varus. Practitionner 134: 225

Browne D (1936) Congenital deformities of mechanical origin. Proc R Soc Med 29: 1409

Browne D (1937a) Modern methods of treatment of club foot. Br Med J 2: 570

Browne D (1937b) Talips equino-varus. Postgrad Med J 13: 349

Bruce J, Walmsley R (1938) Some observations on the arches of the foot and flat foot. Lancet 235: 656–659

Bruni L (1838) Sopra la sezione del tendine d'Achille. Napoli

Bruno G (1933) Come si comporta il pede considerato come una leva durante la marcia. Chir de Organi Mov 18 (3): 286–288

Bruno G (1951) Le superfici d'appogio e i punti di maggiore pressione nella pianta del piede umano. Rass Clin Sci IBI 27: 43–48

Bryniczka GC, Pascente RW (1977) Arthrose de l'articulation sous-astragalienne. J Am Podiatry Assoc 67/2: 115–117

Buchet R, Picard JM, Dubost E (1961) La maladie de Freiberg-Köhler. Les entretiens de Bichat 1961 spécialités. Expansion Scientifique Française

Buchholz HW, Engelbrecht E, Siegel A (1973) Totale Sprunggelenksendoprothese Modell "St Georg". Chirurg 44: 241

Buchholz HW, Engelbrecht E, Rottger J, Siegel A (1976) Experience with the total ankle joint replacement: a four year follow-up review. Ann Soc Belg Med Chir Pied 125–137

Buetas E (1960) Secuela de algunos tratamientos quirurgicos del hallux valgus. Rev Ortop Traumatol 4 (1): 271

Buetas E (1965) Estudio del pie en Indios centroamericanos. Podologie 4: 5

Bureau G (1945) Pied creux: notions de base et rappel des différentes thérapeutiques non chirurgicales. Rev Orthop 38

Bureau G (1954) Le port de semelles orthopédiques: un leurre dans le traitement du genu valgum. Conc Méd 4: 1509

Bureau G (1960) Hallux valgus. Ann Chir 14 [1–2]: 81–89

Bureau G (1981) Prévention et traitement opératoire de l'hallux valgus. Med Prat 4: 37–42

Bureau Y, Barriere H (1955) Acropathies pseudo-syringomyéliques des membres inférieurs. Essai d'interprétation nosographique. Sem Hop Paris 31 (25)

Bureau Y, Delaunay, Jarry, Barriere H (1954) Acropathies mutilantes des pieds, pseudo-syringomyéliques. Bull Soc Franc Dermatol Syphil 61: 176–178

Bureau Y, Barriere H, Kerneis JP, Ferron A (de) (1957) Acropathies ulcéro-mutilantes pseudo-syringomyéliques non familiales du membre inférieur (à propos de 23 observations). Presse Med 94: 2127–2131, Bull Soc Fr Dermatol Syphil 64 (2): 187–192

Bureau Y, Barriere H, Litoux P, Bureau B (1965) Les ostéo-arthropathies neurotrophiques. Presse Médic 73: 547–550

Burke G (1948) Le pied bot congénital. J Int Surg (NY) 2 (1)

Burkle de la Camp H (1927) Die Gefahren der gewaltsamen Umformung des Klumpfußes. M M W 974

Burutaran JM (1967) Grundgliedverkürzung der Großzehe und proximale Osteotomie (MI bei Hallux valgus). Med Dissertation, San Sebastian

Burutaran JM (1968) La arthrorisis posterior en el pie equino espatico. Podologie 6: 109

Burutaran JM (1971) Fisiopatologia del antepie. Podologie 6: 135

Burutaran JM (1973) Retroposicion de los sesamoideos. Podologie 8: 199

Burutaran JM (1976) Hallux valgus y cortedad anatomica del primer metatarsiano (correción quirurgica). Actual Med Chir Pied 9: 261–266

Burutaran JM (1977) Correción quirurgica para el valgo del hallux y del 5 metatarsiano. Congrès du collège international de podologie, Turin

Busch LF (1947) The use of homogenous bone grafts: a preliminary report of the bone bank. J Bone Joint Surg 29: 620–628

Butel J, Faure C, Francois M, Plas F (1978) Entorses de la tibiotarsienne. Encyclop Med Chir Appl Locom 14089 B 10

Butilin WE (1974) Modifications of the McBride procedure for correction of hallux valgus. J Am Podiatry Assoc 64: 585

Butturini V (1968) Les lésions osseuses du pied diabétique. Podologie 6: 343

Byers PD, Cotton RE, Lowy M, Sissons HA, Thompon AD (1968) The diagnosis and treatment of pigmented villonodular synovitis. J Bone Joint Surg 50-B: 290

Bywaters EGL, Dixon A St Y (1965) Paravertebral ossification in psoriasic arthritis. Ann Rheum Dis 24: 313–331

Cabanac J, Petit P, Maschas A (1952) Traitement du pied bot varus congénital. Rev Chir Orthop 38: 314–351

Cabitza A (1965) Intérêt de l'intervention de Miller dans le pied plat de l'adolescent. Rev Podol 4: 199

Cabot JR, Vilaseca JM (1950) La osteopatia dinamica del metatarso en la pratica civil. Rev Esp Reum Enferm Osteoartic 6: 539

Cadet D (1967) Les lésions du pied dans la spondylarthrite ankylosante. Thesis, University of Montpellier

Caffiniere JY (de la), Mazas F, Seringe R (1972) Résultats du traitement fonctionnel dans les fractures articulaires du calcanéum. Rev Orthop 58 (3): 217–228

Cahuzac M (1960) La chirurgie du pied. Toulouse Med 721–727

Cahuzac M, Claverie P, Ollie R, Mansat C, Hichil J, Delpech R (1972a) Notre expérience de la chirurgie du pied chez l'enfant. IMC Chirurg 98: 680–688

Cahuzac M, Mansat M, Cahuzac JP, Mansat C (1972b) Etude sur les résultats thérapeutiques dans le traitement des pieds bots varus équins. Actual Med Chir Pied 8 (1): 63

Cailliet R (1971) Tobillo y pie. El manual moderno. Mexico

Cailliet R (1976) Le pied. Collection de rééducation fonctionnelle et de réadaptation. Masson, Paris

Calafat F (1975) L'appareillage des lésions statiques du pied. Kine Scient 121/254: 42-50

Calcagni V (1965) La solidarisation des tendons jambiers dans le traitement du pied plat valgus. Rev Podol 4: 203-205

Camera R (1945) La double ténodèse des extenseurs du pied dans le traitement du pied équin paralytique. Rev Orthop Chir 35 (3-4)

Camera U (1949) Contributo al trattamento del piede piatto valgo congenito o piede piatto reflesso. Arch Ortop 3: 3-7

Campbell WC (1923) An operation for correction of drop foot. J Bone Joint Surg 5: 815

Campbell WC (1930) Block operation for drop foot. J Bone Joint Surg 12: 317

Campell's Operative Orthopedies (1963) Maladie de Morton. Mosby, St Louis, p 1616

Camus JP (1965) Spondylarthrite ankylosante et maladie périodique. Rev Rhumat 32: 614

Canadell J (1960) Tratamiento del hallux valgus. Rev Ortop Traumatol 4 (2): 234

Canadell J, Jimeno E, Villas C (1979a) Wedge-shaped resection of the base of metatarsal for the treatment of mechanical metatarsalgia. Chir Piede 3: 39-44

Canadell J, Villas C, Ayala H (1979b) Substitution of metatarsals with implants of flexible silicon. Chir Piede 3: 45-50

Cangialosi CP (1978) Primary epidermoid carcinoma of the foot. J Am Podiatry Assoc 68 (10): 691-692

Capecchi V, Cicala G, Crisafulli A (1968) Le ossa soprannumerarit del piede. Acta Ortop Ital 10: 1

Carbonnier J (1976) Etat clinique et radiologique des métatarso-phalangiennes dans la polyarthrite rhumatoïde. Mémoire d'Internat de Nanterre

Carboz H, Pons JG. Le pied bot varus équin congénital. Sociéte Francaise de Chirurgie Orthopédique et Traumatologique, vol 3. Expansion Scientifique Française, Paris

Carli M, Bardelli D (1977) L'artrite reumatoide nel piede: aspetti radiologici e soluioni chirurgiche. Congress of College International de Podologie, Turin

Carnevali (1937) Sur l'apophysite calcanéenne des adolescents. Arch Ortop 51 (4): 730-763

Caron P (1939) Contribution à l'étude clinique de la sclérose tubéreuse de Bourneville. Thesis, University of Paris

Carreno Martinez A, Amirola Barrenengoa A, Cervantes Soto A, López García A (1965) Roturas subcutáneas del tendón de Aquiles. Rev Hosp Gen 5 (1)

Carret JP, Schnepp J (1981) Etude cinématique des articulations de la cheville et du pied. In: Claustre J, Simon L (eds) Pied normal et methodes d'exploration du pied. Masson, Paris, pp 38-43

Carret JP, Schnepp J (1983) Notions de biomécanique du pied. XXXe Semaine de Rhumatologie, Aix-les-Bains, April, p 50

Carret JP, Bejuy J, Fischer LP, Herdzberg, Crochet, Schnepp J (1981) Luxation sous-astragalienne et medio-tarsienne. Travail de l'hopital Edouard Herriot, du Laboratoire d'anatomie, du Centre du Val Rosay. Lyon Chir 77 (4): 226-227

Carrol AT, Laurin (1962) Une nouvelle technique pour le diagnostic d'entorse grave de la tibio-tarsienne. Rev Med Mond

Cartesegna M, Indemini E, Gallinaro P (1979) La nostra esperienza nel trattamento chirurgico dell'alluce valgo. Chir del piede, 3 (1): 59-64

Casalis F (1958) Les verrues plantaires, un problème social. Presse Med 66: 968

Casalis F (1964) Les mycoses des pieds, clinique et moyens thérapeutiques actuels. Ann Podol 3: 153-161

Cassagne P (1972) Inégalité de longueur des membres inférieurs. Rev Podol May/June: 9

Castaing G (1968a) Tibio-tarsienne. Entorse à répétition. Ligamentoplastie externe. Rev Chir 54 (8): 789-791

Castaing G (1968b) Les entorses de la cheville. Orthopédie traumatologique. Conférences d'Enseign. SOFCOT. Expansion Scientifique Française, Paris

Castaing J, Buchet C (1960) Entorse à répétition ou "luxation récidivante de la tibiotarsienne". Rev Médic Tours I: 71-73

Castaing J, Delplace J (1972a) Entorses de la cheville: recherche radiographique du tiroir astragalien antérieur. Rev Chir Orthop 1-11 58 (1): 51-63

Castaing J, Delplace J (1972b) A propos de 62 cas de rupture du tendon d'Achille. Ann Orthop Ouest 4: 25

Castaing J, Le Chevalier PL, Meunier M (1961) Entorse à répétition ou "luxation récidivante de la tibiotarsienne". Une technique simple de la ligamento-plastie externe. Rev Chir Orthop 47: 598-608

Castaing J, Castellani L, Delplace J (1967) Les instabilités de la cheville par insuffisance musculo-ligamentaire externe. Ann Chir VIII-IX 21 (15-16): 947-958

Castaing J, Delplace J, Dien F (1975) Instabilites chroniques de la cheville. Rev Chir Orthop 61: 167-174

Castellana A (1952) L'allongement d'achille et la capsulotomie postérieure dans le pied bot congénital. Minerva Orthop 2

Castellana A (1973) Cura dell'alluce valgo. Acta Med Chir Pied 8 (2): 179

Caulay RMC (1947) Le traitement opératoire des pieds bots. NY J Med 47 (3)

Cayla G (1972) L'ostéonécrose de l'astragale. Actual Rhum 9: 229

Cayla G, Denis A (1973) Nécrose de l'astragale. Encycl Med Chir App Locomot 15741 D: 10

Ceccaldi A (1967) Pratique de la rééducation du pied. Masson, Paris

Cecile JP, Descamps C, Regnier G, et al. (1973) L'arthrographie du pied diabétique. J Radiol Electrol 54 (4): 313-318

Cesari M (1966) Le metatarsalgia d'appoggio. Pologie 5: 98

Chambers EFS (1946) An operation for the correction of flexible flat feet of adolescents. West J Surg Obstet Gynecol 14 (3)

Chamaillard (1912) Vices de conformation de l'ongle. Thesis, University of Paris
Chaouat Y, Benichou C, Pioline G (1964) Ostéoarthrite destructive des articulations métatarso-phalangiennes au cours d'une spondylarthrite akylosante. Rev Rhum Mal Osteoartic 31: 354
Charcot JM (1868) Sur quelques arthropathies qui paraissent dépendre d'une lésion du cerveau ou de la moëlle épinière. Arch Physiol Norm Pathol 1: 161-178
Charlesworth F (1961) Chiropody. Theory and practice, 5th edn. Actinic, London
Charpentier J (1971) Le liège et la chaussure orthopédique. Cah Assoc Fr Appar
Charry R (1970) La technique de DuVries dans les gros traumatismes de l'avant-pied (fractures métatarsiennes multiples et luxation du 1er métatarsien). Bull Mem Soc Chir 60 (4): 240
Chatelain E (1896) Précis iconographique des maladies de la peau, 2e ed. Maloine, Paris
Chatignoux G, Braun S (1973) Conceptions actuelles de la chirurgie de l'hallux valgus. Soc Fr Med Chir Pied (B Aires) 10
Chausse JD, Pottier P (1971) Etude de 86 cas d'arthropathies psoriasiques. Bord Med 4: 93-106
Cherlinzoni (1943) Opération de Codivilla dans la cure du pied bot congénital. Chir Organi Mov 29 (4)
Chevrot A (1981) Incidence de ¾ externe du pied en charge rayon horizontal. J Radiol 62 (5): 315-319
Chevrot A, d'Izarn JJ, Pallardy G, Forest M (1976) Tumeurs glomiques et kystes épidermoides des phalanges. J Radiol Electrol 57 (8-9): 645-647
Chiappara P (1965) Le valgus du talon. Podologie 4: 139-144
Chiappara P (1973) La funzione delle articolazioni astragalo calcaneari. Minerva Ortop 24 (1): 6-10
Chiappara P (1975) Alluce rigido. Minerva Ortop 26: 101-107
Chiappara P (1976) Metatarsalgia e alte razioni biomeccaniche negli anziani. Med Geriatr [Suppl 1]: 1-46
Chiappara P, Berardi GC (1963) La caduta della testa dell'astragalo nelle genesi dell'abbassamento della volta plantare. Podologie 2: 73-87
Chiappara P, Berardi GC (1966) Le artrodesi nel piede poliomielitico. Podologie 5: 243-260
Chiappara P, García M (1958) Piede torto sperimentale. Minerva Ortop 9
Chiappara P, Guidi P (1969) L'intervento di fibroplastica nelle correzione dell'alluce valgo. Atti Mem SOTIMI 20: 116-122
Chiappara P, Baruffaldi O, García M (1959) Osteocondrodisplasia sperimentale. Minerva Ortop 10 (4): 143-159
Chigot P (1965) Les maladies des jeunes danseuses. Cinésiologie 4: 11-28
Chigot P, Esteve P (1965) Pied paralytique. Encycl Méd Chir 15730/A10
Chigot P, Garnier C, Cloutier M (1952) Contribution à l'étude anatomo-pathologique et au traitement chirurgical des ruptures sous-cutanées du tendon d'Achille. Rev Chir Orthop 38 (5-6): 512-513
Chigot P, Hermelont, Fournier (1957) Traitement des ruptures du tendon d'Achille par autoplastie avec le plantaire grêle. Bull Mem Acad Chir 83: 45
Cholmeley JA (1958) Hallux valgus in adolescents. Proc R Soc Med 51: 903-906
Chrysospathes J (1938) Cyrtopodie (Forme de pied plat valgus congenital) Z Orthop 68 (3, 14): 257
Chuinard EG, Baskin M (1973) Claw-foot deformity, treatment by transfer of the long extensors into the metatarsals and fusion of the interphalangeal joints. J Bone Joint Surg [Am] 55: 351
Claret F (1960) El tratamiento quirúrgico del hallus valgus. Rev Ortop Traumatol 4 (2): 264
Claustre J (1982a) Le syndrome du canal tarsien. In: Simon L, Rodineau J (eds) Cheville et médecine de rééducation. Masson, Paris, pp 257-262
Claustre J (1982b) Les tendinites autour de la cheville. In: Simon L, Rodineau J (eds) Cheville et médecine de rééducation. Masson, Paris, pp 199-209
Claustre J (1983) Le syndrome du canal tarsien. Med Hyg 41: 1130-1133
Claustre J, Azema MJ (1982) Le traitement physique de l'algodystrophie réflexe de la cheville. In: Simon L, Rodineau J (eds) Cheville et médecine de rééducation. Masson, Paris, pp 263-266
Claustre J, Simon L (1976) Le pied équin en milieu rhumatologique. Ann Med Physique 19: 383-391
Claustre J, Simon L (1978) Aspects de la pathologie sésamoïdienne du premier métatarsien. Rev Rhum Mal Osteoartic 45: 479-486
Claustre J, Simon L (1977) Le pied rhumatoïde. J Agréges 10: 483-490
Claustre J, Simon L (1979) Le syndrome du nerf musculo-cutané du pied. Rhumatologie 31: 45-48
Claustre J, Simon L (1981) Pied normal et méthodes d'exploration du pied. Masson, Paris
Claustre J, Simon L (1982a) Troubles congénitaux et statiques du pied: orthèses plantaires. Masson, Paris
Claustre J, Simon L (1982b) Le pied hyperostosique. Rev Rhum Mal Osteoartic 49: 629-633
Claustre J, Simon L, Blotman F (1976) Les atteintes du pied au cours de la maladie osseuse de Paget. Rev Rhum Mal Osteoartic 43: 45-49
Claustre J, Simon L, Barrault JJ (1979a) Le traitement médical des séquelles de fractures du calcanéum. Rhumatologie 31: 17-19
Claustre J, Simon L, Serre H (1979b) Le pied rhumatoïde: problèmes podologiques pratiques. Rev Rhum Mal Osteoartic 46: 673-678
Claustre J, Simon L, Allieu Y (1980a) Le syndrome du sinus du tarse existe-t-il? Rhumatologie 31: 45-48
Claustre J, Simon L, Allieu Y (1980b) Le syndrome du sinus du tarse existe-t-il? Chir Piede 4: 67-166
Claustre J, Houlez G, Azema MJ, Izard MH (1982a) Traitement non chirurgical de la cheville rhumatoïde. In: Simon L, Rodineau J (eds) Cheville et médecine de rééducation. Masson, Paris
Claustre J, Delagoutte JP, Simon L (1982b) Hallux rigidus. In: Claustre J, Simon L (eds) Troubles congénitaux et statiques du pied: orthèses plantaires. Masson, Paris, pp 144-152

Claustre J, Bonnel F, Constans JP, Simon L (1983) L'espace intercapito-métatarsien: aspects anatomiques et pathologiques. Rev Rhum Mal Osteoartic 50 (6): 435-440

Clark K (1960) Peripheral nerve injuries associated with fractures. Postgrad Med 27: 476-479

Clavel M, Escribano A (1965) Enfermedades de Köhler I y II. Acta Ortop Traumatol Iber 3: 353

Clayton ML (1959) Surgery of the forefoot in rheumatoid arthritis. Arthritis Rheumatism 3: 84

Clayton ML (1960a) Surgery of the forefoot in rheumatoid arthritis. Clin Orthop 16: 136-140

Clayton ML (1960b) Surgery of the forefoot in rheumatoid arthritis. J Bone Joint Surg [Am] 42: 523

Clayton ML (1963) Surgery of the lower extremity in rheumatoid arthritis. J Bone Joint Surg [Am] 45: 1517

Clayton ML, Trott AW, Ulin R (1961) Recurrent subluxation of the ankle with special reference to peroneal nerve block as a diagnostic aid. J Bone Joint Surg 33-A: 502-504

Cleveland M, Winant EM (1950) An end result study of the Keller operation. J Bone Joint Surg [Am] 32: 163

Cohen M (1954) Contribution à l'étude des talalgies. Thesis, Paris

Colin R, Amar E, Lapeyrie H (1964) Luxation-fracture du métatarse. Montpellier Chir 10 (1): 45

Collard JJ, Debas E, Bourlond A (1974) Sclérose tubéreuse de Bourneville: valeur de cannelure unguéale. Arch Belg Dermatol 30 (4): 289-290

Collard M, Wullaert E (1976) Le diagnostic physique différentiel de l'arthrose et de l'arthrite du cou de pied. Ann Soc Belg Med Chir Pied, Charleroi, p 29

Colomb D, Racouchot J, Jeune R (1976) Les lésions des ongles de la sclérose tubéreuse de Bourneville isolées et associées à la tumeur de Koenen. Ann Dermatol Syphiligr 103 (4): 431-437

Colombani C, Forte M (1962) Sulla cura chirurgica dell'alluce valgo. Arch Putti Chir Organi Mov 17: 119-125

Comter JJ, Loras JP (1974) Les paralysies traumatiques du sciatique poplité externe. Cah Med Lyon 50: 1685-1690

Cormier F (1955) Traitement de l'ostéoporose algique post-traumatique par l'hydergine. Thesis, University of Bordeaux

Coscia PL, Dettoni A, Mina A (1982) Il piede dismorfico infantile. Chir Pied 6 (4): 423

Cosentino R (1956) Lésions ligamentaires de l'articulation tibiotarsienne. Rev Orthop 42: 211-226

Costa Bartani G (1944) Reumatismos cronicos y afecciones concomitantes. Ateneo, Buenos Aires

Coste F (1946) Pathologie médicale, vol 6. Masson, Paris

Coste F (1955) Le rhumatisme, études cliniques, biologiques et thérapeutiques, 4th edn. Expansion Scientifique Française, Paris

Coste F, Piguet B (1956) Dystrophie réflexe indolente des membres inférieurs. Rev Rhumatol 23: 153-155

Coste F, Piguet B, Cayla G (1956) Nouveau cas de dystrophie réflexe indolente des membres inférieurs. Rev Rhumatol 23: 581-584

Coste F, Braun S, Montonnet J, Panahi F (1968) L'avant-pied rhumatoïde. Ann Radiol 2: 8

Courriades H (1971) L'hypermobilité du 1er rayon. Podologie 6: 146

Courriades H (1973a) Numéro spécial sur la pathologie du pied. Bord Med 3: 265-326

Courriades H (1973b) Celui dont on parle trop "le pied plat". Bord Med 6 (3): 287-290

Courriades H (1975) Les pieds contracturés. Rhumatologie 27 (2): 87

Courriades H (1979) Clinique du pied creux. Cours International Méd et Chir du Pied de Nantes, vol 3. Imprimeries réunies, Rennes: 148-155

Courriades H, Khalef M (1965) Variations morphologiques de la mortaise tibio-péronière et du tenon astragalien. Déductions thérapeutiques. Ann Podol 6: 9-16

Courriades G, Degabiel J (1977) Le pied plat congénital élément d'un syndrome d'inadaptation. Déductions thérapeutiques. Bord Med 10 (30): 2155-2162

Courtois B (1968) La greffe pédiculée dans la nécrose post-traumatique de l'astragale. Podologie 6: 31

Courtois B, Masse P (1961) Le traitement du pied polio myélitique. Concours Med 5: 2545

Courtry A Etude sur l'architecture du calcanéum, considérations physiologiques, conséquences chirurgicales. Rev Orthop 31 (10): 1945

Couvelaire, Baumann, Delinotte (1938) Résection tibiotarsienne totale. J Chir 51 (3)

Coventry MB (1965) Resection of the metatarsal heads to relieve pain and deformity. Mayo Clin Proc 40: 240-247

Cralley JC, Mc Gonagle W, Fitch K (1976) The role of adductor hallucis in bunion deformity: part I. J Am Podiatry Assoc 66 (12): 910-8

Creer WS (1939) Treatment of hammer toe. J Bone Joint Surg 21: 977

Creff P (1952) Contribution à l'étude des acropathies ulcéro-mutilantes. Thesis, University of Paris

Crego CH, Ford LT (1952) An end-result study of various operative procedure for correcting flat-feet in children. J Bone Joint Surg [Am] 34: 183-195

Crenshaw AM, Milford L (1966) Traité de chirurgie orthop de la clinique Campbell. Maloine

Crespo-Neches A (1971) Biomecanica del pie. Podologie 6: 65

Crispils C, Brissot R (1978) La constitution des chaussures orthopédiques. Cah Reed Readapt Fonct 13 (2): 43-50

Cruickshank B (1960) Pathology of ankylosing spondylitis. Bull Rheum Dis 10: 211

Cser I (1969) A modified Keller-Brandes operation. Arch Orthop Unfallchir 65 (1): 79-82

Dabee M (1976) Contribution à l'étude du traitement chirurgical de l'hallux valgus. Thesis, University of Lyon

Dalla Vedova R (1911) Di alcune ricerche sperimentali sul trapianto libero osteoarticolare. Policlinico Sez Chir 18: 529

Dal Monte A (1976) Il piede torto congenito nell 'età' pediatrica. Correzione chirurgica. Esperienza sull'intervento di Codivilla. G Ital Ortop Traumatol 2: 165-175

Dal Monte A, Manes E, Araoz S, Zajia A (1983) Piede torto congenito: risultati e indirizzi di cura. G Ital Ortop Traumatol 9 (1): 25-38

Dalton E, McGlamry ED (1969) Metatarsal shortening osteoplasty of head or osteotomy of shaft. J Podiatry Assoc 59 (10): 394-398

Dandoy M (1970) Quelques notions de technique de chirurgie plastique appliquée en chirurgie du pied. Podologie 6: 262

Danet F (1964) Le pied dans la polyarthrite rhumatoïde. Mémoire pour le CES de rhumatologie. Paris

Daniels L, Worthingham C (1973) Evaluation de la fonction musculaire. Le testing. Maloine, Paris

Da Paz Campos AJ, De Souza N, De Souza DC (1979) La forma congenita del piede valgo convesso. Orthop Clin 4: 263

Dastugue J (1982) Les maladies de nos Ancêtres. Recherche 13: 21

David-Chausse J, Pasquier P (du), Dehais J, Bullier R, Delmas M (1980) La maladie de Fiessinger-Leroy-Reiter vue dans un service de rhumatologie. A propos de 71 cas. Rev Rhumatol 47: 243-250

Davidson MR (1974) V-osteotomy for correction of metatarsal head pathology. J Foot Surg 13: 23

Davies H (1949) Metatarsus quintus varus. Br Med J 1: 664

Davies-Colley N (1887) Contractions of the metatarso-phalangeal joint of the great toe (hallux flexus) Br Med J 1: 728

Davis LA, Hatt WS (1955) Congenital abnormalities of the foot. Radiology 64: 818-825

Debeyre N, Denis A (1966) Le pied douloureux inflammatoire (polyarthrite rhumatoïde et pelvispondylite rhumatismale) lère journée de podologie médico-chirurgicale du centre Viggo-Petersen. Expansion Scientifique Française, Paris

Debeyre N, Roumignieres, Leger L, Camus (1947) Névrome plantaire. Rapport de F. Poilleux. Mem Acad Chir 65 (31-32): 627

Debrunner H (1936) Der angeborene Klumpfuß. Enke, Stuttgart

Debrunner H (1957) Die Therapie des angeborenen Klumpfußes. Enke, Stuttgart

Debrunner H (1960) Das Sinus-tarsi-Syndrom. Schweiz Med Wochenschr 93: 47

Debrunner H (1963) Das Sinus-tarsi-Syndrom. Schweiz Med Wochenschr

Decoulx P, Duquennoy A (1968) Les cals vicieux du cou de pied. Rev Prat 18 (31): 4593-4604

Decoulx P, Razemon JP, Soulier A (1960) L'ostéonécrose post-traumatique de l'astragale. Ann Chir 14: 771-783

Defilippi Novoa ECA (1963) Semiología quirúrgica del aparato locomotor. Bibliográfica Argentina, Buenos Aires

Defilippi Novoa ECA (1968) Podología práctica. Loras, Buenos Aires

Dega W (1968) Ortopedia i rehabilitcja. Edit PWL, Warszawa

Dega W (1971) Pied plat convexe par verticalité congénitale de l'astragale (une technique chirurgicale). Rev Podol 8 (1): 261-266

Dega W, Swiderski G, Zuk A (1962) La stabilisation du pied paralytique de l'enfant par blocage intra-articulaire. Ann Podol 1: 121-134

Dei Poli G, Dei Poli N, Forcheri V, Rosso P (1970) Hallux valgus. Minerva Chir 25 (13): 934-953

Delagoutte JP (1974) Hallux valgus surgery: human joint prosthesis. Rev Chir Orthop 60 [Suppl 2]: 168-170

Delagoutte JP (1975) Utilisation de l'implant en silastic dans la cure de l'hallux valgus et des déformations métatarso-phalangiennes du gros orteil. Rhumatologie 27 (3): 67-69

Delagoutte JP, Hoeffel JC (1976) Intérêt de l'incidence de Walter-Muller dans le syndrome de dysharmonie d'appui des têtes métatarsiennes. Rhumatologie 28: 151-152

Delahaye RP (1951) Contribution à l'étude de l'ostéochondrite disséquante de l'astragale. Thesis, University of Paris

Delahaye RP, Jolly R. Pied. Technique radiologique et aspects normaux. Encycl Med Chir Radiodiagn 30400 A 10, 30400 A 20

Delahaye RP, Jouffroy J, Laurent H, Loze PC (1966) Les fractures de fatigue. J Radiol Electrol 47: 525-534

Delahaye RP, Doury P, Pattin S, Metges PJ, Mine J (1976) Les fractures de fatigue des métatarsiens. Rev Rhum Mal Ostéoartic 43 (12): 707-713

Delbet M (1896) Traitement de l'hallux valgus par la résection et la vaginoplastie. Bull Mem Soc Chir 22: 181

Delcambre B (1976) Les synoviorthèses à l'acide osmique dans le traitement de la maladie rhumatoïde. Remarques et bilans de cinq années d'utilisation. Lille Med 21 (10): 813-820

Delchef J, Soeur R (1936) Le traitement du pied plat statique. J Chir Bruxelles, June 28

Delitala F (1921) Gli apparecchi otopedici. Bologna

Delitala F, De Gennaro R (1950) Trattato di tecnica ortopedica et traumatologia. Vallardi, Milano

Del Sel JM, Grand NE (1959) Cubo-navicular synostosis. J Bone Joint Surg (Br) 41: 149

Dengler S (1935) Zur Histologie beim angeborenen Plattfuß. Z Orth Chir 63 (1): 43-47

Dengler S (1937) Clinique et traitement du pes adductus. Z Orth 65 (2, 6): 121-129

Dengler S (1937) Revue d'orthopédie, vol 24/2. Masson, Paris, pp 3-4

Denis A (1961) Le pied inflammatoire. Rev Rhum Mal Osteoartic 7-8: 376

Denis A (1962) Les affections inflammatoires au niveau de l'arrière-pied. Podologie 1: 35

Denis A (1968) Les Ostéonécroses aseptiques du pied chez l'adulte. In: De Sèze S, et al. (eds) L'actualité rhumatologique 1968 présentée au praticien. Expansion Scientifique Française, Paris

Denis A (1970a) L'électromyographie du syndrome du tunnel tarsien. In: De Sèze S, Dreyfus P, Hamonet C (eds) Podologie, vol 1. Masson, Paris

Denis A (1970b) La maladie de Morton, son devenir, son traitement. In: De Sèze S, et al. (eds) L'actualité rhumatologique 1970 présentée au praticien. Expansion Scientifique Française, Paris

Denis A (1970c) Les podalgies statiques. Fueill Prat 35 (10): 7–53

Denis A (1970d) L'hallux rigidus. In: De Sèze S, et al. (eds) L'actualité rhumatologique 1971 présentée au praticien. Expansion Scientifique Française, Paris, pp 75–85

Denis A (1971a) Tendinite nodulaire du tendon d'Achille. Incidences thérapeutiques. Rev Rhum Mal Osteoartic 6–7: 472–473

Denis A (1971b) Fractures de fatigue du métatarse. Encycl Med Chir 2: 15740

Denis A (1971c) Metatarsalgies statiques. Encycl Med Chir 2: 15740

Denis A (1971d) Métatarsalgie de Morton. Encycl Med Chir 2: 15740

Denis A (1972a) La pathologie des orteils. Encycl Med Chir 3: 15742–A10,6

Denis A (1972b) L'hallux valgus. In: De Sèze S, et al. (eds) L'actualité rhumatologique 1972 présentée au praticien. Expansion Scientifique Française, Paris

Denis A (1973) Les pied plats, les vrais, les faux, les bénins, les graves. In: De Sèze S, et al. (eds) L'actualité rhumatologique 1973 présentée au praticien. Expansion Scientifique Française, Paris

Denis A (1974a) Le pied douloureux, vol 1. Ciba Geigy, Basel (Folia rheumatologica)

Denis A (1974b) Arthropathie du gros orteil et implant phalangien en silicone. Rev Rhum Mal Osteoartic 41: 251

Denis A (1974c) La pathologie médiotarsienne. In: De Sèze S, et al. (eds) L'actualité rhumatologique 1974 présentée au praticien. Expansion Scientifique Française, Paris

Denis A (1974d) Approche physiopathologique des anomalies morphologiques de l'avant-pied. Presented at Symposium Troubles statiques de l'avant-pied. 47th annual meeting of SOFCOT. Rev Chir Orthop 2 [Suppl 2]: 19

Denis A (1975a) L'ostéonécrose aseptique du sésamoïde du 1er orteil (ONAS) maladie de Renander. Rhumatologie 27 (3): 113–117

Denis A (1975b) Aspects rhumatologiques du pied creux. In: De Sèze S, et al. (eds) L'actualité rhumatologique 1975 présentée au praticien. Expansion Scientifique Française, Paris

Denis A (1975c) A propos de la maladie de Freiberg-Köhler (ostéonécrose primitive juvénile de la tête du 2e metatarsien). Acta Orthop Belg 31: 579–597

Denis A (1976a) Contribution à la connaissance du syndrome douloureux aigue du 2e espace inter-métatarsien. In: De Sèze S, et al. (eds) L'actualité rhumatologique 1976 présentée au praticien. Expansion Scientifique Française, Paris

Denis A (1976b) Arthrose astragalo-calcanéenne et astragalo-scaphoïdienne et osteonécrose aseptique. Soc Belg Med Chir Pied, Charleroi, 16–17 Oct 1976

Denis A (1977a) Le traitement du pied plat statique. Rev Chir Orthop 63: 740–744

Denis A (1977b) Arthropathie métatarso-phalangienne du gros orteil avec implant en silicone en cas d'avant-pied rhumatoïde. In: Simon L, Claustre J (eds) Le pied inflammatoire. 2e colloque de pathologie locomotrice. Montpellier, Maloine, Paris

Denis A (1978) Diagnostic d'une arthropathie isolée de la cheville. In: De Sèze S, Ryckewaert (eds) Le diagnostic en rhumatologie, vol 1. Masson, Paris, p 385

Denis A, Froin-Denuçausse M (1980) Le diagnostic des douleurs de l'avant-pied, le gros orteil étant exclu. Rev Prat 30: 38

Denis A, Huber-Levernieux C (1976) La rééducation fonctionnelle des métatarsalgies statiques. Journée de rééducation. Expansion Scientifique Française, Paris

Denis A, Huber-Levernieux C (1980) Les bursites du talon postérieur. In: De Sèze S, et al. (eds) L'actualité rhumatologique 1980 présentée au praticien. Expansion Scientifique Française, Paris

Denis A, Lacan G (1976) Hallux rigidus et nécrose aseptique de la tête du 1er métatarsien. Soc Belg Med Chir Pied, Charleroi 16–17 Oct 1976

Denis A, Samuel J (1981) La marche. In: Pied normal et méthodes d'exploration du pied. Masson, Paris (Monographie de podologie, vol 1, p 180)

Denis A, Djian A, Annonier C, Baudoin P (1967) La radiopodométrie. In: De Sèze S, et al. (eds) L'actualité rhumatologique 1967 présentée au praticien. Expansion Scientifique Française, Paris

Denis A, Huber-Levernieux C, Levi-Valeusin G, De Sèze M (1977) Les ostéomes ostéoides du pied chez l'adulte. In: De Sèze S, et al. (eds) L'actualité rhumatologique 1977 présentée au praticien. Expansion Scientifique Française, Paris

Denis A, Huber-Levernieux C, David A (1978) Le syndrome douloureux aigu dul le rayon métatarso-phalangien. In: De Sèze S, et al. (eds) L'actualité rhumatologique 1978 présentée au praticien. Expansion Scientifique Française, Paris

Denis A, Lacan G, Cywiner-Golenzer C (1979) Maladie de Ledderhose. In: De Sèze S, et al. (eds) L'actualité rhumatologique 1979 présentée au praticien. Expansion Scientifique Française, Paris

Denis A, Huber-Levernieux C, Debeyre J, De Sèze S, Goutallier D (1980) Notre expérience de la chirurgie de l'avant-pied rhumatoïde (150 interventions) Rev Rhum Mal Osteoartic 47 (1): 9–14

Dennyson WG, Bear JN, Bhoola KD (1977) Macrodactyly in the foot. J Bone Joint Surg 59-B: 355–359

Derot M, Rathery M (1967) Syndrome du scaphoïde tarsien. Diabéte 15: 131–138

Derot M, Rathery M, Defranoux A (1962) Fratture spontanee dello scafoïde tarsale nei diabetici. Bull Mem Soc Med Hop Paris 113: 1108–1112

Desfachelles JL (1979) Cals vicieux du cou de pied. Etiologies, traitements, résultats. A propos de 35 cas. Thesis, University of Reims

Desse A (1973) Epiphysite des phalanges et triphalangie du pouce. Podologie 8 (1): 28

Destot E (1911) Traumatismes du pied et rayons. Masson, Paris

Destot E (1938) Traumatismes du pied et rayons, malléoles, astragale, calcanéum, avant-pied, 2e ed. Masson, Paris

Deuil R, Contamin F (1960) Le pied diabétique. Bull Mem Soc Med Hop Paris: 11-12

Deutschländer C (1921) Über eine eigenartige Mittelfußerkrankung. Z Chir 39: 1422

Deutschländer C Zur Klinik der angeborenen Talusverlagerung. 26e Congrès allemand chirurgie orthopédique

Devan WT, Carlton DC (1954) The march fracture persists. A report of 145 cases during a 15 month period at an infantry Basic Training Center. Am J Surg 87: 227-231

Devine LA (1972) Collectomy: lesser metatarsal neck resection. J Am Podiatry Assoc 62 (12): 447-458

Dick W, Henche HR (1976) The McBride operation of hallux valgus in adolescents (author's transl). Z Orthop 114 (3): 388-93

Dickson FD, Diveley RL (1953) Functional disorders of the foot, 3d edn. Lippincott, Philadelphia

Dillwyn E (1975) Calcaneo valgus. J Bone Joint Surg (Br) 57 (3): 270

Dimeglio A, Pons JC (1976) Le pied bot varus équin, un conflit autour de l'articulation médiotarsienne, du traitement orthopédique au traitement chirurgical. Cahiers Enseign SOFCOT, vol 3. Expansion Scientifique, pp 73-86

Diveley RL (1934) Foot imbalance. JAMA 103: 1510-1515

Dixon A (1970) The rheumatoid foot. Proc R Soc Med 63: 677-679

Djian A, Annonier C (1967) Exploration radiologique du pied. Journée de podologie. Expansion Scientifique Française, Paris, pp 21-28

Djian A, Annonier C, Denis A, Baudoin P (1968) Radiopodométrie. J Radiol Electrol 49: 769-772

Dodd H (1933) Pied forcé or march foot. Br J Surg 21: 131

Domeniconi S (1952) L'opération de Codivilla dans le pied bot. Minerva Orthop 3

Domselier van F (1945) Application des gouttières de Denis Browne dans le pied bot varus équin. Rev Orthop Traumatol (B Aires) 3

Donayre R, Huanuco M, Fukunga L, Garcia-Buca R, Javier LT (1968) Importance of elasticity of foot joints. Podologie 6: 231-239

de Doncker E (1956) Le pied plat valgus de l'enfant. Acta Orthop Belg 22: 561-579

de Doncker E (1970) Pathogénie et traitement de l'avant-pied convexe. Rev Orthop 56 (3): 279

de Doncker E (1974) Anatomie, physiologie et cinésiologie des articulations du Lisfranc. Rev Kinesither Sci 119: 252

de Doncker E, Kowalski C (1970) Le pied normal et pathologique. Acta Med Belg 36: 4-5

de Doncker E, Kowalski C (1979) Cinésiologie et rééducation du pied. Masson, Paris

de Doncker E, Lacheretz M (1977) Symposium: traitement du pied plat statique. Rev Chir Orthop 63 (8): 733-787

Dorriotz L (1939) L'utilisation de l'os humain conservé en chirurgie orthopédique de reconstruction. Thesis, University of Bordeaux

Dossa J (1976a) Explorations arthrographiques du pied. Rhumatologie 28 (5): 165-169

Dossa J (1976b) Médecins rééducateurs et chirurgiens face aux fractures articulaires du calcanéum. Cah Reed Readapt Fonct 11 (1): 21-30

Doury P, Patin S (1978) Le pied dans le syndrome de Fiessinger-Leroy-Reiter. Rhumatologie 30 (7): 233-237

Doutaud B (1975) Semelles destinées à soulager les affections épidermiques. Kinesitherap Scient 121/254: 51-57

Dremann JC, Sharrard WJW (1971) The pathological anatomy of convex pes valgus. J Bone Joint Surgery [Br] 53 (3): 455-461

Drouhet E (1955a) Traitement des infections mycosiques à Candida albicans par un nouvel antibiotique antifongique: la Nystatine. Presse Med 63 (1): 620

Drouhet E (1955b) Action de la Nystatine (fungicidine) "in vitro" et "in vivo" sur Candida albicans et autre champignons levuriformes. Ann Inst Pasteur 88: 298-314

Drouhet E (1960) Aspects mycologiques, pathogéniques et thérapeutiques des candidoses. Bull Soc Fr Dermatol Syphil 67: 638-645

Drouhet E (1965) Les actualités thérapeutiques des mycoses chez l'homme. Rev Pathol Comp 65: 177-185

Dryll A (1967) Psoriasis et rhumatismes inflammatoires du pied. 2e Journée de podologie médico-chirurgicale du Centre Viggo Petersen. Expansion Scientifique Française, Paris

Dryll A, Kuntz D, de Sèze S (1973) Etude comparative de 35 cas de pelvispondylite psoriasique apparus à 35 cas de pelvispondylite rhumatismale. Sem Hop Paris 49: 2439-2444

Dubois JP (1959) Indications et techniques des semelles orthopédiques dans la correction du pied plat interne. Conc Med 22: 2557-2564

Dubois JP (1968) Traitement de l'hallux valgus. Gaz Med Fr 75: 1

Dubois JP (1970) Les pied plats. Cah Reeduc Readapt Fonct 4 (5): 141-164

Dubois JP (1971) Étude radiologique du pied. Rev Podol 2: 11-21

Dubois JP (1972) Conduite à tenir devant une déformation de l'avant-pied et des orteils. Gaz Med Fr 79: 4

Dubois JP (1974) Le pied douloureux statique (Extrait). Rev Kinesither Sci 119 (252): 43-49

Dubois JP (1977) Principales déformations du pied et leur traitement. Perf Prat 10 (245): 41-46

Dubois JP, Durafourg MP (1972) Physiologie et rééducation fonctionnelle du pied. Masson, Paris

Dubois JP, Levame JH (1966) Anatomie descriptive du pied humain. Maloine, Paris

Duchenne de Boulogne (1867) La physiologie des mouvements. Baillères, Paris

Duckwarth T, Smith TWD (1964) Congenital vertical talus. Surgical treatment. J Bone Joint Surg 46-A (5): 342

Duckwarth T, Smith TWD (1974) The treatment of paralytic convex pes valgus. J Bone Joint Surg [Br] 56 (2): 305

Ducroquet C, Launay (1909) Arthrodèse du pied. Presse Med 17

Ducroquet R (1960) Marche normale et marche pathologique. Ann Med Physiol [Suppl]

Ducroquet R, Lescouer J (1948) Hallux valgus. L'arthroplastie par interposition du cartilage appliquée à la cure de l'hallux valgus. Presse Med 22

Ducroquet R, Lescouer J (1949) L'arthrodèse tibio-tarsienne extra-articulaire. Presse Med 81

Dufourmentel C, Mouly F (1958) Place de la chirurgie dans le traitement des verrues des durillons plantaires. Presse Med 66: 1517

Duhamel B (1966) Morphogenèse pathologique, Masson, Paris

Duhamel B, Haegel P (1973) Malformations et déformations du pied. Acta Med Chir Pied, 8 (1): 24-27

Duparc J, Cafiniere de la JY (1970) Mécanisme, anatomopathologie, classification des fractures articulaires du calcanéum. Ann Chir 24: 289-301

Duquennoy A, Padovani JP, Bourets JC et al (1975) Entorses graves de la tibiotarsienne. Rev Chir Orthop [Suppl 2]: 123-187

DuVries HL (1959) Surgery of the foot. Mosby, St Louis

DuVries HL (1978) Surgery of the foot, 4th ed. Mosby, St Louis

Duyck JP (1977) Place des ostéotomies métatarsiennes dans le traitement des troubles statiques de l'avant-pied. Thesis, University of Marseille

Dwyer FC (1954) A new approach to the treatment of pes cavus. 6e Congrès Chir Orthop de Berne. SICOT 551. Lielens, Bruxelles

Dwyer FC (1959) Osteotomy of the calcaneum for pes cavus. J Bone Joint Surg [Br] 41: 80-86

Dwyer FC (1963) The treatment of relapsed club foot by insertion of a wedge into the calcaneum. J Bone Joint Surg [Br] 45: 67-75

Dwyer FC (1964) The relationship of variations in the size and inclination of the shape and function of the whole foot. Ann R Coll Surg Engl 34: 120-137

Echeverri AJ (1947) Cirugía del aparato locomotor, enfermedad de Köhler II en el tercer metatarsiano. Col 4 (20): 145

Echeverri AJ (1958) La vascularizacíon del segmento mediodistal del miembro inferior. Rev Orthop Traumatol 2 (1): 229

Ecoiffier J, Geerts (1956) Aspects radiologiques des ostéoporoses post-traumatiques. 10e Congrès Belg Chir

Economou C (1978) Les prothèses en silastic dans le traitement de l'hallux rigidus. Chir Piede 2 (3): 117-119

Edmonds J, Morris RI, Metzger AL, Bluestoner R, Terasaki PI, Ansell B (1974) Follow-up study of juvenile chronic polyarthritis with particular reference to histocompatibility antigen W27. Ann Rheum Dis 33: 289-292

Edwards G, Lincoln C, Basset H (1969) The tarsal tunnel syndrome. Diagnosis and treatment. JAMA 207: 716

Efther G (1975) Kinésithérapie des lésions statiques du pied. Rev Kinésitherap Sci 122/255: 5-14

Elbanna J, Lauwer M (de), Raynal L (1978) Les fractures de la cheville. Revue de 136 cas. Acta Orthop Belg 44/3: 403-415

Elftmann H (1934) A cinematic study of the distribution of pressure in the human foot. Anat Rec 59 (481): 491

Ellis VH (1951) A method of correction of the metatarsus varus primus. J Bone Joint Surg [Br] 33: 415-417

Elmslie RC (1934) Recurrent subluxation of the ankle joint. Ann Surg 100: 364-367

Emmel HE, Le Cocq JF (1958) Hamstring transplant for the prevention of calcaneo-cavus foot in poliomyelitis. J Bone Joint Surg [Am] 40: 911

Emmert C (1869) Operations for ingrown toenail. Arch Klin Chir 11: 268

Endler F (1955) Der kontrakte Pes valgus, seine Behandlung und Spätprognose. Z Orthop 86: 181-210

Engle T, Morton DJ (1931) Notes on foot disorders among natives of Belgian Congo. J Bone Joint Surg 13 (2): 311-318

English M (1976) Nails and fungi. Br J Dermatol 94: 697-701

English M, Atkinson R (1973) An improved method for the isolation of fungi in onychomycosis. Br J Dermatol 88: 237-241

Enjalbert, Gedeon A, Arlet J, Allegre de la Sougeolle C (1951) Heureux effet de la sympathectomie lombaire dans un cas d'acropathie ulcéro-mutilante non familiale. Toulouse Médical, Toulouse

Enriquez del Corral A (1960) Anatomia patologica y radiologia del hallux valgus. Rev Ortop Traumatol 4 (1-2): 228

Erb (1868) Zur Pathologie und pathologischen Anatomie peripherischen Paralyse. Dtsch Arch Klin Med 4: 539

Erlacher P (1943) Zur Begriffsbestimmung des angeborenen Hackenfußes und angeborenen Plattfußes. Z Orthop 74: 93-96

Escarpenter J (1978) Tarsalgias secundarias a la enfermedad dismetabolica. Actual Méd Chir Pied 12: 40

Estanove B (1973) Abord radiologique de la pathologie du pied. Cah Med Lyon 49 (16): 1671-1680

Esteban Mujica B (1960) Etiopatogenia del hallux valgus. Rev Ortop Traumatol 4 (1-2): 211

Estève P (1971) Pieds plats valgus congénitaux. Rev Podol 8 (1): 70-72

Estève P (1972) Pieds bots neurologiques congénitaux. Rev Podol 8 (1): 112-116

Evans DL (1953) Recurrent instability of the ankle. A method of surgical treatment. Proc R Soc Med 46: 343-344

Evans DL (1961) Relapsed club foot. J Bone Joint Surg [Br] 43: 722-733

Eyre-Brook AL (1967) Congenital vertical talus. J Bone Joint Surg [Br] 49: 618

Faber A (1934) Au sujet de l'os inter-métatarsien. Z Orthop Chir 61 (2): 186-197

Fahlung TR (1946) Suture of the posterior tibial nerves below the knee with a follow-up study of the clinical results. J Neurosurg 3: 223-233

Faraboeuf LH (1893-1895) Précis de manuel opératoire, 4th edn

Favreai JC, Caballe P (1957) Hallux valgus et hallux rigidus. J Bone Joint Surg 33: 792-793

Faye C (1961) A propos de 50 observations de pieds creux. Etude étiologique et thérapeutique (traitement chirurgical). Thesis, University of Paris

Fehr K (1967) Le rhumatisme psoriasique. Folia Reum 15: 7-16

Feray C, Roy-Camille R (1968) La transplantation des tendons extenseurs sur le col des métatarsiens dans les troubles statiques de l'avant-pied. Actual Chir Orthop Hop R Poincaré 6: 193

Feriz H (1925) Makrodystrophia lipomatosa progressiva. Virchows Arch Pathol Anat Physiol Klin Med 260: 308-368

Fernandez Cruz A, Barraquer Bordas L, Rotes-Querol J, Kuprian RM (1958) Los perfiles sindromicos y el contenido etiopatogenico de la acropatia ulcero mutilante. Med Clin 31: 237

Ferrier P, Ferrier S, Stalder G, Buhler E, Bamatter F, Klein D (1964) Congenital asymmetry associated with diploid-triploid mosaicism and large satellites. Lancet 1: 80-82

Fersatl A (1932) Erfahrungen mit der operativen Behandlung des Plattfußes. Z Orthop 57: 276-277

Ficat C (1976) Les contusions du cartilage articulaire. Etude expérimentale. Rev Chir Orthop 62: 493

Ficat P (1966) Acropathie ulcéro-multilante. Rôle possible du tunnel tarsien. Ann Chir 20: 1355-1360

Ficat P (1966) Syndrome du tunnel tarsien. Rev Ann Podol 5: 38-59

Figner G (1974) Surgical treatment of hallux valgus and hallux rigidus. Ther Umsch 31 (1): 23

Finochietto E (1904) El pie bot varus equino congenito. Buenos Aires

Finochietto E (1932) Pied creux. Bol Trab Soc Cir, Buenos Aires

Fitzgerald J (1969) A review of long-term results of arthrodesis of the first metatarso-phalangeal joint. J Bone Joint Surg [Br] 51: 488

Flint MH, Mackenzie JG (1962) Anterior laxity of the ankle. A cause of recurrent paralytic drop foot deformity. J Bone Joint Surg 44-B: 377-383

Fontanillas JL (1965) Osteocondrosis dissecante bilaterale della testa del 1er metatarso. Podologie 4: 61

Forestier J (1926) Le bracelet métatarsien pour la cure de la métatarsalgie statique et du pied plat métatarsien. Rev Orthop

Forestier J, Robert P (1940) X-ray diagnosis in chronic arthritis. Proc R Soc Med 33: 707

Forestier J, Jacquelin F, Rotes-Querol J (1951) La spondylarthrite ankylosante. Masson, Paris

Forrester DM, Nesson JW (1973) The radiology of joint disease. Saunders, Philadelphia

Forrester-Brown MF (1932) Flat foot. Br Med J 3

Forrester-Brown MF (1938) Tendon transplantation for clawing of the great toe. J Bone Joint Surg 20: 56

Forster E, Mole L, Muller J (1960) Etude critique du traitement des fractures du calcanéum (à propos de 98 observations). Rev Chir Orthop 46 (3): 348-368

Fournié A (1975) Le pied dans le rhumatisme psoriasique. Le pied inflammatoire. Maloine, Paris, p 73

Fournié A, Putois J (1966) Tumeurs des gaines et des tendons. Ann Podol 5: 177-184

Fowler AW (1957) The surgery of fixed claw toes. J Bone Joint Surg [Br] 39: 585

Fowler AW (1965) Forefoot reconstruction operation modification. J Bone Joint Surg [Br] 47: 586

Franchin F, Quagliarella L, Galante VN, Boccia G (1982) Protes FQ del seno del tarso. Chir Pied 6 (4): 415-421

Francillon MR (1959) Traitement des entorses récidivantes du cou de pied par réflection du ligament latéral externe par greffe dermique. Acta Orth Belg 25: 559-561

Francillon MR (1961) Lésions ligamentaires dans l'entorse du cou de pied. Répercussions cinétiques. Atti SIOT 46: 110

Francillon MR (1961) Transplantation tendineuse au niveau des extrémités inférieures; considérations physiologiques. Rev Chir Orthop 47: 196-200

Francon F, Exertier J (1959) De nouveau sur la maladie de Ledderhose: épaississement fibreux de l'aponévrose plantaire. Rev Med Suisse Romande 79: 616

Franke D (1961) Le traitement de la fracture-luxation au niveau de l'articulation de Lisfranc. Monatsschr Unfallheilkd 64 (6): 225

Freeman MAR, Dean MRE, Hanhar IWF (1965) The etiology and prevention of functional instability of the foot. J Bone Joint Surg [Br] 47 (4): 678-685

Freiberg AH (1914) Infraction of the second metatarsal bone. Surg Gynecol Obstet 19: 191

Freiberg AH (1926) The so-called infraction of the second metatarsal bone. J Bone Joint Surg 8: 257

Freiberg AH (1923) Osteochondritis dissecans. J Bone Joint Surg 5: 3

Freiberger RH, Hersh A, Harrison MO (1970) Radiology of the normal foot. Sem Roentgenol 5: 341-354

Fried A, Hendel C (1957) Paralytic valgus deformity of the ankle. J Bone Joint Surg [Am] 39a: 921-932

Friedl E (1924) Das Os intermetatarseum und die Epiphysenbildung und Processus trochlearis calcanei. Dtsch Z Chir 188: 150

Friedreich N (1863) Über degenerative Atrophie der spinalen Hinterstränge. Virchows Arch Pathol Anat 26: 1 and 27: 391, 433 (traduit dans les Archives Gén de Méd de Paris, décembre 1863)

Friedreich N (1873) Über progressive Muskelatrophie, über wahre und falsche Muskelhypertrophie

Friedreich N (1876) Über Ataxie mit besonderer Berücksichtigung der hereditären Formen. Arch Pathol Anat Berlin 68: 145-245

Frieh JM (1974) Etude critique des résultats de la chirurgie courante de l'hallux valgus et des déformations associées de l'avant-pied (à propos de 245 observations). Thesis, University of Tours

Froehlich E (1932) Pieds plats valgus. Revue Méd de l'Est

Froehlich E (1939) Heilungsergebnisse der Hallux-Valgus-Operationen. Arch Orthop Unfallchir 39: 624

Frost L (1950) Root resection for incurvated nail. J Natl Assoc Chirop 40: 19

Frost L (1956) A definite surgical treatment for some lateral nail problems. J Natl Assoc Chirop 47: 10, 493

Frykberg RG et al (1978) Neuropathic arthropathy in the diabetic foot. Am Fam Physician 17 (5): 105-13

Gagnal R (1939) Le traitement de l'hallux valgus par la résection de la tête du 1er métatarsien. Thèse de doctorat en médecine, Université de Lyon
Gagnon PA (1968) L'ostéotomie métatarsienne oblique dans le traitement de la keratose plantaire. Podologie 6: 215–230
Galeazzi V (1927) Sul piede piatto reflesso. Arch Ital Chir 18: 697
Galien (1541) Anatomie des os du corps humain. Trad. Sehan Canappe. Dolet, Lyon, p 41
Galmiche F (1972) La lyse radiologique de la tête du 5. metatarsienne au cours de la polyarthrite rhumatoïde. Thesis, Paris
Galmiche P (1962a) Le pied dans la polyarthrite chronique évolutive. Scalpel 115: 539
Galmiche P (1962b) Notions de podologie pratique. Podologie 1: 148–160
Galmiche P, Martin B (1983) Les tumeurs de Koenen. Act Med Chir Pied, 14: 128–136
Gamble FO (1957) Applied foot roentgenology, William and Wilkins, Baltimore
Gandin J (1966) Rupture du tendon d'Achille (d'après 25 cas opérés). Traitement chirurgical. Ann Podol 5: 165
Gandolfi M, Baltar Tojo F, Seral Inigo F (1964) La resección de las cabezas de los metatarsianos. Rev Ortop Traumatol Iber 8 (3): 467
Garceau GJ, Brahms MA (1956) A preliminary study of selective plantar muscle denervation for pes cavus. J Bone Joint Surg [Am] 38a: 553–562
Garelli R (1976) Presupposti per il trattamento chirurgico dell'alluce valgo. Minerva Ortop 27: 573–580
Garelli R (1978) Presentazione del podoscopio operatorio. Chir Pied 2 (1–2): 29–31
Garelli R, D'Onofrio M (1976) Studio scintigrafico del piede dopo interventi correttivi sull'avampiede. Minerva Ortop 27 (6): 315–317
Garelli R, Regnauld B (1976) Sul trattamento chirurgico delle metatarsalgia. Minerva Ortop 27: 431–438
Gaunel C (1972) Diagnostic des troubles statiques de la voûte osseuse du pied. Indices de caviation et de prono-supination. Masson, Paris, pp 331–363
Gaunel C (1979) Chaussures orthopédiques et appareils spéciaux. In: L'appareillage des handicapés moteurs. Enseignement inter-universitaire du CES de rééducation et réadaptation foncionnelle, Nancy, pp 265–287
Gaunel C, Louyot P, Treheux A (1971) New radiological data on plantar statics. J Radiol Electrol 52 (8): 528–529
Gaunel C, Louyot P, Annonier CI (1973) Codification radiologique de la statique du pied. Actual Med Chir Pied 8 (1): 191–199
Gauthier G (1971) Pied bot varus équin congénital. Vie médicale 22 (2): 2725–2738
Gauthier G (1979) Thomas Morton's disease: a nerve entrapment syndrome. Clin Orthop 142: 90–92
Gauthier G (1982) Ostéomie cylindrique du calcanéum. Cinésiologie 21 (83 bis): 14–16
Gauthier G, Dutertre P (1975) La maladie de Morton: syndrome canalaire: 74 cas opérés sans résection du névrome. Lyon Med 223: 917–921
Gay R, Mansat C, Martínez C, Fournier A (1970) Chirurgie de l'avant-pied rhumatoïde. Rev Med Toulouse 6: 575–586
Gechwend N (1971) Tratamiento quirúrgico de la poliartritis crónica progresiva. Toray, Barcelona
Geckeler EO (1957) Resección metatarsiana para incapacidad funcional del pie. Ortop Clin Venezuela
Gentles JC (1971) Laboratory investigations of dermatophyte infections of nails. Sabouraudia 9: 149–152
Geoffroy J, Hoeffel JC, Pointel JP, Brouin P, Debry G, Martin J (1978) Les lésions ostéo-articulaires chez le diabétique. Etude systématique de 1501 dossiers radiologiques. J Radiol Electrol 59 (10): 557–562
Gerbert J (1981) Textbook of bunion surgery. Futura, New York
Gerbert J, Mercado OA, Solokoff TH (1973) The surgical treatment of hallux-abducto-valgus and allied deformities. Futura, New York
Gervis WH (1970) Flat foot. Br Med J 1: 479–481
Geyer (1958) Beiträge zu den Synostosenbildungen der Hand- und Fußwurzel. Z Orthop 90: 395–408
Ghisellini F, Manaresi C (1961) Il piede piatto reflesso congenito. Chir Org Mov 1 (1): 37
Giani R (1905) Die Funktion des M. Tibialis anticus in Beziehung zur Pathogenese des statisch-mechanischen Plattfußes. Z Orthop 14: 34–51
Giannestras NJ (1954) Shortening of the metatarsal shaft for the correction of plantar keratosis. Clin Orthop 4: 225–231
Giannestras NJ (1958) Shortening of the metatarsal shaft in the treatment of plantar keratosis. An end-result study. J Bone Joint Surg [Am] 40A: 61–71
Giannestras NJ (1973) Foot disorders: medical and surgical management. Lea and Febiger. Philadelphia
Giannestras NJ (1973) The congenital rigid flat foot. Orthop Clin North Amer 4: 49
Gibbs RC (1979) Footnotes: mostly about toenails. J Dermatol Surg Oncol 5 (4): 264–269
Gillet M (1976) Exploration isotopique du pied. Cah Reed Readapt Fonct 11 (3): 87–90
Girdlestone GR, Spooner HJ (1937) A new operation for hallux valgus and hallux rigidus. J Bone Joint Surg 19: 30
Giuntini L (1955) Il trattamento del piede cavo anteriore con l'operazione di Scherb-Giutini. Atti SIOT 40: 215
Giuntini L (1968) Manuale di ortopedia e traumatologie. Universo, Rome
Giuntini L (1971) Physio-pathologie de l'avant-pied. Podologie 6: 109
Giuntini L (1971) Aspetti fisiopatologici delle sindromi morbose dell'avampiede. Podologie 6: 109–112
Glicenstein J, Bensahel H (1978) Traitement chirurgical du pied bot invétéré: intérêt d'une autoplastie cutanée. Nouv Press Med 7: 2469–2470
Gloppe H (1978) Hallux valgus associé ou non à un trouble de la statique de l'avant-pied. Étude comparée des résultats de l'intervention de Regnauld et de Lelièvre. Thesis, University of Lyon
Godebout de J (1976) Le bilan musculaire du pied dans les paralysies périphériques. Cah Reed Readapt Fonct 11 (3): 77–80

Godlewski S (1955) Des déformations des pieds en clinique neurologique. In: Coste F (ed) Le rhumatisme, 4th edn. Expansion Scientifique Française, Paris

Godlewski S (1971) Le pied neurologique. Vie Medicale 22: 2663-2698

Goidanich IF (1961) Compendio di ortopedia e traumatologia. Calderini, Bologna

Goldner JL, Gaines RW (1976) Adult and juvenile hallux valgus: analysis and treatment. Orthop Clin North Am 7 (4): 863-887

Gómez Alonso A, Gonzáles González M, Martínez Diez M, Seral Iñigo F (1971) A propósito de 7 casos de acropatiá ulceromutilante. Rev Cis Osteo 6: 349

Gomez Pellico L, Llanos Alcazar LF (1973) Los factores activos de la boveda plantar. Analisis electromiograficos. Rev Ortop Traumatol Iber 17 (1): 101

Gonzales JC, Puig R, Rochera R, Torner C, Viladot R (1972) Tecnica empleada en el tratamiento quirurgico del pie plano. Resultados, consideracionses estadisticas. Rev Ortop Traumatol [Br] 161 (2): 321

Goodfellow J (1966) Etiologie de l'hallux valgus. Proc R Soc Med 59: 821-824

Goodgold, Joseph, Hopell, Harvey, Spielholz, Niel (1965) The tarsal tunnel syndrome. Objective diagnostic criteria. N Engl J Med 273: 742

Gordon RB (1970) Arthrography of the ankle joint. J Bone Joint Surg [Am] 52: 162-163

Goreux J (1977) Les critères de la bonne chaussure. Per Prat 10/245: 75-86

Gottleib A (1932) Flatfoot and its relation to the triceps sural muscle. Am J Phys Ther 8: 321-323

Gougeon J (1965) Les algoneurodystrophies des membres inférieurs. Ann Med Pharm Reims 2: 111

Gougeon J (1968) L'acropathie ulcéro-mutilante. Cah Coll Med Hôp Paris 9: 145-154

Gougeon J, Seignon B (1978) Ostéoarthropathies nerveuses. Encycl Med Chir Paris, App Locomoteur 14285 A: 10

Goutailler G (1969) Les luxations fractures du Lisfranc. Podologie 6: 244

de Graciansky P (1965) Traitement des mycoses superficielles. Rev Prat 9: 1075-1087

de Graciansky P, Timsit E, Schousboe A, Birman M (1965) Granulome moniliasique. Bull Dermatol Syph 3: 238-240

Graham WC, Riordan DC (1948) Reconstruction of a metacarpo-phalangeal joint with a metatarsal transplant. J Bone Joint Surg 30-A: 848-853

Grassin P (1971) Hallux rigidus: artifice technique de rééducation. Congrès de Paris, CIP Annales 2: 8

Grassin P (1973) Étude comparative des différents traitements d'arthroplastie métatarso-phalangienne. Bull Soc Fr Med Chir Pied 3: 10-13

Grassin P (1973) Artifice technique dans le traitement chirurgical de l'hallux valgus. Ann CIP 8 (2)

Grassin P (1976) Étude comparative des différents traitements de l'hallux rigidus. Bull Soc Belg Med Chir Pied 233-238

Grassin P (1976) Réflexions sur les prothèses métatarsophalangiennes. Minerva Med Ann Podol 12

Grassin P (1977) Traitement du pied plat valgus de l'enfant. Indication chirurgical. Edition du 1er cours du CIP, Dijon

Grassin P (1978) Etio-physio-pathogènie clinique et traitement de la métatarsalgie élective du 1er rayon. Edition du 2e cours du CIP, Rennes

Grassin P (1979a) Indications de l'arthrorise sous-astragalienne. 2e Coll Intern, Charleroi. Chir Piede 3 (4)

Grassin P (1979b) Indication de l'enclavement diaépiphysaire de Regnauld. Edition du 3e cours du CIP, Nantes

Grassin P, Regnauld B (1975) Affections rhumatismales de l'avant-pied. Indications et techniques chirurgicales. Rhumatologie 27 (3): 137

Graver HH (1973) Angular metatarsal osteotomy. J Am Podiatry Assoc 63 (3): 96-99

Graver HH (1978) Cuneiform osteotomy in correction of metatarsus primus adductus. J Am Podiatry Assoc 68 (2): 111-116

Gray (1969) The role of the leg muscles in variations of the arches in normal and flat feet. Phys Ther 49: 1084, 1088

Green WT, MacDermott LJ (1942) Operative treatment of cerebral palsy of spastic type. JAMA 118: 434

Grice DS (1952) Extraarticular arthrodesis of the subtalar joint for correction of paralytic feet in children. J Bone Joint Surg [Am] 34: 927-940

Grice DS (1955) Further experience with extraarticular arthrodesis of the subtalar joint. J Bone Joint Surg [Am] 37: 246

Grigoriu D (1975a) Mycoses des pieds. Med Hyg 1148: 763-767

Grigoriu D (1975b) Mycoses des pieds. Actua 1148: 23-32

Gringrich WD (1962) Keratomycosis. JAMA 179 (8): 602-608

Grob D, Gschwend N (1982) Langzeitergebnisse nach Vorfußkorrektur aus subjektiver Sicht. Orthopäde 11 (4): 245-250

Grossiord A (1958) Les grandes articulations des membres inférieurs dans la marche normale. Ann Med Phys 1: 295

Groulier P (1975) Les métatarsalgies. Médit Med 55: 35-48

Groulier P (1976) Résultats et étude critique de la transplantation des extenseurs sur le col des métatarsiens dans les traitements du pied rond antérieur. Medit Med 117: 5-10

Groulier P, Pinaud JC (1970) Les luxations tarso-métatarsiennes (à propos de 10 observations). Rev Chir Orthop 56 (4): 303

Groulier P, Sassoon D (1982) Les ostéotomies du calcanéum dans les troubles statiques de l'arrière-pied de l'adulte. Cynésiologie 21 (83 bis): 12

Grupper C (1956) Le traitement des dermatoses à levures et de quelques dermatoses non moniliiques par la Mycostatine. Sem Hop Paris 32: 2253

Gschwend N (1958) Die fibulären Bandläsionen - eine oft verkannte Folge der Fußverstauchungen. Praxis 47: 809-813

Gschwend N (1976) Die operative Behandlung der chronischen Polyarthritis, 2. Aufl. Thieme, Stuttgart
Gschwend N, Barbier M, Dybowski WR (1977) Die Vorfußkorrektur - Häufigkeit und Bedeutung der Zehen- und Metatarsal-Indices. Arch Orthop Unfall Chir 88: 75-85
Guaccero A (1925) Piedi torti. STEB Paris
Gueur P (1963) Dernière ressource de traitement du pied paralytique définitif. Congrès Ostende, 1962. Ann Podol 2: 198
Guibal C (1968) Exploration fonctionnelle dynamique du pied par l'électropodographie. Thesis, University of Montpellier
Guillain G, Dubois J (1914) Sur une affection mutilante des extrémités. La valeur séméiologique du signe d'Argyll-Robertson. Ann Med 1: 553
Guillain G, Thevenard A (1929) Mal perforant plantaire familial, syringomyélie lombo-sacrée probable chez deux frères. Ann Med 24: 269
Guillain G, Mathieu P, Lereboullet J (1926) Sur une affection mutilante des extrémités inférieures. Syringomyélie de la région lombo-sacrée. Ann Med 19: 548
Güntz E (1938) Apparatus for taking pictures of entire foot in use and at rest. Röntgenpraxis 10: 16-17
Güntz E (1938) Représentation radiographique des têtes des métatarsiens et des sésamoïdes du pied. Z Orthop 68 (4): 465-473
Güntz E (1939) Die pathologische Anatomie des angeborenen Plattfußes. Z Orthop 69: 219-236
Gutman AB (1967) Gout. In: Beeson W, McDermott (eds) Textbook of medicine, 12th ed. Saunders, Philadelphia, pp 1238-1248
Haegel P (1973) Le pied humain. Anatomie comparée, embryologie, morphologie. Podologie 8 (1): 16-23
Haggart GE (1934) The conservative and surgical treatment of plantar warts. Surg Clin North Am 14: 1211
Haglund P (1923) Prinzipien der Orthopädie. Fischer, Jena
Haglund P (1928) Beitrag zur Klinik der Achillessehne, Z Orthop Chir 49: 49
Haimovici N (1968) Contribution au problème du traitement de l'ulcère trophique plantaire après section de troncs nerveux. Podologie 6: 241-245
Haines RW, McDougall A (1954) The anatomy of hallux valgus. Bone Joint Surg [Br] 36b: 272
Hallgrimsson S (1939) Le pied creux, son traitement, quelques remarques sur son étiologie. Acta Orthop Scand 10 (I, II): 73-118
Hallst A, Hallst J (1947) Le traitement du pied bot varus équin essentiel et réfractaire au cours de la 1ère enfance. Acta Orthop Belg tome 13 (4)
Hamilton J (1955) The short tendo calcaneus. J Bone Joint Surg [Br] 37b: 354
Hammond G (1945) Elevation of the first metatarsal bone with hallux equinus. Arch Surg 13: 240
Hammond WA (1879) Fasting girls: their physiology and pathology. Putnam, New York
Haralsson S (1962) Operative treatment of pes plano-valgus staticus juvenilis. Preliminary communication. Acta Orthop Scand 32: 492-498
Haraldsson S (1965) Pes plano-valgus staticus juvenilis and its operative treatment. Acta Orthop Scand 35: 234-256
Harbeson AE (1938) Further studies on the origin of the first dorsal interosseous muscle of the foot from the tendon of the peroneus longus. J Anat 72: 463-464
Hardy RH, Clamphan JCR (1952) Hallux valgus: predisposing anatomical causes. Lancet 14: 1181-1183
Hark F, Woot (1950) "Rocher-foot" due to congenital subluxation of the talus. J Bone Joint Surg 32-A: 344
Harrel RE, Bocobo F (1960) Modern treatment of the systemic fungous diseases. Clin Pharmacol Ther 1: 104-134
Harris RI (1950) Rigid valgus foot due to talocalcaneal bridge. J Bone Joint Surg [Am] 37: 169
Harris RI (1955) Rigid valgus foot due to talocalcaneal bridge. J Bone Joint Surg [Br] 32: 30
Harris RI (1956) Syme's amputation. The technical details essential for success. J Bone Joint Surg [Br] 38: 614
Harris RI (1963) Retrospect peroneal spastic flat foot. J Bone Joint Surg [Br] 45: 447-461
Harris RI, Beath T (1948a) Pied plat spastique. J Bone Joint Surg: 625
Harris RI, Beath T (1948b) Etiologie du pied plat péronier spastique. J Bone Joint Surg 30 (4)
Harris RI, Beath T (1948c) Hypermobile flat foot with short tendo Achillis. J Bone Joint Surg 30-A: 116-140
Harris RI, Beath T (1949) The short first metatarsal. J Bone Joint Surg [Am] 31: 553
Harrisson MH, Harvey FJ (1963) Arthrodesis of the first metatarso-phalangeal joint hallux valgus and hallux rigidus. J Bone Joint Surg 45: 471-480
Harrisson MJG, Faris IB (1976) Le facteur neurogène du pied diabétique. J Neurol Sci 28 (2): 217-223
Harrold AJ (1967) Congenital vertical talus in infancy. J Bone Joint Surg 49-B: 634
Harry N, Harry J (1940) Denis Browne splint in the treatment of talipes equinovarus. Aust NZ J Surg 117
Harty M (1973) Metatarsalgia. Surg Gynecol Obstet 136: 105-106
Hauser EDW (1950) Diseases of the foot, 2nd edn. Saunders, Philadelphia
Hauser EDW (1962) The sinus tarsi syndrome. Ann Podol 1: 11-15
Hauser EDW (1965) Carcinoma following a plantar wart. Podologie 4: 103-108
Hauser EDW (1966) Congenital clubfoot. Thomas, Springfield
Hauser EDW (1971) Common foot disorders. Podologie 6: 267
Hawkins FB (1971) Acquired hallux varus: cause, prevention and correction. Clin Orthop 76: 169-176
Hederich H (1948) Fracturas de calcaneo. Casals, Barcelona
von Heine J (1840) Beobachtungen über Lähmungszustände der unteren Extremitäten und deren Behandlung. Stuttgart. Second edn. (1860) Spinale Kinderlähmung - Monographie. Stuttgart
Helal B (1975) Metatarsal osteotomy for metatarsalgia. J Bone Joint Surg [Br] 57b (2): 187-193

Helfet AJ (1956) Traitements des pieds plats de l'enfance. Lancet 270: 262

Hendrix G (1932) Traitement des pieds douloureux. La polyclinique 35 (1): 1–4

Hendrix G (1934) Vue d'ensemble sur la pathogénie des déformations statiques des voûtes du pied. Bull Mém Soc Belg Orthop 6 (3): 175–224

Hendrix G (1934) Pathogénie des déformations statiques des voûtes du pied. Bull Soc Belge Orthop 6 (3): 175–222

Hendrix G (1962) La loi de l'interdépendance des arches longitudinales du pied appliquée à la chirurgie du pied bot invétéré du jeune enfant. Acta Orthop Belg 28 (1): 8

Henke PJW (1859) Die Kontrakturen der Fußwurzel. Z Med Leipzig 5: 44

Hernandez López E (1949) Ulceras de las extremidades de origen nervioso. Ponencia oficial del 1 congreso nacional de cirugia, Barcelona

Hernandez López E (1960) Tratamiento del hallux valgus. Rev Ortop Traumatol 4 (1): 261

Herndon CH, Chase SW (1952) Experimental studies in the transplantation of whole joints. J Bone Joint Surg 34-A: 564–578

Herndon CH, Heyman CH (1963) Problems in the recognition and treatment of congenital convex pes valgus. J Bone Joint Surg 45-B: 413

Heyman CH, Herndon CH, Strong JM (1958) Mobilization of the tarsometatarsal and intermetatarsal joints for the correction of resistant adduction of the fore part of the foot in congenital club-foot or congenital metatarsus varus. J Bone Joint Surg [Am] 40: 199

Hilton L, Simpson RR (1978) Differential diagnosis of plantar palmar keratoderma. J Am Podiatry Assoc 68 (8): 578–584

Hincky M (1975) Traitement des mycoses cutanées. Conc Méd 10: 1617–1627

Hiramkite J (1950) Metatarsus varus congenital. Study of 300 cases. J Bone Joint Surg [Am] 32: 500

Hoffa A (1902) Lehrbuch der orthopädischen Chirurgie. Enke, Stuttgart

Hoffa A (1905) Orthopädische Chirurgie. Enke, Stuttgart

Hoffman P (1911) An operation for severe grades of contracted or clawed toes. Am J Orthop Surg 9: 441

Hoffmann H (1936) Die congenitale "Phalanx hallucis valgi". Z Orthop 65 (4): 352–360

Hohmann G (1923) Über Fußwurzelkontrakturen beim statischen Pes valgus und Plano-valgus. (17e congrès allemand d'orthop, 1922) Z Orthop Chir 44 (1–2): 206–220

Hohmann G (1924) Problem der Plattfußfrage. Z Orthop 45: 7–16

Hohmann G (1933) Spiralschieneneinlage zur Stützung und Korrektur gewisser schwieriger Formen des Plattfußes und Hohlfußes. Z Orthop 58: 587–590

Hohmann G (1935) Über angeborene Supinationstellung des Vorfußes. Z Orthop 63: 263–267

Hohmann G (1951) Fuß und Bein, 5th edn. Bergmann, München

Hohmann G (1955) Le syndrome de Sudeck: peut-il être la conséquence d'un traitement? Dtsch Med Wochenschr 80: 280

Hohmann G, Thomsen W, Tangen O (1971) Hallux valgus. The treatment by distal wedge osteotomy of the 1st metatarsal. Acta Chir Scand 137: 151

Hoke M (1921) An operation for stabilising paralytic feet. J Orthop Surg 19: 494

Hoke M (1931) An operation for the correction of extremely relaxed flat feet. J Bone Joint Surg 13 (4): 773–783

Hollingsworth RP (1975) An X-ray study of valgus ankles in spina bifida children with valgus flat foot deformity. Proc R Soc Med 66 (8): 481–484

Hooshmand H, Escobar MR, Kopf SW (1972) Neurosyphilis: a study of 241 patients. JAMA 219: 726–729

Howard (1893) Ingrown toenail, its surgical treatment. NY Med Surg J 57: 579

Horst M (1976) Current treatment of hallux valgus. Hippokrates 47 (4): 395–400

Howe F (1932) March fractures of metatarsal bones. Surg Gynecol Obstet 581

Hsu LCS, O'Brien JP, Yau ACMC, Hodgson AR (1976) Batchelor's extraarticular subtalar arthrodesis. A report on sixty-four procedures in patients with poliomyelitic deformities. J Bone Joint Surg [Am] 58a (2): 243

d'Huart F (1967) Le syndrome du canal tarsien. Ann Chir 21: 2122, 1301–1306

Hubault A (1967) Les maux perforants plantaires. In: la pathologie tégumentaire du pied, vol I. Expansion Scientifique Française, Paris

Hubbard E (1973) Technique for use of the silastic toe prosthesis in hallux valgus surgery (Swanson design). J Am Podiatry Assoc 63 (12): 677–86

Huber-Levernieux C, Denis A (1976) Ostéonécrose aseptique des sésamoïdes du 1er orteil: maladie de Renander. In: De Sèze S et al. (eds) Actual Rhumatol 1975. Expansion Scientifique, Paris, pp 205–209

Hueter C (1976) Klinik der Gelenkkrankheiten mit Einschluß der Orthopädie, vol 3, 2nd edn. Vogel, Leipzig

Hugues JR (1942) Sprain and subluxation of the ankle joint. Proc R Soc Med 35: 765–766

Huriez CI (1971) Maux perforants plantaires, 3rd edn. Lille Med 16 (3): 369

Hussenstein J (1956) Luxations récidivantes du cou-de-pied. Ann Chir 14–15: 1239–1243

Hy H (1968) Hallux valgus. Actual Chir Orthop Hop R Poincaré 6: 204

Inge, Ferguson (1933) Surgery of the sesamoid bones of the great toe. Arch Surg 27: 466

Ingelrans P (1962) L'Arthrodèse sous-astragalienne extra-articulaire selon le precédé de Grice pour pied valgus paralytique. Acta Orthop Belg 28 (6): 654–666

Inman VT (1974) Hallux valgus: a review of etiologic factors. Orthop Clin North Am 5 (1): 59–66

Irani RN, Sherman MS (1963) The pathological anatomy of club-foot. J Bone Joint Surg 45: 45–52

Irles M (1974) Résultat du traitement des fractures du calcanéum. Thesis, University of Tours

Isemein L, Fournier AM (1963) Le pied dans la polyarthrite chronique évolutive. Marseille Med 100: 318
Jack EA (1940) The aetiology of hallux rigidus. Br J Surg 27: 492
Jack EA (1953) Naviculo-cuneiform fusion in the treatment of flat-foot. J Bone Joint Surg [Br] 35: 75-82
Jacoby RK (1973) V-osteotomy for correction of intractable plantar keratoses. J Foot Surg 12: 8
Jacoby RK, Vidigal E, Kirkup J, Dixon AStJ (1976) The great toe as a clinical problem in rheumatoid arthritis. Rheumatol Rehabil 15: 143
Jaffe HL, Lichtenstein L, Sutro CJ (1941) Pigmented villonodular synovitis, bursitis and tenosynovitis. Arch Pathol 31: 731
Jamma (1934) Contributo tecnico-operatorio all'arthrorisi laterali del piede. Chir Organi Mov 20: 444-448
Jansen C (1966) Length-angle determinations on the metatarsus with regard to pes plano-transversus and hallux valgus. Chirurg 37 (12): 553-4
Japas LM (1968) Surgical treatment of pes cavus by tarsal V-osteotomy. Preliminary report. J Bone Joint Surg [Am] 50a: 927
Jazikoff D (1939) Luxation de l'articulation de Lisfranc. Rev Orthop 26 (2): 126
Joachimsthael (1905) Handbuch der orthopädischen Chirurgie. Fischer, Jena
Johnson EW, Ortiz PR (1966) Electrodiagnosis of tarsal tunnel syndrome. Arch Phys Med 47: 776-780
Johnson JC (1976) Peroneal spastic flatfoot syndrome. South Med J 69 (6): 807-809
Jones BS (1975) Flat foot. J Bone Joint Surg [Br] 57b (3): 279
Joplin RJ (1950) Sling procedure for correction of splay-foot, metatarsus primus varus and hallux valgus. J Bone Joint Surg [Am] 32a: 779-785
Joplin RJ (1969) Surgery of the forefoot in the rheumatoid arthritic patient. Surg Clin North Am 49: 847
Jorda López E (1977) Radiologia del pie: análisis de los resultados obtenidos y conclusiones. XIIe Congrès du Collège International de Médecine et de Chirurgie du Pied, Turin. Ann Podol 12
Joron G (1968) Etiopathogénie du pied diabétique. Podologie 6: 322
Joz-Roland P, Kritsikis N, Cyprien JM (1978) Fractures de la cheville: pronostic à long terme en fonction du diagnostic et du traitement. Med Hyg 36 (12-90): 2144-2146
Judet H (1906) Essai sur la greffe des tissus articulaires. CR Acad Sci Paris 146: 193-196, 600-603
Judet H (1976) Raideur post-traumatique de la cheville. Ann Soc Belg Med Chir Pied. Colloque international, Charleroi. CIFOP, Charleroi, pp 183-190
Judet J (1972) Podologie pratique. Gaz Med 79 (4)
Judet J (1973) Les possibilités de correction chirurgicale des malformations des os du pied. Acta Med Chir Pied 8 (1): 91-96
Judet J (1973) Le pied talus. Acta Med Chir Pied 8 (1): 73
Judet J (1975) Résultats du traitement chirurgical de la rupture du ligament latéral externe de la cheville. Rev Chir Orthop 61 [Suppl 2]: 157
Judet J, Judet R, Guignard J (1960) Transplantation du tiers externe du tendon d'Achille à la face externe du calcanéum. Rev Orthop 46: 634
Judet J, Judet R, Padovani JP (1972) Entorses et ruptures du ligament latéral externe de l'articulation tibio-tarsienne. Acta Orthop Belg 38 (6): 667-671
Judet J, Laugier A, Pouliquen JC (1976) Les pieds congénitaux. Actual Chir Ortop F2 (13): 106-139
Judet JR, Lord G (1959) L'emploi de la peau conservée en chirurgie osseuse. Acta Orthop Belg 24 (5): 561-564
Judet R (1937) Traitement chirurgical des pieds bots de l'adulte. Thèse Doct. Med., Paris
Judet R (1966) Fractures of the calcaneum. J Bone Joint Surg 378: 516
Judet R (1972) Le traitement chirurgical des fractures du calcanéum et des cals vicieux calcanéens. Cah Med Lyon 48 (36): 4265-4268
Judet R, Judet J, Rigault P (1966) Possibilités de correction chirurgicale des malformations des os du pied. Presse Med 74 (4): 157-161
Kadanov D, Moutaphov S (1964) Empreintes plantaires. Transition de la forme normale à la forme pathologique de la plante et répartition du poids sur la surface plantaire. Orthop Traumatol Sofia 1 (3): 356
Kalish SR, McGlamry ED (1974) The modified Keller hallux valgus repair utilizing Silastic implants, with some comments on implants in general. J Am Podiatry Assoc 64 (10): 761-73
Kallio E (1963) Osteoid osteoma of the metatarsal and metatarsal bones. Acta Orthop Scand 33 (3): 246
Kamberoglou K, Smirnis P, Tsiboukis B, Mariakakis N, Vayanos ED (1971) Traitement du pied bot varus équin congénital récidivé. Rev Chir Orthop 57 2: 166
Kapandji IA (1965) Physiologie articulaire du membre inférieur. Maloine, Paris, p 2
Kaplan M, Kaplan T (1935) Flat foot. Radiology 25 (4): 485
Kates A (1970) Surgery of the rheumatoid foot. Proc R Soc Med 63: 679
Kates A, Kay A (1971) La chirurgie du pied rhumatoïde. Med Hyg 29 (991): 2060-2063
Kates A, Kessel L, Kay A (1967) Arthroplasty of the forefoot. J Bone Joint Surg [Br] 49: 552-557
Kaye JJ, Ghelman B, Schneider R (1975) Talocalcaneonavicular joint arthrography for sustentacular-talar coalition. Radiology 115 (3): 730-731
Keasbey SE (1953) Juvenile aponeurotic fibroma (calcifying fibroma). Cancer 6: 338-346
Keck (1962) Tarsal tunnel syndrome. J Bone Joint Surg [Am] 44: 180-182
Kelikian H (1965) Hallux valgus. Allied deformities of the forefoot and metatarsalgia. Saunders, Philadelphia
Keller WL (1904) The surgical treatment of bunions and hallux valgus. NY Med J 80: 741-742
Kempf I (1972) L'évolution de nos conceptions dans le traitement chirurgical des fractures thalamiques du calcanéum. Cah Med Lyon 48 (36): 4254-4258
Kempf I, Touzand RC (1978) Les fractures du calcanéum. Masson, Paris

Kerbrat M (1974) Les aspects radiologiques du pied en pathologie générale. Thesis, University of Brest
Kessel L, Bonney G (1958) Hallux rigidus in the adolescent. J Bone Joint Surg [Br] 40: 668
Key JA (1934) Contusion of cartilage as an etiological factor in chronic arthritis. Surg Gynecol Obstet 58: 166
Keyes EL (1934) The surgical treatment of ingrown toenails. J Am Podiatry Assoc 102: 1458
Khuns JG (1960) The foot in chronic arthritis. Clin Orthop 16: 141-151
Kidner FC (1929) The prehallux (accessory scaphoïd) in its relation to flat-foot. J Bone Joint Surg 11: 831-837
Kienböck R, Muller W (1937) Os tibiale externum et lesions du pied. Z Orthop 56 (3): 257-271
Kieffer E (1977) Les troubles trophiques du pied diabétique en milieu chirurgical. Conc Med 99 (1-2): 29-38
Kilberg AJ (1935) Surgical treatment of onychocryptosis. Clin J Chirop Pod Pedic Surg 7: 222
Kimmelstiel, Kremser, Richter (1932) Osteochondrosis necroticans findens des Sesambeins des 1er metatarsale. Arch Klin Chir 172: 3
Kingreen (1933) Etiologie de l'hallux flexus. Zentralbl Chir 36: 2116-2118
Kirk AA, Kunkle HM, Waive HJ (1971) Ledge tenodesis of the extensor hallucis longus. A substitution for the Jones operation. J Bone Joint Surg [Am] 53: 769
Kirkup JR (1974) Ankle and tarsal joints in rheumatoid arthritis. Scand J Rheumatol 3: 50-52
Kirkup JR (1978) Dislocation of the hallux in rheumatoid arthritis. Chir Piede 2 (3): 87-93
Kirkup JR, Vidigal E, Jacoby RK (1977) The hallux and rheumatoid arthritis. Acta Orthop Scand 48: 527-544
Kirmisson (1908) Déviations digitales. Rev Orthop 249
Kirmisson (1920) Le pied bot. J Praticiens 187
Kissel P, Schmitt J, Barrucand D (1967) Les acropathies ulcéro-mutilantes. Rev Prat 17 (12): 1731-1742
Kite JH (1930) Nonoperative treatment of congenital club foot: a review of one hundred cases. South Med J 23: 337-345
Kite JH (1935) The treatment of congenital club foot. Surg Gynecol Obstet 61: 190-200
Kite JH (1942) Principles involved in the treatment of congenital club foot. J Bone Joint Surg [Am] 24: 191-198
Kite JH (1938) Congenital club foot. In: Chormely RK (ed) Orthopedic surgery. Nelson, New York
Kite JH (1940) Some comments on the treatment of congenital club foot. J Med Assoc Georgia 29: 212-216
Kite JH (1945) Congenital deformities of foot. In: Bancroft A, Murray (eds) Surgical treatment of the motor-skeletal system. Lippincott, Philadelphia
Kite JH (1965) Congenital metatarsus varus. J Bone Joint Surg [Am] 49: 388-397
Klages F (1933) Le traitement de l'ongle incanré par une plaque d'argent, methode de Voelker. Zentrabl Chir 30: 1762-1764
Kleiger B (1956) Mechanism of ankle injuries. J Bone Joint Surg 381: 59-70
Kleiger B (1976) Lésions de l'astragale et de son articulation. Clin Orthop 121: 243-266
Koenen J (1932) Eine familiäre, hereditäre Form von tuberoser Sklerose. Acta Psychiatr Neurol 7: 813-821
Köhler A (1923) A typical disease of the second metatarso-phalangeal joint. AJR 10: 705
Kohn Tebner A, Carnevale V (1971) Sindrome del canal tarsiano. Podologie 6: 27
Kojima T (1963) A case of carpal tunnel syndrome associated with tarsal tunnel syndrome. Tohoku J Orthop Traumatol 7 (2): 214-218
Komprda J (1966) Syndrome du sinus du tarse. Étude de 116 observations. Podologie 5 (2): 19
Koniza J (1950) The operative treatment of hallux valgus. Pol Przegl Chir 22: 133
Kopell M, Thompson W (1960) Peripheral entrapment neuropathies of the lower extremities. N Engl J Med 262: 56-60
Koutsogiannis E (1971) Treatment of mobile flat-foot by displacement osteotomy of the calcaneus. J Bone Joint Surg [Br] 53 (1): 96
Kowalski C (1970) In: De Doncker E, Kowalski C (eds) Le pied normal et pathologique. Acta Orthop Belg 36: 4-5
Kramarenko GN (1975) Surgical treatment of static pes planus transversus and hallux valgus. Beitr Orthop Traumatol 22 (3): 183-5
Krasensky JP (1976) Le renfort interne pour le pied plat valgus du jeune enfant hyperlaxe. Rev Podologie 33: 43-44
Laaksonen AL (1966) A prognostic study of juvenile rheumatoid arthritis: analysis of 554 cases. Acta Paediatr Scand [Suppl] 166
Labrousse C, Lathelize H, Andrieu J, Desproges-Gotteron R (1975) Les talalgies. Rhumatologie 27 (2): 75-78
Lacassagne J (1954) Traitement des verrues plantaires. Presse Med 62: 1115
Lacheretz M, Debeugny P (1964) L'arthrodèse sous-astragalienne extra-articulaire selon le procédé de Grice pour pied valgus paralytique. Son utilisation possible dans le pied creux talus. Chir Orthop 50: 87-102
Lacombe M (1962) Lesions traumatiques des nerfs: Le syndrome du canal tarsien. Encycl Med Chir A 10: 5003
Lagier R, Morong E (1958) Contribution à l'étude anatomo-pathologique de la maladie de Ledderhose (épaississement de l'aponévrose plantaire). Press Med 66 (6)
Lai G (1966) Discussione gli esiti fontai dell'intervento di duplice artrodesi nel piede poliomielitico. Ann Podol 5: 291
Lake N (1935) The foot. Baillière, Tyndall and Cox, London
Lake N (1937) The arches of the feet. Lancet 233: 872-873
Lam SJS (1962) A tarsal tunnel syndrome. Lancet 2/7270: 1354-1355
Lambrinudi C (1927) An operation on drop-foot. Br J Surg 15: 193
Lamy P (1930) Traitement du pied bot varus équin congénital par l'évidement sous-cutané. Sem Hôp Paris 168
Lamy P (1934) Pied valgus congénital convexe. Bull et Mémoire, Société Chir de Paris, 26 (12): 484-498

Lamy L, Weissman L (1939) Congenital convex pes valgus. J Bone Joint Surg 21: 79

Lance M (1947) Le traitement orthopédique et cinésique dans la période évolutive de la poliomyélite. Gaz Hop, August 16–23

Lance M (1948) La métatarsalgie et les deux maladies de Morton. Gaz Hop, February 28

Lance M, Lamy L (1938) Orthopédie. Maloine, Paris

Lance P (1936) Le traitement chirurgical de l'hallux valgus par le procédé du Bilboquet. Gaz Hop Civ Mil 109: 1628

Lance P (1939) Traitement des fractures du scaphoide tarsien. J Chir 54 (6)

Lange M (1934) Die Arthrodese des hinteren unteren Sprunggelenkes (Talocalcanealgelenk) zur Behandlung schwerer Fußverbildungen, insbesondere des Platt- und Klumpfußes. Chirurg 16: 569–575

Lange M (1935) Der Plattfuß als soziales Problem, seine Diagnose und Behandlung. Münch Med Wochenschr 47: 1875 und 48: 1912

Lange M (1951) Orthopädische chirurgische Korrektion, Operationslehre. Bergman, München

Langrot, Micheau, Dostagliola, Mansat (1965) A propos du traitement des luxations métatarsiennes. Ann Podol 4: 257

Lantzouris LA (1940) Congenital subluxation of the fifth toe and its correction by a periosteo-capsulo-plasty and tendon transplantation. J Bone Joint Surg 22: 147

Lanz T, Wachsmuth W (1938) Praktische Anatomie, vol 1. Springer, Berlin

Lanzetta A (1975) Le fratture del calcagno. Verducci, Roma

Lapeyre (1894–1895) Le pied bot. Thesis, University of Paris

Lapeyre J (1970) Chirurgie de l'avant-pied rhumatoïde. A propos de 28 cas. Thesis, University of Toulouse

Lapeyre F (1977) Réflexions sur l'examen du pied et la confection des semelles orthopédiques. Bilans, perspectives. Perspectives 4: 53–64

Lapidus PW (1939) Operation for correction of hammer toe. J Bone Joint Surg 21: 977

Lapidus PW (1940) "Dorsal bunion": this mechanics and operative correction. J Bone Joint Surg 22: 267

Lapidus PW (1942) Transplantation of the extensor tendon for correction of over-lapping fifth toe. J Bone Joint Surg 24: 555

Lapidus PW (1946) Spastic flat foot. J Bone Joint Surg 28: 126–136

Lapidus PW (1960) The author's bunion operation from 1931–1959. Clin Orthop 16: 119

Lapidus PW (1963) Kinesiology and mechanical anatomy of the tarsal joints. Clin Orthop 30: 20–36

Laplane D (1969) Diagnostic des lésions nerveuses périphériques. Cah Baillères, Paris

Laplane D, Ricou P (1976) La neurosyphilis. Rev Pratic 26 (57): 4133–4136

Larichelliere R (1962) Étude du scaphoïde sur 2514 radiographies. Podologie 1: 84

Lasagni PM (1958) La terapia del piede piatto valgo mediante la trasposizione astragalo-calcaneare. Acta Ortop Ital 4: 219–241

Lasserre C, Bord B (1940) Pied plat valgus congénital. Soc Med Chir Bordeaux, in J Med Bordeaux 20 avril 1940

Laurence G (1966) Orthopedie du 1er âge, 2nd edn. Baillère, Paris

Lavarde G (1975) Traumatismes de la cheville. Pathol Chir 1326: 228

Lavigne A, Noviel D (1973) Nouvelles thérapeutiques en podologie. Morgan, Paris

Lavigne A, Noviel D (1975) Traité théorique et pratique de la semelle orthopédique. Scerdes, Boulogne

Leache (1974) Metatarsal osteotomy for bunionette deformity. Clin Orthop Relat Res 100: 171–175

Lebeurre R (1963) Les talalgies rhumatismales. Sem Hop Paris 39: 227–228

Leboucq H (1882) Le développement du 1er métatarsien et son articulation tarsienne chez l'homme. Arch Biol 3: 335

Leclerc GC (1963) Traitement du metatarsus varus congénital. Rev Orthop 49 (6): 765–767

Leclerc GC (1966) Résultats thérapeutiques des pieds bots varus équins. Rev Orthop 52 (8): 724

Leclerc GC, Moine CJ (1964) Subluxation récidivante de l'astragale. Ann Podol 3: 13–32

Leclerc GC, Moine CJ (1965a) Subluxations antérieures récidivantes de l'astragale. Rev Chir Orthop 51 (2): 167–176

Leclerc GC, Moine CJ (1965b) Les entorses de la tibiotarsienne. Encycl Med Chir App Locomot 14097: A 10

Leclerc GC, Benard J, Autissier JM (1961) La subluxation chronique de la cheville. Rev Orthop 47 [1]: 68–75

Lecoeur P (1938) La pince malléolaire. Physiologie normale et pathologique du péroné. Thesis, University of Paris

Lecoeur P (1976) La pince malléolaire. Ann Soc Belg Med Chir Pied, CIFOP, Charleroi, pp 5–12

Le Coulant P, Civatte J, Texier L, Regnier (1967) Granulome candidosique du pied. Bull Ste Derm Syph 74 (4): 504–506

Ledos M (1956) Architecture et géométrie du pied. Ledos, Paris

Lee HG (1957) Surgical repair in recurrent dislocation of the ankle joint. J Bone Joint Surg, 39-A: 828–834

Leemans G (1933) Pied plat valgus bilatéral. Bull Mém Soc Belge Orthop 5 (2): 21–26

Lefebvre J, Koiffman A (1956) Étude de l'apparition des points osseux secondaires et détermination de l'âge osseux. Arch Fr Pédiatr 13: 1101–1105

Léger L (1946) Traitement de la métatarsalgie (maladie de Morton) par résection du neurofibrome du nerf plantaire interne. Presse Med 51: 713

Léger L, Olivier C (1945) Entorses du cou-de-pied et entorses du genou. Masson, Paris

Leitner B (1954) Luxation sous-astragalienne interne récente du pied avec subluxation tibiotarsienne de l'astragale. Rev Chir Orthop 40 (2): 232–235

Lejeune E, Bouvier M, Maitrepierre J, Siradj-el-Dine (1966) Le pied décalcifié douloureux ou algodystrophie réflexe du pied. Rhumatologie 18: 377–393

Lelièvre J (1953) Notes sur le traitement de quelques lésion du pied: métatarsectomie. Ann Med Chir Centre Brux 9: 113

Lelièvre J (1954) Notes sur le pied creux essentiel. Gaz Med Fr March: 427

Lelièvre J (1955a) Le pied dans la chaussure. Presse Med 63: 873

Lelièvre J (1955b) Les semelles orthopédiques. Conc Med September: 3441

Lelièvre J (1955c) Traitement médical du pied creux. Conc Med November: 4433

Lelièvre J (1956/1957) Pathologie des orteils, métatarsalgies, pied creux antérieur, mal perforant plantaire, maladie de Ledderhose, tumeur du pied, talalgie, pathologie des ongles. Pathol Chir Gen, vol 2, membres inférieurs. Encycl Med Chir

Lelièvre J (1958) Luxations pathologiques des orteils. Rev Orthop 44: 106

Lelièvre J (1959) Radiothérapie du pied. Conc Med 1: 431

Lelièvre J (1961) Traitement orthopédique et chirurgical des lésions du pied dans le rhumatisme inflammatoire. Rev Rhum Mal Osteoartic 7-8: 357-367

Lelièvre J (1962a) Lesions statiques de l'avant-pied. Acta Orthop Belg 28 (3): 209-217

Lelièvre J (1962b) Schéma clinique et thérapeutique du pied creux antérieur. Ann Podol 1: 45

Lelièvre J (1964a) L'alignement articulaire métatarsophalangien. Nouv Prat Chir Ill 23

Lelièvre J (1964b) Les problèmes de l'hallux valgus. Ann Podol 3: 89

Lelièvre J (1965a) La métatarsectomie pour pied creux. Nouv Prat Chir Illust 24: 241-277

Lelièvre J (1965b) Planus et cavus en cybernétique du pied. Gaz Med Fr 1: 111

Lelièvre J (1965c) Synthese sur le valgus du talon. Podologie 4: 183

Lelièvre J (1966) Cure de l'hallux valgus et de la griffe proximale des orteils. Nouv Prat Chir Illust 25: 232-261

Lelièvre J (1967) Pathologie du pied, 3e ed. Masson, Paris

Lelièvre J (1968a) L'arthroplastie tibiotarsienne. Podologie 6: 23

Lelièvre J (1968b) Mille alignements articulaires métatarso-phalangiens. Podologie 6: 155

Lelièvre J (1958b) Les talalgies plantaires. Conc Med 80: 1053-1054

Lelièvre J, Bertrand P (1968) Traitement chirurgical du pied spastique. Podologie 6: 119

Lelièvre J, Lelièvre JF (1971) Pathologie du pied: physiologie, clinique, traitement médical, orthopédique et chirurgical, 4th edn. Masson, Paris

Lelièvre J, Maschas A (1956) La metatarsectomie, techniques, indications. Rev Orthop 42: 886-887

Lelièvre J, Maschas A (1957) Intérêt de la troformone dans les radiodermites. Presse Med 65: 1034

Lelièvre JF (1969) Maux perforants plantaires. Rev Podol 100: 221-224

Lelièvre JF (1974) Cure de l'hallux valgus par la technique de Petersen. Rev Chir Orthop (Suppl) 60: 162-167

Lelièvre JF, Mamoudy P (1980) Traitement chirurgical des métatarsalgies siégeant sous les métatarso-phalangiennes moyennes. In: Deuxièmes journées d'ortopédie de la Pitié. Masson, Paris, pp 212-219

Lemaire R (1974) Le traitement chirurgical de l'hallux valgus. Rev Med Liege 29 (20): 613-621

Lemoine-Dubois-Bommelaire MCh (1976) Pied plat valgus statique de l'enfant. Thesis, University of Toulouse

Lempereur L (1963) Fibrome juvénile aponévrotique. Ann Podol 2: 123-129

Léonard MH (1960) The sesamoids of the great toe. The pedal polemic. Clin Orthop 16: 295

Léonard MH (1942) Injuries of the lateral ligaments of the ankle (a clinical and experimental study). J Bone Joint Surg [Am] 31 A: 373-377

Lepoutre C (1941) Sésamoïde du gros orteil. J Science Med Lille 59

Leriche R (1923) Déséquilibres vaso-moteurs post-traumatiques primitifs des extrémités. Lyon Chir 20: 746

Leriche R (1924) Ostéochondrite disséquante. Lyon Chir 51

Leriche R (1941) Traitement de l'ostéoporose algique post-traumatique. Presse Med 49: 609

Leriche R, Fontaine R (1930) Des ostéoporoses douloureuses post-traumatiques. Presse Med 37: 617-621

Letterman (1933) Die physikalischen Grundlagen einer exakten Fußkorrektur. Med Welt 4

Levame JH (1971) Anatomie fonctionnelle du pied. Vie Med 21: 2567-2574

Levame JH, Durafourg MP (1975) Appréciation des pressions plantaires par le podogramme. Kinesitherap Scient 121/254: 5-10

Leveuf J (1941) Le traitement du pied convexe valgus congénital. Rev Orthop 27: 3-4

Leveuf J, Bertrand P (1946) Traitement du pied bot varus équin congénital chez le jeune enfant. Acad Chir 72: 29

Leveuf J, Bertrand P (1948a) La réduction sanglante du pied bot varus équin chez l'enfant. Rev Orthop 97: 113

Leveuf J, Bertrand P (1948b) Le rétablissement de l'équilibre musculaire dans le traitement du pied bot varus équin congénital. Rev Med Fr 7: 5

Lewin K, De Wit S, Ferrington RA (1971) Nail involvement in psoriasis: a clinico-pathological study in psoriasis. Farber, Cox (eds) Stanford University Press, Stanford

Lewin P (1930) Prescription blank for modification of shoes. J Bone Joint Surg 12 (3): 668-669

Lewin P (1959) The foot and ankle. Lea and Febiger, Philadelphia

Lewis MR (1952) Roentgen foot. Diagnosis. Von Schill

Lewis OJ (1964) The tibialis posterior tendon in the pronate foot. J Anat 98: 209-218

Libotte M, Klein P, Colpaert H, Alameh M, Blaimont P, Halleux P (1932) Contribution à l'étude biomécanique de la pince malléolaire. Rev Chir Orthop 68 (5): 299-305

Lièvre JA, Cohen M (1954) Étude clinique et étiologique sur les talalgies. Bull Med Soc Med Hop Paris 70 (3-4): 124

Lièvre JA, Leca (1956) Remarques sur la maladie de Morton. Rev Rhum Mal Osteoartic 23: 290-298

Lièvre JA, Merle d'Aubigne R, Busson, Morin (1949) Ostéolyse goutteuse. Rev Rhum Mal Osteoartic 11: 592

Lièvre JA, Auquier L, Lièvre A (1971) Macrodactylie. Rev Rhum 38: 424-426

Lilienfeld A (1931) Zur Behandlung des spastischen Plattfußes mit intramuskulärer Novocaineinspritzung und Vereisung des Nervus peroneus. Dtsch Z Chir 230 (3-5): 301-308

Lindahl O, Nilsson H (1974) Plantar protrusion of the metatarsal heads. Acta Orthop Scand 45: 473-480

Lindemann K (1936) Die juvenile Arthritis deformans des Großzehengrundgelenkes (Hallux rigidus). Z Orthop 64: 391-403

Linquette M, Fossati P, Fourlinnie JC (1974) Le pied et l'angiopathie diabétique. Intérêt de la radiographie osseuse. Rev Fr Endocrinol Clin 15 (4): 321-329

Lippmann HI, Perotto A, Farrar R (1976) Il piede neuropatico nel diabete. Bull NY Acad Med 52 (10): 1159-1178

Lipscomb PR, Kelly PS (1955) Injuries of the extensor tendons in the distal part of the leg and in the ankle. J Bone Joint Surg [Am] 37a: 1206

Lithner F (1976) Skeletal lesions of the feet in diabetics and their relationship to cutaneus erythema with or without necrosis on the feet. Acta Med Scand 200: 155-61

Lloyd-Roberts GC, Clark RC (1973) Ball and socket ankle joint in metatarsus adductus varus. J Bone Joint Surg [Br] 55b: 193-205

Lloyd-Roberts GC, Spence AJ (1958) Congenital vertical talus. J Bone Joint Surg [Br] 40b: 33-41

Lloyd-Roberts GC, Swann M, Catterall A (1974) Medial osteotomy for severe residual deformity in club foot. A preliminary report of a new method of treatment. J Bone Joint Surg [Br] 56b: 37-43

Loison M (1901) Note sur le traitement Chirurgical de l'hallux valgus d'après l'étude radiographique de la déformation. Bull Mem Soc Chir Paris 27: 528-531

Lombard P (1946) Pied bot varus équin. Rev Orthop 32 (5)

Lombard P (1950) Les bases du traitement dans le pied bot varus équin congénital. Rev Orthop 36: 1-2

Lombard P (1956) Le traitement fonctionnel du pied bot varus équin congénital. Rev Orthop 42: 227

López A (1970) Pie rumático. Tratamiento quirúrgico. Podologie 6: 364-373

López A, Zuzuarregui C (1962) Contribución al tratamiento del pie cavus. Ann Podol 1: 25

López A, Zuzuarregui C (1963) Tratamiento del pie plano valgo (estudio tomografico y técnica operatoria). Ann Podol 2: 53

Lord G (1959) Les ruptures sous-cutanées dú tendon d'Achille. Presse Med 67: 1625

Lord G, Marotte JH (1973) Prothèse totale de cheville. A propos de 12 observations. Rev Chir Orthop 59: 139-151

Lorenz A (1883) Die Lehre vom erworbenen Plattfuß. Enke, Stuttgart

Lorenz A (1939) Directives d'orthopédie pratique. Deuticke, Wien

Louria DB (1965) Pathogenesis of candidiasis. Antimicrob Agents Chemother: 417-426

Louyot P, Gaucher A (1967) Lésions destructrices de l'avant-pied dans la spondylarthrite ankylosante. Ann Med Nancy 6: 154-171

Lowett (1903) The physiological flat foot. JAMA 1051

Loyau G (1958) La polyarthrite psoriasique. Thesis, University of Paris

Ludloff PW (1956) A quarter of a century of experience with the correction of metatarsus varus primus in hallux valgus. Bull Hosp Joint Diss 17: 404-421

Lund SH (1965) Arthrorise pour pied plat. Acta Orthop Scand 33: 234

Lundberg BJ, Sulja T (1972) Skeletal parameters in the hallux valgus foot. Acta Orthop Scand 43 (6): 576-582

Lusskin AL (1950) Méthode non rigide de traitement du pied bot traité dès le début. J Int Coll Surg 14 (4)

McBride ED (1928) Conservative operation for bunions. J Bone Joint Surg 10: 735

McBride ED (1963) The surgical treatment of hallux valgus bunions. Am J Orthop 5: 44

McBride ED (1965) La operacion de McBride par el hallux valgus. In: Sanchis, Olmos (eds) Libro homenaje. Serv Traum Rehab Hosp Prov, Madrid, p 205

McBride ED (1967) The McBride bunion hallux valgus operation. J Bone Joint Surg [Am] 49: 1675

McCain LR, Nuzzo JJ (1969) The "sesamoidal ligament" and its employ in the suturing of the Keller bunionectomy procedure. J Am Podiatry Assoc 59 (12): 479-80

MacConaill MA (1977) Pronation and supination of the foot. Physiotherapy 29 (3): 125-130

MacCormick DW, Blount WP (1949) Metatarsus adductovarus. "Skewfoot". JAMA 141: 449

McDaniel WJ, Wilson FC (1977) Trimalleolar fractures of the ankle. An end result study. Clin Orthop 122: 37-45

McElvenny RT (1943) The etiology and surgical treatment of intractable pain about the fourth metatarsophalangeal joint. J Bone Joint Surg 25: 657-679

MacGlamry ED, Kitting RW, Butlin WE (1973) Keller bunionectomy and hallux valgus correction. Further modifications. J Am Podiatry Assoc 63 (6): 237-46

MacGrea JD, Clark WD, Fann T, Venson J (1977) Effects of radiographic technic of the metatarso-phalangeal joints. J Am Podiatry Assoc 67 (12): 837-840

MacGregor IA (1972) Fundamental techniques of plastic surgery and their surgical applications, 5th edn. Williams and Wilkins, Baltimore

Mchacek J (1940) Traitement opératoire dans une vieille maladie de Köhler. Zentralbl Chir (39): 1825-1828

McKeever DC (1952) Arthrodesis of the first metatarsophalangeal joint for hallux valgus, hallux rigidus and metatarsus primus varus. J Bone Joint Surg [Am] 34: 129-134

McKeever DC (1952) Discussion on "Experimental studies of transplantation of whole joint" (Herndon) J Bone Joint Surg 34-A: 578

MacLennan R (1966) L'hallux valgus de la population néolithique de la Nouvelle-Guinée. Lancet, June

Magnusson B (1946) Ostéotomie de rotation employé dans le pied bot varus équin congénital. J Bone Join Surg 2

Maincent P (1939) La maladie de Morton. Vigot, Paris

Maiotti A (1957) Studio radiografico della volta trasversale del piede sotto carico Ortop Od Riabil 2: 533–54(

Maiotti A (1979) La terapia chirurgica dell'alluce valgo associato a metatarsalgia. Minerva Med 20: 1–18

Malerba F, Zagra F (1968) I nostri risultati della cura chirurgica dell'alluce valgo. Podologie 6: 209

Manes E, Costa C, Innao V (1973) La cura del piede torto congenito nel primo anno di vita. Chir Organi Mov 62: 303–314

Manigue (1942) La réintégration non sanglante de l'astragale. Rev Orthop 28: 37–50

Manigue (1945) Examen radiologique des pieds bots. Presse Med: 633

Manigue (1946) Subluxation dans les pieds bots. Presse Med: 411

Manigue (1947) Le traitement du pied bot varus équin congénital. Acta Orthop Belg 13 (4)

Manigue (1951 a) Sur l'utilité du contrôle radiographique du pied bot: tractions calcanéennes. Acta Orthop Belg 17 fasc (6)

Manigue (1951 b) Traction transcalcanéenne dans le pied bot. Rev Chir Orthop Paris 37: 5–6

Mann R, Inman VT (1964) Phasic activity of intrinsic muscles of the foot. J Bone Joint Surg [Am] 46: 469–480

Mann RA, DuVries HL (1973) Intractable plantar keratosis. Orthop Clin North Am 4 (1): 67

Manzoni A (1966) Terapía chirúrgica del pie reumático. Podologie 5: 209

Marchi E (1968) A propos de la technique de l'arthrodèse tibiotarsienne. Podologie 6: 9

Marcondes De Souza (1957) Tratamiento cirurgico di pe varo equino congenito. Sao Paulo

Mareev YUS, Chubakov YUM (1976) L'osteo-artropatia diabetica. Khirurgiya 52 (2): 95–101

Maresca A (1959) Considerazioni sulla lussazione congenita astragalo scafoidea nel quadro del cosidetto piede a dondalo. Ortop Odierna Riab, 4: 187

Marin GA (1968) Arthrodesis of the metatarso-phalangeal joint of the big toe for hallux valgus and hallux rigidus. A new method. Int Surg 50 (2): 175–180

Marjoni D'Intignano MIM (1922) Appareil pour le maintien des pieds bots au cours du traitement par massages. Rev Orthop 9: 148

Marjoni D'Intignano MIM (1947) Réduction sanglante de l'astragale dans le traitement du pied bot varus équin congénital. Rev Orthop 33 (1–2): 130

Marmor L (1964) Surgical treatment of chronic arthritis. Mod Treat 1: 1313

Marneffe R de, Lorthioir J (1966) Le traitement chirurgical de l'hallux valgus. Acta Orthop Belg 32 (5): 673–4

Maroteaux P (1969) Classification des dysplasies osseuses. Ann Radiol 12: 993

Maroteaux P, Bouvet JP, Briard ML (1972) La maladie des synostoses multiples. Nouv Presse Med 1 (45): 3041–3047

Marquardt W (1963) Die Einflüsse der orthopädischen Schuhtechnik auf die Chirurgie des Fußes. Podologie 2: 145

Martens M, Tanghe W, Muller JC, Willems D (1972) Pigmented villonodular synovitis of joints, tendons and bursae. Acta Orthop Belg 38: 233

Martin B (1981) Les tumeurs de Koenen. Thesis, University of Paris

Martini M (1977) Tuberculose osseuse et ostéo-articulaire du membre supérieur, du coude-pied et du pied. Encycl Med Chir Paris App Locomoteur 14185 E 10

Martini M, Got G, Chlap Z (1976) Quatre nouveaux cas d'ostéome ostéoïde du col de l'astragale. Rev Chir Orthop 61: 651–657

Martorell Martorell J (1963) Factores importantes para el tratamiento de las metatarsalgias; su tratamiento por un nuevo concepto de plantillas. Podologie 2: 175–188

Martorell Martorell J (1965) Conceptos básicos para la corrección del pie plano valgo esencial de la infancia. Progr Pediatr Puericultura (3)

Martorell Martorell J (1968) Nouvelle semelle pour métatarsalgie. Podologie 6: 419

Martorell Martorell J (1971 a) Esquema de la etio-patogenia de las metatarsalgias. Podologie 6: 154

Martorell Martorell J (1971 b) Algunos aspectos de la metatarsalgia. Podologie 6: 159

Martorell Martorell J (1971 c) Luxación patológica poco común. Podologie 6: 242

Martorell Martorell J (1971 d) El calzado infantil. Podologie 6: 320

Martorell Martorell J (1973 a) Analyse de la marche grâce à l'aspect de la chaussure et de la semelle orthopédique. Actual Med Chir Pied 8 (2)

Martorell Martorell J (1973 b) Technique personnelle en quartier d'orange glissé. Actual Med Chir Pied 8 (2)

Martorell Martorell J (1973 c) Modification de la technique de Regnauld pour le traitement de l'hallux valgus. Actual Med Chir Pied, 8 (2)

Martorell Martorell J (1973 d) Concepts et études sur la métatarsalgie et son traitement. Actual Med Chir Pied 8 (2)

Martorell Martorell J (1973 e) Nuestros conceptos sobre la metatarsalgia. Rev Inform Med Terap (5–6): 131–150

Martorell Martorell J (1976 a) Corrección del pie plano valgo laxo (no congénito) con tiras de esparadrapo. Ann Soc Esp Med Cir Pie (Podología)

Martorell Martorell J (1976 b) Corrección del pie plano valgo laxo (no congénito) con grapas por via interna. Ann Soc Esp Med Cir Pie (Podología)

Martorell Martorell J (1978 a) Cálculo del calzado y errores. Actual Méd Chir Pied 10: 135

Martorell Martorell J (1978 b) Respuestas al tema "Plantillas para pie plano". Actual Med Chir Pied 10: 147

Martorell Martorell J (1978 c) Introduction au symposium de la marche. Actual Med Chir Pied 10: 3

Martorell Martorell J (1978 d) Particularités des divers types d'alignement frontal en charge. Ann Med Chir Pied 11: 41

Martorell Martorell J (1978e) Études sur le comportement de l'avant-pied dans la marche. Ann Med Chir Pied 11: 57

Martorell Martorell J (1979) Traitement conservateur du pied plat valgus essentiel de l'enfance. Chir Piede 3 (4): 309-310

Martorell Martorell J (1981) Hallux disorder and metatarsal alignment. Clin Orthop 157: 14

Martorell Martorell J (1982a) Métatarsalgie type S1i; sa cure chirurgicale radicale. Actual Med Chir Pied 13

Martorell Martorell J (1982b) Pied creux et alignement frontal en charge. Actual Med Chir Pied 13

Martorell Martorell J (1982c) Hallux valgus et alignement frontal en charge. Actual Med Chir Pied 13

Marziani R (1933) Lussazione congenita dell'astragalo o piede piatto reflesso congenito. Arch Orthop 49 (1): 175-194

Maschas A (1954) Thèse: contribution à l'etude des indications therapeutiques dans le pied bot varus équin congenital du cours de la 1e enfance. Germain, Paris

Maschas A, Bergeron R (1961) Le rétablissement de la statique de l'avant-pied par la résection de têtes métatarsiennes. Rev Chir Orthop 47: 163-183

Massart R (1948) Affections médicales et chirurgicales du pied. Doin, Paris

Masse P (1956) Pieds plats. Conc Med 78 (11): 1207-1209

Masse P, Taussig G, Bazin G (1974) Ostéotomie cunéiforme externe du calcanéum dans le traitement du pied bot varus équin. Rev Chir Orthop 60 (2): 135-149

Masse P, Taussig G, Elberg JF (1975) Techniques chirurgicales en orthopédie pédiatrique. Flammarion, Paris

Masse P, Benichou J, Dimeglio A, Morel JM, Onimus M, Padovani JP, Seringe R (1976) Pied bot varus équin. Rev Chir Orthop [Suppl 2]: 62

Mastromarino (1936) Étude clinique et statique sur le pied bot congénital. Arch di ortop 50, 4: 897-916

Matus S (1937) Recherche d'anthropologie anatomique sur l'astragale. Thèse, Univ. de Bordeaux

Mau C (1940) Eine Operation des kontrakten Spreizfußes. Zbl Chir 67: 667-670

May H (1942) The regeneration of joint transplants and intracapsular fragments. Ann Surg 116: 207-310

Mayo CH (1908) The surgical treatment of bunions. Ann Surg 48: 300-302

Mazzinari S, Filippi E (1974) Podostati-Rxgrafia e pressopodostati. Rxgrafia. Estratto da Minerva Ortop. Minerva

Meary MR (1951) L'opération de Lambrinudi dans le traitement du pied équin paralytique. Rev Orthop 37 (1): 68-83

Meary MR (1956) Sur une forme particulière de défaut d'appui plantaire antéro-interne du pied. Rev Orthop 42: 235

Meary MR (1967) Symposium sur le pied creux essentiel. Rev Chir Orthop 53: 390-466

Meary R (1969) Symposium sur le pied plat. Ann Orthop de l'Ouest 1: 55-71

Meary R, Roger A (1969) Les synostoses congénitales du tarse à propos de 41 cas. Rev Chir Orthop Rep App Mot 55 (8)

Meary MR, Mattei CR, Tomeno B (1976) Tarsectomie antérieure pour pieds creux. Rev Chir Orthop 62: 231-243

Meary MR, Filipe G, Aubriot JH, Tomeno B (1977) Étude fonctionnelle de la double arthrodèse du pied. Rev Chir Orthop 63 (4): 345-359

Megreth H (1966) Verticalisation d l'astragale dans le pied plat valgus du jeune enfant. Thesis, University of Lyon

Melvin H, Jahss MD (1982) Disorders of the foot. Saunders, Philadelphia

Mercado OA (1973) The McKeever operation. Hosp Podiatry Rev 1

Mercado OA (1974) Peg and hole technique for metatarsal shortening. J Podiatr Med 60 (1-4)

Mercado OA (1981) Atlas of foot surgery. Carolando Chicago

Merklen FG (1954) La maladie de Ledderhose (aponévrosite plantaire). Thesis, University of Paris

Merle d'Aubigné R, Lance P (1949) Affections traumatiques des membres. In: Nouveau précis de pathologie chirurgical, vol 1. Masson, Paris

Merle d'Aubigné R, Ramadier JO (1959) Traumatismes anciens: rachis, membre inférieur. Masson, Paris

Merle d'Aubigné R et al (1949) Chirurgie reparatrice. Expansion Scientifique Française, Paris

Merle d'Aubigné R et al (1951) Affections traumatiques. Flammarion, Paris

Merle d'Aubigné R, Benassy J, Ramadier JO (1956) Chirurgie orthopédique des paralysies. Masson, Paris

Meyer JM (1976) Le traitement de l'hallux valgus. Med Hyg 34: 938-940

Meyer JM, Kritsikis N (1978) Traitement chirurgical de l'hallux valgus par l'opération de Brandes Keller. A propos de 92 malades opérés. Med Hyg 36/12 90: 2133-2138

Meyer JM, Taillard (1975) L'arthrographie de l'articulation sous-astragalienne dans les syndromes douloureux post-traumatiques du tarse postérieur. Rev Chir Orthop 60 (4): 321

Meyer JM, Tomeno B (1976) Le défaut d'appui plantaire interne. Rev Chir Orthop 62: 463-476

Meynadier J, Guilhou JJ (1977) L'étude des ongles au cours du rhumatisme inflammatoire. In: Simon L, Claustre J (eds) Le pied inflammatoire. Maloine, Paris, p 99

Michel L (1949) Le pied bot varus équin et son traitement actuel. Rev Orthop 35 (3-4)

Michon J, Delagoutte JP, Jandeaux M (1974) L'utilisation d'une prothèse de Swanson dans le traitement de l'hallux valgus. Ann Chir Plast 19 (1): 23-29

Michon P, Larcan A, Huriez C, Vicari F, Vert P (1961) Le neuropatie diabetiche. Statistiche su 498 casi di diabete. Bull Mem Soc Med Hop Paris 77 (12-13): 433-441

Miller GR (1977) Traitement chirurgical du pied plat hypermobile chez le jeune enfant. Clin Orthop 122: 95-101

Miller LO (1927) A plastic flat foot operation. J Bone Joint Surg 9 (1): 84-91

Miller Walter (1926) Maladie der Sesambeine 1er Metatarsale - ein typisches Krankheitsbild. Brunsw Beitr 134 (2)

Minaker K, Little H (1973) Painful feet in Rheumatoid arthritis. Can Med Assoc J 108: 724-730

Mirouze J (1968) Le pied diabétique (introduction au symposium sur le pied diabétique, congrès de Montréal, 1967). Ann Podol 6: 308

Moine C (1963) Subluxations récidivantes du cou-de-pied. Thesis, University of Lyon

Mole L (1972) La reconstruction arthrodèse dans le traitement des fractures du calcanéum. Cah Med Lyon 48/36: 4261-4263

Mollard S (1978) Conduite à tenir devant un durillon plantaire. Bord Med 11/14: 1263-1264

Mommsen F (1926) Die unblutige Korrektur schwerer Plattfüße. Z Orthop 47: 325-352

Monet JL, Apoil A, Vinceneux JF (1977) Fractures du calcanéum, résultats du traitement par la méthode fonctionnelle de 1962 à 1973. Kinesitherap Scient 153/286: 21-28

Montagne J (1962a) Les incidences de base dans la radiographie du pied. Ann Podol 1: 180-185

Montagne J (1962b) Étude radiologique des déformations de la coupole plantaire. Ann Podol 1: 79-83

Montagne J, Chevrot A, Galmiche JM (1980) Atlas de radiologie du pied. Masson, Paris

Montagne J, Chevrot A, Galmiche JM (1981) Atlas of foot radiology. Masson, New York

Montero Gómez M (1967) Técnicas para el hallux varus congénito. Rev Ortop Traumatol Iber 2 (4): 509

Montgomery RM (1969) Les dermatoses des mains et des pieds. Original article, Cutis Symposium on General Practice Dermatology, San Francisco, California 5 (4): 452-456

Mooney V, Wagner FW (1977) Atteintes neurocirculatoires du pied. Clin Orthop 112: 53-61

Moreau (1936) Contribution à l'étude du pied valgus congénital convexe. Thèse, Univ de Paris

Moreau G (1974) Morphologie du pied. Kinesitherap Scient 119/252: 11-15

Moreau M (1971) Les mycoses du pied. Rev Podologie 2: 49-53

Moreau M, Bertoni GC, Moreau J (1949) Mensurations angulaires dans l'étude radiologique du valgisme et du varisme du pied. Prensa Medico-Argentina 36 (8)

Mori F, Molfetta L (1982) Il piede reflesso congenito astragalo-verticale. Tratamento chirurgico. Chir Pied 6 (4): 397-405

Morris MA (1977) Morton's metatarsalgia. Clin Orthop 127: 203-207

Morton DJ (1924a) Evolution of the longitudinal arch of the human foot. J Bone Joint Surg 6: 56-90

Morton DJ (1924b) Mechanism of normal foot and flat foot. J Bone Joint Surg 6: 368-406

Morton DJ (1935) The human foot. Columbia University, New York

Morton DJ (1937) Physiological considerations in the treatment of foot deformities. J Bone Joint Surg 19: 1052-1056

Morton DJ, Fuller DD (1952) Human locomotion and body form. Williams and Wilkins, Baltimore

Morton TG (1886) On cases of painful affection of the foot. Med Times, Philadelphia

Morton TG (1876) A peculiar and painful affection of the fourth metatarso-phalangeal articulation. Am J Med Sci 71: 37

Morton TG (1893) Metatarsalgia (Morton's painful affection of the foot) with an account of six cases cured by operation. Ann Surg 17: 680

Mossman HW (1950) Le pied bot: étude embryologique des anomalies musculaires associées. J Bone Joint Surg [Am] 23 (4)

Mostini G (1962) Syndromes algodystrophiques et pied creux. Podologie 1: 33-35

Mostini G (1975-1977) Readaptation du pied rhumatoïde. In: Simon L, Claustre J (eds) Le pied inflammatoire. Maloine, Paris, pp 211-213

Mostini G (1979) Étude clinique, traitement et indications chirurgicales du pied goutteux. Coll Intern Med Chir Pied, 3e cours Nantes. Réunies, Rennes, pp 162-176

Motta A (1966) Studio artografio dell'artico lazione tibiotarsico in condizioni normali et patologiche. Ann Coll Podol 5: 60

Mouchet A (1922) Les difformités du gros orteil. Rapp Soc Fran Orthop

Mouchet A (1938) L'épine du 1er métatarsien. J radio et d'électroradiol, 22 (6) 275-278

Mouchet A, Mouthier G (1926) Osselets surnuméraires du tarse (tarsalia). Presse Med 23: 369

Moulonguet P, Cazala JF (1959) Chondromes évolutifs sur exostoses ostéogéniques. Presse Med 67 (26): 1057

Mouly R, Beres J (1971) Radiodermites du pied. Podologie 2 (8): 110

Mounier-Kuhn A (1971) Résultats des interventions pour ruptures du tendon d'Achille. Rev Chir Orthop 57 [Suppl I]: 229-236

Mounier-Kuhn A, Marsan C (1968) Le syndrome des tendons péroniers. Ann Chir V 22 (9-10): 641-650

Moyniham FJ (1967) Arthrodesis of the metatarso-phalangeal joint of the great toe. J Bone Joint Surg [Br] 49b: 544

Mukerjee SK, Pringle RM, Baxted AD (1974) Fracture of the lateral process of the talus. J Bone Joint Surg [Br] 56 (2): 263

Mulder J (1951) The causative mechanism in Morton's metatarsalgia. J Bone Joint Surg [Br] 33: 94

Muller W (1927) Eine eigenartig doppelseitige Veränderung des Os naviculare pedis beim Erwachsenen. Dtsch Z Chir 201: 84

Mullin JFP, Sallis JG (1958) Recurrent sprain of the ankle joint with diastasis. J Bone Joint Surg 40 B: 270-273

Mumenthaler M, Probst C, Mumenthaler B, Weber B, Schnyder J (1964) Das Tarsaltunnelsyndrom. Schweiz Med Wochenschr 94 (11): 373-382

Mumenthaler M, Mosimann W (1969) Neurologische Komplikationen nach Läsionen des Fußes und des Sprunggelenkes. Dtsch Med Wochenschr 94: 995

Mutter TD (1839) A lecture on coxarthrus, or club foot. Hooker and Claxton, Philadelphia
Mygind (1953) Some views on the surgical treatment of hallux valgus. Acta Orthop Scand 23: 152-158
Mynte H (1974) Complicanze osteo-articolari nel piede in corso di diabete. Pol Przegl Radiol Med Nukl 38 (4): 413-420
Napieralski K (1968) Fracture de la base du 5e métatarsien. Zentralbl Chir 93 (13): 466-471
Natiello OB (1969) Classificatión de las metatarsalgias biomecánicas. Rev Ortop Traumatol Lationam 14: 2
Natiello OB (1970) Tratamiento quirúrgico del pie plano. La "tenoplastia de los tibiales". Podologie 6: 82
Natiello OB (1971) Enfermedad de Renander. Rev Orthop Traum Lat Am 15: 73-78
Natiello OB, Bamballi ES, Natiello NH (1973) Nuestra experiencia en el tratamiento quirúrgico del hallux valgus con el procedimiento de J. Lelièvre. Podologie 8 (2): 167
Navarre M (1966) A propos du syndrome du sinus du tarse. Acta Orthop Belg 32 (5): 743-754
Navarro Quilis A (1969) La artrodesis frente a la operación de Keller en el tratamiento hallux valgus y hallux rigidus. Rev Cir Osteo 4 (22): 301
Nayrac P et al (1966) Acropathie ulcéro-mutilante atypique (mal perforant dysraphique) Press Méd 11 (6): 708-711
Nelaton C (1890) Arch Gen Med 9: 386
Nelaton A (1851) Eléments de pathologie chirurgicale. Germer Baillière, Paris
Nelson D (1960) Forced inversion of the ankle. J Bone Joint Surg 42-B: 793
Neuman M (1963) Les antibiotiques antifongiques. EMC Thér Antiinfect Antivirale 006 A 10: 1-4
Neuman M (1966) Les médications antifongiques par voie générale. Gaz Med Fr 88 (43): 6315-6325
Newton C, Anast G (1961) Vertical talus (congenital talonavicular dislocation). Clinical orthopaedics 21. Lippincott, Philadelphia, p 198
Ney GC (1923) An operation for ingrowing toenails. J Am Podiatry Assoc 80: 374
Niederecker K (1959) Der Plattfuß. Enke, Stuttgart
Niethard FU (1974) Die Stabilität des Sprunggelenkes nach Ruptur des lateralen Bandapparates. Arch Orthop Unfall Chir 80: 53
Nilsonne (1930) Hallux rigidus and its treatment. Acta Orthop Scand 193
Nissen KI (1948) Plantar digital neuritis, Morton's metatarsalgia. J Bone Joint Surg [Br] 30: 84-94
Nisonne H (1932) Making a new ligament in ankle sprain. J Bone Joint Surg 14: 380-381
Noack H, Nègre J (1968) Luxations médio-tarsiennes et tarso-métatarsiennes. Actual Chir Orthop 6: 175-192
Noury JY (1972) Pathologie des ongles. Gaz Med Fr 79 (4): 431-434
Noury JY (1977) Pathologie dermatologique du pied. Perf Prat 10/245: 23-36
Nove-Josserand Précis d'orthopédie. Doin, Paris
Nowotny H (1932) Über den kompensatorischen Pes valgus und Pes valgoplanus. Z Orthop 58: 233-242
O'Donoghue DH (1940) Traitement des ongles incarnés de l'orteil. Am J Surg 50: 519
O'Donoghue DH (1957) Impingement exostosis of the talus and tibia. J Bone Joint Surg [Am] 39: 835
Ogston A (1902) A new principle of curing club-foot in severe cases in children of few years old. Br Med J 1 (1): 524
Ombredanne L (1925) Précis clinique et opératoire de chirurgie infantile. Masson, Paris
Ombredanne L, Fevre M (1949) Précis clinique et operatoire de chirurgie infantile, 5th edn. Masson, Paris
Ombredanne L, Mathieu P (1937) Traité de chirurgie orthopédique. Masson, Paris
O'Rahilly R, Gardner E, Gray DJ (1960) The skeletal development of the foot. Clin Orthop 16: 7
Ory M (1962) Les empreintes du pied en relief. Podologie 1: 178-179
Osmond Clarke H (1956) Congenital vertical talus. J Bone Joint Surg, 38-B: 334
Ottolenghi C, Petracchi J, Schajowicz P (1948) Metatarsalgia de Morton. Bol Soc Arg Cir Ortop 13 (7): 262
Outland T, Sherk H (1960) Congenital vertical talus. Clinical orthopaedics 16. Lippincott, Philadelphia, p 214
Owens RE (1962) Surgical correction for onychauxis. J Am Podiatry Assoc 52: 591
Padovani JP (1937) Physiologie du pied, pied plat valgus douloureux. Traite Chir Orthop 5
Padovani JP (1973) Conduite à tenir devant une boiterie de l'enfant. Gaz Med Fr 80 (23)
Padovani JP (1978) Traitement du pied bot varus équin congénital négligé. Chir Piede 2 (1-2): 39
Pagella P (1976) Surgical treatment of hallux valgus (proceedings). Ann Osp Maria Vittoria Torino 19 (7-12): 174-82
Paitre, Boppe (1935) Fractures du calcanéum. J Chir 46 (4): 491
Palazzi SA (1962) Tratamiento quirúrgico de los dedos en martillo y del pie redondo doloroso. Rev Nac Podol 6: 11
Palmer I (1948) Mécanisme et traitement des fractures du calcanéum. Réduction ouverte et greffes d'os spongieux. J Bone Joint Surg [Am] 30: 2
Papadoulos, Sarantis A (1934) La dermosyndesmolyse interne comme intervention de choix contre le pied bot varus équin congénital. Rev Orthop 247
Paparella-Treccia R (1946a) Le formazioni muscolari, legamentose ed aponeurotiche nel quadro del piede piatto statico. Ortop Traumatol App Mot 14: 59-82
Paparella-Treccia R (1946b) Sulla lussazione dorso-laterale congenita del la articolazione astragalo-scafoidea. Ortop Traumatol App Mot 14: 83-89
Paparella-Treccia R (1949) Il Piede piatto. Prog Ter 7/8: 3-7
Paparella-Treccia R (1950) Sviluppo del piede e deformita congenite. Aggior Pediatr 2: 1-8
Paparella-Treccia R (1977) Il piede dell'uomo. Verduci, Roma
Paparella-Treccia R, Rampoldi A (1947) Piede valgo embrionale da assenza di migrazione calcaneare. Ortop Traumatol App Mot 15: 5-12

Pardo-Castello J, Pardo OA (1950) Diseases of the nails. Thomas, Springfield
Parisel (1947) Maladie de Morton. Acta Orthop Belg 15
Parkes JC (1977) Lésions de l'arrière-pied. Clin Orthop 122: 38-36
Parra G (1960) Stress fractures of the sesamoids of the foot. Clin Orthop 18
Pasquali-Lasagni M (1958) Contributo al trattamento del piede valgo reflesso congenito. Acta Ortop Italia 4: 171
Passeri A (1965) Le applicazioni del logetron allo studio della iconografia riguardante la patologia del piede. Podologie 4: 223-236
Patterson RL, Parrish FF, Hathaway EN (1950) Opérations stabilisatrices au niveau du pied. J Bone Joint Surg [Am] 32: 1-26
Patterson WR, Fitz DA, Smith WS (1968) The pathological anatomy of congenital convex pes valgus. Post mortem study of a newborn infant with bilateral involvement. J Bone Joint Surg [Am] 50 (3): 458-466
Paulin M, Tomeno B (1976) Traitement de l'hallux valgus. Limites et indications de l'exostosectomie. Rev Chir Orthop 62 (8): 775-80
Pavlik A (1939) Die operative Behandlung der statischen Plattfüße schweren Grades. Z Orthop 69: 439-445
Peabody CW (1931) The surgical cure of hallux valgus. J Bone Joint Surg 13: 273
Pérez Teuffer A, Ilizaliturii VM, Martínez del Campo F (1972) Ruptures traumatiques du tendon d'Achille. Rev Chir Orthop 58 [Suppl I]: 219-221
Perrin M (1973) Troubles d'appui de l'avant-pied. Traitement chirurgical. Thèse de doctorat en médecine, Université de Dijon
Perrot A (1964) L'hallux valgus (pathogénie et traitement). Med Hyg 22 (645): 539
Perugia L, Del Torto U (1957) Piede normale e piatto in rapporto all'appogio plantare nelle sollecitazioni statiche del piede. Ginn Med 5: 146-148
Perugia L, Ricciardi-Pollini T, Ippolito E (1976) Anatomia patologica del piede torto congenito. Relaz LXI Congrès SIOT 41-55
Perugia L, Ricciardi-Pollini T, Ippolito E (1976) Lo studio radiografico del piede torto congenito. Relaz LXI Congrès SIOT 56-61
Pesle GD, Labeguerie M (1953) Les mycoses, maladies d'avenir. J Fr Med Chir Thor 7: 537
Petit P (1947) Nouveau précis de pathologie chirurgicale
Petit P (1952) Rapport congrès français d'orthopédie, octobre
Petri C (1940) Zur Behandlung von Vorfußdeformitäten. Z Orthop 70: 343-349
Pfister U (1973) Luxation de la ligne articulaire de Lisfranc (tarso métatarsienne). Monatsschr Unfallheilkd 76 (9): 423-425
Phemister DB (1933) Operative arrestment of longitudinal growth of bones in the treatment of deformities. J Bone Joint Surg [Am] 15: 1
Phillips RS (1971) Congenital split foot (lobster claw), and triphalangeal thumbs. J Bone Joint Surg [Br] 53: 5
Picard JJ, Auriach A, Florensa G (1967) Traitement du pied valgus poliomyélitique de l'enfant. Ann Med Phys 10 (1): 77-92
Pick H (1927) Die Technik des Redressements im Schultzeschen Osteoclasten nebst kritischen und epikritischen Betrachtungen. Arch Orth Unfall Chir 26 (2): 323-373
Pierre M (1978) L'ongle. Expansion Scientifique Française, Paris
Pietrogrande V (1965) Technique radiologique personnelle. Note préliminaire. Podologie 4: 208
Piggott H (1960) The natural history of hallux valgus in adolescence and early adult life. J Bone Joint Surg [Br] 42: 749
Pincus A (1950) Intractable Morton's toe. J Natl AM Chir Podol 40: 19
Pisani G (1973a) Nuova metodica di indagine strumentale del piede la podostatigrafia. Minerva Ortop 24
Pisani G (1973b) La semeiottica strumentale del piede in sede di valutazione medico-legale. Minerva Ortop 24
Pisani G (1973c) La podostatigrafia nello studio di routine dell'atteggiamento anatomico e funzionale del piede. Med Sport 26 (9): 248-252
Pisani G (1974a) Podostati-rxgrafia e pressopodostatirxgrafia. Estr Atti Sertot 16: 2
Pisani G (1974b) Esiste un arco metatarsale? Minerva Ortop 25
Pisani G (1975a) La biomeccanica del piede in fuzione del carico metatarseo IV. Minerva Ortop 26 (3): 75-100
Pisani G (1975b) Biodinamica dell'avampiede. Minerva Ortop 26 (12): 590-598
Pisani G (1976a) Piede calcaneale e piede astragalico. Minerva Ortop 27 (3): 110-113
Pisani G (1976b) La sindrome pronatoria dell'avampiede. Minerva Ortop 27 (7-8): 357-364
Pisani G (1977a) Considerationi sull'artrosi della sottoastragalica. Chir Piede 1 (34): 433-440
Pisani G (1977b) Concetti di biomeccanica clinica del piede. Minerva Ortop 28 (1-2): 57-68
Pisani G (1977c) Moderni orientamenti in chirurgia del piede. Chir Piede 1 (3-4): 441-443
Pisani G (1977d) Il Complesso legamentoso periastragalico. Chir Piede 1 (5): 559-561
Pisani G (1978a) Considerationi sul trattamento delle fratture talamiche del calcagno. Chir Piede 2 (1-2): 9-16
Pisani G (1978b) La chirurgia del piede calcaneo-valgo. Atti Soc Emiliana Romagnola Triveneta Ortop Traumatol 20: 2
Pisani G (1978c) Biodinamica dell'avampiede. Actual Med Chir Pied 11: 79-93
Pisani G (1978d) Biomeccanica dell'alluce valgo. Chir Pied 2 (3): 77-85
Pisani G (1979a) L'avampiede, struttura a carico variabile. Chir Piede 3 (2): 80-86
Pisani G (1979b) La chirurgie du pied calcanéo-valgus évolutif de l'enfant. Chir Piede 3 (3): 169-178
Pisani G (1979c) La chirurgie du pied calcanéo-valgus. Chir Piede 3 (4): 335-337

Pisani G (1979d) Pathologie traumatique de la sous-astragalienne et sport. Le pied du sportif. Masson, Paris
Pisani G (1979e) Considerationi sul trattamento delle fratture talamiche del calcagno. Podologie 11
Pisani G (1979f) Indications chirurgicales du valgus de l'enfant. Ann CIP, 3e cours international de Nantes. Réunies, Rennes, pp 41-50
Pisani G (1980) Pathologie traumatique de la sous-astragalienne et sports. Chir Piede 4 (1): 35-40
Pitto E, Giusti E, Santini A (1978) La lussazione traumatica dell'articolazione tarso-metatarsica di Lisfranc (Revisione critica dei casi venuti alla nostra osservazione). Chir Piede 2 (3)
Plas F, Viel E (1975) La marche humaine. Masson, Paris
Poli A (1948) Contributo alla cura chirurgica del piede piatto reflesso. Atti SIOT 33: 44
Poli A (1953) Cura chirurgica precoce del piede piatto reflesso congenito (risultate e metodo personale) Arch Orthop 46: 860
Pollock LJJ, Davis I (1932) Peripheral nerve injuries. Am J Surg 18: 361-401
Ponsetti IV, Becker JR (1966) Congenital metatarsus adductus: results and treatment. J Bone Joint Surg [Am] 48: 702-711
Potter TA (1956) The natural course of rheumatoid spondylitis. Boston Med Q 7: 21
Pous JG, Dimeglio A (1976) La chirurgie neo-natale du pied bot varus équin: pourquois pas? Expansion Scientifique Française
Pouyanne L, Honton JL, Gourdon A, Planes A (1965) Fractures-luxations, dislocations de l'articulation de Lisfranc. Bord Chir 3: 105
Pouzet E (1954) Plastie ligamentaire externe de la tibiotarsienne. Lyon Chir 49: 618-619
Pouzet F (1926) Résultats éloignés de la tuberculose du tarse chez l'enfant. Lyon
Powers J (1934) Les os sésamoides du gros orteil. Lésions traumatiques et anomalies de développement. Am J Surg 23 (2): 315-321
Prignacchi Y, Zanasi R (1957) La technica di Hueter Mayo nella cura chirurgica dell'alluce valgo. Chir Org Mov 64: 234-242
Puissant A (1965) Les mycoses unguéales. Progr Med 14: 567-571
Queipo de Llano E, Queipo de Llano A, Martin J, Cuadros (1975) Anatomía patológica y clasificatión de las fracturas talamicas del calcáneo. Rev Esp Cir Osteoartic 10: 187
Quenu E (1918) Plaies du pied et du cou-de-pied par projectile de guerre. Paris, Alcan
Quenu L, Kuss G (1909) Étude sur les luxations du métatarse (luxations métatarso-tarsiennes) du diastasis entre le 1er et le 2e métatarsien. Rev Chir 1-72: 281-336, 720-791, 1093-1134
Rabischong et al (1937) L'électropodographie. Son intérêt en orthopédie. Montpellier Chir 3: 303
Racker CH (1951) La résection simple de l'exostose et de la première phalange dans le traitement de l'hallux valgus et de l'hallux rigidus. Résultats éloignés. Acta Orthop Belg 17: 181-201
Raiga A (1923) Le canal calcanéen. Presse Med 808-810
Rainatu JJ, Cedard C, D'Hour JP (1966) Les luxations tarso-métatarsiennes. Rev Chir Orthop 52: 449-462
Rall (1954) Zur operativen Behandlung des Plattfußes. Z Orthop 85: 1962-1964
Ramírez A (1968) Técnica quirúrgica para el hallux valgus con metatarsalgia. Rev Cir Osteoartic: 33
Raposo Lence A, Fraga García H (1965) Aportación al tratamiento de la metatarsalgia. Rev Ortop Traumatol Iber 9 (3): 587
Rathery M (1968) Lesioni ossee dei piedi e neuropatie diabetiche. Gaz Med Fr 75 (1): 57-74
Rathery M (1973) Le osteo-artropatie nel diabete mellito. Gaz Med Fr 80 (29): 4589-4599
Ravault PP, Bouvier M (1966) Les algodystrophies (membre supérieur et membre inférieur) Rev Prat 16 (18): 2529-2545
Ravault PP, Maitrepierre J, Riffat G (1959) Le pied décalcifié douloureux idiopathique ou ostéoporose algique essentielle du pied. Rev Rhum 26: 393-407
Ravault PP, Lejeune E, Bouvier M, Jeanne-Ret J, Meunier P, Queneau P, Robillard J (1970) Les formes atypiques de la spondylarthrite ankylosante. Rev Rhum 73: 197-206
Raverdy P (1975) Le diagnostic des démarches neurologiques. Conc Med 10: 5227-5240
Raverdy P, Petit-Pierre de Vesdehlen JC (1979) Syphilis nerveuse en 1979. Concours Méd 101 (21): 3527-3540
Recordier AM, Serratrice G (1968) La part des processus neurologiques dans les altérations du pied diabétique. Podologie 6: 351
Recordier AM, Acquaviva P, Maestracci D, Schiano A (1975-1977) Le pied dans le rhumatisme psoriasique. In: Simon L, Claustre J (eds) Le pied inflammatoire. Maloine, Paris, p 83-86
Recordier AM, Mouren P, Serratrice G (1961) Les ostéo-arthropathies nerveuses. Expansion Scientifique France, Paris
Reggiani G (1965) Le applicazioni delle tomografia allo studio della patologia del piede. Podologie 4: 237
Regnauld B (1956) Contribution à l'étude de la crosse latérale du gros orteil et du deuxième orteil en col de cygne. Thesis, University of Paris
Regnauld B (1962) Problèmes posés par les empreintes plantaires. Ann Podol 1: 161-177
Regnauld B (1963) Corrections prothétiques du pied plat valgus de l'adolescent. Ann Podol 2: 193
Regnauld B (1964) Chaussures physiologiques de traitement. Ann Podol 3: 227-230
Regnauld B (1966) Traitement des fistules rétro-calcanéennes. Ann Podol 5: 34-37
Regnauld B (1968) Technique personnelle de la cure chirurgicale de l'hallux valgus. Ann Podol 6: 395-400
Regnauld B (1970) Correction du pied plat valgus de l'adolescent. Rev Int Pediatr
Regnauld B (1971a) L'enclavement diaphyso-épiphysaire métatarsien. Ann Podol 8 (I): 315-319
Regnauld B (1971b) Chirurgie de l'avant-pied rhumatismal. Acta Ortop Belg 37 (5): 557-560

Regnauld B (1971 c) Terapia chirurgica dell'artrosi metatarso-falangea. Rev Quad Med Chir Pied 10 (1): 7

Regnauld B (1973 a) L'enclavement diaphyso-épihysaire métatarsien. Actual Med Chir Pied 8 (II): 316–325

Regnauld B (1973 b) Autoplasties de glissement plantaire. Actual Med Chir Pied 8 (1): 303–307

Regnauld B (1973 c) Voies d'abord chirurgicales du pied. Actual Med Chir Pied 9: 141–164

Regnauld B (1974) Techniques chirurgicales du pied. Masson, Paris

Regnauld B (1976 a) Genesi e trattamento chirurgico del piede piatto valgo essenziale. Minerva Ortop 27 (5): 254–269

Regnauld B (1976 b) Traitement chirurgical du pied plat valgus. Idelson, Naples

Regnauld B (1976 c) Traitement chirurgical de l'arthrose métatarso-phalangienne. 1er colloque international de Charleroi. CIFoP, Charleroi

Regnauld B (1978 a) Déformations majeures de l'avant-pied. Minerva Med Chir Piede 2 (3): 121–136

Regnauld B (1978 b) Traitement chirurgical du pied valgus. 2e colloque international de Charleroi. CIFoP, Charleroi

Regnauld B (1979 a) Les tarsalgies consécutives aux altérations statiques et dynamiques du membre inférieur et du pied. Actual Med Chir Pied 12: 52–62

Regnauld B (1979 b) Techniques chirurgicales du pied. IIIe Cours du CIP. Rennes, Nantes

Regnauld B (1981) L'avant-pied post-traumatique. Chir Pied 5 (3–4): 291–294

Regnauld B (1982) Das diaphyso-epiphysäre Enclavement der Metatarsalia. Orthopäde 11: 191–199

Regnauld B, Grassin P (1975) Affections rhumatismales de l'avant-pied. Indications et techniques chirurgicales. Rhumatologie 27 (3): 135–138

Regnauld B, Leroux MJ (1965) L'hallux rigidus. Ann Podol 4: 45–60

Regnauld B, Saudreau J (1978) Primauté de l'articulation tibiotarsienne et de sa rééducation dans la cynétique du pied. Actual Med Chir Pied 11: 265–271

Reiter R (1961) Spätresultate nach 1464 Hallux-valgus-Operationen. Z Orthop 94: 178

Renander A (1924) Two cases of typical osteochondropathy of medial sesamoid bone of the first metatarsal. Acta Radiol 3: 521–527

Renier JC (1958) Les algodystrophies du membre inférieur et leur traitement. Rev Prat 8: 3835–3843

Renotte A (1963) La métatarsalgie médio-plantaire. Acta Orthop Belg 29 (6): 840–847

Renotte A (1969) Le traitement de talalgies plantaires. Rev Med Liege 24 (20): 744–746

Renotte A (1976) Hallux valgus. Résultats tardifs de l'opération de Lelièvre. Rev Med Liege 31: 612

Resnick D, Niwayama G, Feingold ML (1977) The sesamoid bones of the hands and feet: participators in arthritis. Radiology, 123: 57–62

Reverdin J (1881) Anatomie et opération de l'hallux valgus. Int Med Congr 2: 408–412

Riaza A, Miralles R, Saura E (1978) Inervacíon y sindrome del seno tarsiano. Actual Med Chir Pied 11: 173

Ribadeau-Dumas C (1941) Troubles trophiques des extrémités des membres inférieurs. Leurs rapports avec la syringomyélie lombo-sacrée et le "status dysraphicus". Rev Neurol March/April

Ricciardi-Pollini PT, Postacchini F (1978) Tenosinovite villonodulare pigmentosa del piede. Chir Pied 2 (4): 191–196

Ricciardi-Pollini PT, Ippolito E (1982) L'importanza dell'anatomia patologica e dello studio radiografico nel trattamento del pied torto congenito. Acta Med Chir Pied (CIP) 13: 60–64

Rice JRD (1977) Digital arthroplasty by power surgery with minimal incision. J Am Podiatry Assoc 67: 811

Richard J (1977) Fractures bimalléolaires – fractures du calcanéum. Vie Med [Suppl] 22: 41–46

Richet A (1957) Traité d'anatomie médico-chirurgicale. Chamerot, Paris

Rigault P (1973) Pied convexe congénital. Acta Med Chir Pied 8: 67–69

Rimbaud MP (1962) Les candidoses cutanées. Doc Med 64

Rimbaud MP (1965) Les eczémas mycosiques. Rev Med May: 553–557

Rinaldi F (1975) Considerazioni sul trattamento operatorio dell'alluce valgo. (Estr) Boll Soc Piemontese Chir 45 (2)

Ringertz N, Unander-Scharin L (1950) Maladie de Morton. Étude clinique et anatomo-pathologie. Acta Orthop Scand 19 (9): 327–348

Riosalido I (1929) De las lesiones de los sesamoideos del dedo gordo. Arch Esp Pediatr

Ripolles J, Henríquez A, Ballaster J (1972) Fracturas del calcaneo. Traumatol Cir Rehabil 2: 9

Rivoalen ME (1982) Étude comparative droite-gauche des 2 premiers orteils. Thesis, University of Bordeaux. Agra

Rix RR (1968) Modified Mayo operation for hallux valgus and bunion. A comparison with the Keller procedure. J Bone Joint Surg 50 (7): 1368–1378

Roaf R (1946) Suture of the external and internal popliteal nerves. Br J Surg 33: 382–385

Robb S (1975) Bunion surgery. Can Nurse 71 (8): 41–44

Robert D'Eshougues J (1972) Les arthrites des psoriasiques. Medicorama 142. Epri, Paris

Robbins H (1976) Naviculectomy for congenital vertical talus. Foot Science 26

Robillard R, Gagnon A, Alarie R (1968) Les Neuroarthropathies diabétiques. Podologie 6: 332

Rocher C (1942) Arthrorise du pied. Rev Orthop 28: 173

Rocher C (1962) Exploracion radiologica de la foncion del teclado metatarsiano POR medio de la incidencia de Rocher-Wangermez (RW) Ann Podol 1: 213

Rocher C (1974) Fonctions et bilans articulaires, 3rd edn. Masson, Paris

Rocher C, Rigaud A (1956) Fonction et bilans articulaires. Masson, Paris

Rocher C, Wangermez, Bonjean (1960) Étude radiologique de la voûte plantaire. J Radiol 34: 162

Rocher H (1978) Appareil métatarsien ou talon antérieur du pied. Anatomie, physiologie et pathologie. Thesis, University of Bordeaux

Rochera Vilaseca R, Viladot A, Folguera JP (1979) Surgical treatment of the flat foot. Chir Piede 3 (1): 17-20

Rodenstein J (1970) Neurología del pie diabético. Actas Trab Com Arg Estud Afecc Pie 31

Rodineau J (1972) Les entorses externes de la cheville. Diagnostic et traitement. Ann Med Phys 15 (4): 439-455

Roederer C, Graffin (1936) Le traitement du pied plat. Bull Med février 1935 (résumé Monde Medical 881: 676-677

Roederer C, Tillier (1936) Pied plat et os tibial externe. Rev Orthop 23 (3): 230-236

Rogers WA, Joplin RJ (1947) Hallux valgus, weak foot and the Keller operation: an end result study. Surg Clin North Am 27: 1295

Rohmer J (1879) Les variations de formes normales et pathologiques de la plante du pied étudiées par la méthode graphique. Collin, Nancy

Roig Puerta J (1965) Exploration du valgus du talon. Podologie 4: 145-158

Roig Puerta J (1968) Radiocontrol en el pie plano valgo. Podologie 6: 389-394

Roig Puerta J, Viladot A (1962) Exploracion del pie cavo con el radiofoto podograma. Podologie 1: 36-44

Rombouts J (1978) Le traitement chirurgical du pied bot invétéré. Chir Piede 2 (1-2): 53-58

Roques E, Arlet J (1949) Les manifestations articulaires périphériques de la spondylarthrite ankylosante. Rhumatologie 4: 168

Rose B (1974) Symposium sur l'avant-pied. Rev Chir Orthop 60 [Suppl II]: 105-202

Rose GK (1958) Correction of the pronated foot. J Bone Joint Surg [Br] 40: 674

Rosenfeld M (1972) A propos de l'ostéochondrite de l'astragale. Rev Rhum Mal Osteoartic 39: 123-127

Rotes Querol J, Múñoz Gómez J (1968) La gota. Toray, Barcelona

Rotes Querol J, Múñoz Gómez J (1971) Tratamiento de las enfermedades reumáticas. Toray, Barcelona

Roux H, Maestracci D, Schiano A, Recordier AM (1975) Les atteintes de la tête du 5e métatarsien au cours de la polyarthrite rhumatoide. In: Simon L, Claustre J (eds) Le pied inflammatoire. Maloine, Paris, pp 43-47

Roy-Camille R (1980) Pathologie traumatique de la cheville et du pied. Masson, Paris

Roy-Camille R, Lelièvre JF (1974) Cure de l'hallux valgus par la technique de Petersen. Nouv Presse Med 6: 299-300

Roy-Camille R, Lelièvre JF, Mamoudy P (1980) Traitement chirurgical des metatarsalgies siegeant sous les metatarso-phalangiennes moyennes. In: Deuxièmes Journées D'orthopédie de la Pitié. Masson, Paris, pp 212-221

Rubens-Duval A, Villiaumey J, Kaplan G, Bisson M, Rondier J (1966) Arthropathie de l'avant-pied à forme destructive au cours de la spondylarthrite ankylosante. Rev Rhum Mal Osteoartic 10: 2799-2804

Rubin, Witten M (1960) The talar tilt angle and the fibular collateral ligament. A method for the determination of the talar. J Bone Joint Surg 42 (1): 311-326

Ruffié R, Fournié A (1970) Le rhumatisme psoriasique. Med Hyg 28: 654-656

Ruffié R, Fournié A, Cuq M, Mansat C (1964) Le pied douloureux, oedémateux, décalcifié. Podologie 3: 177-187

Riggieri F, Damasso R (1954) Sulla lussazione tarsometatarsica di Lisfranc. Riv Inf Mal Prof 41: 97

Rugtveit A (1964) Extra-articular subtalar arthrodesis according to Green and Grice in flat feet. Acta Orthop Scand 34: 367-373

Ruth C (1961) The surgical treatment of injuries of the fibular collateral ligament of the ankle. J Bone Joint Surg 43 (1): 229-239

Rutt (1980) Surgery of the lower leg and foot. Saunders, Philadelphia

Sabatier J, Bertrand P (1975) Les arthroses du pied. Rhumatologie 27 (2): 57-60

Salamon A, O'Sink O, Weisenbach J (1969) Experience with the Mayo hallux valgus operation. Arch Orthop Unfallchir 66 (1): 57-64

Salaverri C, Aranguren M (1965) Comunicacion à la ponencia de metatarsalgia. Rev Orthop Traumatol Iber 9 (1): 193

Samilson RL (1976) Tendon transfer in cerebral palsy. J Bone Joint Surg 58-B: 153

Samman PD (1965) The nail in disease, Heinemann, London

Samson SA (1943) Traitement du pied bot congénital, procédé de Stuart A. Thompson. Ann Med Chir Hop, Montréal 4: 91

Sanchez C (1966) Tecnica de Lelièvre en el hallux valgus. Podologie 5: 89-91

Sanchis Olmos V (1963) Technique personnelle d'arthrodèse tibio-tarsienne par compression. Podologie 2: 21-32

Sardi A, Villani E (1966) L'artrodesi sotto astragalica extra-articolare (operazione di Green-Grice) nel piede paralitico. Podologie 5: 268-276

Sarrafian S (1983) Anatomy of the foot and ankle. Lippincott, Philadelphia

Sarrafian SK, Topouzian LK (1969) Anatomy and physiology of the extensor apparatus of the toes. J Bone Joint Surg [Am] 51: 669

Saussez M, Vertongen P, Deberdt R, Achslogh J, Renoirte P, Bière L de Versyck J (1963) Rapport sur le traitement chirurgical des paralysés cérébraux. Acta Orthop Belg 29: 137

Savill DL (1967) Cirugía del pie en la artritis reumatoidea. Rev Cir Osteo 2: 497

Saxl A (1936) Querplattfuß und Luxation der 2. Zehe. Z Orthop 64: 385-391

Scarfi G (1955) Deformita congenite del piede. Encicl Med Ital 8

Scarpa A (1803) Memoria chirurgica sui piedi torti congeniti. Pavia, Comini

Schaison G, Croisier JC (1971) Pathologie du pied chez le diabétique. Vie Med 52 (22): 2655-2662

Scharling M (1978) Ostéochondritis dissecans of the talus. Acta Orthop Scand 49/1: 89-94

Scharll M (1951) Fußgymnastik mit Kindern. Thieme, Stuttgart
Schede F (1928) Hallux valgus. Zentralbl Chir 55: 1554
Schede F (1928) Indikationen und Methoden in der Behandlung der Fußsenkung. Jahreskurse für ärztliche Fortbildung. Lehmanns, Munich
Schede F (1933) Fußsenkung der Erwachsenen. Ein Leitungswort zum Beispiel Kind und Schulkind. 28e congrès allemand d'orthopédie
Schede F (1935) Hygiene des Fußes. Thieme, Leipzig
Schede F (1955) Betrachtungen zur Detorsion des Vorfußes und den "Detorsions-Einlagen". Z Orthop 86: 582-589
Scheffer JC (1976) Fractures du calcanéum. Gaz Med 83 (18): 1819-1823
Schiano A, Eisinger J, Acquaviva PC (1976) Les algodystrophies. Lab Armour-Montagu
Schnepp J (1973) Intérêt de la radiographie dans le traitement des pieds plats et des pieds creux. Cah Med Lyon 49 (19): 1963-1965
Schnepp J (1976) Angle de flexion dorsale du pied. Appréciations pratiques dans l'ankylose tibio-tarsienne. Cah Reed Readapt Fonct 2: 3
Schnepp J (1979) Le pied creux essentiel - rappel anatomo-clinique - methode et indication therapeutique. Cahiers d'enseignement à la SOFCOT 10: 73-92
Schnepp J (1980) Troubles statiques de l'avant-pied. Entretiens de Bichat. Chirurgie, Expansion Scientifique Française, Paris, pp 59-64
Schnepp J (1981 a) Pied plat essentiel. Rev Prat Podol 31 (15) 1031-1049
Schnepp J (1981 b) Les semelles orthopediques. Lyon Med 245 (10): 675-691
Schnepp J, Carret JP (1982) Formes anatomocliniques des metatarsalgies statiques. Monogr Podol 2: 122-123
Schnepp J, Carret JP (1983 a) Pathologie de l'avant-pied d'origine mecanique. XXXe Semaine de Rhumatologie, Aix-les-Bains, April, p 50
Schnepp J, Carret JP (1983 b) Indication therapeutique dans l'hallux valgus. XXXe Semaine de Rhumatologie, Aix-les-Bains, April, p 62
Schnepp J, et al (1979 a) Chirurgie du pied plat essentiel chez l'adolescent valeur de la chirurgie reparatrice. Chir Piede 3 (4): 351-353
Schnepp J, et al (1979 b) Entorses graves du LLE et de la tibiotarsienne. In: Simon L (ed) Le pied du sportif - actualités en médecine du sport. Masson, Paris, pp 34-41
Schnepp J, et al (1980 a) Possibilites radiologiques actuelles des radiographies standards dans les troubles statiques du pied et de l'avant-pied. LC 76 (1): 38-40
Schnepp J, et al (1980 b) Troubles statiques de l'avant pied - possibilités chirurgicales. Rev Rhumatol 47: 181-186
Schnepp J, et al (1980 c) Chirurgie preventive du pied creux - valeur de l'operation de Stendler. Chir Piede 4 (2): 77-80
Schnepp J, Carret JP, Courcelles P (1983) Analyse des échecs therapeutiques dans les fractures malléolaires. J Lyon Traumatol April: 119-121
Schoenhaus H, DPM Rotman S, Meshon A (1973) A review of normal inter-metatarsal angles. J Am Podiatry Assoc 63 (3): 88-95
Scholder P (1952) Prothèse et appareillages des membres inférieurs. Rev Orthop 38: 437
Scholder P (1970 a) Der Vorfuß. Huber, Wien
Scholder P (1970 b) Anatomie fonctionnelle et biomécanique du pied. Rev Med Occid Mac Prof Zürich 63: 247
Scholder P (1971 a) La fonction élastique de l'avant-pied dans le déroulement de la marche. Podologie 6: 179
Scholder P (1971 b) Remarques thérapeutiques sur le pied bot varus équin congénital. Actual Med Chir Pied 8 (1): 52-62
Scholder P (1983) Le remodelage de croissance dans le pied bot congénital. Acta Med Chir Pied (CIP) 14: 121
Scholder P, Borel H, Ochsner P, Pelet D, Wiasmitinow N, Zollinger H (1978) The treatment of hallux valgus. Chir Piede 2 (3): 95-116
Scholler H (1976) Ostéotomie pour arthrose tibio-tarsienne. Ann Soc Belg Med Chir Pied CIFOP, Charleroi, pp 113-116
Schoolfield MD (1939) Une opération pour le traitement du pied plat. Ann Surg 110 (3)
Schor I (1970) Pie diabético. Actas Trab Com Arg Estud Afecc Pie 21
Schotte M (1935) Fußbeschwerden und ihre Behandlung. Maudrich
Schrader (1932) Die blutige Behandlung des Plattfußes. Rapport au 21e congrès allemand d'orthopédie. Z Orthop Chir [Suppl] 55: 324
Schreiber A, Weber A (1974) Die operative Behandlung des lockeren Spreizfußes. Orthopäde 3: 13
Schumacher ED (1908) Zur Kasuistik der Totalluxationen des Metatarsus im Lisfranc'schen Gelenk. Beitr Klin Chir 59: 510
Schwartz CE (1883) Des différentes espèces de pieds bots et leurs traitements. Thesis, University of Paris
Schwartz RP (1946) Arthrodesis of subtalus and midtarsal joints of the foot. Historical review, preoperative determinations and operative procedure. Surgery 20: 619-635
Schwindt CD, Lulloff RS, Rogers SC (1973) Transmetatarsal amputations. Orthop Clin North Am 4 (1): 31
Searfoss R, Bendana A, Glenking, Miller G (1975) Vertical talus of unusual etiology. J Bone Joint Surg [Am] 57 (3): 409-413
Seigrist H (1970) Technik und Indikation der Hohmannschen Operation. Z Orthop 107: 495
Selig S (1941) Hammer toe: a new procedure for its correction. Surg Gynecol Obstet 72: 101
Seneque J (1937) Précis de diagnostic chirurgical, vol 4, membres. Masson, Paris
Sergeron FH (1943) The treatment of unilateral congenital talipes equinovarus with the Denis Browne splint. J Bone Joint Surg 25: 105
Seringe R (1975) La rééducation des pieds bots varus équins congénitaux. Acta Med Chir Pied (CIP) 11: 251
Seringe R (1976) Traitement du pied bot varus équin congénital chez l'enfant. In: Le pied bot varus équin. Expansion Scientifique Française 3: 57-64

Serra E, Papandrea G (1966) Trattamento chirurgico mediante artrodesi del piede poliomielitico. Podologie 5: 261–262

Serre H, Simon L, Claustre J (1964) Les talalgies plantaires communes. Cah Reed Readapt Fonct 4: 204–218

Serre H, Simon L, Picard JJ, Claustre J, Avila de Azevedo M (1965) Le syndrome du canal tarsien. Rev Rhum Mal Osteoartic 32: 96–106

Serre H, Simon L, Picard J, Claustre J, Avila de Azevedo M (1966) Le syndrome du canal tarsien. Podologie 5: 38–48

Serre H, Simon L, Claustre J (1968) Les algodystrophies réflexes du pied. Podologie 6: 265–284

Serre H, Simon L, Claustre J (1970) Le pied dans la spondylarthrite ankylosante. Rev Rhum Mal Osteoartic 37: 160–167

Serre H, Simon L, Claustre J (1972) Le syndrome douloureux du 2é espace intermétatarsien. Rev Rhum Mal Osteoartic 39: 495–503

Serre H, Claustre J, Simon L (1977) L'algodystrophie réflexe du pied. In: Simon L, Claustre J (eds) Le pied inflammatoire. Maloine, Paris

Sever JW (1930) Calcaneum bifide. Surg Gynecol Obstet 50 (6): 1011

de Sèze S, Ryckewaert A (1954) Maladies des os et des articulations. Flammarion, Paris

de Sèze S, Ryckewaert A (1960) La goutte. Expansion Scientifique Française, Paris

de Sèze S, Lequesne M, Harif V (1965) Les fractures de fatigue vues par le rhumatologue. Rev Rhum Mal Osteoartic 32: 229–236

de Sèze S, Dreyfus P, Denis A, Heuleu JN, Hamonet C, Legeay A (1970) Le syndrome du tunnel tarsien. Étude clinique et électromyographique. Ann Med Phys 13: 2

Sgarlato TE (1970) Transplantation of the flexor digitorum longus muscle tendon in hammer toe. J Am Podiatry Assoc 383

Shaknes IE, Sokolova IM (1980) Periungueal and subungueal fibromatosis. Vestn Dermatol Venerol 4: 33–35

Sharrard WJW, Smith WD (1976) Ténodèse du long fléchisseur du gros orteil pour griffe paralytique du gros orteil dans l'enfance. J Bone Joint Surg [Br] 58: 224–226

Sherman M (1952) Psoriasic arthritis. J Bone Joint Surg 34: 831–852

Sibley WL (1945) Modification de l'opération radicale pour le traitement des ongles incarnés des orteils. Am J Surg 70: 79

Sichère RM (1968) Pied rhumatismal et rééducation. Cah Reed Readapt Fonct 7: 243–246

Sidney JD (1963) A tarsal tunnel syndrome. Lancet 1: 496–497

Siguier M, Caffinière JY (de la), Brunet JC (1972) Fractures thalamiques fraîches du calcanéum. Actual Chir Orthop 10: 15–20

Sigwald (1944) Acropathies mutilantes des membres inférieurs. Encycl Med Chir

Silk FF, Leeds, Wainwright D (1967) The recognition and treatment of congenital flat foot in infancy. J Bone Joint Surg [Br] 49 (4): 628–643

Silver D (1923) Treatment of hallux valgus. J Bone Joint Surg 21: 225

Simeon M, Screve C (1976) Mesure des conditions d'adaptation pied-chaussures. Cah Reed Réadapt Fonct 11 (3): 101–103

Simon L, Claustre J (1977) Le pied inflammatoire. Maloine, Paris

Simon L, Claustre J (1978) La rééducation du pied algodystrophique. In: Actualites de médecine et chirurgie du pied, vol 2. Toray Masson, Barcelona

Simon L, Rodineua J (1982) Cheville et médecine de rééducation. Masson, Paris

Simon L, Blotman F, Claustre J (1975, 1978, 1983) Abrégé de Rhumatologie. Masson, Paris

Simon L, Claustre J, Benezis C (1979) Le pied du sportif. Masson, Paris

Simons GW, Tachdjian MO (1976) Traitement des pieds bots de la naissance à 2 ans. Cah SOFCOT 3: 31–49

Simplet G (1981) Ostéotomie cylindrique du calcanéum. Thèse, Univ. de Lyon

Singer A (1977) Diabetic feet (letter). Br Med J 2 (600078): 48

Sinigallia D (1951) Su di un caso di lussazione tarso-metatarsica. Clin Orthop 3: 80

Sirkis L (1956) Les onychoses à levures et leur traitement par la Nystatine. Thesis, University of Paris

Soeur R (1934) Pathogénie des déformations statiques du pied. Bull et Mémoires Soc Belg orthop, 6, 4: 251–258

Soeur R (1951) L'ostéochondrite disséquante. Réactions de la membrane synoviale. Rev Orthop 37: 5

Soeur R (1959) Le pied contracturé. Rev Orthop 45 (6): 817

Soeur R, Goffin (1933) Pathogénie et traitement de l'hallux valgus. Bull Mém Soc Bel Orthop

Soeur R, Remy R (1975) Fractures of the calcaneus with displacement of the thalamic portion. J Bone Joint Surg [Br] 57: 413

Solac CK (1970) Metatarsalgia por alteraciones mecanicas del arco anterior. Prensa Med Arg 57 (39): 1825–1829

Solimel LC, Rettagliata F, Berardi GC (1959) Problemi tecnici dell'artoclesi tibio tarsica. Atti Sertot 4

Sonnenshein A (1948) Traitement sanglant ou non du pied bot. Acta Orthop Scand 18 (3)

Soren A (1970) Correction chirurgicale de l'hallux valgus. Rev Chir Orthop 56: 355

Sorensen LB (1969) Hyperuricemia and gout – advances. Intern Med 15: 177–201

Sorto LA (1974) Surgical correction of hammer toes: a five year post-operative study. J Am Podiatry Am 64: 930

Soubrane (1936) Transplantations tendineuses au niveau du pied. Thesis, University of Paris

Soule RE (1910) Operation for the cure of hammer toe. NY Med J, page 649

Soulier A (1966) Le traitement chirurgical de l'hallux valgus. Acta Orthop Belg 32 (5)

Soulier A, Duqueunoy A (1969) Arthrodèse tibio-tarsienne par greffons cylindriques. Act Orthop Belg 35 (2): 377

Spiro E (1935) Über den angeborenen Plattfuß. Z Orthop 62: 170-192

Spitzy H (1904) Der Pes planus. Z Orthop 12: 777-797

Stagnara P, Desbrosse J (1961) Arthrodèse sous-astragalienne pour le traitement des pieds plats valgus paralytiques. Rev Chir Orthop 47-5: 641

Stamm TT (1957) The surgical treatment of hallux valgus. Guy's Hospital Rep 106: 273

Steindler A (1929) The supinatory, compensatory torsion of the forefoot in pes valgus. J Bone Joint Surg 11: 272-276

Steindler A (1935) Mechanics of normal and pathological locomotion in man. Springfield, Illinois

Steindler A (1940) Orthopedic operations; indications techniques et résultats finaux. Thomas, Springfield

Steinert (1909) (cited by Tome FMS, Fardeau M) Dystrophie myotonique de Steinert. Encycl Med Chir Paris, Neurologie I, 17178, B10

Steinfort G (1969) Luxation-fracture de l'articulation de Lisfranc. Podologie 6: 236-241

Steinfort G (1975) Podométrie électronique. Rhumatologie 5 (1): 1-10

Stephens (1935) An operation for the correction of pronated feet. J Bone Joint Surg 17: 424-426

Stess RM (1972) A surgical approach to advanced rheumatoid arthritis of the forefoot. J Am Podiatry Assoc 62: 259

Stoffel A (1913) The treatment of spastic contractures. Am J Orthop Surg 10611

Stokes IA, et al. (1975) The neuropathic ulcer and loads on the foot in diabetic patients. Acta Orthop Scand 46 (5): 839-847

Storen H (1959) New method of operative treatment of insufficiency of the lateral ligament of the ankle joint. Acta Chir Scand 24: 117, 501

Storen H (1967) Congenital convex pes valgus with vertical talus. Acta Orthop Scand 94

Stott JRR, Hutton WC, Stokes IA (1973) Forces under the foot. J Bone Joint Surg [Br] 55 (2): 335-344

Stout AP (1954) Juvenile fibromatosis. Cancer 7: 953-978

Stracker O (1943) Entstehung und operative Behandlung des kindlichen Knickplattfußes. Chirurg 15: 4

Straub LR, Smith JW, Carpenter GKJ, Dietz GH (1961) Surgery of gout in upper extremity. J Bone Joint Surg [Am] 43: 731

Straus (1932) Marching fractures of metatarsal bones. Surg Gynecol Obstet 54: 581

Strauss J, Voutey H, Perrin M (1975) Les ténosynovites au niveau du pied. Rhumatologie 27: 79-84

Stringa G, Vigliani F (1958) Trapianti ossei autoplastice nell'uomo. Relaz 43e Congrès Soc Ital Ort Traum, Padova, 21 octobre 1958

Stroescu I (1971) La valeur de la baro-podographie dans le diagnostic fonctionnel podologique et dans la prévention des lésions et des déformations du pied. Podologie 8 (2) 29: 38

Stroescu I (1975) Les traitements podo-orthétiques en rhumatologie. Rhumatologie 5 (1): 47-66

Stucke K (1956) Der Fersenschmerz. Thieme, Stuttgart

Sudeck P (1900) Über die akute entzündliche Knochen-Atrophie. Arch Klin Chir 62: 147

Sudeck P (1902) L'atrophie osseuse aigue après traumatisme des extrémités. Dtsch Med Wochenschr 336

Suppan RJ (1974) The cartilaginous articulation preservation principale and its surgical implementation for hallux abducto valgus. J Am Podiatry Assoc 64 (8): 635-56

Swanson AB (1972) Flexible implant arthroplasty for arthritic finger joints. J Bone Joint Surg [Am] 54 (3): 435

Swanson AB, Herndon J (1977) Flexible implant arthroplasties. J Bone Joint Surg [Am] 59: 362

Sydey JD (1963) A tarsal tunnel syndrome. Lancet 1: 496-497

Taillard W (1952) Le traitement du pied bot par la méthode de Kite. Rev Med Suisse Romande 72 (5)

Taussig G, Hautier S, Maschas A (1969) Les fractures-luxations de l'articulation de Lisfranc. Ann Chir 23 (21-22) C: 1131

Tax HR (1980) Podopediatrics. Williams and Wilkins, Baltimore

Taylor RG (1940) An operative procedure for the treatment of hammer toe and claw toe. J Bone Joint Surg 22: 608

Terrasse J, Rampon S, Gras H, Janny P, Plagne J, Bertrix E (1959) Algodystrophie réflexe des membres. Rev Rhumatol 26: 168-196

Testut L, Latarjet A (1948) Traité d'anatomie humaine, edn. Doin, Paris

Thévenard A (1942) L'acropathie ulcéromutilante familiale. Rev Neurol (Paris) 74: 193-212

Thevenard A (1953) L'acropathie ulcéro-mutilante familiale. Acta Neurol Belg 53 (1): 23

Thiemann H (1909) Juvenile Epiphysen-Störungen. Fortschr Geb A Roentgenstr 14: 79

Thomas A (1947) Pied bot et hémiplégie. Presse Med 75 (18): 191

Thomas BF (1962) Keller's arthroplasty modified. A technique to ensure postoperative distraction of the toe. J Bone Joint Surg 2: 356-365

Thomas WH (1979) Metatarsal osteotomy. Surg Clin North Am 49: 879-882

Thompson FR, MacElvenny RT (1940) Arthrodesis to the first metatarso-phalangeal joint. J Bone Joint Surg 22: 555-558

Thompson TC (1964) Surgical treatment of disorders of the forepart of the foot. J Bone Joint Surg [Am] 46: 1117-1128

Thomsen J (1876) Tonische Krämpfe in willkürlich beweglichen Muskeln in Folge von ererbter psychischer Disposition. Arch Psychiatr 6: 702

Thomsen W (1939) Kampf der Fußschwäche. Lehmann, München

Thomson JE (1946) Treatment of congenital flat foot. J Bone Joint Surg 28: 787-90

Thomson SA (1942) Treatment of congenital talipes equinovarus with a modification of the Denis Browne method and splint. J Bone Joint Surg 24: 291-298

Thomson SA (1946) Attelle pour pied bot récidivant. J Bone Joint Surg 28 (4)

Thomson SA (1969) Hallux varus and metatarsus varus, a 5 years study (1954-1958). Clin Orthop 16: 109

Thornhill HL, Richter RW, Shelton ML, Johnson CA (1973) Neuropathic arthropathy (Charcot forefeet) in alcoholics. Orthop Clin North Am 4 (1): 7

Thys R (1955) A propos des déchirures du ligament malléolaire externe. Brux Med 35 (13): 635-640

Thys R (1965) Traitement chirurgical du calcanéo-valgus chez l'enfant. Podologie 4: 205

Thys R (1972) Arthrographie du cou de pied dans le diagnostic des ruptures musculaires. Acta Orthop Belg 38: 654-668

Thys R (1974a) Traitement des métatarsalgies par dysharmonie de pression. Intérêt de la podométrie. Acta Orthop Belg 40: 77-84

Thys R (1974b) Ostéotomie trapézoidale à base dorsale de la métaphyse proximale des métatarsiens. Acta Orthop Belg 41: 125-132

Thys R (1975) Traitement du pied calcanéo-valgus de l'enfant par élongation du tendon d'Achille. Acta Orthop Belg 41 (2): 125-132

Thys R (1977) L'arthrografia del celle del piede. Chir Piede 1 (6): 717-720

Timal R (1963) Indications opératoires dans le paralysies du pied. Podologie 2: 131-143

Timmer H (1930) Die Behandlung des Hallux valgus. Barth, Leipzig

Tohen A, Carmora J, Chow L, Rosas J (1969) Extra-articular subtalar arthrodesis. J Bone Joint Surg [Br] 51 (1): 45-52

Tomeno B, Aurbriot JH (1974) Traitement de l'hallux valgus par l'intervention de MacBride (modifiée) Rev Chir Orthop Rep 60 [Suppl 2]: 150

Tomeno B, Heurard JC, Dorfmann H (1974) Pied normal et pied pathologique. Cah Int Med 115: 221-260

Tomeno B, Paulin M (1976) Traitement de l'hallux valgus. Limites et indications de l'exostosectomie. Rev Chir Orthop 62 (8): 775-780

Torner CE (1969) Luxación de la articulación de Lisfranc (2 casos). Podologie 6: 192

Torner CE (1970) Luxación de la articulación de Lisfranc. Podologie 6

Torner CE (1971) La marcha en la insuficiencia del primer radio. Podologie 8 (2): 61

Torner CE (1975) El calzado en la edad escolar. Actual Med Chir Pied 9: 113-119

Torner CE (1978) Oscilación y marcha. Actual Med Chir Pied 11: 95-101

Torner CE (1979) Indications chirurgicales du pied creux. IIIe cours du collège international de Médecine et Chirurgie du Pied. Nantes, p 156

Torner CE (1984) Osteotomía hemicilindrica del tarso. Actual Med Chir Pied 15

Torner CE, Mas J (1976) Étude cinématique de l'articulation tibi-tarsienne dans de differents troubles du pied et de la cheville. Colloque international sur l'arthrose du cou de pied et du pied. Charleroi, pp 35-42

Torner CE, Gonzalez JC, Puig R, Viladot R (1972) Bases fisiopatológicas del tratamiento quirúrgico del pie plano exensical. Rev Ortop Traumatol 16: 251

Torner CE, Cervera J-M, Mas J (1976) Pie plano irreductible congénito y síndrome del maullido del gato. Anal Soc Esp Med Cir Pie, pp 69-82

Torner CE, Mas J, Marfany J (1983) Analgesia peridural postoperatoria en cirugía del pie. Actual Med Chir Pied 14: 203-207

Torner CE, Mas J, Bascompte A (1983) Estudio radiográfico de la oblicuidad del calcaneo. Actual Med Chir Pied 14: 91-95

Torto U del (1971) Boveda del antepie y alteración de la acción muscular que la realiza. Podologie 6: 120

Torto U del, Perugia L (1957) Richerche esperimentali sull'anatomia funzionale del piede normale e piatto. Orizz Ortop Od Riabil 11 (2): 213

Toubert J (1890) Le pied plat acquis. Thesis, University of Lyon

Toulon R (1956) Equilibration humaine et évaluation de la posture debout. Maloine, Paris

Toupet (1920) Arthrodèse du pied. J Chir 16: 268

Tournel M (1974) L'hallux valgus. Thesis, University of Nancy

Tramon MP (1978) Conduite à tenir devant un pied creux. Bord Med 11 (14): 1265-1266

Trethowan MU (1923) Hallux valgus. A system of surgery. Hoeber, New York

Trethowan HW (1925) The treatment of hammer toes. Lancet 1: 1257, 1312

Treves A (1925) Rapport au Congrès de la Société Française d'Orthopédie 1931: os surnuméraire du tarse. Rev Orthop

Treves A (1931) Traitement du pied bot varus équin congénital après deux ans. Rapport à la Société Française d'Orthopédie. Rev Orthop 18 (5): 393-456

Treves A (1936) La bosse cunéo-métatarsienne du dos du pied. Bull Mem Soc Chir Paris 28: 460-462

Treves A (1937) Difformités du gros orteil. In Traité d'orthopédie, vol 5. Masson, Paris

Trillat A, Dejour, Brenaut, Grobert (1965) La primauté des lésions ligamentaires internes dans certains traumatismes par abduction-pronation de la cheville. Soc Chir Lyon March: 585

Trillat A, Bousquet G, Lapeyre B (1970) Les fractures séparations totales du col ou du corps de l'astragale. Intérêt du vissage par voie postérieure. Rev Chir Orthop 56 (6): 529-536

Trillat A, Bousquet G, Lapeyre B (1971a) Vissage par voie postérieure de l'astragale. Rev Orthop

Trillat A, Monnier Kuhn A (1971b) Les ruptures du tendon d'Achille. Résultats éloignés. Lyon Chir 67 (5): 34-38

Troisier O (1966-67) A Tendinites et ténosynovites du pied. Podologie 5: 149-154

Trolle D (1948) Os accessoires du pied humain: étude radiologique, histo-embryologique d'anatomie comparée et génétique. Munsgaard, Copenhagen

Troncoso J (1960) Nuestra experiencia en el tratamiento del hallux valgus. Rev Ortop Traumatol 4 (1): 256

Troncoso J, Viladot A (1965) Metatarsalgia. Primera Ponencia al X Congreso Nacional de la SECOT Rev Ortop Traumatol Iber 9: 1

Tschokanow K (1968) Contribution to surgical treatment of severe cases of hallux valgus. Beitr Orthop Traumatol 15 (3): 206

Tupman S (1958) Arthrodesis of the first metatarso-phalangeal joint. J Bone Joint Surg 40: 826

Turco VJ (1971) Surgical correction of the resistant clubfoot. One stage posteromedial release with internal fixation. A preliminary report. J Bone Joint Surg [Am] 53: 477–497

Uro J, Pariente P (1955) Le pied dans la polyarthrite chronique évolutive. Le rhumatisme. Expansion Scientifique France Paris, pp 99–110

Valenti V (1976a) Evoluzione radiologica e clinica de trapianto osteo-cartilagineo secondo Regnauld nell'intervento per alluce valgo. Minerva Ortop 27 (6): 334

Valenti V (1976b) Artrorisi sottoastragalica con protesi acrilica nel trattamento del piede piatto-valgo dell'infanzia. Minerva Ortop 27 (6): 309–314

Valenti V (1976c) Paramorfismi predisponenti e paramorfismi determinanti nella genesi dell'alluce valgo. Minerva Ortop 27 (10): 517–522

Valenti V (1976d) Epoca di sviluppo dei sesamoidi e della cresta intersesamoidea. Minerva Ortop 27 (12): 643–646

Valenti V (1977a) La valutazione della formula metatarsale e dei suoi effetti predisponenti negli atteggiamenti funzionali del piede. Chir Piede 1 (6): 711–715

Valenti V (1977b) La rappresentazione nervosa nella istologia del legamento a siepe. Chir Piede 1 (3–4): 423–428

Valenti V (1977c) Le ortesi del piede. Verduci, Roma

Valenti V (1978) Ortesis del pie. Medicina Panamericana, Buenos Aires

Valenti V (1979) I mezzi di informazione della marcia e loro rapporti con l'economia del passo. Podologie 12: 159

Valenti V (1980a) Anatomie ligamentaire, nerveuse et histologie du sinus du tarse. Chir Piede 4 (2): 101

Valenti V (1980b) Anatomia, histologia, fisiologia e patologia do seno do tarso. Acta do 2° Congresso brasileiro de medicina e cirugia do pé, Canela-Gramado, pp 38–46

Valenti V (1980c) Anatomia geral e biomecanica do pé. As metatarsalgia e seu tratamento cirùgico e com ortese. Principais afeccôes biômecanicas do pé. Volumen del Curso de Podologia Gramado 30/4–3/5

Valenti V (1981) The role of the sesamoid bones in the symptomalogy of the pes cavus. 15e SICOT World Congress (Abstr). Rio de Janeiro, p 110

Valenti V (1982a) Politica del trattamento del piede piatto. Chir Piede 6 (2): 27–29

Valenti V (1982b) Patologia del seno del tarso. Minerva Ortop 33 (3): 303–308

Van Bogaert (1940) Sur les acropathies mutilantes symétriques des extrémités inférieures et leur rapport avec la syringomyélie (contribution à l'étude du mal perforant familial). Presse Med 17.121940 (99)

Van Demark RE, MacCarthy PV (1946) Panner's metatarsal disease: a condition of aseptic necrosis simulating march fracture. J Bone Joint Surg 28: 842–844

Van de Voorde CI, Wulf A de, Vereecken E (1950) Le traitement des séquelles des traumatismes du cou-de-pied. Acta Orthop Belg 16 (4): 119

Van Herpe L, Mitchell CL (1962) Resection of metatarsal heads for painful and intractable plantar callosities. Henry Ford Hosp Med Bull 10: 241–244

Vannoni S, Mezzadra G (1966) La métatarsalgie post-traumatique. Podologie 5: 106

Van Trappen JB, Belenger J (1967) Les fractures des métatarsiens et leur traitement. Acta Orthop Belg 5, 6, 33: 13, 471–486

Veijo Ritsila A (1969) Talipes equino varus and vertical talus produced experimentally in newborn rabbits. Acta Orthop Scand [Suppl] 121

Venning P (1960) Variation of the digital skeleton of the foot. Clin Orthop 16: 26

Venouil J, Vuillard P, Fischer L, Braconnot P (1970) Les luxations traumatiques du pied (toutes les articulations du pied sont envisagées). Cah Med Lyon 46 (4): 281

Venturi R (1960) Metatarsalgia di Morton. Chir Organi Mov 49: 327–339

Verbrugge J (1933) La pathogénie et le traitement de l'hallux valgus. Scalpel 86 (45): 1153

Verbrugge J (1946) Note au sujet du traitement des pieds bots varus équins congénitaux. Acta Orthop Belg 12 (6): 253–259

Verbrugge J (1949) L'ostéotomie et le retournement temporaire du péroné dans la voie d'abord du cou-de-pied. Acta Orthop Belg 14 (5)

Verbrugge J (1965) Remarques au sujet de la double arthrodèse du tarse. Podologie 6: 27

Verhaeghe A (1964) La radiographie de l'avant-pied. Son intérêt diagnostique dans la polyarthrite chronique évolutive de l'adulte. Atlas Radiol Clin 11: 1–4

Verhaeghe A, Le Beurre R (1961) Pied décalcifié douloureux idiopathique. A propos d'un cas bilateral. Lille Med 6: 409–412

Verhaeghe A et al. (1956) Ténosynovite du long péronier latéral. Lille Med 1: 25–28

Verhaeghe A, Lemaire G, Lebeurre R (1961) Les calcanéites de la spondylarthrite ankylosante. Rev Rhum Mal Osteoartic 28: 504–507

Verhaeghe A, Lemaire G, Lebeurre R (1962a) Les calcanéites rhumatismales. J Radiol Electrol 43: 643–646

Verhaeghe A, Lemaitre G, Lebeurre R (1962b) La radiographie de l'avant-pied dans le diagnostic de la polyarthrite chronique évolutive. J Radiol Electrol 43: 634–636

Verne T, Inman VT (1976) The joints of the ankle. Williams and Wilkins, Baltimore

Verola J (1974) Le traitement du pied rond antérieur par l'intervention de R. Judet. Thesis, University of Marseille

Verola J, Groulier P, Bonsignour JP (1976) Place des ostéotomies des métatarsiens dans le traitement du pied rond antérieur. Marseille Chir 114: 77–83

Veyrassat J, Berner A (1943) Résultat anatomique de l'opération de Hueter dans l'hallux valgus. Presse Med 40: 293–294

Vidal R, Arlet J (1973) Cinq cas de neuro-ostéo-arthropathies diabétique. Podologie 8 (1): 231
Vieville R (1962) Podologie et phlébologie. Podologie 1: 109-112
Viladot A (1947) Estudio experimental sobre la hemorragia. Tesis doctoral. Rev Esp Fisiologia 3 (4): 335-350
Viladot A (1952) Lesiones por sobrecarga del segundo metatarsiano. Med Clinica 19: 6
Viladot A (1954) Nuevo metodo de exploracion estatica del pie. Clin Lab 52 (335): 114-117
Viladot A (1957) Protección medicamentosa de la cineseterapia de recuperación en traumatizados. Med Cl 29 (2): 112-124
Viladot A (1958) Un caso de pseudoartrosis post-osteomielitica de radio tratada por el metodo de Hey Groves. Barcelona Quirurgica 3: 1-4
Viladot A (1959a) Principales normas de rehabilitacion en las afecciones del antepie. An Med 45 (2): 241-247
Viladot A (1959b) Estado actual del tratamiento de la tuberculosis osteo-articular. Pract Med Quirurgica Int 1-7
Viladot A (1960a) Acción de un nuevo angiolitico en cirugia del pie. Med Clin 34 (2): 109-111
Viladot A (1960b) Anatomia del hallux valgus. Rev Ortop Traumatol 4 (2): 67-76
Viladot A (1962) Fisiopatologia del antepie. Podologia 1: 87-103
Viladot A (1969-1970) Influencia de los diversos tipos de antepies en la fisiologia del mismo. Podologia 6: 125
Viladot A (1972) Indicaciones quirurgicas en el pie plano. Rev Ortop Traumatol 16 1 B (2)
Viladot A (1973a) Metatarsalgia due to biomechanical alterations of the forefoot. Orthop Clin North Am 4 (1): 165-178
Viladot A (1973b) La evolución del pie. Act Med Chir Pied 9: 37
Viladot A (1975a) Las deformidades del antepie reumatico en fonción de su tipo congenito. Rhumatologie 5 (1): 35
Viladot A (1975b) Patologia del antepie. Toray, Barcelona
Viladot A (1975c) Nouvelle technique pour le traitement chirurgical du pied plat valgus essentiel. Extr Cahier Chir 16, 4e trimestre: 8-10
Viladot A (1975d) Edicion libro "Antepie" - Patologia e clinica dell'avampiede. Verducci, Roma
Viladot A (1976a) La moderna cirurgia del pie. Estratto dagli atti della società italiana di patologia dell'apparato locomotore. I Simposio, Terminillo, Idelson V, Napoli
Viladot A (1976b) Arthrodèse-arthroplastie de la cheville. CIFoP, Charleroi, p 117
Viladot A (1976c) L'arthrodèse dans le pied plat et creux. CIFoP, Charleroi, p 209
Viladot A (1977) Le traitement chirurgical du pied rhumatoide: la chirurgie de l'avant-pied. In: Simon L, Claustre J (eds) Le pied inflammatoire. Maloine, Paris, pp 223-226
Viladot A (1979a) Edición libro "Antepie". Pathologie de l'avant-pied. Expansion Scientifique, Paris
Viladot A (1979b) 10 lecciones sobre patologia del pie. Toray, Barcelona
Viladot A (1980) Alteraciones de la marcha en el nino. MTA 1 (15): 125
Viladot A (1981a) Edición libro "Antepie". Toray, Barcelona
Viladot A (1981b) Dieci lezioni di patologia del piede. Ermes Medica, Roma
Viladot A (1982) Überlegung bezüglich der operativen Behandlung des Hallux valgus und der Hammerzehen. Orthopäde 11: 162
Viladot A, Arandes R (1953) Biomecanica del calcaneo. Med Clinica 21 (1): 25-34
Viladot A, Arandes R (1954) La luxación de los dedos del pie. Cirugia Ginecol Urol 7 (4): 196-204
Viladot A, Gonzalez-Casanova J-C (1972) Malformaciones congenitas del antepie. Podologie 8 (1): 97-110
Viladot A, Moracas A (1965) Enfermedad de Morton. Podologie 3: 233-241
Viladot A, Planell E (1959) Hiperostosis congenita. Presentacion de un caso. An Med 45 (3): 145-149
Viladot A, Planell E (1960) Presentación de un caso raro de osteo-sclerosis familiar. Rev Ortop Traumat 4 (3): 365-376
Viladot A, Roig Puerta J (1962) Exploración del pie cavo con el radiofotopodograma. Podologie 1: 36-44
Viladot A, Sanpera I (1964) Consideraciones sobre la escafoiditis tarsiana. Podologie 3: 37-52
Viladot A, Arandes R, Vilanova X (1956) Clinica y tratamiento de las enfermedades de los pies. Cientifico Medicas, Barcelona
Viladot A, Roig Puerta J, Escarpenter J (1963) Biomecanica de la articulation sub-astragalina. Podologie 2: 33
Viladot A, Viladot R, Rochera R (1972) Tratamiento quirurgico del pie zambo. Podologie 8 (1): 97-110
Viladot R, Torner CE, Rochera R (1976) Nueva técnica quirúrgica para el tratamiento del pie plano. Ann Med 62 (6): 680-687
Viladot Perice R (1971) Tratamiento quirurgico de la artritis. Rev Esp Reum Enferm Osteoartic 14 (3): 216
Viladot Perice R, Valenti Ardanuy J, Palazon de la Barreda M (1978) La astragalectomia nel piede torto infantile (revisione di 9 piedi operati). Chir piede 2 (1-2): 17-23
Vilato P (1953) Fotopodograma. Clin Aux 2: 15
Villani E, Sardi A (1966) La duplice arthrodesi nei moderni orientamenti correttivi del piede Biomielitico. Podologie 5: 278-290
Villiaumey J, Strauss J, et al. (1978) Les monoarthrites rhumatoides. Rev Rhum Mal Osteoartic 40 (11): 627-634
Vinci A (1959) Sindroma di Morton a struttura dello echeleto del piede. Minerva Chir 14 (327): 1302
Volk C (1937) Deux cas d'os naviculare pedis bipartitum. Z Orthop 66 (4): 397-403
Volkow (1902) Bull Soc Anthropol 274-293
Voutey H (1965) Le valgus du talon dans le pied creux. Podologie 4: 160-69
Voutey H (1966) Correction du genu valgum chez l'enfant. Podologie 5: 197-202

Voutey H (1968a) Introduction à l'étude du pied spastique de l'enfant. Podologie 6 (6): 69
Voutey H (1968b) Pathologie du ler rayon. Rev Podol 91-92: 77-80
Voutey H (1969a) Pieds contracturés et pied péroniers spastiques. Approche de traitement. Podologie 6: 74-80
Voutey H (1969b) Métatarsalgies et malformations de l'avant-pied. Rev Med Dijon 4 (8): 553-562
Voutey H (1969-1970) Maladie de Refsum-Thiebaut. Podologie 6: 310-314
Voutey H (1970a) Arthrorise pour pieds plats valgus. Podologie 7: 97
Voutey H (1970b) Ostéotomie du calcanéum pour arrière-pied creux dans les séquelles de pied bot. Rev Pedicur
Voutey H (1970c) Pieds contracturés et pieds péroniers spastiques. Approche de traitement. Ann Podol 6: 74-81
Voutey H (1970d) Troubles d'appui et douleurs de l'articulation métatarso-phalangiennes. Du gros orteil. Rev Med Dijon 5 (1): 13-18
Voutey H (1971a) Séquelles des entorses tibio-tarsiennes. Rhumatologie 23 (3): 69-86
Voutey H, Strauss J (1971b) Synovites subaiguës chroniques des articulations métatarso-phalangiennes. Ann Podol 8 (1): 157-162
Voutey H (1972) Traitement chirurgical du pied plat de l'enfant. Rev Orthop 58 (5): 489-504
Voutey H (1973) Contribution au traitement chirurgical des maux perforants plantaires de l'avant-pied. Podologie 8 (2): 127
Voutey H (1975) Traitement chirurgical des nécroses avancées des têtes métatarsiennes. Rev Rhum Mal Osteoartic 27 (3): 119-123
Voutey H (1978) Manuel de chirurgie orthopédique et de rééducation du pied. Masson, Paris
Voutey H (1979) Tarsalgies par arthrose astragalo-scaphoidienne non traumatique. Podologie 12: 63
Voutey H (1982a) Troubles congénitaux et statiques du pied-ortheses plantaires. In: Claustre J, Simon L (eds) Monographies de podologie, vol 2. Masson, Paris, pp 41-47
Voutey H (1982b) Cheville et médecine de rééducation. In: Simon L, Rodineau J (eds) Collection pathologie locomotricc. Masson, Paris, pp 299-305
Voutey H, Courriades H (1965) Le valgus du talon dans le pied creux. Podologie 4: 160-169
Voutey H, Strauss J, Perrin M (1975) Les ténosynovites au niveau du pied. Rhumatologie 27 (2): 79-86
Vulcan P, Trifu R, Frandin N (1972) Tumeur de Koenen. Derm Venerol 17 (4): 359-360
Vulpius O, Stoffel A (1920) Orthopädische Operationslehre, 2nd edn. Enke, Stuttgart
Wagner FW (1977) Etat actuel des amputations de pied et de cheville. Clin Orthop 122: 62-69
Waill A (1889) Malformations unguéales. Thèse, Univ. de Lyon
Wallet A (1933) Atlas de techniques chirurgicales des affections de l'avant-pied. Maloine, Paris
Wallet A (1942) Maladies et affections douloureuses du pied. Maloine, Paris
Walsham, Hughes (1895) Traité des difformités du pied. London
Ward WC (1948) Posterior tibial nerve injuries. South Surg 14: 124-129
Watkins MB, Jones JB, Ryder CT, Brown TH (1954) Transplantation of the posterior tibial tendon. J Bone Joint Surg 36-A: 1181
Watson Jones R (1943) Fractures and joint injuries, 3rd edn. Williams & Wilkins, Baltimore
Watson Jones R (1955) Fractures and joint injuries. Livingston, Edinburgh
Weigel A (1978) Les fractures et luxations de l'astragale. Thesis, University of Strasbourg
Weil F (1955) Über die Erfahrungen an operativ behandelten kontrakten Plattfüßen. Z Orthop 86: 204-210
Weissback K (1954) Der plastische Ersatz nach Zerreißungen des äußeren Seitenbandes am oberen Sprunggelenk. Chir 25: 465-466
Wenger RJJ, Whalley RC (1978) Total replacement of the first metatarso-phalangeal joint. J Bone Joint Surg [Br] 60 (1): 88-92
Wheeler PH (1933) Os intermetatarseum and hallux valgus. Am J Surg 18: 341
Wheeler Haines R, McDougall A (1954) The anatomy of hallux valgus. J Bone Joint Surg [Am] 36: 272
White H (1886) Thomsen's disease. Brain 4: 86
White JW (1943) Torsion of the achilles tendon: its surgical significance. Arch Surg 46: 784
Wildenauer E (1950) Die Blutversorgung des Talus. Z Anat 115: 32
Wiles P (1934) Flat feet. Lancet 217 (20): 1089-1094
Willis TA (1935) The function of the long plantar muscles. Surg Gynecol Obstet 60: 150
Wilson SAK (1912a) Progressive lenticular degeneration: familial nervous disease associated with cirrhosis of the liver. Brain 34: 295-509; Lancet 1: 1115-1119
Wilson SAK (1912b) Dégénérescence lenticulaire progressive, maladie nerveuse familiale associée à la cirrhose du foie. Rev Neur Paris 1: 230-234
Windfeld P (1953) Treatment of undue mobility of the ankle joint following severe sprain of the ankle with avulsion of the anterior and middle bands of the external ligament. Acta Orthop Scand 105: 299
Winkler H, Feltner JB, Kimmelstiel P (1948) Morton's metatarsalgia. J Bone Joint Surg [Am] 30: 496-500
Winograd A (1936) Results in operations for ingrown toenails III. Med J 70: 197
Wisbrun W (1935) Der Senkungs- und Aufrichtungsmechanismus des Skeletts beim statischen Senkfuß. Z Orthop Chir 64 (1): 64-97
Wisbrun W (1955) Gibt es einen statischen Pes valgus? Z Orthop 86: 334-335
Witvoet J, Butel J (1975) Fractures de l'astragale. Encyclopédie médico-chir. 2: 14065 B 10
Wolf MD (1973) Metatarsal osteotomy for the relief of painful metatarsal callosities. J Bone Joint Surg [Am] 55 (8): 1760-1762

Wolff E (1973) Teratologie expérimentale et podologie. Acta Med Chir Pied 8 (3): 12
Wolff I (1903) Über die Ursachen, das Wesen und die Behandlung des Klumpfußes. Hirschwald, Berlin
Wolkas M (1969) Notre expérience des traumatismes de l'avant-pied. Podologie 6: 197–202
Wolkas M, Mondo A (1966) Pathologie des tendons du pied. Ann Podol 5: 186
Wolkas M, Mondo A, Cludts A (1965) Les thérapeutiques conservatrices du talon valgus statique. Podologie 4: 191
Wolkas M, Mondo A, Dandoy M (1971) Greffe libre de peau totale après exérèse d'un fibrome dermique (Extrait) Actual Med Chir pied 8 (2): 154
Wolun I, Glassmann F, Sideman S, Levinthal DH (1950) Internal derangement in the talofibular component of the ankle. Surg Gynecol Obstet 91: 193–200
Wright V (1961) Psoriasic arthritis: a comparative radiographic study of rheumatoid arthritis and arthritis associated with psoriasis. Ann Rheum Dis 20: 123–132
Wrighton JD (1972) A ten-year review of Keller's operation at the Princess Elisabeth Orthopaedic Hospital, Exeter. Clin Orthop 89: 207–14
de Wulf A (1950a) Le traitement des séquelles des traumatismes du cou-de-pied. Acta Orthop Belg 16 (4): 117–219
de Wulf A (1950b) Considérations pratiques sur le traitement du pied bot varus équin. Acta Orthop Belg 16 (3): 98–101
de Wulf A (1964) La méthode de Denis Browne dans le traitement du pied bot varus équin. Ann Podol 3: 217–221
de Wulf A (1969) L'importance des traumatismes des métatarsiens et des fractures-luxations du Lisfranc. Ann Podol 6: 189–191
de Wulf A (1975) La vascularisation de l'astragale. Acta Med Chir Pied (CIP) 11: 141–154
de Wulf A (1978) Arthroplasties métatarso-phalangiennes par interposition de peau pour la cure d'hallux rigidus pathologique, iatrogène ou post-traumatique (observations personnelles)
de Wulf A (1983) Introduction à l'étiopathogénie des maladies congénitales. Acta Med Chir Pied (CIP) 14: 99
de Wulf A, de Doncker E (1965) Traitement non sanglant du valgus du talon. Ann Podol 4: 169–176
de Wulf A, Lambrecht M (1966a) Le traitement des apophysites du calcanéum. Ann Podol 5: 20–21
de Wulf A, Lambrecht M (1966b) Anatomo-pathologie des tendons du pied. Ann Podol 5: 139–147
de Wulf A, Robyns R (1962a) Albin Lambotte et la podologie. Ann Podol 1: 1–7
de Wulf A, Robyns R (1962b) Vissage des fractures de l'apophyse du Ve métatarsien. Ann Podol 1: 104–107
Young CS (1938) An operation for the correction of hammer toe and claw toe. J Bone Joint Surg 20: 715
Young CS (1939) Operative treatment of pes planus. Surg Gynecol Obstet 68: 1099
Yvars MF (1976) Fractures ostéochondrales du sommet de l'astragale. Clin Orthop 114: 185–191
Zadek J (1935) Transverse wedge arthrodesis for the relief of pain in rigid flat foot. J Bone Joint Surg 17: 453–467
Zadik FR (1960) Arthrodesis of the great toe. Br Med J 2 (15): 73
Zaias N (1972) Onychomycosis. Arch Dermatol 105: 263–274
Zaias N (1980) The nail in health and disease. Spectrum, New York
Zaias N, Taplin D (1966) Improved preparation for the diagnosis of mycologic diseases. Arch Dermatol 93: 608–609
Zanasi R, Bertini S, Modena M (1964) La resezione artrodesi tarso-metatarsica nel piede cavo anteriore. Podologie 3: 53
Zanoli R, Azzini CA (1964) La nostra esperienza sul trattamento chirurgico del quinto dito varo. Podologie 2: 65
Zielke K (1971) Functional result of hallux valgus surgery. Dtsch Med Wochenschr 96 (21): 925–926
Zimbler S, Craig C (1976) Déformations du pied. Orthop Clin North Am 7 (2): 331–340

46 Subject Index

U. Heim, K. M. Pfeiffer

Small Fragment Set Manual

Technique Recommended by the ASIF Group

ASIF: Swiss Association for the Study of Internal Fixation
Translated from the German by R. L. Batten, K. M. Pfeiffer

2nd revised end enlarged edition. 1982. 215 figures in more than 500 separate illustrations. IX, 396 pages.
ISBN 3-540-11143-3

The **Small Fragment Set Manual** was met with enthusiastic critical acclaim in its first edition. Orthopedic and surgical journals the world over heralded it as the future standard textbook in the field, praising its clear and sensible demonstration of the philosophy and mechanical principles involved in internal fixation, its excellent illustrative material, and its comprehensive descriptions of instruments and techniques. The large number of supplementary instruments and methodological modifications introduced into the operative treatment of small bone fractures in the intervening years, however, made a thorough revision of the book necessary.

W. Blauth, F. Schneider-Sickert

Congenital Deformities of the Hand

An Atlas of Their Surgical Treatment

Translated from the German by U. H. Weil
1981. 426 figures (most in color). XV, 387 pages.
ISBN 3-540-10084-9

"The book is clearly written for the hand specialist and in this respect is most welcome. Only those procedures which in the author's view have given consistently good functional results are described. Each procedure is illustrated beautifully by black and red drawings of exceptional quality… they (the authors) have done extremely well in covering most of the problems one would expect to encounter in a surgical lifetime." *British Journal of Plastic Surgery*

Springer-Verlag
Berlin
Heidelberg
New York
Tokyo